Principles and Practice of

7th Edition

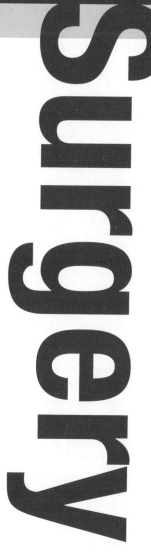

Edited by

O. James Garden

CBE BSc MB ChB MD FRCS(Glas) FRCS(Ed) FRCP(Ed)
FRACS(Hon) FRCSCan(Hon) FACS(Hon) FRCS(Hon)
FCSHK(Hon) FRCSI(Hon)

Regius Professor of Clinical Surgery,
Clinical Surgery, University of Edinburgh;
Honorary Consultant Hepatobiliary
and pancreatic Surgeon,
Royal Infirmary of Edinburgh, UK

Rowan W. Parks

MB BCh BAO MD FRCSI FRCS(Ed)

Professor of Surgical Sciences,
Clinical Surgery, University of Edinburgh;
Honorary Consultant Hepatobiliary and Pancreatic
Surgeon, Royal Infirmary of Edinburgh, UK

ELSEVIER

Edinburgh   London   New York   Oxford   Philadelphia   St Louis   Sydney   Toronto   2018

ELSEVIER

First edition 1985
Second edition 1991
Third edition 1995
Fourth edition 2002
Fifth edition 2007
Sixth edition 2012
Seventh edition 2018

ISBN   978-0-7020-6859-1
IE   978-0-7020-6858-4
Inkling   978-0-7020-6856-0

British Library Cataloguing in Publication Data
A catalogue record for this book is available from the British Library

Library of Congress Cataloging in Publication Data
A catalog record for this book is available from the Library of Congress

Notices

your source for books,
journals and multimedia
in the health sciences
www.elsevierhealth.com

Working together
to grow libraries in
developing countries

www.elsevier.com • www.bookaid.org

The Publisher's policy is to use paper manufactured from sustainable forests

Printed in China
Last digit is the print number: 9 8 7 6 5 4 3 2

Senior Content Strategist: Laurence Hunter
Senior Content Development Specialist: Ailsa Laing / Trinity Hutton
Project Manager: Andrew Riley
Illustration Manager: Nichole Beard
Illustrators: Gillian Lee and Barking Dog Illustrators

Contents

Preface   vii

Acknowledgements   viii

Contributors   ix

International Advisory Board   xi

| SECTION 1 | PRINCIPLES OF PERIOPERATIVE CARE | 1 |

1. **Metabolic response to injury, fluid and electrolyte balance and shock**   3
    Stuart McKechnie, Timothy Walsh

2. **Transfusion of blood components and plasma products**   29
    Rachel H.A. Green, Marc L. Turner

3. **Nutritional support in surgical patients**   40
    Gordon L. Carlson, Ken Fearon[†]

4. **Infections and antibiotics**   48
    Savita Gossain, Peter M. Hawkey

5. **Ethics, preoperative considerations, anaesthesia and analgesia**   60
    Ewen M. Harrison, Michael A. Gillies

6. **Principles of the surgical management of cancer**   86
    Mark A. Potter

7. **Trauma and multiple injury**   98
    Euan J. Dickson

8. **Practical procedures and patient investigation**   112
    Damian James Mole

9. **Postoperative care and complications**   128
    Pawanindra Lal

10. **Evidence-based practice and professional development**   137
    Steven Anderson, Siun Walsh, Arnie D.K. Hill

| SECTION 2 | GASTROINTESTINAL SURGERY | 145 |

11. **The abdominal wall and hernia**   147
    Andrew de Beaux

12. **The acute abdomen**   159
    Simon Paterson-Brown

[†]Deceased

13. **The oesophagus, stomach and duodenum**   179
Richard Hardwick

14. **The liver and biliary tract**   206
Saxon Connor

15. **The pancreas and spleen**   233
C. Ross Carter, Colin McKay

16. **The small and large intestine**   252
Malcolm G. Dunlop

17. **The anorectum**   283
Farhat Din

SECTION 3   **SURGICAL SPECIALTIES**   299

18. **Plastic surgery including common skin and subcutaneous lesions**   301
Patrick Addison

19. **The breast**   326
J. Michael Dixon

20. **Endocrine surgery**   351
Sonia Wakelin

21. **Vascular and endovascular surgery**   375
Hanafiah Harunarashid

22. **Cardiothoracic surgery**   409
Robert R. Jeffrey

23. **Urological surgery**   429
Grant D. Stewart

24. **Neurosurgery**   461
Lynn Myles, Paul M. Brennan

25. **Transplantation surgery**   487
Lorna Marson, John Forsythe

26. **Ear, nose and throat surgery**   502
Janet Wilson

27. **Orthopaedic surgery**   528
John C. McKinley, Issaq Ahmed

Appendix   Laboratory reference ranges   548
Index   551

Preface

This seventh edition of *Principles and Practice of Surgery* builds on the success and popularity of previous editions and its companion volume *Davidson's Principles and Practice of Medicine*. Many medical schools now deliver undergraduate curricula which focus principally on ensuring generic knowledge and skills, but the continuing success of *Principles and Practice of Surgery* over the last 30 years indicates that there remains a need for a textbook which is relevant to current surgical practice. This text provides a ready source of information for the medical student, for the recently qualified doctor on the surgical ward and for the surgical trainee who requires an up to date overview of the management approach to surgical pathology. The content is patient focused and reflects the fact that surgery is often as much about resuscitation and when not to operate as trying to intervene to deliver a better outcome. This book should guide the student and trainee through the core surgical topics which will be encountered within an integrated undergraduate curriculum, in the early years of surgical training and in subsequent clinical practice.

Although it might seem that surgical practice has remained fairly constant in recent years, there have been considerable developments, and sufficient evidence has become available to merit a number of chapters undergoing significant change. We have also taken into account feedback on the presentation of some of the contents. The format of chapters has been made more consistent and evidence based practice has been highlighted where appropriate. A global focus has been maintained throughout. It is our intention that this edition is relevant to doctors and surgeons practising worldwide and a balanced approach has been taken to the presentation where appropriate to ensure that variations in practice are identified. The contributions of our internationally-based contributors and advisors have ensured the book's contents are fit for purpose in those parts of the world where disease patterns and management approaches may differ.

We very much hope that this edition continues the tradition and high standards set by our predecessors and that the revised content and presentation of the seventh edition satisfies the needs of tomorrow's doctors.

OJG, RWP
Edinburgh, 2018

Acknowledgements

We are indebted for the past contributions from former authors who step down with the arrival of this new edition. They include Sunil Agarwal, Derek Alderson, Andrew W. Bradbury, Ari George Chacko, Trevor J. Cleveland, Steven M. Finney, Pranay Gaikwad, Roy John Korula, Thomas W. J. Lennard, Dermot W. McKeown, Douglas McWhinnie, Rachel E. Melhado, M. J. Paul, Colin E. Robertson, Venkatramani Sitaram, Laurence H. Stewart, Sumit Sural, Anubhav Vindal, James D. Watson and Ian R. Whittle.

We would also particularly wish to acknowledge the outstanding contributions made over the years to past editions and to this new edition by our colleague, Ken Fearon, whose death during the preparation of this edition has cast a shadow over British and international surgery.

We have benefited greatly from the strong editorial support of Professors Andrew Bradbury and John Forsythe over past editions and wish them well as they move on to new phases of their careers. We remain indebted to the founders of this book, Professors Sir Patrick Forrest, Sir David Carter and the late Mr Ian Macleod, who established the reputation of the textbook in its early years with students and doctors around the world.

We are grateful to Laurence Hunter of Elsevier for his encouragement and enthusiasm and to Ailsa Laing for keeping our contributors and the editorial team in line during all stages of publication. As always, this has not been easy!

Contributors

Patrick Addison BSc(Hons) MBChB MD FRCS(Plast)
Consultant Plastic Surgeon, St John's Hospital, Livingston;
Consultant Plastic Surgeon, Royal Hospital for Sick Children,
Edinburgh, UK

Issaq Ahmed FRCS(Ed, Tr&Orth)
Consultant Orthopaedic and Trauma Surgeon, Department
of Orthopaedic Surgery, Royal Infirmary of Edinburgh,
Edinburgh, UK

Steven Anderson MB BAO BCh
Department of Surgery, Beaumont Hospital, Dublin, Ireland

Paul M. Brennan BMedSci(Hons) MBBChir PhD FRCS(SN)
Department of Clinical Neurosciences, University of Edinburgh,
Western General Hospital, Edinburgh, UK

**Gordon L. Carlson BSc MBChB MD FRCS FRCS(Gen)
FRCS(Ed)**
Professor of Surgery, Salford Royal NHS Foundation Trust,
Salford, UK

C. Ross Carter MD FRCS
West of Scotland Pancreatic Unit, Glasgow Royal Infirmary,
Glasgow, UK

Saxon Connor MBChB FRACS
Hepatobiliary Surgeon, Department of General Surgery,
Canterbury District Health Board, Christchurch, New Zealand

Andrew de Beaux MBChB FRCS MD
General and Upper GI Surgeon, Department of Surgery, Royal
Infirmary of Edinburgh, Edinburgh, UK

Euan J. Dickson MBChB MD FRCS
Consultant Surgeon, West of Scotland Pancreatic Unit, Glasgow
Royal Infirmary, Glasgow, UK

Farhat Din BSc MBChB MD FRCS
Senior Lecturer, Academic Coloproctology, Western General
Hospital, Edinburgh, UK

**J. Michael Dixon BSc(Hons) MBChB MD FRCS FRCS(Ed)
FRCP(Ed, Hon)**
Professor of Surgery, Breakthrough Research Unit, Western
General Hospital, Edinburgh; Consultant Surgeon, Edinburgh
Breast Unit, Western General Hospital, Edinburgh; Clinical Lead,
Breast Cancer Now Research Unit, Western General Hospital,
Edinburgh, UK

Malcolm G. Dunlop MD FRCS FRSE FMedSci
Professor of Coloproctology, University of Edinburgh, Edinburgh,
UK

John Forsythe MBBS MD FRCS(Ed) FRCS(Eng) FEBS(Hon)
Consultant Transplant and Endocrine Surgeon, Transplant Unit,
Royal Infirmary of Edinburgh; Honorary Professor, Clinical
Surgery, University of Edinburgh, UK

Michael A. Gillies MD
Consultant and Honorary Reader in Anaesthesia, Critical Care
and Pain Medicine, Royal Infirmary of Edinburgh, Edinburgh, UK

Savita Gossain BSc MBBS FRCPath
Consultant Microbiologist, Public Health Laboratory Birmingham,
Heart of England NHS Trust, Birmingham, UK

Rachel H. A. Green MBChB FRCPath BMedBiolFRCP
Associate Medical Director, Scottish National Blood Transfusion
Service, Glasgow; Associate Medical Director, Diagnostics
Directorate, Greater Glasgow and Clyde Health Board, UK

Richard Hardwick MBBS MD FRCS
Consultant Upper GI Surgeon, Cambridge Oesophagogastric
Centre, Addenbrooke's Hospital, Cambridge, UK

Ewen M. Harrison MBChB MSc PhD FRCS
Senior Lecturer, Clinical Surgery, University of Edinburgh;
Consultant HPB Surgeon, Royal Infirmary of Edinburgh,
Edinburgh, UK

Hanafiah Harunarashid BScMed MBChB FRCS(Ed) FRCS(Ire) FRCS(Gen) AM(Mal)
Director, Advanced Surgical Skills Centre, Associate Professor, Consultant Vascular and Endovascular Surgeon, Department of Surgery, Universiti Kebangsaan Malaysia, Kuala Lumpur

Peter M. Hawkey BSc DSc MBBS MD FRCPath
Professor of Clinical and Public Health Bacteriology, Honorary Consultant, Heart of England Foundation Trust; HPA West Midlands Regional Microbiologist, University of Birmingham, UK

Arnie D. K. Hill MBBCh MCh FRCSI
Professor of Surgery, Department of Surgery, Beaumont Hospital, Dublin; Head of School of Medicine, Royal College of Surgeons of Ireland, Dublin, Ireland

Robert R. Jeffrey BSc(Hons) MBChB FRCSEd FRCPEd FRCSGlas FETCS
Honorary Senior Lecturer, Department of Surgery University of Edinburgh, Edinburgh, UK

Pawanindra Lal MS DNB FCLS FRCS(Ed) FRCS(Glasg) FRCS(Eng) FACS
Director Professor of Surgery, Consultant Laparoscopic Gastro-intestinal, Oncology and Bariatric Surgeon, Chairman, Division of Minimal Access Surgery, Head of Clinical Skills Centre, Maulana Azad Medical College (University of Delhi) & Associated Lok Nayak Hospital, New Delhi

Lorna Marson MBBS MD FRCS(Eng) FRCS(Ed) FRCP(Ed)
Reader in Transplant Surgery, Clinical Sciences (Surgery), University of Edinburgh, Edinburgh, UK

Colin McKay MBChB MD FRCS
Consultant Pancreatic Surgeon, West of Scotland Pancreatic Unit, Glasgow Royal Infirmary, Glasgow, UK

Stuart McKechnie MBChB BSc(Hons) FRCA DICM FFICM PhD
Consultant in Intensive Care Medicine and Anaesthetics, John Radcliffe Hospital, Oxford, UK

John C. McKinley BMSc MBChB FRCS
Orthopaedic Consultant, Royal Infirmary of Edinburgh, Edinburgh, UK

Damian James Mole BMedSci MBChB PhD FRCS
Senior Clinical Lecturer and Honorary Consultant Surgeon, University of Edinburgh; Senior Clinical Lecturer, MRC Centre for Inflammation Research, University of Edinburgh, Edinburgh, UK

Lynn Myles MBChB BCS(Hons) MD FRCS(SN)
Consultant Neurosurgeon, Western General Hospital, Edinburgh, and Royal Hospital for Sick Children, Edinburgh, UK

Simon Paterson-Brown MBBS MPhil MS FRCS(Ed) FRCS(Eng) FCS(HK)
Consultant General and Upper Gastro-Intestinal Surgeon, General Surgery, Royal Infirmary of Edinburgh, Edinburgh, UK

Mark A. Potter BSc MBChB MD FRCS FRCS(Ed)
Consultant Surgeon and Honorary Senior Lecturer, Department of Colorectal Surgery, Western General Hospital, Edinburgh, UK

Grant D. Stewart BSc(Hons) FRCS(Ed, Urol) MBChB PhD
University Lecturer in Urological Surgery, Academic Urology Group, University of Cambridge; Honorary Consultant Urological Surgeon, Department of Urology, Addenbrooke's Hospital, Cambridge; Honorary Senior Clinical Lecturer, University of Edinburgh, Edinburgh, UK

Marc L. Turner MB ChB PhD
Medical Director, Scottish National Blood Transfusion Service, Edinburgh, UK

Sonia Wakelin MBChB BSc(Hons) PhD
Consultant Surgeon, Royal Infirmary of Edinburgh, Edinburgh, UK

Siun Walsh MB BAO BCh MD
Department of Surgery, Beaumont Hospital, Dublin, Ireland

Timothy Walsh BSc(Hons) MBChB(Hons) FRCP FRCA FFICM MRes MD
Chair of Critical Care, Anaesthesia and Pain Medicine, University of Edinburgh, UK

Janet Wilson BSc MD FRCSEd FRCSEng FRCSLT(Hon)
Professor of Otolaryngology Head and Neck Surgery, Newcastle University, Newcastle upon Tyne, UK

International Advisory Board

Section 1

Principles of perioperative care

Metabolic response to injury, fluid and electrolyte balance and shock   3

Transfusion of blood components and plasma products   29

Nutritional support in surgical patients   40

Infections and antibiotics   48

Ethics, preoperative considerations, anaesthesia and analgesia   60

Principles of the surgical management of cancer   86

Trauma and multiple injury   98

Practical procedures and patient investigation   112

Postoperative care and complications   128

Evidence-based practice and professional development   137

Stuart McKechnie
Timothy Walsh

1

Metabolic response to injury, fluid and electrolyte balance and shock

Chapter contents

The metabolic response to injury 3

Fluid and electrolyte balance 9

Shock 18

The metabolic response to injury

To increase the chances of surviving injury, all animals have a complex set of mechanisms that act locally and systemically to restore the body to its preinjury condition. While these mechanisms are vital for survival in the wild, in the context of surgical injury they can be harmful. By minimizing and manipulating the metabolic response to injury, surgical mortality, morbidity and recovery times can be greatly improved. An understanding of the metabolic response to injury is therefore fundamental to modern surgical practice. Reduction of the metabolic (or stress) response to surgery has improved clinical outcomes in surgical patients.

Features of the metabolic response to injury

Historically, the response to injury was divided into two phases: 'ebb' and 'flow'. In the ebb phase during the first few hours after injury, patients were cold and hypotensive (shocked). When intravenous fluids and blood transfusion became available, this shock was sometimes found to be reversible and in other cases irreversible. If the individual survived the ebb phase, patients entered the flow phase, which was divided into two parts. The initial catabolic flow phase lasted about a week and was characterised by a high metabolic rate, breakdown of proteins and fats, a net loss of body nitrogen (negative nitrogen balance) and weight loss. Over 2–4 weeks, there then followed the anabolic flow phase during which protein and fat stores were restored and weight gain occurred (positive nitrogen balance). Modern understanding of the metabolic response to injury is still based on these general principles.

Factors mediating the metabolic response to injury

The metabolic response is a complex interaction between many body systems.

The acute inflammatory response

Inflammatory cells and cytokines are the principal mediators of the acute inflammatory response. Physical damage to tissues results in local activation of cells such as macrophages that release a variety of cytokines (Table 1.1). Some of these, such as interleukin-8 (IL-8), attract large numbers of circulating macrophages and neutrophils to the site of injury. Others, such as tumour necrosis factor alpha (TNF-α), IL-1 and IL-6, activate these inflammatory cells, enabling them to clear dead tissue and kill bacteria. Although these cytokines are produced and act locally (paracrine action), their release into the circulation initiates some of the systemic features of the metabolic response, such as fever (IL-1) and the acute-phase protein response (IL-6, see later) (endocrine action). Other proinflammatory (prostaglandins, kinins, complement, proteases and free radicals) and antiinflammatory substances such as antioxidants (e.g., glutathione, and vitamins A and C), protease inhibitors (e.g., α_2-macroglobulin) and IL-10 are also released (Fig. 1.1). The clinical condition of the patient depends on the extent to which the inflammation remains localised as well as the balance between these pro- and antiinflammatory processes.

The endothelium and blood vessels

The expression of adhesion molecules upon the endothelium leads to leucocyte adhesion and transmigration (Fig. 1.1). Increased local blood flow due to vasodilatation, secondary to the release of kinins, prostaglandins and nitric oxide (NO), as well as increased capillary permeability, increases the delivery of inflammatory cells, oxygen and nutrient substrates important for healing. Colloid particles (principally albumin) leak into injured tissues, resulting in oedema.

The exposure of tissue factor promotes coagulation, which, together with platelet activation, decreases haemorrhage but at the risk of causing thrombosis and tissue ischaemia. If the inflammatory process becomes generalised, widespread microcirculatory thrombosis can result in disseminated intravascular coagulation (DIC).

Table 1.1 Cytokines involved in the acute inflammatory response

Cytokine	Relevant actions
TNF-α	Proinflammatory; release of leucocytes by bone marrow; activation of leucocytes and endothelial cells
IL-1	Fever; T-cell and macrophage activation
IL-6	Growth and differentiation of lymphocytes; activation of the acute-phase protein response
IL-8	Chemotactic for neutrophils and T cells
IL-10	Inhibits immune function

IL, Interleukin; TNF, tumour necrosis factor.

Afferent nerve impulses and sympathetic activation

Tissue injury and inflammation lead to impulses in afferent pain fibres that reach the thalamus via the dorsal horn of the spinal cord and the lateral spinothalamic tract, and further mediate the metabolic response in two important ways:

1. Activation of the sympathetic nervous system leads to the release of noradrenaline from sympathetic nerve fibre endings and adrenaline from the adrenal medulla, resulting in tachycardia, increased cardiac output, and changes in carbohydrate, fat and protein metabolism (see later). Interventions that reduce sympathetic stimulation, such as epidural or spinal anaesthesia, may attenuate these changes.
2. Stimulation of pituitary hormone release (see later).

The endocrine response to surgery

Surgery leads to complex changes in the endocrine mechanisms that maintain the body's fluid balance and substrate metabolism, with changes occurring to the circulating concentrations of many hormones following injury (Table 1.2). This occurs either as a result of direct gland stimulation or because of changes in feedback mechanisms.

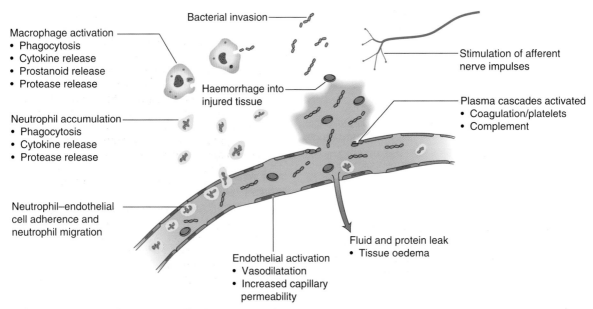

Macrophage activation
- Phagocytosis
- Cytokine release
- Prostanoid release
- Protease release

Bacterial invasion

Stimulation of afferent nerve impulses

Haemorrhage into injured tissue

Plasma cascades activated
- Coagulation/platelets
- Complement

Neutrophil accumulation
- Phagocytosis
- Cytokine release
- Protease release

Neutrophil–endothelial cell adherence and neutrophil migration

Fluid and protein leak
- Tissue oedema

Endothelial activation
- Vasodilatation
- Increased capillary permeability

Fig. 1.1 Key events occurring at the site of tissue injury.

Table 1.2 Hormonal changes in response to surgery and trauma

	Pituitary	Adrenal	Pancreatic	Others
↑ Secretion	Growth hormone Adrenocorticotrophic hormone Prolactin Antidiuretic hormone/arginine vasopressin	Adrenaline Cortisol Aldosterone	Glucagon	Renin Angiotensin
Unchanged	Thyroid-stimulating hormone Luteinizing hormone Follicle-stimulating hormone	–	–	–
↓ Secretion	–	–	Insulin	Testosterone Oestrogen Thyroid hormones

Consequences of the metabolic response to injury

Hypovolaemia

Reduced circulating volume often characterises moderate to severe injury, and can occur for a number of reasons (Table 1.3):

- Loss of blood, electrolyte-containing fluid or water.
- Sequestration of protein-rich fluid into the interstitial space, traditionally termed 'third-space loss', due to increased vascular permeability. This typically lasts 24–48 hours, with the extent (many litres) and duration (weeks or even months) of this loss dependent on the type and severity of tissue injury. For example, it is greater following burns, infection or ischaemia–reperfusion injury.

1.1 Summary

Factors mediating the metabolic response to injury

The acute inflammatory response
Inflammatory cells (macrophages, monocytes, neutrophils)
Proinflammatory cytokines and other inflammatory mediators
Endothelium

Endothelial cell activation
Adhesion of inflammatory cells
Vasodilatation
Increased permeability

Nervous system
Afferent nerve stimulation and sympathetic nervous system activation

Endocrine
Increased secretion of stress hormones
Decreased secretion of anabolic hormones

Bacterial infection

Decreased circulating volume will reduce oxygen and nutrient delivery, and so increase healing and recovery times. The neuro-endocrine responses to hypovolaemia attempt to restore normo-volaemia and maintain perfusion to vital organs.

Fluid-conserving measures

Oliguria, together with sodium and water retention – primarily due to the release of antidiuretic hormone (ADH) and aldosterone – is common after major surgery or injury, and may persist even after normal circulating volume has been restored (Fig. 1.2).

Secretion of ADH from the posterior pituitary is increased in response to:

- Afferent nerve impulses from the site of injury
- Atrial stretch receptors (responding to reduced volume) and the aortic and carotid baroreceptors (responding to reduced pressure)
- Increased plasma osmolality (principally the result of an increase in sodium ions) detected by hypothalamic osmoreceptors
- Input from higher centres in the brain (responding to pain, emotion and anxiety).

ADH promotes the retention of free water (without electrolytes) by cells of the distal renal tubules and collecting ducts.

Table 1.3 Causes of fluid loss following surgery and trauma

Nature of fluid	Mechanism	Contributing factors
Blood	Haemorrhage	Site and magnitude of tissue injury Poor surgical haemostasis Abnormal coagulation
Electrolyte-containing fluids	Vomiting	Anaesthesia/analgesia (e.g., opioids) Obstruction or ileus
	Nasogastric drainage	Ileus Gastric surgery
	Diarrhoea	Antibiotic-related infection Enteral feeding
	Sweating	Pyrexia
Water	Evaporation	Prolonged exposure of viscera during surgery
Plasma-like fluid	Capillary leak/sequestration in tissues	Acute inflammatory response Infection Burns Ischaemia–reperfusion syndrome

Aldosterone secretion from the adrenal cortex is increased by:

- Activation of the renin–angiotensin system. Renin is released from afferent arteriolar cells in the kidney in response to reduced blood pressure, tubuloglomerular feedback (signalling via the macula densa of the distal renal tubules in response to changes in electrolyte concentration) and activation of the renal sympathetic nerves. Renin converts circulating angiotensinogen to angiotensin (AT)-I. AT-I is converted by angiotensin-converting enzyme (ACE) in plasma and tissues (particularly the lungs) to AT-II, which causes arteriolar vasoconstriction and aldosterone secretion.
- Increased adrenocorticotropic hormone (ACTH) secretion by the anterior pituitary in response to hypovolaemia and hypotension via afferent nerve impulses from stretch receptors in the atria, aorta and carotid arteries. ACTH secretion is also increased by ADH.
- Direct stimulation of the adrenal cortex by hyponatraemia or hyperkalaemia.

Aldosterone increases the reabsorption of both sodium and water by distal renal tubular cells with the simultaneous excretion of hydrogen and potassium ions into the urine.

Increased ADH and aldosterone secretion following injury usually lasts 48–72 hours, during which time urine volume is reduced and osmolality increased. Typically, urinary sodium excretion decreases to 10–20 mmol/24 hours (normal 50–80 mmol/24 hours) and potassium excretion increases to >100 mmol/24 hours (normal 50–80 mmol/24 hours). Despite this, hypokalaemia is relatively rare because of a net efflux of potassium from cells. This typical pattern may be modified by fluid and electrolyte administration.

Blood flow–conserving measures

Hypovolaemia reduces cardiac preload, which leads to a fall in cardiac output and a decrease in blood flow to the tissues and organs. Increased sympathetic activity results in a compensatory increase in cardiac output, peripheral vasoconstriction and a rise in blood pressure. Together with intrinsic organ autoregulation, these mechanisms act to try to ensure adequate tissue perfusion (Fig. 1.3).

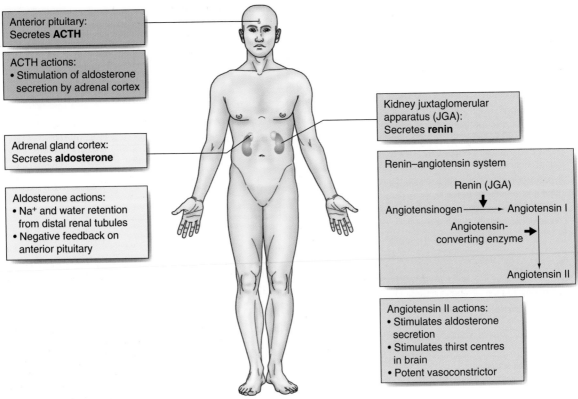

Fig. 1.2 The renin–angiotensin–aldosterone system. *ACTH,* Adrenocorticotrophic hormone.

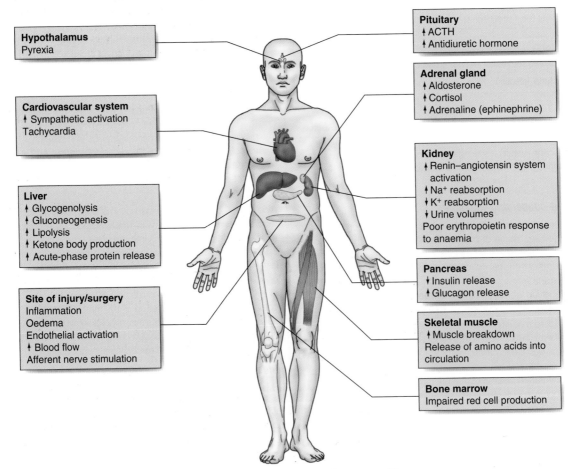

Fig. 1.3 Summary of metabolic responses to surgery and trauma.

> ### 1.2 Summary
> **Urinary changes in metabolic response to injury**
> - ↓ Urine volume secondary to ↑ ADH and aldosterone release
> - ↓ Urinary sodium and ↑ urinary potassium secondary to ↑ aldosterone release
> - ↑ Urinary osmolality
> - ↑ Urinary nitrogen excretion due to the catabolic response to injury.

Increased energy metabolism and substrate cycling

The body requires energy to undertake physical work, generate heat (thermogenesis) and to meet basal metabolic requirements. Basal metabolic rate (BMR) comprises the energy required for maintenance of membrane polarisation, substrate absorption and utilisation, and the mechanical work of the heart and respiratory systems.

Although physical work usually decreases following surgery due to inactivity, overall energy expenditure may rise by 50% due to increased thermogenesis and BMR (Fig. 1.4).

Thermogenesis

Patients are frequently pyrexial for 24–48 hours following injury (or infection) because proinflammatory cytokines (principally IL-1) reset temperature-regulating centres in the hypothalamus. BMR increases by about 10% for each 1°C increase in body temperature.

Basal metabolic rate

Injury leads to increased turnover in protein, carbohydrate and fat metabolism (see below). Whilst some of the increased

metabolic activity might appear to be of limited utility (e.g., glucose–lactate cycling and simultaneous synthesis and degradation of triglycerides), it has probably evolved to allow the body to respond quickly to altering demands during times of extreme stress.

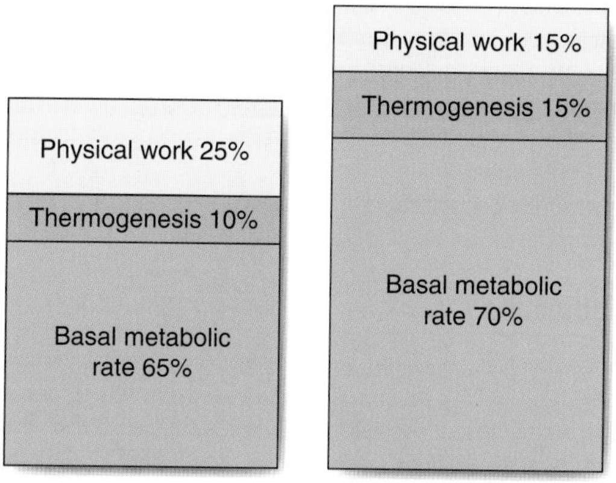

Catabolism and starvation

Catabolism is the breakdown of complex substances to the constituent parts (glucose, amino acids and fatty acids) that form substrates for metabolic pathways. Starvation occurs when intake is less than metabolic demand. Catabolism and starvation usually occur simultaneously following severe injury or major surgery, with the clinical picture being determined by whichever predominates.

Catabolism

Carbohydrate, protein and fat catabolism is mediated by the increase in circulating catecholamines and proinflammatory cytokines, as well as the hormonal changes observed following surgery.

Carbohydrate metabolism

Catecholamines and glucagon stimulate glycogenolysis in the liver, leading to the production of glucose and rapid glycogen depletion. Gluconeogenesis, the conversion of noncarbohydrate substrates (lactate, amino acids, glycerol) into glucose, occurs simultaneously. Catecholamines suppress insulin secretion, and changes in the insulin receptor and intracellular signal pathways also result in a state of insulin resistance. The net result is hyperglycaemia and impaired cellular glucose uptake. While this provides glucose for the inflammatory and repair processes, severe hyperglycaemia may increase morbidity and mortality in surgical patients, and glucose levels should be controlled in the perioperative setting.

Fat metabolism

Catecholamines, glucagon, cortisol and growth hormone all activate triglyceride lipases in adipose tissue, leading to the breakdown of triglycerides into glycerol and free fatty acids (FFAs) (lipolysis). Glycerol is a substrate for gluconeogenesis and FFAs can be metabolised in most tissues to form ATP. The brain is unable to use FFAs for energy production and almost exclusively metabolises glucose. However, the liver can convert FFAs into ketone bodies that the brain can use when glucose is less available.

Protein metabolism

Skeletal muscle is broken down, releasing amino acids into the circulation. Amino acid metabolism is complex, but glucogenic amino acids (e.g., alanine, glycine and cysteine) can be utilised by the liver as a substrate for gluconeogenesis, producing glucose for re-export, while others are metabolised to pyruvate, acetyl coenzyme-A (acetyl-CoA) or intermediates in the Krebs cycle. Amino acids are also used in the liver as substrate for the 'acute-phase protein response'. This response involves increased production of one group of proteins (positive acute-phase proteins) and decreased production of another (negative acute-phase proteins) (Table 1.4). The acute-phase response is mediated by proinflammatory cytokines (notably IL-1, IL-6 and TNF-α), and although its function is not fully understood, it is thought to play a central role in host defence and the promotion of healing.

Physical work 15%

Thermogenesis 15%

Basal metabolic rate 70%

Physical work 25%

Thermogenesis 10%

Basal metabolic rate 65%

Healthy sedentary 70 kg man
- Total energy expenditure about 1800 kcal/day

24 hours following major surgery
- Total energy expenditure increased 10–30%
- Relative reduction in physical work due to inactivity
- Thermogenesis/heat energy increased by mild pyrexia
- Basal metabolic rate increased by raised enzyme and ion pump activity and increased cardiac work

Fig. 1.4 Components of body energy expenditure in health and following surgery.

Table 1.4 The acute-phase protein response
Positive acute-phase proteins (increase after injury)
• C-reactive protein
• Haptoglobins
• Ferritin
• Fibrinogen
• α_1-antitrypsin
• α_2-macroglobulin
• Plasminogen
Negative acute-phase proteins (decrease after injury)
• Albumin
• Transferrin

The mechanisms mediating muscle catabolism are incompletely understood, but inflammatory mediators and hormones (e.g., cortisol) released as part of the metabolic response to injury appear to play a central role. Minor surgery, with minimal metabolic response, is usually accompanied by little muscle catabolism. Major tissue injury is often associated with marked catabolism and loss of skeletal muscle, especially when factors enhancing the metabolic response (e.g., sepsis) are also present.

In health, the normal dietary intake of protein is 80–120 g per day (equivalent to 12–20 g nitrogen). Approximately 2 g of nitrogen are lost in faeces and 10–18 g in urine each day, mainly in the form of urea. During catabolism, nitrogen intake is often reduced but urinary losses increase markedly, reaching 20–30 g/day in patients with severe trauma, sepsis or burns. Following uncomplicated surgery, this negative nitrogen balance usually lasts 5–8 days, but in patients with sepsis, burns or conditions associated with prolonged inflammation (e.g., acute pancreatitis) it may persist for many weeks. Feeding cannot reverse severe catabolism and negative nitrogen balance, but the provision of protein and calories can attenuate the process. Even patients undergoing uncomplicated abdominal surgery can lose ~600 g muscle protein (1 g of protein is equivalent to ~5 g muscle), amounting to 6% of total body protein. This is usually regained within 3 months.

Starvation

This occurs following trauma and surgery for several reasons:
- Reduced nutritional intake because of the illness requiring treatment
- Fasting prior to surgery
- Fasting after surgery, especially to the gastrointestinal tract
- Loss of appetite associated with illness.

The response of the body to starvation can be described in two phases (Table 1.5).

Acute starvation is characterised by glycogenolysis and gluconeogenesis in the liver releasing glucose for cerebral energy metabolism. Lipolysis releases FFAs for oxidation by other tissues and glycerol, a substrate for gluconeogenesis. These processes can sustain the normal energy requirements of the body (~1800 kcal/day for a 70-kg adult) for approximately 10 hours.

Chronic starvation is initially associated with muscle catabolism and the release of amino acids, which are converted to glucose in the liver, which also converts FFAs to ketone bodies. As described above, the brain adapts to utilise ketones rather than glucose, and this allows greater dependency on fat metabolism, so reducing muscle protein and nitrogen loss by about 25%. Energy requirements fall to about 1500 kcal/day and this 'compensated starvation' continues until fat stores are depleted when the individual, often close to death, begins to break down muscle again.

Changes in red blood cell synthesis and coagulation

Anaemia is common after major surgery or trauma because of bleeding, haemodilution following treatment with crystalloids or colloids, and impaired red cell production in bone marrow (because of low erythropoietin production by the kidney and reduced iron availability due to increased ferritin and reduced transferrin binding). Whether moderate anaemia confers a survival benefit following injury remains unclear, but actively correcting anaemia in nonbleeding patients after surgery or during critical illness does not improve outcomes. Evidence from clinical trials suggests that blood transfusions to correct anaemia following surgery are not required unless the haemoglobin concentration has decreased to a concentration of <70–80 g/L.

Following tissue injury, the blood typically becomes hypercoagulable and this can significantly increase the risk of thromboembolism; reasons include:
- Endothelial cell injury and activation, with subsequent activation of coagulation cascades
- Platelet activation in response to circulating mediators (e.g., adrenaline and cytokines)
- Venous stasis secondary to dehydration and/or immobility
- Increased concentrations of circulating procoagulant factors (e.g., fibrinogen)
- Decreased concentrations of circulating anticoagulants (e.g., protein C).

Anabolism

Anabolism involves regaining weight, restoring skeletal muscle mass and replenishing fat stores. Anabolism is unlikely to occur until the processes associated with catabolism, such as the release of proinflammatory mediators, have subsided. This point is often temporally associated with obvious clinical improvement in patients, who feel subjectively better and regain their appetite. Hormones contributing to this process include insulin, growth hormone, insulin-like growth factors, androgens and the

Table 1.5 A comparison of nitrogen and energy losses in a catabolic state and starvation[a]			
	Catabolic state	Acute starvation	Compensated starvation
Nitrogen loss (g/day)	20–25	14	3
Energy expenditure (kcal/day)	2200–2500	1800	1500
[a]Values are approximate and relate to a 70-kg man.			

17-ketosteroids. Adequate nutritional support and early mobilisation also appear to be important in promoting enhanced recovery after surgery (ERAS).

⟳ **1.3 Summary**

Physiological changes in catabolism

Carbohydrate metabolism
- ↑ Glycogenolysis
- ↑ Gluconeogenesis
- Insulin resistance of tissues
- Hyperglycaemia

Fat metabolism
- ↑ Lipolysis
- Free fatty acids used as energy substrate by tissues (except brain)
- Some conversion of free fatty acids to ketones in the liver (used by brain)
- Glycerol converted to glucose in the liver

Protein metabolism
- ↑ Skeletal muscle breakdown
- Amino acids converted to glucose in the liver and used as a substrate for acute-phase proteins
- Negative nitrogen balance

Total energy expenditure is increased in proportion to injury severity and other modifying factors.

Progressive reduction in fat and muscle mass until stimulus for catabolism ends.

Factors modifying the metabolic response to injury

The magnitude of the metabolic response to injury depends on a number of different factors (Table 1.6) and can be reduced through the use of minimally invasive techniques, prevention of bleeding and hypothermia, prevention and treatment of infection, and the use of local or regional anaesthetic techniques. Factors that may influence the magnitude of the metabolic response to surgery and injury are summarised in Table 1.6.

Fluid and electrolyte balance

In addition to reduced oral fluid intake in the perioperative period, fluid and electrolyte balance may be altered in the surgical patient for several reasons:
- ADH and aldosterone secretion, as described earlier
- Loss from the gastrointestinal tract (e.g., bowel preparation, ileus, stomas, fistulae)
- Insensible losses (e.g., sweating secondary to fever)
- 'Third-space' losses, as described earlier
- Surgical drains
- Medications (e.g., diuretics)
- Underlying chronic illness (e.g., cardiac failure, portal hypertension)

Careful monitoring of fluid balance and thoughtful replacement of net fluid and electrolyte losses is therefore important in the perioperative period.

Normal water and electrolyte balance

Water forms about 60% of total body weight in men and 55% in women. Approximately two-thirds is intracellular, one-third extracellular. Extracellular water is distributed between the plasma and the interstitial space (Fig. 1.5A).

The differential distribution of ions (and water) across cell membranes is essential for normal cellular function. The principal extracellular ions are sodium, chloride and bicarbonate, with the osmolality of extracellular fluid (ECF) (normally 275–295 mOsmol/kg) determined primarily by sodium and chloride ion concentrations. The major intracellular ions are potassium, magnesium, phosphate and sulphate (Fig. 1.5B).

The distribution of fluid between the intra- and extravascular compartments is dependent upon the oncotic pressure of plasma and the permeability of the endothelium, both of which may alter

---

Table 1.6 Factors associated with the magnitude of the metabolic response to injury

Factor	Comment
Patient-related factors	
Genetic predisposition	Genotype determines changes in gene expression in response to injury and/or infection
Coexisting disease	Cancer and/or pre-existing inflammatory disease may influence the metabolic response
Drug treatments	Antiinflammatory or immunosuppressive therapy (e.g., steroids) may alter response
Nutritional status	Malnourished patients have impaired immune function and/or important substrate deficiencies. Malnutrition prior to surgery is associated with poor outcomes
Acute surgical/trauma-related factors	
Severity of injury	Greater tissue damage is associated with a greater metabolic response
Nature of injury	Some types of tissue injury cause a disproportionate metabolic response (e.g., major burns)
Ischaemia–reperfusion injury	Reperfusion of ischaemic tissues can trigger an injurious inflammatory cascade that further injures organs
Temperature	Extreme hypo- and hyperthermia modulate the metabolic response
Infection	Infection is associated with an exaggerated response to injury. It can result in systemic inflammatory response syndrome, sepsis or septic shock
Anaesthetic techniques	The use of certain drugs, such as opioids, can reduce the release of stress hormones. Regional anaesthetic techniques (epidural or spinal anaesthesia) can reduce the release of cortisol, adrenaline and other hormones, but has little effect on cytokine responses

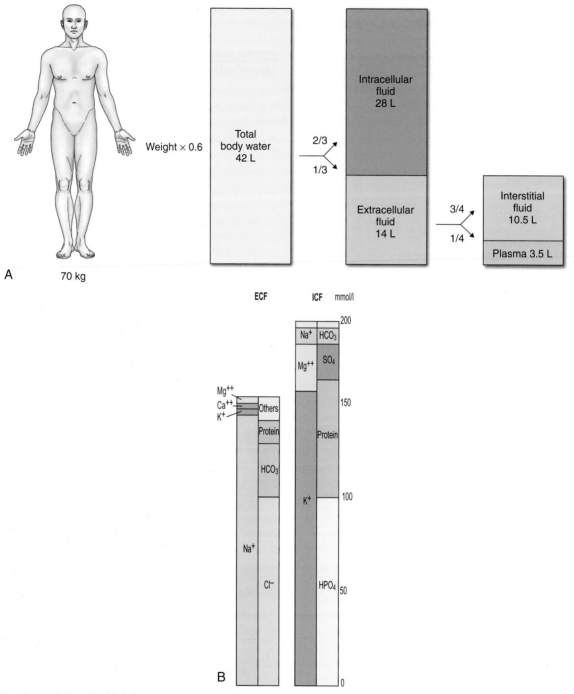

Fig. 1.5 Distribution of fluid and electrolytes between the intracellular and extracellular fluid compartments. (A) Approximate water distribution in a 70-kg man. **(B)** Cations and anions. *ECF,* Extracellular fluid; *ICF,* intracellular fluid.

following surgery, as described previously. Plasma oncotic pressure is primarily determined by albumin.

The control of body water and electrolytes has been described earlier. Aldosterone and ADH facilitate sodium and water retention while atrial natriuretic peptide, released in response to hypervolaemia and atrial distension, stimulates sodium and water excretion.

In health (Table 1.7):

- 2500–3000 mL of fluid is lost every 24 hours from the kidneys and gastrointestinal tract, and through evaporation from the skin and respiratory tract

- Fluid losses are largely replaced through eating and drinking
- A further 200–300 mL of water is provided endogenously every 24 hours by the metabolic oxidation of carbohydrate and fat.

In adults, the normal daily maintenance fluid requirement is ~20–25 mL/kg (~2000 mL/day). Newborn babies and children contain proportionately more water than adults. The daily maintenance fluid requirement at birth is about 75 mL/kg, increasing to 150 mL/kg during the first weeks of life. After the first month of life, fluid requirements decrease and the '4/2/1' formula can be used to estimate maintenance fluid requirements: the first 10 kg of body

Table 1.7 Normal daily losses and requirements for fluids and electrolytes

	Volume (mL)	Na$^+$ (mmol)	K$^+$ (mmol)
Urine	2000	80	60
Insensible losses from skin and respiratory tract	700	–	–
Faeces	300	–	10
Less water created from metabolism	300	–	–
Total	2700	80	70

weight requires 4 mL/kg/h; the next 10 kg 2 mL/kg/h; thereafter each kg of body requires 1 mL/kg/h. The estimated maintenance fluid requirements of a 35-kg child would therefore be:

$$(10 \times 4) + (10 \times 2) + (15 \times 1) = 75\,\text{mL/h}.$$

In the absence of sweating, almost all sodium loss is via the urine and, under the influence of aldosterone, this can fall to 10–20 mmol/24 hours. Potassium is also excreted mainly via the kidney, with a small amount (10 mmol/day) lost via the gastrointestinal tract. In severe potassium deficiency, losses can be reduced to about 20 mmol/day, but increased aldosterone secretion, high urine flow rates and metabolic alkalosis all limit the ability of the kidneys to conserve potassium and predispose to hypokalaemia.

In adults, the normal daily requirement for both sodium and potassium is approximately 1 mmol/kg.

Assessing losses in the surgical patient

Only by accurately estimating (Table 1.8) and, where possible, directly measuring fluid and electrolyte losses, can appropriate therapy be administered.

Insensible fluid losses

Hyperventilation increases insensible water loss via the respiratory tract, but this increase is not usually large unless the normal mechanisms for humidifying inhaled air (the nasal passages and upper airways) are compromised. This occurs in intubated patients (e.g., in the intensive care unit) or in those receiving nonhumidified high-flow oxygen. In these situations inspired gases should be humidified routinely.

Pyrexia increases water loss from the skin by approximately 200 mL/day for each 1°C rise in temperature. Sweating may increase fluid loss by up to 1 L/h but these losses are difficult to quantify. Sweat also contains significant amounts of sodium (20–70 mmol/L) and potassium (10 mmol/L). High ambient temperatures in tropical countries will contribute to increased losses in sweat.

The effect of surgery

The stress response

As discussed above, ADH leads to water retention and a reduction in urine volume for 2–3 days following major surgery. Aldosterone conserves both sodium and water, further contributing to oliguria. As a result, urinary sodium excretion falls while urinary potassium excretion increases, predisposing to hypokalaemia. Excessive and/or inappropriate intravenous fluid replacement therapy can easily lead to hyponatraemia and hypokalaemia in this context.

'Third-space' losses

If tissue injury is severe, widespread and/or prolonged then the loss of water, electrolytes and colloid particles into the interstitial space can amount to many litres, significantly reducing circulating blood volume.

Fluid accumulation in the interstitial space contributes to oedema. Excess fluid moves from this space into the lymphatics only up to a point. Formation of 'oedema fluid' is largely dependent on the net balance of hydrostatic and oncotic pressures inside the capillary and in the interstitium. The hydrostatic pressure on the arteriolar side of the capillary falls from 37 mmHg to 17 mmHg on the venular side. The colloid oncotic pressure throughout the lumen of the capillary is 25 mmHg. The hydrostatic pressure is 1 mmHg in the interstitium. There is a net outward pressure on the arteriolar side (37 − 1 − 25 = 11) and a net inward pressure (25 − 17 − 1 = 9) on the venular side.

This normal arrangement becomes 'disturbed', and excess interstitial fluid accumulates if the hydrostatic pressure increases on the venular side (e.g., heart failure), the colloid oncotic pressure falls (e.g., liver or kidney disease) or endothelial permeability is increased (e.g., sepsis and/or injury).

In recent years, the role of the endothelial glycocalyx in the homeostasis of transvascular fluid exchange has been recognised. The glycocalyx is a web of membrane-bound glycoproteins on the luminal side of endothelial cells. This forms a dynamic interface (~2 μm thick) between blood and the capillary wall. It appears that the integrity of the glycocalyx may be compromised by the rapid infusion of intravenous fluids and in a range of systemic inflammatory states, such as sepsis, surgery and trauma, contributing to the capillary leak.

Minimising 'third-space losses' may increase rates of recovery following surgery. For very sick patients, such as those with sepsis and multiple organ failure in the intensive care unit, there is evidence that very positive overall fluid balance may delay recovery or even increase mortality. The goal of fluid therapy is therefore to provide sufficient fluids to replace losses and to maintain an adequate intravascular circulating volume, but avoid excessive replacement that increases localised or generalised oedema formation.

Table 1.8 Sources of fluid loss in surgical patients

	Typical losses per 24 hours	Factors modifying volume
Insensible losses	700–2000 mL	↑ Losses associated with pyrexia, sweating and use of nonhumidified oxygen
Urine	1000–2500 mL	↓ With aldosterone and antidiuretic hormone secretion; ↑ with diuretic therapy
Gut	300–1000 mL	↑ Losses with obstruction, ileus, fistulae and diarrhoea (may increase substantially)
Third-space losses	0–4000 mL	↑ Losses with greater extent of surgery and tissue trauma

Loss from the gastrointestinal tract

The magnitude and content of gastrointestinal fluid losses depends on the site of loss (Table 1.9):

- *Intestinal obstruction.* In general, the higher an obstruction occurs in the intestine, the greater the fluid loss because fluids secreted by the upper gastrointestinal tract fail to reach the absorptive areas of the distal jejunum and ileum.
- *Paralytic ileus.* This condition, in which propulsion in the small intestine ceases, has numerous causes. The most common is probably handling of the bowel during surgery, which usually resolves within 1–2 days of the operation. Occasionally, paralytic ileus persists for longer, and in this case other causes should be sought and corrected if possible. During paralytic ileus the stomach should be decompressed using

nasogastric tube drainage, and fluid losses monitored by measuring nasogastric aspirates.

- *Intestinal fistula.* As with obstruction, fistulae occurring high in the gut are associated with the greatest fluid and electrolyte losses. As well as volume, it may be useful to measure the electrolyte content of the fluid lost in order to determine the fluid and electrolyte replacement required.
- *Diarrhoea.* Patients may present with diarrhoea or develop it during the perioperative period. Fluid and electrolyte losses may be considerable.

Intravenous fluid administration

When choosing and administering intravenous fluids (Table 1.10) it is important to consider:

- What fluid deficiencies are present
- The fluid compartments requiring replacement
- Any electrolyte disturbances present
- Which fluid is most appropriate.

Types of intravenous fluid

Crystalloids

Dextrose 5% contains 5 g of dextrose (D-glucose) per 100 mL of water. This glucose is rapidly metabolised, and the remaining free water distributes rapidly and evenly throughout the body's fluid compartments. So, shortly after the intravenous administration of 1000 mL 5% dextrose solution, about 670 mL of water will be added to the intracellular fluid compartment (IFC) and about 330 mL of water to the extracellular fluid compartment (EFC), of which about 70 mL will be intravascular (Fig. 1.6). Dextrose solutions are therefore of little value as resuscitation fluids to expand intravascular volume. Dextrose 5% is an isotonic solution in contrast to more concentrated dextrose solutions (10%, 20% and 50%), which are hypertonic. These solutions are an irritant to veins

---

Table 1.9 The approximate daily volumes (mL) and electrolyte concentrations (mmol/L) of various gastrointestinal fluids[a]

	Volume	Na$^+$	K$^+$	Cl$^-$	HCO$_3^-$
Plasma	–	140	5	100	25
Gastric secretions	2500	50	10	80	40
Intestinal fluid (upper)	3000	140	10	100	25
Bile and pancreatic secretions	1500	140	5	80	60
Mature ileostomy	500	50	5	20	25
Diarrhoea (inflammatory)	–	110	40	100	40
Mixed gastric aspirate	–	120	10	–	–

[a]If gastrointestinal loss continues for more than 2–3 days, samples of fluid and urine should be collected regularly and sent to the laboratory for measurement of electrolyte content. For calculation of electrolyte replacement, mixed gastric aspirate composition can be used for ease of calculation. For example, replacement of 2 litres of nasogastric aspirate would require an additional supply of 240 mEq of Na$^+$ and 20 mEq of K$^+$ in addition to the daily requirement.

Table 1.10 Composition of commonly administered intravenous fluids

	Na$^+$ (mmol/L)	K$^+$ (mmol/L)	Cl$^-$ (mmol/L)	HCO$_3^-$ (mmol/L)	Ca^{2+} (mmol/L)	Mg^{2+} (mmol/L)	Oncotic pressure (mmH$_2$O)	Typical plasma half-life	pH
5% dextrose	–	–	–	–	–		0	–	4.0
0.9% NaCl	154	0	154	0	0		0	–	5.0
0.18% NaCl/4% dextrose	31	0	31	0	0	0	0	–	4.0
Ringer's lactate (Hartmann's solution)	131	5	112	Lactate 28[a]	1	1	0	–	6.5
Plasma-Lyte 148	140	5	98	Acetate 27[b] Gluconate 23[b]	0	1.5	0	–	7.4
Haemaccel (succinylated gelatin)	145	5.1	145	0	6.25	0	370	5 hours	7.4
Gelofusine (polygeline gelatin)	154	0.4	125	0	0.4	0.4	465	4 hours	7.4
Human albumin solution 4.5%	150	0	120	0	0		275	–	7.4

[a]The lactate present in Ringer's lactate solution is rapidly metabolised in the body. This generates bicarbonate ions.
[b]The acetate and gluconate present in Plasma-Lyte 148 is rapidly metabolised in the body. This generates bicarbonate ions.
Bicarbonate cannot be directly added to the solutions because it is unstable (tends to precipitate).

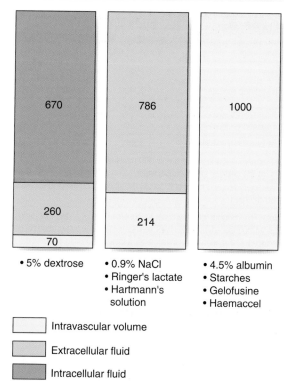

5% dextrose

0.9% NaCl
Ringer's lactate
Hartmann's solution

4.5% albumin
Starches
Gelofusine
Haemaccel

☐ Intravascular volume

▨ Extracellular fluid

▨ Intracellular fluid

Fig. 1.6 Distribution of different fluids in the body fluid compartments 30–60 minutes after rapid intravenous infusion of 1000 mL.

and their use should be limited to the management of diabetic patients or patients with hypoglycaemia.

Sodium chloride 0.9%, Hartmann's solution and *Plasma-Lyte 148* are isotonic solutions of electrolytes in water. Sodium chloride 0.9% (also known as normal saline) contains 9 g of sodium chloride dissolved in 1000 mL of water; Hartmann's solution (also known as Ringer's lactate) has a more physiological composition of sodium, potassium, chloride and calcium. Plasma-Lyte 148 contains physiological concentrations of sodium, chloride and magnesium but does not contain calcium or potassium. All three fluids have an osmolality similar to that of ECF (about 290–300 mOsm/L) and after intravenous administration they distribute rapidly throughout the EFC (Fig. 1.6). Isotonic crystalloids are appropriate for correcting EFC losses (e.g., gastrointestinal tract or sweating) and for the initial resuscitation of intravascular volume, although only about 25% remains in the intravascular space after redistribution (which typically occurs within 30–60 minutes).

Balanced solutions, such as Ringer's lactate and Plasma-Lyte 148, more closely match (or balance) the composition of ECF by providing physiological concentrations of sodium and chloride. These solutions do not contain bicarbonate because this is unstable in solution and may precipitate during storage. The solutions contain a substrate that the body can metabolise to generate bicarbonate ions as part of the metabolic pathway. For Ringer's lactate, lactate is the substrate. For Plasma-Lyte 148, acetate and gluconate are the substrates. These solutions decrease the risk of hyperchloraemia, which can occur following large volumes of fluids with higher sodium and chloride concentrations, such as sodium chloride 0.9%. Hyperchloraemic acidosis can develop in these situations. This has been associated with renal impairment in some studies. Plasma-Lyte 148 is increasingly used as the first-line crystalloid for resuscitation because the risk of hyperchloraemic acidosis is reduced, and it does not contain potassium

(minimizing the risk of hyperkalaemia, especially when renal failure or hyperkalaemia may be present). The use of acetate/gluconate rather than lactate is also an advantage, because lactate is used as an index of shock severity and response to resuscitation, and will be altered by the lactate in Ringer's lactate solution.

Hypertonic saline solutions have an osmolality greater than ECF and induce a shift of fluid from the IFC to the EFC, so reducing brain water and increasing intravascular volume and serum sodium concentration. Potential indications include the treatment of cerebral oedema and raised intracranial pressure, hyponatraemic seizures and 'small-volume' resuscitation of hypovolaemic shock.

Dextrose–saline solutions

A number of dextrose–saline solutions are available. The isotonic solution of 4% dextrose/0.18% sodium chloride is widely used as a solution for maintenance of fluid status when replacement of losses rather than resuscitation are needed, because this combination provides an appropriate replacement of sodium, chloride and glucose when used as a single fluid at 80–100 mL/h for an average-sized adult. Importantly, it reduces the risk of excessive sodium and chloride replacement. 'Half-normal saline' is a commonly used (hypertonic) crystalloid and contains 0.45% sodium chloride in 5% dextrose. Commercially available 5% dextrose with 0.9% normal saline in 500 mL is a hypertonic solution (twice the osmolarity of plasma) and should be used with caution.

Colloids

Colloid solutions contain particles that exert an oncotic pressure and may occur naturally (e.g., albumin) or be synthetically modified (e.g., gelatins, hydroxyethyl starches, dextrans). When administered, colloid remains largely within the intravascular space until the colloid particles are removed by the reticuloendothelial system. The intravascular half-life is usually between 6 and 24 hours and such solutions are therefore appropriate for fluid resuscitation. Thereafter, the electrolyte-containing solution distributes throughout the EFC.

The use of human albumin is discussed in Chapter 2. Synthetic colloids are more expensive than crystalloids and have variable side effect profiles. Recognised risks include coagulopathy, reticuloendothelial system dysfunction, pruritus and anaphylactic reactions. Hydroxyethyl starch in particular appears to be associated with increased mortality and renal failure, and is no longer recommended.

The theoretical advantage of colloids over crystalloids is that, as they remain in the intravascular space for several hours, smaller volumes are required. However, current evidence suggests that crystalloids and colloids are equally effective for the correction of hypovolaemia with comparable patient outcomes (EBM 1.1). As colloids are not associated with improved survival and are more expensive than crystalloids, it is difficult to justify their use in routine surgical practice.

Maintenance fluid requirements

Under normal conditions, adult daily sodium requirements (80 mmol) may be provided by the administration of 500–1000 mL of 0.9% sodium chloride. The remaining water requirement to maintain fluid balance (2000–2500 mL) is typically provided as 5% dextrose. An alternative is to use 0.18% NaCl/4% dextrose solutions (2000–3000 ml per 24 hours according to size and estimated fluid losses). Daily potassium requirements

Table 1.11 Provision of normal 24-hour fluid and electrolyte requirements by intravenous infusion. An alternative approach is to use 0.18% NaCl/4% dextrose solution with addition of potassium as required. The total fluid requirements per 24 hours vary according to patient weight and fluid losses, but are typically 2000–3000 mL per 24 hours

Intravenous fluid	Additive	Duration (hours)
500 mL 0.9% NaCl	20 mmol KCl	4
500 mL 5% dextrose	–	4
500 mL 5% dextrose	20 mmol KCl	4
500 mL 0.9% NaCl	–	4
500 mL 5% dextrose	20 mmol KCl	4
500 mL 5% dextrose	–	4

Table 1.12 Estimating fluid (mL) and electrolyte (mmol/L) requirements in a patient with ileus[a]

	Volume (mL)	Na$^+$	K$^+$
Urine	1500	80	60
Nasogastric aspirate	2000	240	20
Insensible loss	800	–	–
Minus endogenous water	−300	–	–
Net losses/requirements	4000	320	80

2 L of normal saline would supply 300 mmol of Na$^+$.
2 L of 5% dextrose would supply water.
The required 60–80 mmol of K$^+$ could be added as 20 mmol to alternate 500-mL bags.

Note: The 1500 mL of urine is not an abnormal loss. It shows that during this 24-hour period, hydration has been adequate. Urine output need not be replaced. The abnormal loss (nasogastric aspirate 2000 mL) + normal daily requirement (shown in Table 1.11) = 5000 mL is the requirement. The insensible loss and endogenous water have been accounted for in the normal daily requirement.

[a]Assuming that the patient is in electrolyte balance and is losing 2 L/day as nasogastric aspirate and 1.5 L/day as urine, 24-hour losses can be calculated as shown.

(60–80 mmol) are usually met by adding potassium chloride to maintenance fluids, but the amount added can be titrated to measured plasma concentrations. Potassium should not be administered at a rate greater than 10–20 mmol/h except in severe potassium deficiency (see section on hypokalaemia later) and, in practice, 20-mmol aliquots are added to alternate 500-mL bags of fluid.

An example of a suitable 24-hour fluid prescription for an uncomplicated patient is shown in Table 1.11; the process of adjusting this for a hypothetical patient with an ileus is shown in Table 1.12.

In patients requiring intravenous fluid replacement for more than 3–4 days, supplementation of magnesium and phosphate may also be required as guided by direct measurement of plasma concentrations. The provision of total parenteral nutrition should also be considered in this situation.

Treatment of postoperative hypovolaemia and/or hypotension

Hypovolaemia is common in the postoperative period and may present with one or more of the following: tachycardia, cold extremities, pallor, clammy skin, collapsed peripheral veins, oliguria and/or hypotension. Hypotension is more likely in hypovolaemic patients receiving epidural analgesia as the associated sympathetic blockade disrupts compensatory vasoconstriction. Intravascular volume should be rapidly restored with a series of fluid boluses (e.g., 250–500 mL), with the clinical response being assessed after each bolus (see below). Although the evidence in favour of balanced solutions is currently uncertain, Plasma-Lyte 148 or equivalent solutions are widely considered the optimum first-line crystalloid solution for bolus resuscitation of hypovolaemia.

EBM | **1.1 Crystalloid vs colloid to treat intravascular hypovolaemia**

'There is no evidence from randomised controlled trials that resuscitation with colloids reduces the risk of death, compared to resuscitation with crystalloids, in patients with trauma, burns or following surgery.'

Perel P, et al. Colloids versus crystalloids for fluid resuscitation in critically ill patients. Cochrane Database Syst Rev. 2013 Feb 28;(2):CD000567.

Specific water and electrolyte abnormalities

Sodium and water

Sodium is the most abundant extracellular cation (Fig 1.5B) and is the major determinant of ECF osmolality or tonicity. As a consequence, plasma sodium concentration largely determines the relative ECF and intracellular fluid (ICF) volumes. Both hyponatraemia (Na$^+$ <134 mmol/L) and hypernatraemia (Na$^+$ >145 mmol/L) are common in surgical practice, and reflect an imbalance between the sodium and, more often, water content of the ECF.

Water depletion

A decrease in total body water of 1–2% (350–700 mL) causes an increase in blood osmolality. This stimulates brain osmoreceptors, triggering the sensation of thirst. Clinically obvious dehydration, with thirst, a dry tongue and loss of skin turgor, indicates at least 4–5% deficiency of total body water (1500–2000 mL). Pure water depletion is uncommon in surgical practice, and is usually combined with sodium loss. The most frequent causes are inadequate intake or excessive gastrointestinal losses.

Water excess

For reasons explained earlier, this is common in patients who receive large volumes of intravenous 5% dextrose in the early postoperative period. Such patients have an increased extracellular volume and are commonly hyponatraemic (see later). The increase in extracellular volume can be difficult to detect clinically, as patients with water excess usually remain well and oedema may not be evident until the extracellular volume has increased by more than 4 L. In patients with poor cardiac function or renal failure, water accumulation can result in pulmonary oedema. Careful scrutiny of fluid intake and output records should help prevent this complication. Treatment is by restriction of fluids.

Hypernatraemia

Normal sodium levels are in the range of 135–145 mmol/L. Hypernatraemia (Na$^+$ >145 mmol/L) results from either water (or hypotonic fluid) loss or sodium gain. Common causes of net water loss include reduced water intake, vomiting, diarrhoea, diuresis, burns, sweating and insensible losses from the respiratory tract, and diabetes insipidus. It is typically associated with a low ECF volume (hypovolaemia). In contrast, sodium gain is usually caused by excess sodium administration in hypertonic intravenous fluids and is typically associated with hypervolaemia.

Hypovolaemic hypernatraemia is treated with isotonic crystalloid to rapidly restore intravascular volume followed by the more gradual administration of water or hypotonic fluid to correct the relative water deficit. The latter can be administered enterally (oral or nasogastric tube) or intravenously in the form of 5% dextrose. Another option would be the administration of fluids with lower NaCl concentrations such as 0.18% NaCl/4% dextrose or 0.45% NaCl solutions. These will result in a more gradual correction of hypernatraemia.

Cells, particularly brain cells, adapt to a high sodium concentration in ECF, and once this adaptation has occurred, rapid correction of severe hypernatraemia can result in a rapid rise in intracellular volume, cerebral oedema, seizures and permanent neurological injury. To reduce the risk of this, free water deficits should be replaced slowly, with the sodium being corrected at a rate less than 0.5 mmol/h.

Hyponatraemia

Hyponatraemia (Na$^+$ <135 mmol/L) is the most commonly encountered electrolyte disturbance in hospital practice and can occur in the presence of decreased, normal or increased extracellular volume. The most common cause is the administration of hypotonic intravenous fluids to replace sodium-rich fluid losses from the gastrointestinal tract or when excessive water (as intravenous 5% dextrose) is administered in the postoperative period (dilutional hyponatraemia). Other causes include diuretic use and the syndrome of inappropriate ADH secretion (SIADH). Comorbidities associated with secondary hyperaldosteronism, such as cirrhosis and congestive cardiac failure, are potential contributing factors.

Treatment depends on correct identification of the cause:

- If ECF volume is normal or increased, the most likely cause is excessive intravenous water administration and this will correct spontaneously if water intake is reduced. Although less common in surgical patients, the inappropriately high levels of ADH observed in SIADH promotes the renal tubular reabsorption of water independently of sodium concentration, resulting in inappropriately concentrated urine with a high sodium content (osmolality >100 mOsm/L) in the face of hypotonic plasma (osmolality <290 mOsm/L). The urine osmolality helps to distinguish inappropriate ADH secretion from excessive water administration.
- In patients with decreased ECF volume, hyponatraemia usually indicates combined water and sodium deficiency. This is most frequently the result of diuresis, diarrhoea or adrenal insufficiency, and will correct if adequate 0.9% sodium chloride is administered.

The most serious clinical manifestation of hyponatraemia is a metabolic encephalopathy resulting from the shift of water into brain cells and cerebral oedema. This is more likely in severe hyponatraemia (Na$^+$ <120 mmol/L) and is associated with confusion, seizures and coma. Rapid correction of sodium concentration can precipitate an irreversible demyelinating condition known as osmotic demyelination syndrome or central pontine myelinolysis. To avoid this, sodium concentration should not normally be increased by more than 6–8 mmol per 24 hours, particularly in

patients known to have chronic (>48-hour) hyponatraemia. This can usually be achieved by the cautious administration of isotonic (0.9%) sodium chloride, occasionally combined with the use of a loop diuretic (e.g., furosemide). Hypertonic saline solutions are rarely indicated and can be dangerous.

↻ 1.4 Summary

Aetiology of hyper- and hyponatraemia

Hypernatraemia

Hypovolaemic
- ↓ Oral intake (e.g., fasting, ↓ conscious level)[a]
- Nausea and vomiting[a]
- Diarrhoea[a]
- ↑ Insensible losses (↑ sweating and/or ↑ respiratory tract losses)
- Severe burns[a]
- Diuresis (e.g., glycosuria, use of osmotic diuretics)

Euvolaemic
- Diabetes insipidus–central or nephrogenic

Hypervolaemic
- Excessive sodium load (hypertonic saline, TPN, sodium bicarbonate)
- ↑ Mineralocorticoid activity (e.g., Conn's syndrome or Cushing's disease)

Hyponatraemia

Low extracellular fluid volume
- Diarrhoea[a]
- Diuretic use[a]
- Adrenal insufficiency
- Salt-losing renal disease

Normal extracellular fluid volume
- Syndromes of inappropriate ADH secretion (SIADH)
- Hypothyroidism
- Psychogenic polydipsia

Increased extracellular fluid volume
- Excessive water administration[a]
- Secondary hyperaldosteronism (cirrhosis, cardiac failure)
- Renal failure
- Transurethral resection of the prostate (TURP) syndrome.

[a]Causes commonly encountered in the surgical patient.
TPN, total parenteral nutrition.

Potassium

Small changes in extracellular levels of potassium can have profound effects on the function of the cardiovascular and neuromuscular systems. As about 98% of total body potassium (around 3500 mmol) is intracellular, serum potassium concentration (normally 3.5–5 mmol/L) is a poor indicator of total body potassium and there is no absolute formula to determine potassium deficit. Serial monitoring of serum potassium is necessary to guide the appropriate management of potassium disturbances.

Acidosis reduces Na$^+$/K$^+$-ATPase activity and results in a net efflux of potassium from cells and hyperkalaemia. Conversely, alkalosis results in an influx of potassium into cells and hypokalaemia. These abnormalities are exacerbated by renal compensatory mechanisms that correct the acid–base balance at the expense of potassium homeostasis.

Hyperkalaemia (K >5.5 mmol/L)

This is a potentially life-threatening condition that can be caused by exogenous administration of potassium, the release of potassium from cells (transcellular shift) as a result of tissue damage or changes in the Na^+/K^+-ATPase function (e.g., acidosis), or impaired renal excretion.

Mild hyperkalaemia (K^+ <6 mmol/L) is often asymptomatic, but as serum levels rise there is progressive slowing of electrical conduction in the heart and the development of significant cardiac arrhythmias. All patients suspected of having hyperkalaemia should have an electrocardiogram (ECG) for this reason. Tall 'tented' T-waves in the precordial leads are the earliest ECG changes observed, but as hyperkalaemia progresses more significant ECG changes occur, with flattening (or loss) of the P waves, a prolonged PR interval, widening of the QRS complex and, eventually, asystole. Severe hyperkalaemia (K^+ >7 mmol/L) requires immediate treatment to prevent this (Table 1.13).

Hypokalaemia (<3.0 mmol/L)

This is a common disorder in surgical patients. Dietary intake of potassium is normally 60–80 mmol/day. Under normal conditions, the majority of potassium loss (>85%) is via the kidneys and maintenance of potassium balance largely depends on normal renal tubular regulation. Potassium depletion sufficient to cause a fall of 1 mmol/L in serum levels typically requires a loss of ~100–200 mmol of potassium from total body stores. Potassium excretion is increased by metabolic alkalosis, diuresis, increased aldosterone release and increased losses from the gastrointestinal tract—all of which occur commonly in the surgical patient. Muscle weakness, paralytic ileus and flattening of T waves with prominent U waves on ECG are diagnostic features. In hypokalaemia, for

every three potassium ions that come out from the intracellular compartment, one hydrogen and two sodium ions are exchanged, causing extracellular alkalosis and intracellular acidosis.

Oral or nasogastric potassium replacement is safer than intravenous replacement and is the preferred route in asymptomatic patients with mild hypokalaemia. Severe (K^+ <2.5 mmol/L) or symptomatic hypokalaemia requires intravenous replacement. While replacement rates of up to 40 mmol/h may be used (with cardiac monitoring) in an emergency, there is a risk of serious cardiac arrhythmias and rates exceeding 20 mmol/h should generally be avoided. Potassium solutions should never be administered as a bolus. A useful rule of thumb is: not more than 40 mmol of potassium chloride in 500 mL and not more than 15 mmol/h (outside a critical care setting).

Other electrolyte disturbances

Calcium

Clinically significant abnormalities in calcium balance in the surgical patient are most frequently encountered in endocrine surgery (see Chapter 20).

Magnesium

Hypomagnesaemia is common in surgical patients who have restricted oral intake and who have been receiving intravenous fluids for several days. It is frequently associated with other electrolyte abnormalities, notably hypokalaemia, hypocalcaemia and hypophosphataemia. Hypomagnesaemia appears to be

---

↻ 1.5 Summary

Hyper- and hypokalaemia

Hyperkalaemia	Hypokalaemia
Consequences	
• Arrhythmias (tented T waves, ↓ HR, heart block, broadened QRS, asystole) • Muscle weakness • Ileus	• ECG changes (flattened T waves, U waves, ectopics) • Muscle weakness and myalgia
Causes	
Excess intravenous or oral intake	*Inadequate intake*[a]
Transcellular shift—efflux of potassium from cells	*Gastrointestinal tract losses*
• Metabolic acidosis[a] • Massive blood transfusion[a] • Rhabdomyolysis (e.g., crush and/or compartment syndromes) [a] • Massive tissue damage (e.g., ischaemic bowel or liver) [a] • Drugs (e.g., digoxin, β-receptor antagonists)	• Vomiting[a] • Gastric aspiration/drainage[a] • Fistulae[a] • Diarrhoea[a] • Ileus[a] • Intestinal obstruction[a] • Potassium-secreting villous adenoma[a]
Impaired excretion	*Urinary losses*
• Acute renal failure[a] • Chronic renal failure • Drugs (ACE inhibitors, spironolactone, NSAIDs) • Adrenal insufficiency (Addison's disease)	• Metabolic alkalosis[a] • Hyperaldosteronism[a] • Diuretics[a] • Renal tubular disorders (e.g., Bartter's syndrome, renal tubular acidoses, drug-induced)
	Transcellular shift—influx of potassium into cells
	• Metabolic alkalosis[a] • Drugs[a] (e.g., insulin, β-agonists, adrenaline)

[a]Common causes in the surgical patient.
ACE, Angiotensin-converting enzyme; *ECG, electrocardiogram; HR*, heart rate; *NSAID*, nonsteroidal antiinflammatory drug.

Table 1.13 Management of severe hyperkalaemia (K⁺ >7 mmol/L)

1. Identify and treat cause. Monitor ECG until potassium concentration controlled	
2. 10 mL 10% calcium gluconate iv over 3 minutes, repeated after 5 minutes if no response	Antagonises the membrane actions of ↑ K⁺ reducing the risk of ventricular arrhythmias
3. 50 mL 50% dextrose + 10 units short-acting insulin over 2–3 minutes. Start infusion of 10–20% dextrose at 50–100 mL/h	Increases transcellular shift of K⁺ into cells
4. Regular salbutamol nebulisers	Increases transcellular shift of K⁺ into cells
5. Consider oral or rectal calcium resonium (ion exchange resin)	Facilitates K⁺ clearance across gastrointestinal mucosa. More effective in nonacute cases of hyperkalaemia
6. Renal replacement therapy	Haemodialysis is the most effective medical intervention to lower K⁺ rapidly

associated with a predisposition to tachyarrhythmias (most notably torsades de pointes [polymorphic ventricular tachycardia] and atrial fibrillation), but many of the clinical manifestations of magnesium depletion are nonspecific (muscle weakness, muscle cramps, altered mentation, tremors, hyperreflexia and generalised seizures). As magnesium is predominantly intracellular, serum magnesium levels poorly reflect total body stores. Despite this limitation, serum levels are frequently used to guide (oral or parenteral) magnesium supplementation. When hypokalaemia and hypomagnesaemia coexist it may be difficult to correct the former without correcting the latter.

Phosphate

Phosphate is a critical component in many biochemical processes such as ATP synthesis, cell signaling and nucleic acid synthesis. Hypophosphataemia is common in surgical patients, and if severe (<0.4 mmol/L) causes widespread cell dysfunction, muscle weakness, impaired myocardial contractility, reduced cardiac output and altered sensorium. Most hypophosphataemia results from the shift of phosphate into cells and most commonly occurs in chronically malnourished and/or alcoholic patients commencing enteral or parenteral nutrition. The increased carbohydrate load leads to insulin secretion, which results in the rapid intracellular uptake of glucose and phosphate together with magnesium and potassium. For reasons that remain unclear, these changes are accompanied by fluid retention and an increase in ECF volume (refeeding syndrome). To avoid this syndrome, feeding should be established gradually and accompanied by regular measurement and aggressive supplementation of serum electrolytes (phosphate, magnesium and potassium). Phosphate can be supplemented orally or by slow intravenous infusion. Sepsis is another situation in which marked hypophosphataemia can be seen.

Acid–base balance

The pH of blood is tightly regulated, with acid–base homeostasis critical for normal cellular function. This homeostasis is dependent on the interplay of the respiratory system (via control of Paco₂), blood buffers (principally bicarbonate) and the kidneys (through excretion of acid [H⁺] and reabsorption of bicarbonate).

While some meaningful data pertaining to acid–base balance can be derived from the analysis of venous blood, accurate assessment of acid–base disturbance relies on the measurement of arterial blood gases. This is frequently coupled with measurement of blood lactate concentration. Arterial blood gas analysis is a straightforward technique, with samples typically taken from the radial artery (Fig. 1.7) and rapidly analysed by near-patient or laboratory-based machines (Table 1.14).

There are two broad types of acid–base disturbance: acidosis ('acidaemia' if plasma pH <7.35 or H⁺ >45 mmol/L) or alkalosis ('alkalaemia' if plasma pH >7.45 or H⁺ <35 mmol/L). Both acidosis and alkalosis may be respiratory or metabolic in origin.

Metabolic acidosis

Metabolic acidosis is characterised by an increase in plasma hydrogen ions in conjunction with a decrease in bicarbonate concentration. A rise in plasma hydrogen ion concentration stimulates chemoreceptors in the medulla, resulting in a compensatory respiratory alkalosis (an increase in minute volume and a fall in Paco₂). Base deficit is a measure of the amount of bicarbonate required to correct acidosis.

Metabolic acidosis can occur as a result of increased production of endogenous acid (e.g., lactic acid or ketone bodies), referred to as 'increased anion gap acidosis', or increased loss of bicarbonate (e.g., intestinal fistula, hyperchloraemic acidosis), leading to 'normal anion gap acidosis'. The anion gap (normal range of 12–15 mmol/L) is a calculated measure that simply represents the concentration of unmeasured anions in plasma:

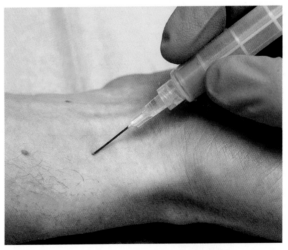

Fig. 1.7 A blood gas sample being taken from the radial artery under local anaesthesia.

Table 1.14 Normal arterial blood gas report

pH	**7.35–7.45**
H⁺	44–36 nm/L
HCO₃	23–28 mmol/L
P_aCO₂	36–44 mmHg (4.8–5.9 kPa)
P_aO₂	80–100 mmHg (10.6–13.3 kPa)

$$\text{Anion gap} = \text{Concentration of measured cations}$$
$$- \text{Concentration of measured anions}$$
$$= ([Na^+] + [K^+]) - ([HCO_3^-] + [Cl^-])$$

The most common cause of metabolic acidosis encountered in surgical practice is shock and impaired tissue oxygen delivery (see section on shock). In these cases plasma lactate is likely to be increased (lactic acidosis). Treatment is directed towards restoring circulating blood volume and tissue perfusion. Adequate resuscitation typically corrects the metabolic acidosis seen in this context. Another common cause of acidosis is acute kidney injury, which will be evident from measurement of urea and creatinine, and clinical signs of oliguria. These two causes of metabolic acidosis frequently occur concurrently.

Metabolic alkalosis

Metabolic alkalosis is characterised by a decrease in plasma hydrogen ion concentration and an increase in bicarbonate concentration. A rise in $Paco_2$ occurs as a consequence of the rise in bicarbonate concentration, resulting in a compensatory respiratory acidosis.

Metabolic alkalosis is commonly associated with hypokalaemia and hypochloraemia. The kidney has an enormous capacity to generate bicarbonate ions and this is stimulated by chloride loss. This is a major contributor to the metabolic alkalosis seen following significant (chloride-rich) losses from the gastrointestinal tract, especially when combined with loss of acid from conditions such as gastric outlet obstruction. Hypokalaemia is often associated with metabolic alkalosis because of the transcellular shift of hydrogen ions into cells and because distal renal tubular cells retain potassium in preference to hydrogen ions.

 1.6 Summary

Metabolic acidosis

Common surgical causes

Increased anion gap acidosis
Lactic acidosis
- Shock (any cause)
- Severe hypoxaemia
- Severe haemorrhage/anaemia
- Liver failure

Accumulation of other acids
- Diabetic ketoacidosis
- Starvation ketoacidosis
- Acute or chronic renal failure
- Poisoning (ethylene glycol, methanol, salicylates)

Normal anion gap acidosis
Increased bicarbonate loss
- Diarrhoea
- Intestinal fistulae
- Hyperchloraemic acidosis

Acid–base findings

Acute uncompensated
- H^+ ions ↑
- $Paco_2$ ↔
- Actual HCO_3^- ↓
- Standard HCO_3^- ↓
- Base deficit < -2

With respiratory compensation (hyperventilation)
- H^+ ions ↔ (full compensation), ↑ (partial compensation)
- $Paco_2$ ↓
- Actual HCO_3^- ↓
- Standard HCO_3^- ↓

The treatment of metabolic alkalosis involves adequate fluid replacement and the correction of electrolyte disturbances, notably hypokalaemia and hypochloraemia, and treatment of the primary cause.

Respiratory acidosis

Respiratory acidosis is a common postoperative problem characterised by increased $Paco_2$, hydrogen ion and plasma bicarbonate concentrations, as in type II respiratory failure with alveolar hypoventilation. In the surgical patient, respiratory acidosis usually results from respiratory depression and hypoventilation. This is common on emergence from general anaesthesia and following excessive opiate administration. Occasionally, respiratory acidosis occurs in the context of pulmonary complications such as pneumonia. This is more usual in very sick patients or those with pre-existing respiratory disease. Patients with this cause of respiratory acidosis frequently require ventilatory support as the hypercapnia observed reflects inadequate respiratory muscle strength to cope with an increased work of breathing.

Respiratory alkalosis

Respiratory alkalosis is caused by excessive excretion of co_2 as a result of hyperventilation. $Paco_2$ and hydrogen ion concentration decrease. Respiratory alkalosis is rarely chronic and usually does not need specific treatment. Patients may present with features of tetany due to a fall in the ionised levels of calcium due to alkalosis. It usually corrects spontaneously when the precipitating condition resolves.

1.7 Summary

Metabolic alkalosis

Common surgical causes

Loss of sodium, chloride and water
- Vomiting
- Loss of gastric secretions
- Diuretic administration

Hypokalaemia

Acid–base findings

Acute uncompensated
- H^+ ions ↓
- $Paco_2$ ↔
- Actual HCO_3^- ↑
- Standard HCO_3 ↑
- Base excess $> +2$

With respiratory compensation (hypoventilation)
- H^+ ions ↔ (full compensation), ↓ (partial compensation)
- $Paco_2$ ↑
- Actual HCO_3^- ↑
- Standard HCO_3^- ↑

Shock

Definition

Shock exists when tissue oxygen delivery fails to meet the metabolic requirements of cells. An imbalance between oxygen delivery (Do_2) and oxygen demand can result from a global reduction in oxygen delivery, maldistribution of blood flow, impaired oxygen utilisation or an increase in tissue oxygen requirements. Left

1.8 Summary

Respiratory acidosis

Common surgical causes

Central respiratory depression
- Opioid drugs
- Head injury or intracranial pathology

Pulmonary disease
- Severe asthma
- COPD
- Severe chest infection

Acid–base findings

Acute uncompensated
- H^+ ions ↑
- Pa_{CO_2} ↑
- Actual HCO_3^- ↔ or ↑
- Standard HCO_3^- ↔
- Base deficit < -2

With metabolic compensation (renal bicarbonate retention)
- H^+ ions ↔ (full compensation), ↑ (partial compensation)
- Pa_{CO_2} ↑
- Actual HCO_3^- ↑
- Standard HCO_3^- ↑↑

1.9 Summary

Respiratory alkalosis

Common surgical causes
- Pain
- Apprehension/hysterical hyperventilation
- Pneumonia
- Central nervous system disorders (meningitis, encephalopathy)
- Pulmonary embolism
- Septicaemia
- Salicylate poisoning
- Liver failure

Acid–base findings

Acute uncompensated
- H^+ ions ↓
- Pa_{CO_2} ↓
- Actual HCO_3^- ↔ or ↓
- Standard HCO_3^- ↔
- Base excess $> +2$

With metabolic compensation (renal bicarbonate excretion)
- H^+ ions ↔ (full compensation), ↓ (partial compensation)
- Pa_{CO_2} ↓
- Actual HCO_3^- ↓
- Standard HCO_3^- ↓

unchecked, shock will result in a fall in oxygen consumption (V_{O_2}), anaerobic metabolism, tissue acidosis and cellular dysfunction leading to multiple organ dysfunction and ultimately death. Although shock is sometimes considered to be synonymous with hypotension, it is important to realise that tissue oxygen delivery may be inadequate even though the blood pressure and other vital signs remain normal.

1.10 Summary

Shock

Shock is an imbalance between oxygen delivery and oxygen demand. This results in cell dysfunction and ultimately cell death and multiple organ failure.

Classification of shock

Hypovolaemic shock

This is probably the most common and most readily corrected cause of shock encountered in surgical practice, and results from a reduction in intravascular volume secondary to the loss of blood (e.g., trauma, gastrointestinal haemorrhage), plasma (e.g., burns), or water and electrolytes (e.g., vomiting, diarrhoea, diabetic ketoacidosis) (Table 1.15).

Septic shock

Septic shock results from circulatory and cellular abnormalities that occur as part of a dysregulated host response to infection. These changes impair tissue oxygen delivery and are associated with significantly increased mortality (>40%). Patients with septic shock can be identified as those with sepsis, persisting mean arterial blood pressure (MAP; <65 mmHg) and an elevated serum lactate (>2 mmol/L) despite adequate fluid resuscitation (~30 mL/kg). The 1992 consensus definitions of sepsis (systemic inflammatory response syndrome [SIRS], sepsis, severe sepsis and septic shock) lack sensitivity and specificity. New consensus definitions (Sepsis-3) have been published (Fig. 1.8). In the new criteria, the quick sepsis-related organ failure assessment (qSOFA) score is used to assess the presence of three symptoms: altered mental status, low blood pressure (<100 mmHg) and tachypnea (respiratory rate >22 breaths per minute). If a patient with infection has two or more of these criteria ('qSOFA positive'), they should be assumed to have sepsis. Importantly, qSOFA-positive status should also prompt clinicians to investigate organ dysfunction and escalate therapy, including critical care referral, as appropriate.

Sepsis usually arises from a localised infection, with gram-negative (38%) and increasingly gram-positive (52%) bacteria being the most frequently identified pathogens. The most common sites of infection leading to sepsis are the lungs (50–70%), abdomen (20–25%), urinary tract (7–10%) and skin (see Chapter 4).

Table 1.15 Causes of hypovolaemic shock
Gastrointestinal haemorrhage
• Oesophageal varices
• Oesophageal mucosal (Mallory–Weiss) tear
• Acute erosive gastritis
• Gastric and duodenal ulceration
• Cancer
• Diverticula
Trauma
Ruptured aneurysm
Obstetric haemorrhage
• Ruptured ectopic pregnancy
• Placentia praevia
• Placental abruption
• Postpartum haemorrhage
Pulmonary haemorrhage
• Pulmonary embolus
• Cancer
• Cavitating lung lesions, e.g., tuberculosis, aspergillosis
• Vasculitis
Major blood loss during surgery

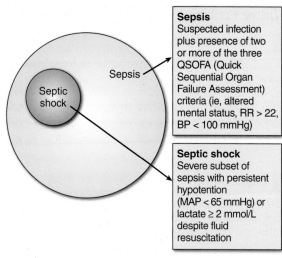

Sepsis
Suspected infection plus presence of two or more of the three QSOFA (Quick Sequential Organ Failure Assessment) criteria (ie, altered mental status, RR > 22, BP < 100 mmHg)

Septic shock
Severe subset of sepsis with persistent hypotention (MAP < 65 mmHg) or lactate ≥ 2 mmol/L despite fluid resuscitation

Fig. 1.8 **The interrelationship between sepsis and septic shock.** Based on third international consensus definition Sepsis-3. *BP,* Blood pressure; *MAP,* mean arterial pressure; *qSOFA,* Quick Sequential Organ Failure Assessment, *RR,* respiration rate.

Infection triggers a cytokine-mediated proinflammatory response that results in peripheral vasodilatation, redistribution of blood flow, endothelial cell activation, increased vascular permeability and the formation of microthrombi within the microcirculation. Cardiac output typically increases in septic shock to compensate for peripheral vasodilatation. However, despite a global increase in oxygen delivery, microcirculatory dysfunction impairs oxygen delivery to the cells. Compounding disturbances in oxygen delivery, mitochondrial dysfunction may block the normal bioenergetic pathways within the cell, impairing oxygen utilisation.

Cardiogenic shock

This occurs when the heart is unable to maintain a cardiac output sufficient to meet the metabolic requirements of the body. This 'pump failure' can be caused by myocardial infarction, arrhythmias, valve dysfunction, cardiac tamponade, massive pulmonary embolism and tension pneumothorax.

Anaphylactic shock

This is a severe systemic hypersensitivity reaction following exposure to an agent (allergen) triggering the release of vasoactive mediators (histamine, kinins and prostaglandins) from basophils and mast cells. Anaphylaxis may be immunologically mediated (allergic anaphylaxis), when IgE, IgG or complement activation by immune complexes mediates the reaction, or nonimmunologically mediated (nonallergic anaphylaxis). The clinical features of allergic and nonallergic anaphylaxis may be identical, with shock a frequent manifestation of both. Anaphylactic shock results from vasodilatation, intravascular volume redistribution, capillary leak and a reduction in cardiac output. Common causes of anaphylaxis include drugs (e.g., neuromuscular-blocking drugs, β-lactam antibiotics), colloid solutions (e.g., gelatin-containing solutions, dextrans), radiological contrast media, foodstuffs (peanuts, tree nuts, shellfish, dairy products), hymenoptera stings and latex.

 1.11 Summary

Sepsis—1992 Consensus definitions[a]

Systemic inflammatory response syndrome (SIRS)
Defined as two or more of the following criteria:
- Temperature >38°C or <36°C
- Heart rate >90 beats per minute
- Respiratory rate >20 breaths per minute or $PaCO_2 < 4.5$ kPa
- White cell count >12 or $<4 \times 10^9$/L or >10% immature neutrophils.

Bacteraemia
- The presence of viable bacteria in the blood. The presence of other pathogens in the blood is described in a similar way; i.e., viraemia, fungaemia and parasitaemia

Sepsis
- The systemic response to infection. Defined as SIRS with confirmed or presumed infection

Severe sepsis
- Sepsis with evidence of organ dysfunction

Septic shock
- Sepsis-induced hypotension and/or tissue hypoperfusion (e.g., oliguria, lactic acidosis) despite adequate fluid resuscitation.

Sepsis-3 Consensus definitions[b]

Sepsis
- Organ dysfunction caused by dysregulated host response to infection
- Organ dysfunction can be identified as an acute change in Sequential Organ Failure Assessment (SOFA) score of ≥2
- Patients with suspected infection can be promptly screened for sepsis using an abbreviated quick Sequential Organ Failure Assessment score (qSOFA) by assessing the presence of three criteria:
  - Respiratory rate ≥22 breaths per minute
  - Altered mental state
  - Systolic blood pressure ≤100 mmHg
- Patients with infection and two or more qSOFA criteria (qSOFA positive) should be assumed to have sepsis

Septic shock
- A severe subset of sepsis where circulatory and cellular changes are associated with a substantial increase in mortality
- Patients with septic shock can be identified as those with persistent hypotension requiring vasopressors to maintain mean arterial blood pressure ≥65 mmHg and serum lactate ≥2 mmol/L despite adequate fluid resuscitation

[a]American College of Chest Physicians & Society of Critical Care Medicine Consensus Conference Committee definitions 1992;[b]Third International Consensus Definitions for Sepsis and Septic Shock (Sepsis-3), 2016.

Neurogenic shock

This is caused by a loss of sympathetic tone to vascular smooth muscle. This typically occurs following injury to the thoracic or cervical spinal cord and results in profound vasodilatation, a fall in systemic vascular resistance (SVR) and hypotension. A temporary drug-induced form can also occur in 'high' spinal anaesthesia.

Pathophysiology

In clinical practice there is often significant overlap between the causes of shock; for example, patients with septic shock are frequently also hypovolaemic. Whilst differences can be detected at the level of the macrocirculation, with the exception of neurogenic shock, most types of shock are associated with increased sympathetic activity and all share common pathophysiological features at the cellular level.

Macrocirculation

When assessing a patient with shock, it is useful to remember that mean arterial pressure (MAP) is equal to the product of cardiac output (CO) and systemic vascular resistance (SVR) (Table 1.16).

Shock (inadequate tissue oxygen delivery) can occur in the context of a low, normal or high cardiac output.

In hypovolaemic shock, a fall in intravascular volume results in a fall in cardiac output. There is catecholamine release from the adrenal medulla and sympathetic nerve endings, as well as the generation of AT-II from the renin–angiotensin system as a consequence. The resulting tachycardia and increased myocardial contractility act to preserve cardiac output, whilst vasoconstriction acts to maintain arterial blood pressure, diverting the available blood to vital organs (e.g., the brain, heart and muscle) and away from nonvital organs (e.g., the skin and gut). Clinically, this 'low cardiac output' state manifests as pale, clammy skin with collapsed peripheral veins and a prolonged capillary refill time. The resulting splanchnic hypoperfusion is implicated in many of the complications associated with prolonged or untreated shock.

In septic shock, circulating proinflammatory cytokines (notably TNF-α and IL-1β) induce endothelial expression of the enzyme NO synthetase and the production of NO that leads to smooth muscle relaxation, vasodilatation and a fall in SVR. The initial cardiovascular response is a reflex tachycardia and an increase in stroke volume resulting in an increased cardiac output. Clinically this manifests as warm, well-perfused peripheries, a low diastolic blood pressure and raised pulse pressure. Fit young patients may compensate for these changes relatively well even though oxygen delivery and utilisation is compromised at the cellular level. However, as septic shock progresses endothelial dysfunction results in significant extravasation of fluid and a loss of intravascular volume. Cardiac ventricular dysfunction also impairs the compensatory increase in cardiac output. As a result, peripheral perfusion falls and the clinical signs may become indistinguishable from those associated with the low cardiac output state described previously.

In neurogenic shock, traumatic disruption of sympathetic efferent nerve fibres results in loss of vasomotor tone, peripheral vasodilatation and a fall in SVR. Loss of cardiac accelerator fibres (T1–4) and anhydrosis as a result of loss of sweat gland innervation also frequently occur, with patients typically presenting with hypotension, bradycardia and warm, dry peripheries.

Cardiogenic shock typically presents with signs of a low-output state, although, unlike hypovolaemic shock, circulating volume is typically normal or increased secondary to increased circulating AT-II and aldosterone levels. If associated with left ventricular failure, there may be pulmonary oedema.

Table 1.16 Haemodynamic and oxygen transport parameters

$MAP = CO \times SVR$
$Do_2 \approx CO \times 1.34 \times [Hb] \times (Sao_2/100)$
$Vo_2 = CO \times 1.34 \times [Hb] \times (Sao_2 - Svo_2)$

CO, Cardiac output; Do_2, oxygen delivery; [Hb], haemoglobin concentration in g/dL; MAP, mean arterial blood pressure; Sao_2, arterial oxygen saturation; Svo_2, mixed venous oxygen saturations (sampled from pulmonary artery); SVR, systemic vascular resistance; Vo_2, oxygen consumption.

Microcirculation

Changes in the microcirculation (arterioles, capillaries and venules) have a central role in the pathogenesis of shock.

Arteriolar vasoconstriction, seen in early hypovolaemic and cardiogenic shock, helps to maintain a satisfactory MAP, and the resulting fall in the capillary hydrostatic pressure encourages the transfer of fluid from the interstitial space into the vascular compartment so helping to maintain circulating volume. As described above, high vascular resistance in the capillary beds of the skin and gut results in a redistribution of cardiac output to vital organs.

If shock remains uncorrected, local accumulation of lactic acid and carbon dioxide, together with the release of vasoactive substances from the endothelium, override compensatory vasoconstriction leading to precapillary vasodilatation. This results in pooling of blood within the capillary bed and endothelial cell damage. Capillary permeability increases with the loss of fluid into the interstitial space and haemoconcentration within the capillary. The resulting increase in blood viscosity, in conjunction with reduced red cell deformability, further compromises flow through the microcirculation, predisposing to platelet aggregation and the formation of microthrombi.

In sepsis, there is upregulation of inducible NO synthetase and smooth muscle cells lose their adrenergic sensitivity, resulting in pathological arterio–venous shunting. Endothelial and inflammatory cell activation results in the generation of reactive oxidant species, disruption of barrier function in the microcirculation and widespread activation of coagulation. Microthombi occlude capillary blood flow, and the consumption of platelets and coagulation factors leads to thrombocytopenia, coagulopathy and DIC (Fig. 1.9).

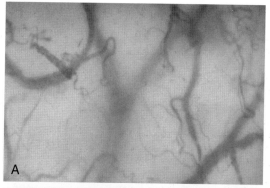

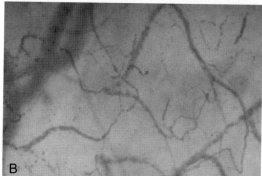

Fig. 1.9 The effect of septic shock on the microcirculation. Photomicrograph from a video clip of the normal microcirculation **(A)** and the microcirculation in septic shock **(B)**. Septic shock is associated with an increased number of small vessels with either absent or intermittent flow.

Cellular function

Under normal (aerobic) conditions, glycolysis converts glucose to pyruvate. Pyruvate is converted to acetyl-CoA and enters the tricarboxylic acid (TCA; also known as the Krebs or citric acid) cycle. Oxidation of acetyl-CoA in the TCA cycle generates nicotinamide adenine dinucleotide (NADH) and flavine adenine dinucleotide, which enter the electron transport chain and are oxidised to NAD^+ in the oxidative phosphorylation of ADP to ATP.

The oxidative metabolism of glucose is energy efficient, yielding up to 38 moles of ATP for each mole of glucose, but requires a continuous supply of oxygen to the cell. Hypoxaemia blocks mitochondrial oxidative phosphorylation, inhibiting ATP synthesis. This leads to a decrease in the intracellular ATP/ADP ratio, an increase in the $NADH/NAD^+$ ratio and an accumulation of pyruvate that is unable to enter the TCA cycle. The cytosolic conversion of pyruvate to lactate allows the regeneration of some NAD^+, enabling the limited production of ATP by anaerobic glycolysis. However, anaerobic glycolysis is significantly less efficient, generating only 2 moles of ATP per mole of glucose and predisposing cells to ATP depletion (Fig. 1.10).

Under normal conditions, the tissues globally extract about 25% of the oxygen delivered to them, with the normal oxygen saturation of mixed venous blood being 70–75%. As oxygen delivery falls, cells are able to increase the proportion of oxygen extracted from the blood, but this compensatory mechanism is limited, with a maximal oxygen extraction ratio of about 50%. At this point, further reductions in oxygen delivery lead to a critical reduction in oxygen consumption and anaerobic metabolism, a state described as dysoxia (Fig. 1.11).

Anaerobic metabolism leads to a rise in lactic acid in the systemic circulation. In the absence of significant renal or liver disease serum lactate concentration is a useful marker of global cellular hypoxia and oxygen debt. Similarly, a fall in mixed venous oxygen saturations may reflect increased oxygen extraction by the tissues and an imbalance between oxygen delivery and oxygen demand.

In septic shock, cell dysoxia and lactate accumulation may reflect a problem with both oxygen utilisation and oxygen delivery. The increased sympathetic activity occurring in sepsis leads to increased glycolysis and an increase in pyruvate generation. Coupled with dysfunction of the enzyme pyruvate dehydrogenase, this leads to accumulation of pyruvate and (hence) lactate. In addition, sepsis is associated with significant mitochondrial dysfunction and marked inhibition of oxidative phosphorylation. The phrase 'cytopathic shock' has been used to describe this condition.

The movement of sodium against a concentration gradient is an active process requiring ATP. Reduction in ATP supply leads to intracellular accumulation of sodium, an osmotic gradient across the cell membrane, dilatation of the endoplasmic reticulum and cell swelling. When combined with the failure of other vital ATP-dependent cell functions and the reduction in intracellular pH associated with the accumulation of lactic acid, the result is disruption of protein synthesis, damage to lysosomal and mitochondrial membranes, and ultimately cell necrosis.

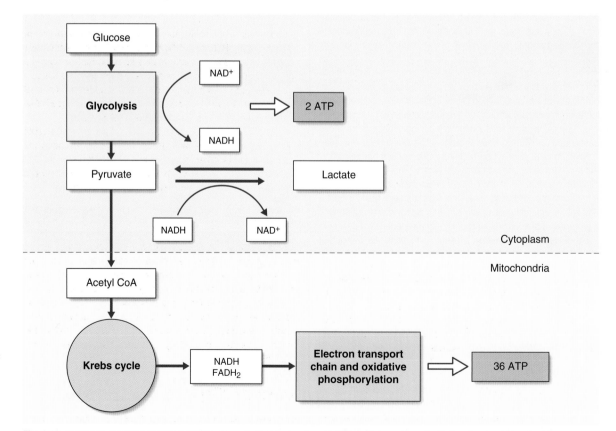

Fig. 1.10 Glycolysis. Simplified diagram illustrating glycolysis, the tricarboxylic acid (TCA) or Krebs cycle, and oxidative phosphorylation. Aerobic metabolism yields up to 38 moles of ATP per mole of glucose oxidised. Anaerobic metabolism is considerably less efficient, yielding only 2 moles of ATP per mole of glucose.

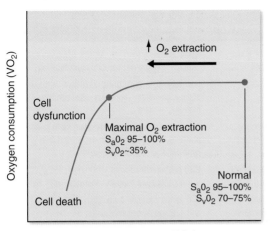

Fig. 1.11 The relationship among oxygen delivery, oxygen consumption and oxygen extraction (S_aO_2–S_vO_2). As oxygen delivery falls in shock, oxygen extraction increases until it reaches maximal oxygen extraction (60–70%). Further reductions in oxygen delivery result in a fall in oxygen consumption and tissue dysoxia. As ATP supply falls below ATP demand this leads to cell dysfunction and ultimately to cell death. S_aO_2, arterial oxygen saturation; S_vO_2, mixed venous saturation.

The effect of shock on individual organ systems

Shock leads to increased sympathetic activity. This results in a rise in cardiac output (CO), systemic vascular resistance (SVR) and mean arterial pressure (MAP). Preservation and redistribution of cardiac output, coupled with intrinsic organ autoregulation, helps to maintain adequate perfusion and oxygen delivery to vital organs (brain, heart, skeletal muscle). However, these compensatory mechanisms have limits, and in the case of severe, prolonged and/or uncorrected shock ('decompensated' shock), the clinical manifestations of organ hypoperfusion become apparent.

Shock also leads to the upregulation of proinflammatory cytokines (TNF-α, IL-1β and IL-6), which clinically are characterised by SIRS, organ dysfunction and multiple organ failure. These complications of shock are determined as much by this host inflammatory response as the disease or injury that caused shock to occur. This emphasises the importance of early recognition and correction of shock to prevent organ failure.

Cardiovascular

As described above, cardiogenic shock results from a fall in cardiac output whilst neurogenic shock results from vasodilatation and reduced SVR. Significant myocardial and vascular dysfunction also frequently occur in other causes of shock.

Despite coronary autoregulation, severe (diastolic) hypotension results in an imbalance between myocardial oxygen supply and demand, and ischaemia in the watershed areas of the endocardium. This impairs myocardial contractility. Hypoxaemia and acidosis deplete myocardial stores of noradrenaline (norepinephrine) and diminish the cardiac response to both endogenous and exogenous catecholamines. Acid–base and electrolyte abnormalities, combined with local tissue hypoxia, increase myocardial excitability and predispose to both atrial and ventricular dysrhythmias. As described above, circulating inflammatory mediators implicated in the pathogenesis of sepsis and SIRS depress myocardial

contractility and ventricular function, increase endothelial permeability (resulting in intravascular volume depletion) and cause widespread activation of both coagulation and fibrinolysis (leading to DIC).

Respiratory

Tachypnoea driven by pain, pyrexia, local lung pathology, pulmonary oedema, metabolic acidosis or cytokines is one of the earliest features of shock. The increased minute volume typically results in reduced arterial PCO_2 and a respiratory alkalosis (see earlier). Initially this will compensate for the metabolic acidosis of shock but eventually this mechanism is overwhelmed and blood pH falls.

In hypovolaemic states, there is reduction in pulmonary blood flow and this leads to underperfusion of ventilated alveolar units and ventilation–perfusion (V/Q) mismatch. In cardiogenic shock, left ventricular failure and pulmonary oedema compromise the ventilation of perfused alveolar units, increasing the shunt fraction (Qs/Qt) within the lung. Increased V/Q mismatch and shunt fraction also occur in sepsis. The net result is hypoxaemia that may be refractory to increases in inspired oxygen concentration.

Sepsis and hypovolaemic shock are both recognised causes of acute respiratory distress syndrome. This is characterised by the influx of protein-rich oedema fluid and inflammatory cells into the alveolar air spaces resulting in significant V/Q mismatch and hypoxaemia. Acute respiratory distress syndrome appears to be cytokine mediated (notably IL-8, TNF-α, IL-1 and IL-6).

Renal

Reduced renal blood flow results in the production of low-volume (<0.5 mL/kg/h), high-osmolality and low sodium content urine. If shock is not reversed, hypoxia leads to acute tubular necrosis, characterised by oliguanuria and urine with a high sodium concentration and an osmolality close to that of plasma. With a fall in glomerular filtration, blood urea and creatinine rise; hyperkalaemia and a metabolic acidosis are also usually present.

Renal failure occurs in about 30–50% of patients with septic shock. In addition to the mechanisms responsible for the simple prerenal failure described above, there is an imbalance in pre- and postglomerular vascular resistance, mesangial contraction and microvascular injury leading to glomerular filtration failure.

Nervous system

Due to the increased sympathetic activity, patients may appear inappropriately anxious. As compensatory mechanisms reach their limit and cerebral hypoperfusion and hypoxia supervene, there is increasing restlessness, progressing to confusion, stupor and coma. Unless cerebral hypoxia has been prolonged, effective resuscitation will usually correct the depressed conscious level rapidly. In septic shock, the clinical picture may be complicated by the presence of an underlying (septic) encephalopathy and/or delirium.

Gastrointestinal

The redistribution of cardiac output observed in shock leads to a marked reduction in splanchnic blood flow. In the stomach, the resulting mucosal hypoperfusion and hypoxia predispose to stress ulceration and haemorrhage. In the intestine, movement (translocation) of bacteria and/or bacterial endotoxin from the gut lumen to the portal vein and hence systemic circulation may occur. This is thought to be an important pathophysiological mechanism in the development of SIRS and multiple organ failure in shock.

Hepatobiliary

Despite its dual blood supply, ischaemic hepatic injury is frequently seen following hypovolaemic or cardiogenic shock. An acute, reversible elevation in serum transaminase levels indicates hepatocellular injury, and typically occurs 1–3 days following the ischaemic insult. Increases in prothrombin time and/or hypoglycaemia are markers of more severe injury. Significant ischaemic hepatitis is more frequent in patients with underlying cardiac disease and a degree of hepatic venous congestion.

1.12 Summary

Clinical effects of shock

Nervous system
- Restlessness, confusion, stupor, coma
- Encephalopathy and/or delirium, common in sepsis

Renal
- Renal hypoperfusion → activation of the renin–angiotensin system
- Oliguria (<0.5 mL/kg/h urine) → anuria
- Acute renal failure → ↑ urea, ↑ creatinine, ↑ K$^+$ and metabolic acidosis

Respiratory
- Tachypnoea
- ↑ Ventilation/perfusion (V/Q) mismatch and ↑ shunt → hypoxia
- Pulmonary oedema (common in cardiogenic shock) → hypoxia
- Acute respiratory distress syndrome → hypoxia

Cardiovascular
- ↓ Diastolic pressure → ↓ coronary blood flow
- ↓ Myocardial oxygen delivery → myocardial ischaemia → ↓ contractility and ↓ cardiac output
- Acidosis, electrolyte disturbances and hypoxia predispose to arrhythmias
- Widespread endothelial cell activation → microcirculatory dysfunction

Gastrointestinal
- Splanchnic hypoperfusion → breakdown of gut–mucosal barrier
- Stress ulceration
- Translocation of bacteria/bacterial wall contents into blood stream → systemic inflammatory response syndrome
- Acute ischaemic hepatitis.

Management

General principles

The management of shock is based upon the following principles:
- Identification and treatment of the underlying cause
- Resuscitation and the maintenance of adequate tissue oxygen delivery.

As with most clinical emergencies, treatment and diagnosis should occur simultaneously with the immediate assessment and management following an Airway, Breathing, Circulation (ABC) approach.

Table 1.17 Clinical assessment of shock

Conscious level	Restlessness, anxiety, stupor and coma are common features and suggest cerebral hypoperfusion
Pulse	Low-volume, thready pulse consistent with low-output state; high-volume, bounding pulse consistent with high-output state
Blood pressure	Changes in diastolic may precede a fall in systolic blood pressure, with ↓ diastolic in sepsis and ↑ in hypovolaemic and cardiogenic shock
Peripheral perfusion	Cold peripheries suggest vasoconstriction (↑ SVR); warm peripheries suggest vasodilatation (↓ SVR)
Pulse oximetry	Hypoxemia common association of all forms of shock and ↓ tissue O_2 delivery
ECG monitoring	Myocardial ischaemia most common cause of cardiogenic shock but common in all forms of shock
Urine output	<0.5 mL/kg/h suggestive of renal hypoperfusion
CVP measurement	Low CVP with collapsing central veins consistent with hypovolaemia
Arterial blood gas	Metabolic acidosis and ↑ lactate consistent with tissue hypoperfusion

In isolation, single measurements are not helpful. Measurements are far more useful when used in combination with the findings of a detailed clinical examination. Observation of trends over time, together with the response to therapeutic interventions (e.g., a fluid challenge) is key to the successful management of shock. CVP, Central venous pressure; SVR, sustained virological response.

The early recognition and treatment of potentially reversible causes (e.g., bleeding, intraabdominal sepsis, myocardial ischaemia, pulmonary embolus, cardiac tamponade) is essential and may be facilitated by a detailed history, a thorough clinical examination (Table 1.17) and focused investigations.

Whilst shocked patients may be more sensitive to the effects of opiates, there is no justification for withholding effective analgesia if indicated and this should be titrated intravenously (e.g., morphine in 1–2-mg increments) to response during the initial assessment and treatment.

Most patients with shock will require admission to a high-dependency or intensive care unit.

Airway and breathing

Hypoxaemia must be prevented and, if present, rapidly corrected by maintaining a clear airway (e.g., head tilt, chin lift) and administering high-flow oxygen (e.g., 10–15 L/min). The adequacy of this therapy can be estimated continuously using pulse oximetry (SpO_2), but frequent arterial blood gas analysis allows a more accurate assessment of oxygenation (PaO_2), ventilation (PaCO_2) and indirect measures of tissue perfusion (pH, base excess, HCO$_3^-$ and lactate). In patients with severe hypoxaemia, cardiovascular instability, depressed conscious level or exhaustion, intubation, and ventilatory support may be required.

Circulation

Initial resuscitation should be targeted at arresting haemorrhage and providing fluid (crystalloid or colloid) to restore intravascular volume and optimise cardiac preload. It is common practice to use blood to maintain a haemoglobin concentration 8–10 g/dL during the initial resuscitation of shock, particularly if there is active bleeding and/or evidence of inadequate tissue oxygen delivery, such as a raised lactate concentration. However, there is little evidence to support any particular transfusion trigger, and evidence from randomised studies suggests a more restrictive trigger (Hb 7 g/dL) is equally effective in the resuscitation of patients with gastrointestinal haemorrhage or septic shock. A reduction in tachycardia, increasing blood pressure, and improving peripheral perfusion and urine output in response to a series of 250–500-mL (~3-mL/kg) fluid challenges indicate 'fluid responsiveness' and suggest that further fluid and optimisation of preload may be required. Once parameters stop improving it is unlikely that further fluid will be beneficial, particularly if there is an associated fall in oxygen saturation or the development of pulmonary oedema. As resuscitation continues, more invasive monitoring (central venous catheter; arterial line) allows the acid–base status, arterial and central venous pressure (CVP), or central venous oxygen saturations (S_cVO_2) to be used to further assess the response to fluid (Fig. 1.12). When more physiological information about circulatory status is required, more advanced methods for assessing cardiac output and intravascular volume may be required (e.g., arterial pulse contour analysis, oesophageal Doppler, ultrasound-based methods or pulmonary artery catheterisation). These are all specialised techniques used in the intensive care unit or operating theatre.

If blood pressure remains low and/or signs of inadequate tissue oxygen delivery persist despite fluid resuscitation and the optimisation of preload, then inotropes and/or vasopressors may be required. Although there is a degree of crossover in their mechanism of action, vasopressors (e.g., noradrenaline) cause peripheral vasoconstriction and an increased SVR, while inotropes (e.g., dobutamine) increase myocardial contractility, stroke volume and cardiac output. The initial choice of inotrope or vasopressor therefore depends upon the underlying aetiology of shock and an understanding of the main physiological derangements (Table 1.18). Adrenaline, which has both vasopressor and inotropic effects, is a useful first-line drug in the emergency treatment of shock. Vasoactive drug administration should be continuously titrated against specific physiological end points (e.g., blood pressure or cardiac output) in an appropriate critical care environment.

Hypovolaemic shock

The most common cause of acute hypovolaemic shock in surgical practice is bleeding (Table 1.15).

Normal adult blood volume is about 7% of body weight, with a 70-kg man having an estimated blood volume (EBV) of around 5000 mL. The severity of haemorrhagic shock is frequently classified according to percentage of EBV lost, where class I (<15%) represents a compensated state (as may occur following the donation of a unit of blood) and class IV (>40%) is immediately life-threatening (Table 1.19). The term 'massive haemorrhage' has a number of definitions including: loss of EBV in 24 hours; loss of 50% EBV in 3 hours; blood loss at a rate ≥150 mL/min.

Arrest of haemorrhage and intravascular fluid resuscitation should occur concurrently; there is only a limited role for inotropes or vasopressors in the treatment of a hypotensive hypovolaemic patient. As described above, fluid therapy should be titrated to clinical and physiological response.

In the emergency situation, before bleeding has been controlled, a systolic blood pressure at which a radial pulse is just palpable (~80 mmHg) is increasingly used as a resuscitation target (permissive hypotension) as it is thought less likely to dislodge clot and lead to dilutional coagulopathy. Once active bleeding has been stopped, resuscitation can be fine-tuned to optimise organ perfusion and tissue oxygen delivery, as described above. It remains unclear whether permissive hypotension is appropriate for all cases of haemorrhagic shock but it appears to improve outcomes following penetrating trauma and ruptured aortic aneurysm.

Rapid fluid resuscitation requires secure vascular access and this is best achieved through two wide-bore (14- or 16-gauge) peripheral intravenous cannulae.

The type of fluid used (crystalloid or colloid) is probably less important than the adequate restoration of circulating volume itself. In the case of life-threatening or continued haemorrhage, blood will be required early in the resuscitation. Ideally, fully cross-matched packed red blood cells (PRBCs) should be administered, but in life-threatening haemorrhage type-specific or O Rhesus-negative blood may be used until this becomes available. A haemoglobin concentration of >7 g/dL may be sufficient to

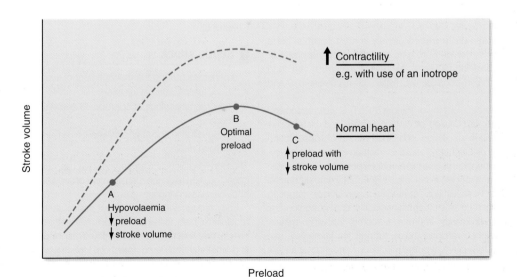

Fig. 1.12 Frank–Starling curve. Demonstrating the relationship between ventricular preload and stroke volume.

Table 1.18 Effects of commonly used vasoactive drugs

Drug	CO	SVR	Main effects
Adrenaline	↑	↑	α- and β-agonist; positive inotrope and vasopressor
Noradrenaline	↔/↓	↑	α-agonist; vasopressor
Dobutamine	↑	↓	β1-agonist; positive inotrope and systemic vasodilator
Dopamine	↑	↓	β1-agonist (at doses >5 μg/kg/minute); positive inotrope and systemic vasodilator
Dopexamine	↑	↓	β1-agonist; positive inotrope and systemic vasodilator
Levosimendan	↑	↓	Calcium sensitiser; positive inotrope and systemic vasodilator
Milrinone	↑	↓	Phosphodiesterase inhibitor; positive inotrope and systemic vasodilator
Glyceryl trinitrate	↑	↓	Nitric oxide-mediated vasodilatation

CO, Cardiac output; SVR, systemic vascular resistance.

Table 1.19 Estimated blood loss and presentation of hypovolaemic shock

	Class I	Class II	Class III	Class IV
Blood loss (mL)	<750	750–1500	1500–2000	>2000
Blood loss (% EBV)	<15	15–30%	30–40%	>40%
Pulse	<100	>100	>120	>140
Blood pressure	Normal	Decreased	Decreased	Decreased
Respiratory rate	14–20	20–30	30–40	>35
Urine output (mL/h)	>30	20–30	5–15	Negligible
CNS symptoms	Normal	Anxious	Confused	Lethargic

CNS, Central nervous system; EBV, estimated blood volume.
Adapted from Committee on Trauma: Advanced Trauma Life Support Manual.

ensure adequate tissue oxygen delivery in most patients, but a haemoglobin target of 8–10 g/dL may be more appropriate in actively bleeding patients. Massive transfusion can lead to hypothermia, hypocalcaemia, hyper- or hypokalaemia, and coagulopathy.

The acute coagulopathy of trauma (ACoT) is well recognised and multifactorial. Dilution of clotting factors and platelets as a result of fluid resuscitation, combined with their consumption at the point of bleeding, results in clotting factor deficiency, thrombocytopenia and coagulopathy. Hypothermia, metabolic acidosis and hypocalcaemia also significantly impair normal coagulation. Resuscitation strategies aggressively targeting the 'lethal triad' of hypothermia, acidosis and coagulopathy appear to significantly improve outcome following military trauma, and observational studies support the immediate use of measures to prevent hypothermia, early correction of severe metabolic acidosis (pH <7.1), maintenance of ionised calcium >1.0 mmol/L and the early empirical use of clotting factors and platelets.

Where possible, correction of coagulopathy should be guided by laboratory results (platelet count, prothrombin time, activated partial thromboplastin time and fibrinogen concentration). Thromboelastography (TEG) or rotational thromboelastometry (ROTEM) provide near-patient functional assays of clot formation, platelet function and fibrinolysis, and are also now widely used to guide the management of coagulopathy. Clotting factor deficiency is normally treated by the administration of fresh frozen plasma (FFP; 10–15 mL/kg), thrombocytopenia or platelet dysfunction by the administration of platelets (usually one 'pool' or adult dose containing $2–3 \times 10^{11}$ platelets). Fibrinogen deficiency (<1.0 g/L) is best treated with cryoprecipitate (usually one 'pool' of 10 single donor units) or FFP. The antifibrinolytic, tranexamic acid, has been shown to reduce mortality from bleeding when used early (<3 hours) following major trauma. It also reduces bleeding associated with surgery. Tranexamic acid should be given to all trauma patients with major haemorrhage as early as possible (1 g over 10 minutes followed by infusion of 1 g over 8 hours). Recommended targets for other important coagulation parameters during resuscitation from major haemorrhage are a fibrinogen concentration >1.5 g/L, platelet count $>75 \times 10^9.l^{-1}$, and an INR <1.5.

In the case of rapid haemorrhage, it is often not possible to use traditional laboratory results to guide the correction of coagulopathy because of the time delay in obtaining these results. This has led to a formula-driven approach to the use of PRBCs, FFP and platelets targeting the early empirical treatment of coagulopathy. Evidence from observational studies supports the use of warmed PRBCs and FFP in a 1:1 or 2:1 ratio as soon as possible during the resuscitation of major haemorrhage following trauma in conjunction with platelet transfusions to maintain platelets $>100 \times 10^9$ (often administered at the same rate as FFP units). This approach, combined with early control of bleeding and the use of tranexamic acid, has been associated with major reductions in mortality from trauma, especially in the military setting.

A recombinant form of activated factor VII (rVIIa) is approved for the management of bleeding in haemophiliacs with inhibitory antibodies to factors VIII or IX. Although rVIIa has been used effectively in the treatment of life-threatening haemorrhage in other patient groups, its use is associated with a significant rate of arterial thromboembolic events. It is not recommended for routine use, and should only be used by experienced clinicians (see also Chapter 2).

Septic shock

The principles guiding the management of septic shock are:

- Early identification of infection
- Early administration of appropriate antibiotics and source control
- Resuscitation and supportive care to ensure adequate tissue oxygen delivery

The Surviving Sepsis Campaign (SSC) has published evidence-based guidelines on the management of sepsis and septic shock: http://www.survivingsepsis.org.

Early recognition of sepsis and septic shock is critical. This requires a high index of suspicion together with a detailed history and examination to identify signs of organ dysfunction and potential sources of infection. Hospital-acquired infection, including intravascular access devices, should always be considered as a cause of clinical deterioration in surgical patients.

As with all forms of shock, the initial assessment and management of septic shock should follow an ABC approach. Resuscitation is time critical and should be started as soon as signs of sepsis-induced tissue hypoperfusion are recognised (e.g., hypotension, prolonged capillary refill, oliguria, elevated lactate and/or low central venous saturations). Following the publication of a landmark single-centre study in 2001, early goal-directed therapy, in which resuscitation in the first 6 hours was guided by CVP and S_cVO_2, became widely adopted as the standard of care. However, several more recent multicentre studies have failed to demonstrate the superiority of CVP and/or S_cVO_2 in guiding the resuscitation of patients who have received timely antibiotics and fluid resuscitation. The current Surviving Sepsis Campaign recommendations for the early resuscitation of septic shock are outlined in Summary 1.13.

1.13 Summary

Early resuscitation of septic shock

To be completed within 3 hours of presentation

1. Measure lactate
2. Obtain blood cultures prior to administration of antibiotics
3. Administer broad-spectrum antibiotics
4. Administer 30 mL/kg crystalloid for hypotension and/or lactate ≥4 mmol/L

To be completed within 6 hours of presentation

1. If hypotension does not respond to initial fluid resuscitation, start vasopressor to maintain MAP ≥65 mmHg
2. If hypotension does not respond to initial fluid resuscitation, reassess volume status and adequacy of tissue perfusion:
   - Repeat focused examination (e.g., vital signs, consciousness level, capillary refill, urine output)
   - Perform dynamic assessment of fluid responsiveness with fluid challenge, or passive leg raise
   - Consider cardiovascular ultrasound (echocardiography) and/or measurement of CVP and S_cVO_2
3. Remeasure lactate if initial lactate elevated

Adapted from Surviving Sepsis Campaign, revised (2015) resuscitation bundle http://www.survivingsepsis.org
CVP, Central venous pressure; *MAP*, mean arterial pressure; S_cVO_2, central venous oxygen saturation.

Septic shock is associated with both relative and absolute hypovolaemia as a result of profound vasodilatation and extravasation of fluid from the intravascular space. Both crystalloid and colloid can be used to restore intravascular volume. As there is little evidence that colloids confer clinical benefit (EBM 1.1), it is both reasonable and pragmatic to use crystalloid (e.g., Plasma-Lyte 148 solution) as the first-line resuscitation fluid. Starch-based colloid solutions appear to be associated with an increase in renal failure and mortality, so should be avoided. Current guidelines suggest the administration of 30 mL/kg crystalloid in patients with hypotension and/or lactate >4 mmol/L. This should be followed by reassessment of volume status and tissue perfusion (Summary 1.13). Persistent hypotension (MAP <65 mmHg) following restoration of circulating volume is best treated with a vasopressor such as noradrenaline in the first instance. While the titration of fluid and vasopressor to a MAP ≥65 mmHg should be sufficient to preserve tissue perfusion in most patients, this may not be the case in all patients (e.g., those with pre-existing hypertension) and

it is important to supplement these simple resuscitation end points with clinical assessment and additional markers of global tissue perfusion (e.g., lactate, S_cVO_2) to determine whether oxygen delivery is adequate. If serum lactate remains elevated (>2 mmol/L) and central venous saturations are low (<70%) in the context of septic shock, this suggests inadequate tissue oxygen delivery with increased oxygen extraction from the blood and anaerobic metabolism. In this situation, interventions that further increase oxygen delivery to the tissues using blood transfusions (if the patient has significant anaemia, e.g., Hb <10 g/dL) and/or inotropic drugs such as dobutamine should be considered. These interventions often require specialised monitoring and clinical judgement based on both chronic comorbidity (e.g., cardiovascular disease) and acute patient status, and should be undertaken in an intensive care unit.

In patients with hypotension unresponsive to fluid resuscitation and vasopressors, intravenous hydrocortisone has been shown to promote reversal of shock. However, this does not appear to translate into a survival benefit and the use of corticosteroids is associated with an increased risk of secondary infections. Because of this, the use of corticosteroids in the treatment of refractory septic shock remains controversial. Vasopressin is an alternative vasopressor to noradrenaline that can be used under specialised supervision, but does not appear to improve survival rates compared with noradrenaline.

Treatment of infection involves adequate source control and the administration of appropriate antibiotics. Source control includes the removal of infected devices, abscess drainage, the debridement of infected tissue and interventions to prevent ongoing microbial contamination such as repair of a perforated viscus or biliary drainage. This should be achieved as soon as possible following initial resuscitation and should be performed with the minimum physiological disturbance; where possible, percutaneous, minimally invasive or endoscopic techniques are preferable to open surgery.

Intravenous antibiotics must be administered as soon as possible (EBM 1.2), preferably in discussion with a microbiologist. The choice depends on the history, the likely source of infection, whether the infection is community or hospital acquired, and local patterns of pathogen susceptibility. Covering all likely pathogens (bacterial and/or fungal) usually involves the use of empirical broad-spectrum antibiotics in the first instance, with these rationalised or changed to reduce the spectrum of cover once the results of microbiological investigations become available. Most hospitals have antibiotic policies to guide which antibiotics to use according to the clinical presentation and suspected source of infection.

EBM 1.2 Early administration of antibiotics

'In the presence of septic shock, each hour delay in the administration of effective antibiotics is associated with a measurable (~8%) increase in mortality.'

Kumar A, Roberts D, Wood KE, et al. Duration of hypotension prior to initiation of effective antimicrobial therapy is the critical determinant of survival in human septic shock. Crit Care Med. 2006;34:1589–1596.

Two (peripheral) blood cultures should be taken 5 minutes apart prior to the administration of antibiotics but this must not delay therapy. Culture of urine, cerebrospinal fluid, faeces and bronchoalveolar lavage fluid may also be indicated. Targeted imaging (chest x-ray ultrasound, computed tomography) may also help identify the source of infection.

Cardiogenic shock

The most common cause of cardiogenic shock in the perioperative period is myocardial ischaemia and acute myocardial infarction. As with other forms of shock, the management of cardiogenic shock is based upon the identification and treatment of reversible causes and supportive management to maintain adequate tissue oxygen delivery. This involves active management of the four determinants of cardiac output: heart rate, preload, myocardial contractility and afterload.

Routine investigations to identify the cause of cardiogenic shock include serial 12-lead ECGs, troponin and a chest x-ray. A transthoracic echocardiogram may provide useful information on (systolic and diastolic) ventricular function and exclude potentially treatable causes of cardiogenic shock such as cardiac tamponade, valvular insufficiency and massive pulmonary embolus.

General supportive measures include the administration of high concentrations of inspired oxygenation. In patients with cardiogenic pulmonary oedema, there is some evidence that continuous positive airway pressure improves oxygenation, reduces the work of breathing and provides subjective relief of dyspnoea. It remains unclear whether these advantages translate into a significant survival benefit.

For patients with acute myocardial ischaemia, intravenous opiates should be titrated cautiously to control pain and reduce anxiety. In addition to providing analgesia, opiates reduce myocardial oxygen demand and reduce afterload by causing peripheral vasodilatation.

As with all forms of shock, correction of hypovolaemia and optimisation of intravascular volume (preload) is of central importance in maximizing stroke volume, cardiac output and tissue oxygen delivery. However, the management of fluid balance in cardiogenic shock can be challenging and should be undertaken by experienced clinicians with access to physiological monitoring. Patients with acute heart failure and cardiogenic shock are usually normovolaemic or relatively hypovolaemic as a result of intravascular fluid loss into the lungs and the development of pulmonary oedema. In contrast, patients with chronic heart failure are usually hypervolaemic as a result of longstanding activation of the renin–angiotensin system and salt and water retention. The key point is that some patients in cardiogenic shock are hypovolaemic and require cautious fluid resuscitation. This is best achieved by careful titration of a fluid challenge and assessment of the clinical response in an appropriately monitored environment (see earlier). Once hypovolaemia has been corrected and cardiac preload optimised, refractory hypotension and/or signs of inadequate tissue perfusion may require treatment with vasoactive drugs. This frequently requires a careful balance of vasodilator, inotrope and vasoconstrictor.

The major derangements in cardiogenic shock are a reduction in cardiac output and a compensatory increase in SVR. The use of a vasodilator such as glyeryltrinitrate may reduce SVR (afterload) and improve cardiac output, but vasodilatation frequently results in a significant reduction in blood pressure, compromising tissue perfusion. Adrenaline, an α- and β-agonist with both inotropic and vasoconstricting actions, is frequently used in the emergency management of cardiogenic shock, increasing both myocardial contractility and SVR. However, while adrenaline may increase blood pressure, it significantly increases myocardial workload, potentially worsening myocardial ischaemia, and profound vasoconstriction further reduces already compromised tissue perfusion. Frequently, the most appropriate choice of vasoactive drug in cardiogenic shock is one that has both inotropic and vasodilating properties such as the β-agonist dobutamine. Alternative ino-dilating agents include the calcium sensitiser levosimendan and the phosphodiesterase inhibitor milrinone.

An intraaortic balloon pump (IABP) can be used as an adjunct in the supportive management of cardiogenic shock in a highly specialised environment, usually supervised by a cardiologist. This device works by inflating a balloon in the thoracic aorta during diastole, with deflation occurring in systole. Inflation during diastole augments the diastolic blood pressure, improving coronary perfusion and myocardial oxygen delivery; deflation in systole reduces afterload. While it still remains unclear which patient groups benefit from insertion of an IABP, they are generally used as a bridge to more definitive treatment such as percutaneous coronary intervention (PCI), coronary artery bypass grafting (CABG) or mitral valve repair.

Anaphylactic shock

The management of anaphylactic shock is illustrated in Table 1.20.

Table 1.20 The management of anaphylaxis

1. Stop administration of causative agent (drug/fluid)
2. Call for help
3. Lie patient flat, feet elevated
4. Maintain airway and give 100% O_2
5. Adrenaline (epinephrine)
   • 0.5–1.0 mg (0.5–1.0 mL of 1:1000) IM or
   • *If experienced using IV adrenaline,* 50–100 µg (0.5–1.0 mL of 1:10,000) IV titrated against response
6. Intravascular volume expansion with crystalloid or colloid
7. Second-line therapy
   Antihistamine: Chlorphenamine 10–20 mg slow IV
   Corticosteroid: Hydrocortisone 200 mg IV

IM, Intramuscularly; IV, intravenously

Transfusion of blood components and plasma products

Chapter contents

Introduction 29

Blood donation 29

Blood components 29

Plasma products 31

Red cell serology 32

Pretransfusion testing 32

Indications for transfusion 33

Blood administration 33

Adverse effects of transfusion 34

Autologous transfusion 35

Transfusion requirements in special surgical settings 36

Methods to reduce the need for blood transfusion 38

Better blood transfusion 39

Future trends 39

Introduction

In the UK currently 35% of all the blood transfused to patients is performed in the surgical setting. Blood transfusion can be life-saving and many areas of surgery could not be undertaken without reliable transfusion support. However, as with any treatment, transfusion of blood and its components carries potential risks, which must be balanced against the patient's need. The magnitude of risk depends on factors such as the prevalence of infectious disease in the donor population, the resources and professionalism of the organisation collecting, processing and issuing the blood and plasma products, and the care with which the clinical team administers these products.

Blood donation

In the UK, whole blood is donated by healthy adult volunteers over the age of 17 years with normal haemoglobin levels. The standard 480 mL donation contains approximately 200 mg of iron, the loss of which is easily tolerated by healthy donors. Blood components (red cells, platelets and plasma) can be separated from the donated blood or obtained from the donor as separate products by the use of a cell separator, in a process called *apheresis*.

Strict donor selection and the testing of all donations are essential to exclude blood that may be hazardous to the recipient, as well as to ensure the welfare of the donor. All donations are ABO-grouped, Rhesus (Rh) D-typed, antibody-screened, and tested for evidence of hepatitis B, hepatitis C, human immunodeficiency virus (HIV) I and II, human T-cell leukaemia virus

(HTLV) I and II and syphilis, using tests for antibody to the virus, viral antigen or nucleic acid. Some donations are tested for antibody to cytomegalovirus (CMV), so that CMV-negative blood can be provided for patients such as transplant recipients and premature infants. Dependent on epidemiology, other testing may be required, e.g., malaria, West Nile virus.

Because of concerns regarding transmission of variant Creutzfeldt–Jakob disease (vCJD) by transfusion, a number of new precautions have been introduced. Since 1999 all blood donated in the UK has been filtered to remove white blood cells (leucodepletion), UK plasma has been excluded from fractionation, and since April 2004 people who have received a blood or blood product transfusion in the UK after 1980 have been excluded from donating blood. Some countries currently exclude donations from individuals who resided in the UK during the time of the bovine spongiform encephalitis (BSE) epidemic. There is currently no blood test for vCJD.

Blood components

The components that can be prepared from donated blood are shown in Fig. 2.1 and their descriptions follow.

Red blood cells in additive solution

Donated whole blood is collected into an anticoagulant (citrate) and nutrient (phosphate, dextrose and adenine) solution (CPDA). Centrifugation removes virtually all of the associated plasma, and a solution of saline, adenine, glucose and mannitol (SAGM) is

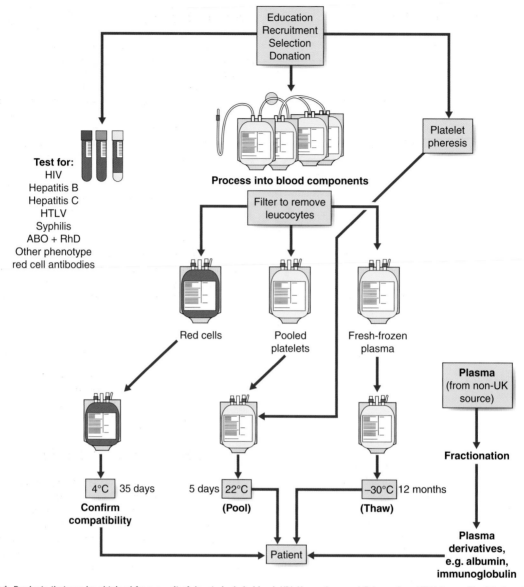

Test for:
HIV
Hepatitis B
Hepatitis C
HTLV
Syphilis
ABO + RhD
Other phenotype
red cell antibodies

Fig. 2.1 Products that can be obtained from a unit of donated whole blood. HIV, Human immunodeficiency virus; HTLV, human T-cell leukaemia virus.

added to provide optimal red cell preservation. The red cell concentrate is run through a leucodepletion filter to reduce the white cells to a concentration of less than 5×10^6/L. The final product has a haematocrit of 55–65% and a volume of approximately 300 mL. The blood cannot be sterilised, so that blood transfusion can transmit organisms not detected by donor screening. Red cell concentrates must be stored at $+4°C \pm 2°C$

Transfused blood must be ABO- and RhD-compatible with the recipient and transfused through a sterile blood administration set with an in-line macroaggregate filter, designed for the procedure. The set should be primed with saline and no other solutions transfused simultaneously. This product is indicated for acute blood loss and anaemia, and is the most widely available form of red cells for transfusion.

Platelets

Platelet concentrates can be made either from centrifugation of whole blood (random donor platelets [RDP]) or from an individual donor using apheresis (single donor platelets [SDP]). An adult dose is manufactured from four separate donations pooled together or one apheresis collection. Platelets are currently concentrated in plasma rather than an optimal additive solution and carry a greater risk of bacterial contamination as they cannot be refrigerated but must be stored at 22°C ± 2°C. For this reason platelet concentrates are now tested for bacterial contamination prior to release.

Platelets are infused through a standard blood-giving set over less than 30 minutes. As the concentrate contains some red cells and plasma, it should ideally be ABO- and RhD-compatible with the recipient. RhD-negative girls and women of child-bearing potential must receive RhD-negative platelets or, if only RhD-positive platelets are available, prophylactic RhD immunoglobulin should also be given. An adult dose should raise an adult platelet count by 20–40×10^9/L.

Platelet concentrates are indicated in thrombocytopenia, when platelet function is defective, and in patients receiving massive blood transfusions when there is microvascular bleeding (oozing from mucous membranes, needle puncture sites and wounds).

Fresh frozen plasma (FFP)

Some 200–300 mL of plasma can be removed from a unit of whole blood and stored frozen at −30°C. FFP contains albumin, immunoglobulins and, most importantly, all of the coagulation factors. FFP can be stored at −30°C for 3 years and is thawed to 37°C before issue. FFP must be ABO-compatible with the recipient and can be transfused after thawing for up to 120 hours if stored at 4°C without losing clinically significant coagulation activity. The average adult dose is 3–4 units. Imported, virally inactivated plasma (treated with methylene blue or solvent detergent) is available for use in children up to the age of 16 years and patients who require repeated exposure to FFP, such as patients undergoing plasma exchange for thrombotic thrombocytopenic purpura.

FFP is used when there are multiple coagulation factor deficiencies (e.g., disseminated intravascular coagulation [DIC]) associated with severe bleeding. It may be indicated in selected patients who are over-anticoagulated with warfarin, but there are now prothrombin complex concentrates that should ideally be used in preference for this purpose. In the case of massive blood loss arising during or after surgery, the decision whether to use FFP and, if so, how much to use, should be guided by timely tests of coagulation. FFP should not be used to correct prolonged clotting times in patients who are not bleeding or who are not about to undergo immediate surgery, for whom vitamin K is preferred.

Cryoprecipitate

A single unit of cryoprecipitate can be removed from 1 unit of FFP after controlled thawing. After resuspension in 10–20 mL plasma, the cryoprecipitate is frozen to −30°C, in which condition it can be stored for 3 years. It is enriched in high molecular weight plasma proteins such as fibrinogen, factor VIII, von Willebrand factor, factor XIII and fibronectin. A normal adult dose is 10 units. ABO-compatible units should be given, and the product infused as soon as possible after thawing. Cryoprecipitate is used when fibrinogen levels are low, as in DIC. However the pooling required for cryoprecipitate manufacture does lead to high donor exposure per dose and many countries do not produce this product, preferring instead to use higher volumes of FFP or fibrinogen concentrates to reverse hypofibrinogenaemia.

Plasma products

Fractionated products are manufactured from large pools (several thousand donations) of donor plasma that undergo some form of viral inactivation stage through the manufacturing process. Virus inactivation processes now mean that these products should not transmit HIV I and II or hepatitis B and C, but this may not apply to heat-resistant viruses that have no lipid envelope (e.g., hepatitis A) or to prions.

Human albumin

Albumin is prepared by fractionation of large pools of plasma that, at the end of processing, are pasteurised at 60°C for 10 hours. There are no compatibility requirements.

Solutions of 4.5% or 5% are used to maintain plasma albumin levels in conditions where there is increased vascular permeability, e.g., burns, and are sometimes used in acute blood volume replacement, although crystalloid or nonplasma colloid solution would be the recommended first-line volume expander. Randomised controlled trials on the use of albumin suggest that there is no clear advantage from the use of albumin solutions in the treatment of hypovolaemia over judicious use of saline or colloid solutions. Resuscitation with crystalloid requires volumes of fluid three times greater than with colloid (see Chapter 7).

Twenty per cent albumin solutions can be used when hypoproteinaemia is associated with oedema or ascites that is resistant to diuretics (e.g., liver disease, nephrotic syndrome). Twenty per cent albumin is hyperoncotic, so that there is a risk of acutely expanding the intravascular space and precipitating pulmonary oedema.

Factor VIII and factor IX concentrates

Factor VIII and IX concentrates have been widely used in the treatment of haemophilia. In the UK these have almost completely been replaced by recombinant products to reduce, among other things, the vCJD transmission risk.

Prothrombin complex concentrates

These products contain factors II, IX and X, and may also contain factor VII (vitamin K-dependent clotting factors). Their use is indicated in the prophylaxis and treatment of bleeding in patients with single or multiple deficiencies of these factors, whether congenital or acquired. They are used to reverse the anticoagulant effect of warfarin when there is major bleeding. Care must be taken in patients with liver disease as this therapy may be thrombogenic.

Immunoglobulin preparations (90% IgG)

These are prepared from fractionation of large pools of plasma from unselected donors or from individuals known to have high levels of specific antibodies. Some products are administered intramuscularly. The indications for some of the more commonly used immunoglobulins are shown in Table 2.1, e.g., hyperimmune globulin against hepatitis B, herpes zoster, tetanus and RhD. Intravenous IgG was originally developed as replacement therapy

Table 2.1 Indications and doses for the most commonly used specific immunoglobulins

Problem	Patients eligible for IgG	Preparation	Dose
Hepatitis B	Needle-stick or mucosal exposure victims. Should also be immunised	Hepatitis B IgG	1000 IU for adults and 500 IU for children <5 years
Tetanus-prone wounds	Nonimmune patients with heavily contaminated wounds. Toxoid should be administered with IgG	Tetanus IgG	250 IU routine prophylaxis 500 IU if >24 h since injury or heavily contaminated wound

for immunodeficiency states, but is also used to treat immune thrombocytopenia and other rare diseases such as Guillain–Barré syndrome.

Red cell serology

The red cell membrane is a bilipid layer that contains over 400 red cell antigens that have been classified into 23 systems.

ABO antigens

Nearly all deaths from transfusion error are due to ABO-incompatible transfusion. ABO are carbohydrate antigens present on the majority of cells of the body. Their presence depends on the pattern of inheritance of genes encoding glycosyltransferases. Since carbohydrate antigens are widely expressed by other organisms including bacteria, individuals who lack A or B antigens will produce anti-A and anti-B antibodies, respectively. These are usually IgM antibodies (naturally occurring) and are present from the age of 3–6 months. ABO antibodies can react at body temperature and activate complement, and are of major clinical significance as a cause of rapid intravascular haemolysis. For example, transfusion of group A blood to a group B patient results in haemolysis of the transfused red cells because of the anti-A antibodies present in the recipient. Similarly, group O individuals have both anti-A and anti-B antibodies in their plasma that will react with any red cells apart from group O (Table 2.2). Group O blood (universal donor) can be used in the majority of recipients because it will not be destroyed by anti-A or anti-B antibodies and because processing removes most of the plasma from the unit and hence reduces the donor antibodies contained within.

Rhesus antigens (RH)

Allelic genes at two closely linked loci on chromosome 1 code for this complex blood group system. Phenotypes termed Rhesus D positive or negative (complete absence of D expression), and biallelic C,c and E,e antigens exist. RhD is by far the most immunogenic of the Rhesus antigens and is the only one for which blood is grouped routinely. Individuals who are RhD-negative do not normally have anti-RhD in their plasma unless they have been immunised by previous transfusion or pregnancy. Antibodies to RhD are IgG antibodies and do not activate complement, although they do cause extravascular haemolysis. RhD antibodies can cause transfusion reactions and haemolytic disease of the newborn (HDN). It is therefore essential that RhD-negative girls and women of child-bearing potential are not transfused with RhD-positive blood to avoid the production of antibodies to RhD.

Other red cell antigens

Many different blood group antigens exist against which antibodies can be formed of varying clinical significance, depending on their propensity to cause intra- or extravascular haemolysis and HDN. The most important of these are those of the Kell, Kidd and Duffy systems.

Pretransfusion testing

Pretransfusion testing consists of three steps:

1. *Blood grouping* involves determining the patient's ABO and RhD type. The donors' blood groups will already be determined by the Blood Service at the time of taking the donation.
2. *Antibody screening* involves the use of a panel of cells to screen a sample of the patient's serum for the presence of clinically significant antibodies. Around 2% of a patient population is likely to have red cell antibodies and where present the specificity of these is identified using further, more detailed, cell panels. The sample is retained for up to 7 days.
3. *Cross-matching* involves checking the compatibility of the donor units with the patient's serum. This can take three forms:
   - If the patient has an antibody, donor blood negative for the offending antigen(s) is identified and an Indirect Antiglobulin Test (IAT) cross-match carried out. This process may take several hours, depending on the population incidence of the antigen(s) in question.
   - If the patient has no abnormal antibodies, then blood can normally be released much more quickly after a rapid-spin cross-match that effectively only checks for ABO incompatibility.
   - Some laboratories are able to release blood by electronic issue where there is accurate patient identification, a historic blood group and antibody screen, no serum antibodies, and a secure blood bank testing and computer system that can reliably select and issue blood of compatible type. These systems allow very rapid release of blood. In the UK there is now guidance that requires a second sample from every patient before issuing blood or components as an added safety feature. Unless secure electronic patient identification systems are in place, a second sample should be requested for confirmation of the ABO group of a first time patient prior to transfusion, where this does not impede the delivery of urgent red cells or other components.

Table 2.2 **The antigens and antibodies of the ABO blood group system**						
Blood group	Frequency (India) %	Positive Rh status % (India)[a]	Frequency (UK) %	Red cell antigen	Plasma antibody	Compatible donor blood
A	23	22	42	A	Anti-B	A or O
B	32	31	8	B	Anti-A	B or O
AB	7	6	3	AB	—	AB, A, B or O
O	38	36	47	—	Anti-A,B	O only
[a]95% Positive for Rhesus factor.						

Maximal surgical blood ordering schedule (MSBOS)

Cross-matched units are allocated to the individual patient and held in reserve for 48 hours either in the hospital blood bank or in a local blood fridge. The hospital MSBOS lists the number of units of blood routinely cross-matched preoperatively for elective surgical procedures. This surgical tariff is based on retrospective analysis of actual blood use. The aim is to correlate as closely as possible the number of units cross-matched to the numbers of units transfused. It does not account for individual differences in blood transfusion requirements of different patients undergoing the same procedure, nor does it identify over-transfusion.

Under electronic cross-match, it is often possible to release blood on an 'as required' basis, again either from the blood bank or from a 'remote issue' blood fridge. In this situation, the MSBOS becomes redundant and blood wastage is reduced.

In an emergency, the laboratory must be told of the urgency and quantity of blood needed as soon as possible, and asked what they can provide in the time available. Group O RhD-negative blood is available in all hospitals for emergencies where the blood group of the patient is unknown. Patient samples can be rapidly ABO- and RhD-typed, and compatible blood released after a rapid test of ABO compatibility while the antibody screen is ongoing and group O RhD-negative blood is being transfused.

2.1 Summary

Ordering blood in an emergency

- Immediately take samples for cross-matching, ensuring that the sample and the request form are clearly and correctly labelled and are the same on subsequent requests. If the patient is unidentified, then some form of emergency admission number is the best identifier
- Inform the blood bank of the emergency, the volume of blood required, and where blood is to be delivered
- One individual should take responsibility for all communications with the blood bank, and should ensure that it is clear who will be responsible for blood delivery
- Do not ask for cross-matched blood in an emergency. In cases of exsanguination, use emergency group O Rh(D)-negative blood.

Indications for transfusion

The decision to transfuse is a complex one. Clinical judgement plays a vital role, as there is no consensus on the precise indications for red cell transfusion. The clinician prescribing any blood component should consider the risks and benefits of transfusion for each individual patient. Tolerance of anaemia is dependent on a number of factors, including the speed of onset, age, level of activity and co-existing disease. In chronic anaemia, fatigue and shortness of breath, although subjective, are still useful in determining the need for transfusion. In acute anaemia (usually secondary to blood loss), the effects of hypovolaemia need to be differentiated from those of anaemia. Healthy adults can tolerate significant blood loss (30–40% of circulating volume) without adverse effects and would not normally require transfusion. This is largely due to adaptive mechanisms such as a compensatory rise in cardiac output and peripheral vasoconstriction, which act to maintain tissue oxygen delivery. The actual haemoglobin

EBM 2.1 **Red cell transfusion in the correction of a low haemoglobin in critically ill patients**

'A single large RCT of red cell transfusion in patients in intensive care showed that patients who were maintained with an Hb in the range of 70–90 g/L had a lower mortality and morbidity compared to those with an Hb maintained in the range of 100–120 g/L. The former groups received approximately half the number of red cell units.'

Hebert PC, et al. with the Canadian Transfusion Requirements in Critical Care Group. N Engl J Med 2004; 340: 409–417.

For further information: www.transfusionguidelines.org.uk
www.sign.ac.uk

concentration is not a reliable clinical indicator in acute haemorrhage and does not in itself indicate a definite need for transfusion; however, it can act as a prompt for the clinician to seek other features that suggest transfusion is required. In a clinically stable situation, red cell transfusion is usually not required with a haemoglobin concentration of ≥100 g/L.

Generally, in healthy individuals, a transfusion threshold of 70–80 g/L is appropriate, as this leaves a margin of safety over the critical level of 40–50 g/L, at which point oxygen consumption becomes limited by the amount that the circulation can supply. For elderly patients or those with cardiovascular or respiratory disease, who may tolerate anaemia poorly, transfusion should be considered at a haemoglobin concentration of ≤80 g/L to maintain a haemoglobin level of around 100 g/L. In the intensive care setting, some studies have shown that maintaining a lower haemoglobin threshold may be associated with better patient outcomes, at least in some patient groups. The best available evidence for this is the randomised, controlled TRICC trial (EBM 2.1), which compared a liberal transfusion strategy (Hb 100–120 g/L) with a restrictive one (Hb 70–90 g/L). Overall in-hospital mortality was significantly lower in the restrictive group, although the 30-day mortality rate was not significantly different. However, the 30-day mortality rate was significantly lower in the restrictive transfusion group for those patients who were less ill (Acute Physiology and Chronic Health Evaluation [APACHE] – ICU scoring system of disease severity < 20) or younger (<55 years of age). These data show that a restrictive strategy is at least equivalent, and in some patient groups is superior, to a more liberal transfusion strategy.

Blood administration

Avoidable errors in the requesting, supply and administration of blood lead to significant risks to patients. Multiple errors contribute to more than 50% of 'wrong blood' incidents reported to the UK Serious Hazards of Transfusion (SHOT) scheme. Of these, 70% occur in clinical areas and 30% occur in laboratories. Acute haemolytic transfusion reactions due to ABO incompatibility can be fatal and are most often caused by errors in identification of the patient at the time of blood sampling or administration (EBM 2.2).

The British Committee for Standards in Haematology has produced a guideline for the administration of blood and blood components and the management of transfused patients. This contains a number of recommendations that should be adhered to in order to minimise transfusion error. These include the following:

1. It is crucial that the identity of the patient is established verbally (if possible) *and* by checking the patient identification wristband before blood is taken. The sample must be labelled

EBM 2.2 Risks of fatal transfusion reactions—cases reported to national reporting systems

'In the UK between 1996 and 2000 there were 33 reports of death attributed to transfusion. During this period approximately 10 million units of blood components were supplied. The largest cause of major morbidity remains transfusion of the incorrect unit of blood, leading to an incompatible red cell transfusion reaction.'

Love EM, Soldan K. Serious hazards of transfusion, Annual report 1999–2000. Manchester: SHOT; 2009.

For further information: www.shotuk.org
www.transfusionguidelines.org.uk

fully (in handwriting) before leaving the bedside. (Sample tubes must never be pre-labelled.)

2. The blood request form should be completed and should provide, as a minimum, the patient's full name, date of birth and hospital number. Each patient must have a unique identification number. The location of the patient, number and type of blood or blood components and time when required, the patient's diagnosis and the reason for the request are also essential.

3. Before transfusion is commenced, the following details must be checked by two individuals, at least one of whom must be a State Registered Nurse (SRN) or medical officer:
    a. Full patient identity on the patient wristband against the compatibility label on the unit of blood.
    b. ABO and Rh(D) type on the pack compatibility label.
    c. Donation number on the pack compatibility label.
    d. Expiry date of the pack.
    e. Examination of the pack to ensure that there are no leaks or evidence of haemolysis.
    If there are any discrepancies, the blood must not be transfused and the laboratory must be informed immediately.

4. As a minimum, the patient's pulse rate, blood pressure and temperature should be recorded prior to commencing the transfusion, 15 minutes after commencement of each unit (as this is when transfusion reactions are most likely), and on completion of the transfusion. The vital signs should be rechecked if the patient feels unwell during the transfusion.

5. A permanent record of the transfusion of blood and blood components and the administration of blood products must be kept in the medical notes. This should include the sheets used for the prescription of blood or blood components and those used for nursing observations during the transfusion. An entry should also be made in the case notes, documenting the date, the indication for transfusion, the number and type of units used, whether or not the desired effect was achieved, and the occurrence and management of any adverse effects.

⟳ 2.2 Summary

Safety checks for blood administration

Before administering blood, two staff members (one of whom must be a doctor or trained staff nurse) must check:

* the patient's full identity (wristband, and verbally if possible)
* the blood pack, compatibility label and report form (noting donation number and expiry date)
* the blood pack for signs of haemolysis or leakage from the pack

Any discrepancies mean that the blood must not be transfused and that the laboratory must be informed immediately.

Adverse effects of transfusion

A voluntary anonymised reporting scheme for serious hazards of transfusion (SHOT) has been in place in the UK since 1996, and the incidence of reported hazards is shown in Fig. 2.2. The greatest concern for most patients is the risk of transfusion-transmitted infection, but by far the most common risk is the transfusion of an incorrect blood component.

Transfusion reactions can be divided into those that occur early (acute transfusion reactions, [ATRs], occurring within 24 hours of commencing but usually during the transfusion) and those that occur late (delayed transfusion reactions [DTRs] occurring more than 24 hours after commencing the transfusion and often once the patient has been discharged). Acute adverse reactions to

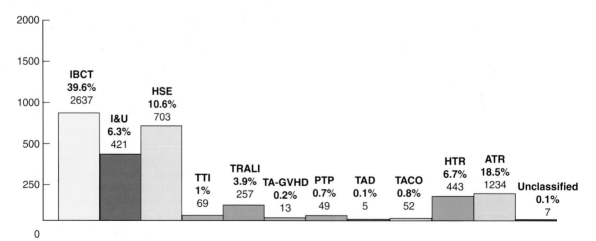

Fig. 2.2 SHOT report for 1996–2009 (*n* = 6653) showing the rate (%) of serious hazards of transfusion reported in the UK. *ATR*, Acute transfusion reaction; *HTR*, haemolytic transfusion reaction; *I&U*, inappropriate and unnecessary transfusion; *IBCT*, incorrect blood component transfused; *HSE*, handling and storage errors *PTP*, post-transfusion purpura; *TACO*, transfusion-associated circulatory overload; *TAD*, transfusion-associated dyspnoea; *TA-GVHD*, transfusion-associated graft-versus-host disease; *TRALI*, transfusion-related acute lung injury; *TTI*, transfusion-transmitted infection.

blood transfusion require urgent investigation and management, as they may be life-threatening. The major acute causes frequently have similar symptoms and signs, and blind treatment may initially be necessary until the exact cause becomes apparent. Acute and delayed adverse effects of transfusion are listed in Tables 2.3 and 2.4, respectively. The risks of infection from blood transfusion are listed in Table 2.5. Management of acute transfusion reactions is illustrated in Fig. 2.3.

2.3 Summary

Transfusion errors

- Almost all deaths from transfusion reaction are due to ABO incompatibility
- Errors in patient identification at the time of blood sampling or administration are the major cause (occurring in at least 1:1000–1:2000 transfusions)
- When taking the initial blood sample:
  Check the patient's identity verbally and on the wrist identification band
  Label the sample fully before leaving the bedside
  Make sure that the blood request form is clearly and accurately completed.

Autologous transfusion

Three main autologous programmes exist.
1. Preoperative donation: blood is taken and stored in advance of planned surgery and is used like volunteer donor blood as required.
2. Isovolaemic haemodilution: blood is taken just before surgery and replaced with fluid and then returned unmanipulated immediately after the operation.
3. Cell salvage: blood is collected from the operative field and replaced during or immediately after the surgical procedure.

Preoperative donation

Autologous blood can be collected from otherwise fit patients preoperatively and stored for 35–42 days. These units are subject to the same testing and processing as allogeneic donations. There is no evidence to show a reduction in allogeneic transfusion in patients who have donated autologous blood and in fact some which may suggest that these individuals require more following autologous donation. The use of autologous predeposit has diminished to such an extent that it is only used now for individuals where they are of such a rare blood type that there is no opportunity to identify fresh units within a reasonable time period.

Isovolaemic haemodilution

This technique is restricted to patients in whom significant blood loss (>1000 mL) is anticipated. Following induction of anaesthesia, up to 1.5 L of blood is withdrawn preoperatively into a clearly labelled blood pack containing a standard anticoagulant, and replaced by saline to maintain blood volume. The fall in haematocrit reduces the loss of red cells (and haemoglobin) during surgical bleeding while maintaining optimal tissue perfusion. The withdrawn blood can be re-infused, either during surgery or postoperatively, with transfusion complete before the patient leaves the

Table 2.3 Acute transfusion reactions

	Cause	Implicated components	Clinical features
Immunological			
Acute haemolytic transfusion reaction	ABO-incompatible transfusion resulting in acute intravascular haemolysis	RCC	Develops within minutes. Chills, fevers, rigors, chest tightness, infusion site pain, hypotension, shock, DIC and acute renal failure. May be fatal.
Transfusion-related acute lung injury (TRALI)	HLA or neutrophil Abs in donor plasma react with recipient leucocytes	Any component containing more than 50 mL plasma (RCC, FFP, cryo, platelets; especially SDP because RDP have less than 50 mL plasma)	Develops within 4 hours of transfusion. Dyspnoea, cough, fever, hypoxia, pulmonary infiltrates (ARDS). With supportive care, improvement over 2–4 days in 80% of patients.
Febrile non-haemolytic transfusion reaction	Neutrophil Ab in recipient plasma reacts with donor leucocytes	RCC Platelets	Develops late in course of transfusion. Usually mild. Full recovery expected.
Allergic reactions	Reaction to plasma proteins	Any plasma-containing component	Urticaria/itch within minutes of start of transfusion. Occasionally severe with anaphylaxis. Usually full recovery with appropriate management.
Nonimmunological			
Bacterial contamination	Contamination during collection or storage. Rarely, bacteraemic donor	Platelets most commonly RCC	Symptoms/signs of sepsis develop early in course of transfusion. May be fatal.
Transfusion-associated circulatory overload	Over-transfusion	Any	Symptoms/signs of acute left ventricular failure. Resolves with appropriate management.

Ab, Antibody; Ag, antigen; ARDS, acute respiratory distress syndrome; Cryo, cryoprecipitate; DIC, disseminated intravascular coagulation; FFP, fresh frozen plasma; HLA, human leucocyte antigen; RCC, red cell concentrate.

Table 2.4 Delayed transfusion reactions

	Cause	Implicated components	Clinical features
Immunological			
Delayed haemolytic transfusion reaction	Patient has non-ABO red cell Ab and extravascular haemolysis develops	Red cells Platelets	May be asymptomatic or develop jaundice, fever and haemoglobinuria with a fall in haemoglobin. Seldom fatal but can result in significant morbidity if the patient is already unwell.
Alloimmunisation	Recipient forms Ab in response to donor Ag	Red cells	Usually not detected until subsequently grouped and saved or cross-matched.
Posttransfusion purpura	Recipient has a platelet-specific Ab and develops secondary immune response on re-exposure, resulting in destruction of donor platelets and, through an unknown mechanism, recipient platelets	Platelets	Sudden development of severe thrombocytopenia associated with bleeding 5–12 days following transfusion. Complications are related to bleeding. Platelet count usually recovers with appropriate management, which includes IV immunoglobulin.
Transfusion-associated graft-versus-host disease (GVHD)	Viable T lymphocytes transfused into immunocompromised recipient	Any cellular product, especially from first degree relative donor to an immunosuppressed host	Fever, desquamating rash, abnormal LFTs and pancytopenia develop 1–4 weeks following transfusion. Mortality rate >90%. Prevent by irradiation of cellular components in patients at high risk.
Nonimmunological			
Transfusion-transmitted infection: Risks shown in Table 2.5			
Iron overload: Chronic red cell transfusion leads to accumulation of iron in tissues, e.g., liver, heart, pancreas			

Ab, Antibody; Ag, antigen; IV, intravenous; LVT, liver function tests.

Table 2.5 Risks of a single red cell unit transmitting disease in the UK

Infection	Estimated risk (per unit transfused)
Hepatitis B	1:1,400,000
Hepatitis C	1:40,500,000
HIV	1:5,700,000
HTLV	1:10,000–100,000
vCJD	Unknown, not zero
Bacterial	1:2000–10,000

HIV, Human immunodeficiency virus; HTLV, human T-cell leukaemia virus; vCJD, variant Creutzfeldt–Jakob disease.

responsibility of the anaesthetist. Blood is maintained at the point of care, minimising the risk of administrative or clerical errors, although standard pretransfusion checks should be carried out to ensure the correct pack(s) are re-infused. This is not common practice in the UK.

Cell salvage

Blood can be collected from the operation site either directly during surgery or by the use of collection devices attached to surgical drains. During surgery, blood can be collected by suction, processed by a cell salvage machine in which it is anticoagulated while the cells are washed to remove clots and debris, and then returned to the patient. The process is contraindicated in patients with malignancy or sepsis, and is only appropriate when there is substantial blood loss. Several litres of blood can be salvaged intraoperatively, far more than with other autologous techniques. Postoperative drainage can be returned to the patient, most commonly not washed. This process does require some positive suction pressure, and in some circumstances this may lead to increased blood loss. The other main disadvantage is that salvaged blood is not haemostatically intact, as there may have been clotting in the wound leading to consumption of clotting factors and platelets. Cell salvage can significantly reduce the exposure of patients to allogeneic blood and is used extensively in cardiac surgery, trauma surgery and liver transplantation.

Transfusion requirements in special surgical settings

Blood component use in major haemorrhage

Major haemorrhage has been arbitrarily defined as the loss of an entire blood volume within a 24-hour period. Alternative definitions of 50% blood loss within 3 hours may be more meaningful. Whatever is used each hospital must ensure a policy that allows early recognition and management of these situations. The therapeutic goal in these situations is to maintain tissue perfusion and oxygenation by restoration of blood volume and haemoglobin, and to stop bleeding by treating the traumatic, surgical or obstetric source.

The use of crystalloid to restore the circulating volume is critical in preventing hypovolaemic shock and the consequent

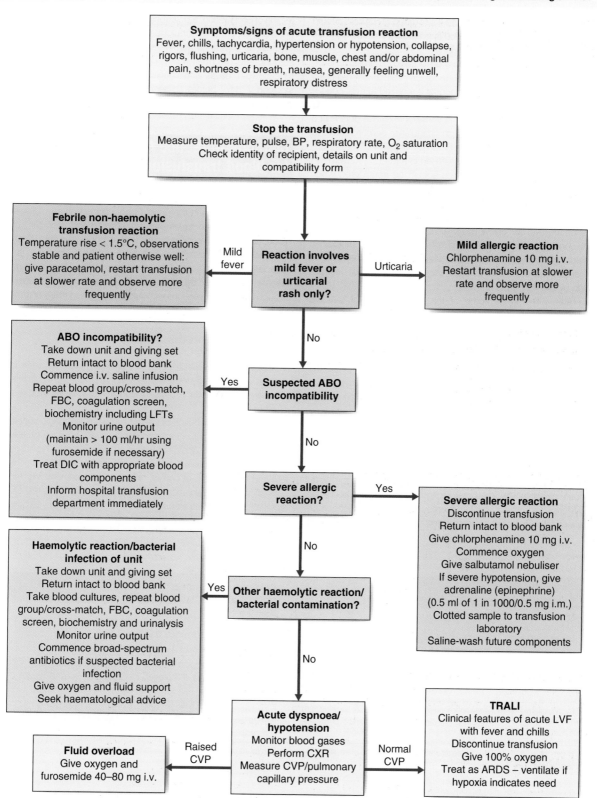

Fig. 2.3 **Management of an acute transfusion reaction.** (*DIC,* Disseminated intravascular coagulation; *LVF,* left ventricular failure; *TRALI,* transfusion-related acute lung injury)

multi-organ failure. Emergency stocks of group O red cells should be used until group-specific blood is available. Fresh blood does not confer any survival advantage.

Access to 24/7 cell salvage may be required in cardiac, obstetric, trauma and vascular centres to rapidly replace lost red cells.

Judicious use of blood components is required to treat coagulopathy that is associated with massive blood loss. In major haemorrhage associated with trauma consider early use of FFP at a ratio of 1:1 with red cells and use coagulation screen results to guide further requirements for FFP. In other cases of major haemorrhage then FFP may be transfused in a ratio of 1:2 with red cells. Fibrinogen supplementation should be considered when the fibrinogen level falls below 1.5 g/L.

Platelets should be maintained at a level of $>50 \times 10^9$/L and platelet transfusion should be ordered in the bleeding patient when the level falls below 100×10^9/L. Adult trauma patients with no contraindications should receive the antifibrinolytic, tranexamic acid 1 g intravenously over 10 minutes. They should then receive maintenance of 1 g over 8 hours. This drug prevents clot destruction by the fibrinolytic pathway.

Table 2.6 outlines some of the complications of massive transfusion.

Cardiopulmonary bypass

Platelets and coagulation factors may be activated or lost in the extracorporeal circulation during cardiopulmonary bypass at open heart surgery, so that FFP and platelet transfusion may be needed to deal with postoperative bleeding. The platelet count may be normal but the platelets are likely to be dysfunctional, having been activated by the extracorporeal circuit. Platelet transfusion is indicated if there is microvascular bleeding, or if the bleeding cannot be corrected surgically after the patient is off bypass and once heparin has been reversed with an appropriate dose of protamine sulphate. Coagulation screens should be performed to assess required therapy prior to infusion of coagulation factors in all but life-threatening haemorrhage. Near-patient testing of coagulation, e.g., thromboelastography, may also guide decisions on the need for blood component therapy.

Aspirin is commonly administered to patients awaiting bypass surgery. This drug has a prolonged inhibitory effect on platelet function (5–7 days), and should therefore, where possible, be stopped 7 days before surgery and commenced immediately postoperatively, when it significantly helps graft patency.

Methods to reduce the need for blood transfusion

Large variations in transfusion practice are due to many factors, including differences in the patient populations treated, surgical and anaesthetic techniques, and attitudes to and availability of blood, as well as differences in pre- and postoperative care. Such differences in transfusion practice have not been shown to be associated with significant differences in mortality. These findings indicate that it may be possible to reduce blood transfusion through various interventions without impacting negatively on clinical outcomes.

Acute volume replacement

Nonplasma colloid volume expanders of large molecules, such as dextran, are a relatively inexpensive colloidal alternative to plasma in first-line management of patients who are volume-depleted as a result of bleeding.

In the initial resuscitation of patients with haemorrhagic shock, the adequacy of volume replacement is usually of much greater importance than the choice of fluid. A reasonable guide in adults is 1000 mL of crystalloid (0.9% saline or Ringer's lactate solution), followed by 1000 mL of colloid, and then replacement with red cells. In the elderly and those with cardiac impairment, red cell replacement should be started earlier to maintain oxygen-carrying capacity without causing fluid overload.

Table 2.6 Complications of massive transfusion

Complication	Mechanism	Management
Thrombocytopenia	Consumption/DIC Dilutional after 1.5–2.0 blood volumes replaced	In patients with acute bleeding, transfuse platelets to maintain count $>50 \times 10^9$/L ($>100 \times 10^9$/L if acute trauma or CNS injury).
Coagulopathy	Consumption/DIC Dilutional after 1.0 blood volume replaced	If continued blood loss and PT or APTT ratio $>1.5 \times$ control levels, give FFP 10–15 mL/kg. If fibrinogen <1.0 g/L, cryoprecipitate is also indicated.
Hypocalcaemia	Citrate anticoagulant binds to ionised Ca, lowering plasma levels (only problematic in neonates and liver disease)	If ECG shows signs of hypocalcaemia, give 5 mL Ca gluconate (or equivalent paediatric dose) over 5 min. Repeat if ECG remains abnormal.
Hyper- or hypokalaemia	Red cell degeneration during storage increases plasma K^+. Following transfusion, red cells rapidly normalise Na/K equilibrium, which may lead to ↑ K^+	Careful monitoring of K^+ levels in massive transfusion.
Hypothermia	Transfusion of blood at 4°C lowers core temperature	Prevent by use of blood warmer when transfusion rate >50 mL/kg/h in adults (15 mL/kg/h in children).
ARDS	Multifactorial	Minimise risk by maintaining tissue perfusion, correct hypotension and avoid over-transfusion.

APTT, Activated partial thromboplastin time; ARDS, acute respiratory distress syndrome; DIC, disseminated intravascular coagulation; FFP, fresh frozen plasma; PT, prothrombin time.

Mechanisms for reducing blood use in surgery

Preoperative

When surgery is elective, significant reductions in blood use can be made by ensuring that the patient has a normal haemoglobin and by correcting any preexisting anaemia, e.g., iron or folic acid deficiency. Drugs that interfere with haemostasis, e.g., nonsteroidal antiinflammatory drugs, aspirin and warfarin, should be stopped where appropriate. An abnormal clotting screen or platelet count should be investigated and corrected prior to surgery. To ensure optimal management, these issues should be addressed 4–6 weeks prior to surgery at preoperative assessment clinics.

Intraoperative

The training, experience and competence of the surgeon performing the procedure are the most crucial factors in reducing operative blood loss. Meticulous surgical technique, with attention to bleeding points, is very important. Other techniques, such as posture, the use of vasoconstrictors and tourniquets, and avoidance of hypothermia, should always be considered, as these can have a significant impact on perioperative blood loss. Certain pharmacological agents, e.g., antifibrinolytics such as tranexamic acid, may significantly reduce the requirements for blood and are indicated in certain operative procedures.

Fibrin sealant mimics the final stage in the coagulation cascade, in which fibrinogen is converted to fibrin in the presence of thrombin, factor XIII, fibronectin and ionised calcium. Freeze-dried sterilised fibrinogen, fibronectin and factor XIII can be delivered from one barrel of a double-barrelled syringe while thrombin, calcium and aprotinin are delivered from the other. If the two mixtures meet at a surgical bleeding site the solution clots almost immediately, the clot resolving over a period of days. Alternatively, fibrinogen and thrombin sealant may be incorporated into an oxidised regenerated cellulose patch that can be applied directly at the bleeding site in patients with impaired coagulation. Fibrin sealants and patches have been used in vascular, cardiac and liver surgery and in situations where even small amounts of bleeding can be problematic (e.g., middle ear surgery).

Acute normovolaemic haemodilution and intraoperative blood salvage are two of the autologous methods of blood conservation that can be employed during surgery to reduce exposure to transfusion. They are described in the section on autologous programmes.

Postoperative

Postoperative cell salvage (see previous discussion) can reduce the need for allogeneic transfusion.

The decision to transfuse postoperatively should depend on several factors (see 'Indications for transfusion'). Blood transfusion should be limited to the amount of blood required to raise the haemoglobin above the transfusion threshold and/or achieve clinical stability, even if this is only 1 unit. Appropriate use of antifibrinolytic drugs such as tranexamic acid and the routine prescribing of iron and folic acid also reduce postoperative transfusion. A reduction in transfusion has been shown to result from the introduction of simple protocols that give guidance on when the haemoglobin should be checked and red cells transfused.

Recombinant human factor VIIa (Novoseven) can be used in patients who continue to bleed despite adequate component therapy, after coagulation parameters are normalised and platelet count is optimised. The current licensed use is in factor VII deficiency, haemophilia A with inhibitors and Glanzmann's thrombasthenia. Its use in trauma is currently not licensed. Concerns about its use include thrombosis and pulmonary thromboembolism.

Better blood transfusion

In recent times, attention has been focused on blood transfusion practice for a number of reasons. These include concerns about the transmission of vCJD by blood transfusion, increased costs associated with new safety measures such as leucocyte depletion, documented variations in transfusion practice and recommendations arising from the SHOT scheme. Better Blood Transfusion (BBT) programmes have been established in many countries with the purpose of promoting the safe, efficient and appropriate use of blood components and plasma derivatives. The aims of BBT are to establish protocols and guidelines to nationally approved standards, implement accredited learning programmes, audit transfusion practice and achieve a reduction in inappropriate blood use.

Future trends

Although the demand for blood has fallen over the past few years, strict donor selection guidelines and social and economic changes are reducing the number of donors. Furthermore it is predicted that demand will rise again over the next few decades as an increasingly elderly population requires more healthcare. This means that blood should be considered a scarce and valuable commodity that should be responsibly prescribed.

Although red cell substitutes are under development, fluorocarbon oxygen carriers have found limited clinical application and concerns have been raised around potential toxicity of haemoglobin solutions. Recombinant human erythropoietin raises haemoglobin levels in patients with chronic renal failure but its use in the wider clinical setting has been limited.

The objective in managing surgical patients should be to minimise anaemia and bleeding and hence the need for transfusion. Although it is clear that no patient should be transfused unnecessarily, it is equally certain that no patient should be allowed to exsanguinate because of concerns regarding blood safety.

Gordon L. Carlson
Ken Fearon[†]

Nutritional support in surgical patients

Chapter contents

Introduction 40

Assessment of nutritional status 40

Assessment of nutritional requirements 42

Causes of inadequate intake 42

Methods of providing nutritional support 42

Monitoring of nutritional support 47

Introduction

The interrelationship between disease and nutrition has been recognised since at least the time of Hippocrates, who is credited with the phrase 'let food be thy medicine'. Attention to and correction of nutritional status remains fundamental to holistic medical care. Nevertheless, approximately one-third of all patients admitted to an acute hospital will have evidence of protein-calorie malnutrition. In many cases, these abnormalities are not adequately recognised or addressed and, worryingly, two-thirds of patients leave hospital with either no improvement or even deterioration in their nutritional status. Malnutrition has damaging effects on psychological status (depression), activity levels and appearance. Paradoxically, in the surgical patient a low body fat content may sometimes be viewed as an advantage, making technical aspects of surgery easier. There is, however, clear evidence that patients with significant protein-energy malnutrition have a significantly greater incidence of postoperative mortality and morbidity, including pneumonia, pressure sores, surgical site infection and prolonged hospital stay.

It is important to recognise that the definition of malnutrition does not simply include nutritional depletion. In Western society there is now a steadily growing epidemic of obesity. Whilst obese individuals generally have a matching increase in lean body mass, some have underlying muscle wasting (sarcopenic obesity) and these patients are at high risk of metabolic syndrome and postoperative complications. Patients with sarcopenic obesity are difficult to recognise clinically due to their muscle wasting being hidden by overlying fat.

Nutritional disorders in surgical practice have two principal components. First, starvation can be initiated by the effects of the disease, by restriction of oral intake, or both. Simple starvation results in progressive loss of the body's energy and protein reserves (i.e., subcutaneous fat and skeletal muscle). Second, there are the metabolic effects of stress/inflammation; namely, increased catabolism and reduced anabolism. These result in

low serum albumin concentration, accelerated muscle wasting and water retention. Although malnutrition may be the result of simple starvation, in the majority of surgical patients it results from a more complex and interrelated combination of increased demand related to the catabolic effects of illness, reduced food intake and metabolic changes that may result in impaired use of available nutrients (Fig. 3.1)

Assessment of nutritional status

The main energy reserves are found in subcutaneous and intra-abdominal fat depots, but loss of fat reserves does not usually impair function. In contrast, there are no true protein reserves in the body. In response to starvation or stress, structural tissues such as skeletal muscle and even the gut are broken down (catabolism) to liberate amino acids for the generation of glucose precursors and results in functional impairment that can impede recovery.

The key elements of nutritional assessment include current food intake, levels of energy and protein reserves, and the patients' likely clinical course (Fig. 3.2). Patients who have not had an adequate dietary intake for 5 days or more require nutritional support, and those with symptoms such as anorexia, nausea, vomiting or early satiety are at risk of a reduced food intake and hence undernutrition. Energy reserves are most easily assessed by examining for loss of subcutaneous fat (skinfolds); whereas protein depletion is most commonly manifest as skeletal muscle wasting (Fig. 3.3). A history of weight loss of more than 10–15% is highly significant, because this level of nutritional depletion is associated with impaired outcome of treatment. Patients can also be assessed according to their body mass index (BMI), which is calculated as weight (in kg) divided by height (in m^2). Normal BMI is between 18.5 and 24.9 kg/m^2. A BMI of less than 18 suggests significant protein-calorie undernutrition. Finally, it is important to recognise that in assessing the nutritional status of patients, knowledge of their likely clinical course is vital (Fig. 3.4). For example, if patients are well nourished, they should be able to withstand the brief period of reduced food intake associated with major surgery. However, if patients are already severely malnourished (e.g., weight loss of

[†]Deceased.

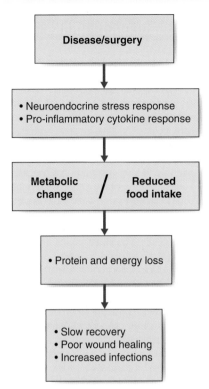

Fig. 3.1 Mechanisms linking the effects of disease/surgery on patient outcomes.

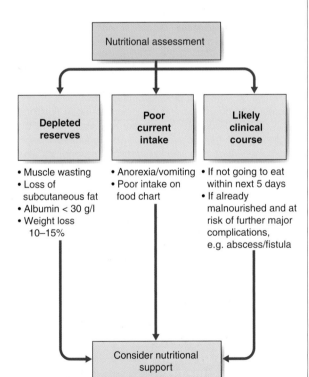

Fig. 3.2 Nutritional assessment in surgical patients.

15%, BMI 17), then even a short period of starvation or catabolism may result in further life-threatening nutritional depletion. Taken together, a patient's food intake, level of reserve and likely clinical course should indicate the need for nutritional support and these

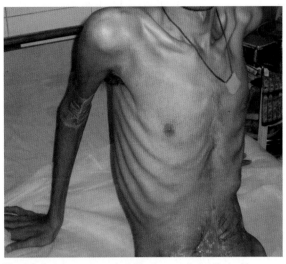

Fig. 3.3 Protein-energy malnutrition in a surgical patient with multiple enterocutaneous fistulae illustrating depleted muscle mass and loss of subcutaneous tissues.

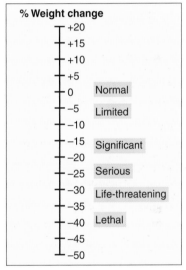

Fig. 3.4 Alterations in nutritional status associated with weight loss.

assessments should form part of the routine daily appraisal of every patient during a surgical ward round.

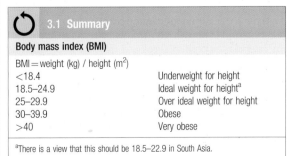

3.1 Summary

Body mass index (BMI)

BMI = weight (kg) / height (m²)

<18.4	Underweight for height
18.5–24.9	Ideal weight for height[a]
25–29.9	Over ideal weight for height
30–39.9	Obese
>40	Very obese

[a]There is a view that this should be 18.5–22.9 in South Asia.

Table 3.1 Estimation of energy and protein requirements in adult surgical patients

	Uncomplicated	Complicated/stressed
Energy (kcal/kg/day)	25	30–35
Protein (g/kg/day)[a]	1.0	1.3–1.5

[a]Grams of protein can be converted to the equivalent amount of nitrogen by dividing by 6.25.

Assessment of nutritional requirements

Energy and protein/nitrogen requirements vary, depending on weight, body composition, clinical status, level of physical activity and dietary intake. For most patients, an approximation based on weight and clinical status is sufficient. Few adult patients require more than 25–30 kcal/kg/day (approximately 1800–2200 kcal in an adult of average body mass; Table 3.1). Additional calories are unlikely to be used effectively and may even constitute a metabolic stress, leading to excessive activation of the sympathetic nervous system (diet induced thermogenesis), that may result in fever and difficulty weaning from mechanical ventilation as a consequence of the excessive carbon dioxide load. Particular caution should be exercised when 'refeeding' the chronically starved patient because of the dangers of potentially fatal cardiac dysrhythmias due to hypokalaemia and hypophosphataemia (refeeding syndrome).

3.2 Summary

Nutritional status

- Nutritional status in surgical patients may be adversely affected by starvation (effects of disease such as oesophageal cancer, restricted intake), the effects of inflammation (increased catabolism) and the effects of the operation itself (stress/inflammatory response)
- Nutritional status is assessed by current food intake, levels of reserves and likely clinical course

The most common method for assessing protein/nitrogen requirement is based on body weight (Table 3.1). Although more accurate assessment for patients receiving nutritional support can be derived from measurement of 24-hour urinary urea excretion, which can be converted to an estimate of 24-hour urinary nitrogen loss, this is seldom necessary in routine clinical practice.

Enteral diets normally provide protein whereas parenteral nutrition delivers nitrogen (N) in the form of amino acids. The nitrogen equivalent of protein is calculated by multiplying protein content (in grams) by a conversion factor of 6.25. In practice, nitrogen requirements are usually estimated based upon predicted calorie intake and the level of metabolic stress. Most patients require 1 g N per 200 kcal of energy daily (typically 10 g N) in the absence of catabolism, but nitrogen requirements increase significantly with the catabolic response to stress and may rise to as much as 18–20 g N/day in critically ill or septic patients. Even if losses exceed this, more than 18 g N/day (equivalent to 112 g protein) is seldom given, however, because it is unlikely to be used effectively because protein is diverted to generate energy precursors associated with the stress response. It is thus impossible to prevent substantial loss of protein reserves and lean body mass in critically ill patients and the aim of meeting requirements under these circumstances is primarily to limit the losses resulting from catabolism.

Causes of inadequate intake

The ideal way for surgical patients to obtain sufficient nutrition is for them to eat or drink an adequate quantity of palatable and nutritious food. Unfortunately, socioeconomic factors may make this difficult. Hospital catering is not traditionally noted for its palatability. In addition, illness is usually associated with a change in eating behaviour, from taking three large daily meals, to frequent consumption of smaller amounts of food, and this is extremely difficult to manage in a hospital environment. Eating is a social activity for most people and lying in solitude in a hospital bed is not conducive to adequate food intake. Other reasons for poor food intake include the patient being too weak and anorexic, poor dentition, having a mechanical problem such as obstruction of the gastrointestinal tract and even the cumulative effects of repeated periods of fasting to undergo investigations. Patients may have difficulty ingesting sufficient food to meet increased metabolic demands. Some patients suffer from 'intestinal failure', i.e., a state in which the amount of functioning gut is reduced below a level where enough food can be digested and absorbed for nourishment. Intestinal failure can be acute (when it is usually reversible) or chronic (when it is usually permanent). Acute intestinal failure is relatively common, especially after abdominal surgery, when it results from the development of surgical complications, whereas chronic intestinal failure is comparatively rare.

The principal causes of acute intestinal failure are mechanical intestinal obstruction and paralytic ileus, frequently associated with abdominal sepsis, as well as intestinal fistula formation, in which bowel content is lost externally or short-circuited (internal fistula) before it can be adequately digested and absorbed. Chronic intestinal failure may result from short bowel syndrome, following extensive small bowel resection, extensive small bowel disease, such as Crohn's disease, and motility disorders, such as chronic intestinal pseudo-obstruction. In some patients with short bowel syndrome, the remaining intestine may adapt over a period of months or years by a process of progressive dilatation and mucosal hyperplasia, allowing the patient to regain nutritional independence. Reconstructive surgery may also improve the function or even be employed to increase the functional length of remaining intestine in selected cases. Increasingly, intestinal transplantation may be undertaken, especially in patients with loss of venous access preventing intravenous feeding, or in those who develop complications of chronic intestinal failure such as liver disease, for which transplantation may be required.

Specialised nutritional treatment is required for intestinal failure if the patient is to remain adequately nourished. The provision of nutrition in such patients is further complicated by the metabolic consequences of ongoing inflammation or sepsis. As a general rule, this results in increased energy requirements and impaired ability to use administered nutrients, rendering nutritional support less effective. The overwhelming priority in providing effective nutritional support for such patients is therefore to eliminate sepsis.

Methods of providing nutritional support

Nutrients can be given via the gastrointestinal tract (enteral nutrition) or intravenously (parenteral nutrition) (Fig. 3.5). Parenteral nutrition is indicated only for the few patients in whom enteral feeding is not feasible. Enteral feeding is both safer and cheaper than parenteral nutrition (EBM 3.1), particularly relevant in

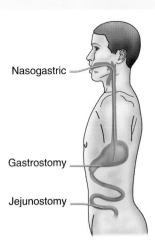

Nasogastric

Gastrostomy

Jejunostomy

Fig. 3.5 Routes of enteral nutrition.

EBM	**3.1 Enteral vs parenteral nutrition in surgical patients**

'Enteral nutrition should be first choice for nutritional support in the critically ill surgical patient.'

Gramlich L, et al. Nutrition 2004;20:843–848.

developing countries where the cost of parenteral nutrition is prohibitive and availability limited. All patients with a normal length of functioning gastrointestinal tract, and most with reduced length, can be fed adequately by the enteral route. Furthermore, the ingestion of even suboptimal amounts of food may help maintain the gut function and may have beneficial metabolic and immunological consequences. A flexible and pragmatic approach employing a combination of enteral and parenteral nutrition is optimal, tailoring the route of nutrient provision to the patient's ability to tolerate and benefit from it.

Enteral nutrition

Oral route

It is essential to provide warm, appetising food in hospital, and elderly/infirm patients may need help to take their food and the assistance of family members can be useful. All staff should be aware of the nutritional needs of all patients. It is against this basic background of nutritional care that the need for artificial nutritional support should be considered.

Many patients suffer from early satiety (feeling full after a meal). Encouraging patients to eat small amounts frequently or to sip an oral supplement between meals can help overcome this symptom. Oral supplements need to be palatable and are available in cartons of approximately 250 mL (approximately 250 kcal and 10 g of protein). Supplements should be available to all patients who require them. They are usually available in a selection of flavours and may be more palatable if chilled. Most patients manage to consume one or two cartons per day, but fatigue with such supplements is commonplace and leads to reduced efficacy. They tend to replace rather than supplement food intake unless used carefully.

Table 3.2 Causes of anorexia in surgical patients
• Intestinal obstruction
• Ileus
• Cancer anorexia
• Depression, anxiety, pain
• Drugs, e.g., opiates
• Oral ulceration/infection
• General debility/weakness

There are numerous reasons why surgical patients may suffer from anorexia (i.e., poor appetite) (Table 3.2). Before embarking on tube enteral feeding, it is important to actively manage any symptoms that can be treated (e.g., oral thrush with nystatin, nausea with antiemetics, provision of adequate dental hygiene or artificial dentures) and thus boost spontaneous oral intake. For patients who are unable to swallow, or for those whose anorexia is resistant to other therapy, nasoenteral feeding via a fine-bore tube should be used.

Methods of administration of enteral feeds

Nasogastric or nasojejunal tubes

If patients cannot drink or sip a liquid feed for mechanical reasons, or if they are unconscious or on a ventilator, enteral nutrition can be given by a fine-bore nasogastric or nasojejunal tube. When carried out at home, this is known as home enteral nutrition. Nasojejunal tubes are weighted or inserted under fluoroscopic guidance until the tip has gone beyond the duodenojejunal flexure. The position of the tube tip should be checked radiologically, or by aspirating gastric content and confirming the presence of acid by litmus paper (in the case of nasogastric tube feeding) before nutrients are infused in order to avoid inadvertent intubation of the respiratory tract with potentially fatal consequences.

Gastrostomy and jejunostomy

If nasoenteric feeding is impossible due to disease or obstruction of the upper alimentary tract, or is clearly likely to be required for 6 weeks or more, nutrients may be given through a tube placed into the gastrointestinal tract below the lesion (Fig. 3.6). Thus a patient with pseudobulbar palsy or an oesophageal fistula or

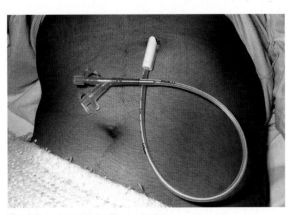

Fig. 3.6 Patient with feeding gastrostomy.

Table 3.3 Preparation of jejunostomy feeds

One unit feed = total volume 300 mL, energy 300 calories, protein 9 g

Ingredients	Amounts
Rice flour	25 g (2.5 tablespoons)
Complan	15 g (2 tablespoons)
Proteinex	15 g (2 level tablespoons)
Coconut oil	5 g (1–1.5 teaspoons)
Sugar	5 g (1 teaspoon)

Method of preparation

1. Make a paste from the rice flour in 50 mL water (approx. 3.5 tablespoons).
2. Boil 150–200 mL water; to this add the rice flour paste, stirring continuously to prevent lumps. Cook well and add oil and sugar, mix thoroughly.
3. Mix Complan in boiled warm water. Add Proteinex and blend well. Add to the cooked rice-flour mixture. Make volume up to 300 mL with cooled boiled water.

stricture can be fed through a gastrostomy, and a patient with a gastric or duodenal fistula can be fed through a jejunostomy. Jejunostomy is preferred in cases where the stomach may be required for surgical reconstruction of the proximal lesion.

Specially designed gastrostomy tubes can now be inserted by a combined percutaneous and endoscopic (PEG) method, and are particularly valuable for prolonged feeding when there is no impairment of gastric emptying (e.g., stroke patients). Feeding jejunostomy tubes can be inserted at the time of laparotomy if the surgeon anticipates that prolonged nutritional support will be needed postoperatively (e.g., in patients undergoing oesophagectomy and gastrectomy for cancer or necrosectomy for severe pancreatitis). The method of securing the tube around the enterotomy can be done using circumferential seromuscular sutures (Stamm's) or making a seromuscular tunnel (Witzel's). The bowel should be securely anchored to the parietal peritoneum circumferentially around the tube (see later). As a rule, 2000–3000 kcal should be provided, of which carbohydrates and fats provide 30–40% each. Enteral feeds can be prepared by the hospital kitchen or may be available commercially according to the calorie and protein, carbohydrate and fat requirement.

Fine-bore nasogastric/nasojejunal/gastrostomy/jejunostomy tubes require a feed that is a homogeneous smooth emulsion and only commercially available proprietary preparations satisfy these requirements. In resource-poor environments these preparations are expensive. An example of a 'home-made' enteral feed is shown in Table 3.3, but requires a larger bore tube.

Complications of enteral nutrition

Complications of enteral nutrition may be at least as common as with parenteral nutrition and can be equally life-threatening. Diarrhoea is more common with nasogastric than with nasojejunal feeding and can be managed by reducing the rate of infusion and by avoiding broad spectrum antibiotic therapy. Selection of lower osmolarity feeds may help. Vomiting can be managed by reducing the rate of feeding and by the use of prokinetic drugs such as metoclopramide or erythromycin. Monitoring of fluid and electrolyte balance is important, at least in the acute phase

of a patient's illness (for metabolic complications, see 'Parenteral nutrition'). It can be extremely difficult to monitor the adequacy of enteral feeding, particularly in the presence of diarrhoea and/or vomiting. A significant proportion of patients receiving enteral feeding cannot tolerate the rate of calorie infusion required for effective nutritional support. Excessive infusion of nasogastric feed may cause marked abdominal bloating, resulting in splinting of the diaphragm and impaired respiratory function. Fine-bore tubes should be flushed thoroughly if rest periods are employed as they block quickly if feed is left in them. Complications may also arise because of difficulty in placing feeding tubes. Examples include a fine-bore nasogastric tube inserted wrongly into the respiratory tract (or even through the cribriform plate into the anterior cranial fossa), early accidental removal of a jejunostomy tube with intraperitoneal leakage, or peritubal leakage with resultant intraperitoneal contamination. The fixation of the jejunal loop to the abdominal wall, required to minimise the risk of intraperitoneal leakage associated with feeding jejunostomy, may in turn increase the risk of small bowel volvulus, though this is extremely rare. Enteral feeding in critically ill patients, usually on inotropic support, who may already have a degree of splanchnic hypoperfusion, has rarely been associated with precipitating acute extensive mesenteric infarction, possibly because of the increased metabolic requirements of the gastrointestinal tract in response to the delivery of nutrients (nonocclusive mesenteric ischaemia). The condition is, unfortunately, almost universally fatal.

 3.3 Summary

Enteral nutrition

- If patients cannot eat adequate amounts of food they should be reviewed by the dietitian
- If oral supplements fail, a fine-bore tube nasogastric/nasojejunal can be used for supplemental or total enteral nutrition
- Most patients tolerate a whole-protein feed (1 kcal/mL), which can be escalated to 100 ml/hour and thus supply about 2400 kcal/day and 14 g N/day
- If a tube cannot be passed down the oesophagus, gastrostomy and jejunostomy feeding should be considered
- The main complications of enteral feeding relate to patient tolerance (nausea, vomiting and diarrhoea) and to the insertion site (gastrostomy or jejunostomy)

Parenteral nutrition

Parenteral nutrition can provide the patient's total needs for protein, energy, electrolytes, trace metals and vitamins, i.e., total parenteral nutrition (TPN).

Indications for total parenteral nutrition

The chief indication for TPN is intestinal failure. TPN can be both effective and life-saving when postoperative complications develop, especially when these prevent enteral nutrition or are associated with infection. Situations in which TPN is invaluable include prolonged paralytic ileus, high output proximal small intestinal fistulas, abdominal sepsis, and in dealing with the increased metabolic demands that follow severe injury, including burns.

TPN should continue until intestinal function has recovered sufficiently to allow nutrition to be maintained by the oral or enteral route. In cases of a high-output stoma, or proximal small bowel fistula, parenteral feeding is continued until the fistula has closed spontaneously or has been closed surgically.

Composition of total parenteral nutrition solutions

TPN is usually provided in preprepared all-in-one bags containing 3 L or more. TPN is compounded in the pharmacy under strictly aseptic conditions, and its contents usually infused over 18–24 hours using a volumetric infusion pump. Most pharmacies have three or four standard regimens available for compounding, according to requirements. The solutions contain fixed amounts of energy and nitrogen, and typically provide 1400–2400 kcal (50% glucose, 50% lipid) and 10–14 g nitrogen.

Fluid and electrolyte needs are also catered for. Many patients on TPN need additional water, sodium and potassium because of excess loss from, for example, a high-output fistula. Trace elements and vitamins can also be incorporated, and the demands created by infection and excessive loss can thus be met. An example of a standard TPN regimen is given in Table 3.4.

Administration of total parenteral nutrition

TPN solutions are typically hypertonic and acidic (because of the glucose and amino acid content). Thus, they have to be infused relatively slowly into a vein with a high blood flow to prevent chemically induced thrombophlebitis and secondary venous thrombosis. Vascular access to the superior vena cava is normally obtained directly through the internal jugular or subclavian vein, or indirectly via a peripherally inserted central (PIC) line. The catheter tip is usually sited, using radiological guidance, at the junction of the superior vena cava and right atrium, as the blood flow is

maximal at that point. The catheter tip should not be placed within the atrium itself as this may predispose to atrial thrombosis.

Cannulae are made of silastic or polyurethane and are of fine bore. For longer-term feeding, catheters are tunnelled subcutaneously to reduce the risk of infection. For very long-term (including home) parenteral feeding a Hickman catheter is used; this type of silastic catheter has a Dacron cuff, which secures it in the subcutaneous fat. With good care, a correctly positioned Hickman catheter can remain in place for many years without infection or occlusion (Fig. 3.7).

Table 3.4 Standard parenteral nutrition regimen

Constituent	Quantity
Nonprotein energy	2200 kcal
Nitrogen	13.5 g
Volume	2500 mL
Sodium	115 mmol
Potassium	65 mmol
Calcium	10 mmol
Magnesium	9.5 mmol
Phosphate	20 mmol
Zinc	0.1 mmol
Chloride	113.3 mmol
Acetate	135 mmol
(Adequate vitamins and trace elements)	

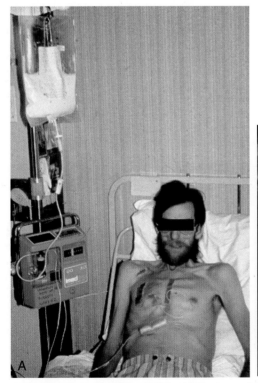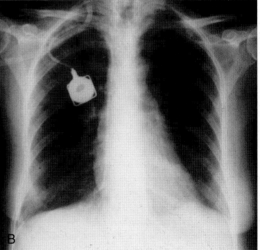

Fig. 3.7 Total parenteral nutrition (TPN). (A) Malnourished patient receiving TPN. **(B)** Chest x-ray of patient with indwelling Portacath for long-term TPN. The subcutaneous catheter hub is accessed using a Huber needle.

Complications of total parenteral nutrition

Catheter problems

Percutaneous insertion of a catheter may damage adjacent structures and can cause pneumothorax, air embolus and haematoma. Ultrasound guidance should always be used for catheter placement, as it enables such problems to be avoided almost completely. Incorrect catheter positioning is excluded by taking a chest x-ray prior to commencing infusion.

Thrombophlebitis

Thrombosis is common when long lines are used, when the catheter tip is not in an area of high flow, and when very hypertonic solutions are infused. The telltale signs are redness and tenderness over the cannulated vein, together with swelling of the whole limb and engorgement of collateral veins if the thrombosis is more proximal. Occasionally, a superior mediastinal syndrome develops in patients with superior vena cava thrombosis. If major vessel occlusion is suspected, the diagnosis is confirmed by venography and anticoagulation is commenced with heparin. If vascular access has to be maintained, an attempt can be made to lyse the clot with urokinase or plasminogen activator given through the catheter as well as systemic anticoagulation. If the clot cannot be dissolved, the cannula must be removed and a new one positioned in a patent vein. The patient may need to remain on long-term anticoagulation.

Infection

Catheter related sepsis and blood stream infection (CRBSI) are the most frequent complications of TPN. The usual offending organisms are skin bacteria; coagulase-negative staphylococci, *Staphylococcus aureus* and coliforms, but the incidence of fungal infection is increasing, possibly because many of the patients requiring TPN are immunocompromised or receiving broad-spectrum antibiotics. Catheter infections are entirely avoidable and are almost always the result of poor line care, with infection usually introduced via the catheter hub as a result of deficient aseptic technique. Although CRBSI rates of 1–5 episodes per 1000 catheter days are regarded as acceptable, it is entirely possible to provide TPN for decades without a single episode, given rigorous attention to asepsis. The insertion site must be protected with an occlusive dressing and should be cleansed on alternate days with an antiseptic agent. The line must only be used for infusion of nutrients and never for taking or giving blood, or administering drugs.

Great care is taken to avoid contamination when changing bags. A nutrition support nurse is invaluable in avoiding CRBSI and supervising all aspects of catheter care. If the patient receiving TPN develops pyrexia, the protocol outlined in Table 3.5 should be followed. While CRBSI in short-term TPN is generally managed by removing the catheter, an attempt is usually made to salvage the catheter and treat the infection with antibiotics in patients receiving long-term TPN via tunnelled catheters, because repeated catheter removal eventually results in loss of venous access. Provided there is no evidence of septic shock, polymicrobial or fungal catheter infection (in which case the catheter is removed), the catheter is salvaged by 'locking it' twice daily for up to 14 days with a solution of vancomycin and urokinase, while intravenous antibiotics appropriate to the causative organism are continued. An alternative route for provision of TPN is employed until serial cultures confirm that the catheter infection has

Table 3.5 Detection and treatment of catheter related sepsis

If a pyrexia >38°C develops, or there is a further rise in temperature if already pyrexial • Stop parenteral nutrition and check for other sources of pyrexia (e.g., chest or urinary tract infection) • Take peripheral and central line blood cultures • Administer intravenous fluids • Heparinise catheter • Consult senior medical staff
If blood culture is negative • Restart parenteral nutrition and continue to monitor for signs of sepsis
If blood culture is positive • Remove catheter and send tip for bacteriological analysis • Administer appropriate antibiotic therapy • If necessary, replace catheter and restart parenteral nutrition within 24–48 hours
Where central access must be preserved • Seek specialist advice from hospital nutrition team

resolved. Such regimens have been shown to salvage at least 60% of episodes of CRBSI.

Metabolic complications

Metabolic complications include under- or overhydration. Patients with co-existing medical conditions (e.g., cardiac failure) should be carefully monitored. There is a physiological upper limit to the amount of glucose that can be oxidised (4 mg/kg/min) and prolonged glucose infusion in excess of this rate may lead to hyperglycaemia and fatty infiltration of the liver with disordered liver function. Mildly abnormal liver enzymes in patients receiving TPN are common. However, severe and progressive abnormalities and, in particular, biochemical or clinical jaundice should lead to a prompt re-evaluation of the feeding regimen. Excessive administration of glucose may also aggravate respiratory failure as a consequence of the need to eliminate larger amounts of carbon dioxide consequent upon increased carbohydrate oxidation. Intolerance of glucose is particularly likely in sepsis and critical illness as a result of insulin resistance. Hyperglycaemia may require a reduction of the glucose load, concomitant infusion of insulin via a separate pump, or both.

3.4 Summary

Parenteral nutrition

- Parenteral feeding is indicated if the patient cannot be fed adequately by the oral or enteral route
- The need to restrict volume when using total parenteral nutrition (TPN) means that concentrated solutions are used, which may be an irritant and thrombogenic. TPN is therefore infused through a catheter in a high-flow vein (e.g., superior vena cava)
- TPN is usually given in an 'all-in-one' bag with a mixture of glucose, fat and L-amino acids combined with fluid, electrolytes, vitamins, minerals and trace elements
- The major complications with TPN can be classed as catheter-related, septic or metabolic. A multidisciplinary approach to the management of TPN patients by a nutrition team will minimise such complications

Hypokalaemia and hypophosphataemia are common when severely malnourished patients are re-fed after a long period of starvation because of the large flux of potassium and phosphate into the cells ('refeeding syndrome'). This can be avoided by gradual administration of feeds and careful monitoring. Abnormal liver function tests may occur in severely stressed or septic patients. If the changes are marked and progressive, the overall substrate load should be reduced and discontinuation of parenteral nutrition considered.

Peripheral venous nutrition

TPN solutions can be compounded specifically to facilitate administration via a peripheral vein, using lipid emulsions and less hypertonic solutions of amino acids. These solutions are less likely to provoke thrombophlebitis, but are still usually suitable only for short-term use and conventional techniques should be employed if long-term nutritional support is needed. Peripheral catheters require the same level of care as central catheters, and the patient must still be monitored for signs of infection or metabolic complications. It is usually not possible to deliver more than 3 L of feed via a peripheral cannula and peripheral feeding usually requires the delivery of nutrients over 24 hours, resulting in impaired mobility.

Monitoring of nutritional support

Patients receiving nutritional support are monitored to detect deficiency states, assess the adequacy of energy and protein provision and anticipate complications. Patients receiving enteral feeding require less intensive monitoring, but are prone to the same metabolic complications as those fed intravenously.

Pulse rate, blood pressure and temperature are recorded regularly, an accurate fluid balance chart is maintained (including insensible losses), and the urine is checked daily for glycosuria. Body weight is measured twice weekly. Serum urea and electrolytes are measured daily, as are blood glucose levels if there is glycosuria. Full blood count, liver function tests, and serum albumin, calcium, magnesium and phosphate are monitored once or twice weekly. In patients where there is a concern about failure to respond to an apparently adequate nutritional regimen or there is ongoing electrolyte imbalance, urine may be collected over one or two 24-hour periods each week to measure nitrogen or electrolyte losses respectively. For patients on long-term enteral nutrition or TPN (i.e., longer than 2–3 weeks) less intense monitoring is appropriate once they are stable.

4

Savita Gossain
Peter M. Hawkey

Infections and antibiotics

Chapter contents

Importance of infection 48

Biology of infection 48

Preventing infection in surgical patients 50

Prophylactic use of antibiotics 52

Management of surgical infections 53

Specific infections in surgical patients 55

Infections primarily treated by surgical management 57

Healthcare-associated infections 59

Importance of infection

By 1847, Semmelweis noted that hand washing with chlorinated lime reduced the incidence of puerperal sepsis. In the latter half of the 19th century, Louis Pasteur hypothesised that bacteria caused infection by being carried through the air (germ theory of disease). Aware of Pasteur's work, in 1865 Joseph Lister first used carbolic acid (phenol) as a spray in the operating theatre to successfully prevent and treat infection in compound fractures. In the early part of the 20th century, with the advent of sterilised instruments, surgical gowns and the first rubber gloves, antisepsis was replaced by modern aseptic surgical techniques, which were championed by Birmingham surgeon Robert Lawson Tait. Penicillin was discovered by Alexander Fleming in 1928 and first used clinically in 1940 by Howard Florey. The prevention and treatment of surgical infection was further transformed by the many different classes of antibiotics that were discovered through the latter part of the 20th century. Nevertheless, control of infection in surgical practice remains an important and challenging issue due to the emergence of antibiotic-resistant organisms, and the rise in the numbers of elderly, comorbid and immunocompromised patients undergoing increasingly complex surgical interventions that frequently involve the use of implants. The risk of infection is related to the type of surgery. Postoperative infections impact on patient outcomes and increase the length of hospital stay, which in turn increases the cost of surgery. In the UK, there is now a legal duty on hospitals to do all they can to minimise the risk of healthcare-associated infections (HCAI) in patients.

Biology of infection

Many body surfaces are colonised by a wide range of microorganisms, called commensals, with no ill effects (Fig. 4.1). However, once the normal defences are breached in the course of surgery, such as skin (e.g., *Staphylococcus aureus*) and bowel (e.g., *Bacteroides* spp. and *Escherichia coli*), commensals can then cause infection. Infection is defined as the proliferation of microorganisms in body tissue with adverse physiological consequences. The factors involved in the evolution of infection are shown in Fig. 4.2.

Bacterial factors

The size of the inoculum is important with smaller numbers of bacteria being more easily removed by the host's immune response. Bacteria with greater pathogenic potential (virulence) in soft tissue (e.g., *Streptococcus pyogenes* versus *Escherichia coli*) will require a lower inoculum to establish infection. Pathogenic bacteria release a wide variety of exotoxins that can act locally, regionally and systemically, having spread via the bloodstream, lymphatics and along nerves (e.g., tetanospasmin, which causes tetanus). Other bacterial pathogenicity factors that are released include haemolysins, which destroy red blood cells, and streptokinase, elastase and hyaluronidase, which damage connective tissues. Endotoxin (lipopolysaccharide [LPS]), a component of the cell wall, is liberated when gram-negative bacteria break up (lysis). LPS stimulates endothelial cells and macrophages to release cytokines, which mediate the inflammatory response and produce septic shock. Lipoteichoic acid is the equivalent molecule in gram-positive bacteria.

Host defence systems

Commensals limit the potential virulence of pathogens by depriving them of nutrients, preventing their adherence and by producing various cell signalling substances that interfere with their activities. Administration of broad-spectrum antibiotics can lead to the replacement of commensals with a pathogen; for example, *Clostridium difficile* in the colon, which is a common cause of potentially life-threatening diarrhoea in postoperative patients.

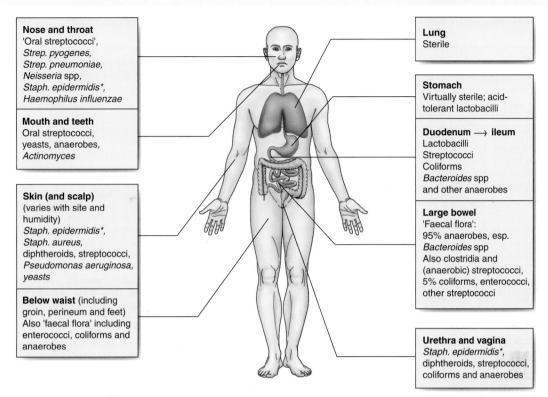

Nose and throat
'Oral streptococci',
Strep. pyogenes,
Strep. pneumoniae,
Neisseria spp,
Staph. epidermidis,*
Haemophilus influenzae

Mouth and teeth
Oral streptococci,
yeasts, anaerobes,
Actinomyces

Skin (and scalp)
(varies with site and
humidity)
Staph. epidermidis,*
Staph. aureus,
diphtheroids, streptococci,
Pseudomonas aeruginosa,
yeasts

Below waist (including
groin, perineum and feet)
Also 'faecal flora' including
enterococci, coliforms and
anaerobes

Lung
Sterile

Stomach
Virtually sterile; acid-
tolerant lactobacilli

Duodenum → ileum
Lactobacilli
Streptococci
Coliforms
Bacteroides spp
and other anaerobes

Large bowel
'Faecal flora':
95% anaerobes, esp.
Bacteroides spp
Also clostridia and
(anaerobic) streptococci,
5% coliforms, enterococci,
other streptococci

Urethra and vagina
Staph. epidermidis,*
diphtheroids, streptococci,
coliforms and anaerobes

Fig. 4.1 Distribution of normal adult flora. Mucosal or skin breaches may allow normal flora to infect usually sterile sites. Overgrowth by potentially pathogenic members of the normal flora may occur with changes in normal composition, e.g., after antimicrobial treatment, local changes in pH (vagina and stomach) or defective immunity (e.g., AIDS or immunosuppressive treatment). The most common yeast is *Candida albicans*. **Staphylococcus epidermidis* is the most common 'coagulase-negative *Staphylococcus*' frequently found on skin. Density of colonisation varies greatly with age and site.

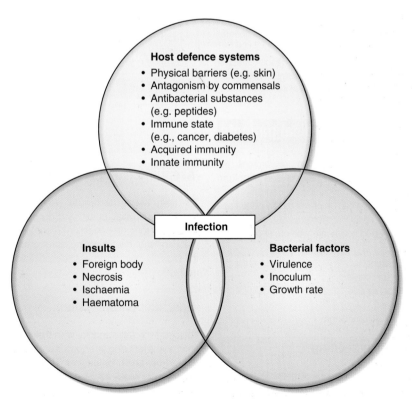

Host defence systems
• Physical barriers (e.g. skin)
• Antagonism by commensals
• Antibacterial substances
  (e.g. peptides)
• Immune state
  (e.g., cancer, diabetes)
• Acquired immunity
• Innate immunity

Infection

Insults
• Foreign body
• Necrosis
• Ischaemia
• Haematoma

Bacterial factors
• Virulence
• Inoculum
• Growth rate

Fig. 4.2 Factors important in the development of infection and their interrelationship.

Humans have evolved a wide range of defences that act at the interface with the surrounding environment. Skin provides a dry, inhospitable mechanical barrier to organisms and also secretes fatty acids in the sebum that kill or suppress potential pathogens. Tears and saliva contain a range of antibacterial substances such as lysozyme; and the low pH of gastric secretions kills many ingested pathogenic bacteria. Many mucosal surfaces are covered in secreted mucus, which both acts as a physical barrier and binds bacteria via specific receptors.

Macrophages, neutrophils and complement provide innate immunity through phagocytosis and bacterial lysis. The complement system (a cascade of bioactive proteins), which is activated when required, attracts the phagocytic cells, directly lyses pathogens and increases vascular permeability. Immunity can also be acquired through antibody- and cell-mediated mechanisms. There are two types of T-lymphocytes involved in cell-mediated immunity: CD4 help macrophages kill phagocytosed bacteria and CD8 kill cells infected with intracellular pathogens, especially viruses. The five classes of antibody (immunoglobulin [Ig]A, IgM, IgG, IgD and IgE) are secreted by B-lymphocytes, usually following stimulation via T cells. Antibodies, with or without complement, bind to and opsonise, lyse or kill the pathogen.

Cytokines (small peptide molecules) are released by leucocytes and facilitate the interaction between immune cells. Overactivation of this cytokine cascade leads to the systemic inflammatory response syndrome (SIRS). Typically, a patient presents with signs of severe infection, but instead of improving with antibiotic treatment develops worsening fever, hypotension, tissue hypoxia, acidosis and multiple organ failure.

A number of host factors make infection more likely:

- Old age, obesity, malnutrition, cancer and immunosuppressive agents, and diabetes
- The presence of dead tissue; e.g., burned flesh or haematoma provide a rich source of nutrients for bacteria and hamper the local immune response
- Poor vascularity; in the leg this is associated with peripheral arterial disease and diabetes
- Foreign material present in tissues either as a result of trauma (e.g., broken glass, clothing, shrapnel) or surgical procedure (e.g., joint replacements, heart valves, vascular prostheses).

Preventing infection in surgical patients

All hospitals should have infection prevention programmes that include measures to minimise risks to patients and staff from infections which may be acquired during and after surgery. Most healthcare-associated infections can be prevented by adherence to good hand hygiene. The WHO five moments of hand hygiene defines the five moments when healthcare workers should clean their hands, i.e.:

- Before touching a patient
- Before clean/aseptic procedure
- After body fluid exposure risk
- After touching a patient
- After touching patient surroundings

Preoperative MRSA screening

Most hospitals screen patients for carriage of methicillin-resistant *Staphylococcus aureus* (MRSA) prior to surgery. Carriers receive decolonisation treatment (nasal mupirocin cream and an antiseptic skin wash) and appropriate antibiotic prophylaxis, usually a

glycopeptide antibiotic (e.g., teicoplanin) prior to surgery. This policy has been shown to reduce MRSA transmission in surgical wards (EBM 4.1). Screening for nasal carriage of *Staph. aureus* followed by decolonisation can also reduce surgical wound infection (EBM 4.2). Screening of emergency surgical admissions may also be performed, although the timing of available results will determine whether this has an impact on management and outcomes.

EBM 4.1 Preventing methicillin-resistant *Staphylococcus aureus* transmission in surgical patients by rapid polymerase chain reaction screening for methicillin-resistant *Staph. aureus*

'A prospective, cluster, two-period cross-over design trial where all MRSA positive patients were decolonised and isolated (only for 17% patients). Infection control practices were the same in both groups. 13,952 patient wound episodes included and results showed that patients on wards using conventional screening were 1.49 times ($p = 0.007$) more likely to acquire MRSA. It was concluded that rapid PCR screening and decolonisation reduces transmission of MRSA.'

MRSA, Methicillin-resistant *Staphylococcus aureus*; PCR, polymerase chain reaction.

Hardy K, et al. Reduction in the rate of methicillin-resistant *Staphylococcus aureus* acquisition in surgical wards by rapid screening for colonisation: a prospective, cross-over study. Clin Microbiol Infect. 2010; 16:333–9.

EBM 4.2 Preventing surgical site infections in nasal carriers of *Staphylococcus aureus*

'A randomised, double-blind, placebo-controlled, multicentre trial over 20 months where a total of 6671 patients were screened for Staph. aureus nasal carriage using PCR. The subgroup of surgical-site infections caused by Staph. aureus was reduced by 60% among those in the active treatment group (nasal mupirocin ointment plus chlorhexidine wash) as compared to those in the placebo group.'

Bode LG, et al. Preventing surgical-site infections in nasal carriers of *Staphylococcus aureus*. N Engl J Med. 2010; 362:9–17.

Aseptic technique

The term 'aseptic technique' refers to specific practices performed immediately before and during a surgical procedure to reduce postoperative infection. These include patients showering preoperatively, hand washing, surgical scrub, skin preparation of the patient, maintaining a sterile operating field and using safe operating practices.

Hand decontamination

The operating team should wash their hands prior to each operation on the list using an aqueous antiseptic surgical solution, with a single-use brush for the nails. The 'six-step hand hygiene technique' is now widely adopted (Fig. 4.3). Hospitals will have policies for which antiseptic agents are used. Where hands are not soiled, alcohol hand gel is a suitable alternative for decontamination on the wards.

Wet hands under warm running water, apply soap, then follow this procedure

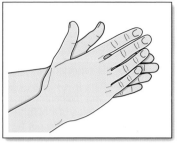
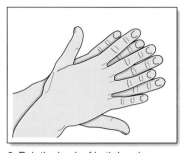
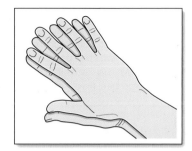

1. Rub palm-to-palm

2. Rub the back of both hands (right palm over left back and then *vice versa*)

3. Rub palm-to-palm interlacing the fingers

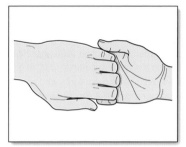
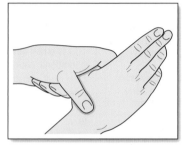
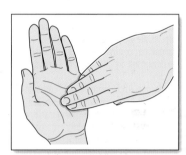

4. Rub the backs of fingers by interlocking the hands

5. Rub the thumbs (rotational rubbing of right thumb clasped in the left palm, and then *vice versa)*

6. Rub palms with fingertips (rotational rubbing of right fingers on left palm, and then *vice versa*)

Rinse the hands under running water, and **dry thoroughly**

Technique based on that of Ayliffe et al. J. Clin. Path. 1978; 31:923

Fig. 4.3 Six-step hand hygiene technique.

Personal protective equipment for staff

The operating team should wear appropriate personal protective equipment (PPE; sterile gowns, gloves, visors, goggles) during the operative procedure. In addition, double gloving and maintaining sharps safety is important for patients known or suspected to be infected with blood-borne viruses (e.g., HIV).

Enhanced PPE including respiratory-protective equipment is necessary for patients at risk of having viral haemorrhagic fever (VHF), e.g., Ebola. This includes water-repellant coveralls, full-length disposable apron over the coverall, fluid-repellant footwear, wearing double gloves as a minimum, and power-assisted personal respirator with P3 filter and full hood. Special attention must be paid to donning and removing PPE in a designated area to minimise the risk of acquiring VHF infection.

Skin preparation

Although it is not possible to sterilise the skin, antiseptics such as chlorhexidine or povidone-iodine applied to the surgical site prior to incision reduce the number of resident organisms and thereby the risks of wound infection. Antiseptics containing alcohol must be allowed to evaporate completely before using diathermy.

Surgical instruments

To prevent cross-infection only sterile or disposable, single-use instruments are used. Sterilisation for reusable instruments is usually undertaken in Sterile Services Departments (SSD) and is the process for complete destruction of all microorganisms, including spores.

Used surgical instruments are first thoroughly washed in automated washer disinfectors that reach temperatures of 85–95°C (thermal disinfection), remove organic matter and kill most microorganisms except spores. Instruments can then be packed and processed in a steam steriliser or autoclave to destroy any remaining microorganisms and their spores. Pressures above atmospheric are used so that higher temperatures can be achieved (e.g., 121°C for 20 minutes; 134°C for 5 minutes).

Maintaining patient homeostasis

Maintaining a normal patient temperature (unless active cooling is part of the procedure), optimal oxygenation and adequate perfusion during surgery are important in reducing the risk of postoperative infection. If a patient's temperature is below 36.0°C before, during or in the immediate postoperative period, they should be actively warmed using forced air warming.

Creutzfeldt–Jakob disease and other prion diseases

Normal decontamination processes do not destroy prions (infectious agents composed only of protein), and so patients known to have, or who are at risk of, Creutzfeldt–Jakob disease (CJD) must be identified prior to surgery. Wherever possible, disposable surgical instruments are used. Whether disposable or not, all instruments used on such patients must be subsequently destroyed by incineration.

4.1 Summary

Prevention of infection

- Preoperative screening of patients for MRSA, and subsequent decolonisation of carriers, is now an integral part of surgical care
- The routine practices of hand washing, surgical scrub, skin preparation of the patient and maintaining a sterile field are collectively known as 'aseptic technique', and is an important component in preventing surgical site infections
- Maintaining normothermia before, during (unless active cooling is part of the procedure) and after surgery lowers the risk of postoperative wound infection
- Sterility of surgical instruments is critical to preventing cross-infection. This may be achieved by decontamination of instruments in Sterile Services Departments or by using sterile, disposable instruments.

Prophylactic use of antibiotics

Antibiotic prophylaxis refers to the prevention of infective complications by the administration of antibiotics (Table 4.1).

Timing and dose

The aim is to achieve high concentrations of drug at the surgical site at the time of incision. A single intravenous dose at induction has been shown to be as effective as multiple doses with the

Table 4.1 Classification of operations on the basis of susceptibility to infection and use of antibiotics

Class	Definition
Clean[a]	Operations in which no inflammation is encountered and the respiratory, alimentary or genitourinary tracts are not entered. There is no break in aseptic operating theatre technique
Clean – contaminated[a]	Operations in which the respiratory, alimentary or genitourinary tracts are entered but without significant spillage
Contaminated[b]	Operations where acute inflammation (without pus) is encountered, or where there is visible contamination of the wound. Examples include gross spillage from a hollow viscus during the operation or compound/open injuries operated on within 4 hours
Dirty[b]	Operations in the presence of pus, where there is a previously perforated hollow viscus, or compound/open injuries more than 4 hours old

[a]Prophylactic antibiotic.
[b]Use therapeutic antibiotics for up to 5–7 days.
See www.sign.ac.uk/pdf/sign104.pdf and www.bnf.org

exception of arthroplasty, when a large observational study supported 24-hour treatment. If the surgery is prolonged >4 hours or blood loss is high then a second intraoperative dose may be given. A comprehensive guideline is available at www.sign.ac.uk/pdf/104.pdf.

Antibiotic choice

The antibiotic chosen must cover the expected pathogens for the type of surgery. Most hospitals have policies that take into account local resistance patterns, and propensity to cause *C. difficile* infection (CDI). Patients with a history of anaphylaxis, urticaria or other signs of allergy to penicillin should not be given β-lactam antibiotic prophylaxis. Information on antibiotic prophylaxis in special circumstances (e.g., prevention of endocarditis, joint prostheses and dental treatment) may be found at www.bnf.org.

Carriage of resistant organisms and prophylaxis

This is a risk factor for surgical site infection (SSI) after high-risk operations, especially when a surgical implant is used, (e.g., vascular graft, prosthetic joint, etc.). Surgical patients who are recognised preoperatively to be carrying MRSA should be decolonised. The significance of carriage of multiresistant gram-negative bacilli (e.g., extended spectrum β-lactamase [ESBL]-producing or carbapenemase-producing Enterobacteriaciae) is not clear, but the advice of a microbiologist should be sought and an appropriate antibiotic used.

Prophylaxis for immunosuppressed patients

The choice of agent will depend on individual circumstances, and expert microbiological help should be sought. Splenectomised patients are at increased risk of infection with encapsulated bacteria and protozoa, and should be:

- Commenced on lifelong antibiotic prophylaxis with penicillin or amoxicillin
- Immunised against *Streptococcus pneumoniae*, *Haemophilus influenzae* type b (Hib), and *Neisseria meningitides* groups A, B, C and W135 (depending on local epidemiology).

Travelers to areas with risk of malaria transmission should consider appropriate precautions.

For elective splenectomy, the vaccines should be given 2–4 weeks prior to the procedure, and for emergency procedures 2–4 weeks after.

4.2 Summary

Prophylactic antibiotics

- Antibiotic prophylaxis in surgical practice aims to prevent infection by achieving high concentrations of antibiotic at the incision and site of operation during surgery
- The choice of antibiotic must cover the likely pathogens for the operation site
- A single dose of antibiotic is usually adequate for prophylaxis, although during prolonged procedures or where there is excessive blood loss, a second dose may be required
- In some circumstances, e.g., colonisation with multiresistant bacteria or immunocompromised patients, the antibiotic choice may need to be modified and expert advice should be sought.

Management of surgical infections

Surgical infections are of two types; those that occur in patients who:

- Have undergone a surgical procedure
- Present with sepsis and require surgery as part of their management.

Diagnosis

Infections in the early postoperative period (>48 hours) are most likely to be respiratory or urinary, with wound infections usually becoming evident later. Implant-related infections may not be evident for weeks, months or even years. Leakage of a gastrointestinal (GI) anastomosis usually presents after 5–6 days with low-grade pyrexia and abdominal symptoms and signs; there may also be leakage of bowel content from surgical drains.

Ask about:

- Cough, dysuria, abdominal pain.

Look for:

- Tachycardia, tachypnoea, pyrexia
- Tenderness at or around the surgical wound
- Signs of peritonitis in postabdominal surgery patients
- Signs of shock – hypotension, pallor, sweating, rigors, confusion – and if present contact the critical care outreach team for urgent resuscitation.

Identify the focus of infection:

- Urine for dipstick test and culture
- Sputum culture
- Pus from wound or deep aspiration for Gram staining and culture
- Blood culture in febrile/septic patients.

Serious sepsis in the surgical patient often arises from intra-abdominal infections (IAI). Approximately 30% of patients admitted to the intensive care unit (ICU) with IAI die, and if peritonitis develops mortality rises to 50%. Early diagnosis and treatment is essential but clinical examination is often unreliable, even misleading. Computed tomography (CT) or magnetic resonance imaging (MRI), preferably with contrast, should be performed to detect peritoneal leaks and collections of pus, and can be life-saving. An integrated and logical approach to patient management should be followed as described in the surviving sepsis guidelines, which are summarised in Tables 4.2 and 4.3. Three recent studies of invasive haemodynamic monitoring have shown that protocol-based, early goal-directed therapy confers little survival advantage over standard care.

Antibiotic therapy

Antibiotics are almost always needed in addition to surgical treatment in surgical infections, e.g., drainage of abscesses, debridement, excision of infected tissue or lavage of a serous cavity.

- Antibiotic policies: each hospital has its own antibiotic formulary and this should be consulted; the principles behind such policies are shown in Table 4.4.
- Specimens for culture and sensitivity testing should always be obtained if possible and then specific antibiotics used as suggested in Table 4.5. It is not always possible to await these results if the patient is seriously ill, and empirical therapy should be started immediately according to Table 4.6.
- When using some antibiotics such as gentamicin and vancomycin, therapeutic drug monitoring is needed to

Table 4.2 Screening for sepsis and severe sepsis	
Are any two of the following present?	
• Temperature <36°C or >38.3°C • Heart rate >90 bpm • WCC >12 or <4 × 10⁹/L **If yes:**	• Respiratory rate >20 breaths/min • Acutely altered mental state • Hyperglycaemia in the absence of diabetes
Does the patient have a history or signs suggestive of a new infection?	
• Cough/sputum/chest pain • Abdominal pain/distension/diarrhoea • Line infections **If yes**, patient has **SEPSIS**	• Dysuria • Headache with neck stiffness • Cellulitis/wound infection/septic arthritis
Are there any signs of organ dysfunction?	
• SBP >90 mmHg or MAP >65 mmHg • Urine output >0.5 ml/kg/h for 2 h • INR >1.5 or APTT >60 s • Bilirubin >34 mmol/L	• Lactate >2 mmol/L • New need for oxygen to keep Sp_{O_2} > 90% • Platelets >100 × 10⁹/L • Creatinine >177 mmol/L
NO: Treat for SEPSIS	YES: Patient has SEVERE SEPSIS
• Oxygen • Blood cultures • IV antibiotics • Fluid therapy • Reassess for SEVERE SEPSIS with hourly observations	Start SEVERE SEPSIS CARE PATHWAY (Table 4.3)
APTT, Activated partial thromboplastin time, INR, international normalised ratio; IV, intravenous; MAP, mean arterial pressure, SBP, systolic blood pressure; WCC, white cell count. http://www.survivingsepsis.org/	

Table 4.3 Severe sepsis care pathway

1. **Oxygen:** high-flow 15 L/min via non-rebreathe mask. Target saturations >94%
2. **Blood cultures:** take at least one set plus all relevant blood tests, e.g., FBC, U&E, LFT, clotting, glucose
Consider urine/sputum/swab samples
3. **IV antibiotics:** as per hospital guidelines
4. **Fluid resuscitate:** if hypotensive give bolus of 0.9% saline or Hartmann's 30 mL/kg
5. **Serum lactate and haemoglobin:** Ensure Hb >7 g/dL
6. **Catheterise** and commence fluid balance chart

PLUS

a. Call outreach team if appropriate
b. Discuss with consultant

FBC, Full blood count; Hb, Haemoglobin; IV, intravenous; LFT, liver function test; U&E, urea and electrolytes.
http://www.survivingsepsis.org/

Table 4.4 Principles underlying antibiotic policy

- Antibiotics should be avoided in self-limiting infections, and due consideration should be given to expense, toxicity and the need to avoid the emergence of resistant strains
- Choice of therapy is determined positively by knowledge of the nature and sensitivities of the infecting organism(s). Therapy may be initiated on clinical evidence, but must be reviewed in light of culture/sensitivity reports
- Restrict the use of antibiotics to which resistance is developing (or has developed)
- Single agents are preferred to combination therapy, and narrow-spectrum agents are preferred to broad-spectrum agents whenever possible
- Adequate doses must be given by the recommended route at correct time intervals
- Antibiotics that are used systemically must not be used topically
- Antibiotics used for prophylaxis are not used for treatment
- The side effects of antibiotics should be known by the prescriber and monitored
- Expensive antibiotics are not used if equally effective and cheaper alternatives are suitable
- With few exceptions (e.g., lung abscess), antibiotics should not be used to treat abscesses unless adequate surgical or radiological drainage has been achieved
- Policies may include automatic 'stop' orders

Table 4.5 Antibiotics in surgery: suggestions for specific therapy

Organism	First choice	Alternative
Methicillin-sensitive *Staphylococcus aureus*	Flucloxacillin	Clarithromycin[b]
Methicillin-resistant *Staph. aureus*[a]	Vancomycin[b]	Linezolid[b] or daptomycin[b]
Coagulase-negative staphylococci	Vancomycin	Linezolid[b] or daptomycin[b]
Streptococcus pneumoniae	Benzylpenicillin	Clarithromycin[b]
Streptococcus pyogenes (group A β-haemolytic streptococcus)	Benzylpenicillin Clindamycin	Clarithromycin[b]
Enterococci	Amoxicillin	Vancomycin[b]
Bacteroides species	Metronidazole[b]	Co-amoxiclav
Escherichia coli		
1. Sepsis, including bacteraemia	Piperacillin-Tazobactam	Meropenem[b]
2. Urinary tract infection	Trimethoprim[b]	Co-amoxiclav
Haemophilus influenzae	Amoxicillin	Co-amoxiclav
Klebsiella spp.	Co-amoxiclav	Meropenem[b]
Proteus spp.	Co-amoxiclav	Meropenem[b]
Pseudomonas aeruginosa	Piperacillin-Tazobactam	Meropenem[b]
Clostridium spp.	Benzylpenicillin[b] Metronidazole	Metronidazole[b]
Clostridium difficile	Stop predisposing antibiotic metronidazole	Vancomycin[b] (oral) for either Fidaxomicin[b] or faecal microbiota transplant relapse

These suggestions should be considered in light of local antibiotic resistance patterns. In countries where ESBL-producing Enterobacteriaceae are common carbapenems (e.g., meropenem) are used 1st line. Patients infected with CPE will require the use of 'last-resort' antibiotics, e.g., colistin or tigecycline.
[a]Gould FK, et al. Guideline (2008) for the prophylaxis and treatment of methicillin-resistant *Staphylococcus aureus* (MRSA) infections in the UK. J Antimicrob Chemother 2009; 63: 849–861.
[b]Suitable for penicillin-allergic patients.

(i) establish adequate serum concentrations and (ii) identify toxic concentrations before renal or neurological damage develops. Specific protocols are available from microbiology/pharmacy departments at individual hospitals.

- Advice should be sought early about antibiotic treatment regimens from microbiologists/infectious diseases specialists, particularly when the diagnosis is not certain and/or the patient is critically ill.

Table 4.6 Empirical therapy for acute infections		
Type of infections	**Antimicrobial**	**Alternative**
Chest infection		
Uncomplicated	Amoxicillin	Clarithromycin
Community-acquired pneumonia	Benzyl penicillin + clarithromycin	Levofloxacin or clarithromycin
'Aspiration' pneumonia	Co-amoxiclav	Levofloxacin + metronidazole
Hospital-acquired/postoperative	Piperacillin-tazobactam	Meropenem + vancomycin
Urinary tract infection		
'Lower' infection	Trimethoprim	Amoxicillin
Acute pyelonephritis	Co-amoxiclav	Gentamicin
Prostatitis	Ciprofloxacin	
Wound infection		
Cellulitis	Penicillin + flucloxacillin	Clarithromycin
Abscess	Drain collection	Flucloxacillin
Intraabdominal sepsis	Amoxicillin + metronidazole + gentamicin	Meropenem
Cholecystitis-cholangitis	Co-amoxiclav	Meropenem
Pelvic inflammatory disease	Azithromycin + metronidazole + gentamicin	Doxycycline + piperacillin-tazobactam
Amputations and gas gangrene	Benzylpenicillin + metronidazole	Metronidazole
Septicaemia and septic shock	Amoxicillin + metronidazole + gentamicin/ciprofloxacin	Piperacillin-tazobactam + meropenem
Severe *Pseudomonas* infections	Piperacillin-tazobactam + gentamicin	Meropenem ± gentamicin
***Candida* sepsis**	Fluconazole	Echinocandins, e.g., caspofungin

The suggestions are for occasions when immediate treatment is necessary. Amendments may be necessary in the light of local epidemiology of hospital-acquired pathogens and antibiotic resistance patterns.

Specific infections in surgical patients

Surgical site infection (SSI)

All surgical wounds are contaminated by microbes but in most cases infection does not develop because of innate host defences. A complex interplay between host, microbial and surgical factors ultimately determines whether infection takes hold and how it progresses (Fig. 4.2, EBM 4.3, and see Table 4.1).

Diagnosis

Superficial SSIs can be identified by pyrexia, local erythema, pain and excessive tenderness, and sometimes discharge. Deeper infection may present more insidiously with pyrexia, leucocytosis, and organ dysfunction, such as prolonged postoperative ileus. Diagnosis may require radiological imaging and sometimes exploratory laparotomy.

Treatment

Cellulitis can be treated with antibiotics but an abscess will require drainage as antibiotics will not penetrate pus. Drainage may involve simply laying open the wound and healing by secondary intention. Deeper, more complex collections will need formal drainage either radiologically (under ultrasound or CT guidance) or by means of open surgery.

EBM **4.3 Surgical site infection (SSI) classification**

'Superficial incisional SSI: *Infection involves only skin and subcutaneous tissue of incision.*
Deep incisional SSI: *Infection involves deep tissues, such as fascial and muscle layers. This also includes infection involving both superficial and deep incision sites and organ/space SSI draining through incision.*
Organ/space SSI: *Infection involves any part of the anatomy in organs and spaces other than the incision, which was opened or manipulated during operation.'*

Horan TC, et al. CDC definitions of nosocomial surgical site infections, 1992: a modification of CDC definitions of surgical wound infections. Infect Control Hosp Epidemiol. 1992;13:606–8.

Prevention

The risks of SSI can be reduced by:
- Careful surgical technique to minimise tissue damage, bleeding, anastomotic leaks and haematoma
- Appropriate antibiotic prophylaxis.

Urinary tract infections

Urinary tract infections (UTIs) are common and may range from simple cystitis to pyelonephritis or even perinephric abscess. Catheterised patients are at increased risk of infection. The most common organisms are *Escherichia coli*, *Klebsiella* species, *Enterococcus faecalis* and *Pseudomonas aeruginosa*. Multiresistant organisms such as ESBL-producing *E. coli* and MRSA are increasingly being seen and can be difficult to treat.

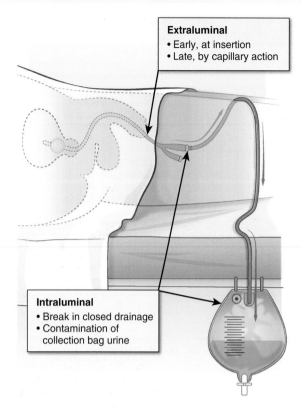

Extraluminal
- Early, at insertion
- Late, by capillary action

Intraluminal
- Break in closed drainage
- Contamination of collection bag urine

Fig. 4.4 Routes of entry of uropathogens into the catheterised urinary tract.

Ask about:
- Fever/rigors
- Dysuria
- Urinary frequency
- Lower abdominal pain
- Loin pain.

Look for:
- Pyrexia
- Suprapubic tenderness
- Tenderness in the renal angle.

Send:
- Midstream sample of urine (MSU) or catheter sample of urine (CSU) for microscopy, culture and sensitivity
- Blood cultures if pyrexia.

In catheterised patients the urine frequently contains organisms but not white cells. This does not require antibiotics unless there are signs of systemic illness. The urine will not become sterile until the catheter is removed. First-line empirical treatment should be guided by local epidemiology; suggestions are included in Table 4.6. Expert advice should be sought in the case of multidrug-resistant pathogens. Aseptic introduction and meticulous care of the urinary catheter helps to prevent bacteria entering the urinary tract (Fig. 4.4).

Emergence of multiresistant bacteria

β-Lactam antibiotics like penicillins and cephalosporins may be rendered ineffective by β-lactamase enzymes produced by gram-positive and gram-negative bacteria. However, extended spectrum cephalosporins (e.g. cefotaxime) remain effective against such pathogens. ESBLs are β-lactamases usually produced by *Klebsiella* spp. and *E. coli* that hydrolyse the extended spectrum β-lactam antibiotics like second- and third-generation cephalosporins, thereby conferring resistance to these antibiotics. Cultures from high-risk patients on these antibiotics in surgical ICUs and high-dependency wards need to be reviewed for the presence of ESBLs in cases of nonresponse to therapy. Carbapenems are the treatment of choice for serious infections due to ESBL-producing bacteria. Recently, carbapenem-resistant strains of particularly *Klebsiella* spp. and *E. coli* have emerged and treatment with carbapenems will fail. Treatment will require the use of specialised antibiotics advised by an expert in infection.

Respiratory tract infections

This comprises upper and lower respiratory tract infection, lung abscess and empyema. Likely pathogens include:
- *Streptococcus pneumoniae*
- *Haemophilus influenzae*
- Gram-negative bacteria, e.g., *E. coli*, *P. aeruginosa* (especially during or after mechanical ventilation)
- *Staph. aureus* (including MRSA)

Ask about:
- Fever
- Cough
- Increased respiratory secretions
- Breathlessness

Look for:
- Pyrexia
- Confusion
- Tachypnoea
- Chest signs, e.g., dullness of percussion, bronchial breathing, coarse crepitations

Diagnosis is made on the basis of history, examination, arterial blood gases, chest x-ray, cultures (blood, sputum and bronchial washings) and sometimes specialist radiology (e.g., CT). A positive sputum culture without clinical symptoms and signs of infection does not automatically merit antimicrobial therapy. Antibiotic treatment should follow the local hospital policy until culture and sensitivity results become available. Abscess or empyema should be drained. Patients should be taught breathing and coughing exercises preoperatively. They should become familiar with the use of an incentive spirometer (Fig. 4.5). Physiotherapy, early mobilisation and adequate pain relief in the postoperative period will help prevent respiratory infection.

C. difficile infection (CDI)

This occurs when the normal colonic microflora is disturbed by the administration of antibiotics in patients either pre-colonised with or exposed after antibiotic treatment to *C. difficile* (an anaerobic spore-forming bacillus). The bacterium produces two cytotoxins, A and B (some strains only produce B), that destroy the colonic mucosal cell cytoskeleton.

A spectrum of disease is seen, ranging from abdominal discomfort to profuse watery diarrhoea (one of the most common features), severe abdominal cramps and rarely toxic dilatation of the colon leading to rupture. At colonoscopy characteristic yellow

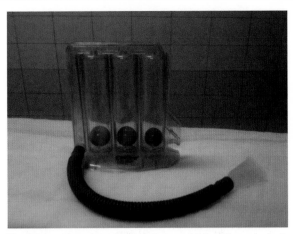

Fig. 4.5 Incentive spirometer. The balls rise on inflation of increasing levels of tidal volume, with all three balls rising on maximum inspiratory effort. The patient is self-motivated to raise the maximum number and keep them afloat for the longest period of time.

plaques, bleeding mucosa and islands of normal tissue are seen, which is called pseudomembranous colitis. Surgical patients can acquire CDI as a consequence of antibiotic treatment or prophylaxis. Infrequently patients with severe CDI may require urgent surgical referral. Emergency colectomy in patients with fulminant colitis can be life saving, although mortality is high.

Diagnosis

Test liquid sample of faeces for the presence of toxin by enzyme imunoassay and/or detection of the toxin gene by polymerase chain reaction (PCR).

Treatment

Mild/moderate disease:	Oral metronidazole 10–14 days
Severe disease:	Oral vancomycin 10–14 days Fidaxomicin
Recurrent disease:	Oral vancomycin (consider longer course) Faecal microbiota transplant (FMT)

Infection control

- Isolate all patients with diarrhoea
- Thorough cleaning of environment and equipment (using hypochlorite solution or hydrogen peroxide vapour)
- Good antibiotic stewardship.

Fungal infections

Invasive fungal infections are increasing in incidence. Invasive candidiasis (most commonly due to *Candida albicans*), in particular, is now recognised as a major cause of morbidity and mortality in the healthcare environment.

Risk factors

- Immunocompromised (e.g., neutropaenia, HIV infection)
- Prolonged ICU stay

- GI surgery, especially anastomotic leaks or recurrent GI perforation
- Central venous catheters and use of total parenteral nutrition (TPN)
- Prolonged use of multiple or broad-spectrum antibiotics.

Distinction needs to be made between colonisation with *Candida* spp. and invasive infection.

Nystatin can be given orally to treat mucocutaneous candidiasis of the oropharynx. Systemic antifungal agents such as triazoles (e.g., fluconazole, voriconazole) or echinocandins (e.g., caspofungin) are available for invasive infections. Empiric antifungal therapy should be considered in critically ill patients with risk factors for invasive candidiasis and no other known cause of fever.

Infections of prosthetic devices

In many fields of surgery the use of implants has become routine and affords huge clinical benefit. Nevertheless, there is a small risk of device-related infection, which can be catastrophic for the patient. Bacteria, often commensals such as coagulase-negative staphylococci, can be introduced at the time of surgery and form a biofilm of extracellular material (glycocalyx) around the device, which is resistant to the body's defences and the penetration of some antibiotics. Alternatively, the implant can be 'seeded' via the bloodstream months, even years, later from a bacteraemia arising from another source; e.g., *Staph. aureus* skin sepsis or *E. coli* UTI. Antibiotics alone are often unsuccessful and removal of the device is frequently necessary to eradicate the sepsis. Such surgery may be difficult and is associated with significant morbidity and mortality.

 4.3 Summary

Management of surgical infection

- The risk of surgical site infection rises in direct proportion to the degree of microbial contamination of the wound
- Whenever possible, the focus of infection should be identified by careful history-taking, clinical examination, imaging and microbiological culture
- Collections of pus should be drained
- In many surgical infections, antibiotics are often needed in addition to surgical treatment, e.g., drainage of abscesses, debridement, excision of infected tissue or lavage of a serous cavity. Surgical treatment is more important than antibiotics
- Tetanus immunisation status of patients must be determined prior to elective surgery or following trauma.

Infections primarily treated by surgical management

Abscess

This is a localised collection of pus containing neutrophils, dead tissue and organisms that can develop anywhere in the body. The most common pathogen is *Staph. aureus*. Abscesses in the abdomen or pelvis often contain a mixture of gut bacteria, e.g., *E. coli*, enterococci and anaerobic bacteria. Abscesses close to the skin are often painful and the overlying skin will be raised, red and hot to the touch. Large or multiple skin abscesses may cause systemic upset. Deeper abscesses may present with a 'swinging' pyrexia, systemic upset and symptoms relating to pressure on surrounding tissues. The pus must be drained and sent for microscopy and culture. This can be achieved through needle aspiration (e.g., breast), radiologically under ultrasound or CT guidance (e.g., subphrenic), or via open surgery (e.g., perianal). Antibiotics do not usually penetrate into abscesses but may be required for treatment if the patient is systemically unwell or for prophylaxis if a surgical wound is being made in the course of drainage.

Necrotising fasciitis

This is an uncommon but severe, life-threatening infection of skin and subcutaneous tissues characterised by necrosis of deep fascia (Fig. 4.6). There are two main types depending on causative organisms:

- Type I: Polymicrobial aetiology, which is also known as synergistic bacterial gangrene; Fournier's gangrene is a special type affecting the perineal area
- Type II: Single-organism infection, usually by β-haemolytic Group A streptococci (S. pyogenes).

The infection usually starts at a site of (often minor) trauma and can spread very quickly, as bacterial exotoxins and enzymes lead to necrosis of fat and fascia and eventually overlying skin. The patient is usually febrile, toxic and in severe pain. Initially, the overlying skin may appear deceptively normal, but as the infection progresses there is oedema, discoloration and crepitus (due to gas production). Urgent surgical debridement of all necrotic tissue is essential and several visits to theatre may be required. Initial antibiotic choice is usually empirical with a combination of broad-spectrum agents against likely pathogens, e.g., carbapenems, clindamycin and metronidazole. Antibiotic therapy can later be tailored according to the results of pus and tissue cultures.

Diabetic foot infections

Infections involving the lower extremities in diabetic patients range from cellulitis to complex skin and soft tissue infection to osteomyelitis. Clinical diagnosis is based on the presence of cellulitis, purulent discharge, pain, tenderness and gangrene. Signs of systemic toxicity may be present in severe infection. Infections are often polymicrobial. Microbiological diagnosis is best achieved by culture of tissue and bone biopsy samples, as culturing surface swabs from ulcers merely indicates which microorganisms are colonising the ulcer/wound. Radiological investigation for osteomyelitis includes plain x-rays and MRI. Antibiotic therapy is usually

the first line of treatment, although a multidisciplinary team approach is required to ensure appropriate wound management: good nutrition, appropriate antimicrobial therapy, glycaemic control, and fluid and electrolyte balance. Surgical involvement is required for debridement, drainage of abscess and/or amputation in chronic osteomyelitis.

Gas gangrene

- Rare
- High mortality
- Causative organisms: Clostridium perfringens, Clostridium novyi and Clostridium septicum (sporing organisms found in soil)
- Risk factors: Contact with soil, especially in the battlefield; presence of devitalised tissue
- Symptoms and signs are toxin mediated and include rapid deterioration, sepsis, spreading muscle necrosis; skin discoloration and oedema; crepitus of tissues (Fig. 4.7)
- Management: Urgent extensive surgical excision of necrotic tissue AND high-dose antibiotics (penicillin and metronidazole).

Infections following trauma

The risk of infection will be related to the amount of tissue damage and contamination with extraneous material (e.g., soil, clothing, etc.). Heavily contaminated wounds need thorough cleaning and debridement of all nonviable tissue; failure may lead to severe infections including gas gangrene. A short course of broad-spectrum antibiotics has been shown to reduce the incidence of early infection in open limb fractures. It is essential to determine the patient's tetanus immunisation status.

Tetanus

This is caused by Clostridium tetani, a spore-forming anaerobic organism that enters the body through soil or animal faecal contamination of a wound, injury or burn, and then multiplies anaerobically in tissues if the wound is not adequately cleaned or debrided. The incubation period varies from 4 to 21 days.

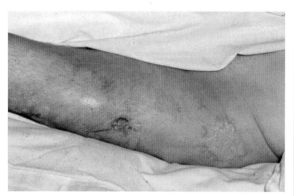

Fig. 4.6 Necrotising fasciitis of the lower limb. (Courtesy Medical Microbiology Dept., University of Edinburgh.)

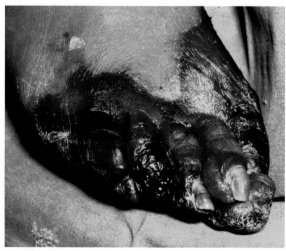

Fig. 4.7 Gangrene developing in the foot of a diabetic. (Courtesy Mr A.S. Whyte FRCS.)

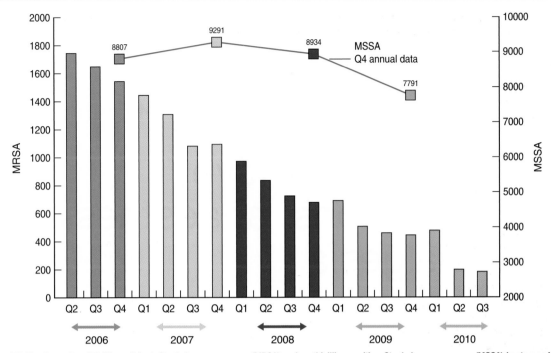

4

Fig. 4.8 Numbers of methicillin-resistant *Staphylococcus aureus* (MRSA) and methicillin-sensitive *Staphylococcus aureus* (MSSA) bacteraemia (quarterly) in England, derived from Health Protection Agency (HPA) surveillance data.

Tetanospasmin (a neurotoxin) spreads along nerves from the site of infection and causes generalised rigidity and spasm of skeletal muscles. The muscle stiffness usually involves the jaw (lockjaw) and neck, and then becomes generalised. Mortality ranges from 10% to 90%, and is highest in infants and the elderly. Antibiotic treatment is with penicillins or, for penicillin-allergic patients, clarithromycin, but is only an adjunct to correct surgical care of wounds and further specialised medical treatment. Tetanus can be prevented by immunisation.

In the UK (a low-risk area), all young children are offered the tetanus vaccine as part of the routine NHS childhood vaccination programme (www.nhs.uk/conditions/Tetanus); current advice is to have five doses over a life time. Details of vaccination in high-risk areas are available at www.who.int/immunisation/topics/tetanus/en/. For nonimmune individuals who have suffered a tetanus-prone injury, Human Tetanus Immunoglobulin (HTIG) is given to provide immediate protection together with wound debridement, active immunisation (three doses of tetanus toxoid at monthly intervals) and antibiotic treatment.

Healthcare-associated infections

In 2006, a survey of 190 acute hospitals in England showed that 8.2% of patients had developed a HCAI (previously known as a nosocomial infection), most commonly SSI, GI infections, UTI and pneumonia. The hospital infection control team are most closely involved in the design and delivery of the HCAI programme, and will liaise with the microbiology laboratory to ensure that infections caused by important pathogens are identified at an

early stage and that trends in antibiotic resistance are monitored. However, all staff members and students have a duty to take responsibility for this very important aspect of patient care. In recent years, there has been a national focus in the UK on reducing MRSA and *C. difficile* infections in England using a multifaceted approach. The use of carriage screening, decolonisation, patient isolation, and improved handwashing and environmental cleaning has reduced cases of bacteraemia from 6000 per annum to 400 per annum (Fig. 4.8). Monitoring SSI is an important quality indicator. Systematic collection of infection data (surveillance) can be by nurse follow-up of all patients who have undergone surgery during a given period. Surveillance nurses will inspect surgical wounds for any signs of infection and often also follow-up the patient once discharged home to detect infection. This enables the early identification of increased incidences of infection so that measures can be taken to prevent further infections. These measures could include suspension of further surgery; deep cleaning of theatres; change in antibiotic treatments and isolation of infected patients.

 4.4 Summary

Healthcare-associated infection (HCAI)

- All hospitals must have effective programmes for prevention and control of HCAI
- The hospital infection control team design and deliver the HCAI programme, but all staff working in healthcare must take responsibility for preventing HCAI
- Monitoring for trends in surgical site infection is an important indicator of the quality of patient care.

5

Ewen M. Harrison
Michael A. Gillies

Ethics, preoperative considerations, anaesthesia and analgesia

Chapter contents

Ethical and legal principles for surgical patients 60

Preoperative assessment 64

Anaesthesia and the operation 79

Day surgery 83

Ethical and legal principles for surgical patients

Patients trust surgeons absolutely when they submit to a surgical procedure. This is unique in society. Surgeons may cause harm to the patient in the course of their treatment; there is also a potential for exploitation. It is therefore important that the practice of surgery is subject to ethical and legal principles that include the rights of patients and the duties of surgeons within the context of varying societal expectations. Medical ethics is a complex area and there should be sufficient latitude within any framework to accommodate differing views in resolving ethical dilemmas. Table 5.1 describes ethical standards upheld by regulatory bodies such as the General Medical Council and the Surgical Royal Colleges in the United Kingdom. Medical ethics is a practical and rigorous discipline that applies to surgical practice on a daily basis.

Principles in surgical ethics

Surgeons regularly make decisions that require broad understanding of medical ethics. Obtaining proper informed consent is the most common example, but surgeons are often involved in ethical dilemmas in acute situations involving unconscious and critically injured patients, as well as in surgical research and in surgical publication.

Principalism

Principalism is a widely adopted approach to medical ethics and judges all possible actions in a particular ethical dilemma against four principles: autonomy, beneficence, nonmalfeasance and justice. All the principles are linked and do not simply cover four unrelated issues. Protagonists of this approach to bioethics suggest that it provides a practical framework for working through ethical dilemmas, allowing identification of important issues, and is universally applicable, with its four principles widely acceptable irrespective of culture or religious beliefs. The principles can be applied to most surgical clinical scenarios and if each element is given due consideration it is unlikely that the resulting decision will be unethical.

Autonomy

Autonomy is a basic aspect of humanity – a right to determine how we live with fundamental respect for dignity, integrity and authenticity. Central to this is the principle that the doctor should never impose treatment upon an individual, except where necessary to prevent harm to others. Autonomy respects the individual's right to opinions, make choices and act on personal values and beliefs. For example, if a competent Jehovah's Witness declines a life-saving blood transfusion based on strongly held beliefs, this should be upheld even if it seems foolish to those treating them. Autonomy does not, however, give the patient the right to treatment on demand.

Beneficence: doing good

This encompasses the moral obligation surgeons have to their patients, to do them good in treating or attempting to cure their diseases. Historically, the surgeon made the judgement, with little input from the patient as to what was in their best interest. Nowadays, the course of action that will result in the most patient good is agreed. The principle of beneficence dictates that surgeons are well placed to do good by being competent, keeping up to date, performing audits, and undergoing accreditation and revalidation as part of an assurance to the patients and society that they serve.

Nonmalfeasance: avoiding harm

This important principle, *primum non nocere* ('first do no harm') has been enshrined in medical practice since the Hippocratic Oath. Many treatments have inherent risks with real complications where harm can result. As long as the risk is in proportion to the potential benefit of a proposed treatment from the competent patient's perspective, and consent to that treatment has been

Table 5.1 The duties of a doctor registered with the General Medical Council		
Patients must be able to trust doctors with their lives and health. To justify that trust you must show respect for human life and you must:		
Make the care of your patient your first concern		
Protect and promote the health of patients and the public		
Provide a good standard of practice and care	Keep your professional knowledge and skills up to date	
	Recognise and work within the limits of your competence	
	Work with colleagues in the ways that best serve patients' interests	
Treat patients as individuals and respect their dignity	Treat patients politely and considerately	
	Respect patients' right to confidentiality	
Work in partnership with patients	Listen to patients and respond to their concerns and preferences	
	Give patients the information they want or need in a way they can understand	
	Respect patients' right to reach decisions with you about their treatment and care	
	Support patients in caring for themselves to improve and maintain their health	
Be honest and open and act with integrity	Act without delay if you have good reason to believe that you or a colleague may be putting patients at risk	
	Never discriminate unfairly against patients or colleagues	
	Never abuse your patients' trust in you or the public's trust in the profession	
You are personally accountable for your professional practice and must always be prepared to justify your decisions and actions.		

given on the basis of reasonable information, then the principle of nonmalfeasance is not violated.

Justice: promoting fairness

The principles that healthcare should be fair and available to all is topical, particularly as treatments become more sophisticated and expensive. As long as demand outstrips supply and exceeds what society can afford, debate on this subject will continue. The resulting process of rationing requires a system of justice that does not discriminate on the basis of race, sex, age, gender or religion to administer resources. Doctors should aspire to give the best possible care within available resources. The focus for the surgeon is more likely to involve individual patients and how their interests should be prioritised, for example, when managing a waiting list for surgery. Resources may be allocated on clinical grounds such as threat to life or degree of pain. These perceptions of clinical need consider the timeliness of intervention to achieve a favourable outcome (e.g., emergency surgery), or the severity of the condition and its consequences if left untreated (e.g., cancer, abdominal aortic aneurysm).

 5.1 Summary

Four tenets of principalism

1. Autonomy: Respecting the individual's right to self-determination
2. Beneficence: The surgeon's obligation to do good
3. Nonmalfeasance: The surgeon's obligation to avoid harm
4. Justice: Treating all patients equally.

Informed consent

General considerations

Informed consent is central to the practice of surgery, and has to be obtained for surgical procedures, other treatment modalities, investigations, screening tests and prior to patient participation in research. Informed consent is not only ethically correct but also a legal right and should be respected even if the patient's wishes are at variance with the surgeon's opinion. Informed consent can only be obtained from patients with 'capacity'. This should be assumed for all conscious adults unless there is evidence to the contrary. The patient's views must be respected and upheld after an information-sharing process that conveys all the information the patient needs and wants in order to make a decision. The surgeon must maximise the opportunity for patients to consent and facilitate the process wherever possible.

Capacity exists if a patient can:

- Understand and retain the information presented
- Weigh up the implications, including risk and benefit of the options
- Communicate their decision.

Circumstances where the capacity to consent may not exist:

- Children
- Mental illness
- Fluctuating or irreversible loss of cognitive function
- Patients subject to undue coercion.

Other important considerations in obtaining consent relate to who should obtain consent and when, and what information should be shared withheld and in what format. In general terms, the surgeon performing the procedure is responsible for obtaining consent, but this can be delegated provided the person to whom it is delegated:

- Is suitably trained and qualified
- Has sufficient knowledge of the proposed procedure including risks
- Understands the process of consent (in the UK as laid out by the General Medial Council [GMC]).

The information that should be shared with a patient to obtain consent should start from a mutual understanding by both doctor and patient of the medical condition, as well as the patient's views, beliefs and prior knowledge. All treatment options should be detailed, including the option of no treatment alongside the risks, side effects, potential benefits and burdens, and the risk that the treatment will be unsuccessful. All potential serious adverse outcomes, no matter how rare, should be discussed, along with more frequent minor complications. Risks and benefits should, wherever possible, be quantified in percentage terms. These figures should derive from audited local/personal practice and not simply plucked from the literature. It is acceptable for the surgeon to give the patient advice; but in such circumstance, any conflict of interest must be declared. A recent UK legal ruling (Montgomery vs. Lanarkshire) expects that the treating surgeon takes *'reasonable care to ensure that the patient is aware of any material risks involved in any recommended treatment, and of any reasonable alternative or variant treatments.'*

If a patient expresses the wish that they do not want the information required for informed consent and understands the potential consequences, then information can be withheld on the basis of nonmalfeasance, but only when serious psychological harm might ensue and not simply because the patient may be upset or refuse treatment. This is called 'therapeutic privilege'. The provision of procedure-specific patient information sheets can supplement the process of informed consent, but does not negate the doctor's responsibility to ensure the patient understands the procedure.

Consent may be implied or explicit. Implied consent is considered adequate for routine interventions with negligible risks where patient consent is implied by their cooperation (e.g., venepuncture). The majority of interventions require explicit consent; this may be oral or written. It is perhaps surprising that although written consent is obtained for the majority of procedures, it is only a legal requirement for organ donation and fertility treatment in the UK. Nevertheless, the existence of a written, dated form of consent provides evidence that a consultation covering specific issues was likely to have taken place.

Where the surgeon and patient are unable to communicate effectively because of language barriers, the consultation and consent process should not be considered via a family member or friend acting as an informal interpreter. It is best practice to use the services of a professional translator. Written information should be available in a range of languages that may be reasonably encountered; if this is not possible the translator should read it out to the patient who then has an opportunity to ask questions back through the translator. The medical records should clearly document that this process has taken place, but patients may require time to reflect on any written information. The surgeon must also be sensitive to, and respect other social and cultural differences. Other challenging situations may arise where close family want to hide unpleasant diagnoses from a patient with the idea of protecting the patient.

5.2 Summary

Informed consent

- Establish patient's capacity
- Gather information on the patient's views, attitudes and wishes regarding their health
- Provide information on treatment options (including no treatment), and the risks and benefits of each and their likely outcomes
- Respect the patient's decision.

Consent in specific circumstances

Children

Children should be involved in the discussions surrounding their treatment wherever possible. In the UK, patients aged 16 years and over are presumed to be competent to consent with legal frameworks guiding treatment of 16- and 17-year-olds who do not have capacity to consent. In children under the age of 16, their mental ability to understand, retain, weigh up and use information, as well as communicate their decision, is more important than their age in determining their capacity to consent. It should be borne in mind that while capacity may exist for simple procedures, this does not necessarily translate into the ability to weigh up more complex treatments. In the UK, the term 'Gillick Competence' is used to describe whether a child under the age of 16 years possesses sufficient understanding to consent to medical treatment without parental consent. For those that lack capacity, treatment can be provided with the consent of parents or the courts. Where either a competent child or the parents refuse life-saving treatment, or where disagreement exists between parents, legal advice should be sought. Procedures undertaken on cultural or religious grounds, such as circumcision, are usually permissible if it is in the patient's best interests taking psychological, cultural and social benefits into account.

Mental illness

Patients with mental illness may retain the capacity to consent. In emergency or urgent situations, treatment may be provided with their compliance if the patient lacks capacity to consent. Although treatment may be administered compulsorily for the treatment of mental illness, treatment for other medical disorders must not be imposed even where mental illness means that the patient lacks capacity. Legal advice is frequently needed in this setting.

Transient/irreversible cognitive impairment

The emergency situation is relatively straightforward; life-saving treatment and intervention necessary to prevent deterioration may be provided in the patient's best interests. In general, the patient's involvement in treatment decisions should be maximised, and in making a treatment decision the surgeon should take into account their own knowledge of the patient's beliefs, views, and previously expressed preferences and advanced directives, as well as those close to the patient, those with legal authority over the patient, appointed representatives and the views of those the patient wishes to be considered. Decisions should always be taken in the patient's best interest, should maximise the patient's future options and be consensual, involving all relevant parties listed previously. If a consensus cannot be reached, then legal advice should be sought or the case referred to the courts to decide.

Confidentiality

Confidentiality is a central element in the doctor–patient relationship. There are certain exceptions where confidentiality can be breached, e.g., for the protection of other individuals or the greater public, but these situations can be complex and expert advice should be sought. In the context of multidisciplinary team working, only information necessary to enable treatment by a third party should be divulged. When patients are discussed for the purposes of teaching or publication, patient identity must be concealed. Confidentiality is not just an important principle; it may be legally enforceable; for example, by the Data Protection Act.

See Table 5.2 for important sources of information regarding ethics in medicine.

Table 5.2 Sources of further information on ethics
Publications
• Guidelines published by the General Medical Council (also available online) include: ○ Good Medical Practice, 2006 ○ 0–18 years: guidance for all doctors, 2007 ○ Consent: patients and doctors making decisions together, 2008 ○ Confidentiality, 2009 ○ Treatment and care towards the end of life, 2010 ○ Good practice in research and consent to research, 2010 • Jonathan Herring. Medical Law and Ethics. 2nd edition, Oxford University Press, 2008 • Margaret Brazier and Emma Cave. Medicine, Patients and the Law. Penguin, 2007
Websites
• www.gmc-uk.org/guidance • Human Tissue Act: https://www.hta.gov.uk/guidance-professionals/codes-practice • Research governance: http://www.hra.nhs.uk/ • Declaration of Helsinki: www.cirp.org/library/ethics/helsinki/ • Declaration of Geneva: www.cirp.org/library/ethics/geneva/

or health of the mother is endangered. Although surgeons are only infrequently involved in decisions around abortion, understanding the law is important, especially in the context of trauma or acute abdominal pain in the early stages of pregnancy.

Negligence

In order for a surgeon to be found negligent three prerequisites must be fulfilled. First, it must be demonstrated that the surgeon owed the patient a duty of care (this is usually assumed). Second, it must be shown that the doctor breached that duty of care; and, third that, on the balance of probabilities (more likely than not), the breach of duty resulted directly in harm (causation). Medical negligence can relate to diagnosis, treatment and the failure to warn a patient of risks that would have resulted in the patient refusing an intervention. The standard against which a doctor's performance is measured was established in UK case law in 1957 (the Bolam case); a doctor is not guilty of negligence if he has acted 'in accordance with a practice accepted as proper by a responsible body of medical men skilled in that particular area.' In practice, Bolam defends a doctor's practice if a body of medical opinion can be found to support that doctor's actions. It facilitates the defence of minimal acceptable practice rather than ideal practice. A subsequent House of Lords ruling went further, stating that, 'the court has to be satisfied that the exponents of the body of opinion relied on can demonstrate that such an opinion has a logical basis … that the experts have directed their minds to the question of risks and benefits and have reached a defensible conclusion.' This updated ruling (Bolitho) provides the legal basis for most complaints that result in an allegation of negligence in the UK.

Human Tissue Act

This was in response to inadequacies in preceding legislation brought to light by inquiries into the storage of human tissue in the Alder Hey and Bristol inquiries. The Human Tissue Act (2004) in the UK (and separate legislation in Scotland) places consent as the fundamental principle in the storage of human tissue, whether from living patients or the deceased, and issues legislation and guidance regarding the removal, storage and use of human tissue.

Completion of a death certificate

Following the death of a patient, it is a legal requirement that a death certificate be completed before the body is released for cremation or burial. Death certification must be completed by the doctor who has attended the deceased during their last illness and includes a record of the patient's name and age, as well as the date, time and place of death. The cause of death has to be recorded, as well as any contributing conditions that have led directly to the cause of death and significant conditions that contributed to the death but are unrelated to the disease causing it. In certain situations, a death has to be referred as a legal requirement to the coroner's office in England, Wales and Northern Ireland or to the Procurator Fiscal in Scotland for consideration of a postmortem examination to establish the cause of death. These include: recent surgery; where death may be due to abortion; accidental death; death in suspicious/violent/unnatural circumstances; death due to suspected poisoning, self-neglect, negligence or suicide; death occurring in prison or police custody; where the death may be due to industrial disease or related to the deceased person's employment; where the cause of death is unknown and where the death is unexpected.

Specific topics

Euthanasia and 'end-of-life' issues

Euthanasia is described as a deliberate intervention undertaken with the express intention of ending life, to relieve intractable suffering due to an incurable, progressive disease. It is usually requested by the patient and is illegal in the UK, as is assisted suicide.

Other 'end-of-life' issues such as withholding and withdrawing futile treatments or any treatments at the request of a competent patient are separate issues and should not be confused with euthanasia. Where treatment with 'double effect' is used, such as opiate analgesia (relieves pain and anxiety while shortening life), this is acceptable because the primary intention was to relieve pain, distinguishing it from euthanasia.

Abortion

In the UK, legal abortion is permitted under the terms of the Abortion Act 1967; amended by the Human Fertilisation and Embryology Act 1990 that reduced the gestational age at which abortion could be carried out from 28 to 24 weeks. The conditions for performing abortion up to 24 weeks of gestation are that continuing the pregnancy would cause greater risk of injury to the mental or physical health of the woman, or any existing children of her family. Abortion can be carried out after the 24th week of pregnancy if it is necessary to save the mother's life, or if there is grave risk of permanent injury to the mental or physical health of the woman by continuing the pregnancy, or if there is substantial risk that the child would have severe physical or mental problems that would render them seriously handicapped. In all cases, two registered medical practitioners have to agree the criteria and appropriateness of the abortion. While a doctor has no obligation in UK law to be involved in abortion if he/she has a conscientious objection, they must refer the patient to a doctor who is. This conscientious objection does not extend to emergency situations where the life

Where cremation is requested, a separate cremation form has to be completed by a doctor who attended the deceased during their last illness and a second doctor who is of at least 5 years full registration. Care must be taken to identify the presence of pacemakers and other potential explosive devices in the body. The cremation of foetal remains of less than 24 weeks' gestation does not require a cremation certificate.

Postmortem examination

A postmortem is carried out in two situations. There may be a legal requirement to establish the cause of death prior to a death certificate being issued as detailed earlier. This mandatory postmortem does not require the consent of the deceased person's family when order by the coroner or fiscal in the UK. Alternatively, the deceased's next of kin, relatives or doctors may request a postmortem to provide information about the deceased's illness or cause of death. In this instance, consent from the next of kin should be obtained to proceed with postmortem examination and should include details of the possible outcomes of postmortem. Specific legal recommendations should be followed for the handling and storage of tissues and organs removed at postmortem.

Research governance

Research governance serves to 'improve research quality and safeguard the public by enhancing ethical and scientific quality, promoting good practice, reducing adverse incidents and ensuring lessons are learned, and preventing poor performance and misconduct.' All of this is achieved through a broad range of regulations, principles and standards of good practice, originally enshrined in the Declaration of Helsinki in 1964. Research governance applies to everyone involved in medical research whether as chief investigator, care professional, researcher, the employing institution or sponsor. This governance safeguards participants, protects researchers and investigators, minimises risk, and enables the monitoring of practice and performance. Surgical journals place great emphasis on research governance. Work that does not demonstrate adherence to satisfactory ethical and quality standards is likely to be rejected.

Ethics committees

Research on human subjects is necessary to advance medical knowledge and treatment. Ensuring that it is carried out in a safe and ethical way is the remit of the ethics committee. All clinical trials involving human subjects or tissue must receive ethical approval prior to commencing recruitment. Ethical approval is obtained in the UK through the Integrated Research Application System (www.myresearchproject.org.uk) and may be through local or multicentre research ethics committees (REC). The composition of ethics committees is important and should reflect societal diversity in terms of age, gender, ethnicity and disability, and embody a broad range of experience and expertise so that the scientific, clinical and methodological aspects of a research proposal can be reconciled with the welfare of the research participants.

Ethics committees take into consideration a whole range of aspects of a research proposal before giving approval. Their primary consideration is to safeguard the rights, safety and wellbeing of research subjects. They examine the recruitment process, including informed consent, the quality of information given to subjects, payments to subjects, the risks of the research protocol including safety measures and information, compensation procedures and indemnity. The likelihood and capability of the trial design to answer the research questions is considered, as well as adequacy of resources, plans for data processing, storage and protection.

Preoperative assessment

Careful preoperative assessment is fundamental to achieving good surgical outcomes. This applies to emergency and elective situations, the only difference being the extent to which time available for full assessment and investigation must be compromised when an emergency condition requires urgent intervention.

Assessment of operative fitness and perioperative risk

Elective preoperative assessment takes place in several stages beginning at the point of referral. A good referral letter should include details not only of the presenting complaint but also of the patient's general health, comorbidities and current medication. The first contact with the surgical team is usually in the outpatient clinic and this consultation may lead to a decision to offer surgery. In reaching such a decision, the surgeon should consider not only the physical fitness of the patient to withstand the proposed surgery, but also the likely impact on their social and emotional well-being. When making the decision to operate, the risks and potential benefits of surgery should be weighed against those of alternative or no treatment. The purpose of preoperative assessment is to prepare the patient for surgery, identify comorbid conditions, estimate perioperative risk and optimise the patient's physical condition. Preoperative assessment may take place in a dedicated assessment clinic a few weeks before surgery and culminates in the admission on the morning of surgery.

The first priority is to establish the severity and extent of the condition requiring surgery by employing appropriate imaging and other investigations. For example, it is important to know that both recurrent laryngeal nerves are functional prior to thyroid surgery as damage is a recognised complication; on the other hand, malignant conditions require appropriate staging to establish the disease extent. The second objective is to obtain a general medical history and carry out an examination to identify comorbid conditions through careful clinical assessment and, through optimisation, minimise perioperative risk. Fig. 5.1 details the areas of potential perioperative risk and Fig. 5.2 shows a logical sequence of preoperative assessment. Details of previous operations and anaesthetics should be sought, as well as drug, alcohol and smoking history, specific allergies and concerns. Investigations to assess the surgical condition, comorbid conditions and general health should be arranged as soon as possible to minimise surgical delay. Thorough and timely preoperative assessment is essential to avoid the expense and delay of cancelled or delayed surgery. Good quality assessment and appropriate optimisation prior to admission mean that many patients can be admitted on the day of surgery. Preoperative assessment of patients with minimal comorbidities undergoing low-risk surgery is often done by a preassessment nurse and may be performed by telephone or even be self-administered using an online questionnaire. However, a review by a specialist anaesthetist at a preassessment clinic should be requested prior to admission where there is increased risk (e.g., advancing age or comorbidity), fitness for

Direct surgical risk
Technical problems with surgery and anaesthesia
Surgical complications, e.g. wound infection
Can be measured from audit of practice or from
published data

Physiological stress of surgery
Mostly involves the cardiovascular and respiratory systems
Often difficult to predict. Depends on the nature of the
surgery, the technical success of surgery, and the
physiological fitness or reserve of the patient

Psychological
Anxiety in relation to proposed surgery and anaesthesia
Sources of anxiety may be unexpected; for example,
a patient may have little concern about the surgery itself
but be terrified of postoperative nausea or of being
'aware' during the operation

Fig. 5.1 Areas of perioperative risk.

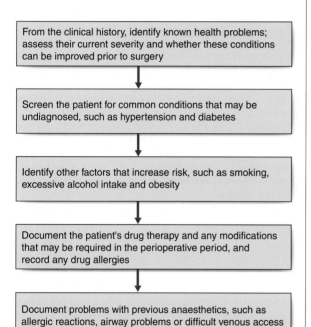

From the clinical history, identify known health problems;
assess their current severity and whether these conditions
can be improved prior to surgery

Screen the patient for common conditions that may be
undiagnosed, such as hypertension and diabetes

Identify other factors that increase risk, such as smoking,
excessive alcohol intake and obesity

Document the patient's drug therapy and any modifications
that may be required in the perioperative period, and
record any drug allergies

Document problems with previous anaesthetics, such as
allergic reactions, airway problems or difficult venous access

Fig. 5.2 A logical approach to assessing perioperative and
anaesthetic risk.

surgery is in doubt, where there are specific anaesthetic issues
requiring assessment or if the surgery itself is particularly high risk.

On the morning of surgery, both the surgeon and anaesthetist
should reassess the patient and identify outstanding issues and
any changes in their condition. All investigation results should
be available, as well as necessary blood products and special
equipment. Details of the anaesthetic should be discussed, and
postoperative analgesic strategies, taking into account patient
preferences wherever possible.

In the emergency situation this process is condensed. Judging
the timing of surgery is crucial. The surgeon must determine which
interventions will optimise the patient's condition while avoiding
deterioration due to unnecessary delay.

Perioperative medicine

Perioperative medicine involves expertise from a multidisciplinary
team including doctors from other specialties outwith anaesthesia
and surgery, including cardiology, respiratory medicine, acute
medicine or care of the elderly. These teams can improve the perioperative management of high-risk patients, reducing the likelihood
of complications and optimising the management of complex disease and its interaction with major surgery. Surgeons and anaesthetists may not have detailed knowledge of the management of
complex disease and this approach ensures patients have access
to the best possible care perioperatively. Perioperative medicine
encompasses not only specialist preoperative investigation and
optimisation, but also intraoperative management and postoperative care, including enhanced recovery programmes.

Oxygen delivery in minimising operative risk

Postoperative morbidity and mortality may in part be related to
inadequate oxygen delivery to the tissues, resulting in hypoxia.
Oxygen delivery (Do_2) is dependent on cardiac output (CO) and
the oxygen content of arterial blood (Cao_2).

$$Do_2 = CO \times Cao_2$$

The arterial oxygen content in turn depends on the delivery of oxygen to the alveoli, its efficient transfer from alveoli into blood, adequately functioning haemoglobin, the arterial partial pressure of
oxygen and arterial haemoglobin oxygen saturation. In an
average resting adult an oxygen requirement of approximately
250 mL/min is exceeded by delivery of around 1000 mL/min,
resulting in a considerable reserve. When oxygen demand increases cardiac output may rise and tissue oxygen extraction
may increase by 50–60% to compensate. If this does not meet
tissue oxygen demand, hypoxia with anaerobic metabolism
ensues. If uncorrected, this can cause local and remote organ
damage, dysfunction, multiple organ failure and ultimately death.
The duration of oxygen debt correlates with the presence and
magnitude of postoperative complications and mortality. Patients
with poor cardiovascular and respiratory reserve or anaemia are
less able to increase oxygen delivery and are at higher perioperative risk. Optimising their condition and oxygen delivery will
minimise that risk.

Goal-directed haemodynamic therapy (HT) uses cardiac output
monitoring to guide intravenous fluid administration, inotropic
therapy, blood transfusion and supplemental oxygen. Modern
noninvasive techniques, such as oesophageal Doppler, pulse
contour analysis or bioimpedance, are now used; however, older
techniques such as pulmonary artery catheters are still used in
certain settings such as cardiac surgery or liver transplantation.
Current evidence does not support routine use of goal-directed
therapy in major surgery, although some studies have reported
a reduction in complications and length of hospital admission.

Systematic preoperative assessment

Cardiovascular system

The severity of cardiovascular disease should be assessed
and signs of undiagnosed or inadequately treated disease sought.
A full history should include exercise tolerance, existing

cardiovascular disease or risk factors (e.g., hypertension) and symptoms associated with cardiovascular disease (e.g., chest pain, intermittent claudication, or syncope). A history of angina and previous myocardial infarction may indicate significant coronary artery disease. Patients may have undergone percutaneous coronary interventions (PCI; e.g., angioplasty, stenting) or even bypass grafting. Shortness of breath on exercise (exertional dyspnoea), on lying flat (orthopnoea) and on waking from sleep (paroxysmal nocturnal dyspnoea) may indicate left ventricular failure, whilst significant dependent oedema could signify right-sided heart failure. Drug history may alert to the presence and severity of cardiovascular disease. Blackouts and dizzy spells may be a sign of arrhythmias, valvular heart or cerebrovascular disease. Clinical examination should detect arrhythmias, heart murmurs, hypertension and signs of cardiac failure. Antiplatelet agents and anticoagulants are widely prescribed in the general population, and these or other cardiovascular medications may need to be stopped or modified prior to surgery (see later).

Respiratory system

A history of new or increased cough, sputum production, and shortness of breath or wheeze may indicate unsuspected respiratory disease or an exacerbation of preexisting pulmonary disease. In patients with asthma, chronic obstructive pulmonary disease (COPD) or fibrotic lung disease, purulent sputum may indicate an infective exacerbation. In asthmatics, previous intensive therapy unit (ITU) and hospital admissions, as well as steroid dependency indicate severe disease. Functional respiratory reserve is best assessed by exercise tolerance; for example, by how far a patient can walk on the flat, up an incline, or how many stairs they can climb before needing to rest because of shortness of breath. Significant dyspnoea should be investigated with pulmonary function tests.

Patients with acute respiratory illness should have surgery postponed where possible due to the increased risk of bronchospasm and susceptibility of the respiratory epithelium to postoperative bacterial pneumonia. General anaesthesia exacerbates the problems by depressing ciliary activity and reducing the clearance of secretions and pathogens.

Smoking

All patients should be offered support to quit smoking, particularly once the decision to operate has been made. The benefits of preoperative smoking cessation should be explained to the patient (Table 5.3). Some of the benefits occur within hours (reduced circulating nicotine and carboxyhaemoglobin) while others take much longer. Many patients are unable or unwilling to stop smoking, and referral to specialist services that support patients to stop smoking may help.

Table 5.3 Benefits of preoperative smoking cessation

- Reduced airway hyper-reactivity bronchospasm
- Reduced sputum production reduces the risk of atelectasis
- Improved ciliary function results in increased sputum clearance, helping to protect against infection
- Reduced carboxyhaemoglobin increases oxygen-carrying capacity of blood
- Reduced nicotine-related systemic and coronary vasoconstriction

Preoperative exercise

Surgically enhanced recovery programmes aim to reduce the length of hospital stay following surgery and expedite return to normal activity. Preoperative exercise may reduce perioperative morbidity by improving cardiorespiratory performance. Research in this area has been conflicting, but some early studies, particularly in the field of orthopaedic surgery, have shown improved preoperative functional status and muscle strength resulting in reduced inpatient rehabilitation requirements.

Alcohol

A history of significant alcohol consumption can impact surgical planning. With chronic alcohol excess, liver enzymes are induced, increasing hepatic drug metabolism. Consequently increased doses of hepatically metabolised drugs, including anaesthetic agents, are required to achieve therapeutic effect. Conversely in acute alcohol intoxication reduced anaesthetic doses are required. Aspiration pneumonia should be anticipated and preventive measures taken. The risk of alcohol withdrawal should also be anticipated and in habitual alcohol consumers prevented with use of detoxification protocols. In patients with a significant alcohol history, the risk of alcohol-related liver and cardiac disease and coagulopathy should be anticipated.

Nutritional status

All patients should have their height and weight measured and body mass index (BMI) calculated. A history of weight loss should be sought and quantified as a percentage of the patient's starting weight. It is important to look for signs of malnutrition such as low BMI, bodyweight 20% weight loss, hypoproteinaemia and hypoalbuminaemia as they have all been associated with increased rates of postoperative complications including delayed anastomotic and wound healing. Preexisting hypoalbuminaemia compounded by perioperative fasting and haemodilution results in oedema, which may delay recovery. Malnutrition should be treated preoperatively if time permits (see Chapter 3).

Obesity

Obese patients are at increased risk from surgery and anaesthesia, and special equipment may be required. Table 5.4 details some of the technical difficulties, perioperative risks and comorbid conditions associated with obesity. If the risks of intervention are outweighed by its potential benefits, surgery may be postponed. In practice, the majority of patients cannot lose weight without support and referral for weight-loss programmes, including supervised exercise, may be beneficial. Weight-loss (bariatric) surgery may result in significant weight loss, reduction in cardiovascular risk and remission of type II diabetes.

Drug therapy

A comprehensive drug history should be recorded prior to admission for surgery. In general, patients should take their routine medication right up to the time of surgery. The perioperative management of diabetes mellitus and patients on anticoagulation is considered separately.

Long-term steroid therapy

Long-term steroid therapy may result in hypoadrenalism and the inability to mount an effective response to surgical stress. Patients taking significant doses of steroids must receive steroid

Table 5.4 **Significance of obesity in the perioperative period**
Cardiovascular system
• Hypertension and ischaemic heart disease more common
• Accurate blood pressure measurement difficult
• Increased risk of right-sided heart failure associated with obstructive sleep apnoea
Respiratory system
• Airway management more difficult
• Reduced lung volumes
• Increased incidence of obstructive sleep apnoea
• Increased risk of perioperative hypoxia
• Increased risk of atelectasis, pneumonia and pulmonary embolism
Surgical
• Surgical access difficult
• Increased wound infection and dehiscence
Other
• Venous access difficult
• Increased incidence of diabetes mellitus
• Increased risk of hiatus hernia and aspiration pneumonia

supplementation throughout the perioperative period. An increased dose is usually necessary to counter surgical stress and the exact amount depends on the procedure. Higher doses (i.e., >100 mg hydrocortisone/day) may be needed if postoperative complications including infection supervene. Signs of hypoadrenalism include hypotension/shock, hyponatraemia and hyperkalaemia, and should be sought in any steroid-dependent patient who is unwell in the postoperative period. Urgent steroid treatment may be needed to avoid an Addisonian crisis.

Antiplatelet therapy and anticoagulants

Antiplatelet therapy with aspirin and clopidogrel is common, especially in patients with cardiovascular disease. There are risks of thromboembolic events, particularly myocardial infarction if antiplatelet therapy is withdrawn. If patients have coronary artery or peripheral stents, then these risks may be high. Antiplatelet agents should not be withdrawn prior to stent endothelialisation, which takes up to 6 months. In all cases these risks should be weighed against the risk of surgical haemorrhage if treatment is continued or epidural haematoma if neuraxial blockade is planned. If feasible, surgery should be postponed and antiplatelet agents withdrawn only after consultation with a cardiologist or vascular surgeon.

Anticoagulation with warfarin is commonly used for prevention of embolic events in atrial fibrillation and for treatment of deep-vein thrombosis and pulmonary embolism. The risk of a thromboembolic event with anticoagulant suspension has to be balanced against the risk of bleeding in an anticoagulated patient undergoing surgery. The use of bridging anticoagulation should be considered and is discussed in more detail in the section on abnormal coagulation (see later).

Oral contraceptives and hormone-replacement therapy

Depending on the type of surgery being planned and the patient's other risk factors for venous thromboembolism (VTE), it may be advisable to discontinue oestrogen-containing drugs (combined oral contraceptive pills [OCP] and hormone-replacement therapy [HRT]) 4–6 weeks beforehand. However, opinions on this vary and

the decision taken has to balance the possible increased risk of thromboembolism against those of unwanted pregnancy.

Psychiatric drugs

Concurrent use of serotonin-selective reuptake inhibitors (SSRIs), lithium, monoamine oxidase inhibitors (MAOIs) and tricyclic antidepressants have implications for general anaesthesia. There is a risk of serotonin syndrome if SSRIs are given concurrently with tramadol. There is also an increased risk of bleeding if coadministered with nonsteroidal antiinflammatory drugs (NSAIDs) or warfarin. Lithium has a narrow therapeutic index and is eliminated by the kidneys, so may accumulate in renal dysfunction and also interact with anaesthetic agents and muscle relaxants. Side effects include arrhythmias and gastrointestinal disturbance. It is not essential that tricyclic antidepressants be stopped preoperatively, but the anaesthetist should be alerted as they may cause hypotension and arrhythmia. MAOIs interact with opiates and vasopressor agents with the potential of neurological and cardiovascular complications. Ideally, they should be stopped 2–3 weeks prior to surgery, but in an emergency opiates and pressor agents should be avoided.

Allergies

Adverse and idiosyncratic reactions to drugs and other substances should be recorded and steps taken to avoid the allergen, as a second exposure may result in a life-threatening hypersensitivity reaction. Common examples include antibiotics, iodine, adhesive dressings and latex. Full-blown anaphylactic reactions to latex are rare but some degree of latex sensitivity is common. Special care has to be taken to clear the patient environment of latex for those with severe allergic responses as it is common in gloves and other surgical and anaesthetic equipment.

Pregnancy

Elective surgery should be avoided in the first and third trimesters of pregnancy. The risk of miscarriage and potential teratogenicity is high in the first trimester and this is usually encountered in relation to surgery for an acute condition in the abdomen. Third-trimester surgery is associated with significant maternal risks and premature labour (Table 5.5). If surgery is necessary, it is best undertaken in the second trimester in conjunction with the obstetric team. Surgery in pregnancy is usually an emergency or related to the pregnancy. Early involvement of the anaesthetist is essential as much of the excess risk relates to the general anaesthesia.

Table 5.5 **Perioperative risks associated with surgery in pregnant patients**
• Spontaneous abortion or premature labour
• Hypotension on supine position (inferior vena caval compression in second and third trimesters)
• Gastrooesophageal reflux (increased risk of aspiration)
• Hypoxia (due to high metabolic rate and reduced lung functional residual capacity)
• Teratogenic effects of drugs (particularly in first trimester)
• Preeclampsia/eclampsia
• Amniotic fluid embolism

Previous operations and anaesthetics

Details of previous anaesthetics including complications, side effects and reactions should be sought. Previous anaesthetic charts are a useful source of information and should alert the anaesthetist to potential anaesthetic challenges including a difficult endotracheal intubation.

The most common complaint after general anaesthesia is postoperative nausea and vomiting (PONV). This causes significant patient distress, and delays recovery and discharge following day case procedures. Risk factors include opioid administration, female gender, nonsmoker status and a prior history of PONV. Steps to minimise PONV include the use of short-acting anaesthetic agents and potent centrally acting antiemetic drugs (e.g., ondansetron), as well as opiate avoidance.

Previous major anaesthetic complications or a family history of anaesthetic problems should alert to the possibility of an inherited abnormality, such as pseudocholinesterase deficiency and malignant hyperpyrexia.

Pseudocholinesterase deficiency, also known as suxamethonium apnoea, is characterised by prolonged neuromuscular blockade following administration of suxamethonium chloride, often necessitating a prolonged period of ventilation. Diagnosis is confirmed by demonstrating decreased plasma cholinesterase activity.

Malignant hyperpyrexia is an inherited autosomal-dominant condition characterised by life-threatening hyperpyrexia as a result of abnormal muscle metabolism after exposure to volatile anaesthetic agents or suxamethonium. Diagnosis is complex and investigations should be carried out in specialist centres.

 5.3 Summary

Key factors in the anaesthetic history

- Adverse drug reactions
- Difficult intubation (more common in patients with restricted neck movement, limited mouth opening, a short neck or a receding chin)
- Damaged/loose teeth, crowns, poor dentition
- Previous postoperative nausea or vomiting
- Previous postoperative pain problems
- Needle or mask phobia
- Family history of adverse reactions to anaesthetics

Preoperative investigations

Preoperative investigations commonly include haematological, biochemical, radiological, cardiovascular and respiratory tests. Most surgical units will have local protocols guiding the use of preoperative investigations.

Haematology

Full blood count

The oxygen-carrying capacity of blood (haemoglobin concentration) is of paramount importance, but the platelet and white cell count are also important considerations in terms of haemostatic capacity and where sepsis is suspected. Full blood count is required in any patient undergoing surgery with the potential for significant blood loss, as should those with signs or symptoms of anaemia, patients with significant cardiorespiratory disease, and those with overt or suspected blood loss (e.g., gastrointestinal tract symptoms). Patients who are anaemic by World Health Organization (WHO) definition (men 13 g/dL, women <12 g/dL)

prior to elective surgery should be investigated and treated appropriately.

 5.4 Summary

Preoperative investigation

Preoperative investigations should be tailored appropriately to avoid unnecessary tests and comprise of both those assessing the patient's fitness for surgery and those specific to the condition requiring surgical intervention.

Haematological: Full blood count, coagulation screen, cross-match group and save

Biochemistry: Urea and electrolytes, liver function tests

Microbiology: Sputum, methicillin-resistant *Staphylococcus aureus* screen, virology (patients at high risk of blood-borne viruses, e.g., HIV)

Radiological: Plain x-ray, ultrasound scan, computed tomography, magnetic resonance imaging, contrast and radionucleotide studies

Respiratory: Pulmonary function tests, arterial blood gases

Cardiovascular: Electrocardiogram, echocardiogram, exercise testing, thallium scan, cardiopulmonary exercise testing.

Wherever possible, anaemia should be corrected preoperatively to optimise oxygen delivery to the tissues. A perioperative transfusion threshold of 7 g/dL is appropriate but patients with coexisting cardiac disease may be at increased risk of ischaemic events and a higher threshold (9 g/dL) may be preferred.

The threshold for transfusion should be lower (because lower haemoglobin concentrations are tolerated) in patients with chronic anaemia (such as renal failure patients) where compensatory mechanisms such as increased red blood cell 2,3-diphosphoglycerol and reduced blood viscosity increase oxygen delivery (EBM 5.1).

EBM **5.1 Red cell transfusion trigger**

'A systematic review with meta-analyses of 31 randomised clinical trials (9813 patients) comparing liberal transfusion strategies (typically haemoglobin <9 g/dL) with restrictive transfusion strategies (haemoglobin of <7 g/dL) showed no difference in mortality, overall morbidity, or myocardial infarction rate. Restrictive transfusion strategies are safe in most clinical settings. Liberal transfusion strategies have not been shown to convey any benefit to patients.'

Holst Lars B, et al. BMJ 2015;350:h1354

An abnormally elevated white cell count should be investigated preoperatively. Thrombocythaemia increases the risk of thromboembolism and prophylactic measures should be taken. Thrombocytopenia may need to be corrected to reduce the risk of bleeding. Most blood transfusion services recommend transfusing to a platelet count of 50×10^9/L for lumbar puncture, epidural anaesthesia, endoscopy with biopsies and surgery in noncritical sites, and to 100×10^9/L for more major surgery including critical sites such as neurosurgery or ophthalmic surgery. Advice from a haematologist may be helpful.

Coagulation screen

The indications for coagulation studies (Table 5.6) include suspected abnormal clotting, anticoagulation treatment and consideration of epidural anaesthesia. When disseminated intravascular coagulation (DIC) is suspected, fibrinogen, fibrinogen degradation products (FDP) and D-dimers should be measured.

Table 5.6 Indications for preoperative coagulation studies
Patient factors
• Liver disease, including jaundice and excess alcohol consumption
• Haematological disease affecting coagulation
• Anticoagulant therapy
• Shock, risk of disseminated intravascular coagulation, e.g., sepsis
• Suspected coagulopathy: excessive bleeding or bruising
• Suspected prothrombotic disorder: history of thromboembolic events
Surgical factors
• Major hepatobiliary surgery
• Surgery involving anticoagulation: cardiopulmonary bypass, major vascular surgery
• High risk of major blood loss
• Consideration of epidural anaesthesia

Cross-matching

This test is performed prior to the administration of a blood transfusion to determine if the donor's blood is compatible with that of the intended recipient. In the past, a number of units of blood were physically cross-matched prior to a major surgical procedure to ensure blood was available in the event of significant bleeding. Hospitals have local policies governing the requirement for performing a group-and-save or full cross-match of blood for a given procedure. Electronic cross-matching uses a computer analysis on the donor and recipient blood to determine compatibility, removing the need for a full physical cross-match. Electronic cross-matching is only suitable if the intended recipient does not exhibit unusual antibodies. For rare blood groups and patients with known antibodies, it is important to allow adequate time for full cross-matching as blood may not be available locally. Blood transfusion and blood products are discussed in more detail in Chapter 2.

Biochemistry

Urea and electrolytes

Analysis of serum urea and electrolytes (U&E) is not necessary in young patients presenting for minor surgery. Routine blood chemistry analysis should be performed on elderly patients, those presenting for major surgery, those with renal dysfunction, cardiovascular disease, or fluid balance problems, and patients on diuretic therapy or any drug therapy that may affect electrolyte balance or renal function. Potassium homeostasis is of particular concern as hypo- and hyperkalaemia can cause arrhythmias. Abnormalities in electrolyte concentrations and renal function should be corrected preoperatively. A detailed discussion of fluid and electrolyte disorders can be found in Chapter 1.

Liver function tests

All patients with known liver disease, significant alcohol consumption or signs of liver disease should have liver function tests including coagulation measured.

Cardiac investigations

Electrocardiography (ECG) is of limited value in predicting the risk of ischaemic events and generally should only be performed in the elderly (over 65 years) to detect occult rhythm disorders or signs of previous cardiac events. In younger patients, ECG should be restricted to those with signs of, or known, cardiovascular disease and those with risk factors for ischaemic heart disease. Chest x-ray should only be performed in the context of cardiovascular assessment where congestive cardiac failure is suspected. Echocardiography is used to assess cardiac function (left ventricular ejection fraction) and may be indicated prior to major surgery and with suspected valvular disease and heart failure. A 24-hour ECG is useful in patients with a history suggestive of paroxysmal arrhythmias or heart block (usually syncopal attacks). Tests of cardiovascular physiological reserve include exercise ECG, thallium scan, stress echocardiography and cardiopulmonary exercise tests (CPEX). The involvement of a cardiologist is advisable if anything more than basic cardiac evaluation is required. The significance of common arrhythmias is listed in Table 5.7.

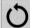

5.5 Summary

History, symptoms and signs associated with elevated perioperative cardiovascular risk
• Myocardial infarction within the past 6 months
• Poor left ventricular function
• Poorly controlled cardiac failure
• Resting diastolic blood pressure >110 mmHg
• Poorly controlled/untreated arrhythmia
• Age >75 years
• Significant aortic stenosis.

Table 5.7 Significance of common arrhythmias in the perioperative period	
Arrhythmia	**Significance**
Uncontrolled atrial fibrillation	May compromise cardiac function Underlying cardiac disease should be sought Exclude metabolic causes, e.g., electrolyte abnormality, thyrotoxicosis Cardioversion or ventricular rate control prior to surgery
Controlled atrial fibrillation	Rarely causes severe perioperative problems unless associated with other significant heart disease Patient may be on anticoagulants; if not, consider thromboprophylaxis
Ventricular extrasystoles	Usually of little significance May indicate ischaemia in patients with ischaemic heart disease
First-degree heart block, asymptomatic bi- or trifascicular block, or asymptomatic second-degree heart block	Little significance Previously considered an indication for temporary pacemaker insertion Now usually managed by careful monitoring in the perioperative period
Third-degree heart block	Requires pacemaker insertion prior to anaesthesia

Respiratory investigations

Preoperative chest x-ray is a useful baseline in patients with known or suspected pulmonary disease, and may demonstrate consolidation, atelectasis and pleural effusions. Routine chest x-ray is not indicated, having poor sensitivity to detect new respiratory disease. Patients with purulent sputum and suspected of having a chest infection should have sputum culture and antibiotic sensitivity performed.

Pulmonary function tests are useful to gauge severity and reversibility of the obstructive component of respiratory disease, and may help guide therapy to optimise function. Pulmonary function tests are indicated in preexisting significant pulmonary disease, patients with significant respiratory symptoms and in patients undergoing thoracic surgery. Table 5.8 lists the commonly performed pulmonary function tests. Although commonly used, the evidence that preoperative pulmonary function tests are predictive of postoperative complications is not convincing. Indications for preoperative arterial blood gas analysis are given in Table 5.9.

Cardiopulmonary exercise testing

In recent years the formal assessment of functional capacity has been used increasingly to stratify perioperative risk. Assessment of functional status has been part of routine preoperative history taking for many years and self-reported poor exercise tolerance has been shown to correlate with increased perioperative risk. Many hospitals now offer cardiopulmonary exercise testing (CPEX or CPET) as part of their assessment for major or high-risk surgery. It provides a safe assessment of cardiac, pulmonary and metabolic function, the patient's ability to respond to the stress of major surgery, and allows stratification of risk according to cardiopulmonary reserve. Physiological variables, usually ECG and respiratory function, are monitored during incremental exercise, e.g., on a treadmill or an exercise bike. The patient wears a nose clip and exhaled gases are collected and analysed to allow calculation of oxygen consumption and carbon dioxide production. The anaerobic threshold marks the threshold at which anaerobic metabolism occurs due to inadequate oxygen delivery. Patients with a low anaerobic threshold may be at risk of postoperative complications and so may be electively admitted to high-dependency or intensive care units postoperatively.

Table 5.9 Indications for blood gas analysis in the preoperative period

Surgical presentation	Useful features
Elective surgery	
Chronic respiratory disease: Moderate-to-severe COPD Fibrotic lung disease Bronchiectasis and cystic fibrosis Severe chest wall deformity, e.g., ankylosing spondylitis Lung malignancy	Degree of hypoxaemia (respiratory failure) Distinguish type I (characterised by normocapnia) from type II (characterised by hypercapnia) respiratory failure Detect degree of compensation of hypercapnia (uncompensated, acute hypercapnia results in respiratory acidosis)
Emergency surgery	
As above Acute respiratory disease: pneumonia, pleural effusion, ARDS, pneumo- or haemothorax, suspected pulmonary embolism Dyspnoea, decreased SaO_2 Shock	As above Measure lactate as part of 'sepsis six' Document acid–base disturbance including the presence and degree of metabolic acidosis indicating inadequate tissue perfusion and to guide resuscitation

ARDS, Acute respiratory distress syndrome; COPD, chronic obstructive pulmonary disease.

Table 5.8 Respiratory function tests commonly carried out preoperatively

Respiratory function test	Significance
FEV1	**Forced expire volume.** Volume of air forcibly expelled in one second
FVC	**Forced vital capacity.** Volume of air forcibly expelled from full inspiration to maximal expiration
FEV1/FVC ratio	**Restrictive** lung disease (fibrosing alveolitis or scoliosis): the FEV1 and FVC are reduced proportionately with an unchanged FEV1/FVC ratio **Obstructive** pulmonary disease (asthma and COPD): the FEV1 is reduced by a greater extent than the FVC, resulting in a reduced FEV1/FVC ratio. A ratio of <70% indicates obstructive pulmonary disease and bronchodilator therapy is indicated
PEFR	**Peak expiratory flow rate.** Maximum speed of expiration. PEFR <70% of expected indicates poorly controlled obstructive lung disease
Gas transfer factor	An estimate of the lungs' ability to transfer gases. Usually performed by inhaling a gas mixture containing a small amount of carbon monoxide Reduced in conditions that reduce the surface area available for gas transfer (emphysema), conditions that thicken the alveolar membrane (fibrosis), interstitial lung disease, asbestosis and anaemia Increased in polycythaemia (some laboratories adjust for haemoglobin concentration)

Patients where there is increased risk of transmission of blood borne viruses or other infection

Blood-borne viruses (hepatitis B, C and HIV) all pose risk and precautions should be taken to minimise the risk of inoculation. Similar precautions are also recommended for patients with known or suspected diagnosis of Creutzfeldt–Jakob disease (CJD) or vCJD (variant CJD), and patients at increased risk of hepatitis B, C or HIV where their viral status is not known. High-risk patients include intravenous drug users, recipients of multiple blood transfusions and blood products, including haemophiliacs and those from HIV endemic areas, particularly sub-Saharan Africa. The adoption of universal precautions for all patients is recommended and helps minimise risk of inoculation injury.

All members of the team should be immunised against hepatitis B. All blood-exposure incidents should be reported to occupational health according to local protocol for assessment and consideration of postprocedure prophylaxis. Theatre staff should be notified of high-risk patients. Precautions include wearing goggles, waterproof gowns and protective footwear, double gloving, and the use of disposable surgical and anaesthetic equipment where possible. Meticulous surgical technique is important, with minimal sharps handling and avoidance of direct tissue contact with hands. Stapling devices should replace sutures where possible and sharp needles replaced by blunt ones where practicable. Specimens from high-risk patients should be appropriately labelled and transported separately.

Where patient testing for blood-borne viruses is indicated, i.e., post-blood exposure incident or in high-risk patients where viral status is not known, it should be performed only after appropriate consent and counselling.

Preoperative screening for methicillin-resistant *Staphylococcus aureus* or other resistant organisms

Infection with methicillin-resistant *Staphylococcus aureus* (MRSA) causes significant in-hospital morbidity and mortality, prolongs hospital stay, and increases cost. Preoperative MRSA screening has been shown to be an effective strategy to decrease MRSA infection rates by identifying asymptomatic carriers and allowing decolonisation treatment prior to hospital admission, reducing the risk of transmission and clinical infection. Preoperative MRSA screening involves swabbing the areas (nostrils, perineum and axillae) regularly colonised by *Staph. aureus*. MRSA carriers should undergo preoperative decolonisation prior to admission using daily antibacterial shampoo, body wash and nasal cream three times daily for 5 days. Although this regimen is only 50–60% effective, in the remainder reduced bacterial shedding reduces the risk of transmission and infection. Where possible, MRSA-positive emergency admissions should be nursed in single-room isolation until decolonisation is complete.

Vancomycin-resistant *Enterococcus* is also associated with prolonged hospitalisation, multiple courses of antibiotics and multiple surgical procedures. Carbapenemase-producing enterococci are increasingly prevalent in some areas of the world and patients with a recent hospital contact in such an area should be screened.

Assessment of the patient for emergency surgery

The principles of assessment, investigation and preparation of patients for elective surgery apply equally to the emergency setting, but may be curtailed by a lack of time and information. As a result, emergency surgery is often associated with increased morbidity and mortality compared with elective surgery. Emergency patients often require resuscitation prior to surgery; assessment and management of airway, breathing and circulation should be the first priority. Particular care should be taken to restore circulating volume wherever possible prior to surgery, with the exception of life-threatening haemorrhage penetrating trauma or where haemodynamic stability cannot be maintained. This is because anaesthesia is associated with attenuation of normal cardiovascular compensatory mechanisms and significant hypotension can result.

Over-zealous attempts to restore biochemistry, haematology and coagulation to normal at the expense of a marked delay in surgery are also to be avoided. This is particularly the case in the timing of surgery for sepsis, where need for adequate surgical source control may outweigh small benefits associated with investigations or interventions that delay surgery (e.g., the

correction of modest hyperglycaemia in the diabetic patient with peritonitis).

Preoperative review

The purpose of preoperative review is to ensure that the patient has been adequately assessed and prepared for surgery, and involves both surgeon and anaesthetist. Consideration should be given to the appropriate administration of drugs in the perioperative period as well as a comprehensive, multidisciplinary approach to the perioperative period. Patient questions should be addressed and full explanations of the surgical procedure, anaesthesia, postoperative analgesia, as well as the use of catheters, drains and postoperative monitoring should be given.

 5.6 Summary

Principles of perioperative management

Preoperative
- Optimisation of chronic conditions
- Optimisation of acute physiological disturbances
- Information-sharing psychological preparation/informed consent
- Surgical strategy planning investigations specific to surgical indication

Intraoperative
- Patient safety: monitoring and positioning
- Equipment: available and functioning
- Operative team: expertise correct

Postoperative recovery
- Analgesia
- Nutrition
- Physiotherapy mobilisation
- Rehabilitation occupational therapy
- Further treatment planning

Drug-management considerations
- Deep-vein thrombosis prophylaxis
- Antibiotic prophylaxis
- Preoperative anxiolytics
- Continuation of regular medication including route of administration
- Glycaemic control
- Reversal of anticoagulation
- Analgesia
- Fluid and electrolyte requirements

Nutrition
- Where there is going to be a prolonged period of reduced oral intake, enteral or parenteral nutrition should be considered.

Venous thromboembolism prophylaxis

In the United Kingdom, 25,000 people die each year from venous thromboembolism (VTE) (EBM 5.2). A substantial proportion of these are surgical patients. In addition to death from pulmonary

EBM 5.2 **Venous thromboembolism**

'Each year, it is estimated that 25,000 die from venous thromboembolism in the UK.
Mechanical methods of prevention are effective.
Pharmacological prophylaxis is cost effective.'

NICE Clinical Guideline 92: Venous thromboembolism – Reducing the risk (2010).; SIGN Clinical Guideline 122: Prevention and management of venous thromboembolism (2010).

embolism (PE), deep-vein thrombosis (DVT) causes substantial morbidity which may persist to cause the chronic health problems of postthrombotic syndrome with leg ulceration and swelling, with huge healthcare costs.

All patients should have their risk of VTE assessed prior to, or on, admission to hospital to enable prophylactic measures to be taken. The patient's risk of bleeding should be taken into consideration and balanced against the risk of DVT when deciding on thromboprophylaxis. The magnitude of the risk of DVT relates to patient and operative factors (Table 5.10). Measures should be taken to reduce the risk of VTE, in addition to thromboprophylaxis; these include maintaining hydration and encouraging mobility, and in patients at very high risk of VTE the use of an inferior vena caval filter. Women should consider stopping oestrogen-containing contraceptives and HRT 4 weeks prior to surgery.

Mechanical and pharmacological thromboprophylaxis is available (Table 5.11). All surgical patients with increased risk of VTE should be offered mechanical VTE prophylaxis at admission and pharmacological VTE prophylaxis if the risk of bleeding is low. Thromboprophylaxis should be continued until mobility is not significantly reduced, usually for 5–7 days, with the exception of orthopaedic lower limb surgery, where it should be continued for 2–4 weeks after surgery.

Table 5.11 Thromboprophylaxis

Mechanical

- Antiembolism stockings (knee or thigh length)
- Foot impulse devices
- Intermittent pneumatic compression devices (knee or thigh length)

Pharmacological

- Low-molecular-weight heparin
- Unfractionated heparin (renal failure)
- Fondaparinux

Antibiotic prophylaxis

Antibiotic prophylaxis refers to the use of antibiotics perioperatively to reduce the incidence of surgical site infections (SSI; EBM 5.3). SSI refer to infections of the wound, tissues involved in the surgery, or devices where surgery involves the insertion of implants or surgical devices. SSI is responsible for approximately 16% of hospital-acquired infections and causes considerable morbidity, prolonged hospital stay and increased costs. Every surgical patient should be assessed for the risk of SSI and its potential severity to allow appropriate prophylactic antibiotic selection. The risk of SSI depends on patient and operative risk factors, including the wound class (Table 5.12). SSI risk should be balanced against the risks of antibiotic prophylaxis such

Table 5.10 Patients at risk of venous thromboembolism

Medical patients	Surgical patients
- Significantly reduced mobility ≥3 days or - Expected ongoing reduced mobility with a VTE risk factor.	- Total anaesthetic + surgical time >90 minutes or - Pelvic or lower limb surgery with total anaesthetic + surgical time >60 minutes or - Acute surgical admission with inflammatory or intraabdominal condition or - Reduced mobility expected or - Any VTE risk factor.

VTE risk factors

- Active cancer or cancer treatment
- Age >60 years
- Intensive care admission
- Dehydration
- Known thrombophilia
- BMI >30 kg/m²
- Presence of significant medical comorbidity (heart disease, metabolic, endocrine or respiratory pathology, or acute infectious or inflammatory conditions)
- Personal history of or first-degree relative with VTE
- Hormone-replacement therapy
- Oestrogen-containing contraceptives
- Varicose veins with phlebitis

Pregnancy

Women admitted during pregnancy or up to 6 weeks postpartum:
- If surgery is planned mechanical plus pharmacological VTE prophylaxis
- Surgery not planned, use mechanical VTE prophylaxis and consider pharmacological prophylaxis if VTE risk factors present

BMI, Body mass index; VTE, venous thromboembolism.
Adapted from: Venous thromboembolism: reducing the risk. NICE Clinical Guideline 92, 2010, with permission.

EBM 5.3 Antibiotic prophylaxis

'A single therapeutic dose of antibiotic is sufficient in most circumstances with enough half life to achieve activity throughout the operation.
Prophylactic antibiotics should be given intravenously.
Intravenous prophylactic antibiotics should be given ≤30 mins before the skin is incised.
The choice of antibiotic should cover the expected pathogens for that operative site.'

SIGN Clinical Guideline 104: Antibiotic prophylaxis in surgery – principles (2008).

Table 5.12 Degree of contamination

Class	Definition
Clean	Operations in which no inflammation is encountered and which do not breach the respiratory, gastrointestinal or genitourinary tracts. Operating theatre technique is continuously aseptic
Clean–contaminated	Operations that breach the respiratory, gastrointestinal or genitourinary tracts but without significant spillage
Contaminated	Operations where acute inflammation is encountered or where the wound is visibly contaminated, e.g., gross spillage from a hollow viscus or compound injuries less than 4 hours old
Dirty	Operations in the presence of pus, a perforated hollow viscus or a compound injury more than 4 hours old

as allergy, and the increasing prevalence of resistant bacteria and infection with organisms such as *Clostridium difficile*. A single dose of intravenous antibiotics is adequate, provided the half-life permits activity throughout surgery. A repeat dose will be required if the duration of operation is more than 4 hours and/or if there is significant bleeding. For a detailed discussion on antibiotic prophylaxis, see Chapter 4.

Preoperative anxiolytic medication

The use of preoperative anxiolytics is at the anaesthetist's discretion. The aim is for the patient to arrive in the anaesthetic room in a relaxed, pain-free state. This can often be achieved by adequate explanation of the planned procedure and reassurance. Very anxious patients may require an anxiolytic. Oral benzodiazepines are commonly used as they have a relatively long duration of action, meaning accurate timing of administration with regard to anaesthetic induction is not required.

Preoperative fasting

The purpose of fasting preoperatively is to try to ensure an empty stomach and minimise the risk of regurgitation and aspiration during induction of anaesthesia. Extended periods of fasting prior to surgery are usually not required, and this is an important component of 'enhanced recovery after surgery' pathways. Where possible, patients should be starved of food for 6 hours and of clear fluids for 2 hours (EBM 5.4). This may not be possible in the emergency setting, in which case anaesthetic technique is adjusted to minimise the risk of aspiration. There are situations where an empty stomach cannot be guaranteed, despite fasting. These include pregnancy, gastric outlet or bowel obstruction, and any condition that causes a functional gastroparesis (autonomic neuropathy with delayed gastric emptying is common in long-standing diabetes). In such patients, a nasogastric tube may be indicated.

EBM **5.4 Perioperative fasting**

'Water and drinks without milk allowed up to 2 hours prior to induction of anaesthesia.
In children, breast milk allowed up to 4 hours prior to induction of anaesthesia.
Food, including sweets and drinks containing milk up to 6 hours prior to anaesthesia.
Chewing gum not permitted on the day of surgery.
Routine medication continued, can be taken with 30 mL fluid or 0.5 mL/kg in children.'

Perioperative fasting in adults and children, Royal College of Nursing 2005.

Perioperative implications of chronic disease

Some of the more important and common chronic diseases are discussed below.

Cardiovascular disease

Cardiac complications occur in 5% of patients aged 40 years or above undergoing major surgical procedures.

Ischaemic heart disease

Ischaemic heart disease is common in the developed world and its incidence increases with age. It is increasingly encountered at preoperative assessment and many patients may be asymptomatic. Clinicians should focus on the assessment of existing disease but also aim to identify undiagnosed disease.

The risk of perioperative myocardial infarction increases with symptom severity in patients with angina. This should be assessed by the frequency of symptoms, duration of attacks and precipitating factors. In particular, the limitation on everyday activities is a good guide to disease severity. Results of previous cardiac investigations, including coronary angiography, taking into account the time elapsed since they were performed, may help gauge disease severity. Cardiology input may be useful to optimise patients prior to general anaesthesia.

Unstable angina occurs when ischemia is severe enough to cause frequent symptoms but without resulting in measurable cardiac injury. Patients with unstable angina are at high risk of perioperative myocardial infarction (MI). In the elective situation these patients should be referred to a cardiologist for investigation and management. Risk of perioperative MI may be reduced by medical therapy and patients may require coronary angiography, PCI such as angioplasty or stenting, or even coronary artery bypass grafting (CABG). The decision to proceed with noncardiac surgery depends upon the indication, weighing the risk of perioperative MI against that of delaying for angiography, PCI or CABG, or cancelling surgery.

Myocardial infarction

MI is classified according to the 'Third Universal Definition' (http://www.escardio.org). To satisfy the requirements of the universal definitions patients must have an elevated cardiac biomarker (troponin) with at least one of: chest pain, ECG changes or wall motion abnormality on echocardiography. In unselected patients over 40 years of age, the risk of true myocardial infarction in the perioperative period is approximately 1% and this can rise to 3% in the presence of risk factors. Myocardial injury after noncardiac surgery (MINS) is troponin elevation within 30 days of noncardiac surgery that does not satisfy the definitions for MI; i.e., may not occur with associated chest pain or ECG changes. This is much more common than MI (as high as 19% in patients over 45 years of age having major surgery) and carries increased risk of cardiac complications and mortality. Risk factors for perioperative MI and MINS are outlined in Table 5.13.

Table 5.13 Risk factors for death or myocardial infarction following surgery (Revised Cardiac Risk Index)

- High-risk surgery (e.g., vascular major abdominal, thoracic)
- History of ischaemic heart disease
- History of heart failure
- History of cerebrovascular disease
- Diabetes requiring insulin therapy
- Creatinine >180 μmol/L

Number of risk factors	Rate of death or myocardial infarction	Rate of major cardiac complication
0	0.4%	0.5%
1	1.0%	1.3%
2	2.4%	3.6%
3+	5.4%	9.1%

Heart failure

Heart failure is increasingly common in patients presenting for noncardiac surgery, and hypertension, diabetes, ischaemic heart disease (IHD) and advancing age are frequently associated. Cardiac failure is typically due to left ventricular systolic or diastolic dysfunction, but may be due to any structural disease of the heart including valves or pericardium.

The clinical syndrome of heart failure is the result of either poor pump function (i.e., failure of the heart to provide adequate blood flow or cope with venous return), the neurohumoral response or underlying cardiac disease. Heart failure may be asymptomatic, compensated, decompensated or end-stage. Potential perioperative complications associated with heart failure are outlined in Table 5.14. Uncontrolled heart failure indicated by peripheral oedema, paroxysmal nocturnal dyspnoea or orthopnoea is associated with very high perioperative risk. Patients with new or symptomatic heart failure should be fully evaluated by clinical examination and echocardiography so that treatment can be optimised prior to elective surgery.

Valvular heart disease

The severity of valvular heart disease should be assessed by clinical evaluation and echocardiography because affected patients are at increased risk of associated arrhythmias and cardiac failure. All patients with new or suspected valvular

Table 5.14 Increased perioperative risk in patients with cardiac failure

Mechanism	Complication
Poor 'pump function'	Pulmonary oedema
	Cardiogenic shock
	Renal failure
	Organ ischaemia, e.g., bowel ischaemia
	Deep venous thrombosis
Cardiac disease	Arrhythmias
	Myocardial infarction
	Venous thromboembolism

disease should undergo formal assessment including echocardiography. Patients with existing moderate or severe valvular stenosis or regurgitation should undergo preoperative echocardiography if there has been a change in clinical condition or no examination has been carried out within a year. In adults who meet indication for valve intervention (i.e., repair, replacement) this should be undertaken where possible prior to elective surgery to reduce the risk (Fig. 5.3). Antibiotic prophylaxis guided by local protocol will depend on the risk of bacterial endocarditis according to the surgical procedure and the presence and type (metallic or bioprosthesis) of prosthetic heart valve.

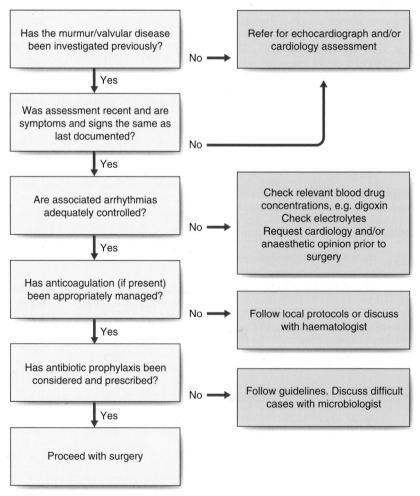

Fig. 5.3 An algorithm for managing patients with known or suspected valvular heart disease.

Pacemakers

Pacemaker function may be affected by anaesthetic equipment and diathermy. Prior to surgery, it is important to establish the indication for pacemaker insertion, the date of insertion and last check, the pacemaker type prior to surgery, and to seek advice from the pacemaker clinic. Referral may be necessary for preoperative device reprogramming or for a check if more than 3 months have elapsed since the last check. Bipolar diathermy or ultrasonic energy devices are preferred to monopolar diathermy. Care should be taken when placing the patient return electrode to direct the electrical current away from the pacemaker if monopolar diathermy cannot be avoided.

Hypertension

Uncontrolled hypertension increases the risk of perioperative myocardial infarction and cerebrovascular accident. A diagnosis of hypertension requires repeated, accurate blood pressure measurements which should be interpreted with respect to the patient's age. An elevated diastolic pressure is of greater significance than the systolic pressure, contributing most of the excess risk. Organ blood flow is tightly regulated over a range of blood pressures; in hypertensive patients, this range is elevated, rendering them vulnerable to organ hypoperfusion even with modest intraoperative hypotension.

Hypertension should be controlled in the elective setting for a few weeks prior to surgery. This is to enable the autoregulatory mechanisms that control organ blood flow to reset and maintain organ perfusion at the lower blood pressure, a process that takes several days. Elective surgery should usually be postponed when the diastolic pressure exceeds 110 mmHg. In the emergency situation, a modest reduction in blood pressure to minimise cardiovascular risk whilst maintaining adequate organ perfusion can be achieved intraoperatively by careful titration of antihypertensives. Regional anaesthetic techniques offer an alternative approach in the emergency setting, by avoiding the potentially large swings in blood pressure associated with general anaesthesia that may cause dysregulation of organ perfusion.

Perioperative management of patients with cardiovascular disease

Drug therapy

In general, cardiac medications should be taken right up to the time of surgery and re-introduced as soon as possible postoperatively. Where the oral route is not available postoperatively, an alternative should be found.

β-Blockers Perioperative use of β-blockers may reduce the incidence of perioperative MI but increase overall mortality. Hence, routine use of perioperative β-blockers cannot be recommended in high-risk patients. Patients already established on a β-blocker should continue because of the risk of rebound tachycardia increasing myocardial oxygen demand with increased risk of myocardial ischaemia.

Angiotensin-converting enzyme (ACE) inhibitors These drugs are commonly used to treat cardiac failure and hypertension. Due to the significant risk of intra- and postoperative hypotension, the anaesthetist may decide whether to omit these drugs perioperatively.

Perioperative haemodynamic therapy

Overt or covert failure of oxygen delivery may be implicated in the development of postoperative complications and mortality following major surgery. This has generated interest in using goal-directed HT in high-risk surgical patients. This approach involves using cardiac output monitoring and giving fluid to maximise cardiac output and hence oxygen delivery. In some algorithms low-dose inotropic agents are also added. The aim is to maximise oxygen delivery to the tissue with the aim of reducing complications after surgery and reducing mortality and length of hospital stay. Use of HT routinely for all high-risk surgical patients remains controversial, and whether aspects of the intervention, e.g., cardiac output monitoring-guided fluid therapy or low-dose inotropic support, are harmful or beneficial remains the subject of debate (Table 5.15 and EBM 5.5).

> **EBM** 5.5 **Optimising high-risk patients using invasive monitoring and resuscitation targets**
>
> 'In study of a cardiac output guided haemodynamic therapy (HT) algorithm in 734 patients undergoing major surgery on the gastrointestinal tract there was no reduction in a composite outcome of death or complications at 30 days after surgery. An updated meta-analysis of 38 trials included in this paper suggested that HT is associated with fewer complications (RR 0.7 [95%CI 0.71 − 0.83]).'
>
> Pearse et al. JAMA 2014;311: 2181.

Respiratory disease

Patients with significant respiratory disease require close monitoring, preferably in a high-dependency or intensive care unit, particularly after thoracic or major abdominal surgery where hypoventilation, atelectasis and pneumonia are common. Adequate analgesia and physiotherapy must be provided to enable the clearance of secretions and avoid atelectasis by coughing to avoid hypoxia and pneumonia.

Table 5.15 Cardiovascular monitoring during the perioperative period

Monitor	Information given
Arterial catheter	Continuous measurement of blood pressure
Central venous catheter	Central venous pressure (estimate of cardiac preload with important exceptions)
Minimally invasive cardiac output monitoring e.g., LiDCO, PiCCO, oesophageal Doppler	Cardiac output, preload indices (e.g., stroke volume, flow time, intrathoracic blood volume)
Pulmonary artery catheter	Pulmonary artery pressure, pulmonary capillary wedge pressure (a measure of left atrial pressure) and cardiac output (by thermodilution). Now seldom used except in special circumstances
Transoesophageal echo	Increasingly used in major cardiovascular and thoracoabdominal surgery. Allows full cardiac and hemodynamic assessment

LiDCO, Lithium Dilution Cardiac Output; PiCCO, Pulse index Continuous Cardiac Output.

A small proportion of patients with chronic hypercarbia rely on hypoxic drive for ventilation and high concentrations of inspired oxygen may cause hypoventilation and respiratory failure. In these patients, close observation in a high-dependency setting may be required, especially if they are hypoxic and require supplemental oxygen or noninvasive ventilation. They are particularly vulnerable to postoperative complications such as respiratory failure and pneumonia, requiring respiratory support including ventilation. The perioperative management of patients with respiratory disease is discussed in the following sections.

Anaesthetic technique

General anaesthesia is associated with a risk of respiratory complications, in part due to altered respiratory function caused by general anaesthesia. This is of particular concern in patients with preexisting respiratory disease and reduced respiratory reserve. Regional anaesthetic techniques may reduce or eliminate the need for general anaesthesia in this group.

Intraoperative ventilatory management

The use of an intraoperative 'lung protective' ventilator strategy, i.e., low tidal volume ventilation, use of positive end expiratory pressure (PEEP) recruitment manoeuvres, may reduce postoperative respiratory complications in high-risk patients undergoing abdominal surgery. This is similar to the ventilator strategy applied to patients with acute respiratory distress syndrome (ADRS) in the ICU.

Postoperative analgesia

Effective postoperative analgesia is important to maintain adequate cough, sputum clearance and ventilation to avoid atelectasis, particularly in patients who have undergone thoracic and major abdominal surgery. Regional anaesthetic techniques, particularly epidural analgesia or other regional techniques, are effective in this regard. Parenteral opiates are effective analgesics but care should be taken not to cause respiratory depression or obtund the conscious level.

Physiotherapy

Pre- and postoperative chest physiotherapy is important in patients with respiratory disease. Manoeuvres that facilitate maximal inspiratory effort, positive airway pressure and the use of incentive spirometry are particularly useful in minimising the risk of atelectasis and guarding against hypoxia and pneumonia.

Postoperative ventilation

Postoperative ventilation may be indicated for respiratory failure as a result of insufficient respiratory reserve or complications such as pneumonia. Meticulous attention to analgesia and regular chest physiotherapy may avoid the need for ventilation. The duration of endotracheal intubation should be minimised because it also increases the risk of pneumonia. The use of noninvasive respiratory support with either noninvasive ventilation (NIV), continuous positive airway pressure (CPAP) via a face mask or high flow nasal oxygen may avoid the need for ventilation, reduce postoperative respiratory complications or be useful in weaning intubated patients from ventilator support.

▌ Diabetes mellitus

The increased perioperative risk associated with diabetes mellitus is attributable to related comorbidities and poor glycaemic control, which is exacerbated by surgical stress.

Diabetic comorbidity

Vascular disease

Diabetics develop both a specific microangiopathy (typified by diabetic retinopathy and nephropathy) and macrovascular disease with accelerated atherosclerosis that results in increased risk of ischaemic heart disease, cerebrovascular accident, peripheral vascular disease, renovascular disease, hypertension and delayed wound healing.

Renal disease

Diabetes is the single most common cause of chronic renal failure in the UK. Due to a lack of renal reserve, diabetics are particularly vulnerable to acute renal failure resulting from hypotension, nephrotoxic drugs, radiological contrast agents and sepsis. A significant proportion of patients developing postoperative renal failure will remain dialysis dependent. It is therefore imperative that care is taken to protect against further kidney insult.

Neuropathy

Diabetic neuropathy is most commonly encountered by the vascular surgeon in association with limb ischaemia as a component of nonhealing ulceration. Autonomic neuropathy should be anticipated and can result in delayed gastric emptying with risk of aspiration during induction of anaesthesia. A lack of sympathetic cardiovascular compensation to anaesthetic-induced hypotension or bleeding can result in severe hypotension.

Infection

Diabetic patients are at increased risk of infective complications, particularly if glycaemic control is poor.

Effect of surgical stress on diabetic control

Part of the metabolic response to surgery involves glucose mobilisation and lipolysis with increased circulating insulin levels to maintain homeostasis and normoglycaemia. The net result in diabetics is a tendency towards hyperglycaemia and ketoacidosis following surgery, which is exaggerated if complications such as sepsis develop. Glycaemic control should be monitored closely and insulin or oral hypoglycaemic drug doses titrated accordingly. The metabolic response to surgery is discussed in more detail in Chapter 1.

Principles of perioperative diabetes management

The aim of perioperative diabetic management is to maintain stable circulating glucose levels, ensuring an adequate fuel supply to the cells. A circulating glucose concentration of 6–10 mmol/L is a reasonable target range. As hypoglycaemia is more dangerous to the patient than hyperglycaemia, moderate hyperglycaemia is acceptable. Care should be taken to administer sufficient potassium when insulin is administered as insulin increases cellular potassium uptake, with a tendency towards hypokalaemia. The approach used to achieve perioperative glycaemic control depends on a number of factors including:

* Whether the diabetes is usually diet, tablet or insulin controlled
* The magnitude of the surgical stress
* The presence of sepsis or other complications
* Whether the patient is 'nil by mouth'.

In practice, many units have protocols for the perioperative management of diabetes, which can be tailored to the individual patient. Table 5.16 gives examples of the typical approach to diabetic control.

Table 5.16 Typical scenarios for diabetic patients presenting for surgery

Patient	Procedure	Management
Diet-controlled diabetic	Elective laparoscopic cholecystectomy (moderate stress response)	Monitor blood glucose until eating
Patient on oral hypoglycaemics	Hernia repair (minor stress response)	Omit oral hypoglycaemic on morning of surgery Monitor preoperatively for hypoglycaemia Monitor postoperatively until eating normally Restart oral hypoglycaemics when on normal diet
Normally well controlled	Elective aortofemoral bypass (major stress response)	Omit oral hypoglycaemic on morning of surgery Monitor perioperatively for hypo- or hyperglycaemia If blood glucose >10 mmol/L, commence glucose/insulin/potassium infusion
Normally poorly controlled blood sugar >10 mmol/L	Emergency aortofemoral bypass (major stress response)	Commence glucose/insulin/potassium infusion prior to surgery Stop oral hypoglycaemics perioperatively
Insulin-dependent diabetic		
Well controlled	Cataract surgery (minor stress response)	Omit morning insulin Monitor blood sugar for hypoglycaemia Restart regular insulin when eating
Normally well controlled	Elective coronary artery bypass graft (major stress response)	Convert to glucose/insulin/dextrose prior to surgery Monitor blood sugar perioperatively Convert to subcutaneous short-acting insulin and then regular insulin as diet reintroduced
Blood sugar >20 mmol/L or ketones in urine	Emergency laparotomy for diverticular abscess (major stress response)	Treat as diabetic ketoacidosis and stabilise *prior to* surgery Ensure adequate volume resuscitation Continue glucose/insulin/potassium infusion perioperatively Convert to intermittent short-acting and then normal insulin as diet reintroduced

Methods of insulin administration

For patients with poor glycaemic control or not established on their usual diabetic medication because normal dietary intake has not been established, sliding scale insulin is normally administered. Sliding scale insulin regimens consist of intravenous insulin, glucose and potassium that can be given as a single mixed infusion (the Alberti regimen) (Table 5.17) or as separate infusions of insulin and glucose with potassium. Single mixed infusions are simple, cheap and safer, with less risk of hypoglycaemia, but at the expense of greater flexibility and tight glycaemic control that can be achieved with separate insulin and glucose infusions.

Chronic renal failure

Patients with chronic renal failure are at increased risk of complications in the perioperative period (Table 5.18). Management of fluid balance and specific arrangements for dialysis should be undertaken in conjunction with a nephrologist.

Table 5.17 The Alberti regimen

- 500 mL 10% dextrose *plus* 10 U short-acting soluble insulin *plus* 10 mmol KCl
- Run 500 mL every 4–6 hours via a controlled infusion pump
- Check blood glucose every 2–6 hours (depending on stability) and potassium 1–2 times daily
- On average, give 250 g glucose daily (1000 kcal) and 50 U insulin
- Adjust insulin and potassium according to results

Dialysis-dependent patients

Considerations in dialysis-dependent patients include:

- Fluid balance. The majority of these patients are anuric and depend on dialysis to remove excess water. Intravenous fluid should be administered with extreme caution.

Table 5.18 Risk factors in patients with renal failure undergoing surgery

Cardiovascular
- Frequently have ischaemic heart disease
- Hypertension
- Left ventricular dysfunction

Respiratory
- Pulmonary oedema and fluid overload (impaired water clearance)

Gastrointestinal
- Delayed gastric emptying

Biochemical
- Electrolyte disturbance (especially hyperkalaemia)

Haematological
- Anaemia
- Impaired coagulation (platelet dysfunction)

Miscellaneous
- Malnutrition
- Multiple drug therapies
- Abnormal drug metabolism
- Vascular access

- Access for dialysis. Patients will either have venous access for haemodialysis (fistulae or large intravenous cannulae) or peritoneal dialysis catheters. Care should be taken to protect this life-preserving access. An arteriovenous or dialysis access graft should never be used for intravenous access or phlebotomy.
- Electrolyte imbalance, particularly hyperkalaemia, is common. Frequent monitoring should be undertaken.
- Timing of dialysis. This should be decided after liaison with a nephrologist. Preoperative dialysis may be advised to optimise the patient for surgery.

Nondialysis-dependent patients

This group of patients have adequate renal function but have minimal functional reserve. They are at risk during the perioperative period of deteriorating renal function that renders them dialysis dependent. The risk of further deterioration in renal function can be reduced by:

- Optimising fluid balance directed by central venous pressure monitoring
- Avoiding nephrotoxic drugs (e.g., aminoglycosides and NSAIDs) and radiological contrast agents
- Treating sepsis aggressively
- Protecting renal perfusion by avoiding hypotension.

Drugs excreted by the kidney may accumulate and should be avoided where possible.

Jaundice

Preoperative diagnosis of the cause of jaundice is important because it will impact management. The risks of surgery in jaundiced patients relate to the following factors:

Hepatitis

The possibility of hepatitis B or C should be considered in patients with elevated aminotransferases or cirrhosis. Patients at increased risk of blood-borne viruses such as hepatitis B and C include patients who have received multiple blood transfusions, intravenous drug abusers, those engaged in high-risk sexual activity, as well as travel from an endemic area. Their viral status should be ascertained after appropriate consent in order to take appropriate measures to protect the healthcare staff.

Coagulopathy

Patients with obstructive jaundice and hepatocellular dysfunction are at risk of coagulopathy due to a lack of vitamin K and synthetic capacity. Adequate vitamin K depends on the presence of bile salts in the gut lumen for absorption. As a result, the function of

vitamin K-dependent coagulation factors II, VII, IX and X is reduced with a prolonged prothrombin time and a bleeding tendency. Clotting should be corrected preoperatively by administration of intravenous vitamin K or fresh-frozen plasma if urgent.

Acute renal failure

Acute renal failure commonly accompanies jaundice and is referred to as hepatorenal syndrome. Although the pathogenesis is not fully understood, multiple mechanisms are probably involved. An imbalance in vascular tone exists, with disturbances in systemic haemodynamics, increased vasoconstriction, and a reduction in the activity of the vasodilator systems. Patients with hepatorenal syndrome typically have an increased cardiac output, low blood pressure, reduced systemic vascular resistance, and increased renal vasoconstriction. Prevention and treatment is with fluid loading using physiological crystalloids.

Cirrhosis

Cirrhotics have significantly increased perioperative morbidity and mortality, which is related to the degree of hepatic decompensation and type of surgery. Nonalcoholic fatty liver disease is increasingly recognised as part of the metabolic syndrome. It is associated with obesity and has been demonstrated to convey an excess risk for postoperative morbidity and mortality in patients undergoing major liver resection. A number of algorithms have been used to estimate postoperative mortality in this patient group, including the modified Childs score (see Chapter 14). This stratifies prothrombin time, albumin, the presence of ascites, encephalopathy and bilirubin to generate a score. Scores of A, B and C are associated with perioperative mortalities of 10, 30 and 80%, respectively, for abdominal surgery. If the balance of risk favours surgery, hepatic function should be optimised. Postoperatively the patient will require intensive care monitoring.

Abnormal coagulation

Patients with abnormal coagulation fall into three categories.

Anticoagulant therapy

Patients receiving oral anticoagulants may require reversal of anticoagulation, bridging anticoagulation to cover the perioperative period and reanticoagulation. Advice from a haematologist or cardiologist may be helpful. Warfarin should be stopped 4–5 days before surgery to achieve an international normalised ratio (INR) <2 for minor surgery and <1.5 for major surgery. The risk of thromboembolism during the perioperative period without anticoagulation should be assessed (Table 5.19). Where the risk is high or medium, bridging anticoagulation with

---

Table 5.19 Risk stratification of conditions requiring consideration of continuous perioperative anticoagulation

High risk	Intermediate risk	Low risk
• Older mechanical mitral valve • Recently placed mechanical heart valve • Atrial fibrillation plus mechanical heart valve • Atrial fibrillation with history of thromboembolism • Recurrent arterial or idiopathic venous thromboembolic events • Venous or arterial thromboembolism in preceding 3 months • Hypercoagulable state	• Newer mitral mechanical valve • Older aortic mechanical valve • Cerebrovascular disease with multiple ischaemic episodes • Atrial fibrillation with risk factors for cardiac embolism • Venous thromboembolism >3, <6 months ago	• Atrial fibrillation without risk factors for thromboembolism • Remote venous embolism >6 months ago • Cerebrovascular disease without recurrent ischaemic events • New model prosthetic aortic valve
Bridging anticoagulation required	**Bridging anticoagulation may be required**	**Bridging anticoagulation not required**

intravenous unfractionated heparin or subcutaneous low molecular weight heparin should be administered. Bridging anticoagulation is not required for patients at low risk of thromboembolism. Oral anticoagulation should be reintroduced as soon as the risk of haemorrhage has subsided and the patient is tolerating oral medication. Bridging anticoagulation should only be stopped once the INR is therapeutic.

Vitamin K can be used to reverse warfarin anticoagulation in patients requiring urgent surgery; it takes 24–48 hours to reverse anticoagulation. Where more rapid correction of coagulation is required, fresh-frozen plasma and prothrombin complex concentrates are indicated. The use of prothrombin complex concentrates usually requires the approval of a haematologist. A rebound increase in INR should be sought. Protamine can be used to reverse the effects of heparin if urgent reversal is required (coagulation normalises without treatment 4–6 hours after heparin cessation).

Inherited disorders of coagulation

The most common inherited disorder of coagulation is haemophilia A (factor VIII deficiency), followed by haemophilia B (factor IX deficiency) and von Willebrand's disease (von Willebrand factor deficiency). These patients require factor infusions to achieve haemostatic levels at the time of surgery and throughout the immediate postoperative period until the risk of bleeding subsides. This should be organised in close collaboration with a haematologist.

Acquired coagulopathy

Acquired coagulopathy may be the first sign of DIC with associated thrombocytopenia. The triggers for DIC include sepsis, malignancy, surgery, trauma, burns, anaphylaxis and blood transfusion reactions. DIC is characterised by microvascular coagulation, intense fibrinolysis, tissue ischaemia, and the consumption of clotting factors and platelets. The diagnosis is based on clinical and laboratory findings. The typical laboratory findings include thrombocytopenia, elevated prothrombin time (PT) and activated partial thromboplastin time (APTT), low fibrinogen, elevated fibrin, and fibrinogen degradation products and D-dimers. Management is complex but focuses on the treatment of the underlying cause; further treatment depends on whether bleeding or thrombosis predominate and should involve a haematologist.

Anaemia

The type and cause of anaemia should be ascertained, enabling preoperative correction where possible. Iron deficiency anaemia commonly encountered in surgical practice is usually as a result of gastrointestinal blood loss or menorrhagia. Where anaemic patients are scheduled for surgery with the potential for blood loss requiring transfusion, consideration should be given to blood-conserving surgical techniques such as cell salvage.

Musculoskeletal disease

Careful handling and positioning of the unconscious, anaesthetised patient is mandatory to avoid injury. Patients with deformity, rheumatoid arthritis and those with proven spinal instability or with a potentially unstable spine demand special attention. Atlantoaxial subluxation can result in an unstable cervical spine in rheumatoid patients leading to spinal cord damage if not protected. Plain cervical spine radiographs should be taken as a minimum requirement and the anaesthetist informed so that excessive neck movements during intubation can be avoided. The use of a neck collar can be used to highlight the potential danger to theatre staff.

Table 5.20 Relevance of some medical conditions in the perioperative period

Condition	Considerations
Rheumatoid arthritis	Neck may be 'unstable', careful positioning necessary, difficult intubation, complex drug therapy, associated chronic diseases, e.g., renal failure, lung disease
Multiple sclerosis	Reduced respiratory reserve; stress of surgery can cause relapse or worsening of disease
Epilepsy	Drugs may interact with anaesthetics; surgical stress and some drugs may precipitate seizures
Scoliosis or spondylitis	Can significantly reduce respiratory reserve; difficult endotracheal intubation
Myasthenia gravis	Risk of respiratory failure or aspiration; anaesthetic technique needs modifying
Sickle-cell anaemia	Stress of surgery, hypoxia, hypothermia, dehydration or hypovolaemia can all precipitate sickle cell crisis

Miscellaneous conditions

Table 5.20 gives an overview of some of the other diseases requiring particular consideration in the perioperative period.

Anaesthesia and the operation

Prior to the induction of anaesthesia, a preoperative check should be completed by the ward nursing and theatre staff, anaesthetist and surgeon. This is to guard against incorrect and wrong site surgery, and prevent poor planning and adverse events.

The recent introduction of the WHO Surgical Safety Checklist has formalised this process. The preoperative check covers patient identity, proposed surgery and site, availability of clinical records, investigation results, consent and patient allergies, as well as equipment availability and anaesthetic concerns. The side to be operated upon should be clearly marked with indelible ink before premedication is administered. This should be visible after the patient is painted and draped; it should not be in the line of the proposed skin incision to avoid the risk of a tattoo.

Anaesthesia

General anaesthesia

The aims of general anaesthesia are to produce a safe, reversible loss of consciousness, optimise the physiological response to surgery and provide good operating conditions. General anaesthesia has three components: loss of consciousness (hypnosis), analgesia and muscle relaxation.

Local anaesthetic agents

Local anaesthetic agents such as lignocaine and bupivacaine exert their effect by causing a local, reversible blockade of nerve conduction by reducing nerve membrane sodium permeability. They are nonspecific and act on autonomic, motor and sensory nerves equally. Their duration of action depends on the local anaesthetic agent used, dose, whether adrenaline has been coadministered and the proximity of local anaesthetic to the nerve.

Maximum local anaesthetic doses are shown in Table 5.21. A patient receiving large doses of local anaesthetic should be

Table 5.21 Safe maximum doses of commonly used local anaesthetics

Drug	With adrenaline (epinephrine) (mg/kg)	Without adrenaline (epinephrine) (mg/kg)
Lidocaine	7	3
Bupivacaine	2	2
Prilocaine	Maximum 600 mg	

Table 5.22 Signs of local anaesthetic toxicity

Early

- Numbness/tingling of the tongue
- Perioral tingling
- Anxiety
- Lightheadedness
- Tinnitus

Late

- Loss of consciousness
- Convulsions
- Cardiovascular collapse
- Apnoea

monitored with ECG, pulse oximetry and noninvasive blood pressure measurement. Local anaesthetic toxicity as a result of inadvertent injection into the blood stream or overdose may be heralded by perioral tingling and altered mental status culminating in arrhythmias, convulsions and cardiovascular collapse (Table 5.22). Intravascular injection should be avoided by aspirating on the needle prior to injection. In the case of suspected toxicity, stop administering the agent. Treatment is supportive; however, if the patient is in cardiac arrest they should be managed according to standard guidelines. Recovery from a cardiac arrest may take more than 1 hour. The airway should be secured, ensuring adequate ventilation, and conventional therapies should be used to treat hypotension and arrhythmias (not lidocaine), recognising that arrhythmias in particular may be very resistant to treatment. Seizures should be controlled with small increments of intravenous benzodiazepines. Lipid emulsion, e.g., intralipid, should be administered in circulatory arrest or severe toxicity, as it can reverse the cardiovascular and neurological toxicity.

Local anaesthetics can be used to provide surgical anaesthesia and postoperative analgesia in a variety of techniques that are discussed in more detail subsequently. Patients undergoing major surgery under regional anaesthesia should always be fasted as for a general anaesthetic in case conversion to general anaesthetic or sedation is required.

Spinal and epidural anaesthesia

Spinal anaesthesia

Spinal anaesthetic is the introduction of local anaesthetic, usually lidocaine or bupivacaine, into the subarachnoid space to block the spinal nerves before they exit the intervertebral foramina (Fig. 5.4). To protect against damage to the spinal cord, spinal anaesthesia is administered below L2, either at the L3/4 or L4/5 level. At this level, the cauda equina nerves acquire their perineural coverings and myelin sheath as they exit the dura, making them exquisitely sensitive to the effect of local anaesthetic. As

a result, 2–4 mL of local anaesthetic produces a dense block up to T6 level, with a rapid onset of action, giving 2–3 hours of surgical anaesthesia. The addition of 6–8% glucose increases the density of the spinal anaesthetic solution, making it easier to control the level of the block using gravity. Aspiration of subarachnoid fluid confirms the correct site of the spinal block needle.

Epidural anaesthesia

Epidural anaesthesia involves the injection of local anaesthetic into the epidural space, which extends along the entire vertebral canal between the ligamentum flavum and dura mater (Fig. 5.5). Local anaesthetic spreads craniocaudally, penetrating the meningeal sheaths containing the nerve roots and causing an anaesthetic block affecting several dermatomes. The level of epidural anaesthetic is therefore dictated by the proposed site of surgery and the dermatomes involved. The nerve roots are fully covered and myelinated as they traverse the epidural space, and therefore a larger volume (10–20 mL) of local anaesthetic, compared with spinal anaesthesia, is required to achieve anaesthesia. The technique by which a needle is introduced into the epidural space depends on sensing a loss of resistance as the needle passes through the ligamentum flavum; aspiration ensures that the needle is not advanced too far into the subarachnoid space, termed a 'dural tap'. An ongoing cerebrospinal fluid (CSF) leak following a dural tap can lead to loss of CSF volume and headache. As well as adequate hydration, the CSF leak may be managed by the use of a blood patch. This involves using the patient's own blood injected into the epidural space to seal the leak. If a dural tap goes undetected with the injection of local anaesthetic into the subarachnoid space, a profound block of all spinal nerves will result, with the potential of respiratory arrest and profound hypotension. A catheter is often left in the epidural space to provide access for ongoing analgesia. Table 5.23 details some common complications of epidural anaesthesia.

Both spinal and epidural anaesthesia block spinal cord sympathetic outflow. Rapid vasomotor paralysis with peripheral vasodilatation is an early sign of a successful spinal or epidural anaesthetic due to the rapid onset of blockade in these small unmyelinated fibres. Conversely, the resulting peripheral vasodilatation can be a nuisance with unwanted hypotension requiring treatment with intravenous fluids, vasoconstrictors or reduction in the rate of the epidural infusion.

Peripheral nerve block

Peripheral nerve blockade requires a detailed working knowledge of the target nerve's surface anatomy, adjacent structures, as well as the cutaneous area supplied by it. Use of a nerve stimulator and insulated block needle can improve the accuracy of placement of the nerve block catheter. A list of commonly performed nerve blocks and their indications are detailed in Table 5.24.

Local infiltration

Local anaesthetics can be used to infiltrate the surgical field, either as the sole anaesthetic to allow minor surgery to be performed or as an adjunct to provide postoperative analgesia. Their effectiveness is impaired in inflamed or infected tissues due to increased acidity and increased absorption due to vasodilatation, and alternative anaesthetic techniques may be necessary. Local anaesthetics may be coadministered with adrenaline, which prolongs their action by causing vasoconstriction resulting in decreased systemic absorption. Local anaesthetic with adrenaline should never be used at a site that has an end arterial supply, i.e., the digits or penis, as ischaemia and gangrene may ensue.

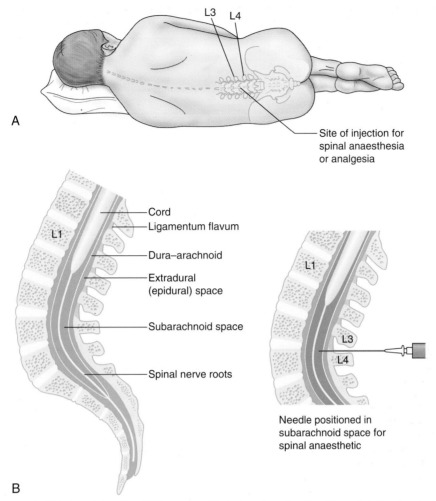

Fig. 5.4 Spinal anaesthesia. (A) Position of the patient. **(B)** The anatomy of the lumbar spine and position of the needle in the subarachnoid space as for spinal anaesthesia.

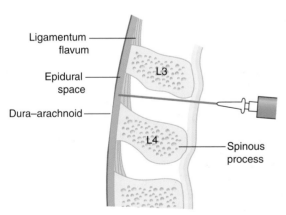

Fig. 5.5 Epidural anaesthesia.

Table 5.23 Complications of epidural anaesthesia and analgesia

Complication	Steps to avoid complication
Epidural abscess (0.015–0.05%)	Avoid if skin or systemic sepsis
Epidural haematoma (0.01%)	Correct coagulopathy, reverse anticoagulation, care in patients who have received recent heparin including thromboprophylaxis
Respiratory depression	Avoid high epidural block (C3–5 innervate diaphragm)
Cardiac depression	Mid-thoracic epidurals may block cardiac sympathetic outflow. May result in bradycardia
Hypotension	Vasodilation resulting from blockade efferent sympathetic outflow commonly results in drop in blood pressure. Fluids and vasoconstrictors may be required

Topical anaesthesia

Due to the mucosal and, to a lesser extent, cutaneous absorption of local anaesthetics, topical anaesthesia has a role in procedures involving the oral cavity, pharynx, larynx, urethra and conjunctiva. Cutaneous anaesthesia can also be achieved in children and needle-phobic adults prior to cannulation or venepuncture; tetracaine (Ametop) and prilocaine/lidocaine (Emla) creams are available for this purpose. Lignocaine is the most commonly used topical anaesthetic and is available as a gel, ointment, cream or

Table 5.24 Commonly performed peripheral nerve blocks	
Block	**Indication**
Axillary or supraclavicular	Upper limb surgery
Interscalene	Shoulder and upper limb
Femoral	Lower limb surgery
Sciatic	Lower limb surgery
Intercostal nerves	Thoracotomy, fractured ribs
Ilioinguinal/iliohypogastric	Inguinal hernia
Penile	Circumcision

spray. The use of cocaine as a topical anaesthetic in otolaryngology has been largely phased out due to the intense sympathomimetic effect.

Postoperative analgesia

Good postoperative analgesia is essential in ensuring surgical success by minimising psychological and physiological morbidity, enabling early mobilisation and optimising respiratory function. Despite this, approximately 20% of patients will have inadequate analgesia. Successful postoperative analgesia requires preoperative planning, taking into account the nature of the proposed surgery, patient factors and preferences, and their comorbidity. Knowledge of pain physiology, assessment and analgesic drugs, including routes of delivery and pharmacology, is essential. The pain pathway is illustrated in Fig. 5.6. Many hospitals have acute pain teams involving doctors and specialist nurses to deliver improved patient analgesia.

Pain assessment

Adequate analgesia requires regular assessment of pain and the adequacy of analgesia. The patient's own subjective experience of pain should always be used. The method of pain assessment varies between institutions. Examples include nonlinear scales such as: no pain, mild, moderate pain and severe pain; and linear scales where a pain score out of ten or a visual analogue scale (1–100 mm) is used.

Postoperative analgesic strategy

Multimodal analgesia, using several analgesics that act at different parts of the pain pathway, is more effective than the use of single agents and reduces the dose required of individual analgesics, minimising side effects. Epidural analgesia and patient-controlled parenteral opiate analgesia are commonly used for major surgery. Limb surgery lends itself to the use of postoperative peripheral nerve blocks or oral morphine regimens may be sufficient for less major surgery. In all cases paracetamol and NSAIDs, where appropriate, should be used alongside opiate analgesia. A step-down regimen should be in place to minimise the use of potent opioid analgesia, as the requirement for them lessens with time elapsed from surgery. Individual analgesic techniques are discussed below.

Epidural analgesia

Epidural analgesia is commonly achieved by a continuous infusion of local anaesthetic, usually in combination with an opiate, into the epidural space. A typical regimen of 0.1% bupivacaine with 2 mg/mL fentanyl running at a rate of up to 16 mL/hour is used

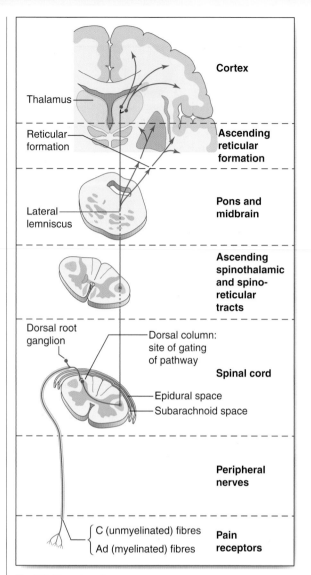

Fig. 5.6 The pain pathway.

for thoracic, abdominal and major lower limb surgery. Inserted prior to surgery, an epidural catheter can safely remain in place for up to 5 days. Pain relief is superior to parenteral opiates but careful patient monitoring in an appropriate environment by trained staff is needed. There is a rate of epidural failure due to misplacement, displacement, inadequate analgesia or intolerable side effects, which should be managed with timely epidural replacement or substitution with another analgesic technique. In addition to the complications discussed above as per epidural anaesthesia, permanent neurological damage (0.005–0.05%) is a devastating but rare complication. Epidural haematoma may cause this, and care must be taken to ensure that patients have normal coagulation and platelet count prior to removal or insertion of the catheter. When patients are receiving unfractionated or low-molecular-weight heparin, care must be taken to remove the epidural catheter at least 6 hours after a dose. Respiratory depression due to cephalad spread of opiates may also occur.

Patient-controlled analgesia

Patient-controlled analgesia (PCA) involves the use of a preprogrammed pump to deliver a small, predetermined dose of drug, usually an opiate, with a minimum time period between doses (lock-out period). The lock-out period allows the patient to feel the effect of the opiate bolus before administering a subsequent dose, minimising the amount of opiate consumed and the risk of respiratory depression, which occurs in up to 11.5% of patients. A typical regimen would involve 1 mg morphine at 5-minute intervals, although this may vary according to patient size, age and history of opiate exposure. Background opiate infusions are not routine due to the increased risk of respiratory depression, but may be useful in chronic opioid users. Similar to epidurals, PCA requires expensive pumps, and to be successful the patient must understand how it works and have the manual dexterity to use the pump. Care must be taken in correct pump programming as deaths from respiratory depression have been reported.

Parenteral and oral opioid regimens

Strong opioids Examples of strong opioids include buprenorphine, fentanyl, oxycodone and pethidine, as well as morphine. In the absence of evidence of superiority of one strong opioid over another, morphine is the most commonly used, particularly in the postoperative period. Strong opioids, either oral or parenteral, are used as the primary analgesia for more minor surgery and on stepping down from an epidural or PCA in order to avoid an analgesic gap. Typical regimens of 10 mg morphine, either subcutaneously or orally, as required at 4–6-hour intervals are used, although the dose should take the age, weight and history of opiate use into account. Opioid side effects include respiratory depression, dysphoria, constipation, nausea and vomiting, pruritus, urinary retention, and depressed conscious level. Opioids can be reversed with naloxone, an opioid antagonist.

Weak opioids Examples of weak opioids, useful in the management of mild pain, include codeine, dihydrocodeine and tramadol. Codeine and dihydrocodeine are available in preparation with paracetamol. In addition to being an opioid agonist, tramadol inhibits serotonin and noradrenaline reuptake, and is effective in neuropathic pain as well as in the acute pain setting.

Paracetamol and NSAIDs

Paracetamol is effective in the management of postoperative pain and can be administered by the oral, intravenous and rectal routes. Regular use has been shown to reduce opioid requirements by 20–30% and, in combination with NSAIDs, the combination is more effective than NSAIDs alone. Paracetamol should therefore be prescribed to all postoperative patients except in the rare instance of contraindications.

NSAIDs are also an important component of multimodal postoperative analgesia. In combination with opioids, NSAIDs increase analgesia and have an opioid-sparing effect, reducing consumption, PONV and sedation. Their use is limited by their side-effect profile, including renal impairment, impaired platelet function with the potential for increased postoperative bleeding, peptic ulceration and bronchospasm in individuals at risk. Asthma is not an absolute contraindication, and previous use without adverse effects permits their use.

Ketamine

Ketamine is a noncompetitive agonist of the *N*-methyl-D-aspartic acid (NMDA) receptor. It has a role in multimodal analgesia for postoperative pain where it is used in low doses by intravenous infusion. It can also be used in trauma particularly in the emergency department or prehospital setting.

Neuropathic pain

Acute neuropathic pain in the postoperative period occurs in at least 1–3% of patients and is probably underestimated. It is a risk factor for chronic neuropathic pain, which may be reduced by early intervention. Expert advice should be sought as neuropathic pain does not respond well to conventional analgesia regimens. Intravenous lidocaine infusions and gabapentin reduce pain, and reduce opioid requirements. Tricyclic antidepressants are used on the basis that they are effective in chronic neuropathic pain, although their efficacy in reducing acute neuropathic pain has not been proven.

5.7 Summary

Postoperative pain control

Regional techniques
- Epidural analgesia (including local anaesthetics and opioids)
- Other catheter-based techniques; e.g., brachial plexus block, wound catheters

Parenteral analgesia
- Patient-controlled analgesia
- Opiates (morphine/pethidine), paracetamol
- Ketamine

Oral analgesia
- Paracetamol
- Nonsteroidal antiinflammatory drugs
- Weak opiates (tramadol, codeine)
- Strong opiates (morphine)

Neuropathic pain
- Tricyclic antidepressants
- Gabapentin
- Lidocaine

Postoperative nausea and vomiting

PONV affects 20–30% of patients. It is very distressing and is a significant factor in causing delayed discharge from day case surgical units. Risk factors include female sex, type of surgery (e.g., gynaecological and laparoscopic surgery), not smoking, a history of previous PONV or motion sickness, and opioid use. Anaesthetic technique is also important; inhalational anaesthetic agents, especially nitrous oxide, are associated with PONV, whereas intravenous anaesthesia with propofol has a lower incidence. Management of PONV centres on identifying high-risk patients and instituting preventative measures. Ondansetron and dexamethasone are particularly effective in the prophylaxis and treatment of PONV.

Day surgery

Facilities

Day surgery units provide an effective setting for surgery and their benefits rely on a well-defined and streamlined pathway. A hospital admission of only a few hours minimises the risk of hospital-acquired infection and early mobilisation reduces the risk of VTE. Patients like day surgery and prefer to recover from their procedure in the comfort of their own home. The economic benefit of shortening the postoperative length of stay in surgery relates to the closure of in-patient beds.

5.8 Summary

Clinical effectiveness of day surgery

- The surgical outcomes of a procedure performed on a day case basis or as an in-patient should, in theory, be identical, as it is the patient pathway and not the surgery that is different
- In practice, surgical outcomes from patients undergoing day surgery rather than in-patient surgery are often better, as day surgery patients are a preselected cohort of healthier patients with fewer comorbidities.

Cost–effectiveness of day surgery

- Same-day admission and discharge avoids the costs of an overnight in-patient bed
- Criteria-based pre-assessment reduces unnecessary investigations
- Dedicated day or ambulatory theatre lists maximise surgical throughput
- Protocol-based discharge with comprehensive patient information reduces unplanned hospital readmissions.

Day surgery facilities all require a day ward, operating theatres and a recovery area. Free-standing day units can be built within the community they serve. These have the advantage of minimising patient travelling distances but a lack of overnight facilities constrains both patient eligibility and case mix. Most hospitals now have dedicated day ward facilities. Day surgery theatres can either be separate or part of the existing theatre complex. Separate theatres can require duplication of specialised equipment but list cancellation is less likely from emergency or urgent elective cases.

Patient pathway

An efficient and effective ambulatory pathway (Fig. 5.7) requires the patient to arrive at the day unit on the day of surgery fully prepared for their procedure both physically and mentally. Day surgery remains an efficient and safe surgical process as long as only specified patients are accepted for operation. Each hospital has its own set of admission criteria dependent on the day unit facilities available and the type(s) of operations to be undertaken. Standalone units require more strictly defined criteria than hospital-integrated units to minimise unplanned overnight admissions requiring transfer to another hospital.

Preassessment of a patient's fitness for elective surgery is best performed by a specialised team of surgeons and anaesthetists. The role of the preassessment team is to allocate patients safely and accurately for day, 23-hour or in-patient surgery, as well as ensuring they have adequate social support. Preassessment provides an opportunity to answer patient questions and allay fears, and has been shown to reduce the rates of cancellation and non-attendance for surgery. The American Society of Anaesthesiologists' Physical Status Classification System (ASA status) is a simple and useful tool to summarise the comorbidity of a patient (Table 5.25).

Preassessment is usually offered to the patient at the surgical outpatient clinic. Where a number of surgical clinics are running concurrently, it is cost effective to offer patients a 'one-stop' preassessment service. Patients requiring more complex preassessment can be deferred to a planned preassessment clinic at a later date.

 5.9 Summary

Preassessment

- All elective surgical patients should be preassessed
- All patients undergoing a procedure suitable for day surgery should initially be defaulted to day surgery, and only if not clinically fit should they be allocated to an overnight stay
- The preassessment team should be empowered to allocate the appropriate length of stay to each individual patient
- Preassessment should be performed early in the patient pathway to avoid late cancellation for surgery. This can occur if the patient is found to be unfit for day surgery, with insufficient time to optimise their health.

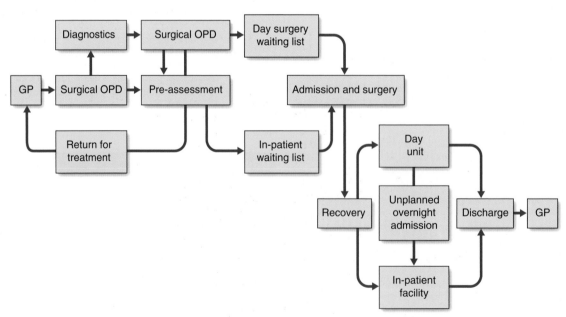

Fig. 5.7 The ambulatory patient pathway.

	Table 5.25 American Society of Anaesthesiologists' classification of physical status
ASA I	Normal healthy patients. Little or no risk for surgery
ASA II	Patients with mild systemic disease. Minimal risk during treatment. Examples include well-controlled noninsulin-dependent diabetes, mild hypertension, epilepsy or asthma
ASA III	Patients with severe systemic disease that limits activity but is not incapacitating. These patients need medical input before surgery. Examples include insulin-dependent diabetes or a history of myocardial infarction, congestive heart failure or cerebrovascular accident in the preceding 6 months
ASA IV	Patients with severe systemic disease limiting activity and is a constant threat to life. Elective surgery is contradicted and emergency surgery requires urgent medical input. Examples include unstable diabetes, hypertension and epilepsy or a recent myocardial infarction
ASA V	Patients who are moribund and not expected to survive more than 24 hours without an operation

Admission for day surgery

An efficient and effective ambulatory pathway requires the patient to arrive at the day unit on the day of surgery fully prepared for their procedure both physically and mentally (Fig. 5.8). Admission administration is minimal. Patients can sign their consent form to confirm they wish to proceed with their operation at any appropriate point before their procedure. If the patient signs the form in advance, a health professional involved in their care on the day should also sign it to confirm the patient still wishes to proceed. The diagnosis and planned surgery should be confirmed as still appropriate and the operation site marked. Although consent remains valid indefinitely unless withdrawn by the patient, many hospitals time-limit consent forms to 3 months after dating on safety grounds.

Discharge criteria

The decision as to when a patient is fit for discharge from the day unit should be taken after a postoperative visit by the surgeon and anaesthetist at the end of the operating list using agreed discharge criteria protocols (Table 5.26). A postoperative visit by the surgeon and anaesthetist is encouraged at the end of the operating list, but awaiting a member of the busy surgical team to discharge the patient usually results in delay.

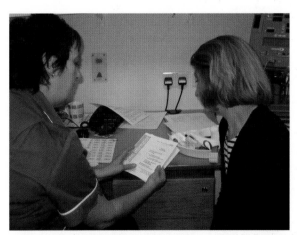

Fig. 5.8 Successful day surgery depends on careful explanation to the patient in advance of the surgical appointment.

Table 5.26 Discharge criteria for day surgery

- Vital signs stable and comparable to those recorded on admission
- Orientation to time, place and person
- Pain controlled and oral analgesics supplied
- Understands the use of medications issued and written information supplied
- Ability to dress and walk (if appropriate)
- Minimal nausea or vomiting
- Minimal wound bleeding
- Has a responsible adult to take them home
- Has a carer at home for the next 24 hours

The criterion of being able to take oral fluids before discharge has now been abandoned as encouragement to drink postoperatively increases the incidence of PONV. Oral intake remains necessary in selected patients such as those with diabetes. Voiding before discharge in patients with a low risk of urinary retention is also considered unnecessary.

When the discharge criteria are met, the patient and their carer should be offered both generic and procedure-specific written discharge information to encompass:

- Medication
- Wound care dressing renewal and suture removal (if required)
- Bathing or showering
- Return to normal activities including work, sexual activities and exercise
- Signs and symptoms that may indicate a problem
- Contact emergency telephone number and follow-up arrangements
- Travel after day surgery.

Patients may return to driving a minimum of 48 hours after general anaesthesia due to impaired reaction times. The procedure undertaken and its surgical site will also determine resumption of driving, which can only occur when the patient can safely perform an emergency stop. It is unclear after what time period patients can safely fly after surgery and it will vary with the complexity and extent of the procedure. Air travel where trapped gas or air may still remain within a body cavity as in laparoscopic or middle-ear procedures requires extra caution, as retained gas expands in flight due to the lower atmospheric pressure. The immobility associated with continuous travel of more than 3 hours within 4 weeks of surgery raises the risk of VTE.

 5.10 Summary

Principles of day surgery care

- Patient information
- Patient counselling
- Exclusion criteria
- Preassessment
- Optimisation of health
- Day of surgery admission
- Theatre scheduling
- Minimally invasive surgery
- Preemptive analgesia
- Regular analgesia
- Avoid opiate analgesia if possible
- Minimise postoperative nausea and vomiting
- Fluid therapy
- Early mobilisation
- Discharge criteria
- Discharge information
- Surgeon/anaesthetist-led discharge.

6

Mark A. Potter

Principles of the surgical management of cancer

Chapter contents

The biology of cancer 86

The management of patients with cancer 90

The biology of cancer

A neoplasm or new growth consists of a mass of transformed cells that does not respond in a normal way to growth regulatory systems. These cells serve no useful function and proliferate in an atypical and uncontrolled way to form a benign or malignant neoplasm. In normal tissues, cell replication and death are equally balanced and under tight regulatory control. However, when a cancer arises, this is generally due to genomic abnormalities that either increase cell replication or inhibit cell death (Fig. 6.1). The mechanisms by which this abnormal growth activity is induced (carcinogenesis) are complex and can be influenced in many ways.

6.1 Summary

Mechanisms of carcinogenesis

- Inherited genetic make up
- Diet
- Residential environment
- Work environment
- Life style choices
- Exposure to ionising radiation
- Exposure to carcinogens
- Viral infection
- Hormonal factors
- Increasing age.

These cellular insults give rise to alterations in the genomic DNA (mutations) that lead to cancer. Mutations can lead to disruption of the cell replication cycle at any point and lead to either activation or overexpression of oncogenes, or the inactivation of tumour suppressor genes, or a combination of the two (Table 6.1). Defining which genes have been mutated in the primary and metastatic cancers may ultimately help predict prognosis. For example, the amplification and over expression of *C-erbB-2* oncogene can give an indication of the aggressiveness of breast cancer. Identification of new genes and hence proteins involved in the formation of cancer will eventually lead to a greater understanding of the development of cancer, and new treatments (EBM 6.1).

Changes within the cellular genome occur frequently and do not necessarily result in cancer. Natural protective mechanisms repair errors in DNA replication; similarly, immune surveillance, simple wastage (i.e., loss of cells from the surface) and programmed cell death (apoptosis) destroy mutant cells before they proliferate. For persistence of growth and cancer formation, these protective mechanisms must break down (e.g., failure of mismatch repair due to mutations in genes such as *MLHI* and *MSH2*, or failure of apoptosis). The host's internal environment may also have a role in the 'promotion' of tumour growth. Examples are the 'hormone-dependent' cancers of the breast, prostate and endometrium, which require a 'correct' balance of hormonal secretion from the endocrine glands of the host for their continued growth. The natural history of a tumour is also related to its growth rate, which in turn is determined by the balance between cell division and cell death. Some tumours are slow-growing (e.g., prostate) and years may pass before deposits reach a size that threatens organ function. Others grow rapidly from a high rate of cell proliferation, and some expand rapidly (despite a relatively normal rate of cell proliferation) if cell death is slow to occur.

6.2 Summary

Factors leading to loss of cell cycle regulation

Growth of a cancer is due to loss of cell cycle regulation, which is dependent on:

- Increased cell proliferation
- Decreased programmed cell death (apoptosis)
- A combination of the two.

EBM **6.1 Cell cycle and cancer**

'Cancer cells are unstable and have many genetic alterations. Cell cycle regulators are frequently mutated in human tumours, increased expression of cyclin D1 is one of the most frequent abnormalities in human cancer occurring in 60% breast cancer, 40% colon cancer, 40% squamous cancer of head and neck. Many effective neoadjuvant and adjuvant treatments are cell cycle directed agents.'

Moon-Park T, Lee S-J. Cell cycle and cancer J Biochem Mol Biol. 2003;36:60 – 5. Williams GH, Stoeber K. The cell cycle and cancer. J Pathol. 2012;226:352–64.

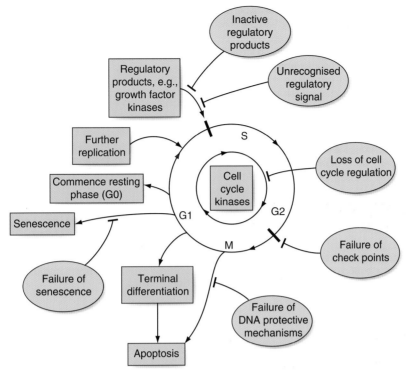

Fig. 6.1 Cell replication and cancer formation. Normal cell replication is under tight regulation by endogenous growth factors *(green boxes)*. Mutations that result in abnormal growth factor proteins can lead to cancer formation *(yellow ellipses)*.

Table 6.1 Examples of gene mutations that can lead to cancer formation	
Gene	**Point of action in cell cycle**
p16, CDK4, Rb	Cell cycle check point
MSH2, MLH1	DNA replication and repair
p53, fas	Apoptosis
E cadherin	Cellular adhesion
erb-A	Cellular differentiation
Ki-ras, erb-B	Regulatory kinases
TGF-β	Growth factors

Carcinogenesis

Neoplasms may be benign or malignant. The cells of benign tumours do not invade surrounding tissues but remain as a local conglomerate. The cells of malignant tumours can directly invade adjacent tissues or enter blood and lymphatic channels, to be deposited at remote sites. This malignant genotype develops as a result of the progressive acquisition of cancer mutations (by point mutation, chromosomal loss or translocation). This progressive accumulation of mutations may lead to the formation of cancer stem cells (Fig. 6.2). These cancer stem cells are

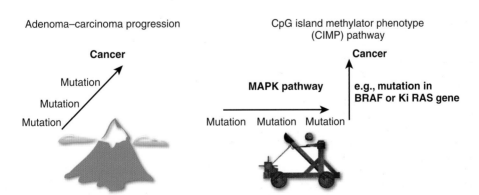

Fig 6.2 Accumulation of mutations. Accumulation of mutations may lead to a stepwise progression form normal cell to cancer cell as in the adenoma–carcinoma progression. Alternatively the mutations may be held in check until a specific mutation catapults the normal cell to a cancer cell as is believed to be the case in the CpG island methylator phenotype (CIMP) pathway. *MAPK*, mitogen-activated protein kinase.

pluripotent (i.e., able to give rise to more than one cell type) and produce cells that form the epithelial, structural and vascular components needed for cancer formation. However, cells arising from a cancer stem cell lack the normal response to the normal cell cycle controls and are, therefore, tumour forming. Such cancer stem cells could explain why cancers can relapse or metastasise. The acquisition of the malignant phenotype can be recognised histologically as a tumour develops from a benign adenoma through to a dysplastic lesion, and finally into an invasive carcinoma (Fig. 6.3). The concept of tumour progression from benign to malignant phenotype provides the rationale behind screening and early detection programmes. Removing benign or preinvasive lesions will prevent invasive disease.

 6.3 Summary

Carcinogenesis

- Acquisition of genetic mutations to produce pluripotent cancer stem cell which lack normal response to cell cycle controls
- Possible pathways
  - Chromosomal instability
  - Microsatellite instability
  - Epigenetic instability (e.g., promoter hypermethylation)

Invasion and metastasis

Benign tumours rarely threaten life but may cause a variety of cosmetic or functional abnormalities. In contrast, malignant tumours invade and relentlessly replace normal tissues, destroying supporting structures and disturbing function; they can spread to distant tissues (metastasise), eventually causing death. Metastases are cancer deposits similar in cell type to the original cancer found at remote (secondary) sites in the body.

The process of invasion and metastasis is complex (Fig. 6.4) and is dependent on the biology of the tumour. For metastases to occur it would appear that further mutations need to occur in

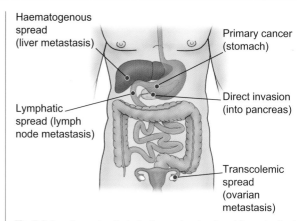

Fig. 6.4 Invasion and metastasis. Cancers invade adjacent tissues by direct infiltration. Spread to distant sites (metastasis) is via the bloodstream or lymphatics, or across body cavities (transcoelomic spread). Following initial growth, cancer cells lose local adherence and invade blood vessels. They are then transported via the bloodstream to adhere in distant organs and grow into secondary tumours.

the cancer cells (the metastatic signature). Some tumours metastasise earlier in their clinical course than others. This variation may depend on the tissue of origin of the primary tumour, but can also vary widely according to the phenotype of individual tumours. For example, cancer of the breast is thought to metastasise early, and micrometastases are often present but not detectable when the patient first presents. Some patients with apparently localised colorectal cancer are cured by radical surgery, but others receiving the same treatment deteriorate rapidly with metastatic disease.

The mechanisms that control invasion and metastasis are obscure (Fig. 6.5). A variety of enzymes and growth factors are secreted by the tumour cells (Table 6.2), their action facilitates tumour cell invasion and metastasis by degrading extracellular collagens, laminins and proteoglycans.

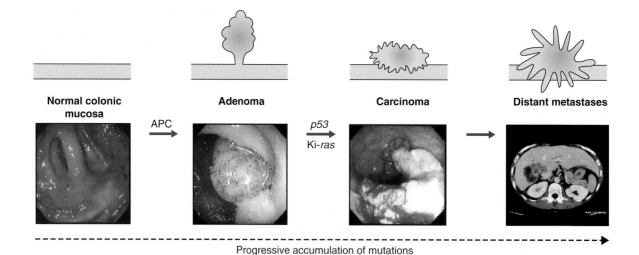

| Normal colonic mucosa | Adenoma | Carcinoma | Distant metastases |

APC → p53 Ki-*ras* →

Progressive accumulation of mutations

Enhanced by mutations in 'protective' genes, such as mismatch repair genes MSH2 and MLH1

Fig. 6.3 Colorectal adenoma–carcinoma progression. By the progressive acquisition of genetic mutations, normal colorectal epithelium forms a benign polyp, which can progress to an invasive or metastatic cancer.

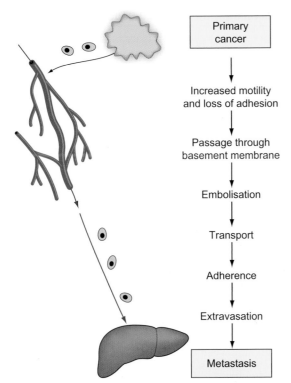

Fig. 6.5 Metastasis. Following initial growth, cancer cells lose local adherence and invade blood vessels. They are then transported via the bloodstream to adhere in distant organs and grow into secondary tumours.

Table 6.2 Mechanisms of invasion and metastasis	
Factors promoting invasion and metastasis	**Factors inhibiting invasion and metastasis**
Local pressure from expanding tumour	Angiostatin/endostatin
Increased motility of tumour cells	
Matrix metalloproteinases	
Endoproteinases	
Urokinase	
Plasminogen-activating factor	
Cathepsins	
Vascular endothelial growth factor	
Fibroblast growth factors	
Prostaglandins	

Clumps of cancer cells can embolise to distant tissues and form metastases. The location for the development of metastases could be a simple mechanical property with organs that have fine capillary beds, such as liver and lung, trapping circulating malignant cells. The survival of metastatic deposits depends on angiogenesis, which is mediated by an imbalance between positive and negative regulatory molecules released by the tumour cells and surrounding normal cells. Cancer cells also secrete prostaglandins, which can induce osteolysis and may promote the development of skeletal deposits.

Natural history and estimate of cure

Calculations based on an exponential model of tumour growth suggest that three-quarters of the lifespan of a tumour is spent in a 'pre-clinical' or occult stage, and that the clinical manifestations of the disease are limited to the final quarter. For cure, every malignant cell must be eradicated and no recurrent tumour should be present during the patient's lifetime, or evident at death. This rigid definition is rarely attainable and a normal duration of life without further clinical evidence of disease is generally accepted as evidence of cure, even though microscopic deposits of tumour may still be present.

Measuring and comparing the outcome(s) of cancer treatment can be difficult. Cancer survival data are not normally distributed but skewed, with many events happening early in the study period. Survival data are generally expressed as a time from a predefined starting point (e.g., surgery) to a similarly defined end point (e.g., disease relapse). Other time points may also be used and so a careful and precise definition of the time period used is essential. In addition, not all patients will have experienced the defined end point by the end of the study period. This phenomenon is known as censoring, and mean survival time will be unknown for a subset of the study group. Other confounding factors such as age and the stage of disease also need to be considered. Hence special methods of data interpretation are required. These various statistical methods of cancer data interpretation and comparison are termed survival analysis.

Measures used in survival analysis include: survival and hazard probabilities, Kaplan–Meier equations and graphs (Fig 6.6), Cox's proportional hazard models, univariate and multivariate analysis. Survival is the probability that a subject survives from the starting point to the end point of the study period. Hazard is the probability that the subject has a specified event at one particular moment in time. 'Cure' rates of individual cancers are assessed by survival rates at various times after treatment. Conventionally, 5- and 10-year intervals are used. Cure rates vary according to the aggressiveness of the disease and the success of treatment. In some patients with cancer (e.g., stomach and lung), metastases grow rapidly and cause death within a few years of clinical presentation. In others (e.g., breast and melanoma), many years may elapse before metastatic spread becomes evident and, even when metastases have occurred, life may be long. It is for this reason that 5-year survival rates cannot provide a satisfactory estimate of cure for all tumours.

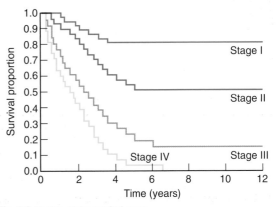

Fig. 6.6 Kaplan–Meier survival curve.

The management of patients with cancer

The goals of treating cancer can be broadly grouped as prevention, cure and palliation. Prevention seeks to modify behaviour to prevent cancer formation. For example, the avoidance of smoking or direct sunlight may prevent the formation of lung or skin cancer. Taking a small dose of aspirin on a regular basis may protect against colorectal cancer (chemoprevention). When a cancer has formed, treatment is aimed at cure for early-stage disease. When a cancer is locally advanced or has metastasised, the chance of cure reduces. In cancers that are felt to be incurable, treatment is then aimed at palliation of troublesome symptoms.

Screening

If cancer can be detected before it causes symptoms, then it is generally smaller, has less chance of having metastasised and is therefore more amenable to cure. Detecting benign lesions with malignant potential, preinvasive cancer, and invasive malignancy before it becomes symptomatic is called screening (Fig. 6.7). Screening is expensive and its effectiveness in relation to cost must be critically evaluated before routine use (EBM 6.2). Screening is most effective when targeted at specific risk groups and when the screening test has a high level of acceptability to the target population. For successful screening, the test used must be able to detect the cancer at a stage when earlier treatment will lead to fewer deaths from the cancer. In any given population, the likelihood of a cancer being present is generally low (<1%); hence, the test must be sensitive to detect these relatively rare lesions. The test must also be specific (i.e., have a low false-positive rate); otherwise, individuals will undergo unnecessary investigation or inappropriate treatment. Finally, the proposed treatment of a cancer patient detected by a screening programme must be effective. In the UK, cervical cytology is offered to women on a 3-yearly basis until the age of 60, and mammographic screening (Fig. 6.8) is offered to women between 50 and 64 years on a 3-yearly basis. Other tumour types that might be amenable to screening are listed with their relevant screening tests in Table 6.3.

Screening for inherited cancer

Some forms of cancer can be inherited; for example, about 5% of patients with colorectal cancer develop the disease because of an autosomal dominant inherited mutation either in the *APC* gene (polyposis coli) or in the mismatch repair genes such as *MSH2* and *MLH1* (hereditary nonpolyposis colorectal cancer, or HNPCC). Alternatively, about 5% of women develop breast cancer as a result of an autosomal dominant inherited mutation on the *BRCA1* or *BRCA2* genes. In these instances, closely related family members should be offered the appropriate tests to detect these specific mutations. Carriers of the mutation can then be offered prophylactic surgery, e.g., bilateral mastectomy (for *BRCA1* and *BRCA2* carriers).

EBM 6.2 Recent screening trials

'Studies in Sweden in the late 1980s established that screening for breast cancer allowed for early detection and improved cancer-specific survival. Recent studies have shown that these benefits can be achieved in the context of national screening programmes and for other cancers such as colorectal cancer.'

Blanks RG, et al. Br Med J 2000; 321:665–9.
Further reading on the breast cancer screening debate: US Preventative Services Task Force. Screening for breast cancer: US Preventive Services Task Force recommendation statement. Ann Intern Med 2009; 151:716–26 and related articles pp 727 and 738.
MG Marmot, et al. The benefits and harms of breast cancer screening: an independent review. Br J Cancer, 2013;108:2205–40.

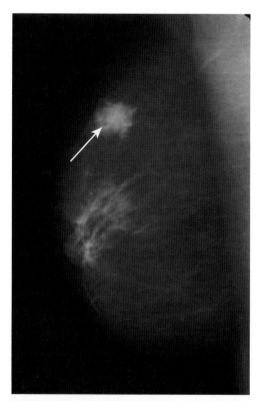

Fig. 6.8 Single mammogram showing malignancy (*arrow*) in peripheral breast tissue. (Courtesy Mr M. Barber, Consultant Breast Surgeon, Western General Hospital, Edinburgh.)

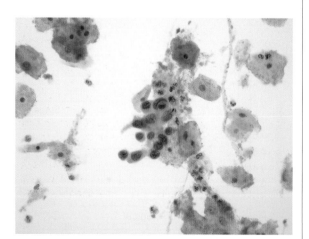

Fig. 6.7 Cervical cytology. A group of severely dyskaryotic squamous cells in a ThinPrep liquid-based cytology preparation. (Courtesy Prof. A.R.W. Williams, University of Edinburgh.)

6.4 Summary

Criteria for screening programmes (http://www.screening.nhs.uk/screening)

A test for use in cancer screening must be:

- Sensitive
- Specific
- Acceptable
- Able to detect cancer at a stage when early treatment is beneficial
- Cost-effective.

Table 6.3 Examples of cancer types that are or could be the subject of screening programmes

Cancer	Screening test
Breast	Mammography
Cervix	Smear cytology
Colon	Faecal occult blood test and flexible sigmoidoscopy or colonoscopy
Prostate	Prostate-specific antigen (PSA)

The cancer patient's journey

The management of cancer frequently involves surgery, whether it is radical for cure or palliative to relieve distressing symptoms. Modern cancer management is organised around a multidisciplinary team approach. (Table 6.4). Good communication with the patient and between team members forms the basis of optimal patient care. The aim is to tailor the best possible treatment for each individual patient based on current medical evidence.

There are several key stages in the management of the patient with cancer, which can be regarded as a journey from the onset of symptoms to definitive treatment and subsequent follow-up (Fig. 6.9). The exact sequence of events may differ from one patient to the next. For example, it may be necessary to remove the tumour to obtain full information on staging before an adequate treatment plan can be evolved. Patients usually begin their

Table 6.4 Multidisciplinary team involved in cancer care

Medical staff

- Surgeon
- Physician
- Radiologist
- Oncologist
- Radiotherapist
- Palliative care physician
- General practitioner

Nursing staff

- Ward nurse
- Chemotherapy nurse
- Clinical nurse specialist
- Hospice nurse

Paramedical staff

- Oncology dietitian
- Physiotherapist
- Occupational therapist
- Clergy

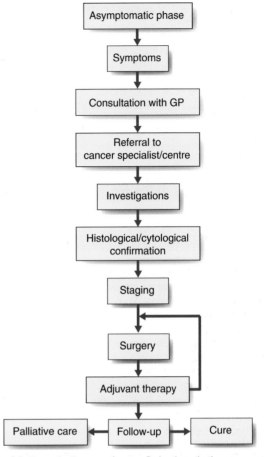

Fig. 6.9 The patient's cancer journey. During the patient's management, several key stages are encountered, from symptoms to diagnosis and treatment.

'cancer journey' by deciding that a new symptom or symptoms are serious enough to merit consultation.

Symptoms that may initiate a patient's 'cancer journey'

Local effects

A tumour that lies on the surface of the body may become visible, change in shape or pigmentation, bleed, or discharge mucus or pus. A hollow viscus or duct may be obstructed by a tumour, e.g., a bronchus (causing pulmonary collapse), a segment of bowel (causing intestinal obstruction) or the bile duct or pancreatic duct (causing jaundice or pancreatitis). A tumour within a closed space may cause pressure symptoms such as increased intracranial pressure (intracerebral tumour). Invasion of an organ by a tumour may compromise its normal functions and cause organ failure. Invasion of tissues such as the pancreas, bone or nerves can cause severe pain. A cancer can also mimic the pain of benign disease: for example, dyspeptic symptoms in stomach cancer.

Systemic effects

Weight loss is often the key symptom that may alert to the possibility of malignant disease and some patients become severely emaciated. This syndrome is known as cancer cachexia, and is clinically characterised by anorexia, severe weight loss, lethargy, anaemia and oedema.

The secretory products of some tumours can produce characteristic clinical syndromes appropriate to the organ of origin. Thus, a tumour of the adrenal cortex may secrete excess corticosteroid (Cushing's syndrome), a parathyroid tumour may secrete excess parathormone (hypercalcaemia) and an islet cell tumour of the pancreas may secrete excess insulin (hypoglycaemia). On the other hand, secretory products may be inappropriate to the site of a tumour. Such 'ectopic' secretion occurs predominantly in tumours of neuroendocrine origin, and produces a variety of endocrine syndromes.

Consultation with the GP

Distressing or dramatic presenting symptoms such as rectal bleeding normally result in prompt referral to a hospital specialist. Frequently, the initial presenting complaint (e.g., general malaise) is nonspecific. Other symptoms, such as epigastric pain, are common complaints in general practice and are usually associated with benign disease. It can be difficult for the GP to decide which patient needs urgent referral. Such nonspecific symptoms may result in several consultations to their GP. Persistence of such nonspecific symptoms should raise the index of suspicion towards neoplastic disease and lead to specialist referral.

 6.5 Summary

Symptoms that should initiate investigation

- Weight loss
- Rectal bleeding/melaena
- Haemoptysis/persistent cough
- Haematuria
- Breast lump
- Dysphagia/dyspepsia
- Persistent headache
- Persistent nonspecific symptoms.

Referral to a specialist/cancer centre

Patients with a suspected diagnosis of cancer are often referred to the surgical outpatient clinic appropriate to the probable site of tumour origin. It is important to spend time undertaking a full and detailed history and examination as well as addressing patient anxiety, providing a clear management plan. Other multidisciplinary team members, such as the clinical nurse specialist, can assist greatly. Increasingly, 'one-stop' clinics are available, allowing the initial consultation and investigations to be performed at one attendance, such as for suspected breast cancer.

Investigations

Investigations serve two main purposes. First, they are aimed at histological or cytological confirmation of the diagnosis of cancer. Second, they are used to assess the extent of the primary disease (local invasion) and to look for evidence of metastatic spread, known as 'staging' the disease.

Diagnostic investigations

Initial investigations to make the diagnosis should proceed in a logical order, starting with simple blood tests and progressing through more complex imaging investigations, with the ultimate aim of obtaining histological or cytological confirmation of the diagnosis (Table 6.5). Serum tumour markers such as carcinoembryonic antigen (CEA), prostate-specific antigen (PSA) and cancer antigen 125 (CA 125) can prove useful for diagnosis and monitoring treatment but their sensitivity and specificity are limited and a normal tumour marker level does not exclude the diagnosis of cancer. Plain radiology may demonstrate a soft tissue tumour, e.g., tumours of the lung or bone, but for tumours of the stomach or intestine, contrast studies are necessary. For some deep-seated tumours, e.g., those of the pancreas or brain, other methods of imaging such as angiography, radioactive scintigraphy and ultrasonography (US), computed tomography (CT) (Fig. 6.10), magnetic resonance imaging (MRI) and positron emission tomography (PET) are required. Neoplastic disease can be

---

Table 6.5 Investigations for the diagnosis of cancer

Blood tests

- *Haematology* Full blood count (FBC)
- *Biochemistry* Liver function tests (LFTs), tumour markers

Radiology

- Plain x-rays, chest x-ray
- Contrast-enhanced, barium enema
- Ultrasound, including endoscopic ultrasound
- Computed tomography (CT)
- Computed tomography/positron emission tomography (CT/PET)
- Magnetic resonance imaging (MRI)

Endoscopy

- Upper gastrointestinal tract endoscopy
- Colonoscopy
- Endoscopic retrograde cholangiopancreatography (ERCP)

Cytology/histology

- Body fluids, e.g., sputum and urine
- Fine-needle aspiration (FNA), e.g., breast and thyroid cancer
- Radiologically guided FNA
- Endoscopic brushings or biopsy

Operative

- Examination under anaesthetic and biopsy
- Excision biopsy, e.g., lymph node
- Diagnostic laparoscopy and biopsy
- Laparoscopic ultrasound

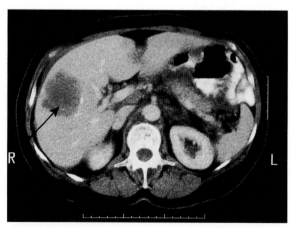

Fig. 6.10 Staging computed tomography of the abdomen showing a large solitary liver metastasis (*arrow*) in a patient with colorectal cancer.

confirmed cytologically, e.g., by the demonstration of malignant cells in secretions, in washings from hollow viscera or in needle aspirates. Biopsies obtained at gastrointestinal endoscopy can provide material for histology, as can US- or CT-guided Tru-cut needle biopsies. It may be necessary to perform an examination under anaesthetic or diagnostic laparoscopy (Fig. 6.11) to obtain suitable diagnostic material. In general, a patient treatment plan cannot be formulated until histological or cytological diagnosis has been made. However, there are circumstances in which this is not possible (e.g., in some pancreatic cancers), and radiological evidence may be relied upon instead.

Staging investigations

Staging investigations will depend on the site of the primary cancer and the relevant common sites of metastasis. Local invasion can be assessed (e.g., oesophageal cancer) by endoscopic ultrasound or by CT and MRI. Metastatic spread can be determined by numerous investigations, e.g., bone scan, CT, PET, MRI and laparoscopy. When combined with CT, PET can be a particularly powerful way to detect metastatic disease (Fig. 6.12). Often, staging investigations will have been undertaken as part of the diagnostic process, e.g., CT.

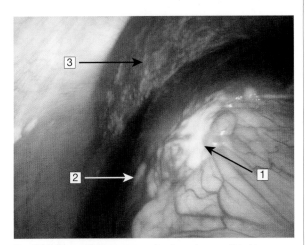
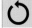

Fig. 6.11 Diagnostic laparoscopy showing primary gallbladder cancer invading the omentum (*1*), a liver metastasis (*2*) and peritoneal metastases (*3*).

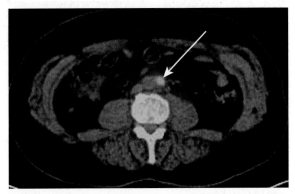

Fig. 6.12 Computed tomography/positron emission tomography (CT/PET) scan highlighting metastatic paraaortic lymph node. Fused CT/PET image clearly showing metastatic node (*arrow*). (Courtesy Dr J Brush, Consultant Radiologist, Western General Hospital, Edinburgh.)

Staging defines the extent of the disease, assesses its likely prognosis and permits the development of an appropriate multidisciplinary treatment plan. The Union for International Cancer Control (UICC) has described a system of staging (TNM) in which three components are assessed. These are the extent of the primary tumour (T), the presence and extent of metastases in regional lymph nodes (N), and the presence of distant metastases (M). The addition of numbers to each component indicates the extent of the disease within that category. The bigger the number, the more advanced the disease.

In the initial TNM system, only clinical, radiological and endoscopic investigations were used. Such clinical staging defines the extent of disease and may be used to plan the initial management of a patient but, without histological confirmation, can sometimes be highly inaccurate. For example, the palpability of regional lymph nodes is a poor indicator of their involvement by tumour. Impalpable nodes may still contain metastases, whereas palpable nodes may be the seat of reactive hyperplasia (sinus histiocytosis). Small tumour deposits in viscera and bones cannot be detected by routine radiology, and thus many patients who appear to have localised disease on clinical and radiological grounds, may have unrecognised microscopic tumour deposits. For this reason, the TNM system has been modified to include a postsurgical pathological classification, denoted as pTNM. In some skin tumours, and in cancer of the bladder and large bowel, histological assessment of the depth of tumour penetration provides important information about the extent and prognosis of the disease. Excision of regional lymph nodes may provide additional information. Staging has its limitations and such systems are therefore used to provide a 'best-guess' scenario upon which patient treatment is based.

Prognosis is also affected by the biological characteristics of a tumour. The degree of nuclear and cellular atypia, the extent of lymphocytic infiltration, inflammatory response, and perineural and vascular invasion all influence outcome. These factors, as well as biochemical indices (e.g., oestrogen receptor status in breast cancer), and genetic profile (EBM 6.3) can be used in the management plan.

⟳ 6.6 Summary

Purpose of staging

- Define the extent of disease
- Assess likely prognosis
- Allow the development of a treatment plan

EBM **6.3 How genetic profiling could indicate prognosis**

'Knowledge of genetic alterations in disease is always advancing. Increasing knowledge about genetic alterations in diseases, particularly cancer, highlight the crucial role of epigenetic alterations—such as DNA methylation—for future diagnosis, prognosis and prediction of response to therapies.'

Heyn H, Esteller M. DNA methylation profiling in the clinic: applications and challenges. Nat Rev Genet. 2012;13:679–92.

Treatment

Following initial diagnosis, staging, and multidisciplinary team discussion, the patient may proceed to surgery, where the primary tumour, surrounding tissue and locoregional lymph nodes are excised and then sent for histopathology. The clinical staging is translated into histopathological staging which facilitates multidisciplinary treatment planning with the maximum available information. Improved staging, progress in chemotherapy agents and regimens, and improved surgical techniques have widened treatment to patients with advanced disease and resulted in improvement in survival rates.

Benign tumours

A benign tumour is cured by local excision provided sufficient surrounding tissue is excised to ensure its complete removal. Some benign tumours (e.g., parotid pleomorphic adenoma) extend beyond their apparent macroscopic limits and removal of the involved segment of the gland or organ is required.

Malignant tumours

A radical cancer operation implies complete removal of the tissue bearing the tumour, together with a margin of unaffected surrounding tissue. Sometimes, it is necessary to give preoperative radiotherapy and/or chemotherapy to 'downstage' the primary cancer to allow radical excision and give a better chance of cure (e.g., some advanced rectal cancers, Fig. 6.13). The use of therapeutic modalities such as chemotherapy, hormonal treatment, immunotherapy or radiotherapy prior to definitive surgical treatment of the primary cancer is known as neoadjuvant therapy. In some tumours, there is sequential spread, first locally, then to lymph nodes, and then to distant organs such as the liver and lungs. In this situation, careful local removal, along with the locoregional lymph nodes ('en bloc resection') can be curative. However, the spread of a tumour may be more unpredictable and the removal of local lymph nodes is simply to provide information for the stage of the cancer, rather than being of true therapeutic benefit. The management of regional lymph nodes thus depends on the site and type of the tumour. With some tumours (e.g., gastrointestinal tract) regional lymph nodes are resected routinely on the basis that sequential spread may have occurred. In other tumours (e.g., breast cancer and melanoma), lymph node sampling or sentinel node biopsy (the lymph node closest to the cancer) may be more appropriate, especially if en bloc lymph node resection may be associated with significant morbidity (e.g., limb lymphedema). This information (nodal status) is then used to decide adjuvant treatment (EBM 6.4).

EBM	6.4 Sentinel node biopsy

Sentinel Lymph node biopsy in breast cancer has emerged as a method for breast cancer staging to reduce morbidity such as arm lymphoedema. However there is still debate as to the accuracy of the technique.

Bonnema J, van de Velde CJH. Sentinel lymph node biopsy in breast cancer. Ann Oncol. 2002;13:1531–7.
Lyman GH et al. Sentinel lymph node biopsy for patients with early-stage breast cancer: American Society of Clinical Oncology Clinical Practice Guideline Update J Clin Oncol. 2014;32:1365 – 83.

Complete radical excision, confirmed by histological examination carries a high chance of surgical cure in the absence of lymph node metastasis, such as with regional lymphadenectomy for colon cancer (Fig. 6.14). During any cancer operation, care must be taken to avoid spillage of malignant cells, which may cause cancer recurrence. In some sites (e.g., testis), it is usual to ligate the draining vessels before the tumour is mobilised so as to minimise shedding of malignant cells into the circulation. Overall, a careful and meticulous approach to all aspects of the operation is vital to improve the outcome of surgery.

Data suggest that surgery performed in 'high volume' specialist centres produces better survival rates than surgery in nonspecialist centres. Hence, surgeons are increasingly subspecialised and concentrate on performing selected operations (EBM 6.5). One of the recent advances in surgical techniques is minimally invasive surgery (sometimes referred to as keyhole or laparoscopic surgery). The trauma related to surgery can be significantly reduced using minimally invasive surgery thereby enhancing the postoperative recovery. These techniques are being increasingly employed in the treatment of cancer. Early results suggested an increased risk of surgical wound metastases; however, it is now recognised

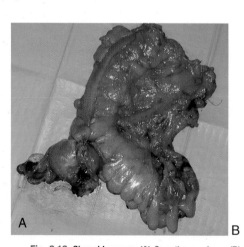

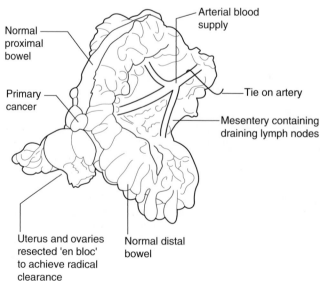

Fig. 6.13 Sigmoid cancer. (A) Operative specimen. **(B)** Diagram shows the structures that have been removed with this en bloc resection.

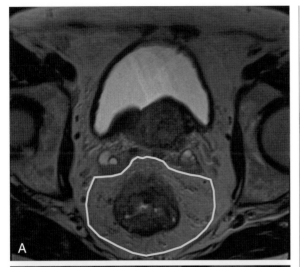

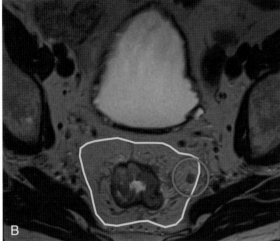

Fig. 6.14 Neoadjuvant therapy. (A) Magnetic resonance imaging (MRI) of rectal cancer where the resection margin (yellow line) is not threatened and surgery with no preoperative radiotherapy is required. **(B)** MRI of a rectal cancer where the resection margin is threatened by and involved lymph node (encircled in red), and neoadjuvant radiotherapy is recommended.

EBM 6.5 Improved outcome with subspecialisation

'The treatment outcomes for cancer patients have improved with the advent of subspecialisation among cancer surgeons (e.g., specialist breast surgeons for breast cancer, colorectal surgeons for colorectal cancer etc.). This benefit seems to be due to the integration with multidisciplinary teams rather than simply due to case volume.'

McArdle CS, Hole DJ. Influence of volume and specialization on survival following surgery for colorectal cancer. Br J Surg. 2004;91:610–7.
Parks RW, et al. Benefits of specialisation in the management of pancreatic cancer: results of a Scottish population-based study Br J Cancer 2004;91:459–65.
Markar SR et al. Volume-outcome relationship in surgery for esophageal malignancy: systematic review and meta-analysis 2000-2011. J Gastrointest Surg. 2012;16:1055 – 63.
Dikkena JL et al. Effect of hospital volume on postoperative mortality and survival after oesophageal and gastric cancer surgery in the Netherlands between 1989 and 2009. Eur J Cancer 2012;48:1004–13.

EBM 6.6 Evidence for laparoscopic colorectal surgery

'Laparoscopic surgery for colorectal cancer allows for shorter hospital stay and is as good as the open technique in terms of short-term survival and recurrence rates.'

MRC CLASSIC trial. Lancet. 2005;365:1718–26.
COLOR trial. Lancet Oncol. 2005;6:477–84.
Laparoscopic versus open surgery for rectal cancer (COLOR II): short-term outcomes of a randomised, phase 3 trial. The Colorectal cancer Laparoscopic or Open Resection II (COLOR II) Study Group. Lancet Oncol. 2013;14:210–8.
COST trial. N Engl J Med. 2004;350:2050–9.
MRC CLASSIC five-year follow up. Br J Surg. 2010;97:1638–45.

6.7 Summary

Strategy for cancer surgery

- Possible neoadjuvant therapy to render primary cancer operable
- Radical surgery for primary cancer
- Treatment of lymph nodes: radical excision (e.g., gastric cancer) or lymph node sampling (e.g., breast cancer)
- Adjuvant therapy based on pathological staging after surgery (e.g., chemotherapy for lymph node metastases)
- Radical surgery for distant metastases (e.g., excision of liver or lung metastases)
- Palliative surgery for the relief of symptoms if no cure possible.

that minimally invasive techniques can be used in cancer treatment with no detriment to their outcome (EBM 6.6).

Adjuvant treatment

The multidisciplinary team can plan the need for further therapy after accurate pathological staging of the cancer. It is sometimes not possible to remove all local disease and early systemic dissemination may have occurred. Thus an adjuvant to surgery is needed to provide both local and systemic control. Adjuvant chemotherapy may prevent local recurrence and distant metastasis, and is commonly used in patients with colorectal or breast cancer with lymph node involvement. Adjuvant radiotherapy or chemotherapy must not be regarded as a safety net for poor surgical practice. In some cancers, such as ovarian cancer, transcoelomic spread occurs early and radical surgery is impossible, but surgical reduction of the tumour burden may contribute to the success of systemic treatment, which is aimed at controlling the disease.

Achieving a balance between the relief of symptoms and the morbidity induced by radical cancer therapy is often difficult, and quality of life is as important as the duration of survival. Chemotherapy is potentially toxic and may result in morbidity and poor quality of life.

The success of adjuvant chemotherapy is dependent on the histological type of cancer. Drugs are given in combination over a variable period and toxicity, such as mouth ulcers, diarrhoea, weakness and alopecia, is common but generally tolerable. In colorectal and breast cancer, the likelihood of death from recurrent cancer is reduced by 20–30% in patients with evidence of lymph node metastasis.

Radiotherapy is normally administered to reduce the chances of local recurrence rather than of distant metastasis. It may be given prior to surgery or postoperatively where the chances of local recurrence are thought to be high (e.g., resection specimen margins are involved with tumour). When tumours are relatively radiosensitive, radiotherapy can reduce the need for radical surgery and a more cosmetic, conservative operation is possible (e.g., lumpectomy and radiotherapy instead of mastectomy).

The impact of intensive chemo- and radiotherapy on growth in children can be significant. The potential for cure, which is possible in many childhood malignancies, has to be balanced against the long-term morbidity of growth failure.

Other modes of adjuvant therapy include less toxic therapies, such as administration of the antioestrogen tamoxifen in women with breast cancer (hormone therapy). Experimental models have shown that monoclonal antibodies, synthetic peptides, antisense oligonucleotides and soluble adhesion molecules can inhibit tumour growth (immunotherapy). These treatments use immune modulators to induce, enhance or inhibit the immunological reaction and can be used in addition to adjuvant chemotherapy in breast and colorectal carcinoma. Gene therapy carries the potential to restore the function of altered tumour suppressor molecules. Matrix metalloproteinase (MMP) inhibitors and angiogenesis inhibitors offer other potential avenues for novel anticancer therapy.

6.8 Summary

Principles of surgery for cancer

- Multidisciplinary team approach
- Accurate pre- and postoperative staging
- En bloc radical surgery
- Appropriate pre- and postoperative adjuvant therapy
- Good communication with patient and relatives
- Audit of results.

Surgery for metastases

Advances in surgical technique and improved chemotherapeutic agents have opened the possibility of submitting a small number of patients (10–20%) with metastatic disease to surgical treatment. Resection of colorectal liver metastases in selected patients has been shown to result in 30 – 40% 5-year survival rates. Following multidisciplinary discussion, patients are increasingly offered liver or lung resection for treatment of metastatic disease, normally in conjunction with second- and third-line chemotherapy (EBM 6.7).

EBM 6.7 Resection of metastases

'The liver represents a common site for metastasis. Better patient selection and surgical techniques have led to improved outcomes with 5 and 10 year overall survival rates of 40% and 20%, respectively.'

Frankel TL, D'Angelica MI. Hepatic resection for colorectal metastases. J Surg Oncol. 2014; 109:2–7.

Follow-up

In most patients with tumours amenable to surgical treatment, it is important to check subsequently that there is no local recurrence of disease and that the patient is symptom-free (EBM 6.8). Patients are reviewed more frequently in the early months after surgery to detect and treat noncancer-related postoperative complications, and since recurrence is most likely at this time. Patients undergoing palliative surgery will have different follow-up requirements from those undergoing curative surgery. It is often difficult to detect recurrence or metastasis in the asymptomatic postoperative patient, and the value of routine investigation in the detection of metastatic disease has been questioned. Once the primary therapy has been undertaken, some patients may be discharged back to their GP for follow-up with re-referral to the multidisciplinary team as necessary.

EBM 6.8 Need for follow-up

'The value of 'aggressive' follow-up of postoperative cancer patients is controversial. Some have shown that systematic postoperative follow-up using a variety of techniques such as tumour markers, regular radiology and endoscopy can increase the number of patients with recurrence that is amenable to further surgery with curative intent.'

Castells A, et al. Dis Colon Rectum 1998; 41:713–4.; Lewis RA. Br J Gen Pract. 2009;59:525–32.

Palliation of advanced cancer

The management of patients with incurable disease involves the relief of distressing symptoms (palliative care). The palliative care physician and the associated team play an important and specialist part in the overall management of the cancer patient. The terminal stages of malignancy can be prolonged, and pain and other distressing symptoms are common. Effective palliation may require local and/or systemic adjuvant therapy to induce tumour regression (e.g., reducing pressure effects of cerebral metastases). Surgery can be employed to resect symptomatic metastases or bypass a malignant obstruction. When a palliative operation is performed, the patient and family should understand that its object is to prevent additional suffering, and not to attempt cure. Medical treatments are used to relieve symptoms such as pain, nausea, depression and infections. A wide range of analgesic and narcotic drugs is available to relieve pain. The choice depends on the type of pain, its severity and the stage of the illness. The aim is to achieve complete analgesia without impairing mental clarity or inducing side effects. It is essential never to let the patient wait for the next dose of analgesic. The psychological, social and ethical aspects of care for both the patient and the family should also be addressed.

Prognosis and counselling

Honesty is the basis of the doctor–patient relationship and it is almost always best to tell patients that they have cancer. In so doing, one should reveal as much of the truth as the patient wishes to have or can understand. In some cultures this may be difficult; close relatives may want to shield the patient from distressing information. Tact is required to ensure patient autonomy. When therapy is undertaken with curative intent, this should be emphasised as the goal. Radical cancer surgery followed by radiotherapy or chemotherapy can be very arduous, and maintenance of morale is essential. When palliation is the objective, it is important not to remove the patient's hope, as 'the end of hope is the beginning of death'. It is usually best to speak to patients in a quiet, private room with one of the nursing staff present.

Care of the dying

Death from malignant disease is usually a gradual process of withdrawal. A sympathetic doctor can greatly help patients and their relatives. A dying patient must never feel abandoned in a surgical ward, and doctors and nursing staff must be prepared to spend time to help the patient die with dignity. Normally, the palliative care team should be involved early since most patients may wish to die at home with appropriate support, or in a hospice, where the level of quiet and care is appropriate to the situation. Palliative care of children with terminal malignant disease is as important and children's hospices will provide great support, not only to affected children, but to their families.

Euan J. Dickson

Trauma and multiple injury

Chapter contents

Introduction 98

Mechanisms of injury 99

Injury severity 99

Trauma scoring systems 100

Trauma systems, centres and teams 101

Shock 102

Resuscitation 102

Imaging 105

Critical decision-making 106

Surgery for trauma 107

Junctional zone trauma 111

Introduction

The importance of trauma

Trauma is the leading cause of death in developed countries in individuals under the age of 40 years. It also ranks third behind cardiovascular disease and cancer as a major cause of death across all age groups worldwide. The morbidity in survivors of major injury has a significant impact on healthcare resources. Trauma is a global epidemic and it places an additional burden on society, as this is often a disease of the young and economically productive. Most preventable deaths following trauma in the United Kingdom occur following failure to recognise, and therefore treat, intracavitary haemorrhage.

The 'golden hour'

The term 'golden hour' was coined by R. Adams Cowley, a US Army surgeon, to describe the period immediately after major injury during which prompt and coordinated care within a trauma system could save lives. In 1975 he stated, 'the first hour after injury will largely determine a critically injured person's chances for survival'. While there is no evidence to support a strictly defined period of 60 minutes from injury to definitive care, it remains a useful concept to reinforce the time-critical nature of early deaths in particular.

The 'platinum 10 minutes'

An analogous concept, the 'platinum 10 minutes', serves to focus on significantly limiting scene times by the prehospital team. The absolute priority is to address immediately life-threatening physiology followed by rapid transport to definitive care. This 'scoop and run' approach includes airway control and temporisation of massive bleeding, rather than the 'stay and play' philosophy, which often results in futile attempts at on-scene 'stabilisation' in the face of rapidly deteriorating physiology.

Temporal distribution of trauma deaths

Death following major injury is classically described as having a trimodal distribution.

Immediate deaths occur within *seconds to minutes after injury*. They are usually the result of catastrophic injury to the brain or high spinal cord, or following exsanguination due to disruption of the great vessels. These deaths are generally considered unsurvivable. Strategies to impact on this cohort should focus on effective prevention policy including seat-belt legislation and gun control.

Early deaths occur within *minutes to hours after injury*. They are often the consequence of potentially survivable shock physiology including tension pneumothorax, cardiac tamponade and massive haemorrhage from thoracic or abdominal vascular injury. Trauma systems, which limit time from injury to definitive care through rapid transport, assessment and intervention, dramatically improve survival and reduce subsequent morbidity in this cohort.

Late deaths occur *days to weeks after injury* as a result of multi-organ failure or sepsis. Early optimal management, including appropriate and aggressive resuscitation, and meticulous continuing care may help to reduce this peak.

This classic description is controversial. The introduction and development of trauma systems has had a profound effect on the cause, and therefore timing, of death following injury. Improvements in prehospital care, resuscitation, trauma surgery strategies and critical care have changed the epidemiology of trauma deaths to a predominantly bimodal distribution. The first peak (immediate deaths) is not impacted by these developments. The second peak (early deaths) has reduced in magnitude through rapid and effective care. The third peak (late deaths) is no longer recognised, and although late deaths still occur they do not form a cluster as originally described.

7.1 Summary

Background

- Trauma is a global epidemic and the leading cause of death in the young
- The 'golden hour' emphasises the time-dependent nature of managing major injury
- The 'platinum 10 minutes' emphasises the 'scoop and run' approach to prehospital care
- Trauma systems have changed the classic trimodal distribution of deaths to a bimodal model.

Mechanisms of injury

Trauma is characterised by structural alteration or physiological imbalance as a result of energy transfer from an external agent to the host. The mechanism of injury may be broadly subdivided into blunt, penetrating and miscellaneous trauma. This distinction is critical for several reasons. Firstly, the anatomical and physiological consequences of different mechanisms of injury to a given body region or organ system vary significantly. Secondly, the investigation and management of these injuries is largely determined by injury mechanism. Thirdly, injury patterns and associations are determined largely by the wounding mechanism.

Blunt trauma

Blunt trauma occurs as a direct result of crushing or shearing mechanisms.

Crushing mechanisms may involve three phases of energy transfer: direct impact between object and patient (e.g., striking the patient with a blunt object), impact between patient and surrounding environment (e.g., contact with the road surface after a motor vehicle versus pedestrian collision) and contact between internal organs and supporting structures (e.g., brain striking the skull).

Shearing mechanisms are usually deceleration injuries between the mobile portion of an organ and an adjacent fixed portion (e.g., the descending thoracic aorta shears at the ligamentum arteriosum).

Mechanisms of injury resulting in blunt trauma include:

- motor vehicle collision
- motor vehicle versus pedestrian collision
- fall from height
- interpersonal assault.

Penetrating trauma

Penetrating trauma occurs when an object transfers energy to the tissue by passing through it. Although wounding objects do not always follow a straight trajectory, penetrating injuries are usually more predictable than blunt force mechanisms.

Mechanisms of injury resulting in penetrating trauma include stab wounds from a sharp implement, most commonly a knife, and from gunshot wounds.

A basic understanding of ballistics is helpful in managing gunshot wounds. The biomechanics of wounding are based on two factors: firstly the kinetic energy of the projectile, and secondly the elasticity and density of the target tissue. Kinetic energy is in turn a function of projectile mass and velocity. Most civilian gunshot wounds are inflicted by low-velocity weapons (<500 m/s). In contrast, military assault weapons are high velocity (>1000 m/s) and result in devastating injury.

The clinical relevance of this distinction is in the energy transfer and consequent tissue damage. Low-velocity weapons produce a permanent cavity as a bullet or missile tract as it passes through creating relatively local damage by crushing the tissues. High-velocity weapons also produce a permanent cavity, but of more concern is the large temporary cavity created as part of the blast effect. This results in massive tissue damage at some distance from the permanent cavity through shearing forces as a result of tissue displacement and recoil.

Miscellaneous trauma

Blast injury as result of detonated explosives causes injury through several mechanisms

- penetrating injury from fragments
- tissue disruption from shock waves
- evisceration and burns
- traumatic amputation.

Burn trauma is a leading cause of accidental death and mechanisms include

- thermal injury
- scalds
- chemical burns
- electrical burns
- frostbite.

7.2 Summary

Mechanism of injury

- Trauma is broadly divided by mechanism into blunt and penetrating injury
- Blunt trauma is frequently caused by motor vehicle collision, falls and assault
- Penetrating trauma is frequently caused by stab wounds or gunshot wounds
- The mechanism of injury plays a significant role in determining investigation and management.

Injury severity

Injury severity scores are used in an effort to bring a degree of reproducible objectivity to a complex, dynamic and often evolving situation. They are based on physiological or anatomical data or, preferably, both.

Purpose

One of the main functions of any severity score is to categorise patients rapidly and allow appropriate triage. Triage attempts to assess severity of injury and prioritise care. In the military field this facilitates transport to the most appropriate level of care. Under triage occurs when a severely injured patient is taken to a facility without adequate resources. Over triage occurs when the less severely injured patient is taken to a high-level trauma centre, bypassing a closer and adequate facility. Injury severity scores attempt to predict the risk of morbidity and mortality for individual patients. They may be used to stratify patient cohorts when planning resource allocation or inclusion into clinical studies, and they are a useful benchmark to analyse outcome and performance improvement strategies.

Limitations

All trauma scoring systems have limitations and are influenced by incomplete or inaccurate data. They are not absolute predictors of outcome and some can only be applied retrospectively when detailed information is available for all injuries. Scoring systems should be regarded as broad estimates of likely outcome rather than definitive values on which to base critical decisions. They should be used as an adjunct to clinical experience, pattern recognition and protocol-driven care.

Trauma scoring systems

Physiological scores

The Glasgow Coma Scale (GCS)

The GCS, described in 1974 by Teasdale and Jennett, is the most commonly used method of evaluating conscious level and is based on the best response in three categories. It is important to note that 'a GCS of 11' is meaningless. The score must be described in component parts, e.g., E3 V3 M5 (see Table 7.1).

Revised Trauma Score (RTS)

The RTS incorporates the GCS, systolic blood pressure and respiratory rate with a coded value applied to each of these (see Table 7.2). It is more accurate in predicting outcome in the hospital than in the field. The score ranges from 0 to 12, with higher scores predicting better outcome (Table 7.2).

Table 7.1 Glasgow Coma Score: total is the cumulative score in the three categories

Eye opening	Score (E)
Spontaneous	4
To voice	3
To pain	2
None	1
Verbal response	**Score (V)**
Orientated	5
Confused	4
Inappropriate words	3
Incomprehensible sounds	2
None	1
Motor response	**Score (M)**
Obeys commands	6
Localises pain	5
Withdraws from pain	4
Flexion to pain	3
Extension to pain	2
None	1

Total GCS > 12 = mild brain injury;
GCS 9–12 = moderate brain injury;
GCS < 9 = severe brain injury

Table 7.2 Revised Trauma Score (RTS)

GCS score	Systolic blood pressure (mmHg)	Respiratory rate (breaths/min)	Coded value
13–15	>89	10–29	4
9–12	76–89	>29	3
6–8	50–75	6–9	2
4–5	1–49	1–5	1
3	0	0	0

Anatomical scores

Anatomical scores define injury severity within each body region either individually or collectively. The most commonly used scores are the Abbreviated Injury Scale (AIS), which quantifies injury within distinct anatomical areas, and the Injury Severity Score (ISS), which is in turn a function of multiples of the AIS. These scores can only be applied when the full extent of injury is known. They are therefore retrospective tools with which to evaluate processes of care and to gather information of epidemiological value.

Abbreviated Injury Scale (AIS)

The AIS is a list of several hundred injuries that are assigned arbitrary values based on severity from 1 (minor) to 6 (usually fatal). It characterises the severity of individual injury and summarises these as a combined score.

Injury Severity Score (ISS)

The ISS summarises multiple anatomical injuries in a single patient. It is calculated as the sum of the squares of the three highest AIS scores of different body regions. For example, an abdominal AIS of 3, chest AIS of 2 and extremity AIS of 3 would give an ISS of $9+4+9=22$. The ISS is a useful predictor of mortality but does not take into account the impact of injuries outwith the three most severely injured regions.

Combination scores

Trauma Related Injury Severity Score (TRISS)

TRISS is a combination anatomical and physiological score using RTS, ISS, mechanism of injury and age. It allows calculation of probability of survival for an individual patient. This helps to benchmark care against other facilities and allows early detection of deviation in outcome for a given injury severity. It is particularly useful in identifying unexpected survivors and, more importantly, unexpected deaths.

7.3 Summary

Trauma scoring systems

- Trauma scoring systems are designed to aid triage and to objectively 'quantify' injury
- They may be based on anatomical scores, physiological scores or both (combination)
- All scoring systems have limitations and should not be used in isolation to determine treatment
- The most commonly used are the GCS (physiological), ISS (anatomical) and TRISS (combination).

Trauma systems, centres and teams

Trauma system

A trauma system is an organised and coordinated process in a defined geographic area. It delivers the full range of care to the injured patient through the seamless transition between each phase from 'road side to rehabilitation'. It is integrated with the local healthcare system. The preventable death rate before implementation of a trauma system is approximately 40%. This rapidly falls to 5% after implementing a trauma system, and to less than 2% as the system matures. Trauma systems save lives and reduce the associated morbidity of survivors (EBM 7.1).

There are four major components of a trauma system:

1. Injury prevention offers the greatest opportunity to reduce the both the healthcare and societal burden of trauma care
2. Prehospital care is critical to delivering the right patient to the right facility at the right time.
3. Trauma Centres are the hub of the network of care
4. Posthospital care to support physical and psychological rehabilitation thereby allowing patients to achieve independence, functionality and a facilitated return to productivity.

EBM 7.1 **Trauma systems**

'Patients managed within a trauma centre had a lower preventable mortality, received more aggressive neurosurgical input and had fewer missed or untreated injuries than those managed outwith a dedicated trauma system.'

West JG, Trunkey DD, Lim RC. Systems of trauma care. A study of two counties. Arch Surg. 1979;114:455–60.

Trauma Centres

A trauma centre is an acute hospital that receives injured patients. The American College of Surgeons has the most clearly structured approach to defining the level of trauma centre based upon its in-house capabilities:

Level 1 A comprehensive regional resource that is a tertiary care facility central to the trauma system. A Level I Trauma Centre is capable of providing total care for every aspect of injury, from prevention through rehabilitation.

Level II Able to initiate definitive care for all injured patients.

Level III Has demonstrated an ability to provide prompt assessment, resuscitation, surgery, intensive care and stabilisation of injured patients and emergency operations.

Level IV Has demonstrated an ability to provide advanced trauma life support (ATLS) prior to transfer of patients to a higher level trauma centre. It provides evaluation, stabilisation, and diagnostic capabilities for injured patients.

Level V Provides initial evaluation, stabilisation and diagnostic capabilities and prepares patients for transfer to higher levels of care.

Trauma team

The trauma team is a well-rehearsed, organised group with explicit task allocation under the supervision and direction of the team leader. Ideally, this core team assemble prior to arrival of the injured patient and performs the initial assessment and

Table 7.3 Resuscitation protocols task allocator

Task	Sub-tasks	Allocation
1. Transfer patient to hospital stretcher		All
2. Listen to handover		All
3. Primary survey	Airway control	D1/N2
	Two (2) IV lines	D2/D1
4. Patient undressed		N2
5. Initial monitoring	ECG	N2
	Pulse oximeter	N2
6. Log roll		N2/D2
7. Re-evaluate		
8. Final monitoring	NIBP	N2
	OGT/NGT	N2
	Urine catheter	N2
9. X-rays	C-spine	Radiology
	AP	
	Lateral	
	Swimmers	
10. Secondary survey		D1
11. Central line		D2
12. Definitive x-rays	Erect chest (if c-spine clear)	Radiology
	PEG (if required)	
	Other views	
13. DPL		D1

AP, Anteroposterior; c-spine, cervical spine; DPL, diagnostic peritoneal lavage; NIBP, noninvasive blood pressure; NGT, nasogastric tube; OGT, orogastric tube; PEG, percutaneous enteral gastrostomy.

resuscitation according to strictly defined protocol. The structure will vary in each institution but it may include trauma surgeons, emergency department physicians, anaesthetists, nursing staff, radiographers and a scribe. These individuals should be clearly identified by their roles displayed on badges or lead coats. Other disciplines may be called upon as required but should not detract from the function and responsibilities of the core team.

Trauma team activation criteria are also institution-dependent and should be the focus of continued audit to ensure appropriate thresholds are in place. Strong leadership and clear communication in a controlled, quiet and calm environment are critical to the efficiency and safety of the process. Resuscitation is **not** a democratic process: a very definite hierarchy is required to facilitate rapid and appropriate decision-making. This is not the time to be debating task allocation or devising management strategies from first principles. An example of this is shown in Table 7.3 where D is Doctor and N is Nurse.

 7.4 **Summary**

Systems of trauma care

- A trauma system delivers organised and coordinated care from the time of injury to rehabilitation
- Trauma Centres are designated by capability and defined by the American College of Surgeons
- The trauma team members have clearly defined task allocation supervised by the team leader
- Trauma systems save lives, reduce the morbidity in survivors and utilise resources efficiently.

Shock

Definition

Shock may be defined as inadequate tissue perfusion to maintain normal cellular function and structure. Untreated it leads to cellular hypoxia, organ dysfunction and death. A potential error trap is to equate shock with hypotension: whilst they may co-exist shock is not the same as low blood pressure. Conversely, 'normal' haemodynamics do not exclude occult hypoperfusion.

Classification of shock

Hypovolaemic shock is caused by decrease in circulating volume.

Haemorrhagic shock is a form of hypovolaemic shock, occurring as a result of acute blood loss and is the most common form of shock in the injured patient. It should be assumed that the trauma patient with shock physiology is bleeding until proven otherwise.

Cardiogenic shock is a reduction in cardiac output as a result of pump failure. It may occur following direct cardiac injury (e.g., myocardial contusion), or as a consequence of cardiac disease (e.g., myocardial infarction).

Vasogenic shock follows changes in vascular tone and resistance such that a normal circulating volume fails to maintain adequate circulatory perfusion.

Neurogenic shock is a form of vasogenic shock following high spinal injury. Loss of sympathetic vascular tone produces peripheral vasodilatation

Septic shock is a form of vasogenic shock following release of proinflammatory mediators. Peripheral vasodilatation with decreased arterial resistance and increased venous capacitance results in hypoperfusion.

Obstructive shock follows mechanical obstruction that impairs cardiac function and output. It may occur after injury as a result of cardiac tamponade or tension pneumothorax.

Management of shock

The definitive management of shock is determined by the aetiology. This is established through history, examination and diagnostic tests. Regardless of the underlying aetiology of shock the initial management is the same and starts with **resuscitation**.

7.5 Summary

Shock

- Shock may be defined as inadequate tissue perfusion
- Untreated, shock will result in death
- There are various different types of shock but the initial management is always the same
- The most common cause of shock in trauma is haemorrhagic shock.

Resuscitation

Definition

Resuscitation is a dynamic and intense period of medical care guided by the initial and continuous assessment of the patient.

It combines diagnostic and therapeutic manoeuvres to rapidly identify and treat life-threatening disorders in order of clinical priority. This systematic approach to the care of the injured is exemplified by the Advanced Trauma Life Support (ATLS) course.

ATLS history

On 17 February 1976 Dr Jim Styner, an orthopaedic surgeon, was flying his light aircraft from Los Angeles, California, to Lincoln, Nebraska. His wife Charlene and his four children were on board with him on the return trip from a family wedding. Five hours into the flight he became disoriented and lost altitude. They flew over a pond and into a row of trees at 168 miles per hour. Mrs Styner was ejected from the airplane and was killed instantly. Three of the four young children sustained head injuries and were unconscious. The fourth child had a fractured right forearm and a serious laceration to his right hand. Dr Styner had fractured ribs, a fractured zygoma and several lacerations to his head and face.

After 8 hours in sub-freezing conditions Dr Styner flagged down a car. He and family were transported to the local hospital, which was closed. When hospital staff arrived it was immediately apparent that they had very little experience and training in the management of major trauma. Dr Styner contacted his colleague and the family were airlifted to Lincoln General Hospital.

Styner was later to observe:

'When I can provide better care in the field with limited resources than my children and I received at the primary facility, there is something wrong with the system and the system has to be changed.'

In 1978, 2 years after the plane crash, Styner and colleagues held the prototype Advanced Trauma Life Support course in Auburn, Nebraska. ATLS has since become the foundation of care for injured patients by teaching a common language and a standardised, systematic approach. It is a measurable, reproducible and comprehensive system of care and has changed the initial management of trauma worldwide.

ATLS in practice

ATLS was designed as a single-provider resuscitation course but it is applicable to every trauma patient in every scenario, from the prehospital arena to the trauma team in a Level I centre. It comprises three protocol-driven phases with the aim of identifying and addressing injuries in life-threatening order of priority using an ABCDE approach.

ATMIST handover from prehospital team to trauma team

While commencing the ATLS primary survey the prehospital providers should handover to the trauma team using the ATMIST system (Table 7.4) to describe the patient and events.

Primary survey

The survey (Table 7.5) focuses on rapid identification of life-threatening conditions in a prioritised sequence, based on the effect of injuries on patient physiology. This should take less than 30 seconds to perform.

Table 7.4 ATMIST handover of trauma patient

	Index	Example
A	**Age** of patient	26-year-old male
T	**Time** of injury	16:35 hours
M	**Mechanism** of injury	Gunshot wound to abdomen
I	**Injuries** from top to toe	Bullet wound × 2: right upper quadrant of abdomen and left flank
S	vital **Signs**	Airway maintained, sats 93% on 10 L O_2, pulse 124 bpm, blood pressure 84/66 mmHg
T	**Treatment** given prehospital	10 L O_2 via mask, 250 ml IV fluid, 3 mg IV morphine

Table 7.5 Primary trauma survey

Airway and cervical-spine control	Quality of voice, air exchange, added noises, e.g., grunting, while maintaining control and immobility of the cervical spine
Breathing	Breath sounds, chest wall movements, neck veins, tracheal deviation
Circulation and haemorrhage control	Mentation, skin colour and temperature, pulse, blood pressure, neck veins, external bleeding
Disability (neurological)	Pupils, GCS, extremity movement, voice
Exposure and environment	Remove all clothing to allow full external inspection, check temperature, avoid hypothermia Log roll with spinal precautions to allow inspection and palpation of the spine

GCS, Glasgow Coma Score.

Catastrophic haemorrhage

One relatively recent modification to the ABC approach is the <C>ABC approach adopted by the military, where <C> reminds us to gain, 'temporary control of external catastrophic bleeding'. This is a paradigm shift to rapidly deal with avoidable exsanguination while addressing A or B issues. It is achieved through simple manoeuvres such as direct manual pressure, tourniquets, dressings or novel topical haemostatic agents.

The primary survey includes generic resuscitation adjuncts:

- High-flow oxygen via a trauma mask or definitive airway
- The cervical spine (c-spine) is protected initially with in-line manual stabilisation (i.e., it is held still by one member of the team using both hands) and if it cannot be cleared clinically it is immobilised with a collar
- Large-bore intravenous access—preferably two 14G peripheral lines in the antecubital fossae
- Blood is drawn for laboratory studies and cross-match at the time of gaining IV access
- Arterial blood gas provides a rapid window on haemoglobin and haematocrit, acid–base balance and gas exchange
- Additional tubes such as urinary catheters and nasogastric tubes should be used when indicated and only after addressing life-threatening issues
- Basic monitoring: electrocardiogram (ECG), pulse oximetry, blood pressure cuff

- Analgesia: small doses of carefully titrated intravenous opiate should not be withheld on the fallacy of 'masking clinical signs' (one of the primary duties as a physician is to relieve pain and distress)
- Temporary splinting of long bone fractures reduces pain, minimises blood loss, and may restore the anatomical position to reduce adjacent vessel compromise and associated distal ischaemia
- Pelvic binders are useful temporising adjuncts to reduce blood loss and pain associated with pelvic fractures
- Warming devices including hot-air blankets to maintain core temperature.

Practical tips and tricks

There is a quick and simple way to assess the trauma patient in the first 10 seconds:

- Introduce yourself to reassure the patient then ask their name and what happened
- An appropriate response implies that there is no immediate ABC or D issue
  - airway patency sufficient to permit speech
  - breathing sufficient to generate air movement
  - circulation sufficient to perfuse brain
  - disability—conscious level sufficient to process information.

Note that that this does not exclude a major or evolving injury—this is a dynamic process and the key word here is 'sufficient'.

Secondary survey

This involves a full clinical examination and a focused history.

- Head-to-toe examination
  - including spine and digital rectal exam
  - take care to inspect the 'hidden zones' such as axillae, perineum and natal cleft.
- AMPLE history
  - Allergies
  - Medications currently taking
  - Past medical history
  - Last ate/drank
  - Events related to injury.
- Imaging
  - determined by physiology, mechanism and anatomy of injury and the clinical question.

The secondary survey may be delayed until after life-saving procedures are performed, including surgery or interventional radiology.

Tertiary survey

The primary and secondary surveys are repeated within 24 hours to identify evolving or previously missed injuries. A 'problem list' is then created for each injury with a coherent management plan and the details of involved specialties.

Airway management in the trauma patient

There are three goals of airway management

- Ensure adequate oxygenation
- Ensure adequate ventilation
- Protect from aspiration.

There are three levels of airway management

1. Basic
   * Airway positioning, e.g., chin lift and jaw thrust to relieve obstruction caused by tongue and soft palate
   * 100% oxygen via non-rebreather mask
   * Suction to clear blood and secretions.
2. Advanced
   * Bag and valve masks
   * Laryngeal masks
   * Endotracheal intubation under direct vision
   * Cricoid pressure to limit risk of aspiration.
3. Surgical
   * Cricothyroidotomy is the preferred option in trauma
     - may be percutaneous with Seldinger approach or open surgical
     - needle cricothyroidotomy using a large gauge cannula is at best a temporising manoeuvre.

A definitive airway is a tube in the trachea with the cuff inflated to prevent aspiration.

Vascular access in the trauma patient

Successful resuscitation is absolutely dependent upon rapidly establishing reliable large-bore venous access for volume replacement, blood component therapy and drug administration. This can be challenging in a high-pressure environment with a distressed or combative patient. In addition, the shocked patient with peripheral venous collapse presents a further technical challenge.

There are three options for vascular access:

1. Peripheral venous access. The first choice for access in the trauma patient.
   - Two large-bore catheters are placed, preferably 14G, in the antecubital fossae
   - Surgical cut down onto relatively constant peripheral veins (e.g., long saphenous vein – 1 cm proximal and 1 cm anterior to the medial malleolus) is an option, but has been largely replaced by central access if standard peripheral access fails
2. Central venous access. The Seldinger technique with commercially available kits makes this a relatively safe and rapid alternative when conventional peripheral access fails. There are three options, each with relative advantages and disadvantages.
   - Subclavian vein, the preferred choice – access to this vein is often easier in the shocked patient as the enveloping fascia tends to hold it open and provides a reliable target. Cannulation at this site does not interfere with airway or c-spine manoeuvres.
   - Internal jugular vein. Access to this site is often limited in the blunt trauma patient by a c-spine collar but it remains a useful option in penetrating injury that does not involve the neck.
   - Femoral vein. This vein is easy to access and has a lower immediate complication rate than subclavian or internal jugular access (e.g., pneumothorax, dysrhythmia, superior vena cava injury). Its use is limited by access to the groin in pelvic trauma, or in the patient with major torso vascular injury, as it does not guarantee fluid or drugs will reach the central circulation above the diaphragm.
3. Intraosseous access. Intraosseous access (IO) is an effective alternative to venous access, which can be particularly challenging in children. In general, this route can deliver safely any IV drug or fluid required during paediatric resuscitation when IV options fail. The preferred IO access site is the anteromedial surface of the tibia 1–3 cm below the tibial tuberosity. Commercially available kits make this a relatively simple procedure but the complications include osteomyelitis and it should be replaced by IV access as soon as the initial resuscitation is complete.

ABCDE: initial management options of the common life-threatening conditions

Airway compromise

Management follows this sequence until an airway is established:

* 100% O_2 by facemask in the patient who can maintain their airway
* Suction to clear blood and foreign bodies
* Airway manoeuvres: chin lift or jaw thrust in the obtunded patient
* Oral or nasopharyngeal airway as airway adjuncts
* Endotracheal intubation in the patient who cannot maintain a definitive airway
* Surgical cricothyroidotomy when endotracheal intubation fails.

Breathing compromise

There are four conditions that require immediate management

* Tension pneumothorax secondary to an unrelieved build up of air in the pleural space
  - immediate treatment by finger thoracostomy
  - this involves a surgical cut down where a chest drain would be sited
  - a finger is used to penetrate and decompress the pleural space
  - this is followed by chest drain through this site as definitive management
  - needle thoracostomy is recommended by ATLS but has significant disadvantages over finger thoracostomy, including bleeding, air embolism and inadequate decompression.
* Open pneumothorax secondary to penetrating chest injury with collapse of the lung
  - immediate treatment with an occlusive dressing taped on three sides to allow air out of the chest but not in
  - definitive treatment with a chest drain.
* Massive haemothorax defined by blood in the pleural cavity
  - immediate management with a chest drain
  - may require surgical control with emergency thoracotomy.
* Flail chest secondary to at least two fractures per rib in at least two ribs.
  - immediate management with intubation and ventilation is only required in cases of significant respiratory distress
  - subsequent management includes analgesia, regional anaesthesia (e.g., nerve block or epidural) and aggressive physiotherapy with pulmonary toilet.

Circulation compromise

There are two conditions which require immediate management

1. Massive haemorrhage
   - acute blood loss may be in one of five places
   - 'on the floor or four more'
   - i.e., external bleeding or in the chest, abdomen, pelvic fracture or long bone fracture

- it is managed with a < C > ABC approach to resuscitation, blood and blood component therapy and control of bleeding. Remember, the treatment of bleeding is to **stop the bleeding**.

2. Cardiac tamponade
   - blood in the tight, fibrous pericardial space results in poor atrial filling, reduced ventricular filling and decreased cardiac output: a form of obstructive shock
   - pericardiocentesis is recommended by some to decompress the pericardial space by aspirating blood through a needle
   - this does not stop the bleeding, is ineffective at aspirating clot, may injure the heart or other structures and, in the author's view, should be abandoned
   - the management of cardiac tamponade is thoracotomy with direct cardiac repair
   - the timing and location of surgery, and choice of surgical access are determined by patient physiology but this principle does not change.

Fluid resuscitation

Choice of fluid, rate of administration and endpoints of resuscitation continue to evolve. The previous dogma of 2 L of crystalloid given immediately to the trauma patient has been replaced by a more measured, controlled and individualised approach. This encompasses several key concepts as a cohesive strategy under the umbrella term of 'Damage Control Resuscitation'. The aim is to avoid death and morbidity as a result of the 'lethal triad': coagulopathy, acidosis and hypothermia.

Regardless of which fluids are given, they should be warmed, limited and titrated to physiological endpoints to avoid the iatrogenic consequences of fluid administration. The patient's response or otherwise to carefully titrated boluses will guide resuscitation strategy and falls into three groups: **responders** (time to investigate), **transient responders** (likely on-going blood loss and require urgent investigation and intervention) and **nonresponders** (require immediate intervention to restore physiology).

Damage Control Resuscitation has three principal components:

1. Permissive hypotension
This strategy is applied to the patient with haemorrhagic shock prior to gaining control of the bleeding (EBM 7.2). By 'permitting' lower blood pressure (palpable radial pulse or systolic of less than 80 mmHg) lower volumes of fluid are given. High-volume resuscitation is detrimental to the bleeding patient as it:
   i) Raises the blood pressure and increases the rate of blood loss
   ii) Disrupts immature thrombus and exacerbates bleeding ('popping the clot')
   iii) Dilutes remaining coagulation factors leading to further blood loss. It is important to note than when bleeding is controlled the patient should be resuscitated to accepted physiological and haemodynamic parameters to minimise further insult.

2. Haemostatic resuscitation
Coagulopathy is common in trauma patients, particularly in the context of haemorrhagic shock. In those patients predicted to require massive transfusion, administration of packed red blood cells, fresh frozen plasma and platelets in a 1:1:1 ratio (of individual units) is associated with improved survival. Adjuncts

for treating or preventing coagulopathy include recombinant factor VIIa, cryoprecipitate and tranexamic acid (EBM 7.3). Whilst a 1:1:1 ratio is advised in the initial management of the bleeding patient, further blood component therapy should be guided by laboratory values or, ideally, by real-time point-of-care testing such as thromboelastography (TEG).

3. Damage Control Surgery
DCS is a strategy to rapidly control bleeding and gastrointestinal contamination. The aim is to restore normal physiology rather than definitively reconstruct anatomy at the initial intervention. It is a form of time-limited or 'abbreviated' surgery with the emphasis on temporary control to allow on-going resuscitation in the critical care environment.

EBM 7.2 Permissive hypotension

'Delayed intravenous fluid resuscitation until surgical intervention improves the outcome, including mortality, for hypotensive patients with penetrating torso injuries.'

Bickell WH, Wall MJ Jr, Pepe PE, et al. Immediate versus delayed fluid resuscitation for hypotensive patients with penetrating torso injuries. N Engl J Med. 1994;331:1105–9.

EBM 7.3 Tranexamic acid

'A short course of tranexamic acid given early after injury reduced the risk of death in bleeding trauma patients. There was no increase in vascular occlusive events associated with the use of tranexamic acid in this patient population.'

CRASH-2 trial collaborators. Effects of tranexamic acid on death, vascular occlusive events, and blood transfusion in trauma patients with significant haemorrhage (CRASH-2): a randomized, placebo-controlled trial. Lancet. 2010;376:23–32.

7.6 Summary

Resuscitation

- Resuscitation should follow a rapid but orderly sequence to identify and treat life-threatening issues
- ATLS uses an ABCDE approach to facilitate this process with a primary, secondary and tertiary survey
- Response to resuscitation guides the next phase in clinical management
- Damage control resuscitation has three key components and aims to reduce preventable mortality.

Imaging

Imaging, if required for the trauma patient, is performed to answer specific questions that will facilitate rapid decision-making. There is an inverse relationship between physiological stability and imaging: the sicker the patient the less time there is for imaging. A common error trap is to employ the 'elective mind set' to the emergency scenario. Imaging to confirm what you already know or suspect in the unstable trauma patient is unnecessary and contributes significantly to avoidable deaths by introducing delays in haemorrhage control.

Trauma imaging, at least in the initial phase, is focused, relevant and timely. It informs rather than replaces clinical decision-making, which should be based on experience, pattern recognition and situational awareness. In addition, the decision to image and choice of modality will be influenced by institutional capability. For example, if there is a dedicated trauma CT scanner adjacent to the resuscitation bay this will not only lower the acceptable threshold for moving the patient to CT, but may negate the need for plain radiology.

Plain radiography

Chest x-ray remains a useful study to rapidly identify life-threatening conditions in the majority of trauma patients. It may be performed as part of the ATLS trauma series with c-spine and pelvic x-ray, or combined with abdominal x-ray in the patient with penetrating injury, to identify bullets or other projectiles.

During the secondary survey it may be appropriate to evaluate suspected extremity fractures unless the patient is proceeding to CT.

Ultrasound

The use of point-of-care sonography to evaluate the trauma patient has increased dramatically and in many centres would be considered a standard of care. Focused Assessment with Sonography for Trauma (FAST) looks specifically for fluid in four predetermined locations ('the 4 Ps'):

1. Pericardial
2. Perihepatic
3. Perirenal
4. Pelvic.

The FAST is either positive or negative and any fluid seen is assumed to be blood. A negative FAST does not exclude bleeding and it should not be performed if there is an absolute indication for surgical intervention on that cavity.

EFAST, or Extended Focused Assessment with Sonography for Trauma, also evaluates the pleural spaces ('the 5th P') for air and blood and may facilitate rapid identification of pneumothorax or haemothorax.

One of the major advantages of FAST or EFAST over other imaging is that it may be performed as part of the primary survey without interfering with the initial assessment and management of ABCDE issues.

Computed tomography (CT)

CT has evolved from the 'doughnut of death' to the gold standard for imaging the injured patient. If CT is immediately available it is the modality of choice for imaging evaluation and negates the need for plain radiography and sonography. This paradigm shift has occurred as a result of several factors:

- Modern scanners can perform plain, arterial and venous phase full body scans (vertex to mid thigh) in minutes
- The geographical location of CT adjacent to the emergency department minimises delay
- Availability of radiographers and radiologist to immediately perform and interpret the images with the aid of trauma protocols has greatly enhanced the 'real-time' value of this modality
- Previously patients were 'sent' to the CT scanner, unaccompanied and often unstable; now they are 'taken' by the trauma team with all necessary equipment for continuing resuscitation in the scan room.

Magnetic resonance imaging (MRI)

MRI is superior to CT in evaluating the central nervous system trauma (brain and spinal cord/column), musculoskeletal injury and some vascular injuries that cannot be clearly defined on contrast CT.

It is of limited value, however, in the initial assessment of the trauma patient as it is time-consuming, less readily available than other modalities such as CT, and does not permit access to the patient for on going resuscitation during image acquisition

Interventional radiology (IR)

The diagnostic and, in particular, therapeutic advantages of IR have greatly enhanced the care of the trauma patient. IR now plays a significant role in many aspects of trauma care but predominantly in vascular injury, whether through haemorrhage control (e.g., embolising the bleeding spleen) or restoration of flow (e.g., thoracic stent grafts). These procedures are much less invasive and more targeted than surgical interventions and have dramatically increased the rate of 'selective nonoperative management'.

Specialised imaging studies

The use of gastrointestinal contrast studies, for example to identify oesophageal injury or rectal injury, has been largely replaced by CT. These and other studies may continue to have a limited role in select patient groups but are of less value in the initial assessment of the trauma patient.

 7.7 Summary

Trauma imaging

- Trauma imaging should be focused, relevant and timely
- Plain x-rays and ultrasound have a role in the immediate assessment of the injured patient
- Full-body CT is the gold standard of trauma imaging but this is determined by institutional-capability
- Interventional radiology.

Critical decision-making

Incisions and decisions

Major trauma is absolutely time-dependent pathology. It is punctuated by a series of critical decision nodes, and at each point on the patient journey imaging or intervention may be required. The greatest challenge in this high-pressure scenario is in determining the need for a given intervention rather than in the practical skill itself. The key is not just making the right decision but making the right decision quickly, often with incomplete information.

Managing these complex scenarios effectively requires a combination of acquired knowledge and experience. Acquired knowledge may take the form of algorithms and protocols. Experience leads to enhanced pattern recognition and situational awareness. In other words, one develops a personal system for dealing with the injured patient.

'Bad thoughts lead to good outcomes'

It is helpful to consider and prepare for the worst case scenario during the initial assessment of the injured patient. The default position until proven otherwise is:

1. This patient is bleeding
2. This patient needs an operation, and
3. Think 'damage control'.

This will over triage the majority of trauma patients but it is easier and safer to downgrade the level of response and readiness than to under estimate the gravity of the injury.

Subdivide trauma patients by physiology

It is helpful to subdivide trauma patients according to physiological status determined by the initial ABCDE assessment, as this dictates the next step in their management. The concepts of 'stable' and 'unstable' have been replaced by the terms 'haemodynamically normal' and 'haemodynamically abnormal', respectively. This serves to remind the resuscitation team that 'stable', i.e., unchanging, is not necessarily normal good. Remember, the patients with the most stable vital signs are in the hospital mortuary—they never change.

It is convenient to consider the immediate management of trauma patients in three groups according to clinical status (Fig. 7.1)

1. Haemodynamically normal: work up +/− intervention
2. Haemodynamically abnormal: urgent work up then intervention
3. In extremis: resuscitation concurrent with immediate intervention.

The trauma patient in extremis

This subgroup of the haemodynamically abnormal patient presents with an anatomical or physiological abnormality which if untreated will result in death within seconds to minutes. This profound instability is usually secondary to massive haemorrhage. Unlike almost every other sphere of clinical practice where there is a logical series of steps to determine a diagnosis prior to commencing therapy, these patients require a 'treat then diagnose' strategy in order to save life. There is no time to debate and consider options – the approach to these patients follows the algorithms in Fig. 7.2, which are further divided according to blunt or penetrating mechanism.

Trajectory of the wounding implement or missile is critical to decision-making in the penetrating trauma patient in extremis.

After ABC the patient should be log rolled only to answer one question: where are the holes? For example, a gunshot wound to the left anterior chest with an exit in the left posterior chest defines the left chest as the priority cavity. The same gunshot wound to the left chest exiting via the right buttock is an entirely different scenario and will involve several cavities with potential for blood loss in each. Of note, differentiating entrance and exit wounds is notoriously difficult and is a forensic rather than clinical endeavour. The general principle, however, of determining trajectory based on location of wounds holds true. If there is time to perform rapid plain radiography in the trauma bay it is helpful to place metallic markers (e.g., open paper clips over each wound). This allows the trauma team to 'mentally reconstruct' the trajectories based on external wounds and the missiles seen on x-ray.

Essentially, log roll determines trajectory, and trajectory determines the likely body cavities involved. This information in conjunction with physiological status facilitates decision-making regarding which cavities to open (e.g., chest and abdomen), the order in which to open them (e.g., chest or abdomen first?) and the geographical location for intervention (e.g., surgery in the resuscitation bay or in the operating theatre).

Clearly this strategy is of little or no relevance in the blunt trauma patient in extremis as by definition there are rarely external wounds to identify the priority cavity.

7.8 Summary

Critical decision-making

- Trauma is absolutely time-dependent pathology punctuated by a series of critical decision nodes
- Assume the worst: 'bad thoughts lead to good outcomes'
- Subdivide patients according to physiology: haemodynamically normal, abnormal or in extremis
- Trajectory of bullet/missile in penetrating injury is key to decision-making.

Surgery for trauma

Most trauma patients do not require surgical intervention. The challenge is in deciding who does need surgery or other intervention, and then what to do and where to do it. It is helpful to take a reductionist view to facilitate this decision-making – there are only three options for the trauma patient:

- Observation, e.g., conservative management with serial clinical examination
- Imaging, e.g., CT
- Intervention, e.g., trauma laparotomy

The haemodynamically normal patient may undergo intervention, imaging, observation or all three. The haemodynamically abnormal patient requires intervention +/− imaging. The patient in extremis requires immediate intervention.

Damage control surgery

Damage control surgery (DCS) is a three-phase approach to the patient with profoundly unstable and deteriorating physiology, usually as a result of massive blood loss. It may be applied to any anatomical region but is most commonly used for exsanguinating chest or abdominal injury. This term was used by the United States Navy as 'the capacity of a ship to absorb damage

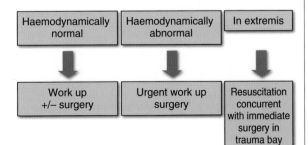

Fig. 7.1 Division of trauma patients by physiology.

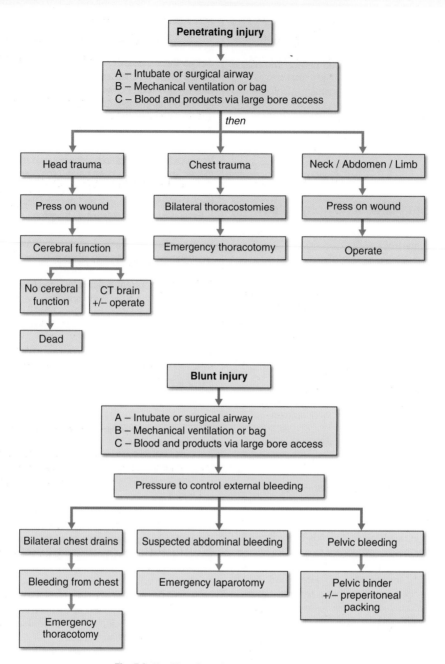

Fig. 7.2 Algorithms for patient treatment in extremis.

and maintain mission integrity'. Whilst packing to control bleeding has been recognised for more than a century, the concept of 'damage control surgery' was not described until 1993 (EBM 7.4).

The principle of DCS recognises that a reduction in mortality is achieved at the cost of sometimes vastly increased morbidity: patients now survive previously lethal injuries and to develop complications.

The three phases of DCS are shown in Box 7.1.

EBM **7.4 Damage control surgery (DCS)**

'Damage control laparotomy appears to offer a survival benefit over conventional surgery in the exsanguinating patient with multiple penetrating abdominal vascular and visceral injuries.'

Rotondo MF, Schwab CW, McGonigal MD, et al. 'Damage control': an approach for improved survival in exsanguinating penetrating abdominal injury. J Trauma. 1993;35:375–82.

Box 7.1 The phases of damage control surgery

Phase 1: Immediate operation concurrent with initial resuscitation

1. Control haemorrhage: packing, ligation, shunts
2. Control GI contamination: suture, staple, soft clamps, tie bowel ends
3. Pack and leave abdomen open: laparostomy

Phase 2: Continue resuscitation in the ICU

1. Restore perfusion, rewarm, correct coagulopathy
2. Monitor for Abdominal Compartment Syndrome, even in the open abdomen

Phase 3: Planned reoperation when physiology restored to normal

1. Remove packs, vascular reconstruction, restore gastrointestinal continuity
2. Close abdomen if possible.

Trauma laparotomy

There are two types of trauma laparotomy: definitive laparotomy and damage control laparotomy. The initial approach is similar and the decision regarding whether to continue with definitive surgery or to abbreviate the laparotomy is absolutely determined by patient physiology.

The aim of the trauma laparotomy is to control bleeding, control gastrointestinal (GI) contamination and identify all injuries. The patient with normal physiology may then proceed to a definitive surgical intervention. However, the surgery is terminated after control of bleeding and contamination in the patient with abnormal physiology, even though this control may be temporary.

It is important to remember:

- The abdomen has two spaces: intraperitoneal and retroperitoneal
- The problem may not be in the abdomen in the patient with penetrating 'abdominal' injury
- It is not necessary to know which structures are injured to make the decision to open the abdomen.

Identification and management of abdominal injury

Abdominal injuries should be identified in life-threatening order of priority, much like the ABC approach to initial assessment. Death is usually the result of uncontrolled bleeding and the structures should be inspected in the order of vascular structures, then solid organs and finally hollow organs. The management of each injury is again dictated by physiology such that the same anatomical injury may be managed entirely differently (Table 7.6).

Table 7.6 Management principles of abdominal injury

	Haemodynamically normal	Haemodynamically abnormal
Vascular injury	Repair/graft	Shunt/ligate
Solid organ injury	Repair/drain	Pack/take out
Hollow organ injury	Repair (excluding rectum)	Staple ends/drain

Table 7.7 Criteria for decision to explore retroperitoneal haematoma

	Blunt injury	Penetrating injury
Zone 1 (Central)	Yes	Yes
Zone 2 (Lateral)	Avoid unless unstable	Avoid unless unstable
Zone 3 (Pelvic)	No	Yes

Retroperitoneal haematoma

The retroperitoneum is divided into three zones:

- Central: contains the great vessels and unpaired mesenteric vessels
- Lateral: contains the kidneys and renal vessels
- Pelvic: contains the iliac vessels.

The decision to explore is based on mechanism (blunt or penetrating) and location (Table 7.7):

Regardless of the zone involved, the retroperitoneum is explored surgically for haemorrhage control, and this necessitates mobilising the viscera for access. It may be best approached for aortic injuries with a left medial visceral rotation (Mattox manoeuvre) and for caval injuries with a right medial visceral rotation (Cattell-Braasch manoeuvre).

Trauma laparotomy sequence

The trauma laparotomy should follow a controlled and predefined sequence to identify life-threatening issues rapidly and to minimise the risk of missed injuries. A suggested series of steps is:

- Scrub before anaesthetising, as induction is often associated with cardiovascular collapse in the hypovolaemic patient
- Have two functioning suction devices and 20 large abdominal packs opened
- Full midline incision
- Four-quadrant packing in order of area most likely to be bleeding
- Stop and discuss findings and physiology with anaesthetic team: 'situational awareness'
- Inform theatre team of the proposed strategy and ensure all equipment is available
- Falciform ligament may be taken down but do not mobilise the liver unnecessarily
- Fixed retractor with several blades and a self-retaining retractor provide excellent exposure
- Remove packs in order starting with area least likely to be bleeding
- Control bleeding, control contamination
- Make the decision regarding damage control early
- Systematic examination in 'life-threatening order' of priority: vascular, solid, hollow
- Examine the entire GI tract from oesophageal hiatus to rectum at least twice.

Trauma thoracotomy

The vast majority of patients with chest trauma do not require surgery. Approximately 10–15% of thoracic injuries require thoracotomy or sternotomy, and the indications and timing of this are determined by the mechanism, physiology and anatomy of injury. There is an unnecessary 'mystique' and even fear of surgery for thoracic trauma probably because most surgeons who deal with trauma in the UK are more comfortable in the abdomen than the chest. The trauma surgery principles and concepts are, however, the same for any anatomical region and it may be helpful to think of the chest as a 'belly with bones'. This serves as a reminder that, for example, the treatment of bleeding is to stop the bleeding, regardless of body cavity.

Surgical access to the chest

The bony thoracic skeleton does pose certain access challenges in the injured patient. The patient with abdominal injury who requires surgery is opened via a full midline laparotomy incision – there is no decision to make.

Decision-making for thoracic injury is more complex for the following reasons:

- The chest cavity is more compartmentalised than the abdomen
- The bony thorax (ribs, sternum, clavicles) makes operative access more difficult
- Large and relatively fixed structures limit exposure of posterior mediastinum.

The choice of chest incision determined by two key factors:

- The expected anatomic injury – based on mechanism, physiology and pattern recognition
- The urgency with which access is required.

There are at least eight routes into the chest:

- Anterolateral thoracotomy – left and right
- Posterolateral thoracotomy – left and right
- Trapdoor – left and right
- Median sternotomy
- Clamshell thoracotomy (bilateral anterolateral thoracotomies joined by dividing sternum).

The safest position for the trauma patient on the operating table is supine: this allows access to most cavities which is critical if more than one cavity is known to be involved from the start of the operation or, of more concern, other injuries become apparent during surgery. Access and position limit the use of anterolateral and posterolateral incisions to specific injuries in the stable patient (e.g., oesophageal). The trapdoor is a morbid incision of little value. The utility incision for trauma is the clamshell, particularly for the unstable patient, as it is easy, rapid and versatile. The median sternotomy provides excellent exposure of the heart, great vessels and thoracic inlet and is a good alternative for these particular injuries.

Surgical strategy in the chest

Once the chest is open, the surgical principles of controlling bleeding and contamination apply. In addition there may be lung or airway injuries that require attention, or cardiac tamponade requiring decompression by widely opening the pericardium. Drains are always placed at the conclusion of surgery in the chest – each opened cavity must have at least one drain (e.g., left pleural space, right pleural space, pericardium).

Emergency room thoracotomy (ERT)

ERT is reserved for the small number of patients presenting in extremis, usually as a result of penetrating injury to the torso. Outcome from this scenario is absolutely dependent upon rapid, protocol-driven decision-making. Fig. 7.3 outlines the approach to this group of patients.

There are five life-saving manoeuvres to perform once inside the chest in the emergency scenario:

1. Open the pericardium, relieve tamponade and control bleeding
2. Divide inferior pulmonary ligament to allow access to the aorta and pulmonary hilum
3. Manually compress the descending thoracic aorta to control bleeding below diaphragm and redistribute remaining circulating volume to heart and brain

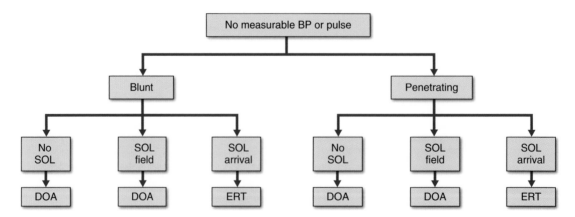

Fig. 7.3 Emergency room thoracotomy. *BP,* Blood pressure; *DOA,* dead on arrival; *ERT,* emergency room thoracotomy; *SOL,* sign of life.

4. Internal cardiac massage if heart in arrest
5. Lung twist: rotate the lung through 180 degrees to control vascular and airway injury.

 7.9 Summary

Surgery for trauma

*   Most injured patients do not require surgery, but this decision can be challenging
*   Trauma laparotomy and thoracotomy should follow a predefined sequence of steps
*   Damage Control Surgery strategies may be applied to any anatomical region
*   ERT should be reserved for the patient in extremis, usually following penetrating torso injury.

Junctional zone trauma

Injury occurring at the junction between anatomically distinct zones is particularly challenging. Examples of junctional zones are demonstrated in Fig.7.4. The clinical significance of junctional zone trauma is:

*   These areas are traversed by major vessels
*   They are therefore usually accessed in trauma for haemorrhage control
*   Proximal and distal control of bleeding may be required in two anatomically distinct regions with fixed musculoskeletal structure limiting access
*   Of note, the chest has three junctional zones (neck, axillae, abdomen).

 7.10 Summary

Take home message for managing trauma

*   Management of trauma requires a combination of data synthesis and prioritisation under pressure
*   Early pattern recognition and protocol-driven care facilitate rapid decision-making
*   Trauma systems reduce preventable mortality and minimise morbidity in survivors
*   Trauma management is simple, it's just not always easy.

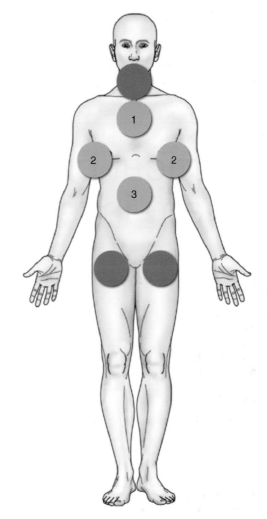

Base of skull = junction between head and neck
Thoracic inlet = junction between neck and chest (1)
Axilla = junction between chest and upper limb (2)
Diaphragm = junction between chest and abdomen (3)
Groin = junction between abdomen and lower limb

Fig. 7.4 Site of trauma junctional zones.

Damian James Mole

Practical procedures and patient investigation

Chapter contents

Introduction 112

General precautions 112

Aseptic technique 112

Local anaesthesia 112

Suturing 113

Airway procedures 114

Thoracic procedures 116

Abdominal procedures 118

Vascular procedures 120

Urinary procedures 124

Central nervous system procedures 125

Excision of lumps and swellings (e.g., sebaceous cyst, lipoma, dermoid, lymph node) 126

Imaging 126

Introduction

Every practical procedure performed on any patient should be with their explicit consent, where this is obtainable, and should be in written form where appropriate. In conscious patients, it is good practice to explain to the patient beforehand what to expect they will feel, including the reasons for the procedure and exactly what it will entail. Appropriate reassurance should always be given. Many patients find comfort in continuing reassurance throughout the procedure, and most are helped by a description of sensations they are likely to experience before these occur. A record that the procedure was performed should be made in the case notes in all but the most minor of procedures (e.g., venepuncture for routine blood sampling).

General precautions

It is important to be aware of the risk of infection or trauma to the patient, operator and assistant during any practical procedure. These risks are minimised by following simple rules:

- Needles should not be resheathed and all disposable sharp instruments discarded by the operator should be placed in an appropriate container to minimise the risk of needle-stick injury. It is best practice to bring the sharps container to the bedside.
- Drapes and other soiled equipment should be placed in appropriate containers after ensuring that no sharps are inadvertently left amongst the drapes.
- Gloves and gown should only be removed after all used instruments and disposable equipment have been placed in the appropriate containers.

Aseptic technique

Transmission of infection is important to avoid, and the risk of spread should be minimised. As a minimum precaution, the skin should be cleansed with an antiseptic solution before all procedures, and sterile instruments should be used. For some procedures, such as central venous catheterisation, bladder catheterisation, insertion of chest drains and lumbar puncture, a full aseptic technique must be employed. Often, this is best achieved by the use of aseptic 'bundles', which not only include use of sterile or disposable equipment but also include nonprocedural measures, for example, routines and avoidance of interruptions and distractions during the procedure. The steps required for asepsis are outlined in Table 8.1.

Local anaesthesia

Local anaesthetic agents inhibit axonal membrane depolarisation and hence block the longitudinal conduction of electrical impulses along nerves. They may be used topically, i.e., painted or sprayed on mucous membranes and wound surfaces, so that they are absorbed locally to produce analgesia. Areas suitable for topical analgesia include the urethra, eye, nose, throat and bronchial tree. Local anaesthesia is most frequently administered by local infiltration, and this is widely used for minor surgical procedures. Local anaesthetic drugs are potentially toxic and care must be taken to avoid inadvertent intravascular injection. The first sign of toxicity is often numbness or tingling of the tongue or around the mouth, followed by lightheadedness and tinnitus. At higher blood concentrations, there is loss of consciousness, convulsions and apnoea, which may culminate in cardiovascular collapse. In general, local

Table 8.1 Aseptic technique

- An assistant is desirable to open nonsterile packs and 'drop' required instruments or solutions onto the sterile field
- Hand-washing for aseptic techniques ('scrubbing up') should last a full 3 minutes. The hands and forearms are wetted under a running tap and thoroughly washed with an antiseptic solution such as povidone-iodine (Betadine) or chlorhexidine (Hibiscrub)
- A sterile brush is then used to scrub the hands: in particular, the ulnar border, the interdigital clefts and the nails
- After the wash is completed, the hands are rinsed and held hands up/elbows down, so that water from the hands runs from the elbows into the sink
- The hands are dried on a sterile towel and the operator puts on a sterile gown and gloves. Thereafter, the operator must not touch anything other than sterile equipment or instruments
- The operative field is now cleansed with an antiseptic solution such as povidone-iodine or chlorhexidine, using sterile instruments and swabs. The area prepared should be much greater than the anticipated operative field, and cleansing should start from the centre and work outwards
- The operative field is then encircled with sterile drapes, which are secured so as to leave the operative field at the centre and provide the operator with as wide a sterile surrounding as possible.

anaesthetics are most effective when placed accurately in terms of anatomy. It is best practice to calculate the maximum recommended dose for any local anaesthetic and if a larger volume is required (for example to infiltrate a wide area) the maximum recommended amount of local anaesthetic can be diluted with 0.9% saline.

Lidocaine (lignocaine), the most widely used local anaesthetic agent, is available in 0.5–2% strength solutions at a maximum recommended dose of 4 mg/kg. Lidocaine is a short-acting anaesthetic (lasting up to 2 hours) whereas bupivacaine is a longer acting local anaesthetic that lasts up to 8 hours. It is permissible to mix local anaesthetics, although the maximum recommended amount will be correspondingly smaller.

Solutions of local anaesthetic mixed with a 1:200,000 concentration of adrenaline (epinephrine) are available. Adrenaline acts as a vasoconstrictor. It minimises bleeding and reduces redistribution of the anaesthetic agent, increasing its efficacy and duration of action. The maximum dose increases to 7 mg/kg when adrenaline is added. Local anaesthetic agents with adrenaline should not be used in anatomical areas supplied by an end-artery, for example the fingers and toes, penis, ear pinna and nose because of the risk of vasoconstriction that can result in ischaemia and necrosis (gangrene).

Suturing

The purpose of suturing is to approximate tissues to facilitate primary wound healing to take place, or to ligate bleeding vessels to arrest haemorrhage. Needles can be straight or curved. Straight needles and large curved needles are usually hand-held, whereas smaller curved needles are designed for use with a needle holder. The thread is 'swaged' inside the needle to eliminate drag. Needles can be cutting (usually reverse-cutting) or round-bodied. Round-bodied needles push tissue aside rather than cut through and are preferred when stitching blood vessels and bowel.

Cutting needles are generally used to pass through tough tissues e.g., skin. For abdominal wall fascial closure, blunt needles are available which reduce the risk of needle-stick injuries.

Suture materials

Nonabsorbable sutures

Nonabsorbable sutures may be classified into three groups:

1. *Natural braided sutures* (e.g., silk, linen) have good handling qualities and knot easily and securely. Their disadvantage is increased tissue reaction and suture line sepsis, caused by the capillary action of the braided material drawing microorganisms into the suture track. Such materials also lose tensile strength quickly with time, or when wet. These sutures are used less frequently.
2. *Synthetic braided materials* (e.g., Nurolon, Ethibond, Mersilene) cause less tissue reaction than natural materials. They have good handling qualities and knot easily and securely.
3. *Synthetic monofilament materials* (e.g., nylon, polypropylene) have less drag through the tissues and cause little tissue reaction. They are free from the capillary effect of braided sutures and cause less suture track sepsis. However, thicker grades handle less well than braided sutures because of increased 'memory' (i.e., they retain the configuration in which they were packaged). Knots in monofilament sutures are less secure than those in braided or natural sutures, and most surgeons use multiple throws when knotting monofilament sutures.

Absorbable sutures

Absorbable sutures are generally made from synthetic materials. They cause relatively little tissue reaction, retain their tensile strength and are absorbed slowly. They can be multifilament, such as Dexon (polyglycolic acid) and Vicryl (polyglycolic plus polylactic acid), or monofilament, such as Maxon (polyglyconate) and PDS (polydioxonone). These synthetic sutures are commonly used for intraabdominal procedures and subcuticular wound closure. Interrupted sutures with each knot buried are used for small wounds, whereas in longer wounds a continuous subcuticular suture is employed.

Suturing the skin

Skin wounds are sutured under as near-sterile conditions as possible, using a strict aseptic technique. A few basic principles underlie good wound care:

- Tissue should be handled gently. The wound should not be rubbed with swabs. Blood in a wound is removed by gently pressing a swab.
- Haemostasis should be meticulous to prevent wound haematoma.
- All foreign material and devitalised tissues should be removed. Where this is prevented by heavy contamination, delayed primary closure or secondary closure should be considered.
- Potential spaces (dead space) in the wound should be closed using absorbable suture material such as Vicryl. Where this is not possible, a suction drain is led from the potential space before more superficial layers are closed.

Table 8.2 Times recommended for removal of sutures	
• Face and neck	4 days
• Scalp	7 days
• Abdomen and chest	7–10 days
• Limbs	7 days
• Feet	10–14 days

• The tension on sutured wounds is critical. If sutures are knotted too tightly, the suture line may become ischaemic, leading to delayed healing, nonhealing and an increased risk of wound infection, and in extreme situations sutures can cut through. Equally, insufficient tension on the suture may result in failure to appose the wound edges or inadequate haemostasis. This does not apply to the knots themselves, which should always be secure.

Cutting needles are used to suture skin. Nonabsorbable sutures are generally preferred, but require subsequent removal. Interrupted sutures have the advantage over a continuous suture in that the removal of one or two appropriately sited stitches may allow adequate drainage if the wound becomes infected. The sutures should be placed equidistant from one another, taking equal 'bites' on either side of the wound. A sufficient number should be inserted to maintain apposition without the skin edges gaping. The size of bite is determined by the amount of subcutaneous fat and by whether or not the fat has been separately sutured. For abdominal wounds, 5-mm bites are taken on either side of the wound, whereas on the face a 1–2-mm bite is preferred. The wound edge is picked up with toothed dissecting forceps, then the needle is introduced through the skin at an angle as close to vertical as possible and brought out on the other side at a similar angle.

Similar principles apply when using a continuous suture. A subcuticular continuous suture is preferred by some surgeons and avoids the small pinpoint scars at the site of entry and exit of interrupted sutures, or the cross-hatching that results if sutures are tied too tightly or left in too long. Table 8.2 gives the suggested times for removal of sutures. Cosmetic results as good as those achieved by subcuticular suturing can be obtained by removing sutures in half the times listed in Table 8.2 and by replacing them with adhesive strips (e.g., Steristrip). Skin stapling is commonly used for closure of wounds at any site, as it can be undertaken rapidly. The staples are supplied in disposable cartridges for single patient use and are easily removed.

Airway procedures

Maintaining the airway

The ability to maintain the airway is a basic skill that every doctor, nurse, paramedic and indeed member of the general public should have. Its simplicity belies its importance, but it is a life-saving skill, which must be learnt through practice.

In the unconscious patient, muscles that normally maintain a clear airway become lax. The tongue and soft tissue fall backwards, particularly in the supine patient, occluding the airway. Maintaining a clear airway allows the patient to breathe or allows the lungs to be ventilated.

Procedure

The simplest manoeuvre is to place the patient on their side with the neck extended in the so-called 'recovery position'. This allows the tongue and soft tissues to fall clear of the larynx and provide a patent airway. The mouth and pharynx should be checked and cleared of debris, such as dentures, vomit or food.

When the patient has to be kept supine, the neck should be extended. The mouth is opened slightly and the mandible pulled firmly forward by pressure applied behind both angles of the jaw. The mandible is held in this position by closing the mouth and using the teeth as a splint. Forward pressure is maintained behind the angles of the jaw (*jaw-thrust* manoeuvre) or submentally (*chin-lift* manoeuvre), avoiding pressure on the soft tissues (Fig. 8.1). In some cases, particularly in edentulous patients, an oropharyngeal airway helps to maintain a patent airway.

Ventilation by mask

The lungs may be ventilated by mask and bag, using one of two systems. The first is a rebreathing bag with an adjustable valve and fresh gas supply (which should be present in each anaesthetic room, intensive therapy unit and resuscitation room). The second and more widespread is the self-reinflating type of bag, such as the 'Ambu' or 'Laerdal' bags, which do not rely on a

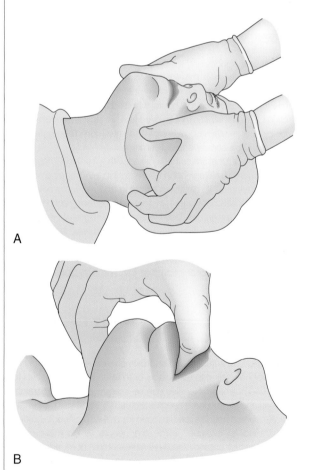

A

B

Fig. 8.1 Maintaining the airway. (A) The jaw-thrust manoeuvre. **(B)** The chin-lift manoeuvre.

gas supply but to which supplemental oxygen can be added. For the inexperienced, this technique is best performed with the help of an assistant.

Procedure

The airway is held patent with the patient supine, as described above. A mask is applied to the face and held in position using the thumb and index fingers of both hands. The little fingers of each hand are placed behind the angles of the jaw and used to lift the mandible forward. The ring and middle fingers are placed on the mandible to help maintain this position. The assistant squeezes the bag to ventilate the lungs. The adequacy of ventilation is assessed by observing appropriate chest movement.

With more experience, it is possible to maintain a patent airway and hold the mask on with one hand, and squeeze the bag with the other.

The laryngeal mask airway

This airway device is designed to be inserted into the pharynx, and has a cuff that, when inflated, forms a gentle seal over the larynx. It is not a replacement for endotracheal intubation and does not protect the airway from aspiration. It does, however, provide a patent airway when positioned correctly, and allows effective ventilation of the lungs. As with other procedures, insertion should be learned under supervision.

Procedure

For men a size 4 laryngeal mask airway is suitable, and for women a size 3, with smaller sizes being available for children. The cuff should be deflated and lubricated with gel. The patient's head is maintained in an extended position using the left hand, and the airway is held in the right hand and introduced into the mouth (Fig. 8.2). The airway is passed backwards over the tongue until resistance is felt. It should then be at the level of the larynx. The cuff is inflated and the airway should be seen to rise slightly out of the mouth. Position is confirmed by the ability to ventilate the lungs.

Endotracheal intubation

Endotracheal intubation can be life-saving; it can maintain a patent airway, facilitate oxygenation and prevent aspiration. Every opportunity should be taken to acquire this skill in the elective situation in the anaesthetic room.

Procedure

The patient's neck is flexed and the head extended at the atlanto-occipital joint, 'sniffing the morning air'. Retaining a pillow under the head but leaving a space free from beneath the shoulders will usually help to attain this position. Failure to position the patient correctly is one of the most common causes of difficulty in intubation.

The laryngoscope is held in the left hand; its blade is inserted into the right side of the patient's mouth and passed backwards along the side of the tongue into the oropharynx. The blade is designed to push the tongue over to the left side of the mouth. Care is taken to avoid damage to the lips and teeth. The laryngoscope is *pulled* upwards and forwards, in line with the handle, *not* used as a lever, to lift the tongue and jaw and reveal the epiglottis (Fig. 8.3). The blade is then advanced to the base of the epiglottis and the laryngoscope pulled further upwards and forwards again in line with the handle to reveal the vocal cords.

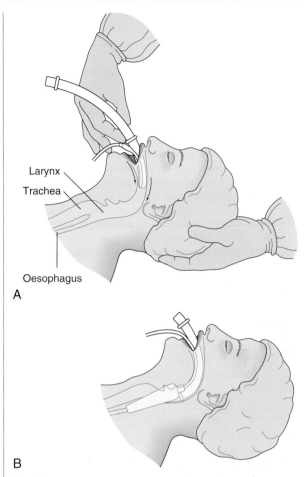

Larynx
Trachea

Oesophagus
A

B

Fig. 8.2 Insertion of a laryngeal mask airway. **(A)** Gentle insertion of airway with head in extended position. **(B)** Advancement of airway.

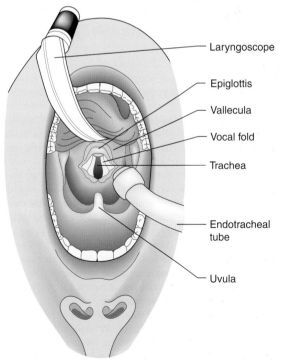

Laryngoscope

Epiglottis

Vallecula

Vocal fold

Trachea

Endotracheal tube

Uvula

Fig. 8.3 Oral endotracheal intubation.

For men, a 9-mm cuffed tube is usually appropriate, and for women an 8-mm tube is generally used. For children, a rough guide to gauge tube size is age divided by 4, +4.5 mm. Normally, an uncuffed tube is used in children.

The endotracheal tube is passed through the vocal cords into the trachea and advanced until its cuff is about 1 cm through. Many endotracheal tubes have a mark to indicate this position. The laryngoscope blade is withdrawn and the cuff inflated to provide an airtight seal in the trachea.

The most serious complication of endotracheal intubation is failure to recognise misplacement of the tube, particularly in the oesophagus or, to a lesser degree, in the right main bronchus. Misplacement is best avoided by direct visualisation of passage of the tube between the vocal cords, inspection of the chest wall for equal movement of both sides of the chest, and auscultation for breath sounds bilaterally in the midaxillary line. Absence of breath sounds or the presence of only quiet ones in the epigastrium is a further reassuring sign. If there is any doubt about the position of the tube, it should be removed and ventilation instituted by mask.

Surgical airway

Inability to intubate the trachea is an indication for creating a surgical airway. In the emergency situation, such as in patients with severe facial trauma or pharyngeal oedema secondary to burns, the insertion of a large-calibre plastic cannula through the cricothyroid membrane (**needle cricothyroidotomy**) below the level of the obstruction can be life-saving. Intermittent jet insufflation of oxygen at 15 L/min (1 second inspiration and 4 seconds to allow expiration) can provide oxygenation for a limited period (30–45 minutes) until a more definitive procedure can be undertaken.

Surgical cricothyroidotomy is performed by making an incision that extends through the cricothyroid membrane and inserting a tracheostomy tube.

In children, care must be taken to avoid damage to the cricoid cartilage, which is the only circumferential support to the upper trachea. Surgical cricothyroidotomy is therefore not recommended for children under 12 years of age.

▍ Procedure

It is important to check all equipment and connections before starting. With the patient in the supine position and the neck in a neutral position, the thyroid cartilage (Adam's apple) and cricoid cartilage are palpated. The cricothyroid membrane lies between the lower border of the thyroid cartilage and the upper border of the cricoid cartilage. The skin is cleansed with antiseptic solution and local anaesthetic infiltrated into the skin, if the patient is conscious. The thyroid cartilage is stabilised with the left hand and a small transverse skin incision made over the cricothyroid membrane. The blade of the scalpel is inserted through the membrane and then rotated through 90 degrees to open the airway. An artery clip or tracheal spreader may be inserted to enlarge the opening enough to admit a cuffed endotracheal or tracheostomy tube (Fig. 8.4). The central trocar of the tube is removed and the tube connected to a bag-valve or ventilator circuit. The cuff is then inflated and air entry to each side of the chest is checked. The tube is secured to prevent dislodgement.

Formal open tracheostomy may be performed as an emergency procedure, but is more commonly undertaken in critically ill patients requiring long-term ventilation, although current practice in most intensive care units is to use percutaneous tracheostomy kits, based on the Seldinger guidewire technique. Open surgical tracheostomy is a procedure for an experienced clinician and involves making an inverted U-shaped opening through the second, third and fourth tracheal rings.

Changing a tracheostomy tube

It is common practice to change a tracheostomy tube every 7 days. Suction must be available.

▍ Procedure

If a cuffed tube is to be inserted, the integrity of the cuff is checked and it is then fully deflated. Lubricant gel is applied to both the cuff and tube. The patient is placed semirecumbent with the neck extended. If replacement is likely to be difficult, a suction catheter inserted into the old tracheostomy tube can be used as an introducer for the new tube.

The cuff of the old tube is deflated. Secretions often collect above the cuff and enter the trachea when it is deflated, causing the patient to cough; both patient and operator should be alert to this. Because the tube is curved, it should be removed with an 'arc-like' movement. The site is then cleansed and any secretions are removed. In the spontaneously breathing stable patient, there is no need for undue haste. The new tube is inserted with a similar movement to that employed for removal, and its cuff inflated.

Any signs of respiratory distress should raise suspicion of the possibility of misplacement or occlusion of the tube. The tube and trachea are immediately checked for patency by passing a suction catheter through the tube. If the catheter passes easily into the respiratory tract, usually signified by the patient coughing as the catheter touches the carina, other causes for respiratory distress should be sought.

When the tracheostomy is no longer needed, an airtight dressing is applied over the site after removing the tube. There is no need for formal surgical closure at this stage, as in most instances the wound will close and heal spontaneously. For the first few days, patients should be encouraged to press firmly on the dressing when they wish to cough, so as to avoid air leakage through the tracheostomy site.

Thoracic procedures

Intercostal tube drainage

Intercostal intubation is used to drain a large pneumothorax, haemothorax or pleural effusion. To drain a pneumothorax, a size 14–16 French (Fr) chest drain tube is inserted, using a lateral approach in the midaxillary line of the sixth intercostal space. Drainage of an effusion or haemothorax requires a larger drain (20–26 Fr), which should be inserted in the seventh, eighth or ninth intercostal space in the posterior axillary line. A slightly higher insertion in the midaxillary line in the fifth intercostal space may be technically easier in supine patients with trauma and other acutely ill patients for pneumothorax or haemothorax or both.

▍ Procedure

If a low lateral approach is to be used, reference should be made to the chest x-ray to ensure that the drain will not be inserted subdiaphragmatically. A strict aseptic technique must be used. The skin, intercostal muscles and pleura are infiltrated with local anaesthetic. If a rib is encountered by the needle, the tip is 'walked' up the rib to enter the pleura above the rib edge. The

8

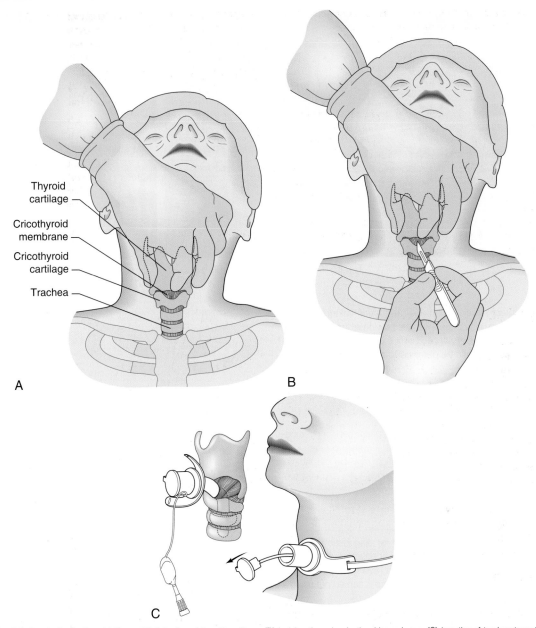

Fig. 8.4 Surgical cricothyroidotomy. (A) Palpation of thyroid cartilage. **(B)** Incision through cricothyroid membrane. **(C)** Insertion of tracheostomy tube.

Thyroid cartilage

Cricothyroid membrane

Cricothyroid cartilage

Trachea

A

B

C

depth at which the pleural space is entered is determined by aspiration with the syringe. A 3-cm horizontal incision is now made in the skin. A tract is developed by blunt dissection through the subcutaneous tissues and the intercostal muscles are separated just superior to the top of the rib to avoid damage to the neurovascular bundle. The parietal pleura is punctured with the tip of a pair of artery forceps and a gloved finger is inserted into the pleural cavity (Fig. 8.5). This ensures the incision is correctly placed, prevents injury to other organs, and permits any adhesions or clots to be cleared. The trocar is removed from the thoracostomy tube, the proximal end is clamped, and the tube is advanced into the pleural space to the desired length. The tube is sutured to the skin with a heavy suture to prevent accidental dislodgement. A 'Z' suture is placed around the incision, wrapped tightly around the drainage tube and tied, thus securing the tube. A sterile dressing and an adhesive bandage are applied to form an airtight seal and prevent aspiration of air around the tube. The drainage tube is attached to an underwater drainage system and a chest x-ray is then obtained. Low-pressure suction may be applied to the drainage bottle to assist drainage or re-expansion of the lung.

Removal of an intercostal drainage tube

The drainage tube may be removed 12–24 hours after cessation of drainage. As a precaution in the case of pneumothorax, the tube can first be clamped for several hours and a chest x-ray taken to ensure that there has been no recurrence, although this practice is variable and some believe this unnecessary.

Procedure

The 'Z' suture is freed from the tube and can be used to close the wound. Where this is not possible, the suture should be removed and a new one inserted around the wound. Patients are asked to

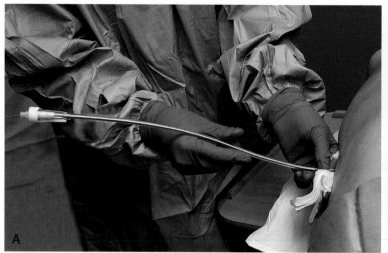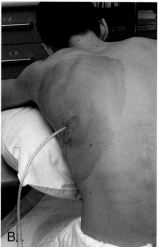

Fig. 8.5 Chest drain. (A) Insertion. (B) In situ.

hold their breath in expiration and the tube is withdrawn, after which the skin is firmly closed with the previously inserted suture. A sterile dressing is firmly applied over the wound. A postprocedure chest x-ray should be obtained to confirm that there is no residual pneumothorax.

Pleural aspiration

Aspiration of fluid from the pleural cavity is performed for diagnostic or therapeutic purposes. Protein or amylase content, and cytological or bacteriological examination may be diagnostic. Complete aspiration of large effusions allows fuller expansion of the lungs and may improve ventilation.

Procedure

Where aspiration is to be undertaken for diagnostic purposes only, a 21-gauge needle and syringe are adequate. For therapeutic aspiration, a larger-bore needle, 50 mL syringe and three-way tap system should be used. The procedure is carried out using a strict aseptic technique.

The patient is positioned sitting up, resting the arms and elbows on a table. The position and size of the effusion should be outlined by percussion and chest x-ray. The lower border of the effusion is determined, particularly on the right to avoid puncturing the liver. In the case of small effusions, ultrasound guidance is helpful.

The skin, intercostal muscles and pleura are infiltrated with local anaesthetic in the seventh or eighth space, in line with the inferior angle of the scapula. The needle is advanced over the upper border of the rib to avoid damage to the neurovascular bundle. Continuous suction should be applied to the syringe and the needle advanced no further than is required to aspirate fluid freely, thereby avoiding damage to the underlying lung.

A three-way tap greatly reduces the risk of air entry during removal of larger volumes and allows the syringe to be emptied into a collection vessel (Fig. 8.6); this avoids having to disconnect the syringe each time it is filled. It is normally recommended that no more than 1–1.5 L of fluid be removed at any one time. This reduces the risk of sudden mediastinal shift or the development of pulmonary oedema associated with rapid re-expansion of a collapsed lung. Coughing or pain on aspiration is an indication

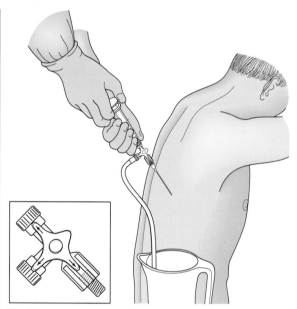

Fig. 8.6 Pleural aspiration.

that visceral pleura is in close contact with the cannula, which should be repositioned or withdrawn.

At the end of the procedure, the needle is withdrawn and a sterile dressing applied. A chest x-ray is taken to assess the amount of residual fluid present and to exclude a pneumothorax.

Abdominal procedures

Nasogastric tube insertion

A nasogastric tube is inserted to drain stomach contents in conditions such as intestinal obstruction, or to administer enteral nutrition. In most situations, a 14–16 Fr single-lumen radio-opaque nasogastric tube with multiple distal openings will suffice. Double-lumen tubes are occasionally used to allow continuous low-pressure suction and to prevent the lumen from becoming blocked by gastric mucosa. Gastric drainage tubes with a jejunal extension to allow distal enteral feeding are also useful in cases of delayed gastric emptying or functional or partial gastric outlet obstruction, for example in acute pancreatitis with external compression of the duodenum due to swelling.

Procedure

Reassurance and a calm approach will make this procedure more acceptable to the patient and increase the chances of successful placement. The nose is inspected for any deformity and the more patent nasal passage is chosen for insertion. The patient is placed in the sitting position vertically upright with the neck flexed with the chin on the chest. A local anaesthetic spray may be used to anaesthetise the nasal passage and the patient can be asked to hold a mouthful of water in their mouth without swallowing. The tube is well lubricated with gel and passed backwards along the floor of the nasal passage (Fig. 8.7). When a slight resistance is felt as the tube passes from the nasopharynx to the oropharynx, or it is detected that the patient senses the tube has passed into the oropharynx, the patient should immediately swallow the mouthful of water. During this time, the tube can be gently passed down the oesophagus in concert with the swallowing cascade.

It is important not to force insertion of the tube in a patient who is retching. The oesophagogastric junction is about 40 cm from the incisor teeth, and ideally, about 10–15 cm of the tube should be placed into the stomach. Most nasogastric tubes have markings to allow measurement of the length inserted. Correct placement of the tube is confirmed by free aspiration of gastric contents, and by auscultation in the epigastrium while 20 mL of air is insufflated. Once in place, the tube is fixed to the nose with adhesive tape.

In patients with head injuries, the nasal route is avoided because of the risk of introducing infection, or even the nasogastric tube itself, into the central nervous system through an open fracture of the skull base. The oral route is also considered in patients with serious coagulopathy, as passage of the tube through the nose may result in significant haemorrhage. Finally, blind passage of a tube in the early period following oesophagectomy should never be attempted, as this may disrupt the anastomosis.

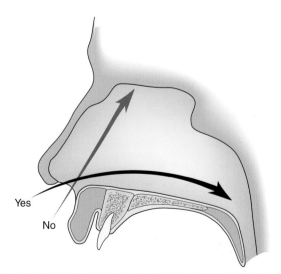

Fig. 8.7 Nasogastric intubation. Note the correct direction for inserting the tube.

Yes

No

Fine-bore nasogastric tubes

Elemental diets tend to have an unpleasant taste and are poorly tolerated when swallowed normally. These are best given by infusion through a fine-bore nasogastric tube, which is more comfortable and less likely to cause oesophageal erosions than a standard nasogastric tube. It does, however, require great care in insertion, as it can easily pass into the respiratory tract. A chest x-ray should be obtained to confirm placement in the stomach and not the lung before feeding commences.

Procedure

Fine-bore nasogastric tubes have a wire stylet to facilitate passage. The tube is passed in the same way as a standard nasogastric tube and it is important not to force passage of the tube. The position of the tube is confirmed by x-ray, and only then is the stylet removed. Once removed, it must never be reintroduced while the tube remains in place, as there is a significant risk of perforating both the tube and the oesophagus. The tube tends to collapse if aspirated, so that aspiration cannot be used to check its position.

It is often advantageous to position the fine-bore feeding tube in the jejunum. This can be achieved using a radiological imaging technique or by the use of an enteral feeding tube with a mercury-filled tip that 'self-propels' into the jejunum, or with the aid of a gastroscope.

Oesophageal tamponade

The Sengstaken tube is a gastric aspiration tube with inflatable gastric and oesophageal balloons, which may be used for emergency treatment of bleeding oesophageal varices. A modification, the Sengstaken–Blakemore or Minnesota tube, has an additional channel to allow the aspiration of saliva from the oesophagus above the level of the oesophageal balloon.

The use of a Sengstaken–Blakemore tube is used as a temporary measure to control haemorrhage prior to definitive treatment, or to allow transfer of the patient to a specialist centre, and can be life-saving. It is advisable to deflate the oesophageal balloon for 5 minutes every 6 hours to avoid the risk of ischaemic necrosis and ulceration of the oesophageal mucosa. The tube is not normally kept in place for more than 24 to 48 hours.

Procedure

The Sengstaken–Blakemore tube should be stored in a refrigerator, as this renders it less pliable and facilitates insertion. The oesophageal and gastric balloons are checked for leaks and completely deflated using an aspiration syringe. The tube is inserted in the same way as a normal nasogastric tube but local anaesthesia and consideration of sedation may be required for nasal passage. Anaesthetic assistance should be sought if there is any threat to the airway through aspiration. An exsanguinating patient will require critical care support. A patient with bleeding varices is unlikely to cooperate fully and the tube may have to be passed with the patient on his or her side. If there is difficulty inserting the tube via the nasal route, the oral route may be used.

The tube is advanced approximately 60 cm and the gastric balloon inflated with 150–200 mL of air or water. The tube is drawn back until this lower balloon is felt to be gently but firmly abutting the gastric cardia. An assistant holds the tube in this position under slight tension, and the oesophageal balloon is inflated with

8

air to a pressure of approximately 40 mmHg, checked by attaching a sphygmomanometer. The tube is secured in position to the cheek with tape, but no additional traction is necessary.

The stomach is aspirated regularly through the main lumen of the tube to check for further bleeding. This lumen may also be used for the administration of medication, such as lactulose and neomycin. A fourth lumen allows aspiration of the upper oesophagus and pharynx and reduces the risk of bronchial aspiration. In patients who are stuporose or comatose, the airway should be protected by an endotracheal tube.

Abdominal paracentesis

Abdominal paracentesis is performed to relieve the discomfort caused by distension with ascitic fluid, or to obtain fluid for cytological examination. The bladder must be emptied, if necessary by preliminary catheterisation, and safe practice often includes marking of a safe target area by ultrasound. A 'Trocath' peritoneal dialysis catheter with multiple side perforations over a length of 8 cm is inserted under sterile conditions.

Procedure

The operator follows the principles of asepsis throughout and a site is chosen for insertion of the catheter. This can be either in the midline (one-third of the way from the umbilicus to the pubic symphysis), or in the right or left iliac fossa (at the junction of the outer and middle thirds of a line drawn from the umbilicus to the anterior superior iliac spine). The vicinity of scars should be avoided, as adhesions increase the risk of bowel perforation. Local anaesthetic is infiltrated through all layers of the abdominal wall. The depth at which the peritoneum is entered is determined by aspiration with the syringe.

A 3-mm stab incision is made in the skin with a scalpel. The trocar is introduced into the catheter and the shaft of the catheter is held firmly between left thumb and index finger some 4–5 cm higher than the estimated depth of the peritoneum. This prevents 'overshoot' as the right hand inserts the trocar and catheter through the abdominal wall into the peritoneum (Fig. 8.8).

The catheter is advanced further with the left hand while the trocar is withdrawn with the right. If any resistance is encountered, the catheter is withdrawn 2–3 cm, rotated 180 degrees and then advanced again. The minimum final length of catheter within the peritoneal cavity must be 10 cm. If this position is not obtained, the side perforations of the catheter may lie within the abdominal wall and allow troublesome extravasation of ascitic fluid into the

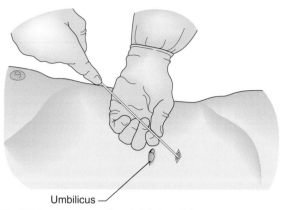

Umbilicus

Fig. 8.8 Insertion of a peritoneal dialysis catheter.

subcutaneous tissues. The catheter is secured to the skin and attached via a connection tube with a flow-control clamp to a sterile drainage bag (Fig. 8.9).

If drainage of large volumes of ascitic fluid is likely or planned, consideration should be given to co-administering intravenous infusion of albumin in order to avoid precipitating a marked shift of fluid from the intravascular compartment into the peritoneal cavity. This prevents significant haemodynamic changes and reduces the risk of developing cardiovascular instability, renal impairment or hepatic encephalopathy.

Vascular procedures

Venepuncture

The antecubital fossa is the most convenient and most frequently used site, as the median cubital vein, median vein of the forearm and the cephalic vein are all easily accessible (Fig. 8.10). Care must be taken to avoid the brachial artery. Sampling from smaller veins on the forearm or the back of the hand may appear attractive, but these veins collapse easily on aspiration and adequate samples are difficult to obtain. In cases of extreme difficulty, the femoral vein should be considered. This vessel lies medial to the femoral artery, which is used as a landmark. In adults, a 21-gauge needle is used; in children, a 23- or 25-gauge will suffice.

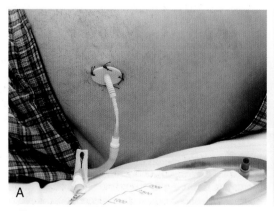
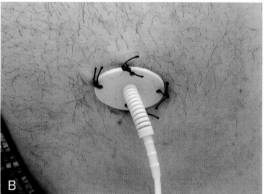

Fig. 8.9 **Abdominal paracentesis catheter in situ. (A)** Catheter inserted in left iliac fossa. **(B)** Flange of catheter secured with sutures.

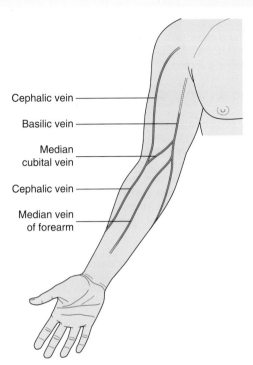

Cephalic vein

Basilic vein

Median cubital vein

Cephalic vein

Median vein of forearm

Fig. 8.10 Venepuncture sites.

Procedure

A venous tourniquet is applied to the upper arm and the patient is encouraged to clench the fist several times to increase venous filling. The position of the vein is identified and the skin cleansed. The needle is advanced through the skin and into the vein, with the needle bevel facing upwards. This manoeuvre is carried out in a 'two-step' fashion, first through the skin and then through the vein wall. Entry through the skin with a decisive action causes much less discomfort than a slow hesitant movement. The needle is advanced 2–3 mm into the vein and the position of the needle and syringe stabilised with one hand. The plunger of the syringe is slowly withdrawn with the other hand until the required amount of blood is obtained. The tourniquet is released before the needle withdrawn and gentle but firm pressure is immediately applied over the site of entry into the vein to prevent haematoma formation, which is painful for the patient and makes subsequent sampling more difficult. The risk of haematoma may be reduced if elbow extension is maintained for several minutes while applying pressure.

The aspirated blood is placed into the appropriate sample tubes after removal of the needle from the syringe. With prevacuumed sample tubes, the needle should be left on the syringe in order to fill the tubes. Haemolysis invalidates some results (for example, potassium and phosphate levels) and is more likely to occur when smaller needles are used or with vigorous ejection of blood from the syringe.

Safety measures

Used needles and syringes should be placed in specially reinforced carriers, marked 'Sharps—for incineration', to avoid the risk of needle-stick injury or blood contamination to staff. To reduce the risk of blood spillage or contamination to staff, sample tubes have been modified so that they may be used as syringes, and sent to the laboratory without the need to transfer blood from syringe to tube.

Venepuncture for blood culture

This procedure is carried out for microbiological culture and identification of organisms that may be present in the blood. The procedure is similar to venepuncture but particular care must be taken to avoid contamination. The adoption of standard protocols and 'care bundles' for taking blood cultures has vastly reduced the false-positive blood culture rate (EBM 8.1).

EBM 8.1

'The use of care bundles has been shown to reduce the contamination rate of peripheral blood cultures and prevent unnecessary antibiotic therapy.'

Department of Health (UK). Saving lives: taking blood cultures. A summary of best practice. Department of Health, London; June 2007.

Procedure

A venous tourniquet is applied, as before, the skin thoroughly cleansed with an appropriate solution, using a sterile swab or cotton wool ball, and venepuncture performed without the operator touching the skin at the site of needle entry. After withdrawal, the needle is removed from the syringe and a second sterile needle substituted and used to introduce the appropriate aliquot of blood into both aerobic and anaerobic culture bottles. The exact volumes of blood and the number of bottles filled will depend on local laboratory policies. All blood culture bottles should be sent immediately to the laboratory or, if this is not possible, placed in an incubator at 37°C until transport is available.

Peripheral venous cannulation

Most intravenous infusions are given into the forearm. The veins of the leg are avoided because of the greater risk of thrombosis. Intravenous cannulas should not be sited over joints as this necessitates splinting and reduces the free use of the arm by the patient. Even with splinting, cannulas are subject to more movement in these positions and are prone to more complications.

All commercially available cannulas consist of an outer flexible sheath and an inner metal needle. A 16- or 18-gauge cannula will suffice for most purposes but where rapid infusions of large quantities of fluid are required, a larger cannula should be used.

Procedure

A venous tourniquet is applied, the site of insertion chosen and the skin is cleansed. Venepuncture is made in the 'two-step' fashion described above and confirmed by a 'flashback' of blood into the cannula. The cannula is initially advanced 2–3 mm into the vein, and the cannula sheath is advanced into the vein with one hand while the metal needle is partially withdrawn with the other.

Once the cannula sheath is fully inserted into the vein, the tourniquet is released and gentle pressure applied over the vein at the tip of the cannula. The metal needle is fully withdrawn from the cannula and disposed of safely in a sharps container. The cannula is fixed in position with adhesive tape or a specially designed sticking plaster. It is common practice to record the date of insertion on the dressing so that the duration of any one cannula is known. An intravenous fluid giving set, previously primed with normal saline, is then connected. The cannula and distal 10–15 cm of the giving set are securely fixed to the skin with adhesive tape.

8

Cannulation sites should be inspected regularly for signs of swelling, erythema or tenderness, which may indicate extravasation, thrombophlebitis or infection. If any of these is present or the patient complains of pain at the site, the infusion must be stopped and the cannula resited. Extravasation may cause tissue necrosis. Thrombophlebitis occurs more readily when small veins are used, or when the pH of the infusate differs significantly from blood pH. The chances of infection increase the longer a cannula is left in situ, and infusion sites must be changed regularly.

Bolus injections through an intravenous cannula should not be made without first ensuring that the cannula is patent and that there is no extravasation.

Venous cut-down

Venous cut-down for fluid replacement is rarely required, except in seriously hypovolaemic patients, usually following trauma and should only be regarded as a temporary measure for resuscitation. The most common site is the long saphenous vein at the ankle (Fig. 8.11) or at the saphenofemoral junction in the groin, the basilic vein in the antecubital fossa or the cephalic vein at the wrist.

Procedure

Using aseptic technique, a transverse incision is made in the skin over the vein, which is then identified by blunt dissection. At the ankle, the site of cut-down is 2–3 cm anterior to the medial malleolus. The vein is cleared for a distance of 1–2 cm and its distal end is ligated with an absorbable ligature. A second absorbable ligature is placed under the proximal end of the exposed vein and is elevated to prevent backflow of blood. Through a transverse incision in the vein, a large-bore cannula is passed through the skin 2 cm below the skin incision and guided into the vein. The cannula is advanced beyond the proximal ligature, which is then tied securely.

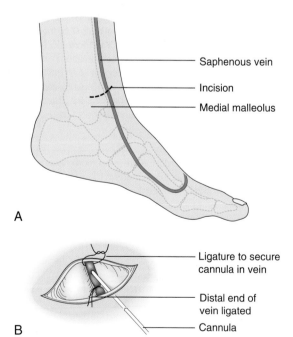

A

B

Fig. 8.11 Saphenous venous cut-down. (A) Incision made anterior to the medial malleolus. **(B)** Cannula inserted in a proximal direction after ligation of the distal vein.

Labels:
- Saphenous vein
- Incision
- Medial malleolus
- Ligature to secure cannula in vein
- Distal end of vein ligated
- Cannula

The intravenous infusion is commenced to ensure free flow, and the wound closed with nonabsorbable sutures. The cannula is sutured to the skin to prevent accidental displacement and a sterile dressing is applied.

Central venous catheter insertion

Placement of a central venous catheter is indicated for monitoring of the central venous pressure (CVP) and for prolonged drug administration or parenteral nutrition. It is recommended that all central lines are placed under ultrasound guidance to reduce complications arising from collateral damage to surrounding structures. Care bundles, incorporating strict asepsis and standard protocols followed on every occasion have been shown to dramatically reduce central line infections and should be used routinely (EBM 8.2).

EBM 8.2

Five evidence-based procedures were implemented to reduce catheter-related septicaemia:

- Hand washing
- Full-barrier precautions during the insertion of central venous catheters
- Cleaning the skin with chlorhexidine
- Avoiding the femoral site if possible
- Removing unnecessary catheters

Practical interventions were:

- Clinician education about central line infection
- Dedicated central-line trolley with necessary supplies
- Checklist to ensure adherence to infection-control practices
- Enforcement if these practices were not being followed
- Removal of central lines discussed at daily ward rounds
- Monitoring and provision of feedback regarding the incidence of catheter-related bloodstream infection at regular meetings.

Pronovost P et al. An intervention to decrease catheter-related bloodstream infections in the ICU. N Engl J Med. 2006;355:2725–32.

Strict aseptic technique is needed and if the catheter is to be used for drug therapy or parenteral nutrition, the procedure should be carried out in the operating theatre. The common sites of insertion of catheters into the superior vena cava are from the internal jugular vein in the neck, from the subclavian vein, or occasionally from a peripheral vein in the antecubital fossa.

Internal jugular vein cannulation

A high approach at the level of the thyroid cartilage carries the least risk. The right internal jugular vein is preferred, as this provides a straighter route into the superior vena cava and avoids the risk of damaging the thoracic duct on the left. A Seldinger technique is normally used with equipment from a commercial kit.

Procedure

The patient is placed in a supine position, with at least 15 degrees head-down tilt to distend the neck veins and reduce the risk of air embolism. The head is turned to the left, unless there is potential for a cervical spine injury following trauma. A wide area on the right side of the neck is cleansed and draped.

The carotid artery is identified at the level of the thyroid cartilage, using the index and middle fingers of the left hand. The internal jugular vein lies just lateral and parallel to it. A bleb of local anaesthetic can be infiltrated into the skin at the proposed puncture site.

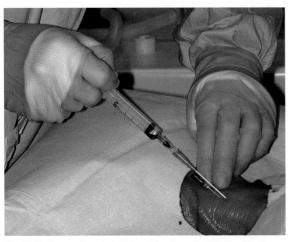

Fig. 8.12 Cannulation of the internal jugular vein. Note the triangle between the sternal and clavicular heads of the sternocleidomastoid muscle.

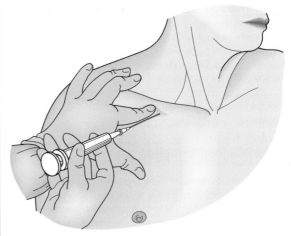

Fig. 8.13 Cannulation of the subclavian vein.

Using ultrasound guidance, an 18-gauge needle on a 10-mL syringe, held in the right hand, is advanced through the skin just lateral to the carotid pulsation, at an angle of 60 degrees to the skin and in the line of the vein (Fig. 8.12). Free aspiration of blood confirms the position of the vein. This manoeuvre is repeated to place a larger (16-gauge) needle in the vein. The flexible 'J' end of the guidewire is passed through this needle into the vein, and the needle removed over it, leaving the guidewire in the vein. A dilator is passed over the wire into the vein and then withdrawn. The catheter is advanced over the wire and the wire is removed, leaving the catheter in situ. In most adults, no more than 15 cm of catheter needs be advanced to ensure correct placement. Blood is aspirated from the catheter to confirm its position in the major vein. Heparinised saline (5 mL) is injected and the catheter is sutured to the skin to fix it in position. A chest x-ray is taken to confirm the position of the catheter and to exclude the presence of a pneumothorax.

Subclavian vein cannulation

Subclavian vein cannulation carries a significant risk of causing a pneumothorax or puncturing the subclavian artery and should only be attempted by an experienced operator.

Procedure

A similar Seldinger technique is generally used under aseptic conditions with the patient in a supine position, with head-down tilt of at least 15 degrees. A small pad placed between the shoulder blades allows the shoulders to drop backwards. Local anaesthetic is infiltrated into the skin and subcutaneous tissue. A large-calibre needle attached to a 10-mL syringe is introduced 1 cm below the junction of the middle and medial thirds of the clavicle. The needle is directed medially, slightly cephalad and posteriorly behind the clavicle towards the tip of a finger placed in the suprasternal notch (Fig. 8.13). Once the vein is accessed, placement of the catheter is identical to that of the internal jugular approach. A chest x-ray is taken and an occlusive dressing applied.

Peripherally-inserted central venous catheter (PICC line)

In theory, this is the safest approach to central venous cannulation, as it avoids the risk of pneumothorax. However, use of a

PICC line is restricted to delivery of total parenteral nutrition and drugs. It is unsuitable for monitoring central venous pressure. Haemorrhage from accidental arterial puncture or as a result of a coagulopathy can be controlled by pressure. Thrombosis and thrombophlebitis are, however, more frequent compared with the internal jugular or subclavian route.

8.1 Summary

Central venous cannulation

- Air embolism is always a risk, even in the head-down position
- When using a guidewire, always keep a secure hold of part of the wire while it remains in the patient
- Blood should be easily aspirated if the catheter is correctly positioned
- A chest x-ray should always be taken to confirm the absence of a pneumothorax and correct positioning. A rough guide to position is that the tip of the catheter should lie at the level of the carina on x-ray
- Cannulas inserted for intravenous nutrition are tunnelled in the subcutaneous tissue to emerge on the chest wall at a distance from the site of entry into the vein (Fig. 8.14). This minimises the risk of sepsis spreading down the tract into the vein.

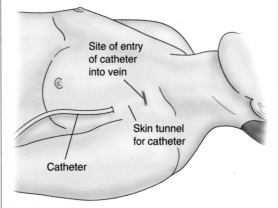

Fig. 8.14 Skin tunnel for central venous catheter.

Procedure

The technique to access a suitable vein in the antecubital fossa is similar to that of peripheral venous cannulation but a large cannula is employed. Once the needle is withdrawn, the long catheter is passed through the cannula into the vein and the venous tourniquet is then released.

The catheter is advanced up the basilic vein and into the superior vena cava. A guide is often provided to gauge the length of catheter inserted. Difficulty is frequently experienced in advancing the catheter past the axilla, and extension and abduction of the arm may help overcome this. The insertion cannula is withdrawn from the vein, leaving the long catheter in place and a chest x-ray performed.

Arterial blood sampling

Arterial blood sampling is undertaken to measure arterial P_{O_2}, P_{CO_2}, [H^+] and standard [HCO_3^-]. The radial artery at the wrist is the site of choice but the femoral artery may also be used. A heparinised sample is required to prevent blockage in the blood gas analyser from coagulation of the sample. Preheparinised syringes are preferred to avoid technical problems with analyser maintenance although local protocol may permit a preheparinised 2-mL syringe.

Procedure

If the syringe is not preheparinised, up to 0.5 mL of 1000 U/mL heparin is drawn into the syringe through a 23-gauge needle. The plunger is fully withdrawn before the air and excess heparin are expelled from the syringe. The residual heparin will be sufficient to anticoagulate the sample.

The course of the artery is defined by palpating the pulse between the index and middle fingers held 2 cm apart. The skin is cleansed and the needle, with its bevel upwards, introduced through the skin at an angle of about 60 degrees and advanced into the artery. Correct positioning is confirmed by blood pulsating into the syringe under pressure; 1–1.5 mL is normally sufficient.

The needle is withdrawn and firm pressure applied over the puncture site for 3 minutes to avoid haematoma formation. The needle is removed from the syringe and any air bubbles are expelled before capping the syringe. The syringe is gently inverted several times to ensure mixing of the heparin. The sample is sent immediately for analysis. Where delay is anticipated, it should be transported in ice.

Needle pericardiocentesis

Cardiac tamponade may result from penetrating or blunt trauma to the chest. Cardiac function may be significantly impaired by a minimal amount of blood within the fixed, fibrous pericardium. The classic signs are elevated CVP, hypotension and muffled heart sounds (Beck's triad). Immediate pericardiocentesis may be life-saving.

Procedure

The patient should be monitored throughout this procedure, with particular reference to the vital signs, CVP and electrocardiogram (ECG). Aseptic technique should be used. The skin is punctured 1–2 cm inferior to the left xiphochondral junction, using a wide-bore plastic-sheathed needle (at least 15 cm in length) with a syringe attached. The needle is angled at 45 degrees and aimed towards the tip of the left scapula (Fig. 8.15). The syringe is aspirated as the needle is advanced, until it easily fills with blood. ECG changes suggest the needle has been advanced too far. Pericardiocentesis must always be followed by a request for an urgent consultation by a cardiologist or cardiothoracic surgeon.

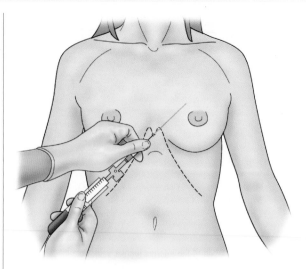

Fig. 8.15 Needle pericardiocentesis.

Urinary procedures

Urethral catheterisation

This procedure may be carried out to relieve urinary retention or to monitor the urine output. Occasionally, catheterisation is necessary to facilitate nursing the incontinent patient. Anatomical obstruction may often be the cause of urinary retention in the male. It is particularly important to avoid forcing the passage of the catheter in this procedure, and if difficulty is experienced, assistance should be sought. A full aseptic technique is required for both male and female catheterisation.

Procedure in the male

The shaft of the penis is held with a sterile swab, the foreskin if present is retracted and the urethral orifice cleansed with a nonalcoholic, noniodine-containing solution. The shaft of the penis is held erect with a sterile swab in the left hand and traction applied to elongate the urethra. Lidocaine gel is instilled into the urethra slowly and carefully, with light but steady pressure. It is important to leave the local anaesthetic agent for a sufficient length of time before proceeding with catheterisation, as difficulty in male catheterisation is often caused by poor analgesia.

The urinary catheter is introduced into the urethra with a 'no-touch' technique and advanced fully to ensure the balloon on the catheter is within the bladder (Fig. 8.16). Correct placement is confirmed by the passage of urine down the catheter. If this does not occur, suprapubic pressure may help. Alternatively, a bladder syringe can be attached to the catheter and aspiration used. With the passage of urine, the balloon on the catheter is inflated with the recommended volume of sterile water (generally, 10–30 mL). The catheter is gently withdrawn until the balloon engages the bladder neck, and it is then connected to the drainage tubing. It is important that the foreskin, where present, is replaced over the glans to prevent paraphimosis.

Procedure in the female

A 16–18-Fr catheter is suitable for this procedure. The labia minora are separated with the thumb and fingers of the left hand to expose the urethral meatus on the anterior vaginal wall.

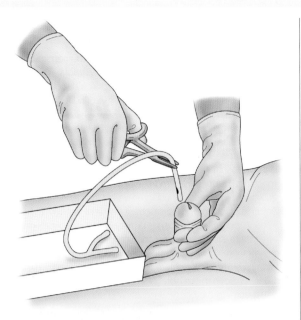

Fig. 8.16 Male catheterisation.

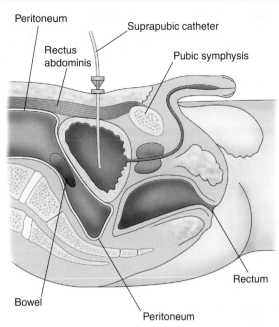

Fig. 8.17 Suprapubic catheterisation.

The pudenda are swabbed with antiseptic solution. Two swabs are used, each being swept once across the pudenda from anterior to posterior and then discarded.

In general, the catheter need only be inserted for half its length before the passage of urine confirms correct placement. The balloon is inflated and the catheter withdrawn until the balloon impacts in the bladder neck.

Suprapubic catheterisation

This procedure is only appropriate when the bladder is distended and urethral catheterisation has failed or is contraindicated.

Procedure

The position of the bladder is determined by percussion. Where available, ultrasound guidance is helpful. Generally, the point of insertion lies two finger-breadths above the pubic symphysis in the midline.

The area is cleansed and draped before local anaesthetic is infiltrated through all layers of the anterior abdominal wall, using an 18-gauge needle. The depth and position of the bladder can be gauged by the free aspiration of urine through this needle. The needle is withdrawn and a stab incision made in the skin. The trocar and catheter are advanced through the incision, into the bladder (Fig. 8.17). Entry into the bladder is confirmed by the loss of resistance, at which point the catheter is advanced as the trocar is withdrawn. Free passage of urine confirms correct placement. The catheter must be advanced far enough into the bladder so that the balloon, when inflated, is well within the bladder. The balloon is filled with 10 mL of water and a sterile dressing is applied.

Central nervous system procedures

Lumbar puncture

Lumbar puncture is carried out to obtain a sample of cerebrospinal fluid (CSF) for diagnostic purposes, to measure the CSF

pressure or to introduce materials into the CSF. It is important to examine the patient beforehand for evidence of raised intracranial pressure, examining the fundi in particular for evidence of papilloedema. Lumbar puncture is contraindicated if raised intracranial pressure is suspected, as it may result in 'coning' in such patients. The advent of computed tomography (CT) has provided a noninvasive aid to the detection of raised intracranial pressure, and in some conditions, such as subarachnoid haemorrhage, has removed the need for lumbar puncture.

Procedure

Patients are placed on one side (usually the left), with their back at the edge of the bed or trolley. They are then asked to curl up as much as possible, to flex the lumbar spine and open up the interspinous spaces (see Fig. 5.4).

The skin is thoroughly cleansed and drapes are applied to ensure strict aseptic technique. The space between the spinous processes of the third and fourth lumbar vertebrae is identified using the point at which a vertical line dropped from the highest point of the iliac crest crosses the spine. Local anaesthetic is infiltrated into the skin and subcutaneous tissues to a depth of about 2 cm. A small stab incision is made in the midline, midway between the two spinous processes.

A 22-gauge spinal needle is inserted through the stab incision and advanced in the midline in a slightly headward direction. Entry into the subarachnoid space is felt with a distinct loss of resistance, and will occur in most adults at a depth of 4–6 cm from the skin.

The stylet is withdrawn from the needle and the position confirmed by the free flow of CSF. If the subarachnoid space is not entered or bone is encountered, the position of the needle in the midline should be checked by observing (from the side) the angle of the needle in relation to the patient's back. If the needle is in the midline, it should be withdrawn and reinserted in a slightly more headward direction. If the patient experiences pain, a nerve has been touched. The needle should be immediately withdrawn and repositioned.

Once the procedure is complete, the needle is withdrawn and a sterile dressing applied. The patient is usually advised to remain supine for at least 12 hours to minimise the risk of developing a 'spinal' headache. Persistent headache may be a result of continued CSF leakage through the puncture in the dura. In these circumstances, an anaesthetist should be asked to advise on an epidural 'blood patch'. With modern needles, the risk of CSF leakage is lessened and the advice to remain supine for 12–24 hours may be unnecessary.

Excision of lumps and swellings (e.g., sebaceous cyst, lipoma, dermoid, lymph node)

The area is cleansed and draped. Local anaesthetic (mixed with a 1:200,000 concentration of adrenaline if appropriate) is used to provide a field block. The skin and subcutaneous tissue is incised in an ellipse to include the swelling and a plane is developed around the swelling. Small blood vessels may be cauterised or ligated. Usually a clean plane of loose areolar tissue is present around these swellings that can be developed by sharp dissection using scissors. Feeding vessels should be deliberately looked for and ligated or cauterised. Special care is required in the case of a sebaceous cyst where skin incision should encircle the punctum to avoid opening the cyst. After excision is completed, haemostasis is ensured and the subcutaneous tissue approximated using absorbable suture. The skin may be closed using subcuticular or interrupted sutures or Steristrips.

Imaging

Radiological imaging has a central role in the management of surgical patients and may guide various therapeutic procedures. A number of imaging techniques are now available that provide information on the structure and function of systems and organs. The principal imaging techniques include radiography (including plain x-rays, contrast studies and CT), ultrasound, magnetic resonance imaging (MRI) and isotope scanning.

Plain radiography

Radiographs account for the highest proportion of all imaging examinations. X-rays penetrate the body and cast an image either on film or on a fluorescent screen. The image is formed by the differences in attenuation of the x-ray beam by various tissues, producing a two-dimensional impression of a three-dimensional structure. On a plain radiograph, bone absorbs most x-rays and appears radio-opaque (white), whereas gas and fat absorb few x-rays and appear radiolucent (dark). If x-ray power (kilovoltage) and exposure time are altered, tissues of varying densities can be visualised. Other calcified tissues, such as most urinary tract stones, old tuberculous lymph nodes and calcified atheromatous plaques, are radio-opaque. Foreign materials, such as metal or glass, are also radio-opaque, but wood and plastic are radiolucent and invisible to x-rays.

Ionising radiation is potentially harmful. Therefore, unnecessary investigations should be avoided and radiation exposure of patients and staff should be minimised. As the inverse square law determines radiation fall-off with distance, workers should maintain a good distance from the x-ray source during exposure. The wearing of x-ray-sensitive film badges is used to monitor the amount of radiation received by staff, and protective lead aprons should be worn when staff are in exposed situations.

Contrast studies

Radio-opaque contrast media may be used to demonstrate the gastrointestinal, biliary, vascular and urinary tracts. They can either be used to outline anatomical structures directly, or else be concentrated physiologically in an organ (indirect imaging). Barium sulphate is insoluble and is used extensively to investigate the gastrointestinal tract. Gastrograffin is a water-soluble contrast medium used if leakage from the gastrointestinal tract into the peritoneal cavity is likely. A barium swallow is used to assess the oesophagus and a barium meal to investigate the stomach and duodenum. Progress of contrast can be observed by fluoroscopic screening, using an image intensifier. The large bowel is studied by giving contrast material rectally (barium enema). A single-contrast enema may be used to determine whether there is a complete mechanical obstruction in the emergency setting; however, improved mucosal detail will be obtained by using a double-contrast technique with barium and gas. Buscopan may be given at the same time to reduce bowel spasm. In the biliary, vascular and urinary tracts, iodine-containing agents are used. The risk of life-threatening anaphylactic reactions with the newer, low-osmolar, nonionic agents is minimal but these are still recognised complications of intravascular administration. Intravenous contrast is also potentially nephrotoxic in patients with impaired renal function and it is important that all patients are well hydrated before intravenous contrast is used.

Computed tomography (CT)

CT involves use of a series of x-rays directed at a narrow transverse section of the body and detected by multiple detectors. More modern machines spiral around the patient (spiral CT), resulting in more rapid image capture and higher resolution of images. Each element of the beam is attenuated according to the density of the tissue it traverses, and is converted into a grey-scale image that is displayed on a screen as a two-dimensional image. Further information can be gained after administration of oral, rectal or intravenous contrast. Three-dimensional reconstruction can be performed to assess relationships between structures and aid in the discrimination of abnormalities. The Hounsfield Unit, named after one of the inventors of CT, is used to measure the radiodensity of tissues (water: zero; air: −1000; fat: −120; muscle: 40; bone: >400). Multislice (MSCT) or multidetector CT that uses a two-dimensional array of detector elements is now standard technology and increases the scan speed and resolution, especially in the abdomen and thorax and for evaluation of cardiac circulation in place of invasive angiography.

Ultrasonography

This is a safe, noninvasive, painless technique that allows the visualisation of solid internal organs. Using 1–15-MHz mechanical vibrations, generated and detected by a piezoelectric transducer, an image is obtained because of differences in the reflection of the transmitted sound at the interface of tissues with different impedance. For transcutaneous ultrasonography, the probe must be 'coupled' to the skin with conduction gel to exclude an air interface. Calcified tissue, such as stones, causes an abrupt and marked change in acoustic impedance, resulting in virtually complete reflection of ultrasound and a posterior acoustic shadow. For biliary ultrasound, the patient should be fasted to ensure the gallbladder is not contracted. Ultrasonography of the pelvis is aided by a full bladder, as this provides a fluid-filled, nonreflective window to scan the pelvic organs.

Special probes have now been developed for insertion into various body orifices, such as rectum, vagina and oesophagus, and also through laparoscopic and endoscopic equipment. These probes can be placed closer to the target organ, allowing the use of higher-frequency sound that has lower penetration but greater resolution. Ultrasound can be employed to study blood flow using the Doppler principle. Ultrasound is reflected from the red blood cells, the movement of which causes a frequency shift related to the velocity. This is used to generate an audible signal that can be used to assess whether flow is normal or abnormal. The term duplex ultrasonography is used when the grey scale conventional ultrasound is combined with Doppler ultrasound.

Magnetic resonance imaging (MRI)

MRI, formerly known as nuclear magnetic resonance, involves the application of a powerful magnetic field to the body that aligns protons (hydrogen ions) in water molecules in one vector plane; emitted radio signals are recorded electronically and deconvoluted using sophisticated computer technology. Images can be displayed in any anatomical plane. T1 and T2 refer to the relaxation phase for the hydrogen ions. On a T2-weighted scan, all fluid containing tissues and water are seen as bright images (mimicking contrast) whereas the fat-containing tissues remain dark. The reverse of this is seen for T1-weighted scans. Intravenous administration of gadolinium-based contrast agents may be used for delineating vascular structures. MRI does not use ionising radiation, is thought to be harmless and provides very good images of soft tissues. Gadolinium contrast agents can cause renal fibrosis and should not be used in patients with decreased renal function (estimated glomerular filtration rate <30 mL/min). Disadvantages of MRI are cost, relatively slow scan times compared with CT, and due to the strong magnetic fields, MRI is unsuitable for patients with pacemakers or metallic implants. An exciting new application of MRI is the study of blood flow and cardiac function. Magnetic resonance angiography (MRA) avoids intravascular injections

and is replacing some conventional techniques. Magnetic resonance cholangiopancreatography (MRCP), a type of T2-weighted scan, has now replaced endoscopic retrograde cholangiopancreatography (ERCP) for diagnostic imaging of the biliary tract, as it avoids the potential complications of pancreatitis and bleeding. ERCP remains a valuable therapeutic tool for intervention of the biliary tree.

Radioisotope imaging

Radioisotope imaging provides more information about function than structure. Suitable tracer agents combine a substance taken up by the target tissue and a radioactive label. Radioisotopes in common usage include ^{99m}Tc (technetium), ^{123}I and ^{131}I (iodine), ^{111}In (indium), ^{133}Xe (xenon), ^{67}Ga (gallium) and ^{201}Th (thallium). Distribution of radioisotopes is visualised using a gamma camera. The investigation is based upon the localisation of the radioactive tracer in the target tissue with the help of the substance specific to the organ (e.g., bi-phosphonates labelled with ^{99m}Tc for bone scan) or the tracer uptake directly (e.g., ^{131}I itself for thyroid). Investigations employing radioisotope techniques include bone scanning, lung scanning to detect pulmonary emboli, renal scanning for detecting cortical scarring (dimercaptosuccinic acid [DMSA]) or renal function (diethylenetriamine pentaacetic acid [DTPA]), red blood cell scan for detection of obscure gastrointestinal bleeding, leucocyte scanning for inflammation and infection, and thyroid scanning.

Positron emission tomography (PET)

PET is based on the detection of gamma photons emitted when positrons emitted by a radioisotope probe (frequently 2-fluoro-deoxy-D-glucose [2FDG]) meet electrons and are annihilated. Metabolically active tissues take up the probe in greater concentrations compared with other tissue (termed PET-avid) and this property therefore may be used to define tumour tissue. However, PET avidity is a measure of tissue metabolic activity rather than the tumour itself and needs clinical correlation. PET images are usually overlaid onto conventional CT images to allow anatomical definition of the site of PET avidity.

9

Pawanindra Lal

Postoperative care and complications

Chapter contents

Introduction 128

Immediate postoperative care 128

Surgical ward care 129

Complications of anaesthesia and surgery 130

Introduction

There are three phases of patient care following an operation. After a short period of immediate postoperative care in a recovery room to ensure the full return of consciousness, the patient is returned to surgical ward care unless there are indications for transfer to a high-dependency or intensive therapy unit. On discharge from ward care, patients may still require rehabilitation and convalescence before they are ready to resume normal activities. The first two phases will be outlined, since these are primarily concerned with regulation of homeostasis and the prevention, detection and management of complications. A timeline for the development of postoperative complications is given in Fig. 9.1.

Immediate postoperative care

Patients who have received a general anaesthetic should be observed in the recovery room until they are conscious and their vital signs are stable. Major life-threatening complications that may arise in the recovery room are airway obstruction, myocardial infarction, cardiac arrest, haemorrhage and respiratory failure. These complications can also arise during ward care, but with few exceptions many of the problems arising do not threaten life and are often specific to the operation performed. The recovery room provides specially trained personnel and equipment for the observation and treatment of acute pulmonary, cardiovascular and fluid derangements, which are the major causes of life-threatening complications.

In general, the anaesthetist exercises primary responsibility for the patient's cardiopulmonary function and the surgeon is responsible for the operative site, the wound and any surgically placed drains. Clinical notes should document the operation and the procedure performed, the anaesthetic record of the patient's progress during surgery, postoperative instructions relating to the administration of drugs and intravenous fluids, and a fluid balance sheet.

Monitoring of airway, breathing and circulation is the priority (EBM 9.1). The nature of the surgery and the patient's premorbid medical condition will determine the intensity of postoperative monitoring required; however, the patient's colour, pulse, blood pressure, respiratory rate, oxygen saturation and level of consciousness will be observed routinely. The nature and volume of drainage into collecting bags or wound dressings, and urinary output are monitored, if appropriate. Continuous electrocardiogram (ECG) monitoring is undertaken and oxygenation is assessed by the use of a pulse oximeter. Monitoring of central venous pressure (CVP) may be indicated if the patient is hypotensive, has borderline cardiac or respiratory function, or requires large amounts of intravenous fluids.

EBM 9.1 Optimal postoperative care

'Optimal postoperative care requires clinical assessment and monitoring; respiratory management; cardiovascular management; fluid, electrolyte and renal management; control of sepsis; and nutrition.'

SIGN guideline 77. Post-operative management in adults; 2004.

The patient may initially remain intubated, but following extubation should receive supplemental oxygen by face mask or nasal prongs, and should be encouraged to take frequent deep breaths. The patient must breathe adequately and maintain a good colour. Shallow breathing may mean that the patient is still partially paralysed. A dose of neostigmine can reverse the residual effects of curariform agents. Cyanosis is an ominous sign indicating hypoxaemia due to inadequate oxygenation, and may be due to airway obstruction or impaired ventilation. Respiratory depression later on in the postoperative period is usually caused by over-sedation with opioid analgesic agents.

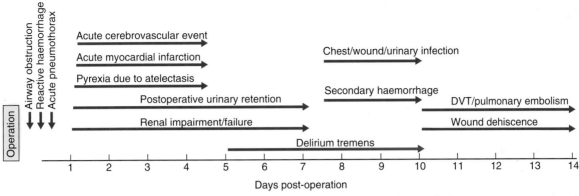

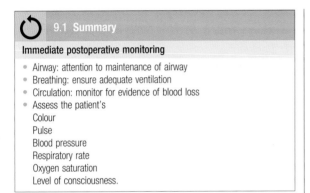

Fig. 9.1 Timeline showing typical times for development of postoperative complications.

9

Airway obstruction

The main causes of airway obstruction are as follows:

- *Obstruction by the tongue* may occur with a depressed level of consciousness. Loss of muscle tone causes the tongue to fall back against the posterior pharyngeal wall, and may be aggravated by masseter spasm during emergence from anaesthesia. Bleeding into the tongue or soft tissues of the mouth or pharynx may be a complicating factor after operations involving these areas.
- *Obstruction by foreign bodies,* such as dentures, crowns and loose teeth. Dentures must be removed before operation and precautions taken to guard against displacement of crowns or teeth.
- *Laryngeal spasm* can occur at light levels of unconsciousness and is aggravated by stimulation.
- *Laryngeal oedema* may occur in small children after traumatic attempts at intubation, or when there is infection (epiglottitis).
- *Tracheal compression* may follow operations in the neck, and compression by haemorrhage is a particular anxiety after thyroidectomy.
- *Bronchospasm or bronchial obstruction* may follow inhalation of a foreign body or the aspiration of irritant material, such as gastric contents. It may also occur as an idiosyncratic reaction to drugs and as a complication of asthma.

Attention is directed at urgently defining and rectifying the cause of airway obstruction. Airway maintenance techniques include the chin-lift or jaw-thrust manoeuvres, which lift the mandible anteriorly and displace the tongue forward (see Chapter 8). The pharynx is sucked out, an oropharyngeal airway is inserted to maintain the airway, and supplemental oxygen is administered. If cyanosis does not improve or if stridor persists, reintubation may be necessary.

Haemorrhage

Significant blood loss into a surgical drain, particularly if associated with hypovolaemic shock, is an indication for immediate transfer of the patient to the operating theatre for reexploration and control of the bleeding source. Reactive bleeding is usually caused by a slipped ligature or dislodgement of a diathermy coagulum as the blood pressure recovers from the operation. Superficial bleeding into the surgical wound rarely requires immediate action; however, patients who have undergone neck surgery must be observed for the accumulation of blood in the wound. If necessary, the wound can be reopened in the recovery room to prevent airway compression and asphyxia.

Late secondary haemorrhage typically occurs 7–10 days after an operation and is due to infection eroding a blood vessel. Rigid drain tubes may also occasionally erode a large vessel and cause dramatic late postoperative bleeding. Secondary haemorrhage associated with infection is often difficult to control. Interventional radiological techniques may achieve temporary control, but surgical reexploration is usually indicated.

Surgical ward care

General care

Monitoring of vital signs and temperature continues on return to the ward along with output from the urinary catheter, nasogastric tube and surgical drains. The frequency of recordings or measurements can be reduced as the patient stabilises. Patients are normally visited morning and evening by medical staff to ensure satisfactory progress. Anxiety, disorientation and minor changes in personality, behaviour or appearance are often the earliest manifestation of complications. The general circulatory state and adequacy of oxygenation are noted, and vital signs recorded on the nursing chart are checked. Temperature readings provide vital information regarding progress and may give early indication of potentially serious postoperative complications.

The chest is examined and sputum inspected. Full chest expansion and coughing are encouraged. Following abdominal surgery, the abdomen is examined for evidence of excessive distension or tenderness. The return of bowel sounds and the free passage of flatus reflect recovery of gut peristalsis. The legs are checked for swelling, discoloration or calf tenderness.

Tubes, drains and catheters

If a nasogastric tube is in place, it is kept open at all times to serve as a vent for swallowed air. Free drainage of gastric contents may be supplemented by intermittent manual aspiration and the tube can be removed once the volume of aspirate diminishes. It is not necessary to wait until bowel sounds have returned or flatus has been passed. Nasogastric tubes are uncomfortable and may prevent coughing with expectoration, and so they should not be retained for longer than necessary. Surgical drains are generally removed when the volume of effluent diminishes. If a urinary catheter has been placed, it should be removed once the patient is mobile.

Fluid balance

Fluid balance is reviewed regularly. Standard intravenous fluid requirement for an adult is 3 L/day, of which 1 L should ordinarily be normal (isotonic) saline and 2 L should be 5% dextrose. In the first 24 hours after surgery, normal saline can be omitted and replaced by 5% dextrose because of sodium conservation as a result of metabolic response. However, this should be judged according to the patient's general circulatory status, the observed fluid losses, and the daily measurement of serum urea and electrolyte levels. Similarly, it is not necessary to replace potassium within the first 24–48 hours after surgery, as potassium is released from injured cells and tissues at the surgical site. Potassium supplements (1 mEq/kg/day, i.e., 60–80 mmol daily) can subsequently be added to intravenous fluids, provided urinary output is adequate (0.5–1.0 mL/kg/h). The daily fluid requirement must take care of extra losses due to environmental temperature in tropical countries where higher insensible fluid loss is not uncommon. Allowance must be made for body fluid losses like nasogastric aspirate and replaced appropriately by Na, K and fluid volume. A mixed gastric aspirate of 1 L must be replaced by 120 mEq of Na and 10 mEq of K over and above the normal requirements for the next 24 hours. Balance fluid is replaced by 5% dextrose. This replacement of abnormal losses should be done every 8 hours in paediatric surgery. Intravenous fluid therapy is discontinued once oral fluid intake has been established.

Blood transfusion

Haemoglobin measurement will be a guide to the need for postoperative blood transfusion. A full blood count should be undertaken within 24 hours of surgery and, as a general rule, blood is administered if the haemoglobin is less than 80 g/L with a low haematocrit (<24). Above this level, patients can be prescribed oral iron, unless they have cardiovascular instability or are symptomatic from their anaemia. Needless transfusion is avoided, especially in patients with colorectal malignancies since it has been linked to recurrence of malignancy. Please refer to Chapter 2 for a detailed account on blood transfusion.

Nutrition

Nutrition in postoperative patients is frequently poorly managed. A few days of starvation may cause little harm, but enteral or parenteral nutrition is essential if starvation is prolonged. Enteral nutrition is preferred, as it is associated with fewer complications and is believed to augment gut barrier function. If a prolonged period of starvation is anticipated in the postoperative period, a feeding jejunostomy tube can be inserted at the time of abdominal surgery. Alternatively, a fine-bore nasogastric or nasojejunal feeding tube can be passed (see Chapter 8). If the enteral route cannot be used, total parenteral nutrition can be prescribed. Dietary intake should be monitored in all patients in the postoperative period, and oral high-calorie supplements given if appropriate.

Complications of anaesthesia and surgery

General complications

Nausea and vomiting can be caused by surgery and/or anaesthesia, and an antiemetic can prove useful and can be considered prophylactically if nausea has been associated with previous anaesthetic procedures. Transient hiccups in the immediate postoperative period are usually no more than a nuisance. Persistent hiccups are more serious, exhausting the patient and interfering with sleep, and may be due to diaphragmatic irritation, gastric distension or metabolic causes, such as renal failure. If no precipitating cause can be found, small doses of chlorpromazine may be helpful.

Spinal anaesthesia may cause headache from leakage of cerebrospinal fluid, and patients should remain recumbent for 12 hours when this occurs. If headache persists, it may be necessary to seal the injection site in the dura-arachnoid with a 'blood patch' (i.e., an extradural injection of the patient's blood, which clots and seals the leak). Myalgia affecting the chest, abdomen and neck is a specific complication of suxamethonium administration, and may last for up to a week.

Intravenous administration of irritant drugs or solutions can cause bruising, haematoma, phlebitis and venous thrombosis. Intravenous cannulae placed in large veins should be securely sealed to guard against air embolism. Sites of cannula insertion should be checked regularly for signs of infection, and the cannula replaced if necessary. Arterial cannulae and needle punctures are the most common cause of arterial injury, and may rarely lead to arterial occlusion and gangrene.

Pulmonary complications

Respiratory complications remain the largest single cause of postoperative morbidity and the second most common cause of postoperative death in patients over 60 years of age. Pulmonary complications are more common after emergency operations. Special hazards are posed by preexisting chronic obstructive pulmonary disease (COPD). Once a patient has fully recovered from anaesthesia, the main respiratory problems are pulmonary collapse and pulmonary infection. Pleural effusion and pneumothorax occur less commonly. Pulmonary embolism (PE) is a major complication of deep venous thrombosis (DVT), which is considered later.

Postoperative hypoxaemia

Hypoxaemia manifests variably with one or more features such as irritability, drowsiness, restlessness, diaphoresis, confusion and dyspnoea. Patients have an increased heart rate, tachypnoea, and may look blue to flushed. Patients are at risk of hypoxaemia immediately after surgery due to ventilation perfusion imbalance, diffusion of anaesthetic gases into lungs, respiratory depression from narcotics and anaesthetic drugs, and shivering (increased muscular oxygen utilisation). As these immediate factors are reversed, hypoxaemia may continue due to old age (loss of elasticity of the lungs, and physiological right to left shunts due to collapse of basal alveoli), preexisting pulmonary disease, COPD, obesity, postoperative pain (especially upper abdominal incisions) and excessive use of opiates. Collapse of lung, hypovolaemic shock (blood loss or inadequate fluid replacement) or pneumothorax, pleural effusion, aspiration of vomitus leading to acute respiratory distress syndrome (ARDS) can all lead to persistent hypoxia. Hypoxaemia 2–5 days after surgery may signify significant preexisting cardiopulmonary disease, retained bronchial secretions and pneumonitis. Persistent paralytic ileus and abdominal distension leading to splinting of the diaphragm, obesity and ARDS further contribute to hypoxia. If hypoxaemia occurs unexpectedly 8–12 days after surgery, massive PE should be considered.

Hypoxia is detected by low oxygen saturation on pulse oximetry with the probe attached to a finger. Values between 95% and 100% are considered normal, while those between 90% and 95% on room air (FIo_2 21%) may be considered normal in some patients depending on their preoperative values. Saturation below 90% is considered low and corresponds to Pao_2 of 60 mmHg, which is dangerously low for a postoperative patient. Supplemental oxygen may need to be administered by a venturi mask or nasal prongs until the patient is able to maintain a saturation of 95% or more on room air. Low values on the finger probe may be due to factors such as vasoconstriction, low pulse volume, low blood pressure and shivering. Nail polish hampers detection of light sensors and should be removed. Pulse oximeters function normally in anaemic patients, but such patients with normal saturation would not be able to deliver oxygen adequately to the tissues due to low haemoglobin levels.

9.2 Summary

Postoperative hypoxaemia: contributing factors

Immediately postoperative
- Persisting ventilation (V)/perfusion (Qc) imbalance
- Anaesthetic gases such as nitrous oxide or halothane diffuse into lungs
- Respiratory depression due to use of anaesthetic drugs and opioids
- Shivering (provokes muscle oxygen utilisation)

24 hours postoperative
- Aging (loss of lung elasticity)
- Preexisting pulmonary disease
- Obesity
- Pain (especially upper abdominal or thoracic incisions)
- Excessive sedation or use of opiates
- Massive collapse
- Hypovolemic shock
- Pneumothorax

2–5 days postoperative
- Preexisting cardiopulmonary disease
- Retained bronchial secretions
- Pneumonitis
- Abdominal distension with diaphragmatic splinting
- Acute respiratory distress syndrome

8–12 days postoperative
- Pulmonary embolism

Pulmonary collapse

Inability to breathe deeply and cough up bronchial secretions is the primary cause of pulmonary collapse after surgery. Contributory factors include paralysis of cilia by anaesthetic agents, impairment of diaphragmatic movement, over-sedation, abdominal distension and wound pain. When there is complete obstruction of a bronchus or bronchiole, air in the lung distal to the obstruction is absorbed, the alveolar spaces close (atelectasis), and the affected portion of the lung contracts and becomes solid. Small bronchioles (1 mm or less) are prone to close when lung volume reaches a critical point (closing volume). The closing volume is higher in older patients and in smokers, owing to the loss of elastic recoil of the lung, which increases the risk of atelectasis. The extent of collapse varies from closure of a small segment to collapse of a lobe or, when a main bronchus is obstructed, the entire lung. Atelectasis is a very common complication of surgery and usually occurs within 24 hours. It is of clinical relevance because it leads to increased work of breathing and impaired gas exchange; if untreated, secondary bacterial infection will supervene, causing lobar or bronchopneumonia.

The clinical signs of pulmonary collapse include rapid respiration, tachycardia and mild pyrexia, with diminished breath sounds and dullness to percussion over the affected segment. Arterial Pao_2 is low and the chest x-ray shows areas of increased opacification.

Preoperative measures to reduce the risk of pulmonary collapse following surgery include cessation of smoking, physiotherapy if COPD exists, and deferring elective surgery for at least 2 weeks in patients with a chest infection. Practising with an incentive spirometer preoperatively will help. Postoperatively, pulmonary collapse is prevented by encouraging the patient to breathe deeply, cough and mobilise. Adequate analgesia and regular chest physiotherapy are of great importance. Placement of an epidural catheter in patients undergoing major abdominal surgery may help alleviate postoperative wound pain. Hypoxia is treated by giving oxygen by mask or nasal prongs, and bronchospasm is relieved by inhalation of salbutamol.

When hypoxia is severe, endotracheal intubation, assisted ventilation and repeated bronchial aspiration may be needed. Posture is important and the patient should initially be placed on the unaffected side to aid expansion of the collapsed lung. Bronchoscopy may be needed to suck out any inspissated secretions.

Pulmonary infection

Pulmonary infection commonly follows pulmonary collapse or the aspiration of gastric secretions. Pyrexia, tachypnoea and green sputum are typical. The chest signs are those of collapse with absent or diminished breath sounds, often in association with bronchial breathing and coarse crepitations from surrounding areas of partial bronchial occlusion. Chest x-ray usually demonstrates patchy opacities.

The patient is encouraged to cough, and antibiotics are prescribed after sputum is sent for bacteriological examination. Most pulmonary infections are caused by the respiratory commensals *Streptococcus pneumoniae* and *Haemophilus influenzae*, but many postoperative pulmonary infections are caused by gram-negative bacilli acquired by aspiration of oropharyngeal secretions. Antibiotics provide the mainstay of treatment. Oxygen is given for hypoxia, and more intensive measures, including

9

bronchoscopy and assisted ventilation, are instituted if respiratory function continues to deteriorate.

Respiratory failure

Respiratory failure is defined as an inability to maintain normal partial pressures of oxygen and carbon dioxide (Pa_{O_2} and Pa_{CO_2}) in arterial blood. Blood gas determinations are the key to its early recognition and should be repeated frequently in patients with previous respiratory problems. The normal Pa_{O_2} is >13 kPa at the age of 20 years, falling to around 11.6 kPa at 60 years; respiratory failure is denoted by a value of less than 6.7 kPa. Severe hypoxaemia may result in visible central cyanosis. In type 1 respiratory failure there is hypoxia and in type 2 there is hypercarbia with hypoxia.

Acute respiratory distress syndrome (ARDS)

ARDS is characterised by impaired oxygenation, diffuse lung opacification on chest x-ray and an increasing 'stiffness' of the lungs (decreased compliance). It may result from pulmonary or systemic sepsis, following massive blood transfusion, or as a consequence of aspiration of gastric contents. The syndrome displays a wide spectrum of severity. Many minor and transient cases recover spontaneously, whereas in a proportion of cases, progressive respiratory insufficiency occurs. Tachypnoea with increasing ventilatory effort, restlessness and confusion develop. Hypoxia initially responds to an increase in the oxygen content of inspired air, but progressively increasing concentrations are required to prevent the Pa_{O_2} from falling. The pathophysiology is unclear, but endotoxin-activated leucocytes may be deposited in the pulmonary capillaries, releasing oxygen-derived free radicals, cytokines and other chemical mediators. Damage to the vascular endothelium results in increased capillary permeability and leakage of fluid, causing widespread interstitial and alveolar oedema. This is seen as bilateral diffuse fluffy opacities on chest x-ray (Fig. 9.2). The lungs become increasingly stiff and difficult to ventilate.

Management includes supportive measures in the form of ventilation with positive end-expiratory pressure (PEEP) and treatment of the underlying condition, i.e., control of infection by antibiotics, drainage of any source of pus and correction of hypovolaemia. The mortality rate of severe ARDS is approximately 50%.

Pleural effusion

Small pleural effusions (Fig. 9.3) are not uncommon following upper abdominal surgery, but are usually of no clinical significance. They may be secondary to other pulmonary pathology, such as collapse/consolidation, pulmonary infarction or secondary tumour deposits. The appearance of a pleural effusion 2–3 weeks after an abdominal operation may suggest the presence of a subphrenic abscess. Small effusions may be left alone to reabsorb if they do not interfere with respiration. Moderate or larger size effusions require pleural aspiration and bacteriological culture of aspirated fluid (see Fig 9.3).

Pneumothorax

The most common cause of postoperative pneumothorax is the insertion of a central venous line, and a chest x-ray is necessary after this procedure to exclude this potential complication. There is also an enhanced risk of pneumothorax in patients on positive-pressure ventilation, presumably owing to rupture of preexisting bullae. The insertion of an underwater seal drain is usually followed by rapid expansion of the lung.

Cardiac complications

The risks of anaesthesia and surgery are increased in patients suffering from cardiovascular disease. Whenever possible, arrhythmias, unstable angina, heart failure or hypertension should be corrected before surgery. Valvular disease, especially aortic stenosis, impairs the ability of the heart to respond to the increased demand of the postoperative period. The administration of fluids to patients with severe aortic or mitral valve disease should be carefully monitored.

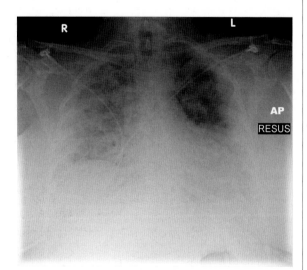

Fig. 9.2 Chest x-ray showing features of acute respiratory distress syndrome (ARDS).

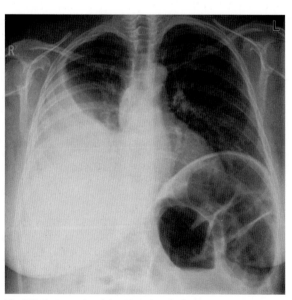

Fig. 9.3 Postoperative right-sided pleural effusion.

Myocardial ischaemia/infarction

Although in most cases there is a history of preceding cardiac disease, myocardial ischaemia or cardiac arrest can occur in an otherwise fit patient. Patients with ischaemia may complain of gripping chest pain, but this is not invariable (particularly in the elderly diabetic patient or in the early postoperative period) and hypotension may be the only sign. The absence of symptoms after operation is thought to be due to the residual effects of anaesthesia and to the administration of postoperative analgesia. If ischaemia is suspected, an ECG is performed urgently and arrangements are made for cardiac monitoring. A sample of blood is withdrawn to estimate concentrations of cardiac enzymes. One-third of postoperative myocardial infarctions are fatal.

Cardiac failure

Although acute cardiac failure occurs most often in the immediate postoperative period, patients with ischaemic or valvular heart disease, arrhythmias or major surgical insult can also go into failure in the subsequent recovery period. Clinical manifestations are progressive dyspnoea, hypoxaemia and diffuse congestion on chest x-ray. Excessive administration of fluid in the early postoperative period in patients with limited myocardial reserve is a common cause, which can be avoided by monitoring CVP. Treatment consists of avoiding further fluid overload, and the administration of diuretics and cardiac inotropes.

Arrhythmias

Sinus tachycardia is common and may be a physiological response to hypovolaemia or hypotension. It is also caused by pain, fever, shivering or restlessness. Tachycardia increases myocardial oxygen consumption and may decrease coronary artery perfusion. Sinus bradycardia may be due to vagal stimulation by neostigmine, pharyngeal irritation during suction, or the residual effects of anaesthetic agents. Atrial fibrillation is the most common postoperative arrhythmia. Fast atrial fibrillation may result in haemodynamic disturbances and may require pharmacological intervention. Refractory cases may require cardioversion.

Postoperative shock

Shock is defined as a failure to maintain adequate tissue perfusion. The three main types are hypovolaemic, cardiogenic and septic shock. Hypovolaemic shock may be caused by inadequate replacement of pre- or perioperative fluid losses, or postoperative haemorrhage, whereas cardiogenic shock is usually secondary to acute myocardial ischaemia/infarction or an arrhythmia. Hypovolaemic and cardiogenic shock are characterised by tachycardia, hypotension, sweating, pallor and vasoconstriction. Septic shock is characterised in the early stages by a hyperdynamic circulation with fever, rigors, a warm vasodilated periphery and a bounding pulse. Later features include hypotension and peripheral vasoconstriction. Without appropriate management, shock will result in oliguria and the development of multisystem organ failure, and may lead to death.

Urinary complications

Postoperative urinary retention

Inability to void postoperatively is common, especially after groin, pelvic or perineal operations, or operations under spinal/epidural anaesthesia (Fig. 9.4). Postoperative pain, the effects of anaesthesia and drugs, and difficulties in initiating micturition while lying or sitting in bed may all contribute. Males tend to be more commonly affected than females. When its normal capacity of approximately 500 mL is exceeded, the bladder may be unable to contract and empty itself. Frequent dribbling or the passage of small volumes of urine may indicate overflow incontinence, and examination may reveal a distended bladder. The management of acute urinary retention is catheterisation of the bladder, with removal of the catheter after 2–3 days (see Chapter 8).

Urinary tract infection

Urinary tract infections are most common after urological or gynaecological operations. Preexisting contamination of the urinary tract, urinary retention and instrumentation are the principal factors contributing to postoperative urinary infection. Cystitis is manifested by frequency, dysuria and mild fever, and pyelonephritis by high fever and flank tenderness. Treatment involves adequate hydration, proper drainage of the bladder and appropriate antibiotics.

Renal failure

Acute renal failure after surgery results from protracted inadequate perfusion of the kidneys. The most common cause of postoperative oliguria is prerenal vascular insufficiency from hypovolaemia, water depletion or extracellular fluid depletion. Hypoperfusion of the kidney may be aggravated by hypoxia, sepsis and nephrotoxic drugs. Patients with preexisting renal disease and jaundice are particularly susceptible to hypoperfusion, and are more likely to develop acute renal failure.

The complication can largely be prevented by adequate fluid replacement before, during and after surgery, so that urine output is maintained at 0.5 mL/kg/h or more. The importance of monitoring hourly urine output means that bladder catheterisation is needed in all patients undergoing major surgery, and in those at risk of renal failure. Early recognition and treatment of

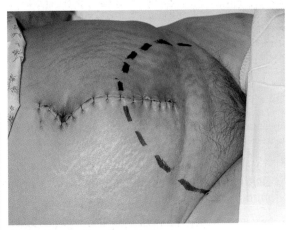

Fig. 9.4 Postoperative urinary retention.

bacterial and fungal infections is also important in the prevention of renal failure.

Urine output below 700 mL in 24 hours (or less than 0.5 mL/kg/h for several hours on catheter drainage) should be considered pathological oliguria. Management involves the restoration of an adequate circulating intravascular compartment by the administration of intravenous fluids. A CVP line is usually required to measure circulating blood volume. Diuretics may be administered only if the patient is well hydrated; however, they should not be continually prescribed if the patient remains oliguric.

Acute postoperative renal failure occurs when the reversible stage of acute renal insufficiency progresses to acute tubular necrosis. Volume loading becomes potentially dangerous with established renal failure, and the mainstays of treatment at this stage are the replacement of observed fluid loss, plus an allowance of approximately 500 mL/day for insensible loss, and restriction of dietary protein intake to less than 20 g/day. Biochemical status is checked by frequent estimations of serum urea and electrolytes. Hyperkalaemia can be treated by intravenous administration of insulin and glucose, or cation exchange resins. Haemofiltration or haemodialysis may be indicated if conservative measures fail to prevent rapid rises in serum concentrations of urea and potassium. Recovery from acute tubular necrosis can be anticipated in survivors after 2–4 weeks. The patient will then enter a polyuric phase, in which fluid and electrolyte balance requires careful monitoring. The mortality rate in patients who develop postoperative renal failure is 50%.

Cerebral complications

Cerebrovascular accidents (CVA)

These are usually precipitated by sudden hypotension during or after surgery in elderly hypertensive patients with severe atherosclerosis. They are a specific complication of carotid endarterectomy, occurring in 1–3% of cases, but may also complicate cardiac surgery.

Neuropsychiatric disturbances

These occur frequently and cover a wide spectrum of disorders. The most common is mental confusion with agitation, restlessness and disorientation, and is known as delirium. It usually occurs in the elderly and may arise on a background of dementia due to cerebral atrophy, but is often precipitated by the use of sedative or hypnotic drugs. Acute toxic confusion state is a well-recognised acute psychiatric disorder that occurs in some patients during a serious illness or after a major surgical intervention. Many factors can contribute, and it is important to look for a treatable cause, such as hypoxia, sepsis, or a metabolic disturbance such as hypoglycaemia, hepatic encephalopathy, uraemia or electrolyte imbalance. Sleep deprivation, particularly in intensive care units, can also cause severe mental disturbance. The primary cause of postoperative confusion needs to be treated and such patients may need management in an intensive care unit.

Delirium tremens (acute alcohol withdrawal syndrome)

Delirium tremens occurs in alcoholics who stop drinking suddenly. In most instances, this can be predicted from a detailed history.

Prodromal symptoms include personality changes, anxiety and tremors. The fully developed condition is characterised by extreme agitation, visual hallucinations, restlessness, confusion and, rarely, convulsions and hyperthermia. If symptoms are mild, treatment involves the prescription of oral diazepam and vitamin B (thiamine). Control of extreme agitation may require intravenous administration of diazepam, or haloperidol.

Venous thrombosis and pulmonary embolism

These complications are discussed in detail in Chapter 21, but the essential details are summarised here for convenience.

Deep venous thrombosis (DVT)

The pathogenesis of venous thrombosis involves stasis, increased blood coagulability and damage to the blood vessel wall (Virchow's triad). The incidence of DVT varies with the type of operation and the associated risk factors, which include increasing age, obesity, prolonged operations, pelvic and hip surgery, malignant disease, previous DVT or PE, varicose veins, pregnancy, and use of the oral contraceptive pill.

Measures to prevent DVT include taking care to avoid prolonged compression of the leg veins during and after the operation; the use of graded compression support stockings (TED stockings); mechanical or electrical compression of the calf muscles during surgery; and low-molecular-weight heparin.

DVT is frequently asymptomatic, but may present with a painful, tender swollen calf. It may be the cause of a postoperative fever. Duplex ultrasonography is now the investigation of choice for diagnosing DVT.

Nowadays, most DVTs are treated with low-molecular-weight heparin injected subcutaneously once daily rather than by means of an unfractionated heparin infusion. Unfractionated heparin is cheaper and a loading dose of 5000 IU intravenously is followed by an infusion of 1000 IU per hour. The rate of infusion is titrated to raise the activated partial thromboplastin time to 70–90 seconds. Heparin therapy is stopped once the patient is fully anticoagulated with warfarin, which is then normally continued for 3–6 months. The dose of warfarin is adjusted to maintain an international normalised ratio at 2–3-times normal.

Pulmonary embolism

Massive pulmonary embolus with severe chest pain, pallor and shock demands immediate cardiopulmonary resuscitation, heparinisation and urgent computed tomography (CT) pulmonary angiography. Fibrinolytic agents, such as streptokinase or urokinase, can be infused intravenously to encourage clot lysis if it is at least 6 days after surgical intervention, or in extreme cases the clot can be removed at open pulmonary embolectomy under cardiopulmonary bypass.

If a PE is suspected in a patient complaining of chest pain, sometimes in association with tachypnoea, haemoptysis and a pleural rub and effusion, a chest x-ray and ECG should be undertaken, mainly to rule out alternative causes of the symptoms. If these are negative, a CT pulmonary angiogram should then be performed, and if this reveals lobar or segmental perfusion defects, the patient is heparinised and monitored carefully (Fig. 9.5). In such cases, it is also important to search for the source of the embolus; warfarin therapy is recommended in all patients who have sustained a pulmonary embolus, and therapy is normally continued for 6 months. If the patient cannot be anticoagulated, or sustains

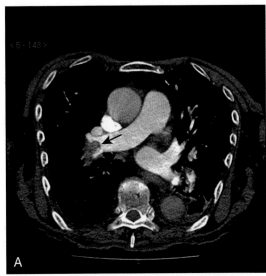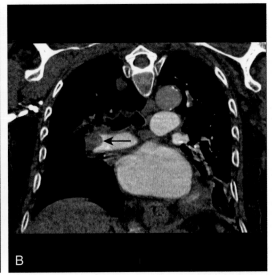

Fig. 9.5 Computed tomography pulmonary angiograms (A, transverse section; B, coronal section) showing pulmonary embolus (black arrow).

further PE despite anticoagulation, then consideration can be given to placing an inferior vena caval filter.

Wound complications

Infection

Infection (Fig. 9.6) is the most common complication in surgery. The incidence varies from less than 1% in clean operations to 20–30% in dirty cases. Subcutaneous haematoma is a common prelude to a wound infection, and large haematomas may require evacuation. The onset is usually within 7 days of operation. Symptoms include malaise, anorexia, and pain or discomfort at the operation site. Signs include local erythema, tenderness, swelling, cellulitis, wound discharge or frank abscess formation, as well as an elevated temperature and pulse rate. If a wound becomes infected, it may be necessary to remove one or more sutures or staples prematurely to allow the egress of infected material. The wound is then allowed to heal by secondary intention. Antibiotics are only required if there is evidence of associated cellulitis or septicaemia. If the wound infection is chronic, the presence of a suture sinus or an enterocutaneous fistula must be excluded.

Dehiscence

The incidence of abdominal wound dehiscence ('burst abdomen') should be less than 1%. Wound dehiscence (Fig. 9.7) may be partial (deep layers only) or complete (all layers, including skin). A serosanguinous discharge is characteristic of partial wound dehiscence. The extrusion of abdominal viscera through a complete abdominal wound dehiscence is known as evisceration. This rare complication usually occurs within the first 2 weeks after operation. Risk factors include obesity, smoking, respiratory disease, obstructive jaundice, nutritional deficiencies, renal failure, malignancy, diabetes and steroid therapy; however, the most important causes are poor surgical technique, persistently increased intraabdominal pressure, and local tissue necrosis due to infection. The wound should be resutured under general anaesthesia. Incisional herniation complicates approximately 25% of cases.

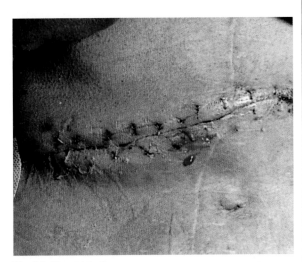

Fig. 9.6 Wound infection.

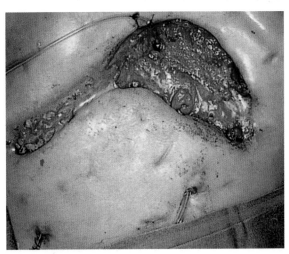

Fig. 9.7 Wound dehiscence.

9.3 Summary

Complications of anaesthesia and surgery

General complications
- Nausea and vomiting
- Hiccups
- Headache

Pulmonary complications
- Pulmonary collapse
- Pulmonary infection
- Respiratory failure
- Acute respiratory distress syndrome (ARDS)
- Pleural effusion
- Pneumothorax

Cardiac complications
- Myocardial ischaemia/infarction
- Cardiac failure
- Arrhythmias
- Postoperative shock

Urinary complications
- Urinary retention
- Urinary tract infection
- Renal failure

Cerebral complications
- Cerebrovascular accidents (CVA)
- Neuropsychiatric disturbances
- Delirium tremens

Venous thromboembolism
- Deep venous thrombosis
- Pulmonary embolism

Wound complications
- Wound infection
- Wound dehiscence.

Postoperative fever

Fever in a patient who has had surgery can be due to a variety of causes related to the primary disease or complications related to the surgical intervention or general anaesthesia. The common conditions that cause fever are listed in Summary 9.4. The cause must be diligently identified and treated appropriately.

9.4 Summary

Postoperative fever

Days 0–2
- Physiological as response to tissue injury: low grade
- Pulmonary collapse, atelectasis
- Blood transfusion
- Thrombophlebitis

Days 3–5
- Sepsis: wound infection
- Biliary or urinary infection: catheter
- Intraabdominal collection
- Pneumonia

Day 5–7
- Deep-vein thrombosis (DVT)
- Enteric anastomotic leak

>7 days
- Intraabdominal collection
- DVT
- Septicaemia.

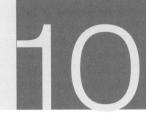

Steven Anderson
Siun Walsh
Arnie D.K. Hill

10

Evidence-based practice and professional development

Chapter contents

Introduction 137

Levels of evidence 137

Care pathways and guidelines 140

Clinical governance 140

Clinical audit 141

Quality improvement 141

Critical appraisal 141

Continuing professional development 141

Introduction

In the past, clinicians relied solely on their experience and the advice of colleagues when making clinical decisions. Modern practice has evolved beyond this as a result of the vast array of information that is now available to clinicians through modern technology. Data and guidelines have become easily accessible through electronic databases such as PubMed and UpToDate. This has led to the evolution of evidence-based practice, which combines up-to-date research with clinical judgement when making clinical decisions (EBM 10.1).

Evidence-based medicine has become ubiquitous in modern-day clinical practice, and so a detailed understanding of what it is, how it is achieved, why it is important, and how it should be interpreted is required of both undergraduates and surgical trainees.

EBM 10.1 What is evidence-based medicine?

'Evidence based medicine is the conscientious, explicit, and judicious use of current best evidence in making decisions about care of individual patients.'

Sackett DL, Rosenberg WMC, Gray JAM, et al. Evidence based medicine: what it is and what it isn't. BMJ. 1996;312:71–2.

Levels of evidence

Many different types of research exist, each with their own strengths and weaknesses. The data from the various research methods can be grouped into a qualitative hierarchy of levels of evidence. Although many different grading methods exist, each designed to answer different questions, one commonly used example is that of the Centre of Evidence-Based Medicine (Table 10.1), which grades evidence on a scale of 1–5, with 1 representing strong evidence and 5 representing weak evidence. The recommendations that develop from these different research methods are also graded A–D, with A being the strongest level of recommendation.

Cochrane review

The Cochrane Collaboration, a global independent network comprising more than 37,000 researchers, professionals, patients and carers from over 130 different countries, was created in 1993 with the aim of improving healthcare decisions. The collaboration gathers and summarises the best evidence available, with a focus on systematic reviews of randomised controlled trials (RCTs) of healthcare-related research. This is done through an explicit protocol that is published in the Cochrane Library. Their results are published in the Cochrane Database of Systematic Reviews (one of their many databases), which are regularly updated and freely available online. The strengths of Cochrane reviews lie in their stringent methodological analysis of high-quality research limiting the risk of bias, the regular intervals at which their reviews are updated, and their ease of access. It has been demonstrated that they are at least of comparable quality to systematic reviews and meta-analyses published in print.

Although they have many clear strengths, Cochrane reviews are not without limitation, the most notable of which is their reliance on volunteers. This results in interest-driven as opposed to priority-driven reviews, making them more susceptible to investigating the most interesting as opposed to the most important healthcare issue. Despite this, Cochrane reviews are considered by many to be the gold standard of healthcare evidence (EBM 10.2).

EBM 10.2 Gold standard of evidence

'Cochrane reviews appear to have greater methodological rigor and are more frequently updated than systematic reviews or meta-analyses published in paper-based journals.'

Jadad AR, Cook DJ, Jones A, et al. Methodology and reports of systematic reviews and meta-analyses: a comparison of Cochrane reviews with articles published in paper-based journals. JAMA. 1998;280:278–80.

Table 10.1 Levels of evidence

Level of evidence	Grading criteria	Grade of recommendation
1a	SR of RCTs (including meta-analysis)	A
1b	Individual RCT with narrow confidence interval	
1c	All-or-none studies	B
2a	SR of cohort studies	
2b	Individual cohort study and low-quality RCT	
2c	Outcome research study	C
3a	SR of case–control studies	
3b	Individual case–control study	
4	Case series and poor-quality cohort and case–control studies	
5	Expert opinion without explicit critical appraisal	D

RCT, Randomised controlled trial; SR, systematic review.

Meta-analysis

A meta-analysis is a statistical method of quantitatively combining data from multiple studies to give an overall summary and estimate of the effect studied. It is usually performed as part of a systematic review. Typically, when conducting a meta-analysis, a clear hypothesis to be investigated is decided upon. In accordance with the Preferred Reporting Items for Systematic Reviews and Meta-analyses (PRISMA) statement, an explicit statement of questions being addressed with reference to participants, interventions, comparisons, outcomes and study design (PICOS) is outlined. A literature search is carried out to identify all relevant studies and is usually limited to RCTs, although nonrandomised cohort studies can also be included. The studies that are ultimately included depend upon the eligibility criteria (a set of criteria defined by the authors that a study must meet in order to be included) of the meta-analysis. Once all eligible studies are identified (usually from a combination of multiple electronic databases and library resources), the data are pooled and analysed through different methods. As the included studies will differ from each other (e.g., with respect to sample size and follow-up), they are weighted accordingly when the data are analysed. As a result, smaller studies ultimately contribute less to the overall result. The principal advantage of a meta-analysis is that it allows a specific clinical question, or range of questions, to be investigated in a larger population than is usually feasible in individual trials. Furthermore, by combining the results of all studies (which often have a wide range of, and sometimes conflicting, results), it can provide a more specific estimate of the effect than a single study. However, despite being graded as the highest level of evidence (level 1a) alongside Cochrane reviews and systematic reviews, the meta-analysis is not without its limitations. One such limitation is that of publication bias (when published research is unrepresentative of all conducted research in that field). This may be as a result of a suboptimal search strategy, or simply because certain types of research are unlikely to be published, such as those with small sample sizes and negative results. One further limitation is that of heterogeneity between studies, which decreases the reliability of summarising results.

Systematic review

A systematic review is a research method in which data from all available evidence, that meets predefined criteria, is collected and summarised to answer a specific clinical question or range of questions, while minimising bias. This is achieved through a detailed literature review, a critical appraisal of the studies identified (which may include performing a meta-analysis, the quantitative assembly of data described above), and a detailed summary of the findings including any limitations of the review. It is grouped together with Cochrane reviews and meta-analyses as highest level of evidence. It shares all the same strengths and limitations as a meta-analysis, with the exception that a systematic review cannot provide a numerical summary of the data that is obtained with a meta-analysis.

Randomised controlled trial

A randomised controlled trial, or RCT, is a type of scientific study in which participants are randomly assigned to one specific treatment arm. They are used to investigate causation between intervention and outcome, as well as effectiveness of a treatment, and are considered to be the most rigorous primary scientific method in doing so. Studies of similar design that do not randomise participants can only establish correlation between intervention and outcome. The important characteristics of RCTs include randomisation, allocation concealment, blinding, placebo controls, and the identical treatment and follow-up of all treatment groups (except for the interventions being investigated).

Randomisation helps to eliminate selection bias, and ensures that all subjects have an equal chance of receiving any given treatment in the study. Many methods of randomisation have been proposed. Simple randomisation is based on a single sequence of random assignments. It ensures complete randomness, but can lead to unequal group sizes in smaller studies. Block randomisation, in contrast, has controlled sample sizes and ensures equal sample sizes across time. Stratified randomisation balances specified covariates between groups but requires knowledge of baseline characteristics of all subjects prior to assignment, which is rarely feasible. Covariate adaptive randomisation addresses covariate imbalances continuously and assigns new patients accordingly and can be achieved using online programmes such as www.graphpad.com and www.randomization.com.

Allocation concealment refers to the process by which the randomisation sequence is implemented. It is important that both the investigators and participants remain unaware of the randomisation sequence. This is because knowledge of the randomisation sequence and upcoming assignments may lead the investigators to, either purposefully or inadvertently, delay inclusion of certain patients until their perceived 'appropriate' assignment appears. It is distinct from blinding, which refers to either the participant, or investigator, or both, not knowing to which treatment arm a particular patient belongs.

Blinding, either the participants alone (single blinding) or in combination with the investigators (double blinding) further minimises bias, decreasing the risk that the outcome can be explained by factors other than the intervention (confounding variables).

Although RCTs are extremely useful research tools, bias can still occur. Furthermore, they are not always feasible due to practical or ethical factors. Practical considerations limiting the use of RCTs are often related to recruitment and cost. Recruitment issues can relate to investigators and participants alike. Clinicians and patients may be unwilling, and understandably so, to investigate the efficacy of a novel intervention when established effective treatments already exist.

Ethical considerations are particularly relevant within surgery, specifically regarding surgical procedures, which are seldom exposed to the extensive evaluation process to which medical interventions are subject. To establish whether or not the benefit of a particular surgical intervention is due to the 'placebo effect', the intervention must be investigated using a placebo-controlled RCT. In surgery, these placebo-controls are referred to as 'sham procedures/surgeries'. These procedures are designed to mimic a surgical intervention, while omitting the perceived therapeutic steps, in order to adequately blind the participants involved in the study. This creates ethical dilemmas not applicable to medical placebos as sham surgeries convey their own risks such as those related to anaesthesia.

A well-known example of sham surgery is Moseley's investigation of the placebo-effect in arthroscopic treatment of osteoarthritis of the knee, comparing arthroscopic debridement and arthroscopic lavage with placebo (sham surgery). This showed no improved treatment outcomes in either intervention group compared with the sham group (who received intravenous sedation, superficial skin incision and debridement simulation without insertion of the arthroscope), which strongly brings into question the validity of arthroscopic interventions for osteoarthritis of the knee.

A recent meta-analysis investigated the effect of invasive procedures beyond the placebo effect and found that, on average, 'the changes in the sham groups accounted for 65% of overall improvement from the treatments', meaning that the improvements seen in the invasive procedures investigated (a mixture of percutaneous, endoscopic and classic surgical procedures) is largely due to the placebo effect. Furthermore, the small treatment-specific effect that was seen disappeared when only large studies (>100 participants) were included, highlighting the need for further high-quality research (EBM 10.3).

EBM **10.3 Sham surgery**

'The non-specific effects of surgery and other invasive procedures are generally large. Particularly in the field of pain-related conditions, more evidence from randomised placebo-controlled trials is needed to avoid continuation of ineffective treatments.'

Jonas WB, Crawford C, Colloca L, et al. To what extent are surgery and invasive procedures effective beyond a placebo response? A systematic review with meta-analysis of randomised, sham controlled trials. *BMJ Open* 2015;5:e009655.

The two most common problems with RCTs are compliance and missing outcomes. Intention-to-treat analysis (ITT) is a strategy to overcome these complications. ITT analysis includes every subject who is randomised according to randomised treatment assignment. It ignores noncompliance, protocol deviations and withdrawal, and is often described as 'once randomised, always analysed'. Patients may drop out or not comply due to the effects of treatments, and therefore ITT ensures that these data are included in the final analysis. ITT analysis minimises type I error. ITT analysis can be criticised for several reasons. The inclusion of dropouts and noncompliers means that information on treatment efficacy may be inaccurate. Also, the mixing of groups of patients who received different treatments introduces heterogeneity. The alternative to ITT analysis is per protocol (PP) analysis. PP analyses exclude all protocol violators, including anyone who did not adhere to treatment, switched groups, or missed follow-up. PP removes patients who do not complete treatment and reflects treatment differences more accurately.

Cohort study

Cohort studies are longitudinal observational studies that are often used to determine the incidence and natural history of a certain disease. They do this by either prospectively or retrospectively observing a group of people over a defined period of time. The advantages of cohort studies are that they are relatively cheap to run, they are not subject to the same ethical concerns as RCTs and that they can investigate multiple outcome variables. The disadvantages are that they cannot be used to determine causation, they are subject to recall bias and confounding variables, and are less effective at studying rare diseases. A well-known example of a prospective cohort study is The Million Women Study, which was performed to investigate the effects of hormone-replacement therapy on women's health, particularly with regards to the effects on breast cancer risk.

Case–control study:

Case–control studies are retrospective studies used to investigate if an exposure is associated with a particular outcome (e.g., if smoking is associated with lung cancer). To do this, a case group who are already known to have the outcome are identified and compared to a control group (a group who are demographically similar to the case group). Both groups are analysed retrospectively to identify and compare the frequency of the exposure in both groups. Case–control studies are relatively quick to complete, cheap, useful for investigating rare diseases and can be used to study multiple exposures in the same trial. They are not subject to the same ethical considerations as RCTs, as for the example above, it would be unethical to randomly assign patients to smoking if it is believed that this may increase their risk of lung cancer. Their disadvantages are that they are subject to bias, they cannot establish causation or generate incidence data, and that they are dependent on participants having well-kept records if their results are to be considered reliable.

Case series and case reports

A case series is a small collection of individual cases, while a case report is a report of an individual case. They are observational, descriptive studies that are at the bottom end of the hierarchy of evidence due their small sample sizes and lack of controls, but remain useful in very rare diseases or in reporting rare, or previously not described, associations between a certain intervention and outcome. As they are descriptive studies, and not analytical studies, they are also useful in developing hypotheses, but not in testing them.

10.1 Summary

Levels of evidence

- *Cochrane reviews*, *meta-analyses* and *systematic reviews* of randomised-controlled trials are the strongest levels of evidence available
- The **PRISMA statement** is a defined standard used in the reporting of systematic reviews and meta-analyses
- Systematic reviews are *qualitative* summaries of data
- Meta-analyses are *quantitative* summaries of data
- The important characteristics of an RCT are *randomisation, allocation concealment, blinding* and *treatment controls*
- Observational studies are useful research tools for investigating the incidence of diseases, their natural progression, as well as rare conditions.

Care pathways and guidelines

Care pathways are locally structured, multidisciplinary, task-orientated care plans that highlight the optimal sequence and timing of essential steps in caring for patients within a particular clinical situation. They generally comprise a single document agreed upon by the multidisciplinary team involved, and are based on the most recent guidelines and evidence. They are designed to optimise patient care by implementing up-to-date guidelines. Care pathways help to improve communication between the multidisciplinary team (MDT) and the patient, ensure that clinical practice satisfies a predefined standard, and reduce in-hospital complications (EBM 10.4).

EBM 10.4 Care pathways and complications

'Clinical pathways are associated with reduced in-hospital complications and improved documentation without negatively impacting on length of stay and hospital costs.'

Rotter T, Kinsman L, James E, et al. Clinical pathways: effects on professional practice, patient outcomes, length of stay and hospital costs. Cochrane Database System Rev. 2010(3):Cd006632.

Clinical guidelines, defined as *'statements that include recommendations, intended to optimize patient care, that are informed by systematic review of evidence and an assessment of the benefits and harm of alternative care options'* have become common place in clinical practice. Although present much earlier, interest in clinical guidelines increased dramatically in the 20th century, most notably following World War II, with the formation of multiple organisations responsible for providing national and international guidance on both promoting health and treating illness.

One such organisation is the National Institute for Health and Clinical Excellence (NICE), which was created in 1999 in the United Kingdom. NICE guidelines are based on the best available evidence with the aim to improve the quality of care while assessing the clinical and cost–effectiveness of treatments within the National Health Service (NHS). They are formulated through a predefined rigorous protocol involving individuals from multiple organisations, with the resulting guidelines being published in a clinical guidance manual. As well as the manual, NICE also publishes detailed care pathways for a vast array of medical and surgical conditions, which can be accessed through their website. Although NICE guidelines are often adopted by many countries, strictly speaking, their guidance is 'England only'. The Scottish Intercollegiate Guidelines Network develops evidence-based clinical practice guidelines for the National Health Service (NHS) in Scotland.

Another prominent example is the National Comprehensive Cancer Network (NCCN) in the United States, which is an alliance of 26 US cancer centres that produces guidelines on the detection, prevention and treatment of a vast array of oncologic disorders.

10.2 Summary

Care pathways and guidelines

- Care pathways and guidelines are based on up-to-date research to provide clinicians with recommendations on how to investigate and manage a certain condition
- They are associated with reduced in-hospital complications
- National Institute for Health and Clinical Excellence (NICE), Scottish Intercollegiate Guidelines Network (SIGN) and the National Comprehensive Cancer Network (NCCN) are notable organisations that provide guidelines that are used across the world.

Clinical governance

Clinical governance is a term used to define the processes by which healthcare organisations maintain and improve the quality of care delivered to patients, while creating a system that is responsible and accountable for the care that is provided. Its surge in popularity in the United Kingdom during the 1990s stems from systematic failures within the NHS that led to significant morbidity and mortality. The most notable event occurred in Bristol in 1995, in which an exceptionally high rate of infant mortality following cardiac surgery over a 7-year period was reported. Three medical practitioners (including two surgeons) were found guilty of serious professional misconduct in the subsequent case, which resulted in a restructuring of NHS trust boards and increased emphasis on clinical governance.

Clinical governance rests on seven key pillars (Fig. 10.1):

1. The continuous education and training of clinicians after qualification

   Clinicians must engage in both formal and self-directed education following qualification to ensure their knowledge remains up to date with recent evidence.

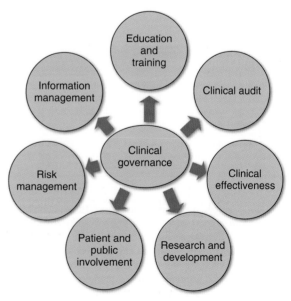

Fig. 10.1 The seven key pillars of clinical governance.

2. The regular use of clinical audit

Clinical audit is a quality assurance process that should be used by clinicians to ensure their current practice adheres to national and local guidelines.

3. Clinical effectiveness

The measure of how much a particular intervention works is referred to as 'clinical effectiveness'. Clinicians should have a good understanding of the clinical effectiveness of the different treatment options available for individual conditions.

4. Participation in research and development

This can be achieved by carrying out novel research or by reviewing established treatments for certain conditions in the form of a literature review.

5. Patient and public involvement through feedback and development of services

Healthcare should be practised within a culture of trust and openness. The public should be involved in discussions regarding adverse event and system changes in order to continuously improve healthcare.

6. The management of risks to patients, healthcare workers and the organisation

Continuous efforts should be made to ensure that healthcare is practised in an environment that is safe to healthcare professionals, patients and the general public.

7. Use and management of information

Information in healthcare, such as patient records, must be used and managed to ensure that systematic errors can be identified, resources can be prioritised and so that confidentiality remains protected.

Clinical audit

Clinical audit is a quality assurance process in which current practice is evaluated and compared to a set standard, with the aim of improving care. When conducting a clinical audit, a six-step cycle is used (Fig. 10.2). The first step involves identifying a potential clinical problem. Audit criteria and standards are then defined. The criteria refer to the questions to be addressed and the exact data to be collected and measured. The standard is usually

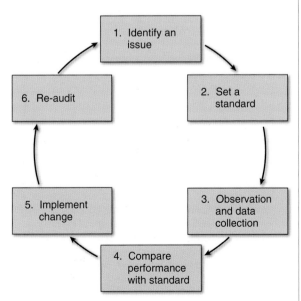

Fig. 10.2 The six-step cycle of clinical audit.

selected from either local or national guidelines pertaining to the clinical issue being audited, as well as the expected level of compliance to these standards. Data are collected, analysed and compared to the chosen standard. If the results show that current practice falls below the expected level of compliance, a change is introduced with the aim of improving compliance. Once the change has been implemented, the audit is repeated to assess whether or not the change has significantly improved compliance, and if so, if it has improved it to an acceptable level. This last step is known as 'closing the audit loop'. Should the audit identify systematic errors in clinical practice, it should prompt an institutional change in local protocols to improve quality of care.

Quality improvement

Quality improvement (QI) has been defined as *'the combined and unceasing efforts of everyone—healthcare professionals, patients and their families, researchers, payers, planners and educators—to make the changes that will lead to better patient outcome (health), better system performance (care) and better professional development'*. It is a process that extends beyond healthcare with a wide range of different models, such as the Six Sigma model first defined in the car industry. Six Sigma uses the Define, Measure, Analyse, Improve and Control (DMAIC) approach. As well as its proven role in business, this five-step approach has been shown to be beneficial in surgery.

Critical appraisal

Critical appraisal is the systematic method by which research is analysed to assess the study strengths and weaknesses, and the validity of data. The high volume of research that is published annually, and the increasing rate at which it is carried out, has resulted in a greater need for clinicians to be able to appraise the available literature critically. Many tools already exist to assist researchers, and even provide different appraisal tools for specific research methods, such as Quality of Reporting of Meta-Analyses (QUORUM) and Assessment of Multiple Systematic Reviews (AMSTAR). The Critical Appraisal Skills Programme (CASP) provides 10–12-point checklists that can be used to appraise different types of research.

Fig. 10.3 outlines a simple checklist to critically appraise all forms of research on a day-to-day basis.

10.3 Summary

Critical appraisal

- Clinical audit is a useful tool used to compare current practice to a defined standard
- Quality improvement projects can be used to improve any aspect of clinical practice, without needing to rely on predefined standards
- Appraising literature is a vital component of evidence-based practice
- QUORUM, AMSTAR and CASP are useful tools to aid in the appraisal of literature.

Continuing professional development

Continuing professional development (CPD) is defined as *'any and all the ways by which doctors learn after formal completion of their training'*. It can be classified into three overlapping categories:

1. Clinical development
2. Professional development
3. Managerial development

Is the research topic relevant?	Will the research add to or reinforce pre-existing knowledge? Will the study address a topic of significant clinical importance?
Has it been studied before, and if so, does this study offer anything new?	Some studies are designed to build on previous research, and some are designed to summarise all evidence that is currently available. However, merely replicating previous studies is of little value
Is the research question clear?	In order to interpret the results, and to critique the research methodology, the readers must clearly understand the research question
Is the study design appropriate for the research question?	For example, if the research question is to assess the effectiveness of a treatment than a well-designed double-blinded RCT is the most appropriate type of research. If the question is to investigate the incidence of a disease then an observational study is the most appropriate type of research
Are the research methods clearly outlined for the readers?	The study should clearly outline information regarding the demographic of the participants, what inclusion and exclusion criteria were used and how the data was collected
Have adequate attempts to reduce bias been taken?	If the methodology is clearly outlined the readers should be able to determine the potential for any systematic bias
Did the study deviate from the original protocol?	A study can deviate from its protocol by failing to recruit the planned number of participants, alterations to inclusion/exclusion criteria or failure to achieve the intended follow-up duration. This can impair the validity of the results by affecting the power of the study or the generalisabilty results
Was the appropriate statistical analysis performed?	This can be difficult for the readers to assess, given that few readers will have an in-depth knowledge of statistics. However, some useful things to know about are how the study was powered, how missing data was dealt with and whether an intention-to-treat or per-protocol analyses were used
Are the results transferable to clinical practice?	If the study investigates the treatment of a condition in a small, homogeneous sample of participants it may not be possible to establish the treatment's effectiveness in a large heterogeneous population that would be expected in clinical practice
Are there any conflicts of interest?	If the investigators have conflicted interests, such as a financial incentive, it predisposes them to systematic biases, and may affect the analysis of the results. Any potential conflict of interest should be clearly disclosed in the study

Fig. 10.3 Checklist to critically appraise all forms of research on a day-to-day basis.

They encompass five key concepts:

1. Innovation. Novel diagnostic methods, management options and surgical techniques are continuously being identified and validated in the literature. As such, it is imperative that surgeons of all levels of seniority update their knowledge if they wish to provide a high quality of care.
2. Lifelong learning. Surgeons must recognise the need to continually update their practice throughout their career to keep up to date with the constantly changing professional environment.
3. Reflective practice and reflective learning. For surgeons to update their practice, they must first review and reflect on their own current practice. This can be done through multidisciplinary team meetings and morbidity and mortality meetings, where clinical decisions are reviewed, discussed and reflected on with colleagues. Organised records, such as logbooks, as well as regular clinical audits are fundamental parts of this process.
4. Relationship between CPD and the principles of 'Good Surgical Practice'. CPD shares many of the same principles outlined in 'Good Surgical Practice'; however, CPD extends beyond these domains as it addresses the managerial and administrative roles in surgical practice.

5. Individual responsibility and accountability. Engaging in CPD is the personal responsibility of each individual surgeon. This extends beyond a moral responsibility, as it has become a professional requirement in many countries.

10.4 Summary

Chapter summary

- Evidence-based medicine should be used in combination with clinical judgement, to ensure patients receive the highest standard of care
- It is the responsibility of each individual healthcare professional to remain up to date with the most recent evidence and guidelines in clinical practice
- Organisations, such as NICE, SIGN and UpToDate, provide detailed guidelines and care pathways on a variety of medical and surgical conditions, and are a valuable reference source for healthcare professionals
- It is vital for healthcare professionals to develop a systematic method of appraising research in order to distinguish between high- and low-quality research
- Clinical audit and quality improvement projects are a central aspect of continuing professional development. Engaging in these research methods early in one's surgical career will help to ensure a career of good surgical practice.

10

Section 2

Gastrointestinal surgery

The abdominal wall and hernia   147

The acute abdomen   159

The oesophagus, stomach and duodenum   179

The liver and biliary tract   206

The pancreas and spleen   233

The small and large intestine   252

The anorectum   283

Andrew de Beaux

The abdominal wall and hernia

Chapter contents

Umbilicus 147

Disorders of the rectus muscle 147

Abdominal hernia 148

Umbilicus

Developmental abnormalities

Persistent vitello-intestinal duct

The vitello-intestinal duct runs in intrauterine life from the apex of the midgut loop to the yolk sac. It is normally obliterated long before birth, but part of it may persist as a Meckel's diverticulum on the antimesenteric border of the ileum. Rarer abnormalities include persistence of a band attaching the umbilicus to a Meckel's diverticulum or a loop of ileum; a patent communication (fistula) between the ileum and umbilicus; an encysted portion of the duct that does not connect with the ileum (enterocystoma); an umbilical sinus; and a persistent umbilical portion of the duct, which forms a polypoidal raspberry-like tumour of the umbilicus (enteroteratoma) (Fig. 11.1). Symptomatic remnants may have to be excised, although a broad-based Meckel's diverticulum is usually left alone if found incidentally at laparotomy. Persisting bands can cause intestinal obstruction.

Urachus

The urachus runs from the apex of the bladder to the umbilicus. It is normally obliterated at birth but may give rise to cysts, a urinary fistula or a discharging umbilical sinus if parts of it remain patent. Symptomatic remnants require excision.

Umbilical sepsis

Umbilical sepsis in neonates may give rise to portal thrombophlebitis, liver abscess formation, jaundice and portal vein thrombosis, which may result in portal hypertension. Tetanus can follow the application of cow dung to the umbilicus, as was once practised in some underdeveloped societies.

In adults, sepsis can result from retention of inspissated sebum within the folds of the umbilicus, and from infection of a pilonidal sinus of the umbilicus. Infection is usually mixed staphylococcal and streptococcal, characterised by erythema, tenderness and swelling. Treatment involves drainage of any pus and the prescription of systemic antibiotics. Rarely, excision of the umbilicus is required.

Umbilical tumours

The umbilicus may rarely be involved by primary neoplasms (e.g., squamous carcinoma or melanoma), or by secondary tumour that has tracked along the ligamentum teres from the liver or lymph nodes in the porta hepatis. Neoplasia is an occasional unexpected finding in an umbilicus that has been excised because of persistent discharge.

Disorders of the rectus muscle

Haematoma of the rectus sheath

Spontaneous or traumatic rupture of a branch of the inferior epigastric artery can result in a painful swelling within the rectus sheath in association with rigidity of the affected side of the abdominal wall. This condition is rare, but may represent an unusual presentation of acute abdominal pain in the elderly patient, especially if they are on anticoagulation therapy. A history of excessive physical exertion may precede the onset of symptoms. Ultrasonography can be used to confirm the diagnosis. Spontaneous resolution is typical but rarely evacuation of clot may be indicated for symptom control.

Desmoid tumour

This rare tumour is thought to arise from fibrous intramuscular septa in the lower rectus abdominis muscle. It is more common in women of child-bearing age and can be associated with intestinal polyposis in Gardner's syndrome. It does not change in size when the abdominal muscles are contracted. The lesion must be excised widely, as it is prone to recur and can become malignant (fibrosarcoma). The resultant defect will need to be reconstructed with a prosthetic mesh after excision.

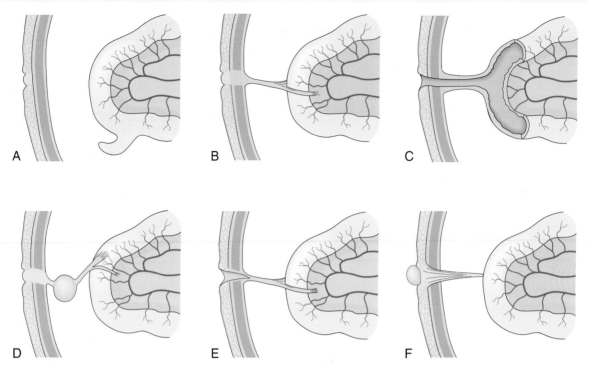

Fig. 11.1 Persistence of the vitello-intestinal duct, giving rise to developmental abnormalities. **(A)** A Meckel's diverticulum. **(B)** A fibrous cord to the ileum. **(C)** An umbilical intestinal fistula. **(D)** An enterocystoma. **(E)** An umbilical sinus. **(F)** An enteroteratoma.

Abdominal hernia

A hernia is an abnormal protrusion of a cavity's contents through a weakness in the wall of the cavity, taking with it all the linings of the cavity, although these may be markedly attenuated (Fig. 11.2). Hernias of the abdominal wall are common. Multiple factors contribute to the development of hernias. Hernias can be considered design faults, either anatomical or through inherited collagen disorders, although these two factors work together in the majority of patients. Hernias may exploit natural openings such as the inguinal and femoral canals, umbilicus, obturator canal or oesophageal hiatus, or protrude through areas weakened by stretching (e.g., epigastric hernia) or surgical incision. In addition to these 'weak' anatomical areas, the collagen make up of the tissues, especially the type I to III collagen ratio, is also important. Type I imparts the strength to the tendon or fascia, type III provides elastic recoil to the tissue. The type I/III collagen ratio varies between individuals but is constant in all the fascia of a particular individual. Hernias can be considered as a disease of collagen metabolism.

The hernia is immediately invested by a peritoneal sac drawn from the lining of the abdominal wall (Fig. 11.2). The sac is covered by those tissues that are stretched in front of it as the hernia enlarges (i.e., the coverings). The neck of the sac is the constriction formed by the orifice in the abdominal wall through which the hernia passes. A hernia may contain any intraabdominal structure, but most commonly contains omentum and/or small bowel. A hernia may involve only part of the circumference of the bowel (Richter's hernia), a Meckel's diverticulum (Littré's hernia) or an incarcerated appendix (Amyand's hernia). A sliding inguinal hernia is defined as one in which a viscus forms a portion of the wall of the hernia sac. Most commonly, the viscus involved is caecum, sigmoid colon or urinary bladder. In the early stages of a hernia, sometimes the hernial contents are preperitoneal fat only, such as a lipoma of the cord, which can mimic an inguinal hernia.

11.1 Summary

Hernia

- A hernia is an abnormal protrusion of a cavity's contents through a weakness in the wall of the cavity, but takes with it all the linings of the cavity
- Hernias of the abdominal wall are common and may exploit natural openings or weak areas caused by stretching or surgical incisions in association with a defect in collagen metabolism
- Abdominal hernias have a peritoneal sac, the neck of which is often unyielding and constitutes a potential source of compression of the hernial contents
- Hernias may be classified as reducible or irreducible, and the contents (e.g., bowel) may become obstructed or strangulated
- Strangulation denotes compromise of the blood supply of the contents and its development significantly increases morbidity and mortality. The low-pressure venous drainage is occluded first and then the arterial supply becomes occluded, with the development of gangrene.

Inguinal hernia

Groin hernias account for three-quarters of all abdominal wall hernias, and inguinal herniorrhaphy is one of the most frequently performed general surgical procedures. The most common types of groin hernia are indirect inguinal (60%), direct inguinal (25%) and femoral (15%) (Fig. 11.3). Most (85%) groin hernias occur in males. Inguinal hernias occur in 1–3% of all newborn males, and in early life an indirect inguinal hernia is by far the most common. After middle age, weakness of the abdominal musculature

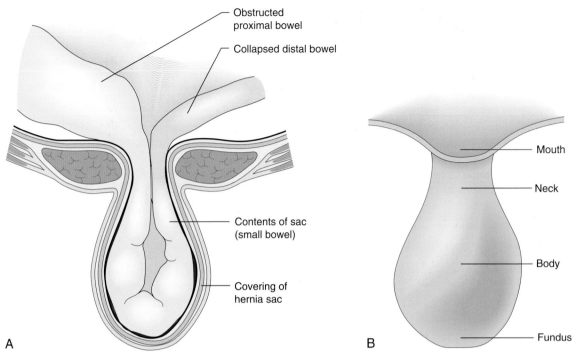

Fig. 11.2 Hernia. (A) Anatomical structure. **(B)** Parts of the hernial sac.

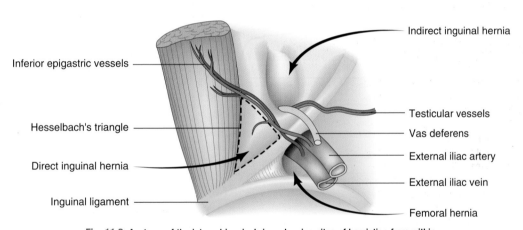

Fig. 11.3 Anatomy of the internal inguinal ring, showing sites of herniation from within.

leads to an increasing incidence of direct inguinal hernias. Femoral hernias are relatively more common in females (possibly because of stretching of ligaments and widening of the femoral ring in pregnancy), but an indirect inguinal hernia is still the most common type of groin hernia in women.

Surgical anatomy

The inguinal canal is an oblique passage 3.75 cm in length, directed downwards and medially in the lower anterior abdominal wall, through which the spermatic cord passes to the testis in the male, or the round ligament in the female. The processus vaginalis traversing the canal is normally obliterated at birth, but persistence in whole or in part presents an anatomical predisposition to an indirect inguinal hernia (Fig. 11.4). The openings of the canal are formed by the internal and external rings. The internal (deep) inguinal ring is an opening in the transversalis fascia, which lies

approximately 1.25 cm above the mid-inguinal point (midway between the pubic symphysis and the anterior superior iliac spine). The internal inguinal ring is bounded medially by the inferior epigastric artery (see Fig. 11.3). The inguinal canal ends at the external (superficial) inguinal ring, which is an opening in the aponeurosis of the external oblique muscle just above and medial to the pubic symphysis.

The testis and spermatic cord receive a covering from each of the layers as they pass through the abdominal wall. The innermost layer is derived from the transversalis fascia (the internal spermatic fascia), the middle layer from the internal oblique muscle (the cremasteric muscle and fascia), and the outer layer from the external oblique aponeurosis (the external spermatic fascia). Within the inguinal canal, the spermatic cord is covered only by the cremasteric and internal spermatic fasciae (see Fig. 11.4). The spermatic cord consists of the vas deferens, the artery of the vas (branch of the inferior vesical artery), the testicular artery (branch of the aorta

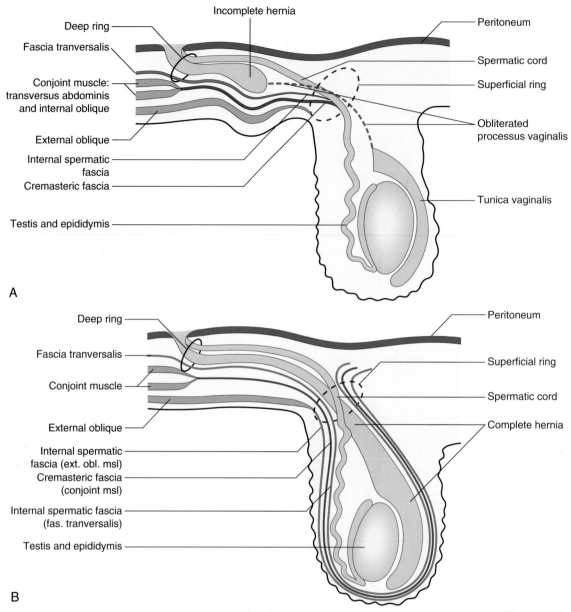

Fig. 11.4 Inguinal hernias. (A) Incomplete inguinal hernia. Note the lack of external spermatic fascia as a covering of the spermatic cord structures within the inguinal canal. **(B)** Complete inguinal hernia. Note the presence of all three layers of coverings over the spermatic cord derived from the abdominal wall muscles after exiting from the superficial inguinal ring.

on the right and renal artery on the left), the cremasteric artery (branch of the inferior epigastric artery), the pampiniform plexus of veins, the ilio-inguinal nerve, the genital branch of the genitofemoral nerve and lymphatics.

Indirect inguinal hernia

An indirect inguinal hernia enters the internal (deep) inguinal ring and descends within the coverings of the spermatic cord so that it can pass into the scrotum, the so-called inguino-scrotal hernia. The hernia may remain within the inguinal canal (bubonocoele), protrude through the external (superficial) inguinal ring (funicular) or extend into the scrotum (complete or scrotal) (Fig. 11.5). Very occasionally, it enlarges between the muscle layers of the abdominal wall to form an interstitial hernia.

Clinical features

Inguinal hernias typically develop over months to years. While such hernias may cause no symptoms, there may be a dragging discomfort in the groin, particularly during lifting or straining, or at the end of the day. Following a period of rest, such symptoms may improve until further strenuous activity. It is not unusual for a patient to present with a lump in the groin rather than because of painful symptoms.

The hernia forms a swelling in the inguinal region, which may be incomplete (appearing as a bulge) or may extend into the scrotum (complete) (Fig. 11.5). It is often readily visible when the patient stands or is asked to cough (Fig. 11.6). However, as the population becomes more overweight, and patients tend to present earlier with symptoms or a small swelling, the diagnosis may not be so obvious on inspection. However, signs of asymmetry between

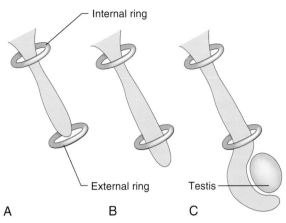

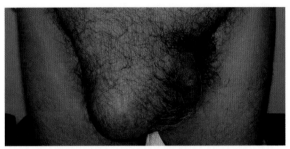

Fig. 11.5 **Types of inguinal hernia sac. (A)** Bubonocoele. **(B)** Funicular. **(C)** Complete or scrotal.

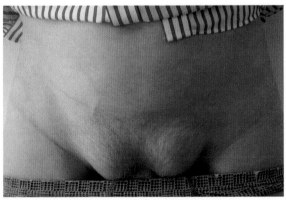

Fig. 11.6 **Unilateral inguinal hernia as inguino-scrotal swelling of long standing.** Note inguino-scrotal extent of the swelling with a prominent bulge in the inguinal region and a 'buried' penis.

Fig. 11.7 **Clinical photograph of bilateral inguinal hernia.**

the two groins may be evident. While bilateral inguinal hernias are not uncommon, it is unusual for both hernias to be of similar size (Fig. 11.7). An inguinal hernia, which passes into the scrotum, passes above and medial to the pubic tubercle, in contrast to a femoral hernia, which bulges below and lateral to the tubercle (Fig. 11.8). In more obese patients, such landmarks can be difficult to palpate with confidence. A cough impulse is normally palpable, and bowel sounds can often be heard within the hernia on auscultation. If there is no visible swelling, a cough impulse is sought with the patient standing. The hernia often reduces spontaneously when the patient lies down.

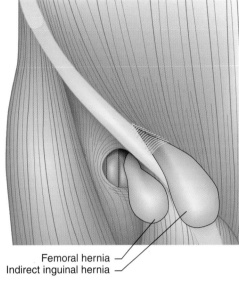

Femoral hernia
Indirect inguinal hernia

Fig. 11.8 **Exit of femoral and inguinal hernias.**

Direct inguinal hernia

Direct hernias are due to weakness of the abdominal wall and may be precipitated by increases in intraabdominal pressure (e.g., obstructive airways disease, prostatism or chronic constipation). The hernia protrudes through the transversalis fascia in the posterior wall of the inguinal canal. The defect is bounded medially by the lateral edge of the rectus abdominis muscle, below by the inguinal ligament, and laterally by the inferior epigastric vessels (see Fig. 11.3). These boundaries mark the area known as Hesselbach's triangle. The hernia occasionally bulges through the external (superficial) inguinal ring, but the transversalis fascia cannot stretch sufficiently to allow it to descend down into the scrotum. The sac has a wide neck, so that the hernia seldom becomes irreducible, obstructs or strangulates. As shown in Fig. 11.3, the neck of the sac of a direct inguinal hernia lies medial to the inferior epigastric vessels, whereas that of an indirect hernia lies lateral to them. A combined indirect and direct hernia may occur on the same side (pantaloon or saddle-bag hernia), with sacs straddling the inferior epigastric vessels.

Clinical features

The hernia forms a diffuse bulge in the region of the medial part of the inguinal canal. It is usually readily reduced by backward pressure, and the edges of the defect may then be palpable. The most commonly performed clinical test to distinguish between a direct and an indirect hernia is to perform the 'deep-ring occlusion test'. With the hernia reduced, digital pressure applied 1.25 cm above the mid-inguinal point is able to control an indirect hernia whereas a direct hernia cannot be controlled. This is not a reliable test, and it is often difficult to distinguish between the two types, leaving the final differentiation to be made on the operating table.

Management of uncomplicated inguinal hernia

The identification of an inguinal hernia in any child is *nearly always* an indication to operate. Elective surgery is usually undertaken as a day case, with liberal use of local anaesthetic blocks for postoperative pain relief.

Adults with a symptomatic inguinal hernia should be offered surgery. Open mesh repair or laparoscopic mesh repair aims to reduce postoperative pain to a minimum, enabling most procedures to be undertaken as day cases (EBM 11.1). Controlling inguinal hernias by the use of a truss is only to be condemned, as this is uncomfortable and causes pressure-induced weakening of the abdominal wall muscles. Furthermore, surgical repair using local or regional anaesthesia can be employed effectively in elderly and higher risk patients.

EBM | 11.1 Laparoscopic inguinal hernia repair

'Laparoscopic inguinal hernia repair is associated with less acute and chronic pain, less nerve injuries such as numbness, quicker return to normal activity and work, and significantly fewer postoperative complications such as infection and haematoma formation than open inguinal hernia repair. Hospital costs are higher for laparoscopic repair and it requires the use of general anaesthetic.'

www.nice.org.uk/TA083guidance, 2010

Indirect inguinal hernia

The first step in the open approach is to open the inguinal canal, free the hernial sac from the spermatic cord (Fig. 11.9), reduce its contents, if any (like bowel or omentum), and excise it after transfixing and ligating its neck. Simple excision of the sac (herniotomy) completes the procedure for infants and young children. An assessment of the strength of the posterior wall can be made at this stage to decide about the use of a prosthetic mesh or a sutured repair. In older children and adults, the internal ring is usually stretched and widened, and it is necessary to tighten the deep ring (Lytle's repair) after herniotomy and/or strengthen the posterior wall with a mesh (herniorrhaphy or hernioplasty). Modified Bassini's herniorrhaphy is a sutured repair that involves approximation of the conjoined tendon with the inguinal ligament using nonabsorbable sutures. Shouldice (Toronto) repair is another form of sutured repair that involves transverse division of the transversalis fascia with double breasting of the loose fascia in two layers followed by repair of the conjoined tendon in two layers. Sutured repairs are associated with

a higher recurrence rate (10%) and increased local pain. These repairs are performed in adolescents and young adults (use of prosthetic mesh can cause fibrosis and infertility), or in emergency inguinal hernia surgery for obstructed or strangulated inguinal hernia where use of prosthetic mesh is contraindicated due to high risk of infection.

Direct hernia

In a direct hernia, the sac, following mobilisation from the spermatic cord, is not normally excised and it is simply invaginated by sutures placed in the transversalis fascia. Insertion of a synthetic mesh is currently used to reinforce the posterior wall of the inguinal canal (EBM 11.2).

EBM | 11.2 Use of mesh in hernia repair

'Mesh reduces the risk of hernia recurrence.'

Scott NW et al. Cochrane Database Syst Rev. 2002;CD002197.

In all hernia repairs, it is important to avoid constricting the spermatic cord by making the deep inguinal ring too tight. This may compromise the blood supply to the testis, particularly in large or recurrent hernias. In older patients, removal of the testis may be considered so that the inguinal canal can be completely obliterated in recurrent hernias.

The most common open surgical procedure now performed for both indirect and direct inguinal hernias is the Lichtenstein open tension-free repair, which involves the insertion of a synthetic mesh underneath the spermatic cord (Fig. 11.10). The mesh is secured to the aponeurotic tissue overlying the pubic bone medially, the inguinal ligament inferiorly, and the internal oblique aponeurosis and conjoint tendon superiorly. Laterally, the mesh is slit to accommodate the spermatic cord and its two sides wrapped around it and sutured in place. This procedure has the lowest recurrence rate (<5%). All open operations can be done under local anaesthesia.

Laparoscopic hernia repair, using a transperitoneal or preperitoneal approach (Fig. 11.11), is increasing in popularity. The technique involves reducing the hernial sac and inserting a large 10 × 15-cm mesh covering the entire musculo-aponeurotic defect. Proponents of these techniques emphasise reduced acute and chronic pain, a rapid return to normal activities and work, improved cosmesis, and fewer infective complications. Critics emphasise the requirement for general anaesthesia, violation of the peritoneal cavity (with the transperitoneal approach), increased hospital costs and the technical difficulty of the surgery. An additional benefit of laparoscopic surgery is that the mesh is larger than that used at open surgery, and covers the direct, indirect and femoral hernial orifices. It is generally accepted that the laparoscopic approach is particularly useful for patients with recurrent inguinal hernias or bilateral inguinal hernias, or exploration of the groin when a symptomatic hernia is suspected from the history but is not obvious on clinical examination.

The asymptomatic inguinal hernia does not always require repair. However, the majority of such hernias become symptomatic within several years, at which time they can be repaired. Hernia recurrence is based on the type of operation performed and the indication. Early recurrence within 2 years is usually a result of an

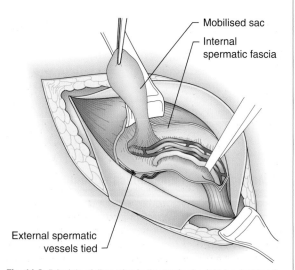

External spermatic vessels tied

Mobilised sac

Internal spermatic fascia

Fig. 11.9 Principle of dissection in the repair of a right inguinal hernia.

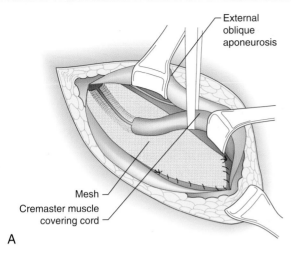

External
oblique
aponeurosis

Mesh
Cremaster muscle
covering cord

A

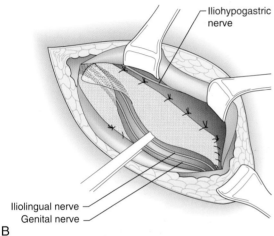

Iliohypogastric
nerve

Iliolingual nerve
Genital nerve

B

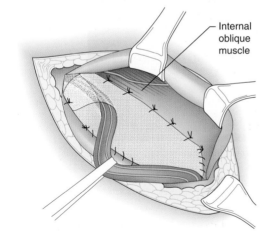

Internal
oblique
muscle

C

Fig. 11.10 Lichtenstein open mesh repair, right-sided hernia. (A) The lower border of the mesh is secured in place with a continuous suture to the inguinal ligament. **(B)** Interrupted sutures are placed between the upper edge of the mesh and the underlying aponeurosis. **(C)** A suture is placed laterally to close the two tails around the internal ring.

inadequate primary operation, whereas late recurrence reflects progression of the underlying muscular weakness. Recurrent hernias can be difficult to repair and the laparoscopic approach may be of particular benefit to these patients, or the open approach if the

first operation was laparoscopic. Chronic pain after surgery, which in 2–3% of patients can be disabling, is a recognised complication of hernia repair (particularly the open approach).

Sportsman's hernia

Groin injury leading to chronic groin pain is often referred to as the sportsman's hernia (EBM 11.3). However, the definition, investigation and treatment of this condition remain controversial. The differential diagnosis includes musculotendinous injuries, osteitis pubis, nerve entrapment, urological pathology, or bone and joint disease. In many cases, clinical signs are lacking, despite the patient's symptoms. Herniography studies have demonstrated a significant incidence of symptomatic impalpable hernia in patients presenting with obscure groin pain. Dynamic ultrasound (ultrasound examination of the groin with the patient at rest and when straining) is replacing herniography as it is noninvasive. Magnetic resonance imaging (MRI) is also used, more to exclude other pathology that might be causing the groin pain rather than to diagnose a sportsman's hernia.

A deficiency of the posterior inguinal wall is the most common operative finding in patients with chronic groin pain. Some authors have described a tear in the conjoint tendon as the cause of the pain, whereas in Gilmore's description, a tear in the external oblique aponeurosis, causing dilatation of the external (superficial) inguinal ring, was implicated. Surgical intervention is recommended only when conservative management has failed. Appropriate repair of the posterior wall of the inguinal canal has proved to be of therapeutic benefit in selected patients.

EBM	**11.3 Chronic groin pain after inguinal hernia surgery**

'A number of factors increase the risk of chronic pain after inguinal hernia surgery **Patient factors:** young, male, painful hernia, other pain syndromes, high preoperative Activity Assessment Scale score and high pain response to a standardised heat stimulus. **Operative factors:** open operation, damage to a nerve(s), acute post-operative pain.'

Aasvang EK et al. Anaesthiology 2010;112:957.

Femoral hernia

Surgical anatomy

A femoral hernia projects through the femoral ring and passes down the femoral canal, which is 1.25 cm long. The femoral ring is 1.25 cm broad and bounded laterally by a thin septum separating it from the femoral vein, anteriorly by the inguinal ligament, medially by the lacunar ligament, and posteriorly by the superior ramus of the pubis and the reflected part of the inguinal ligament (pectineal ligament of Astley Cooper) (Fig. 11.12). As the hernia enlarges, it passes through the saphenous opening in the deep fascia of the thigh (the site of penetration of the long saphenous vein to join the femoral vein) and then turns upwards to lie in front of the inguinal ligament. The hernia has many coverings and may be deceptively small, sometimes escaping detection. It frequently contains omentum or small bowel, but the urinary bladder can 'slide' into the medial wall of the sac.

11

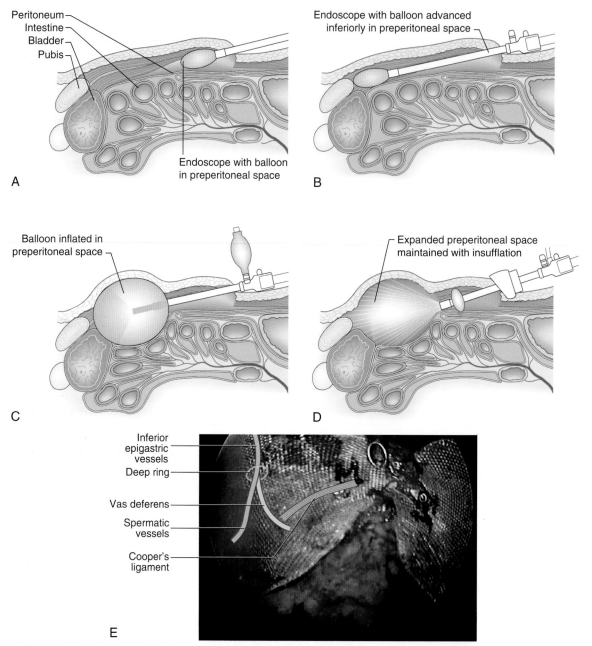

Fig. 11.11 A preperitoneal approach for laparoscopic inguinal hernia repair. Access to the posterior rectus sheath is gained in the periumbilical region. **(A)** A balloon dissector is placed on the anterior surface of the posterior rectus sheath. **(B)** The balloon dissector is advanced to the posterior surface of the pubis in the preperitoneal space. **(C)** The balloon is inflated, thereby creating an optical cavity. **(D)** The cavity is insufflated by carbon dioxide. **(E)** Placement of the mesh. Some surgeons prefer to place the spermatic cord structures and/or the epigastric vessels through a slit in the mesh.

Clinical features

The hernia forms a bulge in the upper inner aspect of the thigh. While a lump or swelling may be the presenting symptom, groin pain related to exercise is also a common presentation. As indicated earlier, it can sometimes be difficult to differentiate between an inguinal and a femoral hernia. Tracing the tendon of adductor longus upwards to its insertion can be a useful guide to the position of the pubic tubercle.

A femoral hernia is frequently difficult or impossible to reduce because of its J-shaped course and the tight neck of the sac. It can be confused with an inguinal lymph node (no cough impulse, irreducible), saphenous varix (positive cough impulse or 'saphenous thrill', which is prominent on standing but disappears on elevating the leg), ectopic testis, psoas abscess, hydrocoele of the spermatic cord or a lipoma. Needle aspiration is not advisable for any such swelling unless the diagnosis has been clearly defined!

Surgical repair of femoral hernia

A femoral hernia is particularly likely to obstruct and strangulate (indeed, 40% of such hernias present this way), and therefore surgical intervention is indicated (EBM 11.4). As with inguinal hernia, repair can be carried out under local or general anaesthesia.

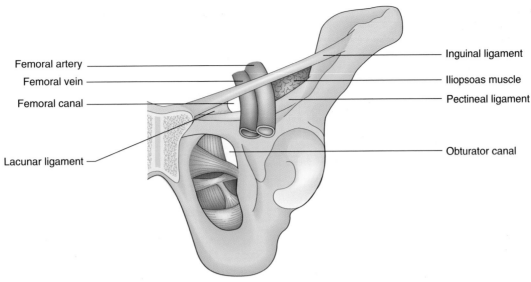

Fig. 11.12 Anatomy of the femoral ring.

11

The aim of operation is to reduce the sac and obliterate the femoral ring by suturing the inguinal ligament to the pectineal ligament. The femoral canal can be approached from below the inguinal ligament (Lockwood), through the inguinal canal (Lotheissen's), or from above by entering the rectus sheath and displacing the rectus abdominis medially. The approach from above (McEvedy approach) gives the best access, and is particularly useful if the hernia contains strangulated bowel and intestinal resection is required. The laparoscopic approach is an alternative 'high' approach.

○ 11.2 **Summary**

Groin hernias

- Indirect inguinal hernias comprise 60% of all groin hernias and commence at the deep inguinal ring, lateral to the inferior epigastric vessels
- Direct inguinal hernias account for 25% of all groin hernias and bulge through a weakness in the back wall of the inguinal canal, medial to the inferior epigastric vessels. They rarely obstruct or strangulate
- Indirect inguinal hernias may pass down within the coverings of the spermatic cord to the scrotum; direct hernias do not descend into the scrotum
- Asymptomatic inguinal hernias do not have to be repaired, especially in the elderly
- Femoral hernias account for 15% of all groin hernias and pass through the femoral canal, emerging below and lateral to the pubic tubercle (in contrast to inguinal hernias, which pass medially to the tubercle and may descend to the scrotum)
- Femoral hernias are often small and easy to miss on clinical examination, but are prone to obstruct and strangulate

Ventral hernia

Ventral hernias occur through areas of weakness in the anterior abdominal wall (Fig. 11.13): namely, the linea alba (epigastric hernia), the umbilicus (umbilical and paraumbilical hernia), the lateral border of the rectus sheath (Spigelian hernia), and the scar tissue of surgical incisions (incisional hernia). Such incisions include scars from laparoscopic surgery, the so-called port-site hernia.

Epigastric hernia

Epigastric hernias protrude through the linea alba above the level of the umbilicus. The herniation may consist of extraperitoneal fat or may be a protrusion of peritoneum containing omentum. The hernia is common in thin individuals and can cause local discomfort. Unless large, an epigastria hernia is rarely visible on

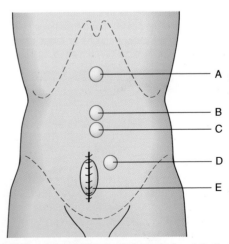

Fig. 11.13 Types of ventral hernia. **(A)** Epigastric: through the linea alba. **(B)** Umbilical: through an umbilical scar. **(C)** Para-umbilical: above or below the umbilicus. **(D)** Spigelian: lateral edge of rectus muscle. **(E)** Incisional: anywhere.

inspection, but is palpable as a firm midline lump. It is repaired by closing the defect with nonabsorbable sutures, by inserting a small mesh, or by laparoscopic intraperitoneal mesh repair.

Umbilical hernia

True umbilical hernias occur in infants. The small sac protrudes through the umbilicus, particularly as the child cries, but is easily reduced. Over 95% of these hernias close spontaneously in the first 3 years of life. Persistence after the third birthday is an indication for elective repair. Surgery involves excision of the hernial sac and closure of the defect in the fascia of the abdominal wall.

Paraumbilical hernia

This hernia is caused by gradual weakening of the tissues around the umbilicus (Fig. 11.14). It most often affects obese multiparous women, and passes through the attenuated linea alba just above or below the umbilicus. The peritoneal sac is often preceded by the extrusion of a small knuckle of extraperitoneal fat through the linea alba. The hernia gradually enlarges, the covering tissues become stretched and thin, and eventually loops of bowel may become visible under parchment-like skin. The sac is often multilocular and may be irreducible because of adhesions that form between omentum and loops of bowel, usually at the apex of the hernial sac. The skin may become reddened, excoriated and ulcerated, and rarely an intestinal fistula may even develop.

Operation is advised because of the risk of obstruction and strangulation. Unless there is a large protrusion of the umbilicus itself, most surgical repairs can be performed preserving the umbilicus. Through a transverse subumbilical incision, the anterior layer of the rectus sheath is exposed. The sac is opened at the neck, which is usually free of adhesions, and the contents are reduced. The defect can be closed using nonabsorbable transverse sutures or the insertion of a mesh. Like epigastric hernias, there is increasing use of laparoscopic intraperitoneal onlay mesh repair.

Incisional hernia

Incisional hernias occur after 5% of all abdominal operations. Over half of incisional hernias occur in the first 5 years after the original surgery. Midline vertical incisions are most often affected. Poor surgical technique, wound infection, obesity and chest infection are important predisposing factors, in addition to the collagen metabolism status of the patient. The diffuse bulge in the wound is best seen when the patient coughs or raises the head and

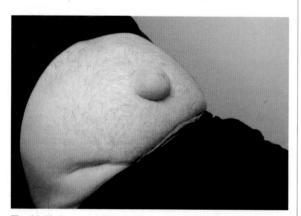

Fig. 11.14 A paraumbilical hernia: note the appendicectomy scar.

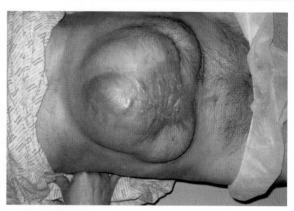

Fig. 11.15 A midline incisional hernia.

shoulders from a pillow, thereby contracting the abdominal muscles (Fig. 11.15). Strangulation is rare, but surgical repair is usually advised.

Open or laparoscopic mesh repair is possible. At open surgery, the mesh can be inserted as an onlay, inlay, sublay or intraperitoneal position (Fig. 11.16). The sublay operation is associated with the lowest incidence of wound complications and recurrence of the hernia. Laparoscopic surgery is associated with less pain, shorter hospital stay and more rapid return to activities. It is difficult to restore the normal anatomy by bringing the muscles together again at laparoscopic surgery, and thus such an approach is mainly used for smaller incisional hernias. Many incisional hernia wounds are cosmetically poor, so laparoscopic surgery for cosmesis is not normally considered. Patients with incisional hernia are at risk for future hernias and laparoscopic repairs, where ports are inserted in the lateral part of the abdominal wall, enable reduction of wound morbidities. Various types of mesh that avoid adhesion to the bowel contents are increasingly used and fixed transfascially.

Parastomal hernia

These occur after the formation of an abdominal wall stoma. The majority of patients with a stoma will develop a parastomal hernia with time. The best way to treat such a hernia includes reversing the stoma, if possible. Otherwise, the techniques for incisional hernia are relevant here including repositioning of the stoma. There is evidence to support the use of mesh reinforcement at the time of creation of the stoma to minimise the risk of parastomal hernia development. Such prophylactic use of mesh is also considered in other high-risk groups, such as midline incisions in the obese. Laparoscopic repairs using meshes that avoid bowel adherence are performed at centres where expertise is available.

Rare external hernias

- A *Spigelian hernia* occurs through the linea semilunaris at the outer border of the rectus abdominis muscle. Treatment is surgical, as the hernia is liable to strangulate
- A *lumbar hernia* forms a diffuse bulge above the iliac crest between the posterior borders of the external oblique and latissimus dorsi muscles. It seldom requires treatment
- An *obturator hernia* is a rare hernia that is more common in women and passes through the obturator canal. Patients may present with knee pain owing to pressure on the obturator nerve; however, the diagnosis is frequently made only when the hernia has strangulated and is discovered at laparotomy.

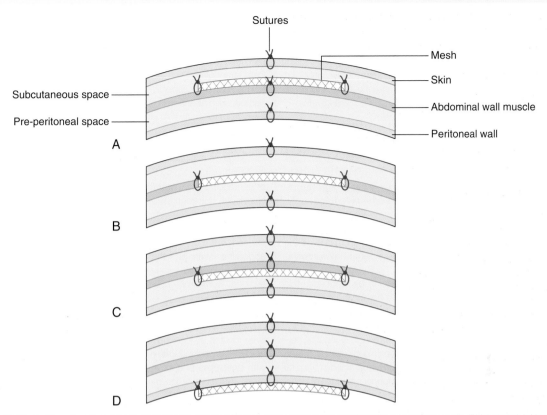

Fig. 11.16 Position of mesh at open incisional hernia repair. (A) Onlay: mesh anterior to the muscles in the subcutaneous space. **(B)** Inlay: mesh bridges the gap in the muscles. **(C)** Sublay: mesh within the muscle layers and/or the preperitoneal space. **(D)** Intraperitoneal onlay mesh (IPOM).

Internal hernia

Herniation of the stomach through the oesophageal hiatus in the diaphragm (hiatus hernia) is a common cause of internal herniation and is considered in Chapter 13. A variety of cul-de-sacs and peritoneal defects resulting from rotation of the bowel and other abnormalities of development may be responsible for the entrapment of bowel and acute intestinal obstruction. For example, herniation may occur through the foramen of Winslow (opening of the lesser sac), paraduodenal/paracaecal fossae and through various openings in the diaphragm, including the oesophageal hiatus (Fig. 11.17). In addition, bowel operations, such as the creation of a Roux loop, can lead to 'iatrogenic' sites for internal hernia formation.

Complications of hernia

▌ Irreducibility

An irreducible hernia is one in which the contents cannot be manipulated back into the abdominal cavity. This may be due to narrowing of the neck of the sac by fibrosis, distension of the contained bowel, or adhesions to the walls of the sac.

▌ Obstruction

An irreducible hernia may progress to intestinal obstruction, signifying compromise to the lumen without any ischaemia to the bowel wall. Colicky abdominal pain, vomiting, constipation and distension signal the need for urgent operation *before* strangulation supervenes.

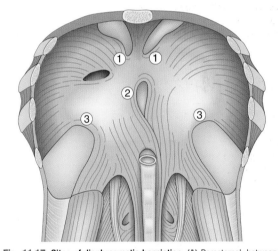

Fig. 11.17 Sites of diaphragmatic herniation. (A) Parasternal, between the sternal and costal slips of the diaphragm (foramen of Morgagni). **(B)** Oesophageal hiatus. **(C)** Pleuroperitoneal canal (foramen of Bochdalek).

▌ Strangulation

The vessels supplying the bowel within a hernia may be compressed by the neck of the sac or by the constricting ring through which the hernia passes. The contents initially become swollen as a result of venous congestion, and there is exudation of a blood-stained fluid. The arterial supply is subsequently compromised and gangrene follows. Bacteria and toxins pass out through the bowel wall, causing local peritonitis.

The patient complains of pain in the hernia and usually has features of intestinal obstruction (vomiting, abdominal distension). The skin overlying the hernia is red, warm to touch and tender, cough impulse is lost, and there may be increasing evidence of circulatory collapse and sepsis. In a Richter's hernia, only part of the circumference of the bowel is strangulated, and there may be no evidence of intestinal obstruction. Strangulation is the main risk factor for death in such cases.

Management of complicated hernia

If there is no evidence of strangulation, an attempt can be made to reduce an apparently irreducible hernia by giving analgesia, putting the patient to bed with the foot of the bed elevated, and applying gentle pressure. Undue force must never be used for fear of rupturing the bowel or returning the entire hernia to the abdomen with the bowel still trapped within it (reduction en masse). If the hernia does not reduce readily, emergency same-day surgery is advised to avoid further complications. Femoral hernias are the least likely hernia (of the common hernias) to be reduced in this way. Following successful reduction of a hernia, the patient can be discharged from the Accident and Emergency department with a plan to repair the hernia within a month.

In infants and children, the majority of 'irreducible' inguinal hernias can be safely reduced by an experienced clinician and then repaired within 72 hours. The child should be detained in hospital pending repair to allow early detection of further episodes of incarceration. Failure to reduce a hernia in this manner necessitates emergency surgery, which is often more difficult than when the hernia has been reduced prior to surgery.

Urgent operation is indicated for all obstructed hernias, since it can never be certain that strangulation is not present, and in clinically strangulated hernias. Occasionally, computed tomography (CT) is indicated especially if an underlying malignancy is suspected, such as anaemia, significant weight loss or palpable mass away from the hernia. At surgery, the hernial sac is opened at the fundus as the adhesions are usually around the neck and the contents are inspected carefully. The gut should be examined for extent of devitalisation. Nonviability of the gut is suggested by bluish or black discoloration, lack of peristaltic activity, loss of peritoneal sheen, and thrombosed mesenteric blood vessels. Nonviable gut requires resection and anastomosis normally requires a midline laparotomy for complete exploration, although this can be achieved from the groin as well. Nonviable omentum is excised. If the contents are viable, they can be returned to the abdominal cavity and the hernia repaired. The use of mesh in potentially infected fields remains controversial and is generally avoided. Sometimes bowel resection and simple suture repair as described above is indicated, with mesh repair reserved if the hernia recurs.

Mesh, like any prosthesis, can become infected. Mesh infection is suggested by local pain, swinging pyrexia, and local redness, tenderness and induration. Mesh infection can often be treated with antibiotics and drainage of any infected fluid around the mesh, but sometimes mesh removal is required to deal with infection.

Simon Paterson-Brown

The acute abdomen

Chapter contents

Introduction 159

Aetiology 159

Pathophysiology of abdominal pain 159

Pathogenesis 161

Clinical assessment 163

Peritonitis 172

Acute appendicitis 174

Nonspecific abdominal pain 177

Gynaecological causes of the acute abdomen 177

Introduction

The 'acute abdomen' is a term used to include a spectrum of surgical, medical and gynaecological conditions, ranging from trivial to life-threatening, which require hospital admission, investigation and treatment. The primary symptom of the condition is abdominal pain. For the purposes of multicentre studies looking at acute abdominal pain, the definition is taken as 'abdominal pain of less than 1 week's duration requiring admission to hospital, which has not been previously investigated or treated'. Acute abdominal pain following trauma is usually considered separately and will not be discussed further.

The acute abdomen is a very common clinical entity. It has been estimated that at least 50% of general surgical admissions are emergencies and, of these, 50% present with acute abdominal pain, which therefore represents a significant part of the general surgical workload. Furthermore, patients with acute abdominal pain have significant morbidity and mortality. Studies have shown a 30-day mortality of 4% among patients admitted with acute abdominal pain, rising to 8% in those who undergo operative treatment. Not surprisingly, the mortality rate varies with age, being the highest at the extremes of age. The highest mortality rates are associated with laparotomy for unresectable cancer, ruptured abdominal aortic aneurysm and perforated bowel, especially the colon.

Individual conditions presenting with acute abdominal pain will not be dealt with in depth in this chapter, but will be covered elsewhere, with the exception of acute appendicitis and nonspecific abdominal pain (NSAP).

Aetiology

The common causes of the acute abdomen presenting to UK hospitals is shown in Table 12.1 and can be subdivided into surgical, medical and gynaecological disorders (Table 12.2). The most common causes in any population will vary according to age, sex and race, as well as genetic and environmental factors (Tables 12.1 and 12.3). The remainder of this chapter will be concerned principally with surgical conditions, rather than gynaecological disorders or medical conditions.

Pathophysiology of abdominal pain

To make an accurate clinical assessment of the patient presenting with acute abdominal pain, it is necessary to understand the pathophysiology. Abdominal pain can be divided into somatic and visceral types.

Somatic pain

The parietal peritoneum covers the anterior and posterior abdominal walls, the undersurface of the diaphragm and the pelvic cavity. It develops from the somato-pleural layer of the lateral plate mesoderm, and its nerve supply is therefore derived from somatic nerves supplying the abdominal wall musculature and the skin (T5–L2). The exception to this is the diaphragmatic portion, which is supplied centrally by afferent nerves in the phrenic nerve (C3–C5), and peripherally in the lower six intercostal and subcostal nerves.

Table 12.1 Common causes of acute abdominal pain in UK adults requiring admission to hospital

Condition	Approximate incidence (%)
Nonspecific abdominal pain	35
Acute appendicitis	30
Acute cholecystitis and biliary colic	10
Peptic ulcer disease	5
Small-bowel obstruction	5
Gynaecological disorders	5
Acute pancreatitis	2
Renal and ureteric colic	2
Malignant disease	2
Acute diverticulitis	2
Dyspepsia	1
Miscellaneous	1

Table 12.3 Common causes of acute abdominal pain in UK children

- Acute appendicitis
- Urinary tract infection
- Mesenteric adenitis
- Gastroenteritis

The parietal peritoneum is sensitive to mechanical, thermal or chemical stimulation, and cannot be handled, cut or cauterised painlessly. As a result of its innervation, when the parietal peritoneum is irritated, there is reflex contraction of the corresponding segmental area of muscle, causing rigidity of the abdominal wall (guarding) and sometimes hyperaesthesia of the overlying skin.

When the diaphragmatic portion of the parietal peritoneum is irritated peripherally, there will be pain, tenderness and rigidity in the distribution of the lower spinal nerves, but when it is irritated centrally, pain is referred to the cutaneous distribution of C3, 4 and 5, i.e., the shoulder area (Fig. 12.1). Somatic pain is classically

Table 12.2 Possible causes of acute abdominal pain

Surgical

Inflammation
- Inflammatory bowel disease
- Acute appendicitis
- Acute diverticulitis
- Acute pancreatitis
- Acute cholecystitis
- Acute cholangitis
- Meckel's diverticulitis

Obstruction
- Intestinal obstruction
- Biliary colic
- Ureteric colic
- Acute retention of urine

Ischaemia
- Mesenteric ischaemia
- Torsion of a viscus

Perforation
- Perforated peptic ulcer disease
- Perforated small bowel (salmonella, cytomegalovirus and tuberculosis infection)
- Perforated diverticular disease
- Perforated appendix
- Toxic megacolon with perforation
- Acute cholecystitis and perforation
- Perforated oesophagus
- Perforated bladder
- Perforation of a length of strangulated bowel
- Ruptured abdominal aortic aneurysm

Medical

Cardiovascular
- Myocardial ischaemia
- Myocardial infarction (inferior)

Gastrointestinal
- Gastritis
- Gastroenteritis
- Mesenteric adenitis
- Hepatitis
- Hepatic abscess
- Curtis–FitzHugh syndrome
- Primary peritonitis

Abdominal wall conditions
- Rectus sheath haematoma

Genitourinary
- Urinary tract infection
- Pyelonephritis

Neurological
- Tabes dorsalis

Haematological
- Sickle cell disease
- Malaria
- Hereditary spherocytosis

Endocrine
- Diabetes mellitus
- Thyrotoxicosis
- Addison's disease

Metabolic
- Uraemia
- Hypercalcaemia
- Porphyria

Infective
- Herpes zoster

Gynaecological
- Ectopic pregnancy
- Ovarian cyst
  Torsion
  Rupture
  Haemorrhage
  Infarction
  Infection
- Pelvic inflammatory disease
- Fibroid degeneration
- Salpingitis
- Mittelschmerz
- Endometriosis

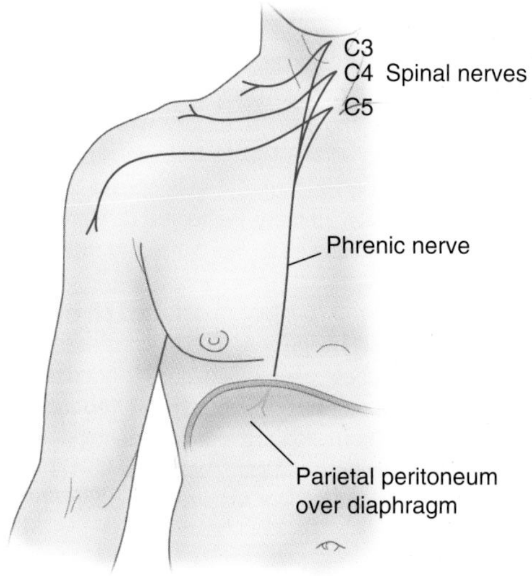

Fig. 12.1 The shared sensory innervation of the shoulder and diaphragm.

described as sharp or knifelike in nature, and is usually well localised to the affected area.

Visceral pain

The visceral peritoneum forms a partial or complete investment of the intraabdominal viscera. It is derived from the splanchnopleural layer of the lateral plate mesoderm, and shares its nerve supply with the viscera (i.e., the autonomic nerves). Visceral pain is mediated through the sympathetic branches of the autonomic nervous system, with afferent nerves joining the presacral and splanchnic nerves, which eventually join thoracic (T6–T12) and lumbar (L1–L2) segments of the spinal cord. The visceral peritoneum and the viscera are insensitive to mechanical, thermal or chemical stimulation, and can therefore be handled, cut or cauterised painlessly. However, they are sensitive to tension, whether due to overdistension or traction on mesenteries, visceral muscle spasm and ischaemia.

Visceral pain is typically described as dull and deep seated. It is usually localised vaguely to the area occupied by the viscus during development, and is referred to the overlying skin of the abdominal wall according to the dermatome level with the sympathetic supply, as mentioned earlier. Therefore, pain arising from the intestine and its outgrowths (the liver, biliary system and pancreas) is usually felt in the midline. Irritation of foregut structures (the lower oesophagus to the second part of the duodenum) is usually felt in the epigastric area. Pain from midgut structures (the second part of the duodenum to the splenic flexure) is felt around the umbilicus. Pain from hindgut structures (the splenic flexure to the rectum) is felt in the hypogastrium/suprapubic area.

Although the division of abdominal pain into visceral and somatic pain is useful, it is important to realise that some pathological conditions will result in a mixed picture. For example, acute appendicitis classically presents with acute abdominal pain that is initially felt in the umbilical area (referred pain) resulting from appendicular obstruction, which gradually localises to the right iliac fossa and becomes sharper in nature as the overlying parietal peritoneum becomes inflamed.

12.1 Summary

Abdominal pain

- Visceral abdominal pain is mediated by the sympathetic nervous system and is typically deep seated and ill localised to the area originally occupied by the viscus during intrauterine life. This is 'referred' pain
- Colic is a form of visceral pain that arises from a hollow viscus with muscle in its walls (e.g., gut, gallbladder and ureter), and results from excessive muscle contraction, often against an obstructing agent
- Patients experiencing colic are usually unable to remain still during the bout of pain but are pain free between attacks. 'Biliary colic' is an exception (and the term colic is a misnomer), in that pain often waxes and wanes on a plateau and there are no pain-free intervals
- Parietal pain, such as that caused by parietal peritonitis, is mediated by somatic nerves and is localised to the area of inflammation
- Parietal pain results in guarding and rigidity of the overlying muscles and the patient is reluctant to move for fear of exacerbating the pain
- Some areas of the peritoneum (e.g., the pelvis, posterior abdominal wall) are 'nondemonstrative' in that parietal peritonitis may be present without tenderness or guarding of overlying muscles.

Pathogenesis

As seen from the list of surgical conditions presenting with acute abdominal pain (Table 12.2), there are two main underlying pathological processes involved, inflammation and obstruction, which may be triggered by a variety of underlying abnormalities. A combination of abnormalities and processes may be involved in any one patient.

Inflammation

Acute inflammation of an intraabdominal organ or the peritoneum may occur as a result of a variety of irritants, which may be broadly classified into infective or noninfective (Table 12.4).

No matter what the trigger of the inflammation, the subsequent pathological process is the same. There is reactive hyperaemia of the injured tissue as a result of capillary and arteriolar dilatation; exudation of fluid into the tissues as a result of an increase in the permeability of the vascular endothelium; and an increase in filtration pressure. Finally, there is migration of leucocytes from the vessels into the inflamed tissues.

Table 12.4 Injurious agents causing inflammation

Infective
• Bacterial
• Viral
• Fungal
• Parasitic
Noninfective
• Chemical
• Ischaemic
• Physical trauma
Heat
Cold
Radiation
Immune mechanisms

The clinical consequences of the inflammatory process depend upon many factors. The underlying condition is the most important: its severity and duration, the organ involved, the patient's age and comorbidity. In general, the patient will complain of abdominal pain and tenderness, which occurs as a result of tissue stretching and distortion, and is due to the release of inflammatory mediators, some of which also mediate pain. On general examination the patient may be pyrexial and have a tachycardia; investigations may reveal a raised white cell count. Examination of the abdomen will reveal tenderness in the affected area, with guarding, rebound and rigidity if the parietal peritoneum is involved.

Peritonitis

Inflammation of the peritoneum (peritonitis) may be classified according to extent (either localised or generalised) and aetiology (Table 12.5). In a surgical setting, the most common cause of generalised peritonitis is perforation of an intraabdominal viscus. Inflammation of the peritoneum results in an increase in its blood supply and local oedema formation. There is transudation of fluid into the peritoneal cavity, followed by accumulation of a protein-rich fibrinous exudate. In the normal state, the greater omentum constantly alters its position within the abdominal cavity as a result of intestinal peristalsis and abdominal muscle contraction, but in the presence of inflammation it will adhere to, and surround, the abnormal organ. The fibrinous exudate effectively glues the omentum to the inflamed viscus, walling it off and preventing further spread of the inflammatory process. In addition, the exudate inhibits intestinal peristalsis, resulting in a paralytic ileus, which limits the spread of the inflammation and infection. As a result of the ileus, fluid accumulates within the lumen of the intestine and, along with the formation of intraperitoneal transudate and exudate, this leads to a decrease in the intravascular volume, producing the clinical features of hypovolaemia.

Clinical features

The clinical features of peritonitis vary considerably but the most common symptom is abdominal pain, which is constant and often described as sharp. The pain is usually well localised if it is secondary to inflammation of an intraabdominal viscus and involves the parietal pertioneum, but may spread to involve the whole peritoneal cavity. Primary peritonitis can present rather more subtly, and as many as 30% of affected individuals may be asymptomatic.

The term 'peritonitis' or 'peritonism detected on clinical examination' is used to describe the collection of signs associated with inflammation of the parietal peritoneum, and includes tenderness, 'guarding' (voluntary), rigidity (involuntary) and 'rebound' tenderness. Evidence of inflammation of the parietal peritoneum in association with inflammation of an intraabdominal viscus is often a strong indication that the patient requires some form of surgical intervention.

Infarction

An infarct is an area of ischaemic necrosis caused either by an occlusion of the arterial supply or the venous drainage in a particular tissue, or by a generalised hypoperfusion in the context of shock (Table 12.6). The typical histological feature of infarction is ischaemic coagulative necrosis. An inflammatory response begins to develop along the margins of an infarct within a few hours, stimulated by the presence of the necrotic tissue.

The consequences of decreased perfusion of a tissue depend on several factors: the availability of an alternative vascular supply, the rate of development of the hypoperfusion, the vulnerability of the tissue to hypoxia, and the blood oxygen content. In the context of acute abdominal pain, intestinal infarction is the most common cause. Other organs that may infarct include the ovaries, kidneys, testes, liver, spleen and pancreas.

Clinical features

In general, the patient will complain of severe abdominal pain and the onset will depend on the nature of the underlying process. Embolisation will result in sudden onset of pain, whereas the onset in thrombosis is likely to be more gradual. Infarction and ischaemia

---

Table 12.5 Classification of peritonitis

Generalised peritonitis

Primary: infection of the peritoneal fluid without intraabdominal disease
- Haematogenous spread
- Lymphatic spread
- Direct spread: usually associated with continuous ambulatory peritoneal dialysis catheters
- Ascending infection: from the female genital tract

Secondary: inflammation of the peritoneum arising from an intraabdominal source
- Infectious
- Noninfectious
  Blood
  Ischaemia
  Bile
  Chemical
  Foreign body
- Perforation

Localised peritonitis
- Usually due to spreading inflammation across the wall of an intraabdominal viscus

---

Table 12.6 Aetiology of infarction

Occlusive

Arterial
- Embolism
- Thrombosis
- Extrinsic compression

Venous
- Thrombosis
- Extrinsic compression

Nonocclusive

Shock
- Hypovolaemia
- Cardiogenic
- Sepsis

Vasoconstrictor drugs

are potent triggers of inflammation of the affected structure, and the clinical features reflect this.

Perforation

Spontaneous perforation of an intraabdominal viscus may be the result of a range of pathological processes. Weakening of the wall of the viscus, which might be associated with a locally advanced malignancy of the bowel, as well as degeneration, inflammation, infection or ischaemia, will all predispose to perforation. An increase in the intraluminal pressure of a viscus, such as occurs in a closed-loop obstruction (Fig. 12.2) when the obstructed bowel cannot decompress itself proximally (obstructing colonic tumours with an intact ileo-caecal valve or a volvulus of either the small or large bowel), will predispose to perforation, as will peptic ulceration, acute appendicitis and acute diverticulitis. Other less common causes are inflammatory bowel disease and acute cholecystitis.

Perforation can also be iatrogenic, and may occur during the insertion of a Verres needle at laparoscopy, because of a careless cut or suture placement during surgery, and during the course of an endoscopic procedure.

Clinical features

Spontaneous perforation of a viscus normally results in the sudden onset of severe abdominal pain, which is usually well localised to the affected area. The resultant clinical picture depends on the nature of the perforated viscus and the relative sterility and toxicity of the material within the abdominal cavity, in addition to the speed with which the perforation is surrounded and sealed (if at all) by the adjacent structures and omentum. The inevitable peritoneal contamination will lead to either localised or generalised peritonitis, and the associated symptoms and signs, as already discussed. Intestinal content, blood and bile are all irritant to the peritoneum.

Obstruction

The term 'obstruction' refers to impedance of the normal flow of material through a hollow viscus. It may be caused by the presence of a lesion within the lumen of the viscus, an abnormality in its wall, or a lesion outside the viscus causing extrinsic compression.

The smooth muscle in the wall of the obstructed viscus will contract in an effort to overcome the impedance. This reflex contraction produces 'colicky abdominal pain', such as seen in 'ureteric colic'. The exception to this rule is 'biliary colic'. The gallbladder and biliary system have little smooth muscle in their wall and attempts at contraction tend to be more continuous than 'colicky'. Similarly 'renal colic' is a misnomer and it should be referred to as 'renal pain'.

If the obstruction is not overcome, there will be an increase in intraluminal pressure and proximal dilatation. The end result depends on the anatomical location of the obstruction, whether it is partial or complete, and whether the blood supply to the organ is compromised. For example, a ureteric calculus in a single functioning kidney can cause urinary outflow obstruction resulting in a dilatation of the proximal ureter and renal pelvis, and subsequent 'postrenal' renal failure. An obstructed inguinal hernia, on the other hand, will not only produce proximal dilatation of the intestine (usually associated with vomiting) but may also result in ischaemia of the bowel wall, leading to infarction and perforation.

Clinical assessment

The ability to make an accurate assessment by taking a good history and performing an appropriate examination is a vital skill in the management of the patient with acute abdominal pain. Although an exact diagnosis is often impossible to make after a detailed history and initial assessment, and often relies on further investigations, it is the formulation of an appropriate, safe and effective management plan that is the most important issue. In most cases,

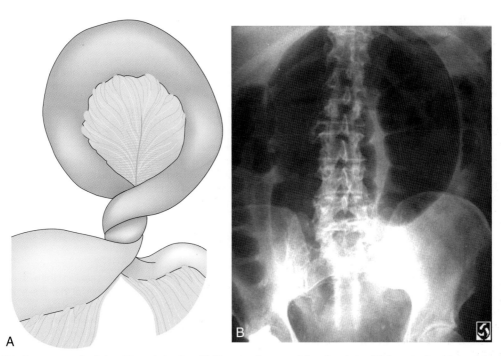

Fig. 12.2 Volvulus: an example of closed-loop obstruction. (A) Diagrammatic representation of a volvulus. **(B)** X-ray showing volvulus of sigmoid colon.

it is possible to take a full history and perform a thorough examination, but this is not always so, and occasionally a rapid evaluation followed by immediate resuscitation is required.

History

The main presenting complaint of patients with an acute abdomen is pain. The characteristics of the pain (Table 12.7) give important clues to the likely underlying diagnosis, and these should be explored in depth. However, the importance of a full history is very important and is essential in all patients.

Site of pain

The site of abdominal pain is perhaps the most valuable pointer to the underlying diagnosis. In order to describe the site of pain, the abdomen is traditionally divided into either quarters or nine regions (Figs 12.3 and 12.4).

Nature of pain

As discussed above, inflammation produces a constant pain made worse by local or general disturbance, and pain which is made worse by movement or coughing suggests inflammation of the parietal peritoneum. In this situation, the patient will often be seen to lie very still to avoid exacerbating the pain.

Obstruction of a muscular viscus produces a colicky pain that comes and goes in 'spasms', often only lasting a few minutes at a

Table 12.7 **Characteristics of abdominal pain**
• Site
• Nature
• Radiation
• Time and mode of onset
• Severity
• Progression
• Duration
• Exacerbating/relieving factors

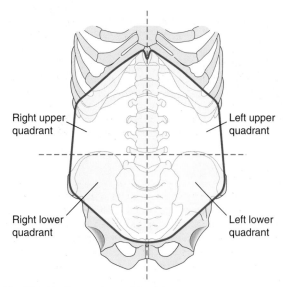

Fig. 12.3 The four quadrants of the abdomen.

Right upper quadrant
Left upper quadrant
Right lower quadrant
Left lower quadrant

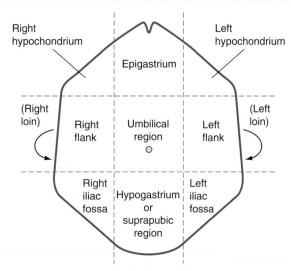

Fig. 12.4 The abdomen divided into nine regions.

Right hypochondrium
Left hypochondrium
Epigastrium
(Right loin)
Right flank
Umbilical region
Left flank
(Left loin)
Right iliac fossa
Hypogastrium or suprapubic region
Left iliac fossa

time but returning at frequent intervals. It may be described as 'gripping' in nature, and between spasms the patient is usually pain free. The pain itself is severe and may be helped by moving around or drawing the knees up towards the chest. Underlying inflammation must be suspected when a colicky pain does not disappear between spasms, or becomes continuous. In the case of intestinal obstruction, this might mean strangulation, for which urgent surgery is required.

Radiation of pain

Radiation is the process whereby pain extends directly from one place to another, while usually remaining present at the site of onset. It is not the same as 'referred' pain, which was described earlier. When a pain radiates, it signifies that other structures are becoming involved. For example, pain from a duodenal ulcer may radiate through to the back, indicating that inflammation has occurred through the wall of the duodenum to involve structures of the posterior abdominal wall, such as the pancreas and retro-peritoneum. Ureteric pain radiates to the tip of the penis in men and to the area around the urethra in women.

Onset of pain

The onset of pain can be sudden or gradual. Typically, pain from a perforation is sudden and that from inflammation is gradual. Patients with the former can usually remember exactly what they were doing at the time of onset, whereas in the latter localisation in time is more difficult.

Severity of pain

A patient's description of the severity of pain is very subjective. Every individual has a different reaction to pain, and this is often more reflective of the patient's personality than of the underlying pathology. A better indication is to assess the effect of the pain on the patients' lives. For example, did they visit a doctor? Were they unable to attend work? Did the pain interfere with their sleep? Furthermore, it is often useful to ask the patient to rate pain severity using a score on a numerical or pictorial scale (visual analogue scale).

Progression of pain

Once a pain has occurred, it may remain exactly the same, may gradually improve or worsen, or may fluctuate.

Movement of pain

It is also useful to note whether the pain moves. Acute appendicitis is a classic example of pain that moves, starting as a vague central 'referred' pain and then moving to the right iliac fossa as the adjacent parietal peritoneum becomes inflamed. The various characteristics of abdominal pain, as shown in Fig. 12.5, are essential in helping the clinician formulate a differential diagnosis.

Examination

During the course of taking a history it is possible to form a general impression of the state of the patient. The unwell patient with acute abdominal pain may look pale and sweaty, lie flat on the bed, be cerebrally obtunded, and be unable to move without

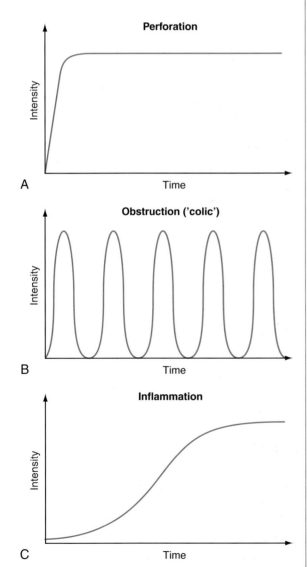

Fig. 12.5 Time versus intensity graphs for acute abdominal pain.

experiencing pain. Others, however, may look surprisingly well, have a good colour, sit up in bed, talk normally and be able to move freely. All these observations should be noted and recorded, along with the temperature, pulse, blood pressure and respiratory rate.

Other important features to look for on general examination include clinical evidence of anaemia, jaundice, cyanosis and dehydration. It is important to bear in mind that physical signs are often less obvious than might be expected in the elderly, the obese, the generally unwell and those taking steroids. As in every emergency patient, a full examination, including the cardiovascular, respiratory and neurological systems, in addition to the abdomen and pelvis, must be carried out and the results documented. Specific details relating to the abdominal examination are described below and in Table 12.8.

In small children with abdominal pain, it is useful to ask the child to 'blow out' and 'suck in' their abdomen and to cough. These three movements will usually elicit pain in the presence of peritonism without laying a hand on the child's abdomen. Rebound tenderness should *never* be elicited in children. Gentle tapping with the percussing finger will elicit the same information (tap tenderness) in a much less cruel way. The history of pain on moving or coughing is also a good indicative as to the presence of rebound tenderness.

Inspection of the abdomen

The patient must be adequately exposed and positioned to examine the abdomen. The full extent of the abdomen should be visible, and by convention the patient should be exposed from 'nipples to knees'. This prevents the common mistake of not examining the breasts, groins and external genitalia. Patient dignity should be maintained and the breasts and genitalia covered once assessed. In some cultures this may be difficult for a male doctor. The presence of a chaperone or a first-degree female relative, tact, good communication skills and a professional attitude will all help to overcome this barrier. Patients should be positioned supine on the bed or trolley with a single pillow behind the head and shoulders, and with the arms resting by their side.

Inspection of the abdomen may reveal a wealth of information. Abdominal swellings due to abnormal enlargement of the liver, kidneys or spleen, and tumours of the bowel, ovaries or other intraabdominal or retroperitoneal structures may be visible. Scars from previous abdominal or pelvic surgery may be observed, and are of importance in the presence of bowel obstruction, which may be secondary to adhesions. All scars should be tested for the presence of herniation. Distended veins on the abdominal wall may be secondary to portal hypertension or occlusion of the inferior vena cava. The abdomen may be generally distended by intraabdominal blood or fluid, or as a result of intestinal obstruction. In cases of obstruction, intestinal peristalsis may be visible, if the patient is thin.

Palpation

Palpation of the abdomen should be carried out in a systematic manner, beginning with gentle superficial examination of the whole abdomen looking for tenderness. This should start away from the site of maximum pain and move towards the tender site, encompassing all areas (Figs 12.3 and 12.4). Palpation over an area of tenderness will cause pain, which in turn will stimulate the patient to contract the overlying muscles (voluntary guarding). If the pain is due to inflammation, the approximation of the parietal

Table 12.8 Checklist for examination of the acute abdomen

Method	Question	Significance
Inspection	What is the abdominal contour?	Distension: intestinal obstruction or ascites
	Does the abdomen move with respiration?	Rigid abdomen: peritonitis
	Can the patient blow out/suck in the abdomen?	Rigid abdomen: peritonitis
	Does the patient lie still or writhe about?	Fear of movement: peritonitis
		Writhes about: colic
	Are there visible abnormalities?	Scars: relevant previous illness, adhesions
		Hernia: intestinal obstruction
		Visible peristalsis: intestinal obstruction
		Visible masses: relevant pathology
Gentle palpation	Is there tenderness, guarding or rigidity?	Tenderness/guarding: inflamed parietal peritoneum
		Rigidity: peritonitis
Deep palpation	Are there abnormal masses/palpable organs?	Palpable organs/masses: relevant pathology
	Is there rebound tenderness?	Rebound tenderness: peritonitis
Percussion	Is the percussion note abnormal?	Resonance: intestinal obstruction
		Loss of liver dullness: gastrointestinal perforation
		Dullness: free fluid, full bladder
		Shifting dullness: free fluid
Auscultation	Are bowel sounds present/abnormal?	Absent sounds: paralytic ileus
		Hyperactive sounds: mechanical obstruction, gastroenteritis
	Is there a bruit?	Bruit: vascular disease

Do not forget to:
Examine the groin
Consider a digital rectal examination
Consider a vaginal examination when appropriate
Examine the chest

peritoneum on to the inflammatory area will result in a reflex contraction of the overlying muscles (involuntary guarding). If the whole peritoneal cavity is inflamed, then there will be generalised peritonitis and the abdominal wall will be rigid (board-like rigidity). When the palpating hand, which has been pushing the parietal peritoneum against the inflamed viscus, is suddenly released, the viscus will bounce back and hit the parietal peritoneum, causing an additional sharp pain (rebound tenderness). This is an excellent indication of underlying peritoneal inflammation (peritonism) but is very painful and is better tested by light percussion or the 'tap test'. As already mentioned earlier, history of pain on coughing or moving is also a good indication of peritoneal inflammation.

If light palpation of the whole abdomen elicits no pain, the process is repeated, pressing more firmly to detect deep tenderness. This will allow for the detection of organomegaly and the presence of any masses.

Analgesia should never be withheld from a patient pending formal examination, as it does not mask important clinical signs. Indeed, the administration of analgesia relaxes the patient and may often help the examination. However, repeated administration of opiate analgesia to a patient with abdominal pain in whom a definite diagnosis has not been made cannot be supported without regular reassessment, as this suggests progression of the disease process and that surgical intervention may be indicated.

During the general examination, particular attention should be paid to the supraclavicular fossae, axillae and cervical regions for the presence of lymphadenopathy. The hernial orifices must also be specifically examined for irreducible inguinal or femoral hernia, as must the male external genitalia, looking for tenderness and masses within the scrotum.

Percussion

Percussion is useful in the localisation and assessment of tenderness, particularly in the assessment of rebound tenderness, in addition to determining the presence of fluid within the peritoneal cavity. The normal abdomen is universally resonant because of the presence of gas-containing bowel lying in front of the solid retroperitoneal structures, and because the normal pelvic viscera lie entirely within the bony pelvis.

The liver gives a dull note to percussion anteriorly from the level of the right fifth rib to the right costal margin, and loss of liver dullness to percussion may represent free intraperitoneal gas. The presence of suprapubic dullness may indicate a full bladder due to urinary retention. If there is free intraperitoneal fluid, the percussion note will be dull in the flanks. The site of the dullness moves as the patient rolls onto his or her side (shifting dullness). Some 1.5 L or more of fluid is required before this sign can be elicited. A 'fluid thrill' may be elicited if there is more than 3 L of free fluid in the peritoneal cavity.

Auscultation

Bowel will only produce gurgling noises if it contains a mixture of fluid and gas. Normal bowel sounds are low pitched and occur every few seconds. Their absence over a 30-second period suggests that peristalsis has ceased, a condition termed *ileus*. This may be due to generalised peritonitis or atony of the bowel smooth muscle, such as might follow a prolonged period of obstruction. Increased peristalsis produces a higher volume, pitch and frequency of the bowel sounds and can be heard in mechanical obstruction (often described as *tinkling*), in addition to conditions such as gastroenteritis. In general, bowel sounds should be described as present and normal, present and abnormal, or absent. Auscultation of bowel sounds are generally not considered reliable in the evaluation of patients with acute abdominal pain.

Auscultation should continue over the course of the aorta and the iliac arteries, listening for the presence of bruits, which are indicative of turbulent flow.

If gastric outlet obstruction is clinically suspected, the patient's abdomen may be shaken from side to side in an attempt to elicit a 'succussion splash'.

Rectal examination

Finally, a rectal examination is performed to assess the pelvis and, if a gynaecological disorder is suspected, a vaginal examination is indicated. Although examination of the rectum has often been considered routine in the past, it is unpleasant for the patient and rarely provides additional helpful information. As such, it may be omitted, particularly in younger patients, when diagnosis and management plans have already been made and unlikely to be influenced by any information obtained. Useful information that might be obtained from a rectal examination includes the presence of masses (in older patients), tenderness from a pelvic source when abdominal signs are not present, faecal impaction and blood.

Specific clinical signs in acute abdominal pain

Murphy's sign

In acute cholecystitis, a deep breath taken by the patient elicits acute pain when the examiner presses downwards into the right upper quadrant. This is caused by the movement of the inflamed gallbladder striking the examining hand.

Boas's sign

In acute cholecystitis, pain radiates to the tip of the scapula and there is a tender area of skin just below the scapula, which is hyperaesthetic.

Grey Turner's and Cullen's signs

In patients with severe acute pancreatitis, bruising and discoloration may be seen around the umbilicus (Cullen's sign) and in the left flank (Grey Turner's sign). Cullen's sign was actually first described in relation to ruptured ectopic pregnancy, but is now often also associated with acute pancreatitis.

Rovsing's sign

In acute appendicitis, palpation in the left iliac fossa produces pain in the right iliac fossa.

Investigations

Following initial clinical assessment, and during assessment in the critically ill, measures should be taken to resuscitate the patient. During this period, further investigations can be organised to help in the diagnostic process. It is important to remember that in all patients a working list of differential diagnoses must be made after clinical assessment so that only appropriate investigations are instituted. There is no point in ordering investigations, the results of which will not influence the clinical management.

The most common investigations carried out on a patient with acute abdominal pain include full blood count (FBC), urea and electrolytes (U&Es), amylase, lipase, C-reactive protein, liver function tests, plain radiology (erect chest and supine abdominal x-rays) and an ultrasound (US) scan.

Blood tests

Blood tests can be very useful in confirming a diagnosis (amylase and lipase for acute pancreatitis), identifying an underlying inflammatory cause for the pain (raised C-reactive protein and leucocytosis) and biliary disorders (liver function tests). It may also be useful to have baseline results for FBC and U&Es for future reference.

FBC, C-reactive protein and U&Es

A single reading of a raised white cell count taken on its own is fairly nondiscriminatory, but a persistent elevation or a rise suggests underlying inflammation and/or infection; similarly for C-reactive protein levels. In the assessment of patients with possible appendicitis, recent studies have demonstrated that, in the presence of a normal C-reactive protein and white cell count, acute appendicitis is very unlikely. Obviously U&Es are essential in patients who might be dehydrated and hypovolaemic in order to monitor renal function and fluid replacement, particularly if surgery is being considered. Similarly, an abnormal haemoglobin level may be significant and require correction.

Serum amylase

A serum amylase greater than three times the upper limit of normal is highly suggestive of acute pancreatitis. Lesser values are nonspecific and can be the result of a wide range of conditions. However, as many as 20% of patients with acute pancreatitis may have normal amylase levels on admission, either because they have presented early and there has not been enough time for the level to rise, or late and the level has returned to within normal limits. Other causes of a raised amylase are shown in Table 12.9. In patients with acute pancreatitis who present more than 48 hours after the onset of pain, the serum amylase may have returned to normal. In these patients, measurement of the urinary amylase or serum lipase may be of value.

Liver function tests

Liver function tests are increasingly becoming available on an emergency rather than a routine basis in many hospitals, as clinicians have recognised their value in the assessment and subsequent management of acute hepatobiliary and pancreatic disorders (see Chapter 14). The measurement of gamma glutamyl transferase (GGT) is a particularly sensitive test for possible stones in the common bile duct (choledocholithiasis).

Blood gas analysis

Arterial blood sampling is often used to monitor the acid–base status and the efficacy of gas exchange in the seriously ill patient. Patients with sepsis and intestinal ischaemia are likely to demonstrate a metabolic acidosis with an elevated lactate level.

12

Table 12.9 Causes of hyperamylasaemia
Pancreatic conditions
• Acute pancreatitis • Pancreatic cancer • Pancreatic trauma
Other intraabdominal pathology
• Perforated peptic ulcer • Acute appendicitis • Ectopic pregnancy • Intestinal infarction • Acute cholecystitis
Decreased clearance of amylase
• Renal failure • Macroamylaseaemia
Miscellaneous
• Head injury • Diabetic ketoacidosis • Drugs (e.g., opiates)

Serum calcium

Patients with hypercalcaemia may complain of abdominal pain as a result of abnormal gastrointestinal motility, nephrolithiasis, peptic ulcer disease, pancreatitis or malignancy. A low calcium level is one of the poor prognostic factors in patients with severe acute pancreatitis.

Sickle tests

Sickle cell crises are a rare cause of acute abdominal pain. Blood should be sent for testing on all at-risk patients.

Blood glucose

Measurement of blood glucose is important, as diabetic ketoacidosis may present with acute abdominal pain, and also because any serious illness can result in poor glycaemic control, particularly in diabetic patients.

Urinalysis

Dipstick testing

Haematuria in the context of acute abdominal pain may indicate a urinary tract tumour, infection or nephrolithiasis. Glucose or ketones in the urine indicate recent starvation or possible diabetic ketoacidosis. Protein, bilirubin or casts in the urine suggest renal or liver disease. In patients with an inflamed retrocaecal appendix, urine testing may demonstrate the presence of protein and white cells, and urgent microscopy (which will confirm or refute the presence of bacteria) should be arranged to determine whether there is an underlying urinary tract infection or whether another condition, such as appendicitis, might be the cause.

Bacteriology

If the clinical picture is suggestive of a urinary tract infection and the urine dipstick demonstrates protein, nitrites and leukocytes, microscopy and culture should be requested. Specimens from any other potential sites of infection should also be submitted for bacteriological analysis (stool, blood, pus etc.).

Pregnancy test

A pregnancy test should be performed in all women of childbearing age who present with acute abdominal pain and in whom the chance of pregnancy cannot be excluded. Not only is this important if x-rays are to be taken, but it will also raise the possibility of an ectopic pregnancy if positive.

Urinary porphobilinogen

Quantitative assay of urinary porphobilinogen is the most important diagnostic test for porphyria, which is a rare condition that may present with acute abdominal pain and should be considered in difficult cases.

Radiological investigations

Plain x-rays

The erect chest x-ray (CXR) is the most appropriate first investigation for the detection of free intraperitoneal gas (Fig. 12.6) and should be carried out in any patient who might have a perforation. If the condition of the patient prevents an erect film being taken, then a left lateral abdominal decubitus film might be helpful. Although a visceral perforation is the most common cause of free intraperitoneal gas, other causes exist and should be considered where appropriate (Table 12.10). An erect CXR is also useful in identifying a respiratory condition that may present with upper abdominal pain. These patients are usually tachypnoeic. Increasingly computed tomography (CT; see later) is replacing erect CXR in patients with a suspected perforation, particularly if they are unwell and a definitive diagnosis is required urgently to decide immediate management.

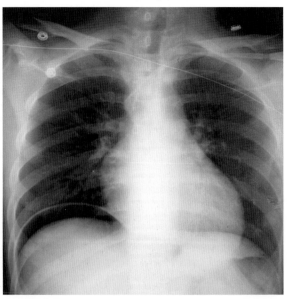

Fig. 12.6 Gas under the diaphragm seen on the erect chest x-ray in a patient with a perforated peptic ulcer.

Table 12.10 Causes of free subdiaphragmatic gas on abdominal x-ray

- Perforation of an intraabdominal viscus
- Gas-forming infection
- Pleuroperitoneal fistula
- Iatrogenic: laparoscopy, laparotomy
- Gas introduced per vaginam: postpartum
- Interposition of bowel between liver and diaphragm

EBM 12.1 Abdominal radiography

'Plain abdominal radiography has a limited role in the assessment of the acute abdomen, particularly when the diagnosis is likely to be peptic ulcer disease, acute biliary disease or acute appendicitis. It is valuable when the diagnosis is uncertain and in patients with other suspected acute gastrointestinal conditions such as obstruction.'

Paterson-Brown S. In: Paterson-Brown S, editor. A companion to specialist surgical practice: core topics in general and emergency surgery, 5th ed. London: Elsevier; 2013: p. 81–99.

The role of plain abdominal radiographs remains controversial, despite many studies that have demonstrated that, with the exception of suspected intestinal obstruction (Fig. 12.7), they rarely help in the diagnosis and have even less of a role in altering the clinical decision (EBM 12.1). However, the supine abdominal x-ray (AXR) can be of use in patients whose diagnosis is unclear and in whom the presence of calcification (e.g., ureteric colic) and abnormal gas shadows (e.g., possible intestinal ischaemia) may be helpful. They should, however, not be performed routinely, and have no role in the investigation of patients with suspected appendicitis.

An erect AXR is only of value in patients with intestinal obstruction, although it is well known that even then the information obtained over and above that from the supine film is small. A good-quality supine AXR can indicate the level of obstruction (concertina jejunal loops or characterless ileal loops, caecal distension, or absence of gas in the rectum), whereas the erect film proves the diagnosis of obstruction by showing air fluid levels.

Contrast radiology

Contrast may be administered orally, by nasogastric or nasojejunal tube, or per rectum to examine the bowel in patients with acute abdominal pain. In the emergency setting, the contrast used is usually water soluble, as free egress of barium into the peritoneal cavity can make subsequent surgery more difficult and will remain for a very long time, making future x-ray examinations more difficult to interpret. As water-soluble contrast does not adhere well to the bowel mucosa, the information obtained is less specific and detailed than with barium, but in the patient with acute abdominal pain, the main issue that requires the use of contrast x-rays is determining the presence or absence of obstruction or perforation.

In up to 50% of patients with a perforated peptic ulcer, no free gas can be identified on plain radiography. If the diagnosis remains uncertain based on clinical assessment, a water-soluble contrast meal might be diagnostic (Fig. 12.8). In patients with small-bowel obstruction, a water-soluble small-bowel follow through can help, not only in confirming or refuting obstruction, but also in predicting which patient is likely to require surgery. Failure of contrast to reach the caecum by 4 hours or longer suggests obstruction, and these patients will not usually settle with nonoperative management (Fig. 12.9). Increasingly CT with oral contrast is replacing contrast radiography for suspected perforations without free air seen on CXR and probable intestinal obstruction without an obvious cause. In patients who have had previous abdominal surgery, and adhesions are considered the likely pathology, contrast radiography still has a role to play.

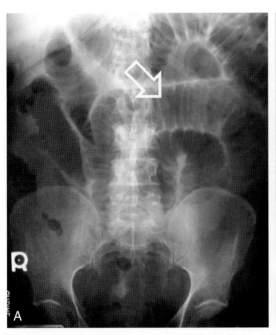 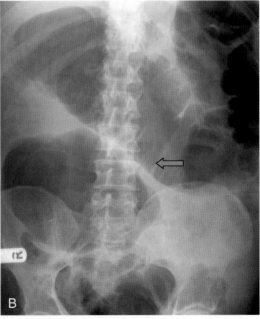

Fig. 12.7 Abdominal c-rays in bowel obstruction. (A) Supine film in a patient with small-bowel obstruction showing valvulae conniventes. **(B)** X-ray demonstrating large-bowel obstruction with *arrow* at a haustration.

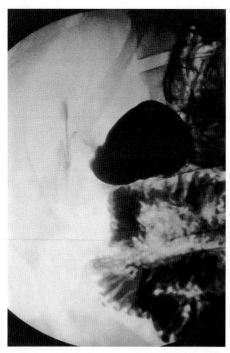

Fig. 12.8 Supine abdominal radiograph taken 20 minutes after oral administration of 50 mL of water-soluble contrast in a patient with suspected perforated peptic ulcer, in whom the erect chest radiograph was normal. Note the small trickle of contrast through the perforation. These findings were confirmed at laparotomy. (Courtesy Ellis BW, Paterson-Brown S, editors. Hamilton Bailey's emergency surgery, 13th ed. London, Hodder Education; 2000, with permission)

CT with rectal contrast is preferred to water-soluble contrast enema in the assessment of patients with large-bowel obstruction in differentiating pseudoobstruction from obstruction caused by a mechanical problem (see Chapter 16). Carrying out an unnecessary operation on a patient with pseudoobstruction is associated with a high morbidity and mortality, and cannot be defended.

Intravenous pyelography confirms the diagnosis of renal obstruction by calculi and may be helpful in the diagnosis of other types of renal pain. A CT focusing on the kidneys, ureters and bladder (CT KUB) is now more commonly used to detect renal tract calculi.

Ultrasonography

US is most commonly used to assess acute abdominal pain. As a general investigation it might reveal small amounts of intraperitoneal fluid in conditions such as perforation and infection, whereas in specific conditions such as acute cholecystitis, biliary obstruction, aortic aneurysms and ovarian cysts it can be diagnostic. Although some studies have reported high levels of sensitivity and specificity in the diagnosis of acute appendicitis, ultrasonography is highly operator dependent and a negative result cannot be relied upon, particularly if the clinical picture suggests otherwise.

Computed tomography

CT is rapidly replacing US as the main diagnostic investigation for patients with acute abdominal pain. Contrast-enhanced CT can reliably identify free intraabdominal gas (Fig. 12.10), ischaemic bowel, the cause of intestinal obstruction, and acute inflammatory conditions such as appendicitis and colonic diverticulitis. However, because of the radiation exposure, the use of CT should still be limited where possible to cases of diagnostic difficulty where the results might alter the surgical management plan. It remains a mainstay of the evaluation of traumatic injuries and intraabdominal sepsis in patients with suspected intraabdominal collection or abscess, in addition to suspected leaking abdominal aortic aneurysms. Contrast-enhanced CT is also used to detect pancreatic necrosis in patients with severe acute pancreatitis (Fig. 12.11). CT should not be used routinely in young patients with suspected appendicitis and magnetic resonance imaging (MRI) can be performed in pregnant patients.

Angiography

Mesenteric angiography has been superseded by CT angiography in the investigation of suspected mesenteric ischaemia. CT angiography can also reliably differentiate arterial from venous causes and distinguish occlusive from nonocclusive disease. It can also be used in the diagnosis and management of lower gastrointestinal haemorrhage, although patients with this condition rarely present with acute abdominal pain. If embolisation is required, formal angiography is necessary.

Endoscopic investigations

Flexible sigmoidoscopy is performed on patients who present with an acute abdomen associated with rectal bleeding and in those patients with large-bowel obstruction to evaluate the anorectum. Additional information can be obtained from a colonoscopy. Both flexible sigmoidoscopy and colonoscopy can be therapeutic in the management of sigmoid volvulus and pseudoobstruction (see Chapter 16). Upper gastrointestinal endoscopy is used to investigate patients with acute upper abdominal pain in whom a perforated peptic ulcer has been excluded.

Peritoneal investigations

Peritoneal lavage

The use of peritoneal lavage in patients suspected of having intraabdominal injury from trauma has now been replaced by CT. Many Emergency Departments use FAST (Focused Abdominal Scans for Trauma) in the immediate assessment of patients with abdominal trauma to identify free fluid (i.e., blood or bowel contents). If free fluid is seen, haemodynamically stable patients should undergo CT; those who are haemodynamically unstable require emergency laparotomy. Occasionally some patients on the intensive care unit requiring large amounts of cardiac support are too unstable to be transferred for CT. In these patients, peritoneal lavage can be helpful in confirming or excluding a surgical cause of a patient's condition. It is carried out by inserting a dialysis catheter into the peritoneal cavity under local anaesthetic and infusing 1 L of normal saline. The effluent is removed and examined for red blood cells, white blood cells, amylase, bacteria and bile.

Laparoscopy

Many studies have demonstrated that laparoscopy (Fig. 12.12) can significantly improve surgical decision-making in patients with acute abdominal pain. It is particularly useful in patients for whom the decision to operate is in doubt and in the elderly

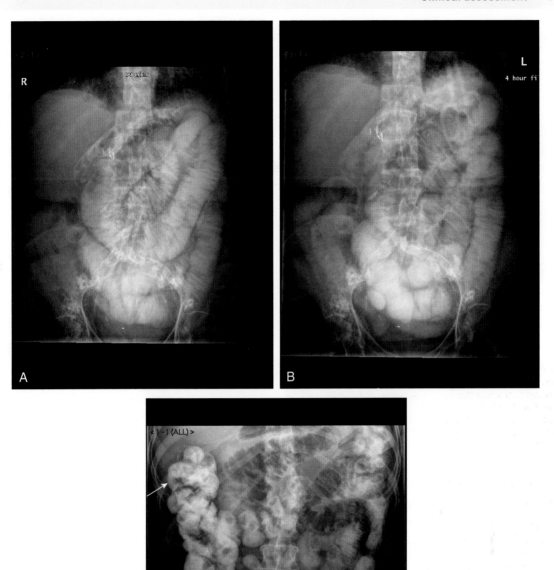

Fig. 12.9 Supine abdominal radiographs taken after oral administration of 50 mL of water-soluble contrast material. (A) Ninety minutes after administration. **(B)** Four hours after. Note failure of contrast to reach the caecum and the obvious small-bowel obstruction. Laparotomy confirmed small-bowel obstruction due to adhesions. **(C)** Ninety minutes after administration of contrast in another patient showing contrast in the large bowel (*arrows*) excluding small bowel obstruction.

when findings from the history and examination can be misleading. Young women probably benefit the most from laparoscopy, as it is often difficult in this group to accurately differentiate (even with a pelvic US) acute appendicitis from acute gynaecological conditions, many of which do not require surgery. As laparoscopic appendicectomy has now almost completely replaced open appendicectomy, most patients will undergo diagnostic laparoscopy first.

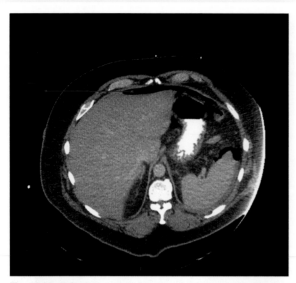

Fig. 12.10 Abdominal computed tomography demonstrating free gas *(arrowed)* due to a perforated peptic ulcer.

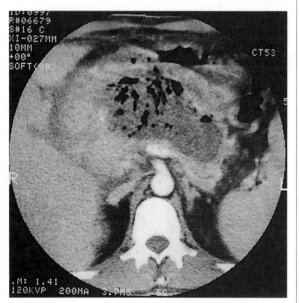

Fig. 12.11 Computed tomography of upper abdomen showing an acute fluid collection with gas in a patient with acute pancreatitis.

Management

All patients admitted with acute abdominal pain require resuscitation and close monitoring, with regular re-evaluation. It is a good clinical rule that initial treatment should be based around the ABC principle (airway, breathing and circulation). Except in the management of overwhelming haemorrhage (e.g., ruptured abdominal aortic aneurysm and ruptured ectopic pregnancy) when resuscitation takes place on the way to the operating theatre, all patients with acute abdominal pain, including those requiring urgent surgery, benefit from adequate resuscitation. This will usually involve the administration of several litres of normal saline. Intravenous antibiotics if sepsis is suspected and oxygen by face mask (see Chapter 1). Monitoring by means of temperature, pulse, blood pressure, urine output and central venous pressure will depend on the clinical circumstances and will not be detailed further here. Good preoperative assessment, resuscitation, monitoring and regular reviewing of the patient with acute abdominal pain (initially every 30 minutes to 2 hours, depending on the state of the patient) is a prerequisite for a satisfactory clinical outcome. Following the first assessment, close observation and regular reassessment should be carried out on all patients without a definitive diagnosis, as their condition may well change and the underlying cause, or the correct management plan, become more obvious. Until this time, it is common practice to keep the patient fasted; if there are signs or symptoms of obstruction, a nasogastric tube is inserted. Appropriate analgesia should be administered early to keep the patient as comfortable as possible. Deep venous thrombosis prophylaxis should also be commenced routinely.

The remainder of this chapter will address the principles that support the management of peritonitis, acute appendicitis, nonspecific abdominal pain (NSAP) and gynaecological causes of the acute abdomen.

Peritonitis

Inflammation of the peritoneum is a common feature of the acute abdomen and can be classified as acute or chronic, septic or aseptic, and primary or secondary. Acute suppurative peritonitis secondary to visceral disease is the most common form of peritonitis in surgical practice and primary peritonitis is rare. Chronic peritonitis due to tuberculosis is rare in the West, but seen often in Asia and Africa. It is also seen in patients undergoing peritoneal dialysis, where it results in abdominal pain, ascites or obstruction due to 'matting' of the bowel by dense adhesions. Treatment is by removal of the dialysis catheter and drainage of any loculated collections, usually under US guidance, but occasionally laparotomy is required. Aseptic peritonitis is generally due to chemical (e.g., urine, bile, gastric contents, blood, meconium) or foreign-body irritants (e.g., starch, talc, cellulose), and is frequently followed by secondary bacterial peritonitis.

The primary objective is to deal promptly and effectively with the underlying cause. For example, perforation of a viscus must be repaired, infarcted bowel must be resected, and infective foci should be removed or drained. Operation is undertaken with minimal delay. The only time that should be spent before operation is that needed to resuscitate an ill patient. It is imperative that extracellular fluid volume is replaced adequately, and central venous pressure monitoring is essential in critically ill and elderly patients. A nasogastric tube should be inserted to empty the stomach and prevent further vomiting, and a urinary catheter should also be placed to monitor urinary output. Antibiotic cover is indicated early in all patients with established secondary peritonitis and is directed against gut flora in the first instance (e.g., piperacillin–tazobactam, or gentamicin, amoxycillin and metronidazole). Thorough peritoneal lavage is an essential adjunct to any operation. Patients presenting late and in a moribund condition may require 'damage limitation surgery', whereby immediate life-saving surgery is carried out and further laparotomies are required for more definitive surgery over the next few days. This will include removal of infarcted or perforated bowel, stapling of the bowel ends, lavage and drainage (see Chapter 7).

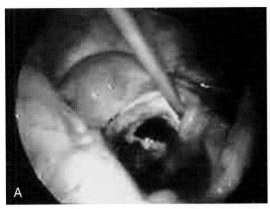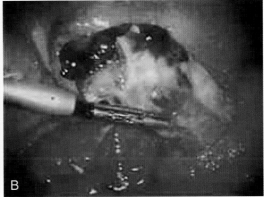

Fig 12.12 Diagnostic laparoscopy. (A) Bleeding ovarian cyst. (B) Acute appendicitis.

Primary peritonitis

Primary peritonitis is uncommon, although in childhood it can account for up to 15% of acute abdominal emergencies. The condition used to be common in young girls following the ascent of pneumococcal or streptococcal infection from the genital tract.

Escherichia coli is now the predominant causal organism and probably gains access through the gut wall, or rarely by bloodborne spread from a distant focus. In adults, spontaneous bacterial peritonitis may occur in patients with the nephrotic syndrome, but is more frequently seen in those with liver cirrhosis and ascites or chronic renal failure (particularly in patients on peritoneal dialysis). The mortality rate for patients with primary bacterial peritonitis varies from 20% to 80%.

Classically, diffuse peritonitis with generalised abdominal tenderness and rigidity develops within 24 hours. Fever and leucocytosis occur early. Abdominal rigidity is relatively uncommon. A sample of peritoneal fluid, which is usually turbid, is sent for microscopy and bacterial culture. Antibiotic therapy is the mainstay of treatment, but either laparoscopy or laparotomy may be needed to rule out a surgical cause, if this is suggested by the culture of enteric organisms.

Postoperative peritonitis

Peritonitis after abdominal surgery may be a residual effect of the original disease or a direct complication of its operative management (e.g., anastomotic leakage). Diagnosis is difficult, as:

- The patient is usually receiving analgesia and/or sedation, and may not complain of pain
- Any pain and tenderness may be attributed to the wound
- There is often a 24–48-hour period after abdominal surgery when bowel sounds are absent and the abdomen is distended.

Persisting abdominal distension or the development of vomiting and distension after an initial return to normality should raise the suspicion of peritoneal infection. Suspicion is heightened if the patient looks unwell and has fever, tachycardia and an altered mental state. Contrast-enhanced CT with oral contrast/rectal contrast is the best investigation to identify anastomotic leakage and any associated collections.

Fluid and electrolyte replacement, nasogastric suction and broad-spectrum antibiotic therapy are instituted, and the need for reoperation is considered. Patients with a small anastomotic leak that is well drained (by drains left at the time of the original surgery) may be managed nonoperatively and intraperitoneal collections can be drained by percutaneous drainage under radiological guidance. Patients with more widespread peritonitis require repeat laparotomy. There is an increasing role for re-look laparotomy in patients with severe sepsis identified at the time of the first operation to allow further washout of the peritoneal cavity, if there are still signs of severe sepsis. This is usually preceded by CT to help identify any collections which may have occurred.

Intraabdominal abscess

An intraabdominal abscess may develop in conjunction with an underlying inflammatory process or be a complication of peritonitis or intraabdominal surgery. The abscess gives rise to pyrexia, tachycardia and clinical signs of toxicity. Leucocytosis and raised C-reactive protein are usual. Common sites for abscess formation are the subphrenic and subhepatic spaces, the pelvis, and between loops of bowel (inter-loop abscess). Complications include rupture with generalised peritonitis, the erosion of blood vessels with potentially catastrophic bleeding and septicaemia. Occasionally, subphrenic abscesses rupture into the pleural cavity and pelvic abscesses sometimes discharge spontaneously through the rectum.

The site of the abscess may be suspected from the history and clinical examination, but localising signs can be surprisingly few, particularly with subphrenic abscess, hence the expression 'pus somewhere, pus nowhere, pus under the diaphragm'. Unexplained fever after peritoneal infection or operation should always raise the suspicion of abscess formation. Tachycardia is usual. Pain and tenderness over the ribcage, shoulder-tip pain and a 'sympathetic' pleural effusion strengthen the suspicion of subphrenic abscess, whereas urgency of defecation, diarrhoea and a boggy swelling in the pelvis on rectal examination are features of a pelvic abscess (Fig. 12.13).

US and/or CT are of immense value in diagnosis, aspiration to obtain material for bacteriological culture and subsequent drainage. However, surgical drainage may still be needed to ensure effective drainage, particularly if the collection is loculated. Pelvic abscesses frequently rupture spontaneously into the rectum, but on occasion may require incision and drainage through the anterior rectal wall. Antibiotic therapy is used in conjunction with drainage of the abscess. Signs usually resolve rapidly following effective drainage.

12

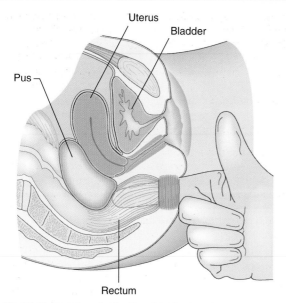

Fig. 12.13 Rectal examination for pelvic abscess.

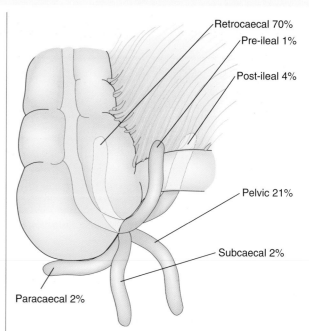

Fig. 12.15 Variations in the position of the appendix.

Acute appendicitis

Anatomy

The appendix is a worm-shaped, blind-ending tube that arises from the posteromedial wall of the caecum 2 cm below the ileocaecal valve. It varies in length from 2 to 25 cm, but is most commonly 6–9 cm long. On the external surface of the bowel, the base of the appendix is found at the point of convergence of the three taeniae coli of the caecum. On the surface of the abdomen, this point lies one-third of the way along a line drawn between the right anterior superior iliac spine and the umbilicus (McBurney's point; Fig. 12.14). The appendix has its own mesentery, the mesoappendix, and its blood supply comes from the appendicular artery, a branch of the ileocolic artery. The appendicular artery runs in the free border of the mesoappendix up to a few centimetres from the

tip, after which it lies on the muscle wall beneath the peritoneum. The position of the appendix is variable, depending on its length and mobility. In cadaveric dissections the most common site is retrocaecal, but data from diagnostic laparoscopy indicate that the pelvic position is probably more common (Fig. 12.15). In children, there are abundant lymphoid follicles in the submucosa, but these atrophy with age.

Epidemiology

In the UK, appendicitis is the most common cause of acute abdominal pain requiring surgery, and it has been estimated that 16% of the population of developed countries will undergo appendicectomy for presumed appendicitis during their lifetime. There has been a decline in the incidence of appendicitis over the last 20 years for unknown reasons. There is an equal incidence in males and females. Appendicitis is uncommon in patients below the age of 2 and above the age of 65, and is most common in the under 40s, with a peak incidence between 8 and 14 years of age. There is a geographical variation in the incidence, being rare in Asia and Central Africa, which is thought to be due to environmental factors. In Western countries, it is seen more frequently in cities than in rural areas.

Aetiology

Despite its prevalence, the aetiology of acute appendicitis remains unclear. Several different mechanisms have been proposed, one of the more popular causes being a diet lacking in fibre, and a consequent slow transit time and alteration in bacterial flora. However, this theory is challenged by a decline in incidence of appendicitis over recent years that has not been matched by an increase in dietary fibre intake. Others have suggested that viral infection may be an aetiological agent, as there is an association between appendicitis and concurrent viral illness and because there is a seasonal variation in the incidence of appendicitis.

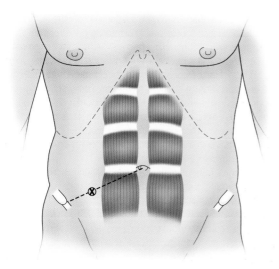

Fig. 12.14 McBurney's point.

Pathogenesis

Obstruction of the lumen of the appendix is thought to play the main role in the initiation of inflammation in about two-thirds of the cases. Faecoliths, foreign bodies or parasites may occlude the lumen; lymphoid hyperplasia, carcinoid tumours, strictures and rarely carcinoma may occlude the wall; while adhesions and kinking outside the wall may also cause luminal obstruction. Following obstruction, the wall of the appendix becomes inflamed, commencing in the mucosa and spreading to involve the submucosal, muscular and serosal layers. A fibrinopurulent exudate forms on the serosal surface and extends to any adjacent peritoneal surface. Perforation is usually at the site of impaction of a faecolith before any adhesions have formed. Within 12–24 hours, the appendix distal to the site of obstruction becomes inflamed and subsequently gangrenous.

In the nonobstructive or catarrhal type (one-third of cases), inflammation of the wall of the appendix causes venous congestion, which may compromise arterial inflow, especially in the distal appendix where the artery lies in a subperitoneal position, leading to ischaemia, infarction and gangrene near the tip of the appendix. Organisms from the lumen of the appendix enter the submucosa through an ischaemic ulcer, causing liquefaction of the wall and ultimately perforation.

As a result of the transmural inflammation, small bowel and omentum adhere to the appendix, creating a localised area of sepsis. If left untreated, this may progress to form an appendix mass or even an abscess. If perforation occurs early in the clinical course, the inflamed area will not have had time to be walled off, and generalised peritonitis follows.

Clinical features

History

Classically, the onset of acute appendicitis is associated with the gradual onset of poorly localised central abdominal pain. After a variable amount of time, the pain moves to the right iliac fossa and changes in character, to become sharper, constant and well localised. It is aggravated by movement and coughing. As described earlier, this change in the nature of the pain occurs when the parietal peritoneum overlying the appendix becomes involved in the inflammatory process. In general, most patients present within 24 hours of the onset of the central abdominal pain. Many patients also admit to anorexia and occasional vomiting.

In children, nonspecific symptoms (anorexia, nausea, vomiting, diarrhoea) and signs (fever, foetor, pallor, abdominal distension) can confuse the inexperienced clinician. The finding of tenderness and guarding in the right iliac fossa usually makes the diagnosis without the need for other investigations.

Examination

The patient with established acute appendicitis looks unwell, is flushed and has a dry, furred tongue with a foetor. The temperature is usually only mildly elevated (37.3–38.5°C) and there is often a tachycardia. Classically, the area of maximal tenderness is over McBurney's point, with guarding and rebound (percussion) tenderness. Palpation in the left iliac fossa may reproduce the pain in the right iliac fossa (Rovsing's sign) and the patient may find it painful to extend the right hip owing to irritation of the psoas

muscle (psoas stretch sign). Although rectal and vaginal examinations are frequently normal, they can be useful when the abdominal signs are vague, particularly if the acutely inflamed appendix lies within the pelvis, when tenderness may be elicited with the examining finger. In women a vaginal examination is extremely useful in helping to differentiate acute appendicitis from acute gynaecological disorders.

Variations in clinical features

The symptoms and signs of acute appendicitis are influenced by a variety of factors, which include age, sex, personality and the position of the appendix. Only 50% of patients with acute appendicitis give a typical history. An inflamed retrocaecal appendix may produce poorly localised abdominal pain and an inflamed pelvic appendix lying close to the bladder may produce symptoms of frequency and dysuria. In this scenario, as with a retrocaecal appendix that overlies the ureter, it may be quite difficult to differentiate between urinary infection and acute appendicitis. Dipstick examination of the urine may reveal microscopic haematuria, proteinuria and leucocytes in both cases. However, urgent microscopy of the urine will demonstrate significant bacteria in urinary tract infection. An inflamed pelvic appendix lying near the rectum causes irritation and diarrhoea, and is commonly mistaken for gastroenteritis. However, gastroenteritis is a dangerous diagnosis to make in the acute abdomen as it almost never causes abdominal tenderness. A very long appendix extending up to the right upper quadrant can mimic acute cholecystitis.

Acute appendicitis is most dangerous in the very young, the very old and the pregnant patient. When it does occur under the age of 2 years, it is often incorrectly diagnosed as gastroenteritis and generalised peritonitis can develop quickly. In contrast, in elderly patients, the onset can be more insidious. The inflamed area tends to wall off, with the development of a mass, and symptoms and signs of obstruction may be present. In the pregnant patient, the appendix is displaced upwards by the enlarged uterus, and the site of the pain and tenderness is high in the abdomen. Appendicitis in pregnancy carries a high rate of morbidity and mortality for both mother and foetus.

A list of conditions that should be considered in the differential diagnosis of acute appendicitis is given in Table 12.11.

Table 12.11 Differential diagnosis of acute appendicitis
• Mesenteric adenitis
• Meckel's diverticulitis
• Regional ileitis (Crohn's disease)
• Carcinoma of the caecum
Gynaecological disorders
• Ruptured ovarian follicle (Mittelschmerz)
• Acute salpingitis
• Ruptured ectopic pregnancy
• Torsion of an ovarian cyst
Genitourinary
• Pyelonephritis
• Ureteric colic
• Urinary tract infection
• Right-sided testicular torsion

12

Complications

Gangrenous appendicitis and perforation tend to occur after a significantly more prolonged period of pain than uncomplicated appendicitis. Generalised peritonitis results if the inflamed area is not walled off by omentum and loops of bowel. If walling off does occur, either an appendix mass or abscess will develop. A perforated pelvic appendix will lead to a pelvic abscess and on examination there may be very little in the way of abdominal signs, but rectal examination may be particularly useful.

Investigations

The diagnosis of acute appendicitis is based on clinical assessment and there are no really specific diagnostic tests except for CT. US might demonstrate a swollen noncompressible appendix, free fluid or even a mass in the right iliac fossa. If, after clinical assessment, the diagnosis remains in doubt, the clinician must proceed along one of two lines: either to carry out a laparoscopy and undertake appendicectomy if indicated, or to institute a short policy of close and repeated observation with reassessment every hour. On occasions when there is diagnostic difficulty, and particularly in the elderly, abdominal CT is helpful in making the diagnosis in addition to excluding other conditions (Fig. 12.16). Due to the radiation involved CT is rarely indicated in younger patients.

Management

The treatment of appendicitis is almost always surgical and now invariably using the laparoscopic technique, especially if a diagnostic laparoscopy has been performed first to establish the diagnosis (EBM 12.2). Open appendicectomy is still performed where expertise for laparoscopic procedures is unavailable or when gross sepsis is found at laparoscopy. The main steps of the operation, whether by laparoscopic or open surgery, involve the electrocoagulation or ligation of the appendicular artery, and division of the base of the appendix between two ligatures. Burying the base of the appendix, popular in the past, is no longer carried out unless there has been a perforation at the base of the appendix and a more formal closure of the caecum carried out. A large number of recent studies have now confirmed the advantage of

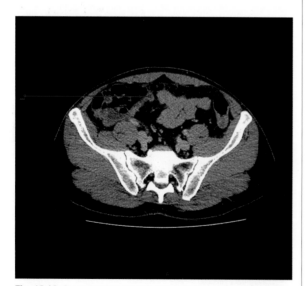

Fig. 12.16 Computed tomography demonstrating acute appendicitis (*arrowed*).

laparoscopic appendicectomy over the open approach with regard to a shorter hospital stay and return to normal activities. There is still some concern as to possible increased postoperative collections in patients with perforated appendicitis in whom there is gross peritoneal soiling following laparoscopic appendicectomy, and in such cases open appendicectomy may be advisable. It is also possible to treat patients who have suspected uncomplicated acute appendicitis (in other words, who do not have overt peritonitis) nonoperatively with antibiotics and this is becoming increasingly popular around the world, especially where easy access to surgery is impossible. The concerns relate to recurrent problems in the future, although recent studies have suggested that these may be less than previously thought. The choice of either laparoscopic appendicectomy or antibiotics in patients with possible appendicitis but with minimal clinical signs are both reasonable and would be part of the informed consent process between surgeon and patient. Early surgery should however be offered to patients at the extremes of age and those with diabetes or other comorbid conditions who are less able to deal with the underlying inflammatory and infective complications.

EBM 12.2 Acute appendicitis

'Patients with symptoms and signs consistent with appendicitis should undergo appendicectomy, preferably using the laparoscopic approach, although in the presence of widespread sepsis the open approach should be considered. In patients with minimal clinical signs non-operative management with antibiotics is an acceptable option although there remain concerns as to recurrent problems in the future.'

Lamb PJ. In: Paterson-Brown S, editor. A companion to specialist surgical practice: core topics in general and emergency surgery, 5th ed. London: Elsevier; 2013: p. 158–78.

Management of an 'appendix mass'

An 'appendix mass' is formed by an inflamed or perforated appendix surrounded by oedematous small bowel, caecum and omentum. It can usually be felt after 24–48 hours of onset of pain. It becomes well defined by the 4th/5th day, and thereafter usually resolves or forms an abscess. Nonoperative management with intravenous fluids and antibiotics is the treatment of choice, provided there are no signs of peritonitis (when an operation should be carried out). During this period of close observation, the patient is monitored for pain, fever, tachycardia, local size of the mass, tenderness and area of rigidity. The presence of worsening symptoms or signs is an indication to abandon the nonoperative regimen in favour of surgical intervention, which will invariably require open rather than laparoscopic surgery. The mass usually begins to reduce in size within 48 hours of treatment and resolves completely in 2–3 weeks. Worsening of symptoms often indicates the formation of an appendix abscess, which can be picked up on US; if one is present, it should be drained either under radiological guidance or surgically. A persistent right iliac fossa lump should always merit investigation for the presence of ileocaecal tuberculosis in African and Asian countries.

Following successful nonoperative treatment of an appendix mass, it used to be traditional practice to carry out an interval appendicectomy 6 weeks later. However, several studies have now confirmed that after the successful nonoperative treatment of either an appendix mass or an abscess, only a few patients develop recurrent problems and most of them do so within the first few months. Current practice is now not to carry out an interval appendicectomy unless the patient experiences further symptoms or complications (EBM 12.3). However, in countries with less ready access to surgery and patients who travel to such places, interval appendicectomy (preferably laparoscopic) is still advised. It is still important, especially in those at risk, to exclude a carcinoma of the caecum by colonoscopy. Such patients will very likely have already had a CT at the time of the original diagnosis. An interval appendicectomy should be undertaken if this course is not pursued.

EBM 12.3 Appendix mass or abscess

'The diagnosis should be confirmed using US or CT. Patients with an appendix mass/abscess should be treated non-operatively with antibiotics and intravenous fluids. Any abscess should be drained by percutaneous means if possible. Routine examination of the colon should be carried out 6 weeks following initial presentation to exclude a colonic cause. Interval appendicectomy (preferably laparoscopic) should be reserved for those patients with recurrent symptoms or those where ready access to surgery is not available.'

Lamb PJ. In: Paterson-Brown S, editor. A companion to specialist surgical practice: core topics in general and emergency surgery, 5th ed. London: Elsevier; 2013: p. 158–78.

Prognosis

The overall mortality of appendicitis is less than 1%, rising to 5% if perforation occurs and increasing with age. The postoperative morbidity is mainly related to wound infection (reduced by prophylactic antibiotics), residual abscess (reduced by a thorough peritoneal lavage), paralytic ileus, bleeding from the appendicular artery, leak from the appendix stump and early intestinal obstruction. Late complications include incisional hernia and adhesive small-bowel obstruction, both reduced by the increasing use of the laparoscopic approach. It used to be thought that fertility in female patients was adversely affected by acute appendicitis, but this no longer seems to be the case.

 12.2 Summary

Acute appendicitis

- Incidence has declined, but appendicitis is still the most common acute abdominal condition in childhood, adolescence and early adulthood
- The typical history is of periumbilical pain (visceral midgut pain), followed within several hours by right iliac fossa pain (somatic pain from parietal peritonitis). This is not, however, always present
- Tenderness and muscle guarding in the right iliac fossa are the most reliable signs of acute appendicitis with rebound or 'tap' tenderness indicative of underlying peritonitis. A tachycardia, high temperature, leucocytosis and raised C-reactive protein are all helpful in reaching a diagnosis
- Once the diagnosis has been made appendicectomy should be undertaken before gangrene and perforation supervene. In uncomplicated cases and minimal clinical signs a nonoperative approach is an option, but recurrent problems can occur in the future
- Gangrene and perforation are common and/or particularly dangerous in infants, during pregnancy and in the elderly.

Nonspecific abdominal pain

This term is often applied to patients in whom no cause can be found for their abdominal pain. Its incidence has been found to be around 40% for all patients admitted with acute abdominal pain, reducing to around 25% if investigations such as laparoscopy are used to improve diagnostic accuracy. The major concern in reaching a diagnosis of NSAP is that a serious underlying condition has been missed. It has been reported that 10% of patients over 50 years of age who are discharged with NSAP from hospital after an acute admission with abdominal pain have an underlying malignancy, of which half are colonic. Another group of patients who tend to be diagnosed with NSAP are young females who may have a gynaecological condition, such as pelvic inflammatory disease or ovarian cyst pathology. With better imaging and the more widespread use of laparoscopy in the investigation of patients with acute abdominal pain, the incidence of NSAP will continue to fall. Pain resulting from abdominal wall problems, such as rectus sheath haematoma, can be confirmed by US.

Gynaecological causes of the acute abdomen

Gynaecological conditions commonly present to the on-call surgical team as 'lower abdominal/pelvic pain', mimicking acute surgical conditions such as acute appendicitis and diverticulitis. A detailed gynaecological and sexual history is essential to help differentiate these conditions, in addition to obtaining urine for microscopy and a pregnancy test. Where gynaecological conditions are suspected or confirmed, discussion and referral to the on-call gynaecological team is indicated. However a general knowledge of the common gynaecological conditions which often present to the on-call surgical team and their treatment is required.

Mittelschmerz and ruptured corpus luteum

The Graafian follicle normally ruptures 10–14 days after the start of the last menstrual period, and release of the ovum may be complicated by bleeding. The follicle normally becomes a corpus luteum, which degenerates before the start of the next period unless conception occurs. Bleeding from the corpus luteum is an occasional cause of pain in the late stages of the menstrual cycle.

Patients with these causes of pain are usually between 15 and 25 years of age, and experience sudden pain in one or other iliac fossa. Tenderness and guarding in the right iliac fossa can simulate acute appendicitis and a few patients bleed sufficiently to suggest rupture of an ectopic pregnancy. Rectal or vaginal examination may reveal tenderness in the rectovaginal pouch. US may demonstrate free fluid in the pelvis.

The patient is treated nonoperatively, unless laparoscopy is required to exclude appendicitis or ruptured ectopic pregnancy.

Ruptured ectopic pregnancy

A fertilised ovum implants at an abnormal site in 1 in 200 pregnancies; the fallopian tube is by far the most common site. The erosive trophoblast may penetrate the wall of the tube, and often ruptures after about 6 weeks. Alternatively, the conceptus may be extruded from the fimbrial end of the tube.

Bouts of cramping iliac fossa pain may be associated with fainting and vaginal bleeding. Rupture produces sudden severe pain, bleeding and circulatory collapse, with the abdominal pain often becoming generalised. Immediate surgery is required. A missed period is reported by most patients and a raised beta human chorionic gonadotrophin (β-HCG) level in the presence of abdominal pain should always raise the suspicion of an ectopic pregnancy.

Complications of an ovarian cyst

Benign ovarian cysts are a common cause of torsion, rupture and bleeding. Dermoid cysts often have a long pedicle and account for around 50% of torsions in young women. Pain from rupture/bleeding can be sudden and severe, and may mimic other causes of lower abdominal peritonitis. Pain from a torted ovarian cyst is often severe and cramp-like, and sometimes associated with a smooth round mobile mass that lies higher in the abdomen than might be expected. Tenderness and guarding may be present. Infarction of a fibroid may produce a similar picture.

At laparoscopy the twisted pedicle is transfixed and ligated, and the cyst is removed. Care must be taken to avoid rupture in case the cyst is malignant. Further radical surgery may be needed if histological examination reveals malignancy. In many cases the cyst has actually resulted in torsion of the whole ovary, and by the time of surgery this is usually necrotic and requires removal, although if caught early, untwisting may result in salvage of the ovary. In all such cases the gynaecology team should be involved in management.

Acute salpingitis

Acute salpingitis is most commonly caused by chlamydial infection, but streptococcal, gonococcal or even tuberculous infection can also be responsible. Both tubes are often involved and adhesions may seal the fimbriated end, producing a pyosalpinx, and subsequent infertility.

Bilateral pain is felt just above the pubis and inguinal ligaments. There may be urinary frequency, irregular menstruation, pyrexia, leucocytosis and raised C-reactive protein. Vaginal examination reveals unusual warmth, a tender cervix and a vaginal discharge. The cervix appears red and inflamed, and a swab reveals the causative organism. Vaginal findings may be less marked when there is a closed pyosalpinx.

Treatment consists of antibiotic therapy. Laparoscopy is helpful if acute appendicitis cannot be ruled out. The tubes appear inflamed and oedematous, and 'milking' them gently produces a purulent discharge from which a bacteriological swab can be taken.

12.3 Summary

Gynaecological causes of pain and the acute abdomen

- Nonspecific abdominal pain (i.e., pain for which no cause is defined) is particularly common in female adolescents and young women, and often mimics acute appendicitis. Laparoscopy is valuable when the diagnosis is in doubt and the need for surgery cannot be excluded
- Rupture of the Graafian follicle may cause midcycle pain (Mittelschmerz) in the iliac fossa in young girls and can be associated with minor intraperitoneal bleeding
- Rupture of an ectopic pregnancy causes intraperitoneal bleeding and more severe abdominal pain, with circulatory collapse. Signs of pregnancy are seldom present and pregnancy testing may be unhelpful. Elevation of the foot of the bed may produce shoulder-tip pain and underline the need for laparotomy
- Torsion of an ovarian cyst often causes cramping lower abdominal pain. Ovarian cysts can become very large and produce visible abdominal swellings that lie higher than might be expected. Some cysts prove to be malignant and care must be taken to avoid rupture at operation
- Acute salpingitis is usually due to *Chlamydia* infection and produces bilateral suprapubic pain, which is often associated with urinary frequency, a tender cervix and vaginal discharge.

Richard Hardwick

13

The oesophagus, stomach and duodenum

Chapter contents

Surgical anatomy 179

Surgical physiology 181

History and symptoms 181

Examination 182

Investigations 182

Diagnosis and management: oesophagus 186

Tumours of the oesophagus 191

Diagnosis and management: gastroduodenal 193

Management of uncomplicated peptic ulcer disease 194

Complications of peptic ulceration requiring operative intervention 195

Gastric neoplasia 198

Miscellaneous disorders of the stomach 203

Miscellaneous conditions of the duodenum 203

Surgical anatomy

Oesophagus

The oesophagus extends from the cricoid cartilage (at the level of vertebra C6) to the gastric cardia and is 25 cm long. It has cervical, thoracic and abdominal portions. The oesophagus passes through the diaphragm at the level of the 10th thoracic vertebra and the final 2–4 cm lies within the peritoneal cavity. The relationships are shown in Fig. 13.1.

The oesophagus has an upper sphincter, the cricopharyngeus, and a lower sphincter that cannot be defined anatomically but is a 3–5-cm high-pressure area located in the region of the oesophageal hiatus of the diaphragm. The oesophagus is held loosely in the hiatus by a thickening of fascia, the phrenooesophageal ligament. The healthy oesophagus is lined by squamous epithelium and its wall can be divided into two principal layers, muscular and mucosal. The muscular layer has two components with longitudinal fibres outside and circular fibres inside; the upper third of the oesophagus is striated muscle and the remainder is smooth muscle. Between the muscle and the mucosa is the submucosa where numerous mucous glands and lymphatics are found.

The oesophagus receives its blood supply from the inferior thyroid artery in the cervical region, the bronchial arteries and branches from the thoracic aorta in the thorax, and the inferior phrenic and left gastric arteries in the abdomen.

Venous drainage is to the inferior thyroid veins in the neck, the hemi-azygous and azygous veins (systemic circulation) in the thorax, and the left gastric (portal circulation) in the abdomen. These venous connections are important in the development of varices in patients with portal hypertension.

Sympathetic nerve supply is derived from preganglionic fibres from spinal cord segments T5 and T6, and postganglionic fibres from the cervical vertebral and coeliac ganglia. Parasympathetic supply comes from the glossopharyngeal, recurrent laryngeal and vagus nerves.

The lymphatics run in the submucosa and drain to the regional lymph nodes, and subsequently to the posterior mediastinal, supraclavicular and coeliac lymph nodes.

Stomach and duodenum

The stomach is an easily distensible viscus partly covered by the left costal margin. The diaphragm and left lobe of the liver lie on its anterior surface. Posteriorly, the stomach bed is formed by the diaphragm, spleen, left adrenal, upper part of the left kidney, splenic artery and pancreas. The greater and lesser curvatures correspond to the long and short borders of the stomach, respectively, and the organ can be further divided anatomically into four distinct areas based on the microscopic mucosal appearance: namely, the cardia, fundus, body and antrum. The stomach is limited at its proximal end by the oesophagogastric junction situated just below the lower oesophageal sphincter, a physiological sphincter that prevents stomach contents from regurgitating into the oesophagus. Distally, the stomach is limited by the pylorus, a true anatomical sphincter. It is composed of greatly thickened inner circular muscle that helps to regulate the emptying of stomach contents into the duodenum.

The duodenum is divided into four parts, which are closely applied to the head of the pancreas. The first part is approximately 5 cm in length; its importance lies in the fact which it is the most common site for peptic ulceration to occur. The second part has on its medial wall the ampulla of Vater, where the

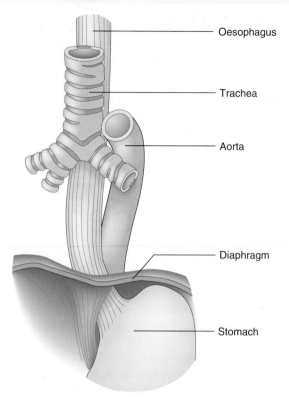

Fig. 13.1 Anatomical relationships of the oesophagus.

The stomach has an extensive blood supply (Fig. 13.2) derived from the coeliac axis. When the stomach is used as a conduit in the chest, as in an oesophagectomy, the left gastric, left gastro-epiploic and short gastric vessels are divided, and the stomach then relies on the right gastric and right gastroepiploic vessels for viability. Ischaemia does not usually result because of the free communication between the vessels supplying the stomach. The blood supply to the duodenum is derived from both the coeliac axis (via the gastroduodenal artery) and branches from the superior mesenteric artery (inferior pancreaticoduodenal artery). The veins from the stomach and the duodenum accompany the arteries and drain into the portal venous system.

The lymphatics from the stomach accompany the arteries, and drainage is to nodes around these vessels. Thereafter, drainage is to other groups around the aorta, liver, splenic hilum and pancreas, and then to the coeliac nodes. The lymphatics of the duodenum drain into the nodes located at the coeliac axis and superior mesenteric vessels.

The parasympathetic nerve supply to the stomach is derived from the anterior and posterior vagal trunks. These pass through the diaphragm with the oesophagus. The anterior trunk gives off branches to the liver and gallbladder and descends along the lesser curvature as the anterior nerve of Latarjet. The posterior trunk gives off a coeliac branch and descends along the lesser curvature of the stomach (as the posterior nerve of Latarjet), going on to supply the pancreas, small intestine and large intestine as far as the distal transverse colon. The parasympathetic system supplies motor fibres to the stomach wall, inhibitory fibres to the pyloric sphincter (thus effecting relaxation of the sphincter), and secretomotor fibres to the glands of the stomach. Sympathetic fibres accompany the gastric arteries to reach the stomach from the coeliac ganglion. These provide motor fibres to the pyloric sphincter. The duodenum receives a sympathetic and parasympathetic supply from the coeliac and superior mesenteric plexuses.

conjoined pancreatic duct and common bile duct deliver their contents to the gastrointestinal tract. The third and fourth parts pass behind the transverse mesocolon into the infracolic compartment.

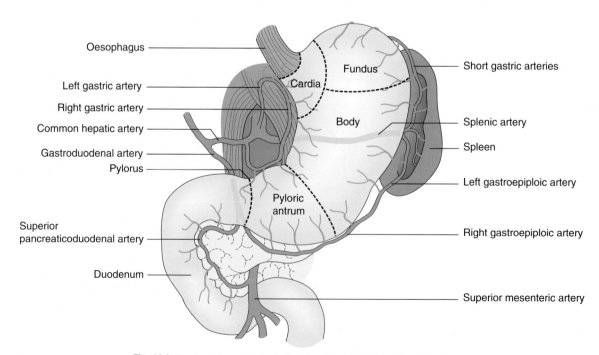

Fig. 13.2 Blood supply and anatomical relationships of the stomach and duodenum.

Surgical physiology

Oesophagus

Oesophageal peristalsis is initiated by swallowing (primary) or luminal distension (secondary) and progresses distally at around 2–4 cm/s, requiring the coordinated contraction and relaxation of oesophageal muscle. The lower sphincter relaxes momentarily 2–3 seconds before the peristaltic wave arrives and pressures of about 80 mmHg are usually generated in the oesophageal body. Disruption of any part of this process can result in difficulties with swallowing and/or pain.

Between the outer longitudinal muscle layer and the inner circular layer is a nerve plexus (Auerbach's or myenteric plexus) receiving parasympathetic motor innervation to smooth muscle cells from vagal nuclei in the dorsal motor nucleus of the brain stem. Between the inner muscular layer and the submucosa is another nerve plexus (Meissner's or submucosal plexus), which relays signals from the numerous free nerve endings in the mucosa and submucosa to vagal afferent fibres. This sensory information is sent back to the brain via the vagus nerve trunks. Sympathetic innervation arrives via preganglionic sympathetic fibres from the spinal cord that synapse with postganglionic nerve cells in sympathetic ganglia before passing with the blood vessels to the oesophagus. Together, the myenteric and submucosal plexuses constitute part of the enteric nervous system of the gut and can be influenced by both neural and hormonal stimuli.

Around 1 L of alkaline saliva is produced each day by the salivary glands, which helps lubricate the food bolus and neutralises refluxed gastric acid.

Stomach

Food is passed from the oesophagus into the stomach, where it is stored, ground and partially digested. As food enters the stomach, the muscles in the stomach walls relax and intragastric pressure rises only slightly. This effect is known as receptive relaxation, and is mediated by the vagus nerve. It is followed by muscular contractions that increase in amplitude and frequency, starting in the fundus and moving down towards the body and antrum. In the antrum, the main role is the grinding of food and propulsion of small amounts (now called chyme) into the duodenum when the pyloric sphincter relaxes.

Gastric emptying is controlled by two mechanisms: hormonal feedback and a neural reflex called the enterogastric reflex. In the former, fat in the chyme is the main stimulus for the production of a number of hormones, the most powerful being cholecystokinin, which exerts a negative feedback effect on the stomach, decreasing its motility. The enterogastric reflex is initiated in the duodenal wall, and this further slows stomach emptying and secretion.

Gastric secretions

Gastric secretion is divided into three phases: cephalic (neural), gastric and intestinal. Mucus is produced by all regions of the stomach. It is composed mainly of glycoproteins, water and electrolytes, and acts as a lubricant protecting the surface of the stomach against the powerful digestive properties of acid and pepsin. Bicarbonate ions are secreted into the mucus gel layer and this creates a protective buffer zone against the effects of the low pH secretions. Alkaline mucus is produced in the duodenum and small intestine, where it has a similar function of mucosal protection.

The parietal cells in the stomach are responsible for the production of acid. Acid secretion by these cells is stimulated by two main factors: acetylcholine, released by the vagus nerve, and gastrin from the antrum. Acetylcholine and gastrin act on neuroendocrine cells located close to the parietal cells. On stimulation, these cells release histamine, which has a paracrine action on the parietal cell, stimulating acid production and secretion. Parietal cells secrete acid via an active transport mechanism, the proton pump. Somatostatin, gastric inhibitory peptide and vasoactive intestinal peptide inhibit acid secretion.

Pepsin is a proteolytic enzyme produced in its precursor form, pepsinogen, by the peptic cells found in the body and fundus of the stomach. Pepsinogen production is stimulated by acetylcholine from the vagus nerve. The precursor is then converted to its active form, pepsin, by the acid contents of the stomach.

Intrinsic factor is also produced by the parietal cells. It is a glycoprotein that binds to vitamin B_{12} present in the diet and carries it to the terminal ileum. Here specific receptors for intrinsic factor exist and the complex is taken up by the mucosa. Intrinsic factor is broken down and vitamin B_{12} is then absorbed into the bloodstream.

History and symptoms

Dysphagia

Dysphagia is defined as a feeling of obstruction while swallowing. It is a serious symptom and requires proper investigation regardless of clinical diagnosis.

- *Onset.* Sudden onset suggests a foreign body. In carcinoma, the dysphagia occurs over a period of weeks, whereas in achalasia and benign strictures, symptoms tend to develop over a number of years.
- *Site.* The actual site of obstruction correlates poorly in general to where the patient feels the discomfort, although some patients who feel the obstruction to be high may have a pharyngeal pouch.
- *Progression.* Dysphagia due to an oesophageal stricture (benign or malignant) tends to be progressive whereas patients with motility disorders will often have intermittent symptoms.
- *Severity.* Difficulty in swallowing solids is initially typical of carcinoma, whereas achalasia and other motility disorders tend to be associated with dysphagia to liquids as well.
- *Causes.* A list of the common causes of dysphagia is shown in Table 13.1.

Odynophagia

This symptom is defined as pain on swallowing. It may occur in patients with oesophagitis or due to oesophageal spasm. The latter may be due to a mechanical obstruction (benign or malignant) or due to intrinsic dysmotility of the oesophageal musculature.

Heartburn

Retrosternal pain is a very common symptom and most people will have experienced it at some time. It is usually associated with

13

Table 13.1 Causes of dysphagia		
Intraluminal	Intramural	Extrinsic
Pharynx/upper oesophagus		
Foreign body	Pharyngitis/tonsillitis Moniliasis Sideropenic web Corrosives Carcinoma Myasthenia gravis Bulbar palsy	Thyroid enlargement Pharyngeal pouch
Body of oesophagus		
Foreign body	Corrosives Peptic oesophagitis Carcinoma	Mediastinal lymph nodes Aortic aneurysm
Lower oesophagus		
Foreign body	Corrosives Peptic oesophagitis Carcinoma Diffuse oesophageal spasm Systemic sclerosis Achalasia Postvagotomy	Paraoesophageal hernia

gastrooesophageal reflux and may be brought on by eating a heavy meal, alcohol or bending over. General practitioners will see many patients in their clinical practice who complain of heartburn and will treat them effectively with acid-suppressing medication such as proton pump inhibitors (PPIs).

Dyspepsia

Dyspepsia is something of a 'catch all' term used to describe the symptoms of indigestion that are very common in the general population. Patients may experience epigastric pain, belching, heartburn, nausea, early satiety or reduced appetite. Guidance from the National Institute for Clinical Excellence (NICE) in the UK, recommends lifestyle advice, medication review and empirical treatment for the majority of patients with dyspepsia but without so-called alarm symptoms (weight loss, progressive dysphagia, iron deficiency anaemia, epigastric mass and persistent vomiting) (EBM 13.1). Unfortunately, the symptoms of early upper gastrointestinal (GI) malignancy are very similar to dyspepsia and only advanced malignancies tend to cause alarm symptoms. Patients with advanced upper GI malignancy have a poor prognosis despite aggressive therapy, which creates a dilemma; which patients with dyspepsia should be referred for endoscopy? NICE

EBM   13.1 NICE guidance on dyspepsia

'Urgent specialist referral for endoscopic investigation is indicated in patients of any age with dyspepsia when presenting with any of chronic GI bleeding, progressive unintentional weight loss, progressive difficulty swallowing, persistent vomiting, iron deficiency anaemia, epigastric mass or suspicious barium meal.'

NICE Guidance CG184, Gastro-oesophageal reflux disease and dyspepsia in adults: investigation and treatment. Sept 2014. Available from www.nice.org/guidance/cg184

---

guidance on dyspepsia should be applied with caution and doctors should recommend gastroscopy in any patient who does not improve quickly with simple treatment. It is also imperative that a careful history is taken and anaemia excluded.

Regurgitation and vomiting

Regurgitation is an effortless (passive) process whereby food is regurgitated into the mouth and is associated with achalasia, hiatus hernia and pharyngeal pouches. Regurgitation can lead to aspiration with coughing/choking, asthma and aspiration pneumonia. Vomiting is an active process whereby the stomach contents are forcefully expelled by powerful contractions of the abdominal musculature at the same time as relaxation of the lower oesophageal sphincter. Potential causes of vomiting include infection, inflammation, endocrine disorders, drugs and medication, gastrointestinal obstruction, and physiological such as morning sickness in pregnancy.

Abdominal pain

Epigastric pain is a common upper gastrointestinal symptom. Pain relieved by eating traditionally suggests a duodenal ulcer whereas gastric ulcer pain is aggravated by food. However, the differential diagnosis for epigastric pain is extensive and includes conditions such as liver metastasis, pancreatic pathology, abdominal aortic aneurysm, gallstones, irritable bowel and even myocardial infarction.

Examination

Physical examination might reveal signs that will aid in the diagnosis of upper GI disorders. A smooth tongue, pallor and koilonychia are signs of iron deficiency anaemia, which can be present in oesophageal carcinoma, oesophagitis and Plummer–Vinson syndrome (see p. 181).

Lymphadenopathy, particularly in the left supraclavicular region (Virchow's node, Troisier's sign), hepatomegaly, abdominal mass, ascites and evidence of weight loss are associated with malignancy. A mass felt in the upper abdomen is usually a bad sign suggesting incurable malignancy. Metastatic deposit in the umbilicus (Sister Joseph nodule) and extra-mucosal nodule on rectal examination (Blummer's shelf) are also signs of advanced upper GI malignancy. Crepitus in the neck of a patient who has been vomiting is a sign of surgical emphysema and suggests an oesophageal perforation. A succussion splash heard over the epigastrium when the patient is gently shaken suggests gastric outlet obstruction.

Investigations

Blood tests

A full blood count may reveal evidence of anaemia or infection. Serum urea and electrolytes tests may show dehydration, renal failure, hypokalaemia and hyponatraemia secondary to dysphagia or vomiting. The electrolyte and acid–base abnormalities associated with prolonged gastric outlet obstruction include hypokalaemic, hyponatraemic and hypochloraemic metabolic alkalosis. Liver function tests might show low plasma proteins, abnormal clotting and elevated enzymes in the presence of metastatic disease, and portal hypertension.

Helicobacter pylori tests

Patients with dyspepsia should normally be tested for infection with *Helicobacter pylori*, the commonest cause of peptic ulceration and gastric adenocarcinoma worldwide. *H. pylori* can be detected in the following ways:

- Blood tests to detect evidence of an immune response to *H. pylori*
- Stool tests looking for *H. pylori* antigens
- Urea breath tests
- CLO tests on endoscopic biopsies
- Histology of endoscopic biopsies.

Chest x-ray

A simple chest x-ray may show any of the following signs: pulmonary consolidation and fibrosis following aspiration in patients with oesophageal motility disorders and oesophageal carcinoma, an air–fluid level behind the heart shadow from a large hiatus hernia with intrathoracic stomach (Fig. 13.3), a mediastinal mass of lymph nodes and pulmonary metastases in oesophagogastric cancer, air in the mediastinum and neck after perforation of the oesophagus (Fig. 13.4) or under the diaphragm from a perforated peptic ulcer (Fig. 13.5).

Contrast swallow/meal

A contrast swallow/meal using barium liquid or water-soluble contrast may be useful:

- As a primary investigation when access to endoscopy is limited (Fig. 13.6)
- In a very frail patient with dysphagia or vomiting who might not be deemed fit enough for endoscopy (rare)
- To exclude a pharyngeal pouch prior to endoscopy
- To complement endoscopy and provide additional anatomical information (i.e., for patients with a large hiatus hernia) (Fig. 13.7)
- To diagnose a suspected upper GI perforation.

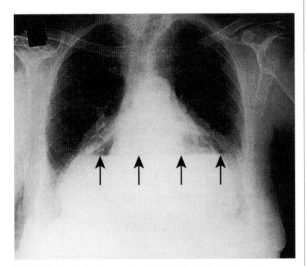

Fig. 13.3 Erect chest x-ray showing an intrathoracic stomach secondary to a giant hiatus hernia. Note the air–fluid level.

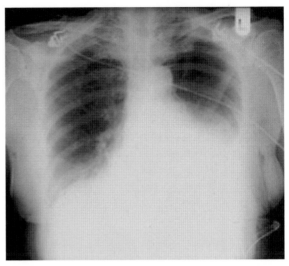

Fig. 13.4 Erect chest x-ray showing left hydropneumothorax in a patient with Boerhaave's syndrome.

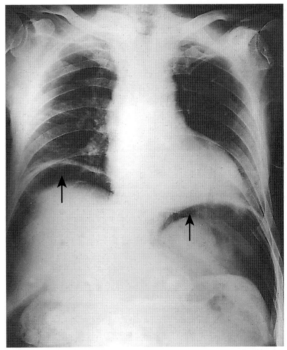

Fig. 13.5 Erect chest x-ray showing free air under both hemidiaphragms secondary to a perforated duodenal ulcer.

Endoscopy

Flexible oesophagogastroduodenoscopy (OGD) is now the first-line investigation for almost all upper GI symptoms. Flexible OGD is carried out with light intravenous sedation or local anaesthetic throat spray alone after a 4 hour fast with pulse and oxygen saturation monitoring to identify and rectify respiratory depression. Endoscopic therapeutic procedures include dilatation of strictures, stent insertion, thermal ablation of tumours, removal of foreign bodies and control of bleeding.

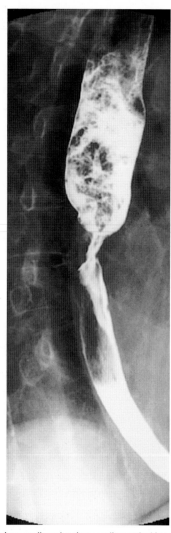

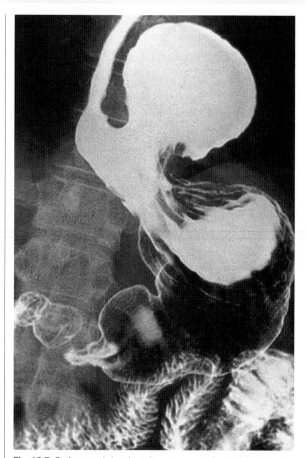

Fig. 13.7 Barium meal showing a large paraoesophageal hiatus hernia.

Fig. 13.6 Barium swallow showing a malignant looking stricture of the mid-oesophagus.

status (positive or negative for cancer) has major implications for treatment (curative or palliative). EUS is also useful for investigating submucosal lesions of the stomach such as gastrointestinal stromal tumours (GISTs) (Fig. 13.9).

Computed tomography

Computed tomography (CT) is used most commonly to investigate end-stage malignancy but may also be helpful when investigating patients with benign conditions such as large hiatus hernias, a suspected gastric volvulus or upper GI perforation. Staging upper GI CT is often done after the patient has drunk water to distend the oesophagus and stomach. Emergency scans looking for evidence of gut perforation will use oral water-soluble contrast.

Endoluminal ultrasound

Endoscopic ultrasonography (EUS) uses a variety of endoscopes containing high-frequency ultrasound probes at their tips to investigate patients with upper GI disorders. By placing the probe within the GI lumen great detail of the underlying structures can be obtained. Linear probes facilitate needle biopsy and radial probes provide a 360-degree circumferential view. EUS is mostly used for staging the 'T' and 'N' component of TNM staging for oesophagogastric cancer (Fig. 13.8). EUS is used increasingly to allow fine-needle biopsy of suspicious lymph nodes since the

Staging laparoscopy

Staging laparoscopy is a superior modality compared with EUS and CT, for detecting small volume peritoneal metastasis and surface liver metastasis when used to stage upper GI malignancy. When staging laparoscopy is used as an additional staging modality, more than 20% of patients with gastric cancers are upstaged due to metastatic disease and therefore unnecessary surgery can be avoided.

Positron emission tomography

Positron emission tomography (PET) is another staging modality used to detect tumour tissue. The tracer used is a radiolabelled glucose analogue, 18-fluoro-deoxyglucose (FDG). As the malignant tissue is metabolically more active, FDG uptake is preferentially greater, compared with normal tissue. PET is commonly used to detect distant metastases in oesophageal malignancy.

Manometry and pH studies

Measurements of lower oesophageal pH can be made over a 24-hour period using an intraluminal electrode placed 5 cm proximal to the lower oesophageal sphincter attached to a catheter passed

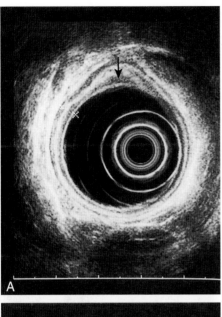

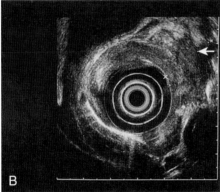

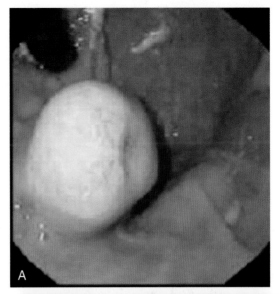

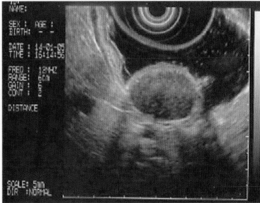

13

Fig. 13.8 Endoscopic ultrasound (EUS). (A) The normal layers of the oesophagus and a small T1 cancer confined to the mucosa marked with an arrow. **(B)** A full-thickness T3 tumour of the oesophagus (*arrow*). Note the complete destruction of the normal oesophageal layers.

Fig. 13.9 (A) Endoscopic view of a 2-cm diameter polypoid submucosal gastric lesion. **(B)** EUS confirms the lesion is arising from the muscularis propria and likely to be a gastrointestinal stromal tumour.

through the nose and pharynx. Alternatively, oesophageal pH can be measured over three days using a Bravo capsule, which is clipped to the oesophageal mucosa and is wireless (Fig. 13.10). Patients can indicate symptom events during the recording and these can be correlated with the pH trace. A composite scoring system (the DeMeester score) is used to diagnose pathological gastrooesophageal reflux disease (GORD). Oesophageal pressure and peristalsis can be analysed during a series of swallows (station manometry) or over a longer period (ambulatory manometry) (Fig. 13.11). Newer techniques for investigating reflux and dysmotility include high resolution manometry, bile reflux probe and oesophageal impedance.

Gastric emptying studies

Nuclear medicine scans require the patient to swallow radiolabelled liquid and solids (a two-phase study). The speed at which the stomach empties can be monitored using a gamma ray detector. Patients whose major complaint is nausea and vomiting but appear to have no structural abnormality of their upper GI tract

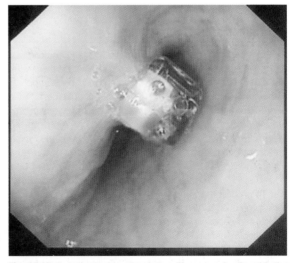

Fig. 13.10 Endoscopic view of a wireless Bravo capsule clipped to the oesophageal mucosa 5 cm proximal to the gastrooesophageal junction. These record for up to 72 hours before falling off and passing harmlessly through the gut.

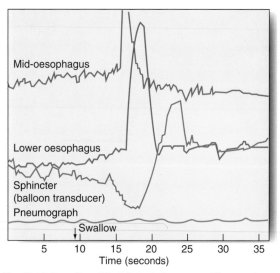

Fig. 13.11 Recording of the intraluminal pressure of the oesophagus.

should undergo a two-phase gastric emptying study to look for gastroparesis, a common condition in diabetics secondary to autonomic neuropathy.

Diagnosis and management: oesophagus

Gastrooesophageal reflux disease and Barrett's oesophagus

Patients typically complain of heartburn, regurgitation of acid into the back of their throat, nausea, waterbrash (hypersalivation), epigastric pain and occasionally vomiting. Reflux symptoms affect up to 30% of the population. The lower oesophageal sphincter usually prevents reflux by maintaining a resting pressure of 15–20 mmHg.

Diagnosis and management

GORD is based on history, endoscopy findings and sometimes a 24-hour oesophageal pH study. In young patients and those without alarm symptoms, empirical treatment may be appropriate without doing any investigations. Patients should be advised about lifestyle changes including weight loss if obese, stopping smoking, eating less fatty and spicy food, and drinking less caffeine and alcohol. Many patients will already have tried over-the-counter remedies such as antacids, alginates or low-dose H_2 antagonists. Definitive treatment, however, is provided by a course of PPIs. Prokinetic agents such as metoclopramide may also help patients by improving the lower oesophageal muscle tone, promoting gastric emptying and reducing nausea.

Barrett's oesophagus is a histological diagnosis made after endoscopic biopsies. GORD can cause oesophagitis and in some patients this leads to a metaplastic change in the mucosa from squamous to columnar type. Barrett's oesophagus may become dysplastic (low and high grade) thereby leading to oesophageal adenocarcinoma. This disease is increasing in incidence and patients with this condition offer a target group for surveillance

to detect early neoplasia. This can be eradicated successfully by endoscopic radiofrequency ablation (RFA) or mucosal resection (EMR) (EBM 13.2).

EBM | 13.2 **Barrett's oesophagus guidelines**

'It is vitally important for accurate diagnosis that the precise sites of biopsies taken are recorded by the endoscopist in terms of distance from the incisor teeth and relation to the oesophagogastric junction (Recommendation grade C).'

Fitzgerald RC, di Pietro M, Ragunath K, et al. British Society of Gastroenterology guidelines on the diagnosis and management of Barrett's oesophagus. Gut. 2014;63:7–42.

Antireflux surgery

Although surgical treatment of patients with severe reflux disease has always been associated with good long-term outcomes, the introduction and refinements of laparoscopic techniques have brought the surgical option to more patients. Surgery may be indicated for those whose symptoms cannot be controlled by medical therapy, those with complicated reflux disease (stricture formation, respiratory complications, other atypical symptoms), and young patients who do not wish to continue taking acid suppression therapy long-term. Symptoms that fail to be brought under control with acid suppression therapy are usually due to high-volume alkaline reflux, and surgery is an extremely effective cure (EBM 13.3). The presence of Barrett's metaplasia alone is not considered a suitable indication for antireflux surgery.

EBM | 13.3 **Surgery for gastrooesophageal reflux disease**

'It has been shown that, following antireflux surgery, quality of life is improved and costs are reduced significantly compared with medical treatment. Antireflux surgery should be offered to patients with proven symptomatic reflux that cannot be controlled symptomatically with medical therapy.'

For further information: www.acg.gi.org/physicians/guidelines/GERDTreatment.pdf

---

Surgery requires reduction of the hiatus hernia if present, approximation of the crura around the lower oesophagus and fundoplication. This involves mobilising the fundus of the stomach from its attachments to the undersurface of the left hemidiaphragm and the left crus, and wrapping it around the oesophagus, either anteriorly or posteriorly. The most common procedure is the Nissen fundoplication, in which the fundus is taken posteriorly around the lower oesophagus and sutured to the left anterior surface of the left side of the proximal stomach as a 360-degree wrap (Fig. 13.12). Other procedures involving a partial (incomplete) fundoplication include the Toupet (posterior 270-degree wrap) and the Watson (anterior 180-degree wrap) repairs. Current data do not demonstrate much difference between the various approaches although early postoperative dysphagia is more common with 360-degree wraps. All procedures have a success rate in curing the symptoms of reflux of around 90% at a year and 70–80% at 10 years. Unwanted complications after surgery include gas bloat (inability to belch), dysphagia, early satiety and increased flatus. These operations are now carried out laparoscopically, with excellent results in skilled hands.

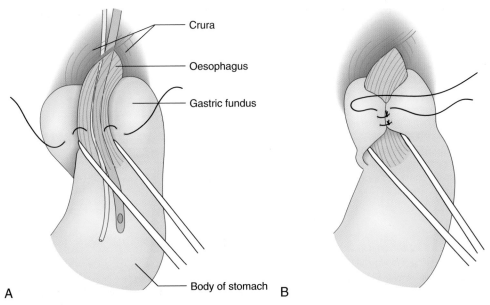

Fig. 13.12 **Fundoplication for gastrooesophageal reflux disease.** (A) Gastric fundus wrapped around the lower oesophagus. (B) Fundal wrap sutured in position.

13.1 Summary

Gastrooesophageal reflux disease

- Reflux type symptoms are very common
- 'Lifestyle' advice to patients is important (i.e., smoking, dieting, etc.)
- Proton pump inhibitors are generally effective treatment
- GORD for >10 years (especially men) is a risk factor for Barrett's oesophagus
- Screening and surveillance for Barrett's patients increasingly relevant
- Laparoscopic antireflux surgery is clinically effective and cost efficient.

Hiatus hernia

A hiatus hernia is an abnormal protrusion of the stomach through the oesophageal diaphragmatic hiatus into the thorax and may be sliding (90%) or rolling (10%) (Fig. 13.13). A sliding hernia occurs when the stomach slides through the diaphragmatic hiatus, so that the gastrooesophageal junction lies within the chest cavity. It is covered anteriorly by peritoneum, and posteriorly is extraperitoneal. A rolling or paraoesophageal hernia is formed when the stomach rolls up anteriorly through the hiatus; the cardia remains in its normal position and therefore the cardiooesophageal sphincter remains intact.

Rolling and sliding hernias are caused by weakness of the muscles around the hiatus. They tend to occur in middle-aged and elderly patients. Women are affected more frequently than men and there is a higher incidence in the obese.

Clinical features

Hiatus hernias are often asymptomatic, but can produce some of or all the following symptoms:

- *Heartburn and regurgitation* owing to an incompetent lower oesophageal sphincter, which is aggravated by stooping and lying flat at night, and can be relieved by antacids.

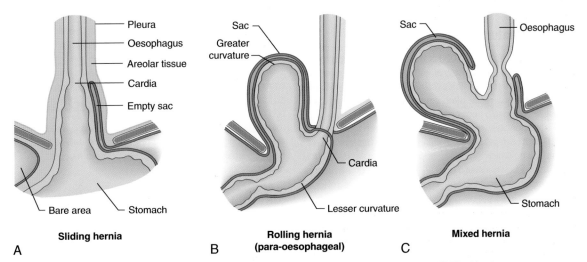

Fig. 13.13 **Types of hiatus hernia.** (A) Sliding hernia. (B) Rolling hernia (paraoesophageal). (C) Mixed hernia.

- *Oesophagitis* resulting from persistent acid reflux, which leads to ulceration, bleeding with anaemia, fibrosis and stricture formation.
- *Epigastric and lower chest pain,* especially in paraoesophageal hernias, as the herniated part of the stomach (usually the fundus) becomes trapped in the hiatus. This can be a surgical emergency owing to the obstruction and strangulation of the stomach.
- *Palpitations and hiccups,* symptoms caused by the mass effect of the hernia in the thoracic cavity irritating the pericardium and the diaphragm. In patients with a large rolling hiatus hernia, displacement of the whole stomach may result in a volvulus into the chest, producing symptoms of vomiting from gastric outflow obstruction.

Management

Treatment is as for GORD, although patients with obstructive symptoms such as vomiting and regurgitation or breathlessness due to reduced lung capacity should be considered for surgical repair. Patients who present as an emergency with an obstructed hiatus hernia should have it decompressed with a nasogastric tube or endoscopically to prevent strangulation. Emergency surgery is occasionally necessary except if conservative therapy fails or gastric necrosis is suspected. Even large hiatus hernias can be repaired laparoscopically although the risk of conversion to open surgery is higher.

Achalasia

This disorder affects the whole oesophagus. The main feature is failure of relaxation of the lower oesophageal sphincter; as the disease progresses, the obstructed lower oesophagus dilates and peristalsis becomes uncoordinated.

Achalasia is thought to be due to a partial or complete degeneration of the myenteric plexus of Auerbach, and in the later stages of the disease loss of the dorsal vagal nuclei within the brain stem can be demonstrated. Infestation with the protozoon, *Trypanosoma cruzi,* which occurs in South America (Chagas' disease), also causes degeneration of the myenteric plexus, leading to a disorder that is indistinguishable from achalasia. Malignancy of the gastrooesophageal junction can sometimes mimic achalasia and is referred to as pseudoachalasia.

Clinical features

The disease affects 1 in 100,000 of the population of developed countries. The patient is typically 30–40 years old and females are affected more often than males (3:2). There is progressive dysphagia over several years, often greater for liquids than solids in contrast to dysphagia from carcinoma. Gravity rather than peristalsis is responsible for food leaving the oesophagus and the patient finds it easier to eat when standing. There may also be retrosternal pain, which gradually decreases in severity as the oesophagus loses peristaltic activity. Other common symptoms include weight loss, halitosis and regurgitation of undigested food, which can lead to aspiration, particularly at night, resulting in bouts of coughing, pneumonia and recurrent chest infections. In the longer term, achalasia can predispose to squamous cell carcinoma of the oesophagus. Barium swallow shows a smooth narrowing (inverted bird beak appearance) with evidence of proximal oesophageal dilatation (Fig. 13.14).

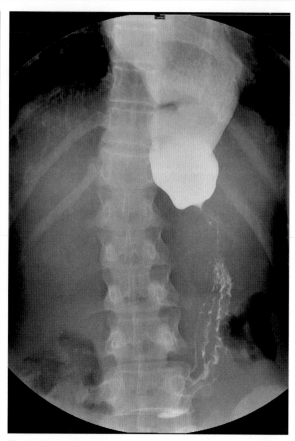

Fig. 13.14 Achalasia cardia. Barium swallow showing smooth narrowing at the oesophagogastric junction along with a massively dilated proximal oesophagus (mega-oesophagus). (Courtesy Dr Bharat Agarwal, New Delhi.)

Management

Treatment comprises balloon dilatation of the lower oesophageal sphincter or surgical myotomy (division of the muscles over the lower oesophagus and proximal stomach). Endoscopic injection of the lower oesophageal sphincter with botulinum toxin gives temporary symptom relief but the effects wear off quite quickly. Balloon dilatation of the gastrooesophageal junction disrupts the lower oesophageal sphincter and improves symptoms in 80–90% of patients, but carries the risk of oesophageal perforation.

Operative treatment involves a laparoscopic Heller's myotomy. The lower oesophageal sphincter is divided down to the mucosa for 5 cm above the oesophagogastric junction and 3 cm down the stomach. Early complications include perforation, and late complications include reflux oesophagitis and recurrent dysphagia from an inadequate myotomy. An anterior partial fundoplication is carried out at the same time to reduce the risk of GORD. A randomised controlled trial comparing myotomy and dilatation did not find any significant difference in outcomes. A new technique for treating achalasia called per-oral endoscopic myotomy (POEM) remains under evaluation.

Diffuse oesophageal spasm

This disorder tends to occur in middle-aged to elderly patients. Complaints are of intermittent dysphagia and retrosternal pain, which can mimic angina. The symptoms are caused by repetitive irregular peristalsis of the oesophageal body and oesophageal manometry is required to make the diagnosis. Diffuse oesophageal spasm can be precipitated by GORD and this should be excluded by 24-hour pH studies.

Management

Surgical treatment involves a long myotomy but results are unpredictable and most patients are treated medically with calcium channel blockers, sublingual GTN and PPIs.

Nutcracker oesophagus

In this uncommon disorder, the symptoms are caused by repetitive forceful peristalsis. Manometry demonstrates normal peristalsis but with excessive amplitudes and pressures exceeding 150 mmHg. Medical treatment is similar to that of diffuse oesophageal spasm, but the results are disappointing. Dilatation and surgical myotomy also have poor results.

Pouches

Pouches are protrusions of mucosa through a weak area in the muscle wall. The most common pouch lies in the pharynx and is associated with raised cricopharyngeal pressure, with the pouch developing through Killian's dehiscence, between the thyropharyngeus and cricopharyngeus muscles. Uncoordination of swallowing and failure of relaxation of the cricopharyngeus muscle cause the herniation. The pharyngeal pouch usually develops posteriorly and is forced by the vertebral column to deviate usually to the left side. Oesophageal pouches can occur around the tracheobronchial tree in relation to pressure from adjacent lymph nodes, if enlarged, and also just above the gastrooesophageal junction in patients with raised lower oesophageal sphincter pressure.

Clinical features

Elderly male patients are more commonly affected. Symptoms include regurgitation of food, halitosis, dysphagia, gurgling in the throat, aspiration and a lump in the neck (pharyngeal pouch) but the patient may be asymptomatic.

Investigations

Barium swallow demonstrates the pouch and uncoordinated swallowing. Endoscopy also confirms the diagnosis but must be performed with care to avoid accidental perforation of the pouch.

Management

Surgical myotomy of the cricopharyngeus and resection of the pouch used to be the surgical treatment of choice, but endoscopic stapling has now superseded this. A special linear stapling device is placed perorally under direct vision with one limb of the device in the oesophageal lumen and the other in the pouch before the stapler is closed and fired. This creates a common lumen between pouch and oesophagus and divides the cricopharyngeal sphincter at the same time.

Perforation

Aetiology

Intraluminal

This is caused by a swallowed foreign body or by its removal during instrumentation, with rigid endoscopy carrying a much greater risk than flexible. The most frequent sites of perforation tend to coincide with the sites of anatomical narrowing. The commonest causes are iatrogenic, occurring during diagnostic endoscopy (rare) or therapeutic procedures such as dilatation (more common).

Outside the wall

These are caused by penetrating injuries such as knife wounds to the neck but are rare.

Spontaneous

This follows episodes of violent vomiting (Boerhaave's syndrome). The perforation is frequently on the left posterolateral aspect of the lower oesophagus. A tear to the oesophageal mucosa only, following vomiting, is known as a Mallory–Weiss tear and causes haematemesis and pain.

Clinical features

Clinical symptoms depend on the site and size of the perforation. Perforation in the cervical region results in neck pain and local tenderness, and surgical emphysema is present. Perforation of the thoracic oesophagus causes retrosternal chest pain and dysphagia. The patient may be shocked, short of breath and cyanosed owing to a pneumothorax or pleural effusion, if the pleural space is involved. Perforation in this area can lead to mediastinitis and septic shock. Perforation of the abdominal oesophagus can lead to peritonitis and a rigid abdomen.

Investigations

The most important factor in diagnosing oesophageal perforation early on is the examining doctor including it in his or her differential diagnosis of any patient who collapses with chest pain, shortness of breath or vomiting.

Erect chest x-ray

In addition to excluding a perforated duodenal ulcer (air under the diaphragm), an erect chest x-ray may show gas in the soft tissues of the mediastinum (surgical emphysema), often extending up to the neck. The mediastinum may also be widened, and if the pleural cavity has been ruptured, there will be a hydropneumothorax.

CT and contrast swallow

The diagnosis is confirmed by a chest CT or water-soluble contrast swallow, which will demonstrate whether the perforation is localised to the mediastinum or open to the pleural or peritoneal cavities (Fig. 13.15). If oesophageal perforation cannot be excluded after radiological imaging and clinical suspicion remains high an experienced endoscopist should perform an OGD. Spontaneous pneumomediastinum can occur in young adults and teenagers after violent vomiting or coughing and is thought to be due to the rupture of a pulmonary bulla. There is no oesophageal injury and the treatment is conservative.

Management

Perforation of the cervical oesophagus can be treated nonoperatively with intravenous fluids, withdrawal of oral fluid and diet, and the administration of antibiotics and antifungals. If an abscess develops in the superior mediastinum, this will require surgical drainage.

Perforation of the thoracic oesophagus has a much higher morbidity and mortality. Localised and small perforations that do not communicate with either pleural cavity can be treated

13

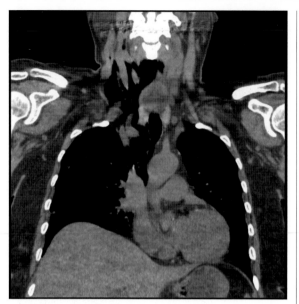

Fig. 13.15 Coronal CT image showing iatrogenic pharyngeal perforation with massive surgical emphysema.

nonoperatively, as outlined above. If the perforation follows the dilatation of a carcinoma in a patient suitable for resection, emergency oesophagogastrectomy may be indicated although longer term survival in this situation is very rare and many specialists would now recommend placing a stent. Small perforations with minimal mediastinal contamination can often be managed conservatively whereas large defects require surgery. If the perforation is detected early a primary repair of the defect may be possible. Late presentation with heavy contamination is best treated by repairing the defect over a T-tube to create a controlled fistula; prolonged mediastinal drainage, antibiotics, antifungals and enteral feeding via a jejunostomy are also required in this life threatening situation. An alternative strategy for late presenting oesophageal

perforations is Endo-vac therapy involving endoscopic placement of a nasogastric tube into the mediastinal cavity via the perforation. Its end is covered by a small piece of Vac sponge to enable suction to be applied and allow the cavity to collapse. Large abscesses may be treated successfully using this method.

Corrosive oesophagitis

Ingestion of strong acid or alkali occurs accidentally, especially in children, and deliberately in attempted suicide. It results in severe chemical burns to the mouth, pharynx and oesophageal mucosa, particularly at the sites of anatomical narrowing. Oedema, ulceration and inflammation follow, which can lead to acute obstruction and perforation. Inflamed tissue heals by fibrosis and stricture formation. Patients complain of severe continuous pain, exacerbated by swallowing. The oropharynx may be inflamed, the patient shocked and the oesophagus perforated.

Ingestion of alkaline solutions tends to result in transmural damage that heals with fibrosis. Acids lead to coagulative necrosis and eschar formation that limits spread to deeper layers.

Investigations and Management

Patients should be resuscitated, given appropriate opiate analgesia and be encouraged to drink water to dilute the corrosive. Endoscopy or barium swallow will demonstrate the extent and severity of the injury, and later can assess stricture formation (Fig. 13.16). Careful, early OGD under general anaesthesia will assess the extent and severity of the injury. Passage of a nasogastric or nasojejunal tube under the same anaesthetic will allow enteral feeding to commence and provide a passage for a guidewire, should subsequent balloon dilatation for stricture formation be necessary.

The patient should be kept nil by mouth subsequently and administered intravenous fluids and antibiotics. The use of steroids remains controversial. If the patient's oropharynx is severely inflamed, a tracheostomy may be required. Appropriate nutritional

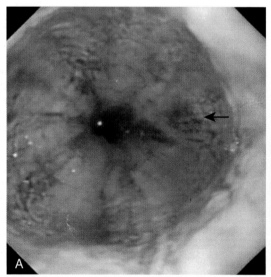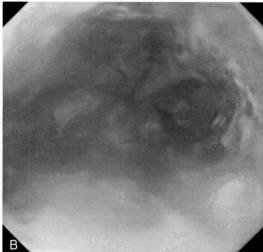

Fig. 13.16 Corrosive oesophagitis. (A) Endoscopic view of the lower oesophagus and oesophagogastric junction 12 hours after inadvertent ingestion of acid. The arrow shows the area of superficial necrosis involving the proximal stomach at the level of the oesophagogastric junction. **(B)** The same endoscopic view after 36 hours, demonstrating mucosal inflammation but no evidence of ongoing necrosis. This patient was lucky and went on to make a full recovery without late stricture formation.

support is established and the patient observed for perforation and later for stricture formation.

Strictures will usually require treatment with balloon dilatation and long-term management may involve resection of the stricture and primary anastomosis, or a more extensive resection with reconstruction using colon, stomach or jejunum. Regular endoscopic surveillance will be required, as corrosive injury predisposes the oesophagus to malignant change.

Tumours of the oesophagus

Benign tumours

These account for less than 1% of oesophageal neoplasms and the most common is leiomyoma that is often asymptomatic but may cause bleeding or dysphagia. It is treated by local enucleation with good results.

Carcinoma of the oesophagus

The incidence of carcinoma of the oesophagus has risen in developed countries over the last two decades and to around 15/100,000 in the UK, due primarily to an increase in adenocarcinoma. The male to female ratio is 3:1. In the Far East and among some black males, there is a greater incidence of squamous cell carcinoma. However, two-thirds of carcinomas are now of the lower one-third (possibly from Barrett's dysplasia) and the remaining are of the upper two-thirds (predominantly squamous) of the oesophagus.

The most important risk factors for adenocarcinoma are reflux and obesity, with a slightly increased risk of cardiac tumours with smoking. Risk factors for squamous cell carcinoma include alcohol, smoking, leucoplakia, achalasia, consumption of salted fish or pickled vegetables, consumption of hot beverages and chewing tobacco and betel nuts. Corrosive injury of the oesophagus is associated with squamous cell cancers. Tylosis palmarum is a rare autosomal recessive disorder, which is associated with a very high incidence of squamous cell carcinoma of the oesophagus.

The tumour may spread by direct invasion across the wall or longitudinally, along the lymphatics or haematogenously. Lymphatic spread is characterised by longitudinal invasion through the submucosal lymphatic channels leading to greater microscopic involvement than what is grossly visible. Regional lymph nodes from the superior mediastinum down to the coeliac axis could be involved. Spread to other organs occurs by the bloodstream in late cases.

Clinical features

Progressive dysphagia to solids, then liquids, is the most common presentation along with regurgitation and weight loss. Additional symptoms like odynophagia (involvement of local nerves), hoarseness of voice (involvement of recurrent laryngeal nerve), Horner's syndrome (involvement of sympathetic chain) and coughing on taking any liquids (tracheo- or bronchooesophageal fistula) suggest locally advanced disease. The average duration of symptoms at the time of presentation is between 3 and 9 months, and as a result, around 70% of patients are not operable at the time of diagnosis.

Occasionally, patients may present with metastatic disease, including enlarged cervical lymph nodes, jaundice, hepatomegaly, hoarseness and chest pain from mediastinal invasion. Other general features of malignancy may be present.

Investigations

The diagnosis may be made initially by barium swallow, but must always be confirmed by endoscopy and biopsy. Endoscopy is the best first-line investigation for anyone with dysphagia. Thereafter, investigations are aimed at accurate staging of the disease to assess resectability, determine prognosis and identify patients who might benefit from neoadjuvant therapy. Local T (tumour) stage and N (nodal) spread are best assessed by endoscopic ultrasonography, and M (metastases) stage by CT and PET (lung, liver and bone metastases, distant lymphadenopathy), and laparoscopy (peritoneal metastases). Routine blood tests may reveal anaemia, liver disease and malnutrition, all of which require full assessment if surgery is to be considered. In those patients with proximal and middle-third tumours adjacent to the tracheobronchial tree, bronchoscopy can be required to assess airway invasion. If enlarged distant lymph nodes are detected, these should be aspirated for cytology, as surgical resection is contraindicated if they are positive for malignancy.

Management

The aim of treatment is to offer radical treatment to those with potentially curable disease and improve the quality of life for the remainder. The overall 5-year survival rate remains low (<10%), although 5-year survival figures of 20–30% are reported when resection is feasible. Multimodal therapy involving perioperative chemotherapy and surgery is the standard of care when the treatment intent is curative. A multidisciplinary team (consisting of surgeons, endoscopists, radiation and medical oncologists, pathologists, palliative care physicians and nutritional therapists) must be involved in the management in a high volume cancer centre.

Surgical resection

Oesophagectomy with palliative intent is not appropriate as few patients recover enough to gain any benefit before they die of their disease. Palliative oesophagectomy may have to be offered if stenting is not available in developing countries if the patient is fit.

- *Ivor–Lewis two-phase oesophagectomy* (Fig. 13.17) involves a laparotomy during which the stomach is fully mobilised on its vascular pedicles, along with the lower oesophagus. A right thoracotomy is carried out to resect the oesophagus, and the mobilised stomach is brought up into the chest and anastomosed to the proximal oesophagus. This is the preferred choice for middle and lower-third tumours.
- *Left thoracolaparotomy* is a good approach for oesophagogastric junction tumours, particularly when the tumour extends down into the proximal stomach and a more extensive gastric resection is required.
- *Trans-hiatal oesophagectomy* involves mobilisation of the stomach via an abdominal incision, the oesophagus (some of it by blunt dissection) through the hiatus, and the cervical oesophagus via a left-sided neck incision. Once the oesophagus is removed, the stomach is brought up into the neck and anastomosed to the cervical oesophagus. This technique is appropriate for tumours of the lower third where adequate lymphadenectomy is possible.

13

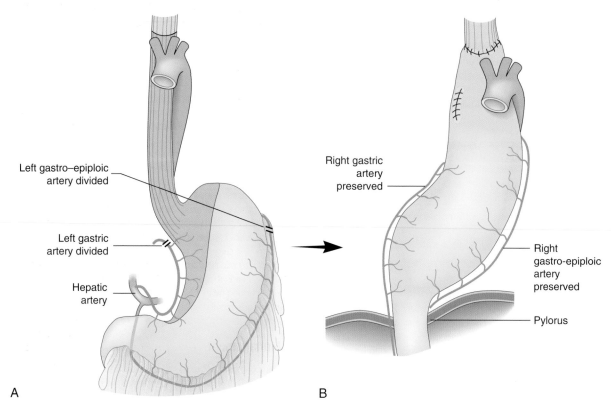

Left gastro–epiploic artery divided

Left gastric artery divided

Hepatic artery

Right gastric artery preserved

Right gastro-epiploic artery preserved

Pylorus

A

B

Fig. 13.17 Reconstruction after Ivor–Lewis oesophagectomy.

- *McKeown three-phase oesophagectomy* involves a laparotomy to mobilise the stomach and lower oesophagus, a right thoracotomy for mobilisation of the thoracic oesophagus and to perform a lymphadenectomy, and a left cervical incision to anastomose the stomach to the cervical oesophagus. The advantages are avoidance of an anastomosis in the chest with its potential complications, and the ability to tackle mid- and upper-oesophageal malignancies due to the high proximal clearance achieved along with adequate lymphadenectomy.
- *Minimally invasive oesophagectomy.* Increasingly surgeons are using laparoscopic and thoracoscopic techniques to mobilise the oesophagus. The commonest technique is to mobilise the stomach laparoscopically and then perform a thoracotomy to resect the oesophagus and perform an anastomosis, a so called 'hybrid technique'. Alternatively, both the abdominal and chest phase of the surgery can be done using minimally invasive techniques.

Postoperative care

Uncomplicated recovery after oesophagectomy hinges on good surgical technique, good pain relief (often by epidural analgesia), avoidance of excess intravenous fluid, early mobilisation and effective chest physiotherapy. Many surgeons place a feeding jejunostomy at the time of oesophagectomy to allow early enteral feeding. The early recognition of postoperative complications and their aggressive management has done much to reduce the perioperative mortality of this major operation to around 5% (EBM 13.4).

EBM 13.4 **National Oesophagogastric Cancer Audit (England & Wales) 2015**

'The 30-day postoperative mortality rate for oesophagectomy and gastrectomy was 2.2% (95 per cent CI 1.7 to 2.8) and 42.3% (95 per cent CI 1.6 to 3.1), respectively.

http://www.hscic.gov.uk/catalogue/PUB19627/clin-audi-supp-prog-oeso-gast-2015-rep.pdf

Radiotherapy and chemotherapy

All patients with locally advanced tumours should be considered for perioperative chemotherapy. Current randomised clinical trials will determine the most effective combination of agents. Chemoradiotherapy can also be used preoperatively, particularly for squamous carcinoma of the oesophagus although postoperative complications for these patients may be higher. Up to a third of patients will have a complete pathological response (no residual tumour when resected) and this has prompted trials of chemoradiotherapy as definitive treatment in squamous cell carcinoma.

Palliation

The majority of patients (about 70%) will have palliative rather than curative treatment. A full range of palliative treatments must be available and an experienced hospital clinician with good specialist nurse support should coordinate care, working closely with community services.

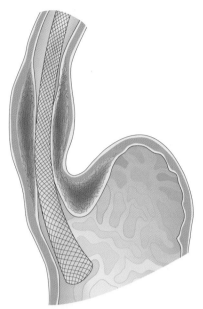

Fig. 13.18 Self-expanding metal stent inserted to relieve dysphagia from an incurable oesophageal tumour.

Best supportive care: Some patients are too frail for any interventional treatment and require a holistic approach to their symptoms involving medication to counter nausea, vomiting and pain. Emotional and dietary support are important.

Endoscopic stent: Patients with significant dysphagia should be considered for a palliative stent as this is a safe and effective method of relieving the distress of not being able to swallow (Fig. 13.18). These are inserted under intravenous sedation endoscopically but can also be screened into position by interventional radiologists. Chest pain for the first few days after insertion is common and patients should be started on a PPI to reduce reflux symptoms. Complications include perforation during insertion, migration of the stent, blockage and tumour ingrowth. The latter can be rectified by laser ablation or placement of a second stent. Stents cannot be used for very proximal tumours involving the cervical oesophagus.

Palliative chemotherapy: This has been shown in a number of randomised clinical trials to improve patients' symptoms (i.e., dysphagia) and double life expectancy for those with advanced oesophagogastric cancer.

Palliative radiotherapy and brachytherapy: Intraluminal radiotherapy (brachytherapy) has been shown to provide a better quality of life for patients with incurable oesophageal cancer than a stent. However, availability of this treatment in the UK is still limited. External beam radiotherapy can provide good palliative care for squamous oesophageal carcinoma but requires more visits by the patient to hospital.

 13.2 Summary

Oesophageal cancer

- Always investigate dysphagia
- GORD, Barrett's and oesophageal adenocarcinoma are linked
- Early diagnosis can allow curative endoscopic or surgical therapy
- Late diagnosis (the norm) results in poor prognosis
- Curative treatment now usually multimodal
- Surgical outcomes better in high volume centres.

Diagnosis and management: gastroduodenal

Peptic ulceration

Peptic ulceration affects areas of mucosa exposed to acidic gastric contents. The main pathology is an imbalance between the acid–pepsin system and the mucosal ability to resist digestion. Duodenal ulcers occur four times more commonly than gastric ulcers.

Pathology

Duodenal ulcers usually occur in the first part of the duodenum and 50% occur on the anterior wall. The majority of gastric ulcers develop on the lesser curvature in the distal half of the stomach. They may coexist with duodenal ulcers in 10% of patients. Duodenal ulcers may be acute (Fig. 13.19) or chronic. Ulcers with a history of less than 3 months' duration and with no evidence of fibrosis are considered to be acute. Gastric ulcers generally run a chronic course.

Gastric ulcers may be benign or malignant. Malignancy was once thought to be a complicating factor of benign gastric ulceration but malignant change in a benign ulcer is rare, and such ulcers are probably malignant from the outset. Duodenal ulcers are very rarely malignant.

Aetiology

Helicobacter pylori

H. pylori is present in around 50% of the world's population, its prevalence increasing with age. It is more prevalent in developing countries, where poor and crowded living conditions are commonplace, and here the infection is probably acquired in early life via the faecal–oral or oral–oral route. Once an individual is infected, *H. pylori* persists; in the majority of patients, there are no symptoms.

H. pylori is detected in 95% of patients with duodenal ulceration. It infects the antral mucosa of the stomach, where it causes an inflammatory response. This gastritis stimulates the gastrin-producing (G) cells of the antrum to increase gastrin production. The subsequent hypersecretion of acid provides an ideal environment for gastric metaplasia of the duodenal mucosa to occur. The

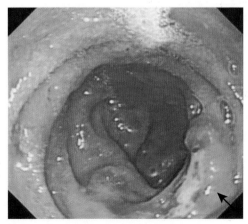

Fig. 13.19 Endoscopic view of an acute duodenal ulcer.

13

colonisation of the metaplastic areas by *H. pylori* further damages the mucosa, and ultimately duodenal ulceration occurs.

H. pylori is found in approximately 75% of patients with gastric ulcers, although its role is less well defined. It may be that the gastritis facilitates the access of acid and pepsin to the stomach mucosa. It seems that the key factor is decreased mucosal resistance, with excess acid having less of a role. Most patients with gastric ulceration have a normal or decreased secretory capacity.

Nonsteroidal antiinflammatory drugs (NSAIDs)

The role of this group of drugs (aspirin, ibuprofen and diclofenac) as antiinflammatory agents centres on their inhibition of the action of cyclooxygenase in prostaglandin synthesis. In the stomach, prostaglandins are responsible for the production of mucus and bicarbonate, which both help to protect the stomach mucosa from acid by maintaining an alkaline buffer zone. NSAIDs are implicated in 30% of gastric ulcers and may also be responsible for the small number of *H. pylori*-negative duodenal ulcers.

Smoking

This aetiological factor is more important in gastric than duodenal ulceration. Smoking delays ulcer healing and increases the likelihood of complications (e.g., bleeding or perforation).

Genetic factors

First-degree relatives of patients with a duodenal ulcer are at increased risk of developing a duodenal ulcer themselves. This risk is further increased if ulcers develop in patients under 20 years of age. First-degree relatives of patients with gastric ulcers are also at increased risk of developing gastric ulcers.

Zollinger–Ellison syndrome

This rare syndrome is caused by a gastrin-secreting tumour (gastrinoma) that is normally found in the pancreas but may occasionally be found in the duodenum or stomach. Approximately 30% of patients have features consistent with multiple endocrine neoplasia syndrome (MEN I). Hypergastrinaemia results in a greatly increased risk of peptic ulceration. Diarrhoea may be a prominent feature, owing to large volumes of acid being secreted into the small intestine. Inactivation of the pancreatic lipase causes steatorrhoea. Complications of ulceration (pain, bleeding and stenosis) are common.

The diagnosis of Zollinger–Ellison is problematic, but ulceration in unusual sites, at an early age, or ulcers persisting despite medical treatment should be reviewed with a high index of suspicion and serum gastrin measured. CT or magnetic resonance imaging (MRI) and selective angiography may be used to localise the tumour; cure is achieved by removal of the tumour wherever possible, although this may be difficult.

Other factors

Other patients at risk of peptic ulceration include those with blood group O and those with hyperparathyroidism. Hyperparathyroidism causes elevated calcium levels, thus stimulating acid secretion. With treatment of the underlying condition, spontaneous ulcer healing usually occurs. Severe illness, trauma, prolonged mechanical ventilation, multiple organ failure, sepsis and major surgery may give rise to stress ulceration. Cushing's and Curling's ulcers are special forms of stress ulceration that occur following central nervous injury and burns, respectively. Ulcers resulting from hypersecretion are usually single and, in common with other forms of peptic ulceration, may be complicated by perforation and bleeding.

Clinical features

Recurrent well-localised epigastric pain is typical of peptic ulcer disease. Classically, the pain of a gastric ulcer occurs during eating and is relieved by vomiting. Patients with duodenal ulceration characteristically describe pain when they are hungry. This pain is relieved by food, antacids, milk and vomiting. Often, however, these well-defined features are not present, and it is usually impossible to differentiate between the symptoms of gastric and duodenal ulceration. Other symptoms associated with peptic ulcer disease include heartburn, anorexia, waterbrash (a sudden flow of saliva into the mouth) and intolerance of certain foods. Intermittent vomiting may occur. Where persistent vomiting is troublesome, the possibility of gastric outlet obstruction should be considered. Such vomiting may be projectile and contain recognisable undigested food eaten many hours previously.

Diagnosis

As already described, endoscopy and biopsy is essential in the diagnosis of peptic ulceration. In addition, *H. pylori* can be diagnosed using the CLO test; a biopsy specimen taken from the antrum is placed in a gel containing urea. Ammonia released by the action of the *H. pylori*-derived urease is detected and causes a colour change (in most kits, from yellow to pink/red). Biopsy of gastric ulcers is particularly important, as malignancy needs to be excluded.

Management of uncomplicated peptic ulcer disease

Medical management

General measures helpful in the management of peptic ulcers include the avoidance of NSAIDs, smoking and excessive alcohol. If NSAIDs cannot be avoided in patients with a history of peptic ulceration PPIs should be prescribed (e.g., omeprazole or lansoprazole). These agents act by irreversibly inhibiting H^+/K^+ ATPase and thus are powerful inhibitors of acid secretion.

Eradication of *H. pylori*

Duodenal ulcers

Eradication of the *H. pylori* has become the mainstay of management in patients with a duodenal ulcer (EBM 13.5). Eradication therapies comprise an antisecretory agent, typically a PPI, together with one or more antibiotics. This 'triple therapy' is usually given for 7 days followed by a healing dose of PPI for 4–6 weeks. Eradication rates of greater than 90% occur with good compliance, although reinfection following successful eradication is possible. Without eradication therapy, approximately 80% of ulcers will recur within 1 year. Complete resolution of symptoms is a good indicator of successful eradication. However, where symptoms persist, it is advisable to recheck the *H. pylori* status.

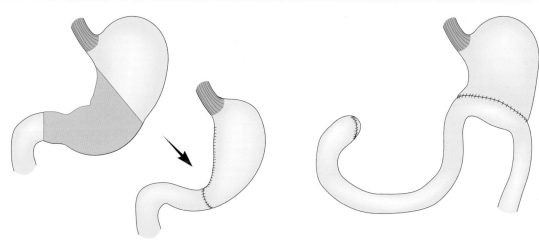

Fig. 13.20 Gastrectomy for peptic ulceration.

Gastric ulcers

Malignancy should be excluded by endoscopic biopsy before a diagnosis of benign gastric ulcer is made. Eradication therapy should be instituted for *H. pylori*-positive patients. Without eradication, the relapse rate is in the region of 50%, but this falls to less than 10% with successful eradication therapy. Endoscopic surveillance of a treated ulcer should continue until healing is complete. Failure to heal warrants further biopsies.

Surgical management

Duodenal ulceration

Surgery for uncomplicated duodenal ulceration is now extremely rare. Operations such as a truncal vagotomy, highly selective vagotomy, or gastric resectional surgery have had little role since the introduction of eradication therapy. The principle of these operations was: no acid, no ulcer. Both vagotomy and antrectomy reduce acid secretion. When combined they had the lowest recurrence rates at the cost of increased morbidity and mortality. Definitive procedures for peptic ulcer in the setting of perforated peptic ulcer are not recommended today.

Gastric ulceration

Failure of conservative therapy to heal a gastric ulcer is an indication for surgical intervention. Where malignancy cannot be excluded or is suspected, resection of the ulcer is the treatment of choice. The extent and type of resection will be determined by the position of the ulcer within the stomach and its suspected malignant potential.

Benign distal ulcers may be treated by a Billroth I gastrectomy, whereby the distal part of the stomach is removed and the proximal stump anastomosed to the duodenum. More proximal ulcers usually necessitate a Polya-type reconstruction involving anastomosis of the gastric remnant to the jejunum (Fig. 13.20).

Many patients who had surgery for ulcer disease in the 1960s and 70s are still alive today and suffer long-term side effects similar to those experienced by patients having a gastrectomy for cancer such as dumping syndrome, abdominal pain after eating and diarrhoea.

Complications of peptic ulceration requiring operative intervention

The complications that necessitate surgery include:
- perforation
- bleeding
- obstruction.

Perforation

Duodenal ulcers

Up to 50% of patients will have had no previous ulcer symptoms and for this reason duodenal ulcer perforation remains a common surgical emergency. The overall incidence of duodenal ulcer perforation is decreasing, probably due in part to improvements in the medical management of duodenal ulcers. Perforation usually occurs in acute ulcers on the anterior wall of the duodenum.

Gastric ulcers

Gastric ulcer perforation is less common than duodenal ulcer perforation. It has a peak incidence in the elderly, and consequently the associated morbidity and mortality are higher. Gastric perforation has a strong association with NSAID use.

Clinical features

The acute onset of severe unremitting epigastric pain is strongly suggestive of the possibility of perforation. Thereafter, the range of symptoms depends on the intraabdominal course. The patient may be pale, shocked and peripherally shut down secondary to

13

generalised peritonitis. Irritant stomach contents in the peritoneal cavity may give rise to shoulder-tip pain, resulting from diaphragmatic irritation. Vomiting may occur. The abdomen does not move freely with respiration, and marked tenderness, guarding, fear of movement and board-like rigidity may be found on examination. Respiration is shallow and bowel sounds are usually absent. Shock is frequently seen in patients presenting late in a moribund state, especially in the developing world.

Generalised peritonitis does not occur in some patients because the perforation seals over with omentum. In others, the fluid tracks down the right paracolic gutter, simulating acute appendicitis. Silent perforations may also occur, and are only found incidentally on a chest x-ray.

Diagnosis

In 60% of cases of perforation, an erect chest x-ray will demonstrate free air under the diaphragm, although the absence of free air does not exclude a perforation (see Fig. 13.5). A lateral decubitus film can be useful where an erect chest x-ray is not feasible, e.g., because of shock or disability.

Moderate hyperamylasaemia may be found with a perforated duodenal ulcer but high amylase levels are more suggestive of acute pancreatitis. Where there is doubt, an emergency water-soluble contrast meal or an abdominal CT may be indicated.

Management

The initial management, as for other causes of peritonitis, consists of resuscitation, oxygen therapy, intravenous fluids, broad-spectrum antibiotics, and the passage of a nasogastric tube. Several litres of fluid may be needed to correct dehydration from 'third space loss'. Intravenous opiate analgesia and PPIs should be given as necessary. A urinary catheter enables close monitoring of urine output.

Operative management is usually indicated although patients who do not have generalised peritoneal signs or systemic sepsis may be successfully managed conservatively so long as frequent reassessment shows no deterioration in their condition. Surgeons are increasingly using a laparoscopic approach to treatment but open surgery should not be considered inferior.

Duodenal ulcers

Surgery involves simple closure, whereby the ulcer is plugged using a pedicled omental patch (Fig. 13.21), coupled with a thorough peritoneal lavage. If the omentum is necrotic in neglected cases, the round ligament of the liver is a good substitute. All patients should receive 72 hours of intravenous PPI therapy and *H. pylori* eradication therapy for 2–3 weeks, followed by a healing course of oral PPIs. OGD is performed 6–8 weeks later to establish healing of the ulcer.

Gastric ulcers

Approximately 15% of perforated gastric ulcers prove ultimately to be malignant. However, current practice suggests biopsy of the ulcer wall, followed by simple closure or local excision of the ulcer, is the least complicated procedure and probably the safest. However, large prepyloric ulcers or those close to the lesser curvature pose a significant challenge due to their size and location, and distal gastrectomy provides a better chance of primary healing. If the ulcer turns out to be malignant, a formal gastric resection should be performed following tumour staging (see later).

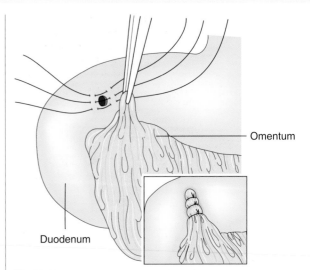

Fig. 13.21 Closure of perforated duodenal ulcer.

Omentum

Duodenum

 13.3 Summary

Peptic ulcer disease

- *Helicobacter pylori* is the most important cause: eradicate it
- NSAID medication next commonest cause
- Surgery now only for complications (bleeding, perforation, gastric outlet obstruction)
- Always biopsy a gastric ulcer: some will be malignant
- If an ulcer fails to heal with medical therapy look for rare causes (i.e., ZE).

Acute haemorrhage

The differential diagnosis of upper gastrointestinal bleeding is summarised in Table 13.2. Upper gastrointestinal bleeding presents with haematemesis (vomiting blood) and/or melaena (the passage of black tarry stool that has a very characteristic smell). Melaena results from the digestion of blood by enzymes and

Table 13.2 Causes of upper gastrointestinal bleeding.

• Peptic ulceration	50%
• Mucosal lesions including gastritis, duodenitis and erosions	30%
• Duodenitis and erosions	
• Mallory-Weiss tear	5–10%
• Varices	5–10%
• Reflux oesophagitis	5%
• Angiodysplasia	2%
• Carcinoma	Uncommon
• Aortoduodenal fistula	Uncommon
• Dieulafoy syndrome (rupture of a large tortuous submucosal artery normally found in the body of the stomach)	Rare
• Coagulopathies	Uncommon

bacteria. Less commonly, melaena may be the result of a bleed from the right colon. Very rarely, if bleeding is very brisk, upper gastrointestinal bleeding may present as fresh rectal bleeding, in which case signs of cardiovascular instability are present. Slow chronic blood loss may be asymptomatic and detected on rectal examination by a positive faecal occult blood test.

Diagnosis

History and examination

Pointers to the diagnosis include the past medical history (peptic ulcer disease, previous bleeding, liver disease, previous surgery, coagulopathies), drug history (most importantly, NSAIDs and anti-coagulants) and social history (alcohol abuse).

Specific features to be looked for include those suggestive of acute substantial blood loss and shock (hypotension, tachycardia, tachypnoea and pallor), and signs of liver disease and portal hypertension (spider naevi, portosystemic shunting and bruising). The latter are particularly important, as variceal haemorrhage necessitates specific treatment.

Blood tests

The full blood count may be normal immediately after an acute bleed but will fall once haemodilution has occurred. The test may show anaemia, suggestive of more chronic blood loss. Urea is often high following a gastrointestinal bleed, due to the absorption of blood and its subsequent metabolism by the liver. Coagulation derangement occurs in the presence of significant liver disease.

Management

Resuscitation

Bleeding is now the most common cause of death from peptic ulcer disease and resuscitation is vital. Following the administration of high-flow oxygen, intravenous access is obtained and blood taken for the investigations noted above. A sample is also taken for blood cross-matching and intravenous fluids started.

A nasogastric tube is passed to monitor the bleeding and prevent aspiration. A urinary catheter is inserted. A central and arterial line may aid resuscitation. Volume replacement is gauged against pulse, blood pressure, urine output and central venous pressure. Over-transfusion or rapid transfusion in those with compromised cardiac function can lead to pulmonary oedema.

Detection and endoscopic treatment

The aims of management of bleeding peptic ulcers are to identify the bleeding point, arrest the bleeding (bleeding ceases spontaneously in 90% of patients) and prevent recurrence. Once resuscitation has occurred, endoscopy is used to detect the site of bleeding (Fig. 13.22), doing so in 80–90% of cases. The endoscopist should also have the necessary experience and training to attempt control of the bleeding using techniques such as adrenaline (epinephrine) 1:10,000 injection and application of heater probes and clips. Bleeding from the ulcer base, the presence of a visible vessel and adherent clot overlying the ulcer are features associated with a significantly increased risk of further bleeding.

If endoscopy does not identify the bleeding point, angiography should be used, but the limitation of this investigation is that it can only detect active bleeding of greater than 1 mL/min. In these

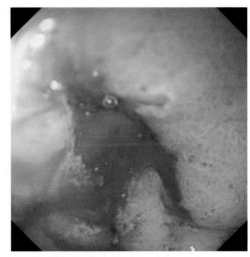

Fig. 13.22 Endoscopic view of bleeding duodenal ulcer.

patients, selective embolisation can be used to stop the bleeding and thus avoid the need for surgery.

Surgical management

Emergency surgery may be indicated if endoscopic therapy is unable to control the bleeding. However, this is becoming less common as hemostatic endoscopic techniques have improved and interventional radiology has become more readily available. Recurrent bleeding after therapeutic endoscopy may be controlled by a further endoscopy, but is associated with significant morbidity and mortality, particularly in the elderly. Continuing bleeding is particularly common in those with a chronic ulcer and is more common in gastric ulceration. The type of operation used depends on the site of the bleeding ulcer and the comorbidity of the patient. A bleeding duodenal ulcer may simply be under-run with sutures, through a duodenotomy (opening of the anterior wall of the duodenum). Once tolerating oral fluids, the patient should be started on *H. pylori* eradication therapy empirically. A bleeding gastric ulcer must always be biopsied to determine its nature. In young fit patients, the ulcer should be excised completely by taking a small wedge resection. In elderly patients or those with significant comorbidity, under-running of the ulcer may be preferable. If the pathology confirms malignancy, the patient should have accurate staging and further treatment as indicated. *H. pylori* eradication is indicated for benign ulcers.

Obstruction

Benign gastric outlet obstruction may be a sequel of peptic ulcer disease and may present with vomiting of undigested food. The vomiting is characteristically non-bile-stained. The clinical features include a palpable dilated stomach, succussion splash in the epigastrium and the presence of visible gastric peristalsis from the left to right in the upper abdomen. Management includes adequate resuscitation, normalisation of electrolyte and acid–base abnormalities, nasogastric suction and washout. A subsequent OGD is mandatory to rule out carcinoma of the stomach. Surgical treatment will involve a gastrojejunostomy, performed by open or laparoscopic access.

Gastric neoplasia

Benign gastric neoplasms

Benign tumours of the stomach may arise from epithelial or mesenchymal tissue. Adenomatous polyps may be single or multiple and are the most common benign epithelial neoplasm. Gastrointestinal stromal tumours (GISTs) arise from the pacemaker cells in the gastric wall and have a variable natural history. Diagnosis is usually by endoscopy and EUS; biopsies are rarely helpful as the lesions are submucosal. Small asymptomatic GISTs (up to 2 cm diameter) can safely be left alone but larger ones should be either kept under surveillance (2–5 cm) or resected (>5 cm). Symptomatic gastric GISTs (bleeding, pain, obstruction) should usually be resected (Fig. 13.23) and laparoscopic techniques are often possible.

Malignant gastric neoplasms

Gastric carcinoma

Epidemiology

Adenocarcinoma is the most common malignancy affecting the stomach. It accounts for 90% of malignant tumours found within the stomach; lymphomas, carcinoids and gastrointestinal stromal tumours make up the rest. The incidence of gastric cancer has decreased substantially in the last 50 years. Gastric cancer

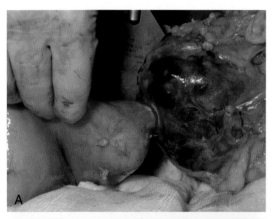

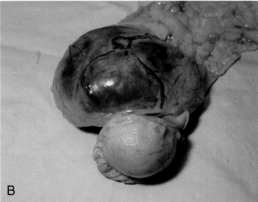

Fig. 13.23 **(A)** Large dumb-bell shaped gastric gastrointestinal stromal tumour lesion in situ. **(B)** Lesion resected showing intact gastric mucosa over its luminal aspect.

principally affects those in the 60–80-year age group, but is not infrequently seen in younger patients. Where once the tumour was more commonly noted in the gastric antrum, its incidence in this region has diminished and a corresponding increase in incidence in the proximal stomach has occurred. The Indian scenario is similar; the incidence of proximal gastric cancers is on the increase but distal gastric cancers are still more common. Although proximal gastric cancers are associated with GORD and Barrett's change, distal gastric cancers have a strong association with *H. pylori* infection. The male/female ratio is 2:1. Gastric cancer has the fifth poorest 5-year survival rate after cancer of the pancreas, liver, oesophagus and lung.

Aetiology

- *Diet.* Gastric cancer is noted more commonly where malnutrition is prevalent. It has also been associated with the use of certain preservatives in food; nitrates, nitrites and nitrosamines have been implicated. Where soils are rich in nitrates or dietary intake is high, gastric carcinoma is more common. A high vitamin intake is thought to be protective against the development of cancer of the stomach. Diets rich in carotene and vitamins C and E have been shown to reduce the incidence of intestinal metaplasia in the stomach, a condition thought to be associated with malignant change.
- *H. pylori infection.* Recent epidemiological studies have suggested that *H. pylori* may be associated with an increased incidence of malignant change within the stomach (EBM 13.6). At the present time, it is thought that its ability to produce ammonia as well as other mutagenic chemicals may play a part in neoplastic transformation of the gastric mucosa. Chronic *H. pylori* infection leads to atrophic gastritis, which is characterised histologically by the loss of specialised gastric glands and thinning of the mucosa. There is also a simultaneous inflammatory response in the gastric mucosa, which leads on to intestinal metaplasia (of colonic type). This is considered as an irreversible change that progresses to malignancy in the presence of favourable factors.
- *Gastric polyps.* Hyperplastic and adenomatous polyps are the most frequently found, but only the latter have significant malignant potential. Studies have shown that over one-quarter of adenomatous polyps may show malignant changes within them. Furthermore, gastric carcinoma is frequently encountered in stomachs affected by polyps.
- *Gastroenterostomy.* Where there has been a previous gastric resection or duodenal bypass for benign disease and the remaining stomach has been anastomosed to the bile-containing upper gastrointestinal tract, the stomach remnant is more vulnerable to malignant change than the intact stomach. The risk of malignant change increases with the time elapsed since surgery. Patients who have had gastric resections with gastroenterostomy may be 4–5 times more liable to develop gastric carcinoma in the stomach remnant than the normal population.

EBM	13.6 The role of *H. pylori* eradication in the prevention of gastric cancer

'RCTs have found that Helicobacter eradication reduces the risk of developing gastric cancer as long as premalignant lesions do not pre-exist at the time of eradication.'

Ley C et al. Cancer Epidemiol Biomarkers Prev. 2004;13:4–10; Wong BC et al. JAMA. 2004;291:187–94.

- *Chronic atrophic gastritis.* This condition is associated with a loss of the gastric glands from the stomach mucosa. It has been noted to be more frequent in patients at increased risk of developing stomach cancer. Chronic atrophic gastritis is associated with pernicious anaemia, which is linked to an increased risk of gastric cancer. Such patients have a four-fold increased risk compared with the normal population.
- *Intestinal metaplasia.* This condition arises when the gastric mucosa is replaced by mucosa containing glands that have features more in common with those found in the small intestine. Such changes are usually found in the distal part of the stomach and are associated with an increased risk of development of gastric carcinoma.
- *Gastric dysplasia.* When the gastric mucosal cells become less uniform in size, shape and organisation, dysplastic changes may result and may be low or high grade. Patients with high-grade dysplasia often have associated malignant change.
- *Hereditary diffuse gastric cancer*: Inherited mutations of the E-cadherin gene can result in an aggressive form of signet ring gastric adenocarcinoma affecting young patients. Once symptomatic these patients are rarely curable. Consequently, patients with a strong family history of gastric cancer should be referred for genetic counselling and, if appropriate, offered endoscopic surveillance and/or a prophylactic total gastrectomy.

Early gastric cancer

Early gastric cancer (EGC) results when neoplastic cells are limited to the mucosa or submucosal layers of the stomach wall. This type of cancer is confined to the most superficial layers of the stomach wall and is independent of the occurrence of lymph node metastasis (which can be present in a small minority of patients). EGCs are classified by their endoscopic appearance according to Murakami as elevated, depressed and combined types. The histologic classification (Lauren) is of intestinal and diffuse types. EGCs are amenable to local therapies such as endoscopic mucosal resection and ablative therapies such as argon plasma coagulation. Surgical treatments include laparoscopic or open resections. Such tumours, if adequately treated surgically, are associated with 5-year survival rates in excess of 90%. The survival rate will depend upon the depth of invasion of the tumour and the presence or absence of lymph node metastases at the time of surgical excision. Early gastric cancer in the UK accounts for approximately 10% of all resected cases of gastric adenocarcinoma whereas in Japan (a high incidence country for gastric cancer) it makes up well over 50%. The explanation for this is multifactorial but includes the Japanese public's awareness of the symptoms of gastric cancer and a national screening programme to detect early disease.

Advanced gastric cancer

The vast majority of malignant gastric tumours found in Western countries are locally advanced gastric adenocarcinomas. These tumours have invaded into the muscularis propria and sometimes through to the serosa. The risk of peritoneal metastases and lymphovascular invasion is much higher than for early tumours. Advanced gastric tumours often invade the adjacent gastric wall via submucosal lymphatics creating a diffusely thickened and rigid stomach (linitis plastica) (Fig. 13.24). Invasion into adjacent structures such as the pancreas can also occur (Fig. 13.25)

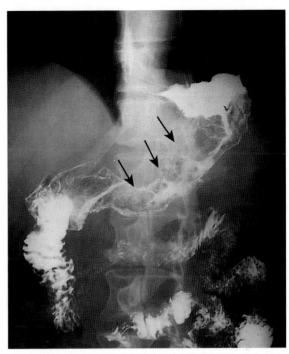

Fig. 13.24 Barium meal showing extensive gastric carcinoma with narrowing of the lumen (*arrowed*).

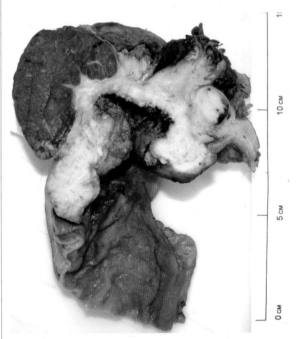

Fig. 13.25 Resection specimen showing invasion of a gastric cancer into the tail of the pancreas. The spleen has been removed en bloc with the stomach and distal pancreas.

Factors affecting survival in advanced gastric cancer

The survival of patients with advanced gastric cancer depends upon the stage of the tumour at presentation and on the general fitness of the patient. Treatment with curative intent implies surgical resection, increasingly combined with perioperative chemotherapy. For surgery to be curative, excision of the primary tumour must be adequate, with margins clear of the tumour and with satisfactory en bloc resection of all possible involved lymph nodes (EBM 13.7).

EBM | **13.7 D1 versus D2 (radical) lymph node dissection in gastric cancer**

'*Subgroup analysis suggests a survival benefit for T_3 and T_4 tumours with more radical surgery. Learning curves of surgeons and centres performing low-volume cancer surgery may confound any benefit of more radical surgery.*'

McCulloch P et al. Cochrane Database Syst Rev. 2004;CD001964.

Poor survival has been correlated with depth of tumour invasion through the stomach wall, involvement of tumour resection margins and the presence of lymph node metastases. Transgression of the tumour through the stomach wall is associated with poor survival, as the tumour is able to spread transperitoneally and therefore seed the peritoneum with malignant cells, making complete surgical excision impossible.

A comprehensive pathological classification of tumours has enabled the prognosis of a particular stage of cancer to be estimated. Such staging is usually classified according to the tumour size (T), the node status (N), and the presence or absence of distant metastases (M) (Table 13.3).

Clinical features of gastric malignancy

The symptomatology of gastric carcinoma may be subtle, and mild symptoms of indigestion, flatulence or dyspepsia may be the early signs of malignancy. Such symptoms should not be overlooked and should not be treated without further investigation, particularly in patients in a vulnerable age group (>40 years). More advanced gastric cancer tends to be associated with weight loss, anaemia, dysphagia, vomiting, epigastric or back pain, or the presence of an epigastric mass. The patient may also manifest signs of more widespread distant metastases, such as jaundice (liver secondaries or compression of the biliary tree by enlarged lymph nodes), ascites, spurious diarrhoea (secondary to pelvic infiltration), and signs and symptoms of intestinal obstruction secondary to malignant deposits on the bowel.

Diagnosis

Diagnosis is made on the basis of a thorough medical history, clinical examination and an upper gastrointestinal endoscopy and biopsy. Following histological diagnosis the patient should meet with an experienced clinician to be told their diagnosis in an appropriate environment preferably with the support of a family member and a specialist upper GI nurse. Patients deemed potentially fit enough for radical therapy should have a series of staging investigations.

Staging of gastric carcinoma

- *CT:* Any patient with a histological diagnosis of gastric cancer should undergo a CT of their chest, abdomen and pelvis unless they are very frail. This should provide information about the M-stage (liver, lung, peritoneum and distant nodes) and can help exclude T4 involvement of adjacent structures such as the pancreas.
- *EUS:* EUS is excellent at determining T-stage. High frequency probes (10 MHz or more) can accurately differentiate between T1–2 disease and add information of local nodal status (N-Stage). EUS is of limited value in advanced gastric cancer.
- *Staging laparoscopy:* This procedure is essential in patients with locally advanced tumours to detect small volume peritoneal and liver metastases that cannot be detected by CT (Fig. 13.26). Peritoneal washings are also helpful as patients with positive peritoneal cytology for malignancy have a very poor prognosis and rarely benefit from surgery.
- *PET-CT:* Gastric adenocarcinomas are not always PET-avid. This limits the application of PET as a routine staging procedure looking for metastatic disease.

Treatment with curative intent

All patients should be discussed by a multidisciplinary upper GI team. Those with potentially curable disease who are deemed fit enough for radical therapy have the following options:

- *Surgery alone*: Patient with early gastric cancer should undergo a distal (subtotal) or total D2 gastrectomy

Table 13.3 TNM classification of gastric carcinoma[a]	
T (Tumour)	
T_1	Tumour invades lamina propria or submucosa
T_2	Tumour invades muscularis propria
T_3	Tumour invades subserosa
T_4	Tumour invades serosa or adjacent structures
N (Node)	
N_0	No lymph node involvement
N_1	1–2 lymph nodes involved by tumour
N_2	3–6 lymph nodes involved by tumour
N_3	More than 7 lymph nodes involved by tumour
M (Metastases)	
M_0	No metastases
M_1	Metastases present (includes positive peritoneal cytology)

[a]AJCC/UICC Classification, 2010.

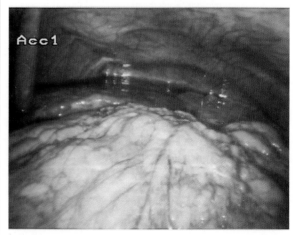

Fig. 13.26 Staging laparoscopy showing omental metastases and ascites secondary to advanced gastric cancer.

(depending upon the site of the tumour) done by an experienced surgeon working in a high-volume cancer centre. The nomenclature of the nodal stations used by the Japanese Research Society of Gastric Cancer (JRSGC) ranges from 1 to 16. Groups 1 to 6 are called N1 nodes (first tier nodes or perigastric lymph nodes) and groups 7 to 12 are N2 nodes (second tier nodes along the named gastric arteries). A 'D2' gastrectomy refers to the excision of both the first tier of perigastric lymph nodes and the second tier of nodes along the gastric arteries (Fig. 13.27). Reconstruction is usually by Roux-en-Y to prevent bile reflux (Fig. 13.28). When oncologically safe to do so, a distal gastrectomy is preferable to a total gastrectomy as it gives a better quality of life.

- *Combined therapy*: Randomised clinical trials in the UK have shown improved survival for patients who have perioperative chemotherapy and surgery compared with those who have surgery alone. The effect seems most pronounced for advanced tumours; the neoadjuvant or preoperative component of the chemotherapy seems to have the biggest impact on survival (EBM 13.8). The chemotherapeutic agents used include epirubicin, cisplatin and 5-fluorouracil. Newer agents such as oxaliplatin, cepcetabine and bevacizamab can improve survival further.

<table>
<tr><td>**EBM**</td><td>**13.8 Combination surgery and chemotherapy in gastric cancer**</td></tr>
</table>

'In patients with operable gastric or lower esophageal adenocarcinomas, a perioperative regimen of ECF decreased tumor size and stage and significantly improved progression-free and overall survival.'

Cunningham D et al. Perioperative chemotherapy versus surgery alone for resectable gastroesophageal cancer. N Engl J Med. 2006;355:11–20.

Palliation

- *Best supportive care*: Some patients are too frail for any anticancer therapy and all focus should be on relieving their symptoms and supporting them and their families through their terminal illness. Nausea and vomiting is treated with antiemetics such as cyclizine or ondansetron. Poor appetite may respond to steroids such as dexamethasone. Pain often requires opiate analgesia. Eating can be particularly difficult for patients with advanced gastric cancer and dietetic support is essential. Towards the end of life, the patient may need medication via a subcutaneous infusion from a portable syringe driver.
- *Palliative chemotherapy*: For patients who are fit enough, valuable improvements in quality of life can be achieved with palliative chemotherapy using combinations of drugs such as epirubicin, cisplatin and 5-fluorouracil. Life expectancy can be extended if the tumour is chemosensitive (EBM 13.9).
- *Palliative radiotherapy*: Bleeding from advanced gastric tumours can be troublesome and can be greatly reduced by a short course of external beam radiation.
- *Stenting*: Patients with gastric outlet obstruction who have persistent vomiting may benefit from the endoscopic placement of a self-expanding metallic stent although results are unpredictable.

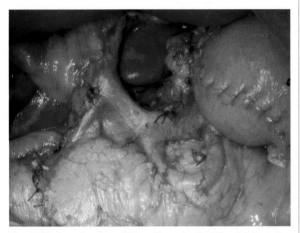

Fig. 13.27 Operative view of the coeliac axis after D2 nodal dissection and removal of all lymph nodes.

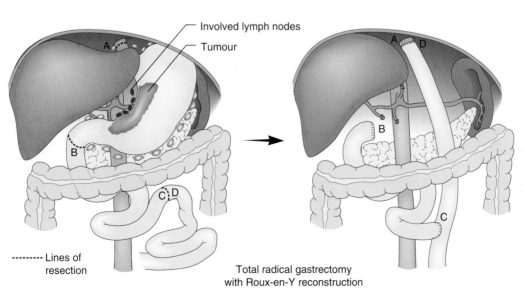

Involved lymph nodes
Tumour
Lines of resection
Total radical gastrectomy with Roux-en-Y reconstruction

Fig. 13.28 Total gastrectomy with curative intent.

202 • THE OESOPHAGUS, STOMACH AND DUODENUM

- *Palliative surgery*: Palliative surgery is indicated for obstruction and bleeding. Options include a gastric bypass (often done laparoscopically) for distal tumours, or palliative resection. The latter is a big undertaking for patients with incurable disease and should only be considered in fit patients with distal tumours who have not benefited from lesser interventions (Fig. 13.29). Palliative surgery should not be attempted in the presence of gross ascites or jaundice because of the poor outcome.

EBM | **13.9 The role of palliative chemotherapy in gastric cancer**

'Systematic reviews show a modest survival benefit for palliative chemotherapy in gastric cancer, with ECF (epirubicin, cisplatin and 5-fluorouracil) regimens currently amongst the more effective. Newer combinations with irinotecan- or taxane-based regimens show promising results.'

Wohrer SS et al. Ann Oncol. 2004;15:1585–95.

Prognosis

When the tumour is confined to the mucosa or submucosa without lymph node or distant metastases, 5-year survival of 95–100% can be achieved. With increasing penetration of the tumour through the stomach wall and increasing numbers of involved nodes, the 5-year survival decreases. When distant metastases are present, 5-year survival is unusual (Table 13.4).

Other gastric tumours

Lymphomas

The stomach represents the most common site for gastrointestinal lymphomas, malignant aggregations of lymphatic tissue. Many are thought to arise from mucosa-associated lymphoid tissue and are frequently referred to as MALT lymphomas. There is a frequent association with the presence of *H. pylori* infection, which is

Table 13.4 Examples of stages of gastric cancer and their prognosis

Stage	5-year survival (%)
$T_1N_0M_0$	95 +
$T_1N_1M_0$	70–80
$T_2N_1M_0$	45–50
$T_3N_2M_0$	15–25
M_1	0–10

thought to bring about lymphomatous change. Tumours are usually low-grade and may respond to eradication of the *H. pylori* infection. Occasionally, lymphomas may transform to a high-grade type of tumour that carries a poorer prognosis and require more aggressive treatment with chemotherapy. Surgery is reserved for specific indications such as perforation or bleeding.

Carcinoid tumours

These are tumours of neuroendocrine origin (classified as NET tumours) that vary enormously in their malignant potential. The majority are benign, but occasionally malignant carcinoids can behave aggressively. When associated with liver metastases, they can result in the carcinoid syndrome, which is related to the overproduction of 5-hydroxytryptamine.

⟳ | 13.4 Summary

Gastric cancer

- Curable if detected early
- Early symptoms similar to peptic ulcer
- Do not wait for 'alarm symptoms' to investigate: it is usually too late
- Multimodal therapy for advanced disease
- Good palliation for incurable disease can be challenging
- Rare inherited cases prevented by prophylactic gastrectomy.

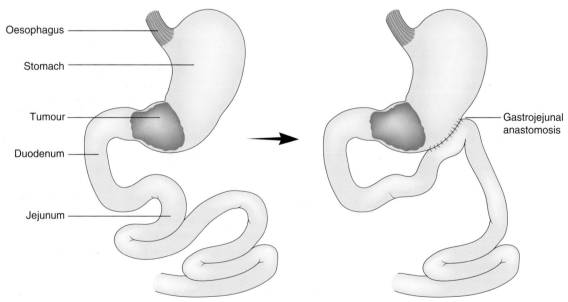

Fig. 13.29 Palliative bypass procedure (gastrojejunostomy) for obstructing distal gastric cancer.

Miscellaneous disorders of the stomach

Ménétrier's disease

This is a condition of gastric mucosal hypertrophy, in which the mucosal rugal folds are grossly enlarged in the fundus and body of the stomach; the antrum is usually spared. Mucosal hypertrophy may lead to abnormally large secretions of mucus or acid. Over-secretion of acid and protein-rich mucus may contribute to symptoms of epigastric pain and hypoproteinaemia.

Ménétrier's disease is associated with an increased incidence of malignancy in the stomach and once diagnosed, total gastrectomy should be considered in the fit patient.

Gastritis

This common condition is due to inflammation of the gastric mucosal lining. It may be caused by a variety of injurious agents, both chemical and bacteriological. It is frequently associated with over-indulgence in alcohol. Biliary gastritis is seen in the presence of bile in the stomach (frequently seen after Polya-type partial gastrectomy).

Gastritis may arise as a consequence of extreme stress resulting from shock, and is more frequently encountered in the intensive care situation. Such gastritis is thought to be a consequence of mucosal hypoperfusion and acidosis secondary to a shock-like state. This leads to mucosal ischaemia and stress gastritis with loss of mucosa causing erosions that may bleed profusely. Gastritis may be prevented by resuscitation, administering mucosal protective agents, and minimising gastric acid secretion. Surgery is undertaken rarely to control massive haemorrhage resulting from gastritis.

Dieulafoy's lesion

A condition of profuse bleeding from an abnormal vessel situated in the gastric mucosa and not associated with ulceration, Dieulafoy's lesion is usually found in the upper stomach. Such bleeding may require open gastrotomy and oversewing of the bleeding point if initial treatment by injection sclerotherapy is unsuccessful.

Bezoars

Accumulations of hair (trichobezoars) or vegetable matter (phytobezoars) or combinations of the two (trichophytobezoars) may form a complete cast of the stomach resulting in reduced nutritional intake and malnourishment. They are usually seen in females who eat their hair, which remains undigested. Diagnosis is made by barium examination and surgical removal of the bezoar through a gastrotomy is the optimum treatment (Fig. 13.30). Patients may need psychiatric evaluation and appropriate medical therapy.

Miscellaneous conditions of the duodenum

Duodenal obstruction

Common causes of duodenal obstruction are pyloric stenosis and carcinoma of the pancreas in developed countries but may include tuberculosis elsewhere. Rarer causes include blockage

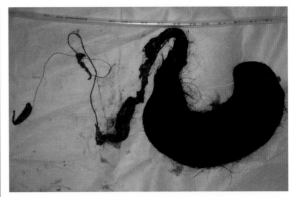

Fig. 13.30 Trichobezoar removed from the stomach of a young girl. Note the extension of the same into the duodenum and jejunum (Rapunzel syndrome).

by mesenteric lymph nodes, duodenal diverticulum, duodenal atresia, annular pancreas and chronic duodenal ileus. If surgical treatment is required, bypass by duodenojejunal or gastrojejunal anastomosis is often appropriate. Diverticula rarely develop before the age of 40 years and symptomatic lesions may have to be excised. Chronic duodenal ileus is an ill-defined entity that may affect visceroptotic females and rapidly growing, thin children. It has been suggested that the duodenum is obstructed by the superior mesenteric vessels as they cross its third part, but most surgeons are sceptical about this explanation. The condition is usually self-limiting in children, but in adults surgical bypass may have to be considered. Duodenal involvement is seen in 2–3% of cases of intestinal tuberculosis. Acute tubercular duodenal ulcers may be seen in the early stages on endoscopy in any part and must be subjected to biopsy. Ulcers heal with fibrosis, leading to stricture formation. Patients may present with features of pain and dyspepsia and in the later stages with symptoms and signs of gastric outlet or duodenal obstruction. A mass due to enlarged lymph nodes may sometimes be palpable. Barium meal and CT are diagnostic. Antitubercular treatment is the mainstay of management (see Chapter 16) with surgery reserved for persistent obstruction due to strictures.

Surgery for obesity

Obesity is an increasing problem worldwide. Previously thought to be a Western disease, affluence, poor eating habits and genetic predisposition have brought this problem to the developing world in large numbers. It is defined as a body mass index (BMI) greater than 30 kg/m^2; morbid obesity represents a BMI greater than 40. (The cut-off values for the Asian population have been modified to 28 and 38, respectively.) The effect of obesity on the respiratory, cardiovascular, locomotor and metabolic systems, as well as on mental health, can be severe. Patients with morbid obesity have a significantly reduced life expectancy; for example, a person with a BMI of 45 at the age of 25 will have a reduction in life expectancy of 11 years.

Prevention is better than cure. Weight reduction programmes combining reduced calorie intake with increased exercise have variable results. Weight loss is slow and the programme often requires to be followed for many, many months. Furthermore, a change in eating and exercising behaviour is necessary if the weight loss is to be maintained long term.

Patients who are morbidly obese can benefit from obesity or bariatric surgery. Such patients need to be assessed very carefully, taking account of their mental state, physical fitness, and

13

the presence of medical conditions that lead to obesity but can be corrected by treatment (e.g., hypothyroidism). The careful selection of patients involves a multidisciplinary team approach.

Current obesity surgery is designed to be restrictive or malabsorptive:

- *Restrictive*: decreases food intake, as the patient suffers early satiety even after small meals. Overeating causes upper abdominal pain, and vomiting may be required to relieve it.
- *Malabsorptive*: alters digestion, leading to food intake being poorly absorbed and eliminated in the stool. Overeating typically leads to excessive diarrhoea and flatulence.
- *Combined restrictive and malabsorptive*: this provides a combined effect of restrictive capacity with bypass of the proximal intestine.

Operations for obesity and related comorbidities

Surgical procedures are offered to patients with very high BMI or with lower BMI up to 35 (32 in Asian population) with severe medical comorbid conditions such as diabetes, hypertension, obstructive sleep apnoea, etc. Their resolution and the potential to 'cure' diabetes is referred to as 'metabolic surgery'. Current options include restrictive procedures like gastric banding and sleeve gastrectomy, a purely malabsorptive procedure such as a duodenal switch procedure, or a combination of a restrictive and malabsorptive procedure such as a gastric bypass procedure.

Increased acceptance of these operations has been seen in the last two decades as they can be performed laparoscopically. However, the technical difficulty of such surgery increases in the order that these operations are listed above. The more complex operations are more likely to lead to better excess weight loss in the short term. However, there is increasing evidence to show that although gastric banding is the safest procedure, it accomplishes lower weight loss and slower resolution of comorbidities in comparison to gastric bypass. Sleeve gastrectomy is presently being compared for its long-term efficacy with the gold standard procedure of gastric bypass. The procedures can be combined; for example, gastric banding is technically easier to perform in the very obese patient who has a BMI greater than 55. Once excess weight loss has plateaued, removing the band and performing a gastric bypass may allow further excess weight loss.

The gastric band is a ring with an inflatable inner cuff, which is placed laparoscopically a short distance below the oesophago-gastric junction, creating a small (approximately 50 mL) gastric pouch (Fig. 13.31A). The cuff can be inflated or deflated via

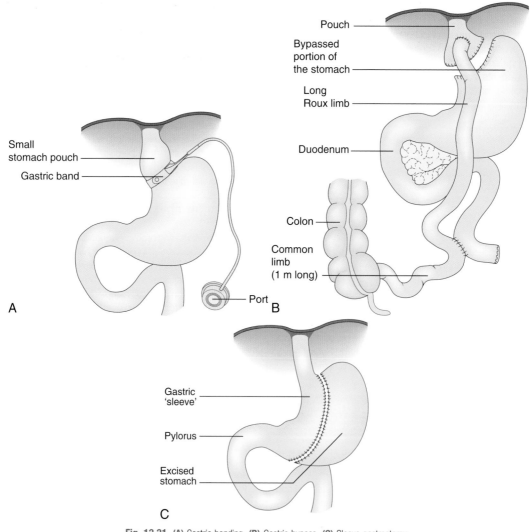

Fig. 13.31 **(A)** Gastric banding. **(B)** Gastric bypass. **(C)** Sleeve gastrectomy.

injections into a port site located in the subcutaneous tissues, in order to tighten or relax the cuff around the stomach. The tighter the cuff, the longer foodstuffs entering the gastric pouch will take to exit through the ring into the remainder of the stomach and intestinal tract, prolonging the feeling of satiety.

Gastric bypass involves stapling the stomach closed a short distance below the oesophagogastric junction (Fig. 13.31B). A Roux limb is brought up and anastomosed to the small proximal gastric remnant. Depending on the size of the pouch and calibre of the anastomosis, there will be a degree of restrictive activity, as well as a major malabsorptive element, as food will enter the distal jejunum and proximal ileum without exposure to bile or pancreatic and other digestive enzymes.

Sleeve gastrectomy has become extremely popular in the last 5 years and involves excision of the fundus and body of the stomach while retaining the pyloric antrum, thereby converting the stomach into a narrow tube with a volume of 100–150 mL (Fig 13.31C). The popularity stems from the ease of this procedure as a restrictive procedure that has shown weight loss comparable to gastric bypass. Most importantly, resolution of comorbidities occurs and there is always a possibility to combine it with a malabsorptive procedure like gastric bypass should the weight loss become static.

Vertical banded gastroplasty is rarely performed. Duodenal switch is a complex operation reserved for a minority of obese patients. Most patients with restrictive-type surgery find that they can eat more with time as the gastric remnant dilates. Hopefully, however, the target weight loss will have been achieved and improved eating habits established to allow maintenance of a healthier weight.

Complications of obesity surgery

Obesity increases the risk of all types of surgery: in particular, chest infection, deep venous thrombosis and wound infection. All procedures involving intestinal anastomoses, are prone to leakage, with resultant sepsis and peritonitis that can be life threatening. Such patients need a high index of suspicion for early recognition, drainage of the collection and relook if required together with intensive care management if necessary. Stricture of the anastomosis is managed with endoscopic dilatation and the use of stents.

Careful follow-up of patients by the multidisciplinary team is necessary, not only to monitor weight loss, but also to ensure that malnutrition of vitamins, trace elements, essential fatty acids and other important constituents of the diet does not occur. Patients who continue to eat chocolate and ice-cream to excess may not lose weight with the restrictive-type operations.

Most patients who lose significant weight will develop gallstones and, in some, cholecystectomy may be indicated at the same time as obesity surgery. Following significant weight loss, plastic surgery procedures may be necessary to remove excess skin, especially from the abdomen, thighs and arms.

13.5 Summary

Obesity surgery

- Different approaches (restrictive vs malabsorptive vs combination)
- Mostly laparoscopic now
- Clinically effective and cost efficient
- Extends life expectancy and improves quality of life
- Can 'cure' diabetes and other medical comorbidities.

13

Saxon Connor

The liver and biliary tract

Chapter contents

The liver 206

The gallbladder and bile ducts 219

The liver

Anatomy

The liver is the largest abdominal organ, weighing approximately 1500 g. It extends from the fifth intercostal space to the right costal margin. It is triangular in shape, its apex reaching the left midclavicular line in the fifth intercostal space. In the recumbent position, the liver is impalpable under cover of the ribs. The liver is attached to the undersurface of the diaphragm by suspensory ligaments that enclose a 'bare area', the only part of its surface without a peritoneal covering. Its inferior or visceral surface lies on the right kidney, duodenum, colon and stomach.

Topographically, the liver parenchyma is smooth and provides few external markings as clues to it underlying segmental anatomy. The leading edge of the falciform ligament running on the cranial surface contains a remnant of the embryological umbilical vein. It acts as external guide to the plane between segments 2/3 and 4. On its visceral surface the porta hepatis contains the draining extrahepatic biliary tree and dual vascular inflow (portal vein and hepatic artery) wrapped in a layer of loose connective tissue that separate segment 4 anteriorly and caudate lobe (segment 1) posteriorly. An imaginary line drawn over the cranial surface from the gallbladder to the termination of the middle hepatic vein into the inferior vena cava acts a guide to the principal plane separating the anatomical right and left hemilivers. (Fig. 14.1A). A detailed knowledge of the liver segmental anatomy, as defined by the distribution of its blood supply is important to the surgeon.

Segmental anatomy

The portal vein, hepatic artery and draining biliary tree are wrapped in a fibrous sheath and divide into right and left branches in the porta hepatis. Occluding the vascular inflow to either hemiliver produces an easily visible line of demarcation demonstrating the location of the principal plane, along which lies the draining middle hepatic vein. Each hemiliver is further divided into sectors and segments by a combination of branches of the vascular inflow and draining hepatic veins. The right hemiliver is divided into the right anterior and posterior sector (separated by the right hepatic vein) and then segments 8/5 (anterior sector) and 6/7 (posterior sector) by branches of the right hemiliver inflow. On the left side, three segments (2, 3, 4) are formed by branches of the left hemiliver inflow and drained by the left and middle hepatic vein. The caudate lobe (segment 1) lies across the inferior vena cava surrounded by the right and left hemiliver and is supplied by the vascular inflow from both hemilivers with corresponding biliary drainage (Fig. 14.1B).

Blood supply and function

The liver normally receives 1500 mL of blood per minute and has a dual blood supply, 75% coming from the portal vein and 25% from the hepatic artery, which supplies 50% of the oxygen requirements. The main venous drainage of the liver is by the right, middle and left hepatic veins, which enter the vena cava (Fig. 14.1B). In 25% of individuals, there is an inferior right hepatic vein. The venous drainage of the caudate lobe is by numerous small veins (short hepatics) emptying directly into the vena cava.

The functional unit of the liver is the hepatic acinus. Sheets of liver cells (hepatocytes) one cell thick are separated by interlacing sinusoids through which blood flows from the peripheral portal tract into the hepatic acinus to the central branch of the hepatic venous system. Bile is secreted by the liver cells and passes in the opposite direction along the small canaliculi into interlobular bile ducts located in the portal tracts (Fig. 14.2).

The liver has an important role in nutrient metabolism and is responsible for storing glucose as glycogen, or converting it to lactate for release into the systemic circulation. Amino acids are utilised for hepatic and plasma protein synthesis or catabolised to urea. The liver has a central role in the metabolism of lipids, bilirubin and bile salts, drugs and alcohol. It is the principal organ for storage of a number of minerals and vitamins, and is responsible for the production of the coagulation factors I, V, XI, the vitamin K-dependent factors II, VII, IX and X as well as proteins C and S and antithrombin. The liver is also the largest reticuloendothelial organ in the body and its Kupffer cells play a role in the removal of damaged red blood cells, bacteria, viruses and endotoxin, much of which enter the body from the gut.

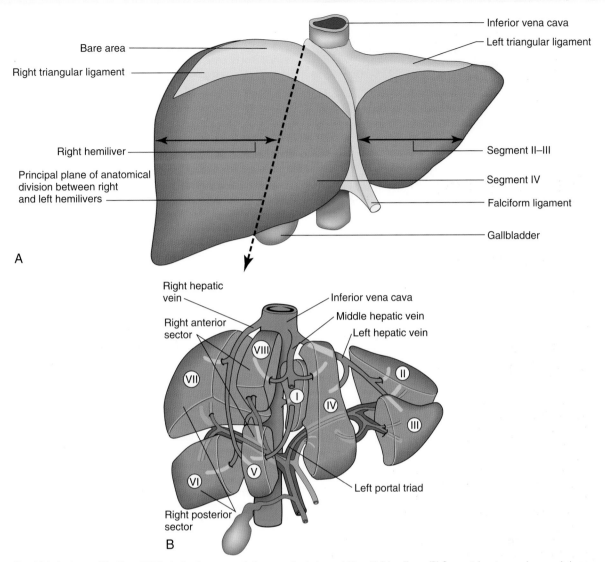

Fig. 14.1 **Anatomy of the liver.** **(A)** The broken line represents the separation between right and left hemilivers. **(B)** Segmental anatomy and venous drainage.

14

> ## ↻ 14.1 Summary
>
> **Surgical anatomy**
>
> - The liver is divisible into right and left hemilivers using a line running from the gallbladder fossa to the inferior vena cava
> - Each hemiliver receives a branch of the hepatic artery and portal vein; 75% of liver blood flow and 50% of its oxygen supply are provided by the portal vein
> - The hepatocytes are arranged in lobules, each of which has a central branch of the hepatic vein and peripheral portal tracts (containing a branch of the hepatic artery, portal vein and bile duct)
> - Understanding segmental liver anatomy allows the surgeon to perform anatomical resections ranging from individual segmentectomy through to extended resections taking up to 70% of the liver parenchyma.

Jaundice

Jaundice is caused by an increase in the level of circulating bilirubin and becomes obvious in the skin and sclera when levels exceed 50 µmol/L (Fig. 14.3). It may result from excessive destruction of red cells (*haemolytic jaundice*), from failure to remove bilirubin from the bloodstream (*hepatocellular jaundice*),

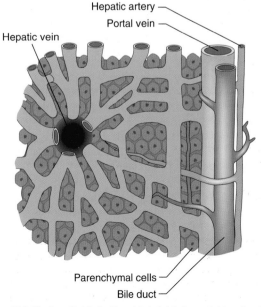

Fig. 14.2 **The hepatic lobule.** Sinusoids drain into the central hepatic vein.

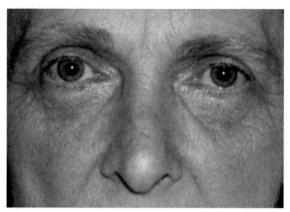

Fig. 14.3 Patient demonstrating the features of jaundiced skin and sclera.

or from obstruction to the flow of bile from the liver (*cholestatic or obstructive jaundice*) (Fig. 14.4). Congenital nonhaemolytic hyperbilirubinaemia (Gilbert's syndrome) is a relatively rare cause of jaundice due to defective bilirubin transport; the jaundice is usually mild and transient, and the prognosis is excellent.

To the surgeon, the most important type of *haemolytic jaundice* is that caused by hereditary spherocytosis, in which splenectomy may be necessary (Chapter 15). Haemolytic jaundice may also occur after blood transfusion and after operative or accidental trauma, when haematoma formation produces a pigment load that exceeds hepatic excretory capacity.

Hepatocellular jaundice is usually a medical rather than a surgical condition, although its recognition in patients presenting with abdominal pain is important, as surgical intervention may aggravate the hepatocellular injury.

Cholestatic jaundice due to intrahepatic obstruction of bile canaliculi may be a feature of acute and chronic liver disease. Examples include drugs such as antibiotics, antituberculosis and HIV therapies. This form of jaundice must be differentiated from that due to extrahepatic obstruction, the causes of which have the most surgical relevance. Extrahepatic obstruction most commonly results from gallstones or cancer of the head of the pancreas. Other causes can be broken down into lesions of the lumen, lesions of the wall or extrinsic compression. Examples of luminal causes include parasitic infection or medically placed stents. Examples of lesions of the wall include primary neoplastic lesions such as cholangio or ampullary carcinoma, inflammatory lesions such as primary sclerosing cholangitis, postsurgical strictures or autoimmune disease or congenital lesions such as choledochal cysts. Extrinsic compression can result from neoplastic lesions such as metastatic nodal disease, inflammatory pseudocysts or chronic pancreatitis.

Diagnosis

History and clinical examination

An accurate, rapid diagnosis of the cause of jaundice allows prompt institution of appropriate treatment (Fig. 14.5). The age, sex, occupation, social habits, drug and alcohol intake, history of injections or infusions, and general demeanour of the patient must be considered. A history of intermittent pain, fluctuant jaundice and dyspepsia suggests calculous obstruction of the common bile duct, whereas a history of weight loss and relentless progressive jaundice favours a diagnosis of neoplasia. Obstructive jaundice is likely if there is a history of passage of dark urine

and pale stools, and if the patient complains of pruritus (owing to an inability to secrete bile salts into the obstructed biliary system). Hepatocellular jaundice is likely if there are stigmata of chronic liver disease, such as palmar erythema, spider naevi, testicular atrophy and gynaecomastia. The abdomen must be examined for evidence of hepatomegaly or gallbladder distension (not usually found with gallstones), and for signs of portal hypertension such as splenomegaly, ascites and large collateral veins (caput medusae) in the abdominal wall.

Biochemical and haematological investigations

Haemolytic jaundice is suggested if there are high circulating levels of unconjugated bilirubin but no bilirubin in the urine. Serum concentrations of liver enzymes are normal in these circumstances and the appropriate haematological investigations should be done.

In jaundice due to biliary obstruction, the circulating bilirubin is conjugated by the liver and rendered water-soluble; it can then be excreted in the urine and gives it a dark colour. As bile cannot pass into the gastrointestinal tract, the stool becomes pale and urobilinogen is absent from the urine. Obstruction increases the formation of alkaline phosphatase from the cells lining the biliary canaliculi, producing raised serum levels. It is believed that bile acids may act to solubilise membranes and thus promote the release of alkaline phosphatase. The increased levels correlate with the severity of luminal obstruction and are used as a better estimate of bile flow patency postoperatively even when bilirubin levels have normalised. This rise precedes that of bilirubin and its fall is more gradual once obstruction is relieved. Serum transaminase and lactic dehydrogenase levels may rise in obstruction. Conversely, swelling of the parenchyma in hepatocellular jaundice frequently produces an element of intrahepatic biliary obstruction and a modest rise in serum alkaline phosphatase concentration.

Full blood count and coagulation screen should be undertaken as a matter of routine and viral status should be determined. Anaemia may signify occult blood loss, and a low white cell or platelet count may indicate hypersplenism due to portal hypertension. Prolongation of the prothrombin time may be present in both hepatocellular and cholestatic jaundice.

Radiological investigations

If the clinical picture and biochemical investigations suggest that jaundice is obstructive, radiological techniques can be used to define the site and nature of the obstruction.

Ultrasonography

In skilled hands, this key investigation is safe, noninvasive and reliable using ultrasound wave echoes reflected from tissues at various depths and described as hyperechoic or hypoechoic compared to that of the liver (or spleen when the liver is abnormal due to cirrhosis). It is used to define whether the patient has bile duct dilatation or gallbladder distension due to obstruction. Obstructive or surgical jaundice is diagnosed by the presence of dilated intrahepatic biliary radicles that the sonologist can follow distally to determine the level of obstruction. The cause of obstruction may also become clear. In the case of tumours, the presence of regional lymphadenopathy, liver metastases and free fluid will help in avoiding expensive and invasive investigations. Ultrasonography will also detect gallstones (seen as a hyperechoic lesion casting a classic 'acoustic shadow') and space-occupying lesions in the liver and pancreas, although overlying bowel gas may prevent a clear view of the pancreas. For the same reason, stones in a dilated common bile duct may not always be seen clearly.

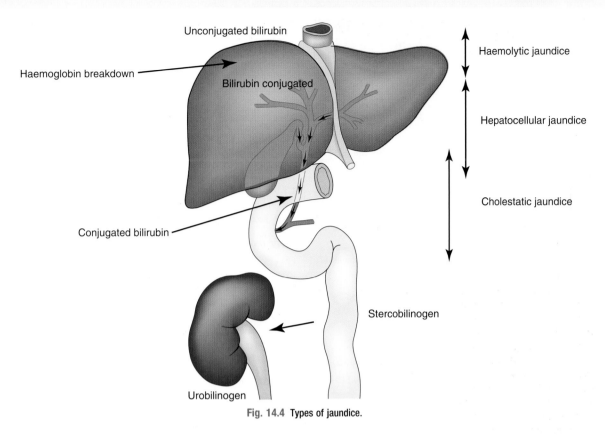

Fig. 14.4 Types of jaundice.

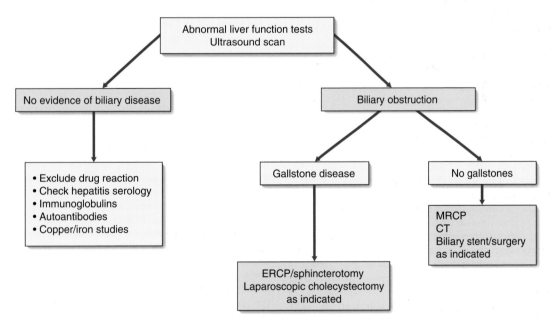

Fig. 14.5 **Investigation of the jaundiced patient.** *CT,* Computed tomography; *ERCP,* endoscopic retrograde cholangiopancreatography; *MRCP,* magnetic resonance cholangiopancreatography.

Magnetic resonance imaging (MRI)

Magnetic resonance cholangiopancreatography (MRCP) has largely replaced other forms of invasive radiological imaging of the bile duct and pancreas. MRI has the advantage that it does not introduce infection into an obstructed biliary system or the pancreatic duct. This is important in patients presenting with symptoms suggestive of malignant obstructive jaundice. The T2-weighted MRI scans are reconstructed by software to show the entire biliary tree with luminal stones or obstruction seen as filling defects amidst the biliary secretions, seen as white in the absence of any contrast (Fig. 14.6). MRCP is performed without contrast and therefore is only useful for assessment of stones. To

14

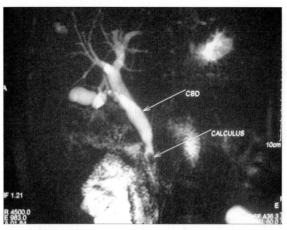

Fig. 14.6 Magnetic resonance cholangiopancreatography showing a stone in the common bile duct seen as a filling defect. *CBD*, common bile duct.

fully stage hepatic, biliary or pancreatic tumours invading the biliary tree, contrast is required to obtain arterial, portal venous and delayed hepatobiliary phases.

Endoscopic retrograde cholangiopancreatography (ERCP)

ERCP is now restricted to therapeutic indications. It outlines the biliary and pancreatic systems by injecting contrast through a cannula inserted into the papilla of Vater by means of a side-viewing endoscope passed into the duodenum. It gives more detailed information than ultrasonography and allows endoscopic extraction of common bile duct stones, biopsy of periampullary tumours, and relief of obstructive jaundice by stent insertion. Distal obstructions are more amenable for stenting than proximal or hilar obstructions. Stenting should be performed only in the presence of uncontrolled sepsis or for malignant lesions when an operation is considered inappropriate. The investigation may be complicated by acute pancreatitis, and prophylactic antibiotics should be administered to reduce the risk of cholangitis for complex interventions. Haemorrhage and perforation are less frequent complications.

Percutaneous transhepatic cholangiography (PTC)

With the advent of MRCP and high level of technical success associated with ERCP, PTC is restricted to a therapeutic role for proximal biliary lesions or when ERCP has failed for distal lesions or cannot be used due to anatomical considerations. Access to the biliary system is achieved by a slim flexible needle passed into the liver under ultrasound and fluoroscopic guidance. Injecting contrast while withdrawing the needle under fluoroscopic guidance achieves access to the dilated intrahepatic biliary radicles. A positioned catheter can provide external drainage of the bile or the obstructing lesion can be crossed with a drain or stent. Alternatively, a wire can be placed through the ampulla allowing a rendezvous procedure to be performed via ERCP. Complications of PTC include bleeding, bile leakage, bacteraemia and renal dysfunction. Hence coagulation status must be checked, antibiotic cover should be given and the patient should be well hydrated prior to the procedure. The procedure is considered unsafe in the presence of ascites, bleeding disorders and hepatic hydatidosis.

Computed tomography (CT)

Contrast enhanced CT can be used to identify and stage hepatic, bile duct and pancreatic tumours in jaundiced patients. It often demonstrates the dilated biliary tree to the level of the obstruction, vascular abnormality or invasion and may show dissemination to adjacent lymph nodes or distant viscera or peritoneum. It is also used to diagnose acute pancreatitis (in cases where there is doubt) and assess viability of pancreatic tissue in severe pancreatitis.

Other radiological investigations

Positron emission tomography (PET-CT) has found an increasing role in staging hepatobiliary and pancreatic (HBP) malignancy. Isotopic liver scanning has been superseded by ultrasonography and CT. Selective angiography has been largely superseded by CT and MRI assessment of vascular anatomy but may be used for embolisation of tumours or haemorrhagic complications of HBP disease.

Liver biopsy

Liver biopsy may be considered in patients with unexplained jaundice, in whom an obstructing lesion has been excluded radiologically. 'Targeted' liver biopsy can be conducted under ultrasound or CT guidance. Prothrombin time, platelet count and hepatitis B surface antigen (HBsAg) status must always be determined, and clotting abnormalities should be corrected before biopsy is undertaken. Ascites remains an absolute contraindication to perform any type of liver puncture.

Laparoscopy

Laparoscopy under general anaesthesia may be used in the evaluation of liver disease. In selected patients with malignancy of the liver, pancreas and biliary tree, it may have a role in the staging of the tumour to exclude peritoneal or hepatic dissemination.

Managing the patient with jaundice

Given the important synthetic and excretory function of the liver, the development of obstructive jaundice can lead to significant metabolic derangement and disrupted haemostatic equilibrium. Medical team members caring for such patients should be aware of potential complications that such patients may develop. The most common abnormality is prolongation of the prothrombin time, but this should readily correct within 36 hours with the administration of parenteral vitamin K when jaundice is cholestatic. Importantly, prolonged prothrombin time does not automatically correlate with bleeding tendency as synthesis of other coagulative factors such as protein C, S and antithrombin III may also be affected, resulting in patients becoming thrombogenic. Prophylactic measures aimed at preventing venous thromboembolism should therefore be considered. Patients with longstanding jaundice can become malnourished and develop steatorrhoea particularly if combined with pancreatic duct obstruction as seen with pancreatic head cancer. Nutritional supplementation and pancreatic enzyme replacement therapy may be indicated. Jaundiced patients are also at risk of renal dysfunction. Although the aetiology is not fully understood it is likely that an enteric endotoxin crosses into the systemic circulation due to the absence of enteric bile salts, leading to renal vasoconstriction. Further contributing factors include cardiovascular depression secondary to jaundice resulting in peripheral vasodilatation. When combined with hypovolaemia or septicaemia this can precipitate acute renal failure and is associated with a high mortality. Ensuring patients are well hydrated, aggressive treatment of suspected sepsis and early biliary decompression are all important preemptive measures. Jaundiced patients are at increased risk of cholangitis and subsequent septicaemia due to bacterial translocation (retrograde or haemotogenous) into the biliary tree or by iatrogenic introduction during interventional procedures (see EBM 14.1). Resuscitation, antibiotic therapy and biliary drainage are key to successful management outcome.

EBM 14.1 Acute cholangitis

'Appropriate antibiotic prophylaxis and effective biliary drainage is the cornerstone of successful management of acute cholangitis.'

Takada et al. TG13: Updated Tokyo Guidelines for the management of acute cholangitis and cholecystitis. J Hepatobiliary Pancreat Sci. 2013;20:1–7.

 14.2 Summary

Jaundice

- Jaundice is a yellowish discoloration of the tissues that becomes clinically apparent when serum bilirubin levels exceed 50 μmol/L (normal <20 μmol/L)
- It may be due to excessive haemolysis, hepatic insufficiency or cholestasis; cholestatic (obstructive) jaundice is the type encountered in surgical practice
- The two most common causes of surgical obstructive jaundice are cancer of the head of the pancreas and stones in the common bile duct (choledocholithiasis)
- In cholestatic jaundice, the bilirubin has been conjugated by the hepatocytes and is therefore soluble in water and can be excreted in the urine; patients with obstructive jaundice typically have dark urine and pale stools and may have pruritus (thought to be due to the accumulation of bile salts)
- Obstructive jaundice is characterised by elevated serum alkaline phosphatase levels in addition to hyperbilirubinaemia, and may be accompanied by modest elevations in transaminase (aminotransferase) levels, reflecting liver damage.

Congenital abnormalities

Up to 5% of the population have simple liver cysts. They are lined by biliary epithelium and contain serous fluid, but never communicate with the biliary tree. They rarely produce symptoms, are associated with normal liver function, and on ultrasound or CT have no discernible wall (Fig. 14.7). In the few patients who develop symptoms, cysts tend to recur following aspiration, and sclerosis by alcohol injection is of little value for large symptomatic cysts. Surgical management consists of deroofing and may be undertaken by laparoscopic means. Polycystic disease is a rare cause of liver enlargement and may be associated with polycystic kidneys as an autosomal dominant trait. In symptomatic patients, it may be necessary to combine a deroofing procedure with hepatic resection or to consider liver transplantation. Such surgical interventions can be associated with significant postoperative morbidity and so patients must be well counselled given it is usually performed for quality-of-life reasons.

Cavernous haemangiomas are one of the most common benign tumours of the liver (up to 5% of population) and may be congenital. Women are affected six times more frequently than men. Most haemangiomas are small solitary subcapsular growths found incidentally at laparotomy or autopsy, but they are sometimes detected on ultrasound examination as densely hyperechoic lesions that mimic hepatic tumours. Centripetal 'filling in' of contrast during dynamic imaging with CT or MRI is seen. These

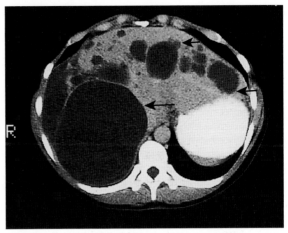

Fig. 14.7 CT demonstrating multiple biliary cysts appearing as hypodense areas within both lobes of the liver (*arrowed*).

lesions rarely give rise to pain. Resection may be considered for symptomatic lesions exceeding 5 cm in diameter.

Liver trauma

After the spleen, the liver is the solid organ most commonly damaged in abdominal trauma, particularly following road traffic accidents. Stab injuries and gunshot wounds of the liver are also increasing in incidence. These are considered in Chapter 7.

Hepatic infections and infestations

Liver abscesses can be classified as bacterial, parasitic or fungal. Bacterial abscess is the most common type in Western medicine, but parasitic infestation is an important cause worldwide. Fungal abscesses are found in patients receiving long-term broad-spectrum antibiotic treatment or immunosuppressive therapy, and may complicate actinomycosis.

Pyogenic liver abscess

Infection from the biliary system is now more common due to the increasing use of radiological and endoscopic intervention. Infection may spread through the portal vein from abdominal sepsis (e.g., appendicitis, diverticulitis), via the hepatic artery from a septic focus anywhere in the body, or by direct spread from a contiguous organ (e.g., empyema of the gallbladder). Abscess formation may follow blunt or penetrating injury, and in one-third of patients the source of infection is indeterminate (cryptogenic). Common organisms are:

- *Streptococcus milleri*
- *Escherichia coli*
- *Streptococcus faecalis*
- *Staphylococcus aureus*
- anaerobes (*Bacteroides* spp).

Clinical features

The onset of symptoms is often insidious and the patient may present with pyrexia of unknown origin. There is sometimes a history of sepsis elsewhere, particularly within the abdomen, and pain in the right hypochondrium. Other patients present with swinging pyrexia, rigors, marked toxicity and jaundice. The liver is often enlarged and tender.

14

Investigations

Plain radiographs may show elevation of the diaphragm, pleural effusion and basal lobe collapse. Leucocytosis is usually present and liver function tests are deranged. Ultrasonography or CT of the abdomen is used to define the abscess (which is often irregular and thick-walled), to facilitate percutaneous aspiration for culture and to exclude a portal source. Abscesses are generally multiple rather than single. ERCP or antegrade tubogram via the abscess cavity may identify a biliary cause if bile is aspirated from the abscess cavity. The underlying microbe may also guide to further investigations such as dental examination or colonoscopy. Patients should be investigated for occult diabetes or other immunosuppressive illnesses depending on the prevalence of such illnesses in the population being treated.

Management

Untreated abscesses often prove fatal because of spread within the liver to multiple sites, and because of septicaemia and debility. The principles of treatment are percutaneous drainage of accessible abscesses under ultrasound or CT guidance, and antibiotic therapy selected on the basis of culture of blood or pus. It is exceptional to resort to surgical drainage. Percutaneously or surgically placed drainage tubes are left in place and the size of the cavity is monitored by CT or serial x-rays following the injection of contrast material. Multiple small abscesses may require prolonged treatment with antibiotics for up to 8 weeks.

Amoebic liver abscess

Entamoeba histolytica is a protozoal parasite that infests the large intestine and is endemic in many tropical regions. Trophozoites released by the cyst in the intestine may penetrate the mucosa to gain access to the portal venous system and so spread to the liver. The abscess is large and thin-walled, is usually solitary and in the right lobe, and contains brown sterile pus resembling anchovy sauce.

Clinical features

Right upper quadrant pain may be accompanied by anorexia, nausea, weight loss and night sweats. Tender enlargement of the liver is invariable, although jaundice is uncommon. Other signs include basal pulmonary collapse, pleural effusion and leucocytosis.

Investigations

Ultrasonography and CT are used to demonstrate the site and size of the abscess, which often has poorly defined margins (Fig. 14.8). The stools should be examined for amoebae or cysts. Direct and indirect serological tests (indirect haem-agglutination [IHA], enzyme-linked immunosorbent assay [ELISA]) to detect amoebic protein are extremely useful, especially in nonendemic areas.

Management

Early diagnosis is important, and treatment may be commenced empirically in areas where the problem is endemic. Treatment consists of the administration of metronidazole (800 mg 8-hourly for 7–10 days) and usually results in rapid resolution. A luminal agent (diloxanide furoate 500 mg 8-hourly for 10 days) is advised to prevent carrier state. The abscess should be aspirated by needle puncture if there is no clinical response within 72 hours. If untreated, an amoebic abscess may rupture into the peritoneal cavity (features of peritonitis), pleural space (pleural effusion), into a bronchus (anchovy sauce expectoration) or rarely into

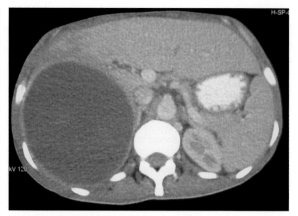

Fig. 14.8 Contrast enhanced (oral and intravenous) CT showing large abscess replacing the right lobe of the liver.

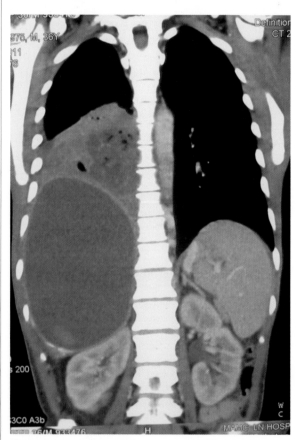

Fig. 14.9 Contrast enhanced CT showing a massive amoebic liver abscess with rupture into pleural cavity and lungs. The patient presented with severe toxic symptoms and anchovy-sauce coloured expectoration.

pericardial cavity (Fig 14.9). Abscess that ruptures into the peritoneal cavity are managed with laparotomy and lavage.

An amoeboma is a chronic granuloma involving the caecum, usually seen in patients with incompletely treated amoebiasis infection of a long duration. The lesion feels like a lump in the right iliac fossa and needs to be differentiated from a malignancy. Fulminant amoebic colitis is rare and may present with peritonitis or lower gastrointestinal bleeding, which is treated appropriately.

Hydatid disease

This less common infestation is caused in humans by one of two forms of tapeworm, *Echinococcus granulosus* and *E. multilocularis*. The adult tapeworm lives in the intestine of the dog, from which ova are passed in the stool; sheep or goats serve as the intermediate host by ingesting the ova, whereas humans are accidental hosts (Fig. 14.10). The condition is most common in sheep- and goat-rearing areas. Ingested ova hatch in the duodenum and the embryos pass to the liver through the portal venous system. The wall of the resulting hydatid cyst consists of the pericyst or adventitia, which is the host tissue formed by the body as a reaction to the parasite, the laminated membrane (ectocyst or the external layer of the cyst) and the germinative layer of laminated membrane on which brood capsules containing scolices develop (endocyst).

Clinical features

The disease may be symptomless, but chronic right upper quadrant pain with enlargement of the liver is the common presentation. The cyst may rupture into the biliary tree or peritoneal cavity, the latter sometimes causing an acute anaphylactic reaction due to absorption of foreign hydatid protein. Other complications include secondary infection and biliary obstruction with jaundice.

Investigations

Eosinophilia is common and serological tests, such as complement fixation, are available to detect the foreign protein. Hydatid cysts commonly calcify and may be seen on a plain film of the abdomen. Alternatively, they can be detected by ultrasound, CT or MRI and are recognisable by their thick trilaminar wall, which may contain multiple daughter cysts. MRI has the advantage of delineating the biliary tree to determine if there is any communication or cyst debris within the duct. The Gharbi classification describes a range from univesicular cyst (grade 1) to reflecting thick walled calcified cyst (grade 5).

Management

In asymptomatic patients, small calcified cysts may require no treatment. Patients can be treated successfully with albendazole or mebendazole, but this may be prolonged. Large symptomatic cysts are best managed by open or laparoscopic deroofing and complete excision of the endocyst. The residual cavity may be filled with hypertonic saline (scolicidal) and closed if uninfected or marsupialised after deroofing, or packed with omentum (omentoplasty) if infected. Caution should be employed in using scolicidal agents if the cyst communicates with the biliary system. A laparoscopic approach is possible for superficial accessible cysts. Selected patients may be suitable for puncture–aspiration–injection–reaspiration (PAIR). More recently, complete excision, together with the parasites contained within, known as pericystectomy, is preferred for superficial lesions, especially those in the left lobe, in centres accustomed to undertaking liver resections. Preoperative chemotherapy and perioperative steroid cover should be used in conjunction with packing off the peritoneal cavity from the cyst to prevent intraoperative anaphylaxis and seeding of live daughter cysts.

Portal hypertension

Portal hypertension results from increased resistance to portal venous blood flow. Rarely, it results primarily from an increase in portal blood flow. The normal pressure of 5–15 cmH$_2$O in the portal vein is consistently exceeded (above 25 cmH$_2$O). Portal vein thrombosis is a rare cause and is most commonly due to neonatal umbilical sepsis. The most common cause of portal hypertension is cirrhosis resulting from chronic liver disease and is characterised by liver cell damage, fibrosis and nodular regeneration. The fibrosis obstructs portal venous return and portal hypertension develops. Arteriovenous shunts within the liver also contribute to the hypertension.

Alcohol and steatohepatitis associated with obesity are the most common aetiological factor in developed countries, whereas in North Africa, the Middle East and China, schistosomiasis due to *Schistosoma mansoni* is a common cause. Chronic active hepatitis and primary and secondary biliary cirrhosis may result in portal hypertension, but in a large number of patients the cause remains obscure (cryptogenic cirrhosis).

Posthepatic portal hypertension is rare. It is most frequently due to spontaneous thrombosis of the hepatic veins and this has been associated with neoplasia, oral contraceptive agents, polycythaemia and the presence of abnormal coagulants in the blood. Inferior vena caval obstruction above the level at which the hepatic veins open into the cava is more common in South and South East Asia. The resulting Budd–Chiari syndrome is characterised by portal hypertension, caudate hypertrophy, liver failure and gross ascites.

Effects of portal hypertension

As a result of gradual chronic occlusion of the portal venous system, collateral pathways develop between the portal and systemic venous circulations. Depending on the site of obstruction with reference to the hepatic sinusoid, portal hypertension is classified as presinusoidal, sinusoidal and postsinusoidal (see

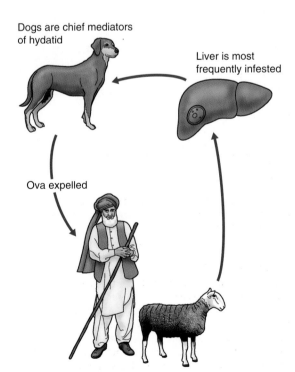

Dogs are chief mediators of hydatid

Liver is most frequently infested

Ova expelled

Fig. 14.10 Life cycle of *Echinococcus granulosus*.

14

Table 14.1 Causes of portal hypertension

Obstruction to portal flow:

Presinusoidal extrahepatic
- Congenital atresia of the portal vein
- Portal vein thrombosis
  Neonatal sepsis
  Pyelophlebitis
  Trauma
  Tumour
  Extrahepatic portal vein obstruction (EHPVO)
- Extrinsic compression of the portal vein
  Pancreatic disease
  Lymphadenopathy
  Biliary tract tumours

Presinusoidal intrahepatic
- Schistosomiasis
- Noncirrhotic portal fibrosis (NCPF)

Sinusoidal
- Cirrhosis

Postsinusoidal
- Budd–Chiari syndrome
- Constrictive pericarditis

Increased blood flow (rare)
- Arteriovenous fistula
- Increased splenic blood flow in hypersplenism

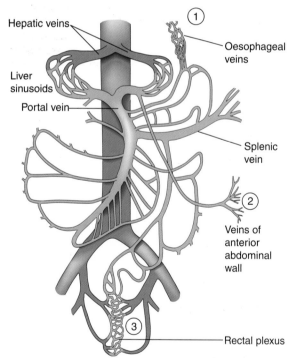

Fig. 14.11 The portal venous system. Sites of portosystemic shunting are marked *1–3*. Retroperitoneal communications also exist.

Table 14.1). Portosystemic shunting occurs at three principal sites (Fig. 14.11). The most important is the development of varices in the submucosal plexus of veins in the lower oesophagus and gastric fundus. The portal side of this communication are the short gastric veins and the left gastric vein. The systemic side (caval side) are the azygos and hemiazygos veins. Oesophageal varices may rupture, causing acute massive gastrointestinal bleeding in about 40% of patients with cirrhosis. The initial episode of variceal haemorrhage is fatal in about one-third of patients, and recurrent haemorrhage is common. Bleeding from retroperitoneal and periumbilical collaterals ('caput medusae') is troublesome during abdominal surgery, and collaterals may develop and cause bleeding at the site of stomas. Anorectal varices are not uncommonly found at proctoscopy but rarely cause bleeding.

Progressive enlargement of the spleen occurs as a result of vascular engorgement and associated hypertrophy. Haematological consequences are anaemia, thrombocytopenia and leucopenia (with the resulting syndrome of hypersplenism). Ascites may develop and is due to increased formation of hepatic and splanchnic lymph, hypoalbuminaemia, and retention of salt and water. Increased aldosterone and antidiuretic hormone levels may contribute. Portosystemic encephalopathy is due to an increased level of toxins such as ammonia in the systemic circulation. This is particularly likely to develop where there are large spontaneous or surgically created portosystemic shunts. Gastrointestinal haemorrhage increases the absorption of nitrogenous products and may precipitate encephalopathy.

Clinical features

Patients with cirrhosis frequently develop anorexia, generalised malaise and weight loss. Clinical manifestations include hepatosplenomegaly, ascites, jaundice and spider naevi. Slurring of speech, a flapping tremor or dysarthria may point to encephalopathy, and this may be precipitated or intensified by the accumulation of blood in the gastrointestinal tract. The serum bilirubin may be elevated and the serum albumin depressed. Anaemia may be present and the leucocyte count raised (or depressed if there is hypersplenism). The prothrombin time and other indices of clotting may be abnormal. Clinical and biochemical parameters are used as the basis of the modified Child's classification (Table 14.2). Patients allocated to grade A have a good prognosis, whereas those in grade C have the worst prognosis.

Patients with portal hypertension need to be assessed for varices (EBM 14.2). Patients with varices may be referred to a surgeon because of uncontrolled bleeding from oesophageal varices, or for consideration of elective surgery for varices that have been resistant to nonsurgical management.

Table 14.2 Assessment of patients with portal hypertension using the Child–Turcotte–Pugh grading system

Points scored

Criterion	1	2	3
Encephalopathy	None	Minimal	Marked
Ascites	None	Easily controlled	Intractable
Bilirubin (μmol/L)	<35	35–50	>50
Albumin (g/L)	>35	28–35	<28
Prothrombin ratio	<1.7	1.7–2.3	>2.3

Grade A = 5–6 points; grade B = 7–9 points; grade C = 10–15 points.

EBM 14.2 Variceal bleeding in cirrhosis: assessment and prophylaxis

'Severity of cirrhosis is best assessed by Child Pugh score. Risk of varices increases with Child Pugh score. Assessment of varices is best done by endoscopy and should be performed for all patients with cirrhosis. Varices should be graded by size (5 mm). For patients with large varices (>5 mm) or small varices and high risk stigmata of bleeding or severe liver disease prophylactic non selective β-blockers should be prescribed. Endoscopic variceal ligation (EVL) can also be used for high risk patients as an alternative to β-blockers. The two treatments have different side effect profiles that should be considered.'

Garcia-Tsao G et al. Prevention and management of gastroeoesophageal varices and variceal haemorrhage in cirrhosis. Hepatology. 2007;46:922–38.

Acute variceal bleeding

Patients presenting with acute upper gastrointestinal bleeding are examined for evidence of chronic liver disease. The key investigation during an episode of active bleeding is endoscopy. This allows the detection of varices and defines whether they are or have been the site of bleeding. It is important to remember that peptic ulcer and gastritis are common complaints that occur in 20% of patients with varices.

Management

The priorities in the management of bleeding oesophageal varices are summarised in Table 14.3 and EBM 14.3.

Active resuscitation

The aim is to replace blood loss quickly with a view to urgent endoscopy. Resuscitation must be done cautiously aiming for haemoglobin (Hb) of 8 g/L as over-resuscitation can increase mortality. Avoid large volumes of saline solutions. Many patients have coagulation defects from the outset, and thrombocytopenia

---

Table 14.3 Priorities in the management of bleeding oesophageal varices

Active resuscitation
- Ensure safe and protected airway
- Group and cross-match blood
- Establish IV infusion line(s) and resuscitate to haemoglobin of 8g/L
- Monitor patient in appropriate high care environment with timely access to appropriately trained staff and interventional therapies
- Commence antibiotic prophylaxis and pharmacological treatments to reduce portal pressures (somatostatin analogues or terlipressin)

Assessment of coagulation status
- Prothrombin time
- Platelet count
- Physiological coagulation screen
- Correct coagulopathies with assistance of haematologist

Urgent endoscopy

Control of bleeding
- Endoscopic banding or injection sclerotherapy
- Tamponade (Minnesota tube) if bleeding uncontrolled
- Pharmacological measures (e.g., vasopressin/octeotide)

Treatment of hepatocellular decompensation

Treatment/prevention of portosystemic encephalopathy
Prevention of further bleeding from varices
- Endoscopic banding or injection sclerotherapy
- Stapled oesophagogastric junction
- Portosystemic shunting/transjugular intrahepatic portosystemic stent shunting (TIPSS)
- Liver transplantation

---

is a common manifestation of hypersplenism. The advice of the haematologist is sought regarding the use of fresh-frozen plasma (FFP), platelet transfusion or other coagulation factors. Antibiotic prophylaxis should be administered using norfloxacin 400 mg twice a day for 7 days or IV ceftriaxone 1 g/day for 7 days. This decreases bacterial infections, reduces rebleeding and improves survival. Pharmacological therapies, such as terlipressin or somatostatin analogues, aimed at reducing portal pressures can be commenced. However, they cannot be regarded as definitive treatments and urgent endoscopy should be arranged.

Endoscopy and control of bleeding

Endoscopy will reveal tortuous varices in three columns most prominent in the lower third of the oesophagus. Haemorrhage usually occurs from varices at the lowest few centimetres of the oesophagus. Rarely, bleeding occurs from varices in the gastric fundus. Endoscopic variceal ligation (EVL) is regarded as the first-line treatment, with sclerotherapy being reserved for those where band ligation is not possible. If haemorrhage is torrential and prevents direct injection, balloon tamponade may be used to stop the bleeding. The four-lumen Minnesota tube (Fig. 14.12) has largely replaced the three-lumen Sengstaken–Blakemore tube. The four lumina allow:

- aspiration of gastric contents
- compression of the oesophagogastric varices by the inflated gastric balloon
- compression of the oesophageal varices by the inflated oesophageal balloon
- aspiration of the oesophagus and pharynx to reduce pneumonic aspiration.

Balloon tamponade arrests bleeding from varices in over 90% of patients, but the tube is not left in place for more than 24–36 hours for fear of causing oesophageal necrosis. Tamponade should be regarded as a holding measure that allows further resuscitation and treatment of hepatic decompensation before more definitive measures are used.

Emergency portosystemic shunting

Shunt surgery carries a high mortality and has been abandoned in most centres. Elective portosystemic shunting is still used occasionally to decompress the portal system and reduce the risk of further variceal haemorrhage in patients with preserved liver function, but portosystemic encephalopathy can be troublesome. In

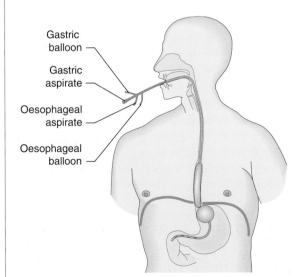

Fig. 14.12 Oesophageal tamponade using a Minnesota tube.

14

severe liver disease, transplantation is more likely to be considered if there is no contraindication.

Types of shunt procedure

Most portosystemic shunts have been replaced by nonsurgical approaches to treatment. In transjugular intrahepatic portosystemic stent shunting (TIPSS; Fig. 14.13) a metal stent is inserted via the transjugular route using a guidewire passed through the hepatic vein to the intrahepatic branches of the portal vein. The technique is a relatively safe means of decompressing the portal system as general anaesthesia and laparotomy are avoided. The risk of encephalopathy is similar to that of a surgical portosystemic shunt, but the procedure is now considered routinely before surgical intervention in both the acute and elective setting. Surgical shunts may be classified into total nonselective shunts (portocaval, mesocaval, conventional splenorenal shunts), selective shunts (distal splenorenal 'Warren', left gastricocaval 'Inoguchi') and partial shunt (low diameter portocaval shunt 'Sarfeh').

EBM | 14.3 Control of variceal bleeding

'Airway protection, controlled resuscitation and correction of coagulopathy should commence immediately. Antibiotics and splanchnic vasoconstrictors should be commenced. Urgent endoscopy within 12 hours should be instituted. EVL is the method of choice for control of variceal haemorrhage, with endoscopic variceal sclerotherapy as second choice. If delays to definitive therapy are likely or if the haemorrhage proves difficult to control endoscopically temporary deployment of a modified Sengstaken tube is indicated. Further endoscopic treatment, transjugular intrahepatic portosystemic stent shunting (TIPSS) or surgical treatment (portosystemic shunt or oesophageal transection) can subsequently be employed as definitive therapy.'

Garcia-Tsao G et al. Prevention and management of gastroesophageal varices and variceal haemorrhage in cirrhosis. Hepatology. 2007;46:922–38.

Prevention of further bleeding

Rebleeding rates are high in patients surviving an acute variceal haemorrhage. Secondary prophylaxis is critical for those in whom the portal pressure has not been definitively lowered (surgery or TIPSS). The treatment of choice is the combination of β-blockers with nitrates and EVL. The dose of β-blocker should be increased to maximal tolerance and repeat endoscopy will be required. Patients who suffer a further bleed after such treatment require definitive intervention in the form of TIPSS, shunt surgery or liver transplantation depending on the severity of the underlying liver disease. For those patients undergoing TIPPS or surgical shunts monitoring for the development of encephalopathy should be performed.

Ascites

Ascites is a common complication of cirrhosis and is a marker of worsening liver disease and portends a poor prognosis. Other causes of ascites should be considered, including but not limited to heart failure, malignancy, nephrotic syndrome and tuberculosis. Paracentesis and fluid analysis can help determine the underlying aetiology. Calculating the serum ascites albumin gradient (serum albumin − ascites albumin) can predict the presence of portal hypertension. A level of ≥1.1 g/dL indicates portal hypertension. If spontaneous bacterial peritonitis is suspected the fluid should be cultured. Ascites associated with portal hypertension due to cirrhosis can be controlled in 90% of patients by cessation of alcohol, salt restriction, and diuretic therapy with spironolactone and frusemide. Long term, liver transplantation should be considered. If refractory, ascites can be treated using serial paracenteses, TIPPS or liver transplantation. The use of a peritoneojugular (LeVeen) shunt, which allows one-way flow between the peritoneum and the jugular vein (Fig. 14.14) is usually restricted to those who are not candidates for liver transplantation.

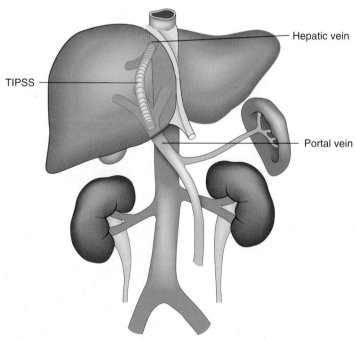

Fig. 14.13 Transjugular intrahepatic portosystemic stent shunting (TIPSS).

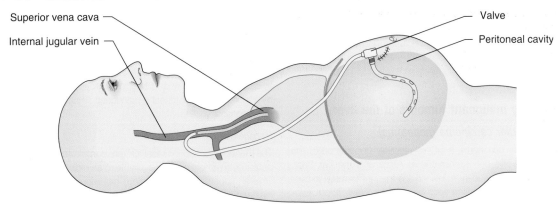

Superior vena cava

Internal jugular vein

Valve

Peritoneal cavity

Fig. 14.14 Peritoneovenous (Le Veen) shunt to relieve ascites.

14.3 Summary

Portal hypertension

- Portal hypertension is almost always due to obstruction to portal flow (rather than increased inflow), and may be presinusoidal, sinusoidal or postsinusoidal
- Cirrhosis of the liver is the most common cause of portal hypertension in developed countries, and alcoholic cirrhosis is most often responsible
- Portosystemic shunts develop between gastric and oesophageal veins, in the retroperitoneum and periumbilical area, and occasionally in the anorectum. Varices in the submucosa of the lower oesophagus are a common source of major bleeding; however, other gastric pathology can be responsible
- Child's grading (A, B or C) is based on encephalopathy, ascites, prothrombin time, bilirubin and albumin levels, and is a valuable prognostic index
- Acute variceal bleeding is most effectively controlled by endoscopic banding and pharmacological splanchnic vasoconstrictors
- For uncontrollable bleeding portosystemic shunts effectively decompress oesophageal varices and reduce rebleeding, but can cause encephalopathy. Surgical shunts have been largely replaced by transjugular intrahepatic portosystemic stent shunting (TIPSS)
- Although EVL and β-blockers reduce the risk of rebleeding and may improve survival rates, long-term outcome is determined by the nature and severity of the underlying liver disease
- Ascites associated with portal hypertension secondary to cirrhosis can usually be controlled with medical interventions such as diuretics, sodium restriction and alcohol cessation.

Tumours of the liver

Hepatic tumours can be benign or malignant, and primary or secondary. Primary tumours may arise from the parenchymal cells, the epithelium of the bile ducts, or the supporting tissues.

Benign hepatic tumours

Cavernous haemangioma

This is the most common benign liver tumour. These lesions rarely reach a sufficient size to produce pain, abdominal swelling or haemorrhage. Heart failure rarely develops, if there is a large arteriovenous communication. Lesions discovered incidentally at laparotomy should be left alone; needle biopsy can be hazardous. Large symptomatic lesions should normally be resected only by an experienced surgeon.

Biliary hamartoma

These are small fibrous lesions that are often situated beneath the capsule of the liver. They can be mistaken for a small metastatic tumour unless a biopsy is obtained.

Focal nodular hyperplasia (FNH)

This is more common in females. The lesion is generally asymptomatic and may regress with time or on withdrawal of the contraceptive pill. Hyperplasia can be differentiated from adenoma by the central fibrous scar, which is often visible on ultrasound or CT (Fig. 14.15). Such lesions do not undergo malignant transformation and do not require excision unless symptomatic.

Liver cell adenoma

This is relatively uncommon and is found almost exclusively in women. The use of contraceptives containing high levels of oestrogen have been implicated causally. The majority present as solitary, well-encapsulated lesions, but malignant transformation has been reported. They may be asymptomatic but generally present with right hypochondrial pain as a result of haemorrhage within the tumour. Superficial tumours may bleed spontaneously and present with symptoms of haemoperitoneum. Adenomas may be detected by ultrasonography or CT. Liver function tests (LFTs) and serum α-fetoprotein levels are usually normal.

Treatment consists of formal hepatic resection because of the difficulties of distinguishing adenoma from a well-differentiated hepatoma, concerns that lesions may undergo malignant transformation and the known risk of spontaneous haemorrhage. There is recent evidence to suggest that cytokeratin 7 and 19

14

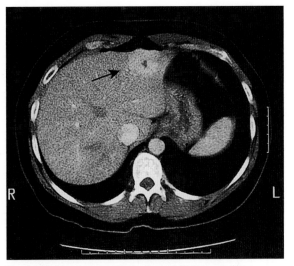

Fig. 14.15 Intravenous contrast enhanced CT demonstrating a hypervascular lesion in the left lobe of the liver (*arrowed*). This symptomatic focal nodular hyperplastic lesion was removed by left lobectomy.

immunostains along with neuronal adhesion molecule taken from liver biopsy can help in differentiating hepatic adenoma from FNH when radiological imaging is inconclusive. However, with the advent of MRI and liver-specific contrast agents, differentiation of the benign liver tumours is rarely an issue.

Primary malignant tumours of the liver

Hepatocellular carcinoma (hepatoma)

Hepatocellular carcinoma (HCC) is relatively uncommon in the developed world but is common in Africa and the Far East. HCC is more common in males and it is thought to result in over 600,000 deaths worldwide each year. In the West, about two-thirds of patients have preexisting cirrhosis and many others have evidence of hepatitis B or C infection. In Africa, 'aflatoxin' (derived from the fungus, *Aspergillus flavus*, which contaminates maize and nuts) is an important hepatocarcinogen.

Clinical features

The diagnosis is usually made late in the course of the disease unless detected incidentally by screening programs in patients with known cirrhosis. In noncirrhotic patients, the tumour may have grown to a considerable size before giving rise to abdominal pain or swelling. In cirrhotic patients, hepatoma may become manifest as sudden deterioration in liver function, often associated with extension of the tumour into the portal venous system. Common presenting features would involve progression of existing liver disease symptoms, and may include abdominal pain, weight loss, abdominal distension, fever and spontaneous intraperitoneal haemorrhage. Jaundice is uncommon unless there is advanced cirrhosis. Examination may reveal features of established liver disease, and hepatomegaly is invariable.

Investigations

LFTs are generally deranged. Although early detection of hepatocellular carcinoma in susceptible individuals can be pursued by a policy of 6-monthly measurement of alpha-fetoprotein (AFP) and ultrasound scanning, this tumour marker is elevated in only one-third of the white population with hepatocellular carcinoma, compared to 80% of African patients with this disease.

The lesion may be detected and characterised by ultrasound scanning. Percutaneous needle aspiration cytology and needle biopsy for histological confirmation should be reserved for patients who are not being considered for hepatic resection, as these investigations carry a small but significant risk of tumour dissemination and haemorrhage. There are accepted criteria based on radiology and tumour marker levels that accept a diagnosis of HCC without the need for biopsy (EBM 14.4).

EBM 14.4 Diagnosis of HCC established

- *If two imaging modalities show a coincidental nodule with arterial hypervascularisation and venous washout regardless of AFP levels, if lesion is 1–2 cm or if one imaging modality shows these features in lesions >2 cm*
- *If a single modality shows a lesion when the AFP is >200 ng/mL*
- *Histological/cytological diagnosis is required if the nodule is less than 2 cm in diameter and imaging is inconclusive with low AFP*
- *NCCN Practice Guidelines in Oncology – v.2.2010.*

Bruix J, Sherman M, Hepatology. 2005;42:1208–36.

Abdominal CT or MRI is valuable in planning resection and excluding the presence of nodal involvement. Hepatocellular carcinoma is seen as an extremely vascular lesion on arteriography, and propagation of tumour thrombus along the portal vein or its branches may be apparent. Pulmonary metastases may not be evident on chest x-ray and their presence should be excluded by a thoracic CT. Peritoneal dissemination may only be excluded by laparoscopy.

Management

The management options for HCC are complex and evolving. The potential treatment options available to an individual patient span several subspecialties including gastroenterology, oncology, interventional radiology, Hepato-biliary-pancreatic (HPB) surgery and transplantation. Therefore, discussion in a multidisciplinary meeting by members conversant with all available treatment options is advised.

In noncirrhotic patients, large tumours (particularly those of the fibrolamellar type) are likely to be amenable to liver resection. Cirrhotic patients have less hepatic functional reserve, and even those with well-preserved liver function may only tolerate limited segmental resection if there is significant portal hypertension. In cirrhotic patients, multicentricity is common and satellite lesions often surround the primary tumour, so that cure is uncommon.

For advanced tumours, sorafenib, a multitargeted oral kinase inhibitor, has been shown to prolong survival in patients with HCC although consideration to the side-effect profile in those with advanced cirrhosis must be considered. Encouraging results have been reported following local embolisation with chemotherapy by selective arteriography (transarterial chemo-embolisation [TACE]) and percutaneous ablation using radiofrequency and microwave energy have been used for small lesions not amenable to surgery. Future efforts may involve a combination of these methods. Antiviral treatment should also be considered for those patients with a viral aetiology and undergoing curative treatments.

The disease is usually advanced at presentation and the 5-year survival rate is less than 10%. Liver transplantation has been used in the treatment of this tumour, but the best results have been reported in cirrhotic patients in whom an incidental hepatoma has been found on examination of the resected specimen following the transplant. If transplantation is not otherwise contraindicated, eligibility criteria have been extended for cirrhotic patients. Traditionally the 'Milan' criteria (single tumour of 5 cm or less in diameter, or with no more than three tumour nodules each one 3 cm or less in size) were employed but these have now been extended in several countries. Transplantation is normally contraindicated if there has been tumour rupture or AFP exceeds 1000 iu/mL.

Cholangiocarcinoma

This adenocarcinoma may arise anywhere in the biliary tree, including its intrahepatic radicals. It accounts for less than 10% of malignant primary neoplasms of the liver in Western medicine, although its incidence is rising. Risk factors include chronic parasitic infestation of the biliary tree in the Far East, and choledochal cysts (see below).

Jaundice, pain and an enlarged liver are the common presenting features, although there may be coexisting biliary infection causing the tumour to masquerade as a hepatic abscess. Resection offers the only prospect of cure but is seldom feasible when cholangiocarcinoma arises in the liver substance. Cholangiocarcinoma arising from the extrahepatic bile ducts is considered below.

Other primary malignant tumours

- *Angiosarcoma* (Fig. 14.16). This rare tumour of the liver may arise after industrial exposure to vinyl chloride or exposure to the previously used radiological contrast medium, Thorotrast.
- *Haemangioendothelioma*. This presents as a diffuse multifocal tumour and is rarely resectable at presentation.
- Hepatic mucinous cystic neoplasm. This rare condition of the liver has a marked female predominance. It usually presents as a large complex cystic lesion within the liver detected on ultrasound. It does not communicate with the biliary tree. It has a high rate of malignant transformation and should be resected. These can be mistaken for biliary intraductal papillary mucinous neoplasms (B-IPMN). Unlike hepatic mucinous cystic neoplasms B-IPMN involve the biliary tree and can occur in both genders.

Metastatic tumours

The liver is a common site for metastatic disease; secondary liver tumours are 20 times more common than primary ones. In 50% of patients, the primary tumour is in the gastrointestinal tract; other common sites are the breast, ovaries, bronchus and kidney. Almost 90% of patients with hepatic metastases have tumour deposits in other sites.

Hepatomegaly and tenderness are distinctive features, and individual deposits characterised by umbilication due to central necrosis may be palpable in advanced disease. The patient may be cachectic, and ascites or jaundice may be present. Pyrexia occurs in up to 10% of patients. The alkaline phosphatase and γ-glutamyl transpeptidase are often raised. Ultrasound and CT may demonstrate multiple solid hypoechoic or hypovascular lesions, respectively. The diagnosis can be confirmed by tumour markers (CEA, CA19-9, Chromogranin A), aspiration cytology or needle biopsy undertaken under radiological guidance. If curative surgical resection is being considered biopsy should be avoided to reduce risk of seeding or haemorrhage.

There is no effective treatment for most patients with hepatic metastases due to the extent of liver involvement and the presence of extrahepatic disease. Nonetheless, for some tumours, notably those arising from the colon and rectum, disease may be confined to the liver and there is strong evidence of survival benefit if these are resected. Assessment of resectability will require a careful search to exclude or assess extrahepatic

disease. This may necessitate colonoscopy, CT of chest, CT or MRI of the abdomen and pelvis and more recently positron emitted tomography (PET) scanning. A more radical approach to resection of liver metastases has resulted from advances in chemotherapy and has been combined with staged resection of liver disease and preoperative portal embolisation to induce hypertrophy of the intended residual liver. In well-selected patients, 5-year survival rates of 30–40% have been reported following resection. Noncurative resection may be considered exceptionally as a means of palliation in patients with symptomatic hepatic metastases such as a carcinoid or other neuroendocrine tumours.

Liver resection

Resection involves mobilisation of the liver from its peritoneal attachments. Following isolation, ligature and division of the appropriate vessels, the devascularised lobe or segment is separated by careful dissection of the parenchyma, which may be facilitated by the use of an ultrasonic dissector. Intervening biliary and vascular channels can be defined and divided between ligatures. The hepatic veins or tributaries are controlled by suture or staple ligation following removal of the resected specimen.

Modern techniques of hepatic resection including the concept of a low central venous pressure have greatly reduced operative blood loss, with a subsequent reduction in morbidity and mortality. Enhanced recovery programmes after liver surgery are associated with reduced use of abdominal drains, immediate restitution of oral intake and early mobilisation in the postoperative period. Postoperative monitoring is undertaken in a high-dependency environment with staff familiar with symptoms, signs and biochemical changes associated with hepatic dysfunction. If clinical concern arises, blood gas, glucose and lactate as well as coagulation screen should be performed. With good preoperative planning and optimisation of the future liver remnant, fatal liver failure should be rare. Complications such as postoperative haemorrhage and intraabdominal/wound infection or bile leak can occur but are uncommon.

Liver transplantation

This is considered in Chapter 25.

The gallbladder and bile ducts

Anatomy of the biliary system

The biliary tree consists of fine intrahepatic biliary radicals that drain individual liver segments before forming the right and left hepatic ducts. The left hepatic duct runs a mainly extrahepatic course and joins the right hepatic duct to form the common hepatic duct, which is 2.5 cm long. This is joined at a variable position by the cystic duct to form the common bile duct, which ends at the ampulla of Vater, usually in the second part of the duodenum (Fig. 14.17). The common bile duct is approximately 7.5 cm long and up to 7 mm in diameter with roughly equal parts being supraduodenal, retroduodenal and intrapancreatic. It lies in the free edge of the lesser omentum before passing behind the first part of the duodenum and through the head of the pancreas. It is usually joined by the pancreatic duct just before entering the

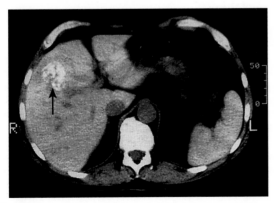

Fig. 14.16 Angiosarcoma. CT demonstrating a lesion in segment V (*arrowed*).

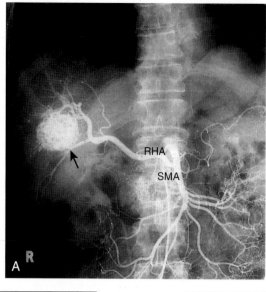

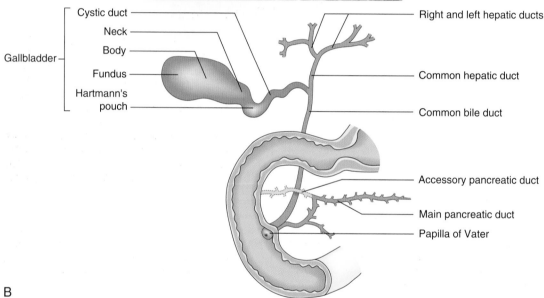

Fig. 14.17 (A) Angiography shows an extremely vascular lesion (*arrowed*) taking its blood supply mainly from an aberrant right hepatic artery (RHA) arising from the superior mesenteric artery (SMA). **(B)** Anatomy of the biliary tree.

duodenum. The blood supply of the bile duct is derived through segmental vessels running as a plexus around it with main vessels at 3 and 9 o'clock positions. Stripping the duct of its adventitia may cause ischaemic stricture at a later date.

The gallbladder lies in a bed on the undersurface of the liver between its right and left halves. It is a muscular structure with a fundus, body and neck. Hartmann's pouch is a dilatation of the gallbladder outlet adjacent to the origin of the cystic duct, in which gallstones frequently become impacted. The gallbladder is supplied by the cystic artery, a branch of the right hepatic artery. The key surgical anatomical landmark is the hepatobiliary triangle. This is defined by the space delineated by three borders: the inferior border of the liver, cystic duct and common hepatic duct. It is covered anteriorly and posteriorly by two layers of peritoneum. The contents include the cystic node, and cystic artery or occasionally the right hepatic artery. This is often erroneously referred to as Calot's triangle; however, Calot described a smaller triangle bounded by the cystic artery, cystic duct and gallbladder fundus.

Physiology

Bile salts and the enterohepatic circulation

Bile acids are synthesised by the liver from cholesterol. The primary bile acids, chenodeoxycholic and cholic acid, are conjugated with glycine or taurine to increase their solubility in water, and the conjugates (e.g., glycocholic and taurocholic acid) form sodium and potassium bile salts. In the intestine, bacterial action produces the secondary bile salts, deoxycholic and lithocholic acid.

Bile salts can combine with lipids to form water-soluble complexes called micelles, within which lecithin and cholesterol can be transported from the liver. Bile salts are also detergents and a reduction in surface tension allows fat to be emulsified in the intestine, thus facilitating its digestion and absorption. On reaching the distal ileum, 95% of the bile salts are reabsorbed, transported back to the liver and passed once again into the biliary system. This enterohepatic circulation (Fig. 14.18) allows a

Hepatic synthesis 0.2–0.6 g/24 h

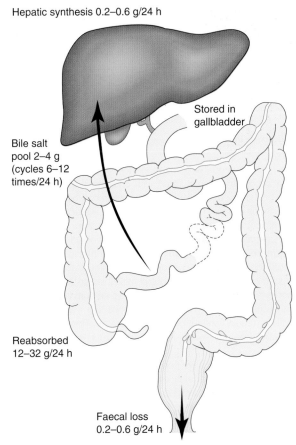

Bile salt
pool 2–4 g
(cycles 6–12
times/24 h)

Stored in
gallbladder

Reabsorbed
12–32 g/24 h

Faecal loss
0.2–0.6 g/24 h

Fig. 14.18 The enterohepatic circulation.

relatively small bile salt pool (2–4 g) to circulate through the intestine some 6–12 times a day. The daily faecal loss equals that of hepatic synthesis (0.2–0.6 g/24 h). When bile is excluded from the intestine, 25% of ingested fat may appear in the faeces and there is marked malabsorption of fat-soluble vitamins, including vitamin K. Urobilin in the urine is derived from urobilinogen reabsorbed through this circulation and is thus absent in obstructive jaundice.

The gallbladder has a capacity of 50 mL and can concentrate bile by a factor of 10. It contracts in response to cholecystokinin (CCK), which is released from the duodenal mucosa by the presence of food, notably fatty acids. Gallbladder contraction is accompanied by reciprocal relaxation of the sphincter of Oddi. The secretion of bile is promoted by the hormone secretin. The vagus nerve also stimulates bile secretion and gallbladder contraction. Some 1–2 L of bile is produced by the liver daily.

Congenital abnormalities

Congenital abnormalities of the gallbladder and bile ducts are common. The gallbladder may be absent (agenesis), double, intrahepatic, partitioned with a fold in the fundus (Phrygian cap), or multiseptate. The cystic duct may be absent or join the right hepatic duct rather than the common hepatic duct, and accessory ducts may be present. The cystic artery may be duplicated or may arise from the common hepatic or left hepatic artery. These anomalies are important in that great care must be taken to avoid the inappropriate division of major ducts and arteries in the course of cholecystectomy.

 14.4 Summary

Bile salts

- The primary bile acids, chenodeoxycholic and cholic acid, are conjugated with glycine or taurine and form sodium or potassium bile salts (e.g., sodium taurocholate)
- Bile salts are vital for the excretion of cholesterol in bile; cholesterol is insoluble in water and must be transported in water-soluble complexes (micelles) with bile salts and lecithin
- Bile salts are detergents, and on reaching the intestine they emulsify fat and facilitate the digestion and absorption of fat and fat-soluble vitamins
- Bile salts must not be confused with bile pigments (e.g., bilirubin), which are waste products and excreted in bile. The small bile salt pool (2–4 g) is conserved by reabsorption of bile salts from the terminal ileum
- Disease or resection of the terminal ileum prevents the enterohepatic circulation of bile and is associated with a high incidence of cholesterol gallstones and diarrhoea (owing to the cathartic action of bile salts on the colon).

Biliary atresia

Failure of development of the duct system occurs once in every 20,000–30,000 births and is the most common cause of prolonged jaundice in infancy. Jaundice usually becomes apparent in the first 2–3 weeks of life and the liver and spleen usually enlarge. LFTs show an obstructive pattern. Liver biopsy reveals cholestatic jaundice, but differentiation from neonatal hepatitis is often surprisingly difficult.

In extrahepatic biliary atresia, a Roux loop of jejunum is anastomosed to the intrahepatic duct system in the hilum of the liver (Kasai operation). A delay in treatment will result in jaundice and cholangitis, allowing cirrhosis to develop, with portal hypertension and ascites.

Choledochal cysts

Cystic transformation of the biliary tree (choledochal cyst) is rare. It is more common in females and in Mongolian races. Five types have been described by Todani (Fig. 14.19). The most common

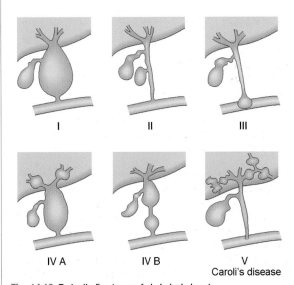

Fig. 14.19 Todani's five types of choledochal cyst.

14

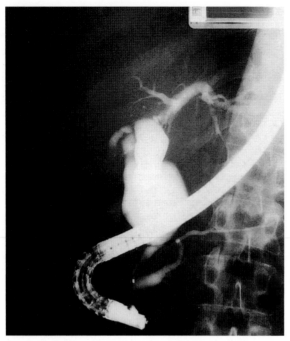

Fig. 14.20 Endoscopic retrograde cholangiopancreatography demonstrating the common type of choledochal cyst involving the common bile duct.

type (1) results in a fusiform dilatation of the common bile duct. Abnormal pancreaticobiliary junction with a long common channel has been implicated in its causation. This may allow reflux into the biliary system, resulting in pain, inflammation, calculus formation and malignant transformation. The abnormalities are probably congenital, although diagnosis may be delayed until adult life.

In the neonate, the cyst may present with jaundice or spontaneous perforation. The adult patient usually presents with intermittent pain and jaundice, and may have attacks of pancreatitis. LFTs show a cholestatic pattern, and ultrasonography and cholangiography (MRCP or ERCP) establish the diagnosis (Fig. 14.20). In view of the significant risk of malignant transformation, excision of the cyst is indicated with reconstruction using a biliary-enteric anastomosis.

Caroli's disease consists of cystic biliary dilatation that is more marked in the peripheral intrahepatic ducts. Recurring infection may progress to cirrhosis and liver failure. When Caroli's disease is found in association with congenital hepatic fibrosis, portal hypertension is often present. Endoscopic, percutaneous and surgical manipulation of the biliary tree is best avoided, and liver transplantation may have a valuable role in management.

Gallstones

Pathogenesis

Gallstones are common in Europe and North America but less so in Asia and Africa. Their incidence increases with age. In developed countries, they occur in at least 20% of women over the age of 40; the incidence in males is about one-third of that in females. The disease has increased markedly in frequency and

cholecystectomy is the most common elective abdominal operation in many Western countries.

Gallstone formation results from an imbalance of the constituents of bile. The majority of stones result from an inability to keep cholesterol in micellar form in the gallbladder; pigment stones are less common. Most cholesterol stones become mixed with bile pigments as they increase in size; such 'mixed' stones are much more common than pure cholesterol stones.

Cholesterol stones

Cholesterol stones are particularly common in middle-aged obese multiparous women. Stone formation is encouraged if bile becomes supersaturated with cholesterol (i.e., lithogenic bile), either by excessive cholesterol excretion or by a reduction in the amount of bile salt and lecithin available for micelle formation. Supersaturation is most likely to occur as the bile is concentrated in the gallbladder, and is favoured by stasis or decreased gallbladder contractility. The formation of cholesterol crystals is the key event, and this 'nucleation' may be due to coalescence of cholesterol molecules or their precipitation around particles of mucus, bacteria, calcium bilirubinate or mucosal cells. Pure cholesterol stones are yellowish-green with a regular shape but rough surface. They are usually solitary, whereas mixed stones are darker and are usually multiple.

Cholesterol stones are particularly common in some tribes of North American Indians, where more than 75% of women over 40 are affected. Such individuals have a small bile salt pool. Conversely, the high incidence of stones in Chilean women reflects high levels of cholesterol excretion. Obesity and high-calorie or high-cholesterol diets favour cholesterol stone formation by producing highly supersaturated gallbladder bile. Drastic weight reduction and diets designed to lower serum cholesterol levels may also promote stone formation by mobilising cholesterol and increasing its excretion.

Disease or resection of the terminal ileum and drugs such as cholestyramine favour cholesterol nucleation by reducing the bile salt pool. Hormonal influences are reflected in an increased incidence of stone formation in women taking oral contraceptives or postmenopausal oestrogen replacement. Pregnancy may also have an effect by increasing stasis within the gallbladder, as does surgical vagotomy.

Pigment stones

Pigment stones consist of calcium bilirubinate and are usually multiple and small. They are more prevalent in those areas of the world where haemolytic blood disorders are most common: for example, Mediterranean countries and malarial regions. Stones found in Western patients are usually composed of black pigment (calcium salts of bilirubin, phosphate and bicarbonate), whereas brown pigment stones are common in people from the Far East (calcium salts of bilirubin, stearates and palmitates, and cholesterol). Pigment stones account for 25% of all gallstones in Western patients, but for 60% of those in some Far Eastern countries such as Japan.

Chronic haemolysis favours pigment stone formation by increasing pigment excretion, and stone formation is common in congenital spherocytosis, haemoglobinopathy and malaria. Cirrhosis and biliary stasis are also important associations. Some patients with brown pigment stones have increased amounts of unconjugated bilirubin in the bile. In Far Eastern patients, this may be due to the action of β-glucuronidase produced by

E. coli, an organism that invades duct systems infested with *Clonorchis sinensis* or *Ascaris lumbricoides.*

Pathological effects of gallstones

Acute cholecystitis and its complications

This is usually produced by obstruction of the neck of the gallbladder or cystic duct by a stone. The obstruction results in increased pressure within the lumen of the gallbladder. This results in bile being forced across the mucosal membrane resulting in an acute chemical inflammatory reaction. Transient obstruction precipitates acute biliary pain (biliary colic) whereas persistent obstruction can lead to acute cholecystitis or its subsequent complications. Bacteria are cultured from the bile in approximately one-half of patients with gallstones, and unrelieved obstruction in the presence of this infected bile may produce an empyema. The persistently obstructed gallbladder becomes intensely inflamed and oedematous. If the obstruction fails to resolve the transmural pressure in the wall of the gallbladder can result in venous ischaemia, leading to gangrene and or perforation. Perforation may be contained by the liver or surrounding viscera leading to localised abscess formation or may result in biliary peritonitis. The common organisms implicated in inflammation of the gallbladder are *E. coli, Klebsiella aerogenes* and *Strep. faecalis.* Staphylococci, clostridia and salmonella are occasionally present. These organisms may be cultured from the blood if there is bacteraemia.

Mucocoele

A mucocoele develops when the outlet of the gallbladder becomes obstructed in the absence of infection. The imprisoned bile is absorbed, but clear mucus continues to be secreted into the distended gallbladder.

Chronic cholecystitis

Repeated bouts of transient gallbladder obstruction (biliary colic) or acute cholecystitis culminate in fibrosis, contraction of the gallbladder and chronic inflammatory change with marked thickening of the wall. The gallbladder ceases to function. Chronic inflammatory change may be present in the absence of gallstones, as is the case in the gallbladders of typhoid carriers. The incidence of carcinoma of the gallbladder is increased in patients with long-standing gallstones.

Fistulation

When large gallstones are present for a long time they can erode by the effect of pressure through the wall of the gallbladder into surrounding structures. Commonly involved structures include the common hepatic or bile duct (Mirizzi's syndrome), duodenum, abdominal wall or colon. Those eroding into the duodenum can pass into the small bowel, resulting in mechanical small bowel obstruction known as gallstone ileus.

Choledocholithiasis

When gallstones (usually small) enter the common bile duct via the cystic duct, they may pass spontaneously or give rise to obstructive jaundice, cholangitis or acute pancreatitis. Gallstone pancreatitis most commonly occurs when a small stone becomes temporarily arrested at the ampulla of Vater.

14.5 Summary

Gallstones

- Most gallstones form because of failure to keep cholesterol in solution. This can result in pure cholesterol stones, but more commonly the stones also acquire a content of bile pigment as they enlarge, forming 'mixed' stones
- Pigment stones are the most common type of stone in some Far Eastern countries, but are less common in Western society, where they are associated with chronic haemolysis, biliary stasis and cirrhosis
- Only 15% of stones contain enough calcium to be seen on a plain film
- The majority of individuals with gallstones are asymptomatic and remain so; the presence of gallstones is not in itself an indication for cholecystectomy
- Gallbladder stones may cause flatulent dyspepsia, biliary colic, acute cholecystitis and gallbladder cancer (although the latter is so rare that this consideration does not affect the decision not to treat asymptomatic stones)
- Gallstones that migrate into the bile duct can cause obstructive jaundice, cholangitis and acute pancreatitis, although they often remain asymptomatic
- Gallstone ileus is a rare form of intestinal obstruction; stones large enough to obstruct the gut are usually too large to pass through the ampulla of Vater and have gained access to the gut by an internal fistula involving the gallbladder

Common clinical syndromes associated with gallstones

14

The majority of individuals with gallstones are asymptomatic or have only vague symptoms of distension and flatulence. Less than a fifth of such patients develop symptoms or complications from their gallstones within 10 years.

Biliary colic

Biliary colic is due to transient obstruction of the gallbladder from an impacted stone. There is severe gripping pain, often developing after meals or in the evening, which is maximal in the epigastrium and right hypochondrium with radiation to the back. Despite being continuous, the pain may wax and wane in intensity over several hours, and vomiting and retching are common. Resolution occurs when the stone falls back into the gallbladder lumen or passes onwards into the common bile duct. The patient then recovers rapidly, but repeated bouts of colic are common. In some patients, the obstruction does not resolve and the patient develops acute cholecystitis.

Acute cholecystitis

Acute cholecystitis is a more prolonged and severe illness. It usually begins with an attack of biliary colic, although its onset may be more gradual. There is severe right hypochondrial pain radiating to the right subscapular region, and occasionally to the right shoulder, together with tachycardia, pyrexia, nausea, vomiting and leucocytosis. The pain in acute cholecystitis is usually constant and continues for 24 hours or more, differentiating this from biliary colic where pain is short-lasting. Abdominal tenderness and rigidity may be generalised but are most marked over the gallbladder. Boas's sign (hyperaesthesia of the region around the tip of the right scapula and Murphy's sign (a catching of the breath at the height of inspiration while the gallbladder area is palpated) are usually present. A right hypochondrial mass may be felt. This is due to omentum 'wrapped' around the inflamed gallbladder.

In 85–90% of patients, the attack settles within 4–5 days. In the remainder, tenderness may spread and pyrexia and tachycardia persist or worsen. The development of a tender mass, associated with rigors and marked pyrexia, signals empyema formation. The gallbladder may become gangrenous and perforate, giving rise to biliary peritonitis. Jaundice can develop during the acute attack. Usually, this is associated with stones in the common bile duct, but compression of the bile ducts due to surrounding inflammation may be responsible. Acute cholecystitis must be differentiated from perforated peptic ulcer, high retrocaecal appendicitis, acute pancreatitis, myocardial infarction and basal pneumonia. Acute cholecystitis can develop in the absence of gallstones (acalculous cholecystitis), although this is rare.

Management of acute cholecystitis

Patients with acute cholecystitis are admitted to hospital to be monitored; analgesics, intravenous fluid and a broad-spectrum antibiotic such as a cephalosporin are prescribed. The majority of patients settle within a few days on this regimen. Failure to settle suggests the presence of an empyema. However, the treatment of choice for patients otherwise fit and well is acute cholecystectomy (EBM 14.5). Provided the operation is carried out by an experienced surgeon and under antibiotic cover, 'early' cholecystectomy is not associated with an increased incidence of complications. The duration of the illness and hospitalisation is reduced, and further attacks of acute cholecystitis during the waiting period for elective surgery are averted. In hospitals serving populations with a high burden of disease, dedicated processes, access to appropriate investigations and facilities alongside experienced surgical staff are key requirements for successfully managing these patients via an acute pathway.

14.6 Summary

Acute cholecystitis

- In the great majority of patients acute cholecystitis is associated with gallstones and results from obstruction of gallbladder outflow
- In contrast to biliary colic, which results from obstruction alone, acute cholecystitis is associated with infection and is a systemic illness
- The patient appears unwell, has pyrexia and tachycardia, and is tender in the right hypochondrium; Murphy's sign is almost always positive
- In 90% of patients, acute cholecystitis will settle with conservative treatment (nil by mouth, intravenous fluids, antibiotics); however, early cholecystectomy by well-trained teams is the treatment of choice
- In 10% of patients, disease progression leads to life-threatening complications: notably, empyema, gangrene and perforation. In such situations emergency cholecystectomy is usually the treatment of choice.

EBM 14.5 Timing of cholecystectomy

'Early cholecystectomy for acute cholecystitis is associated with a better outcome than delayed cholecystectomy.'

Takada et al. TG13: Updated Tokyo Guidelines for the management of acute cholangitis and cholecystitis. J Hepatobiliary Pancreat Sci. 2013;20:1–7.

If the patient is unfit for surgery, has a delayed presentation or disease severity suggests surrounding inflammation, this will make identification of the relevant anatomical structures difficult. Ultrasound-guided percutaneous drainage of the gallbladder may be performed as an interim measure. Elective cholecystectomy is usually performed approximately 2 months later.

Chronic cholecystitis

Chronic cholecystitis is the most common cause of symptomatic gallbladder disease. The patient gives a history of recurrent flatulence, fatty food intolerance and right upper quadrant pain. The pain is worse after meals and is often associated with a feeling of distension and heartburn. The differential diagnosis includes duodenal ulcer, hiatus hernia, myocardial ischaemia, chronic pancreatitis and gastrointestinal neoplasia. Symptoms for mucocoele are the same as those for chronic cholecystitis but a nontender piriform swelling may be palpable in the right hypochondrium. There is little systemic upset and no pyrexia. Treatment is laparoscopic cholecystectomy.

Choledocholithiasis

Stones may be present in the common bile duct of some 5–10% of patients with gallstones. There is little muscle in the wall of the bile duct, and pain is not a symptom unless the stone impedes flow through the sphincter of Oddi. The vast majority of stones in the common bile duct originate in the gallbladder. 'Primary' duct stones are extremely rare.

Impaction of a stone at the sphincter obstructs the flow of bile, producing jaundice, pale stools and dark urine. Obstruction commonly persists for several days but may clear spontaneously, as a result either of passage of the stone or of its disimpaction. Small stones may pass through the common bile duct without causing symptoms. In longstanding obstruction the bile ducts become markedly dilated and the diameter of the common bile duct may exceed its upper limit of 7 mm. Diameter greater than 10 mm is usually strongly suggestive of stone or tumour. A totally obstructed duct system becomes filled with clear 'white bile', as back pressure on the hepatocytes prevents clearance of bilirubin and mucus secretion is increased.

Infection of an obstructed biliary tract causes cholangitis, which is characterised by attacks of pain, pyrexia and jaundice ('Charcot's triad'), frequently in association with rigors. Long-standing intermittent biliary obstruction may lead to secondary biliary cirrhosis. Obstructive jaundice due to stones in the common bile duct has to be distinguished from other causes of obstructive jaundice, notably malignant obstruction and cholestatic jaundice. Acute viral or alcoholic hepatitis may occasionally be confused with obstructive jaundice.

Acute pancreatitis may be associated with a stone in the common bile duct (Chapter 15).

Courvoisier's law

Fibrosed gallbladders that contain stones cannot distend when pressure increases in the obstructed biliary tree. Courvoisier's law states that 'in a jaundiced patient, in obstruction of the common bile duct due to stone, the gallbladder is seldom palpable; the organ usually is already shrivelled; in distension due to other causes, distension is common by comparison'. Simply stated, if the gallbladder is palpable in the presence of jaundice, the jaundice is unlikely to be due to stone and one should think of a malignant cause of the lower extrahepatic biliary tree. However, exceptions to the law are due to double impaction of the cystic duct and the common bile duct due to stone, pancreatic duct calculi, and worm-induced obstruction (ascaris or clonorchis). Distended gallbladders are not always easy to feel but can be detected readily by ultrasound.

Other benign conditions of the gallbladder

Cholesterosis

Cholesterosis or 'strawberry gallbladder' is a condition in which the mucous membrane of the gallbladder is infiltrated with lipid and cholesterol. It affects middle-aged and elderly patients of either sex. Cholesterol stones are found in the gallbladders of half of these patients. Macroscopically, the mucosa is brick-red and speckled with bright yellow nodules. Management is as for chronic cholecystitis.

Adenomyomatosis

This rare condition is characterised by mucosal diverticula (Rokitansky–Aschoff sinuses) that particularly affect the fundus and penetrate the muscular layers to the serosa. Muscular hypertrophy and inflammatory cell infiltrates are present. Clinical presentation can mimic chronic cholecystitis while radiologically it may raise concern about the presence of a gallbladder tumor. The diagnosis may be made on careful imaging but is often only made following cholecystectomy, as the gallbladder normally contains stones.

Acute acalculous cholecystitis

Few patients with acute cholecystitis have acalculous inflammation. The condition may be precipitated by major surgery, bacteraemia, trauma, pancreatitis or other serious illness, and may complicate parenteral nutrition. The condition is best diagnosed using a nuclear imaging hepatobiliary iminodiacetic acid (HIDA) scan. The inflammatory reaction in the gallbladder wall may be intense and severe, leading to gangrene and perforation. In ill patients, percutaneous drainage (cholecystostomy) under ultrasound guidance may be considered, but urgent cholecystectomy is often advisable.

Investigation of patients with suspected gallstones

Blood tests

A full blood count may reveal a neutrophilia in acute cholecystitis or its complications. An elevated serum bilirubin or alkaline phosphatase may signify the presence of common duct stones. Prothrombin time should be measured if there has been a history of jaundice.

Plain abdominal x-ray

As only 15% of gallstones contain enough calcium to be seen on a plain radiograph, this investigation is not used in diagnosis. Gas is rarely seen outlining the biliary tree if there is a fistula between the biliary tract and the gut, as in gallstone ileus or following endoscopic sphincterotomy.

Ultrasonography

Ultrasonography permits inspection of the gallbladder, its wall and its contents, and demonstrates dilatation of the intrahepatic and extrahepatic biliary tree. Stones reflect the ultrasonic wave and are thrown into prominence by the acoustic shadow they produce (Fig. 14.21). The technique is extremely accurate in skilled hands. As it does not depend on hepatic excretion of contrast, it can be used in both jaundiced and nonjaundiced patients. However, it cannot accurately assess the common bile duct with regard to the presence or absence of stones. Further investigations are required if common bile duct (CBD) stones are suspected.

Cholangiography

Cholangiography is used to assess the main biliary tree for causes of obstruction such as stones or strictures. MRCP can assess the biliary tree noninvasively whereas ERCP is reserved for therapeutic interventions. Common bile duct stones can be removed by

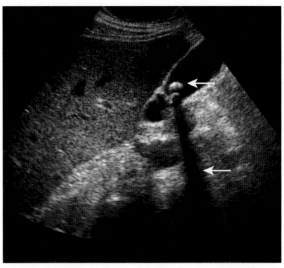

Fig. 14.21 Ultrasound scan of the gallbladder demonstrating the hyperechoic features of a gallstone (*arrowed*) along with the typical acoustic shadow (also *arrowed*).

endoscopic sphincterotomy and subsequent balloon trawling or basket retrieval. Complications occur in up to 7% of patients and may include cholangitis, bleeding and acute pancreatitis.

Surgical treatment of gallstones

Patients with symptomatic gallstones are usually advised to undergo cholecystectomy to relieve symptoms and avoid complications (EBM 14.6). Patients with asymptomatic gallstones are treated expectantly, particularly if they are elderly or suffering from medical conditions likely to increase the risk of surgery. In younger patients, there may be a stronger case for surgery despite the absence of symptoms, particularly if the stones are multiple and likely to cause complications, such as acute pancreatitis or there is a high underlying prevalence of gallbladder cancer within the population being treated.

EBM 14.6 Surgical treatment of gallstones

'*Asymptomatic gallstones do not require treatment. Once a patient with gallstones becomes symptomatic, elective day case laparoscopic cholecystectomy is indicated. For patients with acute cholecystitis, early acute cholecystectomy is indicated. For those patients with common bile duct stones duct clearance and cholecystectomy should be considered irrespective of symptoms. These recommendations should be considered along with individual patient's comorbidities and likelihood to benefit from proposed interventions.*'

Gallstone Disease: Diagnosis and Management of Cholelithiasis, Cholecystitis and Choledocholithiasis. Internal Clinical Guidelines Team (UK). London: National Institute for Health and Care Excellence (UK); 2014 Oct. Available from http://www.ncbi.nlm. nih.gov/pubmedhealth/PMH0070643/

The principles of surgical treatment involve removal of the gallbladder and the stones it contains, while ensuring that no stones remain within the ductal system. 'Open' cholecystectomy has largely been replaced by laparoscopic cholecystectomy, but is still undertaken in up to 10% of patients with symptomatic gallstones and in patients in whom laparoscopic surgery cannot be completed safely. A laparoscopic procedure may not be

14

possible in the patient who has previously undergone multiple abdominal operations but contraindications to laparoscopic surgery are few.

Conversion from a laparoscopic procedure to open cholecystectomy should be seen as a limitation of the minimally invasive technique and not as a failure of the surgeon. Laparotomy is mandatory if uncontrolled bleeding occurs or if a bile duct injury is suspected (EBM 14.7).

EBM **14.7 Complications of cholecystectomy**

'Conversion to an open procedure from a laparoscopic procedure should be considered in the presence of adhesions, difficulty in delineating the anatomy or a suspected complication. Injury to the bile duct during cholecystectomy requires immediate referral to a surgeon or service specialised in the management of such a complication.'

Connor S, Garden OJ. Br J Surg. 2006;93:158–68.

Open cholecystectomy

The gallbladder is usually approached through a right subcostal incision. Good exposure of the porta and anterior surface of the gallbladder is paramount. This can be facilitated by the following manoeuvres: using a self-supporting retractor that can elevate the costal margin, lifting the right lobe of the liver and placing a surgical pack between liver and posterior abdominal wall, dividing the falciform ligament, gentle cephalad retraction of segment IV, packing the stomach medially and counter traction of the duodenum. Using a gallbladder fundal grasper to distract the gallbladder anteriorly and a second grasper to distract Hartmann's pouch inferiorly exposes and triangulates the anterior surface of the hepatobiliary triangle. The peritoneal layer can gently be incised with minimal diathermy and then blunt dissected to expose the contents of the hepatobiliary triangle; this can be repeated for the posterior surface. With the cystic duct and artery clearly identified and skeletonised, intraoperative cholangiography is performed under image intensification by cannulating the cystic duct and following the injection of contrast. The cholangiogram displays the anatomy of the duct system, identifies ductal stones, and confirms that contrast passes freely into the duodenum (Fig. 14.22). The cystic duct and artery are ligated and divided and the gallbladder is removed. A retrograde approach, in which the gallbladder is mobilised 'fundus first', can be used when inflammation makes visualisation of the biliary anatomy difficult but this approach should only be undertaken by surgeons confident with portal anatomy. The surgeon must be very aware of the possibility of fibrosis having drawn in the right portal structures such that they are easily damaged during such dissection. A warning of the presence of this situation is a retracted and shrunken gallbladder with indrawing of the liver capsule (Fig 14.23). A safer approach in such situations is a subtotal cholecystectomy. Here the peritoneal surface of the gallbladder is incised well clear of any potential portal structures, all stones evacuated and the cystic duct orifice identified from within the gallbladder and safely oversewn. Some surgeons pursue a policy of selective cholangiography, obtaining a cholangiogram only in patients at high risk of having ductal stones. The presence of such stones may be suspected if there is a history of jaundice or pancreatitis, if preoperative LFTs are abnormal, or if dilatation of the common bile duct

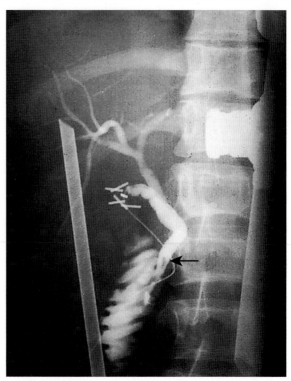

Fig. 14.22 Operative cholangiogram undertaken at laparoscopic cholecystectomy (note the radioopaque ports). The intra- and extrahepatic ducts are seen and there is flow of contrast into the duodenum. A small radiolucent calculus is present at the lower end of the common bile duct (*arrow*).

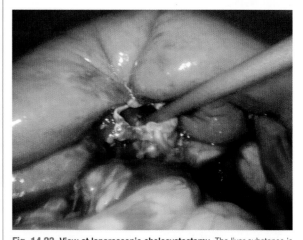

Fig. 14.23 View at laparoscopic cholecystectomy. The liver substance is drawn into the gallbladder fossa. The gallbladder is shrunken. This is a warning sign of severe fibrosis and this situation presents a high risk of duct injury if attempts are made to dissect the hepatobiliary triangle or perform fundus-first cholecystectomy. A safer option is to open the gallbladder as seen here and extract the stones and drain the gallbladder remnant. In event of biliary fistula it can be controlled by endoscopic retrograde cholangiopancreatography and stenting.

or the presence of multiple gallbladder stones has been detected on ultrasound.

The value of routinely placing an abdominal drain has been questioned although its use in difficult surgery may prevent the development of a collection and identify leakage of bile.

Laparoscopic cholecystectomy

Laparoscopic cholecystectomy is now the treatment of choice for symptomatic gallstones, despite having a significantly higher risk of major bile duct injury. Thus it is crucial surgeons performing such surgery create a culture of safety by understanding the steps required for safe cholecystectomy and understanding factors that contribute to bile duct injury. Access to the peritoneal cavity is obtained through three or four cannulae inserted through the anterior abdominal wall and following insufflation of the peritoneal cavity with CO_2. A 30-degree scope should be used to allow changing of the angle of view. Initially the gallbladder fundus is retracted by grasping forceps and reflected cephalad and lateral to the 10 o'clock position (Fig. 14.24). A second grasper is used to lift Hartmann's pouch across toward the falciform ligament. This exposes the posterior surface of the hepatobiliary triangle. Dissection will commence on this surface after having identified Rouvière's sulcus (Fig 14.24). Rouvière's sulcus is a groove in the surface of right liver indicating the right posterior portal pedicle. An imaginary line drawn between here and the base of segment IV indicates the line above which dissection is safe. This posterior dissection is a key difference to the open approach to cholecystectomy. Once completed Hartmann's pouch is distracted inferiorly toward the right iliac fossa and the camera rotated to view the anterior surface of the hepatobiliary triangle. This peritoneal surface is released and any loose areolar tissue cleared from the hepatobiliary triangle including up to the base of the liver. This should leave the cystic duct and artery skeletonised. They should be the only two structures entering the gallbladder. Once obtained this is known as the 'critical view of safety' and the two structures can be clipped safely. The key to avoiding bile duct injury is recognising when it is not safe to persist in trying to obtain the critical view. In such circumstances the surgeon requires a fallback plan that will depend on their personal skill set but should include one of the following: subtotal cholecystectomy, conversion to open, seeking help from a specialist HPB surgeon or abandoning further dissection and referring to an HPB service for definitive management. The routine use of intraoperative cholangiography (IOC) with laparoscopic cholecystectomy is controversial, with most practitioners using a selective approach. Reasons include the widespread availability of good preoperative imaging (MRCP), technical difficulties with IOC and management of subsequently detected CBD stones. Proponents of routine IOC argue it reduces both the incidence and severity of bile duct injury associated with laparoscopic cholecystectomy and therefore should be mandatory.

14.7 Summary

Cholecystectomy

- Cholecystectomy is the standard treatment for symptomatic gallbladder stones; alternatives (stone dissolution, extracorporeal lithotripsy) are now seldom used
- Open cholecystectomy has been largely superseded by laparoscopic cholecystectomy, but conversion to open operation is still sometimes needed
- Cholecystectomy now has a low operative mortality (0.2%); inadvertent injury to the bile duct (0.2% incidence) remains the main source of major morbidity
- Some 5–10% of patients undergoing cholecystectomy have ductal stones, many of which are unsuspected. Opinions vary as to whether intraoperative cholangiography should be undertaken routinely to detect such stones
- In the era of laparoscopic cholecystectomy, there is a growing tendency not to perform routine operative cholangiography, and to extract symptomatic duct stones by nonoperative means (i.e., at endoscopic papillotomy)
- If ductal stones cause symptoms, they frequently give rise to cholangitis and Charcot's triad of pain, jaundice and fever (often with rigors).

Exploration of the common bile duct

This is undertaken much less often with the free availability of therapeutic ERCP (EBM 14.8). At open or laparoscopic surgery, if stones are detected in the main duct system a decision with regard to definitive management needs to be made. In a small nondilated duct a choledochotomy (opening common bile duct) is to be avoided due to risk of postprocedure stricture. Options include flushing the duct with saline after administration of pharmacological smooth muscle relaxants such as glucagon. Transcystic exploration can also be performed using baskets or balloons under radiological guidance or via a fine choledochoscope. If, however, the stones are proximal to the cystic duct insertion or cannot be flushed or retrieved, then an antegrade transsphincteric stent can be placed in preparation for a postoperative ERCP. In some cases it is possible to perform on table ERCP if the equipment and staff are available. In situations where the common bile duct is dilated, a choledochotomy can be performed. It should be opened longitudinally in the supraduodenal portion. The duct can then be explored with forceps, balloons, baskets or choledochoscope. Following exploration, a further check cholangiogram or direct inspection with a fibreoptic choledochoscope should be performed to confirm clearance. Traditionally the opening in the common bile duct is closed around a T-tube, (Fig. 14.25). Nowadays these are rarely required as

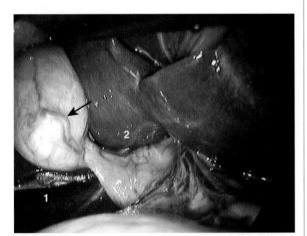

Fig. 14.24 Laparoscopic view of the gallbladder beneath the liver, showing the branches of the cystic artery (*arrow*) on the gallbladder surface. In the background Rouvière's sulcus (*1*) can be seen just below Hartmann's pouch. With Hartmann's pouch lifted up and across towards the falciform ligament, a line drawn between the sulcus and base of segment IV (*2*) indicates the line above which dissection is safe.

EBM   14.8 Exploration of the common bile duct

'Patients undergoing cholecystectomy do not require ERCP preoperatively if there is a low probability of choledocholithiasis. Laparoscopic common bile duct exploration and postoperative ERCP are both safe and reliable in clearing common bile duct stones.'

Nathanson L, et al. Ann Surg. 2005;242:188–92.

14

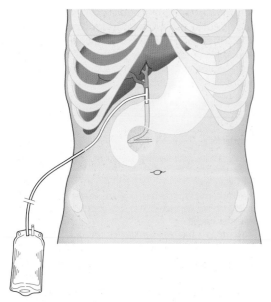

Fig. 14.25 T-tube drainage of the common bile duct.

transphincteric antegrade stents can be placed or a drain left adjacent to the closure and postoperative ERCP be performed in event of persistent bile leak or retained stone.

If, at operation, a stone is firmly impacted at the lower end of the common bile duct, it may have to be removed through the duodenum. Transduodenal sphincterotomy and sphincteroplasty increase the risk of postoperative morbidity and mortality, and are undertaken rarely. Alternatives include using laser or lithotripsy under direct vision via the bile duct using urological scope to fracture the stones.

Complications of cholecystectomy

Intraoperative complications

Bleeding

Although a small amount of bleeding can occur during dissection of the hepatobiliary triangle it will often cease spontaneously with simple pressure. In the event of major bleeding from the hepatobiliary triangle, the surgeon should question if the plane of dissection is correct and must suspect injury to right hepatic artery or portal vein. Hurried attempts to secure bleeding can lead to injuries to major ducts and vessels by injudicious application of clips or haemostats. Instead the Hogarth–Pringle manoeuvre, where the free edge of the lesser omentum is compressed by the surgeon's thumb and finger placed in the epiploic foramen posteriorly, can be used to significantly reduce the bleeding, and localise and ligate the bleeding vessel. Control of the bleeding with small sutures is then possible in a clear field of view. Bleeding can also occur during dissection of the gallbladder off the liver bed. If this plane is hostile it is entirely acceptable to leave the back wall of the gallbladder attached and perform a partial cholecystectomy. Some advocate ablating the remnant mucosa with diathermy. Bleeding while dissecting this plane is suggestive of an injury to the middle hepatic vein. Laparoscopically increasing the intraabdominal pressure may help control the bleeding to allow haemostasis to be achieved. In open surgery the vessel can be simply ligated as compression of the porta will have limited effect.

Bile duct injury

If diagnosed at operation, this should be managed by an experienced hepatobiliary surgeon whose help should be sought and the patient transferred as required. A small lateral injury can be managed by biliary decompression with either placement of a T-tube or antegrade stent. Partial or complete transection of a nondilated duct is best managed by hepaticojejunostomy using a Roux-en-Y loop.

Postoperative course

The use of enhanced recovery programme for patients undergoing open cholecystectomy has significantly reduced hospital stay to 1–2 days. Respiratory complications are not uncommon, particularly in the elderly, and there is a significant risk of wound infection (see later). Operative mortality following elective open cholecystectomy is low (0.2%), but is increased tenfold if there is obstructive jaundice or if the common bile duct has to be explored. In elderly patients similar increases in magnitude of mortality are seen and such patients should be counselled regarding potential risks and alternative options.

Postoperative stay is reduced with laparoscopic cholecystectomy, which in many centres is undertaken as a day-case procedure. Complications resulting from a major abdominal wound are undoubtedly avoided, but there is concern regarding the apparent increased incidence of injury to the bile duct. Failure of the patient to recover quickly following the procedure, the development of abdominal pain or the need for additional analgesia in the immediate postoperative period should cause the surgeon to consider the complications of haemorrhage or bile leakage, and mandates further assessment by LFTs, abdominal imaging or repeat laparoscopy. Mortality and morbidity related to the laparoscopic procedure have also been reported. Nevertheless, the advantages to the patient of this minimally invasive technique have led to its widespread adoption by surgeons.

Haemorrhage

This may originate from the cystic artery or the gallbladder bed. Significant intraabdominal bleeding should be suspected from the development of pain or if the patient exhibits early features of hypovolaemic shock. Blood may issue from the drain, if one is present, and reexploration is mandatory.

Infective complications

Wound infection from organisms present in the bile (notably *E. coli*, *Klebsiella aerogenes* and *Strep. faecalis*) can be reduced following cholecystectomy by the intravenous administration of a cephalosporin at the time of induction of anaesthesia, although the routine use of this group of drugs at laparoscopic cholecystectomy has recently been questioned (EBM 14.9). A longer course of antibiotics may be prescribed when significant bile contamination of the peritoneal cavity has occurred at surgery. Collections of bile and/or blood readily become infected after cholecystectomy. Formal drainage may be needed if this progresses to the formation of a subhepatic or subphrenic abscess.

EBM | **14.9 Antibiotic prophylaxis in laparoscopic cholecystectomy**

'Routine prophylactic administration of antibiotics is unnecessary in patients at low risk of wound or postoperative infection.'

Al-Ghnaniem R, et al. Br J Surg. 2003;90:365–6.

Bile leakage

This may be due to a ligature or clip slipping off the cystic duct, the accidental division of an unrecognised accessory or segmental duct, damage to the common bile duct, or retention of a duct stone after exploration. Bile leakage may be evidenced by the development of abnormal LFTs and localised or generalised abdominal pain. It may be contained if a drain is in place. The key to management is first defining the anatomy of the biliary tree and identifying any injury or distal obstruction. This can be done noninvasively with CT cholangiogram or MRCP using hepatobiliary excreted agents. If biliary peritonitis is present urgent repeat laparoscopy or laparotomy is required to wash out the peritoneum and control the leak. For patients with intact main and sectoral bile ducts or an obstructing distal stone, ERCP with stenting or stone clearance is the treatment of choice. For a more major injury referral to an experienced HPB surgeon is required.

Retained stones

In some patients, unsuspected stones may be left in the bile duct at cholecystectomy or post bile duct exploration. Such stones usually give rise to complications such as jaundice, cholangitis and pancreatitis in the days to years following cholecystectomy. Ultrasonography, MRCP or cholangiogram via T-tube (if used) can be used to confirm the presence of such retained stones (Fig. 14.26) and endoscopic retrograde cholangiography and sphincterotomy are performed to recover them (Fig. 14.27). In this technique, a diathermy wire attached to a cannula is passed through a side-viewing gastroscope and used to divide the sphincter of Oddi. The stones can then be extracted with a Dormia basket or balloon catheter. If the stones are too large to be withdrawn or the patient is unwell, a stent or a catheter can be left in the biliary system (nasobiliary catheter). The stones can be

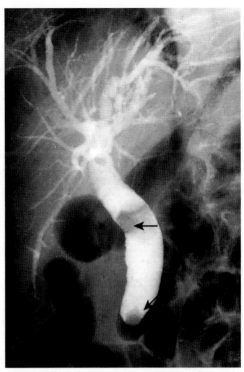

Fig. 14.27 Endoscopic retrograde cholangiography demonstrating multiple stones (*arrows*) within the biliary tree. These calculi were removed from the dilated bile duct by balloon extraction following sphincterotomy.

14

crushed (lithotripsy) and removed at a later date by means of a repeat endoscopic examination. Surgery may be required to retrieve retained bile duct stones that cannot be dealt with in this way. In patients with a T-tube in situ percutaneous extraction can be used using similar instruments as used at ERCP (Fig. 14.28).

Bile duct stricture

About 90% of benign duct strictures result from damage during cholecystectomy, in which the duct is divided, ligated or devascularised. This last mechanism appears to be a common cause of injury at laparoscopic cholecystectomy. Other causes of injury include division of a ligated common bile duct that has been mistaken for the cystic duct, division of the right hepatic duct below the point of anomalous insertion of the cystic duct, and encirclement of the common bile duct by the ligature or clip used to close off the cystic duct. Strictures only occasionally result from abdominal trauma or erosion of the bile duct by a gallstone impacted in the gallbladder (Mirizzi's syndrome).

If the common bile duct is completely occluded, progressive obstructive jaundice develops in the postoperative period. If there is a partial stricture, attacks of pain, fever and obstructive jaundice signal the development of cholangitis. The serum alkaline phosphatase and transaminase concentrations are usually elevated, and blood cultures may be positive during attacks of fever. If left untreated, persistent cholangitis and obstruction progress to hepatic abscess formation and rarely to secondary biliary cirrhosis.

The site and extent of the stricture must be defined radiologically. After ultrasonography has been performed, MRCP, ERCP and/or PTC are undertaken. Reconstructive surgery is carried out in a specialist centre and usually necessitates fashioning a

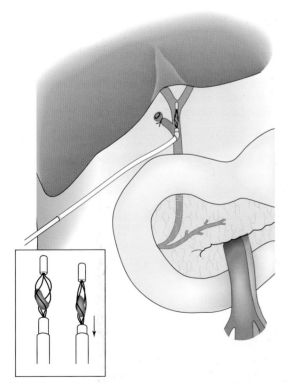

Fig. 14.26 Percutaneous removal of a retained common bile duct stone through a T-tube tract.

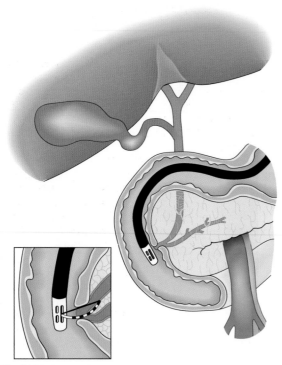

Fig. 14.28 Endoscopic papillotomy to remove retained stones.

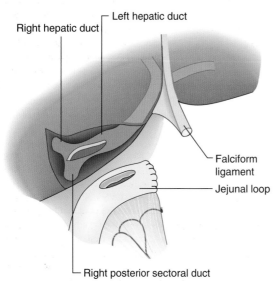

Right hepatic duct

Left hepatic duct

Falciform ligament

Jejunal loop

Right posterior sectoral duct

Fig. 14.29 Relief of bile duct stricture by anastomosis of a limb of jejunum to the distended biliary tree above the stricture (hepaticojejunostomy Roux-en-Y).

Roux loop of jejunum and anastomosing this to the distended biliary system above the stricture (Fig. 14.29).

Postcholecystectomy syndrome

This term is used to embrace a group of complaints such as postprandial flatulence, fat intolerance, epigastric and right hypochondrial discomfort, and heartburn, which may follow cholecystectomy. The complaints tend to be more troublesome when cholecystectomy has been performed in the absence of gallstones. Investigations are usually negative, but some patients

prove to have retained stones or other alimentary disorders such as peptic ulceration, gastritis and chronic pancreatitis. It is possible that some patients develop pain because of functional abnormalities of the sphincter of Oddi (see below).

Atypical 'biliary' pain

More difficulty arises with patients who have attacks of pain consistent with biliary colic but in whom investigations such as ultrasonography, oral cholecystography and ERCP reveal no abnormality. Some of these patients with 'acalculous biliary pain' may eventually prove to have nonbiliary disease, such as peptic ulceration, chronic pancreatitis or irritable bowel syndrome. In the majority, no explanation for the symptoms can be found, although recent evidence suggests that some may be suffering from a functional disorder of the sphincter of Oddi (Fig. 14.30). Endoscopic manometry may be useful in identifying patients who may benefit from endoscopic sphincterotomy; however, there is high risk of inducing pancreatitis and should only be performed by experienced centres.

Nonsurgical treatment of gallstones

Dissolution therapy with bile salts is no longer popular in the management of gallstone disease. Percutaneous extraction or dissolution of gallstones is possible, but the efficacy of this approach has been questioned. Destruction of stones by extracorporeal shock-wave lithotripsy has been used in selected patients but, like the previous treatments, has largely been made redundant with the advent of laparoscopic cholecystectomy and ERCP.

Management of acute cholangitis

This condition is caused by incomplete obstruction of the biliary tree and is more often due to common bile duct stones. It is not frequently observed as a presenting feature of malignancy, but may result from instrumentation of the biliary tree during the investigation or treatment of malignant obstructive jaundice.

The patient is often extremely unwell, with clinical features of Charcot's triad and evidence of septic shock. Treatment involves resuscitation, the administration of appropriate antibiotics, and decompression of the biliary tree. Given the high associated morbidity and mortality of surgical intervention, decompression

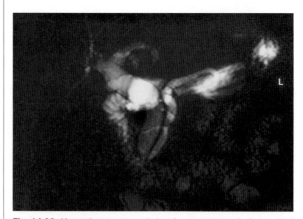

Fig. 14.30 Magnetic resonance cholangiopancreatography in a patient who underwent laparoscopic cholecystectomy 5 years before the development of recurrent right upper quadrant pain. The bile and pancreatic ducts are dilated secondary to biliary dyskinesia.

is normally achieved by endoscopic means. When common bile duct stones are responsible, it may be necessary to drain the biliary tree temporarily by means of a stent, even if sphincterotomy and stone extraction have apparently been successful.

Other benign biliary disorders

Asiatic cholangiohepatitis

There has been a decline in the incidence of this condition, which occurs in the Far East and is particularly common in coastal Chinese and South East Asian communities. The causative organism is *Clonorchis sinensis*, which is a type of liver fluke. Infection occurs due to ingestion of infected fish or snails harbouring the fluke as intermediate host. Man is the definitive host and the adult worm matures in the intrahepatic biliary radicals causing duct thickening, dilatation and periductal fibrosis. Dead worms or eggs form a nidus for formation of stones anywhere in the biliary tree. Suppurative cholangitis develops and pigment stones form in the intrahepatic and extrahepatic biliary tree. Deconjugation of bilirubin glucuronide by bacteria may be implicated in stone formation, and *E. coli* and *Strep. faecalis* can often be isolated from the bile and portal blood.

The clinical features are those of obstructive jaundice, pain and fever, and liver abscesses may form. Stool examination can show the presence of eggs or worms. Ultrasonography shows thick walled and dilated ducts. ERCP can show the presence of worms as filling defects. Cholangitis is treated with antibiotics, and stones in the duct can be removed by percutaneous, endoscopic and operative means. Praziquantel or albendazole remain the drugs of choice for medical management of the worm. Ductal obstruction may be treated by choledochoduodenostomy or hepaticojejunostomy in addition to cholecystectomy. A limb of the Roux loop of jejunum may be left in a subcutaneous position to facilitate subsequent percutaneous manoeuvres to treat residual or recurrent calculi. Hepatic resection may be indicated if suppuration and obstruction have led to regional destruction of liver tissue.

Dysplastic changes have been seen with Asiatic cholangiohepatitis, which leads to an increased preponderance of cholangiocarcinoma and remains the most dreaded complication of this infestation.

Primary sclerosing cholangitis

In this condition, both intrahepatic and extrahepatic bile ducts may become indurated and irregularly thickened. There is a marked chronic inflammatory cell infiltrate and fibrous narrowing of the biliary tree. Its aetiology is unknown, but it may have an immunological basis since most patients have evidence of auto-antibodies. Over three-quarters of patients also suffer from ulcerative colitis; other associated conditions include retroperitoneal fibrosis, immunodeficiency syndromes and pancreatitis. Bile duct carcinoma can develop, and obstruction can give rise to bacterial cholangitis and secondary biliary cirrhosis.

The condition frequently affects young adults and gives rise to intermittent attacks of obstructive jaundice, pruritus and pain. ERCP and liver biopsy are the mainstays of diagnosis. Medical treatment is generally unsatisfactory, and the outlook is extremely variable. Duct strictures can sometimes by treated by surgical bypass or the insertion of stents, but such manoeuvres may compromise the ability to undertake successful liver transplantation, which offers the only prospect of cure.

Tumours of the biliary tract

Carcinoma of the gallbladder

Carcinoma of the gallbladder is rare and almost invariably associated with the presence of gallstones. Stone-induced cholecystitis is considered as the initiating event leading to dysplasia, carcinoma in situ and ultimately leading to invasive carcinoma. The condition is four times as common in females as in males. About 90% of lesions are adenocarcinomas; the remainder are squamous carcinomas.

Direct invasion commonly obstructs the bile duct or porta hepatis, and early lymphatic and haematogenous dissemination is common. Initial symptoms are indistinguishable from those of gallstones and this leads to a considerable delay in presentation. Jaundice, if present, is unremitting and signifies locally advanced or metastatic disease. A mass may be palpable more often due to the malignant gallbladder itself rather than a mucocoele due to obstruction. Many tumours are detected incidentally at cholecystectomy for the treatment of gallstones, on histopathology. TNM staging is used where T1a indicates disease limited to the mucosa, T1b limited to the muscle adjacent to lamina propria, T2 to the perimuscular connective tissue involvement, T3 for involvement of the liver or one adjacent organ, and T4 to spread into the vascular supply of liver or more than one adjacent organ. Disease limited to the mucosa (T1a, N0) in the absence of any other lesion does not warrant any further therapy. T2–3, N0–1, M0 is managed by an aggressive approach of extended cholecystectomy involving resection of segments 4 and 5 of the liver and dissection of the regional lymph nodes. This extended cholecystectomy is also recommended for T1b lesions. Tumours presenting with jaundice are usually unresectable. Palliation of troublesome pruritus can be offered by endoscopic or percutaneous insertion of a stent or a surgical bypass between the left hepatic duct or a segment III duct with a loop of jejunum. The 5-year survival rate is less than 5%.

Carcinoma of the bile ducts

Cholangiocarcinoma is a relatively uncommon cancer that affects the elderly and which is increasing in frequency. Such lesions may arise at any site within the biliary tree and can be multifocal. Tumours can be classified based on the level of involvement of the biliary tree (Fig. 14.31) and are most common at the hilus. Polypoidal tumours are uncommon but carry a more favourable outlook. Sclerotic lesions involving the confluence of the hepatic ducts (Klatskin tumour) pose considerable problems in management. The lesions are said to be slow-growing, but this has been over-emphasised. Cholangiocarcinoma may develop in patients with underlying primary sclerosing cholangitis or choledochal cyst.

Clinical features

Progressive obstructive jaundice, often preceded by vague dyspeptic pain, is the usual presenting feature. The gallbladder may become obstructed because of cystic duct involvement, and mucocoele or empyema can develop, but generally it is impalpable. Anorexia and weight loss are common. Pruritus is often particularly distressing.

Management

The diagnosis may be made on the history and clinical findings. The presence of intrahepatic duct dilatation and a collapsed

14

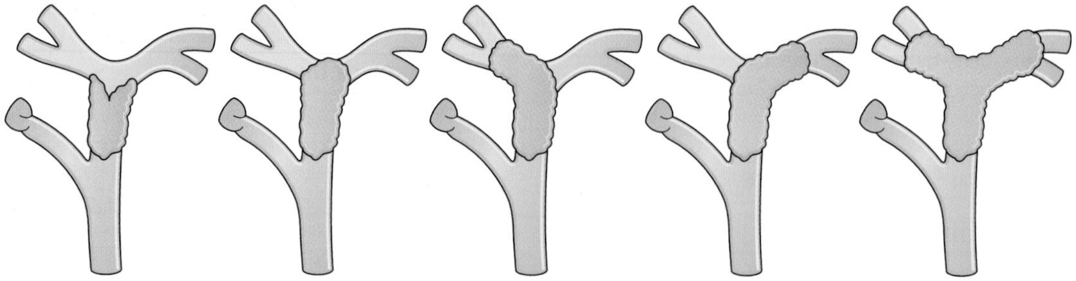

Type 1   Type 2   Type 3a   Type 3b   Type 4

Fig. 14.31 Classification of hilar cholangiocarcinoma.

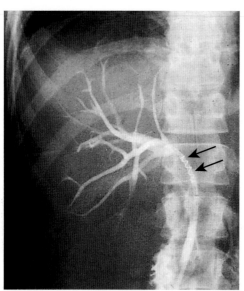

Fig. 14.32 Percutaneous transhepatic cholangiogram demonstrating a stricture at the confluence of the hepatic ducts. This lesion has the typical appearance of a cholangiocarcinoma and has been managed by percutaneous insertion of a stent (*arrowed*).

gallbladder on ultrasound scan are highly suggestive of a tumour involving the common hepatic duct. Resectability is best assessed by CT or MRI to exclude the presence of hepatic metastases and nodal involvement and to determine vascular invasion.

Carcinoma of the lower common bile duct is treated by the Whipple operation (p. 237) if the tumour is localised and the patient is fit for radical resection. Long-term survival following this procedure is better in patients with cholangiocarcinoma than in those with carcinoma of the head of the pancreas.

Carcinoma of the upper biliary tract is resectable in only 10% of patients, some of whom may require hepatic resection to achieve satisfactory clearance of the tumour. Following resection, the divided intrahepatic ducts are anastomosed to a Roux limb of jejunum. Operative mortality is reported in as many as 10% of patients. In the majority of patients not submitted to resection, palliation can be achieved by insertion of a stent by endoscopic or percutaneous transhepatic techniques (Fig. 14.32). Most stents are liable to occlusion, exposing the patient to repeated attacks of cholangitis and/or jaundice. Quality of life is poor and few patients with cholangiocarcinoma survive for more than 18 months. The role of systemic chemotherapy and/or radiotherapy has yet to be established.

C. Ross Carter
Colin McKay

15

The pancreas and spleen

Chapter contents

The pancreas 233

The spleen 248

The pancreas

Surgical anatomy

The pancreas develops from separate ventral and dorsal buds of endoderm that appear during the fourth week of foetal life. The ventral pancreas develops with the biliary tree, and its duct joins the common bile duct before emptying into the duodenum through the papilla of Vater (Fig. 15.1). During gestation, the duodenum rotates clockwise on its long axis, and the bile duct and ventral pancreas pass round behind it to fuse with the dorsal pancreas. Most of the duct that drains the dorsal pancreas joins the duct draining the ventral pancreas to form the main pancreatic duct (of Wirsung); the rest of the dorsal duct becomes the accessory pancreatic duct (of Santorini) and enters the duodenum 2.5 cm proximal to the main duct. In foetal life, the common bile duct and main pancreatic duct are dilated at their junction to form the ampulla of Vater. In extrauterine life, only 10% of individuals retain this ampulla, although most retain a short common channel between the two duct systems.

The pancreas lies in the retroperitoneum, behind the lesser sac and stomach. The head of the gland lies within the C-loop of the duodenum, with which it shares a blood supply from the coeliac and superior mesenteric arteries (Fig. 15.2). The superior mesenteric vein runs upwards to the left of the uncinate process, and joins the splenic vein behind the neck of the pancreas to form the portal vein. The body and tail of the pancreas lie in front of the splenic vein as far as the splenic hilum, and receive arterial blood from the splenic artery as it runs along the upper border of the gland. The intimate relationship of the friable pancreas to these major blood vessels, in addition to the aorta and inferior vena cava, is the reason that bleeding is a significant issue after pancreatic trauma. The close association between the common bile duct and the head of pancreas explains why obstructive jaundice is so common in cancer of the head of the pancreas, and the common channel within the ampulla of Vater why gallstones frequently give rise to acute pancreatitis.

Surgical physiology

Exocrine function

The exocrine pancreas is essential for the digestion of fat, protein and carbohydrate. The pancreas secretes 1–2 L of alkaline (pH 7.5–8.8) enzyme-rich juice each day. The enzymes are synthesised by the acinar cells and stored there as zymogen granules. Trypsin is the key proteolytic enzyme; it is released in an inactive form (trypsinogen) and is normally only activated within the duodenum by the brush border enzyme, enterokinase. Once trypsin has been activated, a cascade is established whereby the other proteolytic enzymes become activated in turn. Lipase and amylase are secreted as active enzymes. The alkaline medium required for the activity of pancreatic enzymes is provided by the bicarbonate secreted by the ductal epithelium.

Pancreatic secretion is stimulated by eating. Hormonal and neural (vagal) mechanisms are involved. Food entering the duodenum (notably fat and protein digestion products) releases cholecystokinin (CCK), which stimulates pancreatic enzyme secretion and contraction of the gallbladder, thereby increasing bile flow into the intestine. Acid in the duodenum releases the hormone secretin, which stimulates the pancreas to secrete watery alkaline juice.

Endocrine function

The islets of Langerhans are distributed throughout the pancreas. Although they account for only 2% of the weight of the gland, they receive 10% of its blood supply. Interaction between the endocrine and the exocrine pancreas is facilitated by the close proximity of islets and acini, and by a local 'portal' system in which blood draining from the islets enters a capillary network around neighbouring acinar cells before entering the tributaries of the portal vein. Four types of endocrine are recognised: A cells produce glucagon; B cells, insulin; D cells, somatostatin; and PP cells, pancreatic polypeptide. Glucagon and insulin have well-established physiological roles; the function of the other islet products is uncertain, but somatostatin and pancreatic polypeptide (PP) may serve as local

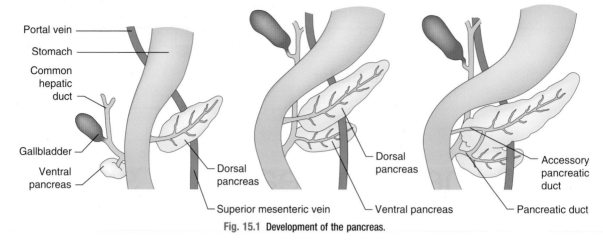

Fig. 15.1 Development of the pancreas.

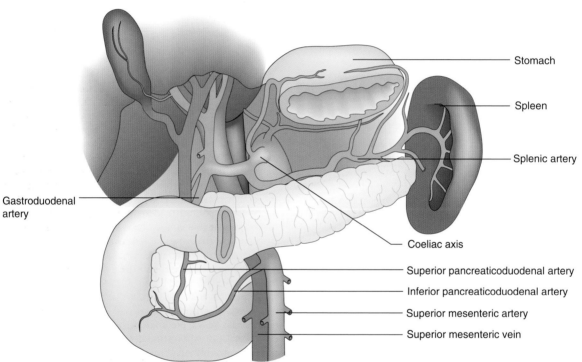

Fig. 15.2 Anatomical relationships of the pancreas.

(paracrine) regulators, rather than as circulating (endocrine) messengers. Gastrin-producing (G) cells are not normally found in the pancreas, except in the rare Zollinger–Ellison syndrome.

Pancreatic pain

The parasympathetic nervous system has no role in the perception of pancreatic pain. Painful stimuli from the pancreas are transmitted by sympathetic fibres that travel along the arteries of supply to the coeliac ganglion, and from there to segments 5–12 of the thoracic spinal cord via the greater, lesser and least splanchnic nerves.

Congenital disorders of the pancreas

Annular pancreas is a rare cause of duodenal obstruction, resulting from failure of rotation of the ventral pancreas. In approximately 5%

of individuals, the ducts draining the dorsal and ventral pancreas fail to fuse, giving rise to pancreas divisum. This means that the secretions of the larger dorsal pancreas have to drain to the duodenum through the smaller accessory duct. There is no evidence to suggest a strong association between pancreas divisum and pancreatitis. Rests of pancreatic tissue may be found at a variety of sites within the gut wall, but are most common in the duodenum, stomach and proximal small bowel. Such heterotopic tissue is usually asymptomatic, but can become a focus of inflammation in the rare condition of cystic duodenal dystrophy ('groove' pancreatitis), causing pain and duodenal obstruction.

Pancreatitis

Pancreatitis may be acute or chronic. After an acute attack, the gland usually returns to anatomical and functional normality, whereas chronic pancreatitis is associated with a permanent derangement of structure and function. Some patients suffer from recurrent acute pancreatitis but enjoy relatively normal health between attacks.

Acute pancreatitis

Acute pancreatitis is a common cause of emergency admission to hospital. The incidence continues to rise, possibly because of an increase in gallstone disease, alcohol misuse and obesity in the population. The disease is relatively rare in children, but all adult age groups may be affected.

Aetiology

Conditions associated with the development of acute pancreatitis are listed in Table 15.1

Gallstone pancreatitis

Gallstones are responsible for nearly three-quarters (75%) of cases of acute pancreatitis in tropical countries in contrast to some 40% of patients in the UK. Tiny gallstones or even

Table 15.1 Causes of acute pancreatitis

Class	Specific causes
Toxic	Alcohol Medication Tropical
Genetic	Cystic fibrosis Hereditary pancreatitis SPINK1 mutation
Metabolic	Hypercalcaemia Hyperlipidaemia

Obstructive	Stone disease
	  Macrolithiasis (bile duct stone)
	  Microlithiasis (sludge)
	Stricture (including postacute
	pancreatitis, trauma)
	Neoplasm
	Infection
	  Parasites
	  Worms
	Anatomical
	  Biliary cystic disease
	  Choledochal cyst/(coele)
	  Duplication cyst
	Duodenal obstruction
	  Afferent limb obstructed
	  Diverticulum
	Congenital anomaly
	  Annular pancreas
	  Anomalous pancreatobiliary junction
	  Pancreas divisum
	  Atresia

Inflammatory	Autoimmune disease
	  Crohn's
	  Polyarteritis nodosa
	  Systemic lupus erythematosus
	  Vasculitis
	  Autoimmune pancreatitis
	Infection
	  Viral

Physiological	Sphincter of Oddi dysfunction

microscopic crystals (so-called microlithiasis) are thought to account for the majority of 'idiopathic' cases. Transient impaction of a gallstone within the common channel between the common bile and pancreatic ducts causes obstruction of the pancreatic duct (Fig. 15.3) and a sequence of events within the pancreatic acinar cells resulting in intracellular activation of pancreatic enzymes, acinar cell damage and pancreatic inflammation.

Alcohol-associated pancreatitis

The proportion of cases linked to alcohol varies in different parts of the world. In Scotland, the figure is around 30%, whereas in some parts of France and North America it may be as high as 50–90%. The mechanism responsible is uncertain. Although there is no direct relationship between the quantity of alcohol consumed and the risk of pancreatitis (in contrast with alcoholic liver disease) alcohol consumption normally exceeds 50 g day (or five standard drinks).

Other causes

Acute pancreatitis occurs in approximately 5% of patients undergoing endoscopic retrograde cholangiopancreatography (ERCP). Such cases are usually mild but can be life-threatening. Trauma, particularly blunt abdominal trauma, may cause pancreatitis or pancreatic duct disruption. Hypercalcaemia is a rare cause of pancreatitis and is usually secondary to hyperparathyroidism. Hyperlipidaemia, due to familial hypertriglyceridaemia, is a rare cause and treatment is directed at the underlying cause. A small number of patients may have a family history of acute pancreatitis.

Viral infections (mumps, Coxsackie virus, rubella, measles and cytomegalovirus) are the most common cause of pancreatitis in children. Bacterial infections are a very rare cause of pancreatitis. Ascaris worms are a relatively common cause of pancreatitis in areas of high prevalence, due to migration through the duodenal papilla from the common bile duct. It is often difficult to prove a causal association with medication, and other causes always need to be considered. Azathioprine, mesalazine and simvastatin are responsible for the best documented cases.

Pancreatic neoplasms may obstruct the pancreatic duct and lead to acute pancreatitis. Such neoplasms can be small and thus easily missed, even by computed tomography (CT). The presence of unexplained pancreatic duct dilatation or other suspicious clinical or radiological appearances should prompt further investigation, usually by CT and endoscopic ultrasound.

Clinical features of acute pancreatitis

Constant, severe or agonising pain in the epigastrium, with radiation through to the back, is usually prominent. Pain can also be experienced in either hypochondrium. Nausea, vomiting and retching are common. Clinical examination often reveals less tenderness, guarding and rigidity than might have been expected from the patient's history, and the presence of generalised peritonism may warrant further investigation by CT to exclude other intraabdominal pathology. Signs of systemic disturbance include tachycardia, hypotension or tachypnoea and suggest severe disease. Obstructive jaundice may result from an impacted gallstone, and if present should raise awareness of the possibility of coexistent cholangitis.

Diagnosis

The key to the diagnosis of acute pancreatitis is a high index of suspicion and measurement of the serum amylase concentration. Serum lipase is an alternative and has some advantages. The usual diagnostic cutoff for serum amylase is three times the upper

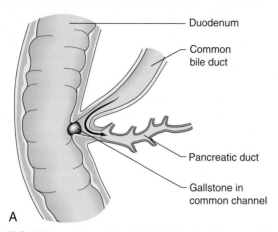

Duodenum

Common
bile duct

Pancreatic duct

Gallstone in
common channel

A

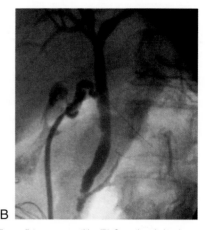

B

Fig. 15.3 (A) Common channel shared by the bile duct and the pancreatic duct may allow gallstone pancreatitis. **(B)** Operative cholangiogram showing a stone in the distal common bile duct and reflux of contrast into the pancreatic duct.

reference limit but the diagnosis should be considered in any patient with a relevant history, even in the context of a nondiagnostic serum amylase. A high serum amylase can be seen in other conditions. The most common of these is mesenteric ischaemia due either to mesenteric vascular occlusion or small bowel strangulation. High serum amylase levels are also seen with perforated ulcer, mesenteric ischaemia or ruptured aneurysm but rarely above the diagnostic threshold for pancreatitis. If the history or clinical examination is atypical for acute pancreatitis, CT should be carried out to clarify the diagnosis.

Serum amylase levels fall rapidly in acute pancreatitis and have no relationship to the severity of the attack or the resolution of the disease. Patients who present some days after the initial onset of abdominal pain may have normal or near-normal serum amylase levels and although urinary amylase or serum lipase can be helpful in such cases, the diagnosis is again best clarified by CT.

Radiology

Initial diagnosis of acute pancreatitis is based on clinical features combined with serum amylase levels. CT is confined to cases where there remains diagnostic doubt, as when serum amylase is nondiagnostic or where the clinical history or examination findings are atypical (for example when there is evidence of generalised peritonitis). In patients with acute pancreatitis, changes will be identified ranging from mild peripancreatic oedema through to extensive pancreatic necrosis (Fig. 15.4) but more importantly

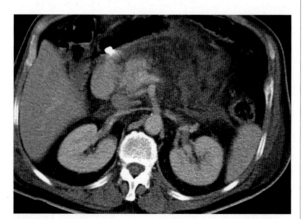

Fig. 15.4 Early computed tomography (CT) with oedema and tail necrosis.

at this stage, other diagnoses that require urgent operative intervention, such as mesenteric ischaemia or perforated viscus, will be excluded.

Differentiation between gallstone- and alcohol-associated pancreatitis

It is important to clarify the aetiology of acute pancreatitis, primarily so that further attacks can be prevented where possible. In the UK, the majority of cases are due to gallstones and these may be present even where there is a clear history of alcohol excess. Therefore, all patients with acute pancreatitis should have an abdominal ultrasound carried out. Even when no stones are identified on ultrasound, other factors may suggest a gallstone diagnosis. In particular, elevated alanine transaminase (ALT) at admission of more than twice the upper reference limit is highly suggestive of gallstone aetiology. In patients where no cause is found, further investigation by endoscopic ultrasound once the acute attack has resolved may detect microlithiasis or a small pancreatic neoplasm.

Assessment of severity in acute pancreatitis

Approximately 80% of patients with acute pancreatitis will have a self-limiting illness, which resolves within 48–72 hours. The focus in these patients is identification and treatment of the underlying cause. The major challenge in the management of this condition is the 20% of patients who have a severe episode of pancreatitis in whom life-threatening complications can occur. Much effort has been directed at the early recognition of severe acute pancreatitis, the aim being to ensure these patients are adequately managed and placed in an appropriate high-dependency or intensive care environment. Many systems have been proposed of which Ranson's Score, Glasgow Prognostic Score, APACHE II score (Table 15.2) and C-reactive protein have been most widely studied. None of these, however, have proved sufficiently accurate to influence management decisions, particularly in the crucial first 24 hours after hospital admission. Other attempts with serum or urine markers of severity have either proved disappointing or have not yet been tested in prospective studies. The challenge is to *recognise* the development of a severe attack, which necessitates a clear understanding of the natural history of the illness.

The most important feature of severe acute pancreatitis is the development of multiple organ dysfunction syndrome (MODS). In most patients, this is identified by the presence of hypoxia, shock or more rarely, renal dysfunction around the time of

Table 15.2 Scoring systems in acute pancreatitis	
Ranson's score	*At admission*: Age in years >55 years White blood cell count >16,000 cells/mm^3 Blood glucose >10 mmol/L (>200 mg/dL) Serum AST >250 IU/L Serum LDH >350 IU/L *At 48 hours*: Calcium (serum calcium <2.0 mmol/L (<8.0 mg/dL) Haematocrit fall >10% Oxygen (hypoxaemia Po_2 < 60 mmHg) BUN increased by 1.8 or more mmol/L (5 or more mg/dL) after IV fluid hydration Base deficit (negative base excess) >4 mEq/L Sequestration of fluids >6 L If the score ≥3, severe pancreatitis is likely.
Glasgow Score (modified)	**P**ao_2 < 60 mmHg/7.9 kPa **A**ge >55 years **N**eutrophils (WBC >15) **C**alcium <2 mmol/L **R**enal function: Urea >16 mmol/L **E**nzymes LDH >600 iu/L, AST >200 iu/L **A**lbumin <32 g/L (serum) **S**ugar BSL >10 mmol/L Three or more positive factors detected within 48 hours of onset suggest severe pancreatitis (refer to HDU/ICU)
APACHE II	**Acute physiology and chronic health evaluation: combined score where**: *Acute physiological indices includes*: Evidence of acute renal failure Age, temperature (rectal), mean arterial pressure, pH, heart rate, respiratory rate, serum levels of sodium, potassium & creatinine, haematocrit, TLC, A–a gradient, Pao_2, Glasgow Coma Scale *Chronic organ insufficiency includes*: Evidence of liver insufficiency, cardiovascular failure, respiratory failure, renal failure and immunosuppression.

admission to hospital. A minority will develop such complications over the next 48 hours and in these patients, the presence of SIRS (systemic inflammatory response syndrome) characterised by tachycardia, raised white cell count and/or tachypnoea is almost always present. It is rare for a patient without SIRS at admission to develop MODS. Where SIRS persists for more than 48 hours, the risk of further deterioration is high and such patients need close monitoring for the development of respiratory and renal complications. It is the group of patients with early persistent SIRS or MODS who are also at greatest risk of developing septic and other local complications of acute pancreatitis.

Contrast-enhanced CT is used in some institutions to identify severe acute pancreatitis, as the presence of pancreatic necrosis or extensive fluid collections identifies a group at high risk of further complications. However, the main determinant of outcome is early systemic organ dysfunction and the role of early CT is now mainly confined to cases of diagnostic doubt. The stratification of patients now includes the category of 'moderately severe' acute pancreatitis, which describes those patients with local complications but no organ failure, or patients with transient systemic organ failure (Table 15.3)

Table 15.3 Severity stratification in acute pancreatitis
Mild acute pancreatitis
• No organ failure • No local or systemic complications
Moderately severe acute pancreatitis
1. Organ failure that resolves within 48 h (transient organ failure) and/or 2. Local or systemic complications without persistent organ failure
Severe acute pancreatitis
3. Persistent organ failure (>48 h) • Single organ failure • Multiple organ failure

Management

Most attacks will settle with conservative management and gradual reintroduction of diet when nausea and vomiting have settled. All patients with SIRS or early systemic organ dysfunction should be managed in a high-dependency or intensive care environment where adequate monitoring and specialist care is available.

Conservative treatment

- *Pain relief.* Severe pain requires the administration of opiates; there is no evidence to support the use of pethidine rather than morphine.
- *Fluid resuscitation.* Patients often require large volumes of fluid to maintain adequate tissue perfusion. Early goal-directed resuscitation is the most important consideration in the initial management. The presence of systemic organ dysfunction necessitates urinary catheterisation, invasive monitoring of venous and arterial pressure, and measurement of biochemical markers of resuscitation including lactate. Patients with MODS or SIRS require oxygen therapy and continuous monitoring of oxygen saturation.
- *Suppression of pancreatic function.* There is no evidence that suppression of pancreatic function improves outcome and nasogastric tubes are not used routinely. Initial nausea and vomiting may initially limit oral intake and when systemic complications or other factors delay recommencement of normal diet, nasoenteric feeding is commenced at an early stage. Suppression of pancreatic secretion with octreotide or somatostatin is of no benefit.
- *Prevention of infection.* Antibiotic prophylaxis has been advocated by some as a means of reducing the risk of infected pancreatic necrosis. Others have been concerned that the more widespread use of antibiotics will result in an increased incidence of severe fungal infection. The most recent consensus is that there is no evidence that prophylactic antibiotics reduce the incidence of infected pancreatic necrosis or mortality (EBM 15.1). It is important to recognise that patients with severe acute pancreatitis often have evidence of SIRS and the presence of a fever and raised white cell count are to be expected, even in the absence of infection. The only definite indication for early antibiotic therapy is when cholangitis is suspected as this may coexist with gallstone pancreatitis. Jaundiced patients with a high fever or rigors are therefore managed with appropriate broad spectrum antibiotics while arrangements are made for urgent ERCP.
- *Inhibition of inflammatory response.* Severe acute pancreatitis is one of many conditions where systemic organ dysfunction

15

is driven by the systemic inflammatory response and there has been much experimental and clinical interest in the role of down-regulation of this response as a potential treatment for acute pancreatitis. Despite encouraging experimental data and promising results from initial clinical trials with the platelet-activating factor (PAF) antagonist, lexipafant, a large international trial, recruiting 1500 patients, showed no difference in mortality.

- *Nutritional support.* Patients with severe acute pancreatitis who are unable to resume normal diet within 48–72 hours require nutritional support. This is best delivered by an enteral rather than parenteral route as trials (EBM 15.2) have demonstrated that total parenteral nutrition (TPN) has a higher rate of complication and mortality. There is no evidence that nasojejunal feeding is better or safer than nasogastric feeding but the nasojejunal route will be required where gastric or duodenal ileus or gastric outlet obstruction prevent effective nasogastric delivery.

EBM   15.1 Prophylactic antibiotics in severe acute pancreatitis

'There is no evidence that supports the routine use of antibiotic prophylaxis in patients with SAP.'

Wittau M et al. Scand J Gastroenterol. 2011;46:261–70.

EBM   15.2 Nutritional support in severe acute pancreatitis

'In patients with severe acute pancreatitis who are unable to return to diet in 48–72 hours nutrition is best given by enteral rather than parenteral (TPN) route.'

Petrov MS, Whelan K. Br J Nutr. 2010;103:1287–95.

- *Other measures.* A randomised trial assessed the role of probiotic therapy as an adjunct to early enteral feeding in the hope that this might reduce bacterial translocation from the gut more than enteral nutrition alone, thus potentially preventing later septic complications. Unfortunately, probiotic therapy actually increased mortality due to gut ischaemia and is no longer used. Other proposed treatments that have been found to be of no benefit in prospective clinical trials include antiprotease therapy and peritoneal lavage.

Endoscopic treatment

There is experimental evidence that the duration of the obstruction at the papilla is an important determinant of the severity of an attack of gallstone-associated pancreatitis and so early removal of an impacted gallstone by ERC and sphincterotomy has long been proposed as treatment. Unfortunately, the results from randomised trials have been conflicting, and differences in study design have made direct comparisons difficult. Patients with evidence of obstructive jaundice and fever/rigors within the first 24 hours are suffering from, or are at least at risk of developing, cholangitis and there is broad consensus that these patients should have urgent ERC with biliary sphincterotomy. However the majority of patients will pass the gallstone spontaneously and in this situation ERC carries additional risk and questionable benefit (EBM 15.3). There is a lack of consensus in published studies regarding the role of ERC in patients with severe acute pancreatitis but not cholangitis. Early ERC with stone removal

can however be life-saving in the patient with cholangitis and it is important to be alert to this possibility in patients diagnosed as having severe acute pancreatitis.

EBM   15.3 ERCP and sphincterotomy in severe acute pancreatitis

'There is consensus in guidelines and meta-analyses that ERCP/ES is indicated in patients with acute biliary pancreatitis (ABP) and coexisting cholangitis and/or persistent cholestasis. Consensus is lacking on the role of routine early ERCP/ES in patients with predicted severe ABP.'

van Geenen EJ et al. Pancreas. 2013;42:774–80.

Surgical treatment

There is no role for surgical intervention in the first 1–2 weeks of an attack of acute pancreatitis, even in the face of deteriorating multiple organ failure. Complications that were managed surgically in the past are now being managed by radiological or endoscopic treatments. Acute pancreatitis is managed conservatively whenever possible, but surgery is indicated under the following circumstances:

1. Where an alternative diagnosis is suggested by CT following initial assessment.
2. Where gallstones are considered the likely cause, cholecystectomy is carried out after recovery from the acute attack. For mild acute pancreatitis, this is best carried out during the index hospital admission but following a severe attack, cholecystectomy is delayed until resolution of the inflammatory process. Even after severe acute pancreatitis it is usually possible to perform cholecystectomy by the laparoscopic route. In patients who have had no prior imaging of the common bile duct by magnetic resonance cholangiopancreatography (MRCP) or ERC, it is important to carry out operative cholangiography to exclude bile duct stones. In patients considered unfit for cholecystectomy, ERC with endoscopic sphincterotomy is carried out to protect against further attacks.
3. When certain complications develop (see later).

Complications

The definition of the local complications of acute pancreatitis is set out in Table 15.4

Infected acute necrotic collection

Infected acute necrotic collection is the most challenging complication of acute pancreatitis and management is complex, requiring input of surgeons, interventional radiologists, endoscopists and the critical care team. Infection occurs in up to 40% of patients with pancreatic necrosis, probably as a consequence of translocation of bacteria from the gut, and usually presents after the second week following symptom onset. The development of infection may be suspected where there is deterioration in systemic organ failure or where new organ failure develops in a patient more than 2 weeks after admission. However, infected acute necrotic collections are not always complicated by organ failure and may present with worsening pain and fever associated with a rise in inflammatory parameters but with little evidence of systemic illness.

An infected acute necrotic collection may be suspected by the presence of gas on CT, but this is not invariable and the diagnosis should not be made on radiological grounds alone. In some

Table 15.4 Local complications of acute pancreatitis

Time scale	Necrosis absent	Necrosis present
<4 weeks	**Acute peripancreatic fluid collection** (peripancreatic fluid associated with interstitial oedematous pancreatitis with no associated peripancreatic necrosis)	**Acute necrotic collection** (a collection containing variable amounts of both fluid and necrosis; the necrosis can involve the pancreatic parenchyma or the extrapancreatic tissues)
>4 weeks	**Pancreatic pseudocyst** (an encapsulated collection of fluid with a well-defined inflammatory wall usually outside the pancreas with minimal or no necrosis)	**Walled-off necrosis** (a mature, encapsulated collection of pancreatic or extrapancreatic necrosis that has developed a well-defined inflammatory wall)
Infection	Each collection type may be sterile or infected	

centres, fine needle aspirates are taken from pancreatic collections under CT or ultrasound guidance to establish whether or not infection is present, with early intervention where infection is proven. Others prefer to act on clinical grounds, and where infection is suspected place a percutaneous drain under CT guidance prior to definitive surgical, endoscopic or radiological management.

There is variation in practice in the management of this life-threatening complication of acute pancreatitis and the variety of approaches reflects local expertise or experience and a lack of good evidence supporting any one approach over another. Where infected acute necrotic collection is confirmed or strongly suspected, the common approaches to management are briefly described later.

Percutaneous drainage/debridement Following initial percutaneous drainage of infected pancreatic necrosis, patients will commonly show signs of initial improvement but subsequently deteriorate as drains block with necrotic debris. Rather than proceeding to conventional surgical debridement, several approaches have been described to facilitate removal of necrotic debris via the percutaneous drain track by radiological, laparoscopic or endoscopic means. A minimally invasive surgical approach through a small flank incision has also been described. Retrospective studies support the view that initial percutaneous drainage followed by definitive intervention if required (the 'step up' approach), is associated with lower mortality and severe systemic complications than conventional surgery alone and this has been confirmed in a prospective randomised trial.

Endoscopic drainage The retrogastric position of the pancreas allows endoscopic transgastric drainage of infected acute necrotic collection, usually under control of endoscopic ultrasound. There is less experience with this approach than open surgery or percutaneous approaches but it is increasingly utilised in selected patients. More than one approach may be used at different times in an individual patient and it is important that patients are managed within a specialist multidisciplinary environment.

Surgical debridement Conventional management involves wide debridement of devitalised pancreatic and peripancreatic tissue (necrosectomy) and either placement of wide-bore drains for

postoperative lavage or abdominal packing and planned re-exploration. If the operation is delayed till the fourth week of illness and the CT is studied carefully, complete removal of all necrotic material may be achieved and avoid the need for re-look laparotomy. This is clearly a major undertaking in the critically ill patient and there has been an increasing trend towards measures to delay surgery until patients are stabilised and organ failure has resolved.

Walled-off pancreatic necrosis

Walled-off pancreatic necrosis (WOPN) is a collection of pancreatic and peripancreatic necrotic material, pancreatic secretions and inflammatory tissue enclosed in a wall of fibrous or granulation tissue. The degree of necrosis is often variable and management depends on symptoms, the anatomical location of the collection(s) and local expertise. By consensus WOPN is differentiated from an acute necrotic collection by persistence for 4 or more weeks from the onset of acute pancreatitis (Fig. 15.5). The commonest sites are between the stomach and transverse colon or liver.

Patients become symptomatic some weeks after the episode of pancreatitis with persistent or intermittent abdominal discomfort and mild to moderate hyperamylasaemia. Larger collections may compress neighbouring structures to cause vomiting and obstructive jaundice. Some collections become so large that they are palpable and, in some cases, visible. Their presence is not in itself an indication for surgical treatment but intervention is normally required if enlarging beyond 6 weeks, if infection develops or in the context of symptoms.

Percutaneous drainage followed by percutaneous necrosectomy or one of the other approaches for infected pancreatic necrosis is employed. Surgical drainage by pancreatic cyst gastrostomy is now commonly achieved laparoscopically. As the tissues holding the sutures must be firm, it is desirable to avoid surgery until at least 6 weeks after the onset of the acute attack to allow the walls of the collection to 'mature'. Endoscopic cyst-gastrostomy or cyst-duodenostomy under ultrasound guidance offers an alternative to surgery (Fig. 15.6). Self-expanding metal stents improve drainage of necrotic debris and facilitate multiple endoscopic cyst lavage and necrosectomy procedures. A plastic double pig-tail stent is sometimes placed through the metal stent to avoid blockage. Haemorrhage is the commonest complication. The selection of the appropriate procedure is often determined by the clinical presentation, anatomical features of the fluid collection,

15

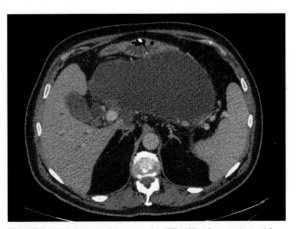

Fig. 15.5 Axial computed tomography (CT) with a large retrogastric postacute inflammatory collection approximately 8 weeks after initial presentation.

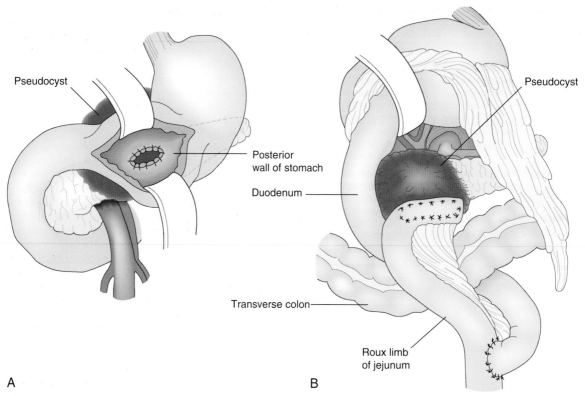

Fig. 15.6 Treatment of pancreatic pseudocyst. **(A)** Transgastric cyst gastrostomy. **(B)** Roux cyst jejunostomy.

the extent of necrosis present and of course, local multidisciplinary expertise.

Pseudocyst/pancreatic abscess

A pancreatic pseudocyst, defined as a collection of fluid persisting for more than 4 weeks but containing no necrosis, is a rare complication as most collections contain some necrotic debris. This may be best appreciated on magnetic resonance imaging (MRI) rather than CT. Pancreatic abscess is a circumscribed intra-abdominal collection of pus, usually in proximity to the pancreas, containing little or no pancreatic necrosis. In effect, this is the result of infection of a pseudocyst and is an indication for drainage as described earlier. However, this is a rare event and the great majority of infected collections will be managed as for WOPN.

Progressive jaundice

Jaundice at presentation suggests that a gallstone is impacted at the lower end of the biliary tree. Such patients may develop ascending cholangitis and early ERC with endoscopic sphincterotomy may therefore be indicated. Where jaundice develops later in the course of acute pancreatitis, this is usually a consequence of compression of the distal bile duct by an inflammatory pancreatic head mass. In such circumstances, treatment is directed towards the underlying pathology and ERCP is challenging due to the degree of duodenal oedema and distortion.

Persistent duodenal ileus

Protracted ileus usually reflects continuing pancreatic inflammation. In the absence of an indication for intervention, conservative management is instituted and nutritional status maintained by nasojejunal feeding or occasionally, if this is not tolerated, by TPN.

Gastrointestinal bleeding

Severe acute pancreatitis may be complicated by bleeding from gastritis, erosions or duodenal ulceration, and prophylactic proton pump inhibitor (PPI) therapy is advisable. Bleeding following treatment of infected pancreatic necrosis is usually a consequence of erosion of a retroperitoneal vessel, often the splenic artery or a major branch of this vessel. In patients with WOPN, bleeding may present with sudden pain and collapse due to rupture of a false aneurysm within the wall of the collection. Control is best achieved by mesenteric angiography with embolisation but surgical control may be necessary. Mortality from bleeding remains high, particularly where surgery is required. Overt evidence of gastrointestinal bleeding in a patient with infected pancreatic necrosis or WOPN commonly indicates a communication between the retroperitoneal collections and the lumen of the gastrointestinal tract (usually stomach or colon) and urgent mesenteric angiography (or CT angiography if the patient is sufficiently stable) (Fig. 15.7) rather than endoscopy is the appropriate course of action.

Gastrointestinal ischaemia/fistulae

Segmental colonic ischaemia requiring resection may be encountered at open necrosectomy, and exteriorisation of the ends following resection is recommended rather than an attempted anastomosis. Local areas of enteric ischaemia do occur, particularly around large peripancreatic collections. Rupture of the collection into the intestine results in an enteric fistula which can either be associated with a clinical deterioration, where the collection remains inadequately drained and the connection results in secondary infection, or a clinical improvement, when fistulation results in decompression of an infected collection into the stomach or duodenum. The presence of gas within a collection does not

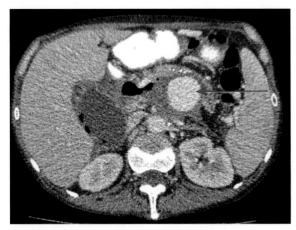

Fig. 15.7 Late computed tomography (CT) with splenic artery pseudoaneurysm (arrow).

therefore mandate intervention. Open surgical or percutaneous drainage of a collection prior to or following internal fistulation will result in an external enteric fistula. Colonic fistulation usually necessitates a defunctioning stoma, whereas gastric or duodenal fistulae may be managed by nasoenteric or parenteral feeding, and adequate local drainage.

Prognosis

Most patients with acute pancreatitis suffer a self-limiting illness and make a full recovery. Further treatment is directed at preventing further attacks by definitive management of gallstones or advising against further alcohol abuse.

Patients with severe acute pancreatitis may be expected to have a more protracted illness and may require many months of hospital care. Overall mortality for such patients is 10–20%, usually as a consequence of multiple organ failure. Death within the first 2 weeks of acute pancreatitis accounts for over 50% of all mortality in this condition, and is more common in patients with extensive necrosis and in the elderly. Late deaths are usually due to complications arising from infected pancreatic necrosis, with mesenteric ischaemia or severe retroperitoneal bleeding being common terminal events. Following recovery from severe acute pancreatitis, return to normal activities can be expected, but full recovery can take many months, requiring nutritional support, management of persistent or recurrent sepsis and definitive management of wound or gastrointestinal complications.

15.1 Summary

Acute pancreatitis

- Gallstones and alcohol are responsible in 70–90%
- Serum amylase three times the upper limit is normally diagnostic
- Abdominal ultrasound scan should be performed in all patients
- CT is undertaken early in the disease only if there is diagnostic doubt
- 80% of patients will have self-limiting illness
- An attempt to assess severity of disease should be performed early following admission
- Multiple organ dysfunction syndrome is a major feature of severe pancreatitis
- If required, nutritional support is best delivered by the enteral route
- Routine antibiotic therapy is not required
- Endoscopic sphincterotomy is indicated if there is coexisting cholangitis
- Percutaneous drainage followed by debridement is associated with better outcomes than conventional surgery.

Chronic pancreatitis

Chronic pancreatitis is a chronic inflammatory condition characterised by fibrosis and the destruction of exocrine pancreatic tissue.

Aetiology

Chronic pancreatitis is a relatively rare disease but its incidence may be increasing with the growing problem of alcohol misuse. Alcohol is the most common aetiological factor, being implicated in some 60–80% of cases. The factors that predispose some patients to develop chronic pancreatitis are poorly understood but cigarette smoking appears to be an important co-factor. The risk of chronic pancreatitis appears to increase when alcohol consumption is greater than 50 g of alcohol (or five standard drinks) per day.

Hereditary pancreatitis is rare with onset in early adult life and is due to one of a variety of identified mutations of the trypsinogen gene. Many patients with idiopathic chronic pancreatitis are now believed to be associated with other gene mutations, such as that of the cystic fibrosis gene, CFTR and SPINK1 gene. Even where there is evidence of alcohol aetiology, there may be complex genetic factors that predispose to the development of chronic pancreatitis and in some, the cause remains unknown.

Pathophysiology

Impaired flow of pancreatic juice leads to inflammation, stricture formation in the duct system and progressive replacement of the gland by fibrous tissue. The secretion of an unduly viscid pancreatic juice may allow protein plugs to form in the duct system, and these plugs subsequently calcify to form duct stones. Loss of acinar tissue is eventually reflected by steatorrhoea and, in time, loss of islet tissue may lead to diabetes mellitus.

Clinical features

Pain is the outstanding feature, is characteristically epigastric with marked radiation through to the back, and is often eased by leaning forward or getting down on all fours. The pain may be precipitated by eating, or the patient learns to avoid certain foods, notably fatty ones. The application of heat sometimes brings relief, and permanent discoloration of the skin (erythema ab igne) may reflect the continued use of heat pads or hot water bottles. The progressive use of powerful opioid analgesics can result in drug dependency and symptoms associated with opiate dysmotility syndromes.

Weight loss is common and reflects a combination of inadequate intake, a poor diet and malabsorption. Steatorrhoea, the bowel motion being pale, bulky, offensive, floating on water, and difficult to flush, may be present but only when exocrine function is less than 10% of normal. Diabetes mellitus develops in about one-third of patients, but islet function is often preserved for some years following the onset of exocrine insufficiency.

Other less common manifestations of chronic pancreatitis include transient or intermittent obstructive jaundice, duodenal obstruction and splenic vein thrombosis (leading to splenomegaly, hypersplenism and gastric and oesophageal varices, segmental or left-sided or sinistral portal hypertension). Many patients also have other comorbidity related to cigarette and alcohol consumption that, particularly when combined with nutritional failure, can make management challenging.

Investigations and diagnosis

CT is the initial investigation and may reveal the speckled calcification typical of chronic pancreatitis, evidence of inflammatory

15

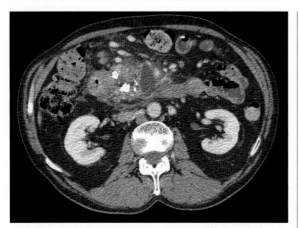

Fig. 15.8 Axial computed tomography (CT) showing extensive calcification and cyst formation within the pancreatic head, duodenal wall thickening and narrowing of the superior mesenteric veins with extensive venous collaterals.

changes, pancreatic duct dilatation or pseudocyst formation (Fig. 15.8). MRCP may reveal the architecture of the pancreatic duct, particularly if surgery or endoscopic therapy is contemplated. It must be borne in mind that cancer of the pancreas may block the duct system and cause pancreatitis, and that the two conditions can coexist. Endoscopic ultrasound is increasingly utilised where diagnostic uncertainty exists, allowing pancreatic fine needle biopsy where appropriate.

Pancreatic endocrine function should be assessed by measurement of blood glucose levels. Exocrine insufficiency may not be detectable until 90% of the pancreatic parenchyma is destroyed. Faecal fat excretion can be measured over 3–5 days while the patient's fat intake is controlled at 100 g/day (normal individuals excrete less than 5 g/day). Faecal elastase is a more convenient method of assessment of exocrine pancreatic function but is less accurate. Where assays of exocrine function are not readily available, a trial of oral pancreatic supplements may be attempted.

Management

The diagnosis of chronic pancreatitis is not in itself an indication for treatment. Clinical judgment is needed to determine the need for, and timing of, intervention. Generally, pain is the most important indication for surgery, but complications such as biliary obstruction or gastric outlet obstruction may also necessitate intervention. Many patients have complex problems and need a multidisciplinary approach to treatment.

Conservative management

This consists of encouraging abstinence from alcohol, relief of pain, treatment of exocrine and endocrine insufficiency, and improvement of nutritional status. Opiates should be avoided but may prove essential to relieve pain. Diabetes mellitus is treated appropriately and nutritional failure is treated by pancreatic exocrine and dietary supplementation. An experienced dietician should be involved, particularly if patients have a combination of diabetes mellitus, fat malabsorption and poor diet, which may require nutritional support.

Endoscopic treatment

Endoscopic management may be considered in the first instance and pancreatic duct stents may be used for dominant pancreatic duct stricture or where there is a pancreatic duct disruption with pseudocyst formation or pancreatic ascites. Aggressive endoscopic treatment with stricture dilatation and stone removal has some advocates. Although endoscopic management can be successful in selected patients, results from randomised trials suggest where feasible, a surgical solution is preferable to repeated attempts at endotherapy.

Surgical treatment

This is indicated if pain is intractable; when neighbouring structures, such as the common bile duct, duodenum, portal or splenic vein, are sufficiently compressed to produce symptoms; when pseudocysts or abscesses develop; when endoscopic therapy has failed; or when cancer cannot be excluded.

The objective is to relieve pain or compression, while at the same time conserving as much healthy pancreatic tissue and function as possible. In about a third of patients, the pancreatic duct is dilated and is amenable to surgical drainage of the obstructed pancreatic duct into a Roux limb of jejunum, usually combined with some form of duodenum-preserving pancreatic head resection. The two most commonly performed procedures are those described by Beger and Frey (Fig. 15.9), the difference between them being the greater extent of pancreatic parenchymal excision and need for formal division of the pancreatic neck in the Beger procedure. No one procedure has been proven to be superior. Approximately 70% of patients remain pain-free or substantially improved when assessed 5 years after surgery for chronic pancreatitis. As with all aspects of chronic pancreatitis treatment, the results of surgery are better in patients who manage to abstain from alcohol.

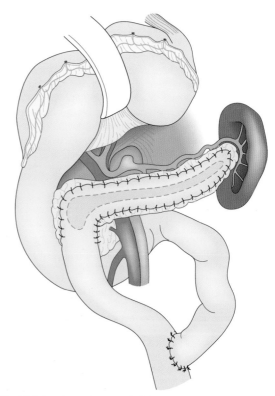

Fig. 15.9 Longitudinal pancreaticojejunostomy.

Tropical pancreatitis

Tropical pancreatitis was thought to be a distinct form of chronic pancreatitis prevalent in many parts of Africa and Asia. The disease has an earlier onset than alcoholic pancreatitis and pancreatic function, both endocrine and exocrine, is said to be more severely affected in these patients; they are also more prone to pancreatic carcinoma. A grossly dilated main pancreatic duct with large calculi is commonly seen. Aetiology is unclear but an increased frequency of gene mutations (SPINK1) has been reported, so genetic factors are likely to play a role.

Neoplasms of the exocrine pancreas

Pancreatic tumours are epithelial in origin, and 80% of these are pancreatic ductal adenocarcinoma (PDAC). Of the remaining pancreatic tumours, there are nearly 20 different histological types, many of which carry a much better prognosis. Careful specialist multidisciplinary assessment and staging of the individual patient is therefore required. Advances in cross sectional imaging (CT/MR) and the widespread availability of endoscopic ultrasound (EUS) allows accurate pretreatment confirmation of the diagnosis in the majority of patients.

Adenocarcinoma of the pancreas

Aetiology

Ductal adenocarcinoma of the pancreas is the 10th (male)/11th (female) most common cancer in the UK, but is now the third most common cause of cancer-related death (after lung and colorectal cancer). There are about 8750 new cases in the UK per annum and the incidence has increased over the last 40 years, with an individual lifetime risk of 1 in 95. Males and females are equally affected. Only 15–20% are resectable and even with multimodality therapy the 5-year survival is only 15–20%. There is an increasing incidence with age but 20% of patients are less than 60 years of age. Although the aetiology is unknown, there is an association with tobacco smoking (20–30% thought to be smoking-related), obesity, race (African–Americans > Hispanics or Caucasians), diabetes, chronic pancreatitis (particularly hereditary pancreatitis) and familial pancreatic cancer.

Pathology

Pancreatic ductal adenocarcinoma

The majority of adenocarcinomas arise from ductal rather than acinar tissue, 60% arising in the head of the gland. The histology (Fig. 15.10) is characterised by groups of infiltrating carcinoma cells often some (histological) distance apart, interspersed by a fibrous stroma, with involvement of nerves, vessels, lymphatics and lymph nodes commonly seen, even when the primary tumour is small. Metastatic spread is most commonly to the liver and lung; 80% of patients present with either locoregional or metastatic dissemination.

Intraductal papillary mucinous neoplasm (IPMN)

Intraductal papillary mucinous neoplasm (IPMN) is a relatively recently recognised entity, and comprises a group of lesions characterised by a papillary growth of the ductal epithelium with rich mucin production and cystic expansion of the affected duct. The widespread availability of cross-sectional imaging has resulted in many being detected incidentally. There is a broad separation into two types; main duct and branch duct. Both subtypes

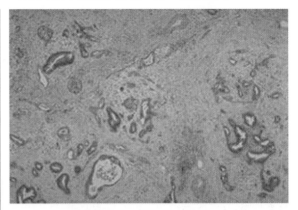

Fig. 15.10 Histology of pancreatic cancer with small groups of epithelial cells attempting to form glands, interspersed with fibrous stoma.

have malignant potential but malignancy or high grade dysplasia is seen more commonly in main duct (70%) than branch duct (15%) IPMN. Resection is recommended for main duct IPMN where clinically appropriate, whereas many branch duct lesions may be observed unless high-risk stigmata are identified. These include nodules within the cyst wall and large cyst size (>4 cm). When malignancy occurs in main duct IPMN, the natural history is different from PDAC in that the majority are resectable, with survival reaching 80–90% for in situ carcinoma, and 50–70% in the presence of invasive carcinoma.

Mucinous cystic neoplasm

Mucinous cystic tumours of the pancreas predominate in the body and tail of the pancreas and almost always occur in women. These multiloculated tumours have a characteristic smooth glistening surface, a dense fibrous wall and occasional calcification (Fig. 15.11). They arise from oversecretion of the mucus by the hyperplastic columnar lining of the ducts and therefore contain thickened viscous material, which can also be haemorrhagic. These tumours should be considered potentially malignant but are classified histologically as benign, borderline or malignant based on degree of dysplastic changes. They can be differentiated from IPMN by the presence of an ovarian-like stroma.

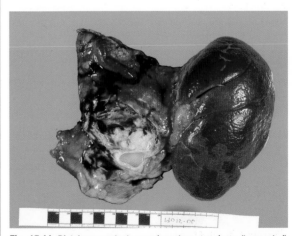

Fig. 15.11 Distal pancreatectomy splenectomy specimen (transected) with mucinous cystic neoplasm (MCN showing cystic and solid components).

15

Serous cystic neoplasm

Serous cystadenoma (SCA) are most commonly microcystic, but can present in an 'oligocystic' or 'macrocystic' form when differentiation from other cystic neoplasms can be difficult. In the presence of multiple serous cysts, Von Hippel–Lindau syndrome should be considered. They often present as incidental findings on CT or MRI but when large can cause pressure symptoms or a palpable mass. Typical SCA has a characteristic radiological appearance with a pancreatic mass characterised by a dense, internal, lacelike, honeycombed matrix and often a central scar, which may be calcified. When the diagnosis can be confirmed preoperatively, resection is usually not required since these tumours have virtually no malignant potential.

Metastases

Isolated metastases in the pancreas are rare, the most common site of origin being renal cell carcinoma, followed by lung, lobular breast carcinoma, melanoma and gastric carcinoma. Some may benefit from resection and so where suspected, endoscopic ultrasound with fine needle cytology is often requested to confirm the diagnosis.

Solid pseudopapillary tumour of the pancreas

This tumour, otherwise known as solid-cystic, or Frantz tumour of the pancreas, is an unusual form of pancreatic carcinoma (Fig. 15.12). Its natural history differs from the more common pancreatic adenocarcinoma in that it is almost always in female patients (10:1), often at a young age (20–30 years), is more indolent, and carries a better prognosis. Pathologically, the tumour is usually well circumscribed with regions of necrosis, haemorrhage and cystic degeneration. Metastatic disease can occur, usually involving the liver, and resection is the preferred treatment.

Acinar cell carcinoma of the pancreas

These are rare tumours accounting for 1% of pancreatic tumours, and arise from the acinar cells of the pancreas. Normal acinar cells are the primary cells of the exocrine pancreas and are responsible for secreting various enzymes; the tumour cells also may secrete pancreatic enzymes, most commonly lipase. Presentation may therefore be confused with acute pancreatitis.

Ampullary tumours

Tumours may arise from the ampulla of Vater, where the pancreatic duct (of Wirsung) and common bile duct merge and exit into the duodenum. They are relatively uncommon accounting for approximately 7% of all periampullary carcinomas, but because of their relationship to the common bile duct, obstruction and jaundice ensues. These tumours therefore present at an earlier stage, with a correspondingly better prognosis.

Cholangiocarcinoma

These tumours are adenocarcinomas that arise in the biliary duct system and may be intrahepatic, extrahepatic (i.e., perihilar) and distal extrahepatic. Those in the distal (intrapancreatic) portion of the biliary tree may be indistinguishable clinically and radiologically from pancreatic carcinomas, although a normal pancreatic duct on imaging is suggestive ('double duct' sign is not seen). These are uncommon tumours with about 2000 cases in the UK per annum. Most are sporadic but inflammatory bowel disease, congenital abnormalities of the bile ducts (choledochal cysts), and chronic infection (parasitic liver fluke [*Clonorchis sinensis*] in Africa and Asia) are thought to increase the risk of developing bile duct cancer. Many proximal tumours are irresectable at presentation but duct obstruction causing jaundice at an early stage can again improve the prognosis for lesions situated in the distal bile duct.

Clinical features of pancreatic neoplasms

Presenting symptoms are dependent on the site of the tumour within the pancreas. For *tumours in the head of the pancreas*, painless progressive jaundice, associated with weight loss is the classic presentation. Involvement of the common bile duct as it runs through the head of the pancreas results in a block to the flow of bile from the liver to the intestine, resulting in obstructive jaundice where the urine is dark and the interruption of the enterohepatic circulation results in pale stools due to the lack of bile pigments. The gallbladder may become dilated and palpable (Courvoisier's sign); it is not tender. This is a worrying sign in a jaundiced patient (Courvoisier's law; Table 15.5). Intense itching may result in skin excoriation from scratching. Loss of taste, poor appetite and weight loss are common.

For *tumours of the body and tail*, biliary obstruction occurs late, and symptoms are often vague with anorexia, weight loss and, with subsequent involvement of the retroperitoneum, the development of back pain. New-onset diabetes may predate the diagnosis. Delay in diagnosis is common, and the diagnosis should be considered at an early stage in patients with unexplained weight loss. Steatorrhoea may result in initial investigations for an alteration in bowel habit. A late manifestation is a malignancy-associated hypercoagulable state, resulting in intravascular clots with vasculitis, named thrombophlebitis migrans (Trousseau's sign, Table 15.5).

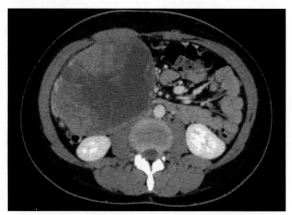

Fig. 15.12 Solid pseudopapillary tumour of the pancreatic head.

Table 15.5 Named signs and laws in pancreatic malignancy	
Courvoisier's Law	
In a jaundiced patient, in obstruction of the common bile duct due to stones, the gallbladder is seldom palpable, the organ usually is already shrivelled; in obstruction due to other causes, distension is common by comparison.	
Interpretation of Courvoisier's Law	**Trousseau's Sign**
In the presence of a nontender palpable gallbladder, painless jaundice is unlikely to be caused by gallstones.	Thrombophlebitis migrans in a patient with pancreatic carcinoma, a nonmetastatic manifestation of malignancy

Investigations and multidisciplinary management (MDM) planning

Patients should be managed by specialist multidisciplinary teams with an interest in pancreatic cancer. Transabdominal ultrasound, along with biochemical confirmation of cholestasis, is the initial investigation for the jaundiced patient, which will confirm intra- and extrahepatic biliary dilatation, exclude gallstones, and may show the mass lesion in the pancreas or liver metastases. It may also identify ascites and regional lymph node enlargement. Even in patients with known gallstones, the diagnosis of periampullary malignancy should be considered and further imaging by MRCP or CT should be carried out.

Abdominal CT (Fig. 15.13), with or without MR/MRCP, is the preliminary investigation if periampullary malignancy is suspected and will define the site of the lesion and the extent of local or distant involvement. Where the diagnosis is confirmed, staging necessitates CT of chest, abdomen and pelvis, with MRI liver and positron-emission tomography (PET) CT sometimes required following multidisciplinary team discussion. Endoscopic ultrasound can provide information on local staging and cytological confirmation of the diagnosis Endoscopic ultrasound and Fine Needle Aspiration (EUS-FNA) without compromising resectability. Circulating tumour markers (e.g., CA 19–9) lack sufficient sensitivity and specificity for diagnosis but a baseline value may be useful in the follow-up of treated patients.

Management should be planned at a regional pancreatic MDM meeting. Biliary intervention (ERCP/percutaneous transhepatic cholangiography [PTC]), before MDM discussion is to be avoided, as optimum treatment may be compromised in some patients, through introduction of infection or procedure-associated morbidity.

Curative management

Surgical resection currently offers the only potential for cure in pancreatic tumours. Tumours localised to the pancreatic parenchyma, or with limited involvement of the peripancreatic fat or lymph nodes may be considered for resection. Many adenocarcinomas of the body and tail are irresectable at diagnosis, but when identified early may be removed by distal pancreatectomy and splenectomy.

For tumours in the head of the pancreas the standard operation is a pancreaticoduodenectomy (Whipple's procedure) (Fig. 15.14), which entails en bloc resection of the head of the pancreas, the distal half of the stomach, the duodenum, gallbladder and common bile duct. Reconstruction is achieved by anastomoses of the pancreatic remnant, the common hepatic duct and the stomach to the jejunum (pancreaticojejunostomy, hepaticojejunostomy, gastrojejunostomy). It is more common to preserve the distal stomach and perform a pylorus-preserving pancreaticoduodenectomy (PPPD). With increased specialisation and the centralisation of these procedures in high-volume centres, surgical mortality is now less than 5%. Removing all of the pancreas or extending the lymphadenectomy beyond locoregional nodes does not improve prognosis. Pancreaticoduodenectomy combined with adjuvant chemotherapy remains the standard of care, and is associated with a median survival of 24 months, although long-term cure is rare. The prospects for patients with other periampullary cancers are better, with 5-year survival rates ranging from 20% to 40%. For patients with borderline resectable tumours, due to early involvement of the portal vein or other vascular structures, neoadjuvant chemotherapy or chemoradiotherapy may be considered.

Palliative treatment

Only 15–20% of patients are candidates for resection through a combination of advanced stage or comorbidity. For the remainder, the primary objective is the optimisation of quality of life through relief of obstructive symptoms (jaundice or duodenal obstruction) and pain control. Chemotherapy can prolong survival in selected patients.

Relief of biliary obstruction is normally achieved by ERCP and biliary stenting. Self-expanding metal stents are usually preferred. Percutaneous biliary stenting (PTC) is sometimes required where ERCP fails due to altered anatomy or duodenal infiltration by tumour. Surgical biliary bypass is only undertaken when patients are found to have inoperable disease at exploratory laparotomy. Patients rarely present with duodenal obstruction until late in the disease and this is usually managed by endoscopic duodenal stenting with self-expanding metal stents. Gastrojejunostomy (usually carried out laparoscopically) is an alternative in patients with good performance status.

For patients with good performance status, palliative chemotherapy should be considered. This requires a cytological (or histological) diagnosis by brush cytology taken at the time of ERCP or by EUS-FNA. A number of benign lesions can masquerade as malignancy and, as discussed earlier, some pancreatic mass lesions may have a significantly better prognosis than pancreatic ductal adenocarcinoma. Quality of life and survival can be improved through palliative chemotherapy. Given the poor outlook for patients with pancreatic cancer, clinical trials where available should be discussed with appropriate patients. Patients often benefit from proactive nutritional support with the addition of pancreatic exocrine supplements to alleviate steatorrhoea, dietary advice and antiemetics. Dexamethasone can be of benefit, but glucose control is needed. Pain is often a late manifestation, but can often be effectively controlled through an analgesic ladder or occasionally coeliac plexus neurolysis or thoracoscopic splanchnicectomy.

15

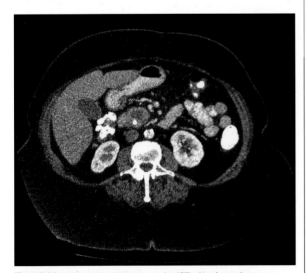

Fig. 15.13 Axial computed tomography (CT) showing a 2-cm hypovascular lesion within the head of the pancreas, apparently clear of the mesenteric vessels. A biliary stent lies within the common bile duct.

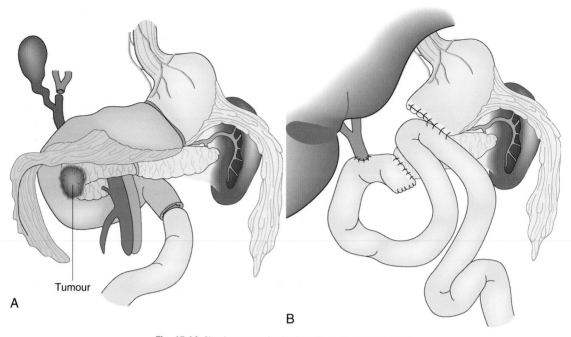

Tumour

A

B

Fig. 15.14 Classic pancreaticoduodenectomy (Kausch–Whipple).

 15.2 Summary

Pancreatic cancer

- 80% of tumours are pancreatic ductal adenocarcinoma (PDAC)
- 80–85% of PDAC are irresectable at presentation
- Intraductal papillary mucinous neoplasm (IPMN) is commonly detected incidentally on abdominal imaging
- Malignancy is more commonly seen in main duct IPMN
- Side branch IPMN may be observed unless high-risk stigmata are present
- Management of pancreatic neoplasia should be multidisciplinary within a high volume centre
- Whipple's resection with adjuvant chemotherapy is the standard treatment for carcinoma of the pancreatic head.

Pancreatic neuroendocrine tumours (pNET)

Pancreatic neuroendocrine tumours are rare tumours (approximately 1/100,000 population/year) of which 60% are nonfunctioning or secrete peptides with low biological impact such as PP or neurotensin. In contrast to insulinoma, the majority of which are benign, approximately 50% of gastrinomas and the majority of nonfunctioning pancreatic neuroendocrine tumours are malignant (Table 15.6). They are usually sporadic but they may also appear among other features of genetic syndromes like multiple endocrine neoplasia type I or von Hippel–Lindau disease. In multiple endocrine neoplasia (MEN1), pancreatic neuroendocrine tumours occur in 40–80% of patients and are mostly nonfunctioning tumours or gastrinomas. Pancreatic neuroendocrine tumours occur in 10–15% of patients with von Hippel–Lindau (VHL) and are frequently multiple (>30%).

Nonfunctioning pNET

Such tumours may express and secrete peptides like neurotensin or chromogranin A (CgA), which are not active. Many nonfunctional pNETs are already metastatic by the time of diagnosis with the liver being the most common site of metastasis. Regional lymph node spread is also common, and pNET may have a 5-year survival as low as 30%. Presentation is related to the mass effect of the tumour and so symptoms are therefore nonspecific. Surgery with curative intent is the mainstay of treatment for localised or locoregional disease (Fig. 15.15). For tumours arising in patients with MEN1 (or VHL), management is more complex as the presence of multiple tumours means that selective resection is indicated. Nonfunctioning tumours should be resected if >2 cm in MEN1 or >2–3 cm in VHL but the decision to operate and choice of procedure in these rare conditions is complex and should be individualised for specific patients as part of the multidisciplinary process.

Debulking surgery as well as other forms of local treatment such as transarterial chemo-embolisation or radiofrequency ablation for liver metastases can improve prognosis. Cellular proliferation index and Ki-67 immunostaining can be obtained from biopsy material and are pointers of aggressive biological behaviour. Systemic therapies have also been better defined and include radionuclide therapy against somatostatin receptors or 123I - iodobenzylguanidine (MIBG) and chemotherapy especially for poorly differentiated tumours. Cytotoxic therapy with compounds like streptozotocin, 5-fluorouracil or doxorubicin can achieve modest outcome.

Functioning pNET

The functioning tumours and syndromes are named according to the hormones they produce: insulinoma, gastrinoma (most gastrinomas are found in the duodenum), VIPoma, glucagonoma and somatostatinoma. The first two (insulinomas and gastrinomas) are the most frequent functioning pancreatic tumours. Presentation of functional pNET is specific and related to the secretion of biologically active peptides like insulin, gastrin, glucagon, somatostatin and vasoactive intestinal polypeptide (VIP).

Table 15.6 Clinical features of pNET

Tumour	Symptoms	Malignancy	Survival
Insulinoma	Confusion, sweating, dizziness, weakness, unconsciousness, relief with eating	10% of patients develop metastases	Complete resection cures most patients
Gastrinoma	Zollinger–Ellison syndrome or severe peptic ulceration and diarrhoea	Metastases develop in 60% of patients; likelihood correlated with size of primary	Complete resection results in 10-year survival of 90%; less likely if large primary
Glucagonoma	Necrolytic migratory erythema, weight loss, diabetes mellitus, stomatitis, diarrhoea	Metastases develop in 60% or more patients	More favourable with complete resection; prolonged even with liver metastases
VIPoma	Werner–Morrison syndrome of profuse watery diarrhoea with marked hypokalaemia	Metastases develop in up to 70% of patients; majority found at presentation	Complete resection with 5-year survival of 95%; with metastases, 60%
Somatostatinoma	Cholelithiasis; weight loss; diarrhoea and steatorrhoea. Diabetes mellitus	Metastases likely in about 50% of patients	Complete resection associated with 5-year survival of 95%; with metastases, 60%
Nonsyndromic pancreatic neuroendocrine tumour	Symptoms from pancreatic mass and/or liver metastases	Metastases develop in up to 50% of patients	Complete resection associated with 5-year survival of at least 50%

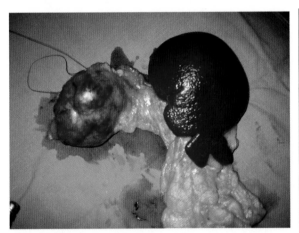

Fig. 15.15 Distal pancreatectomy splenectomy specimen with nonfunctioning pNET.

Insulinomas

Insulinomas arise from the beta cells within the pancreas, are benign in approximately 90% and solitary in 95% of sporadic cases. Beta cells should secrete insulin in response to an increase in blood sugar, but the secretion of insulin by insulinomas is not properly regulated by glucose and the tumours continue to secrete excessive insulin, causing glucose levels to fall further than normal. Patients present with symptoms of low blood glucose (hypoglycaemia), which may be improved by eating or with vague neurological symptoms. The diagnosis of an insulinoma is made biochemically: blood glucose $\leq$2.2 mmol/L (40 mg/dL), associated with an insulin level $\geq$6 µU/mL (36 pmol/L), C-peptide levels $\geq$200 pmol/L, proinsulin levels $\geq$5 pmol/L. Further controlled testing includes the 72-hour fast, which is the criterion standard for establishing the diagnosis of insulinoma, as 98% of patients with insulinomas will develop symptomatic hypoglycaemia within 72 hours. Localisation of the tumour is most commonly achieved with contrast-enhanced CT and endoscopic ultrasound. The definitive treatment is usually surgical enucleation.

Gastrinomas

For gastrinomas (Zollinger–Ellison syndrome), measurements of fasting serum gastrin (1000 pg/mL) and basal gastric acid output are critical. Fasting serum gastrin (FSG) alone is insufficient because of its lack of specificity, making it impossible to distinguish hypergastrinaemia caused by a gastrinoma from that caused by achlorhydric states (i.e., type 1 gastric NETs, use of PPIs, pernicious anaemia, atrophic gastritis). For these measures, a washout period from PPI treatment of 1–4 weeks is recommended. The 2006 European Neuroendocrine Tumour Society guidelines have cutoff values of greater than 10-fold elevation for FSG and gastric pH $\leq$2. Over 90% of gastrinomas are found in the 'gastrinoma triangle' bounded by the third part of the duodenum, the neck of the pancreas and the porta-hepatis. Gastrinomas are multiple in 20–40% of patients and often extrapancreatic, with 20% found in the duodenum. Gastrinomas are frequently malignant with metastatic spread occurring to the liver and local lymph nodes. They tend to be small: 38% of pancreatic and all duodenal tumours are less than 1 cm in diameter at diagnosis. One-third of cases are associated with MEN type I in which multiplicity is the rule and there is a tendency to recurrence. The tumour may be difficult to localise and investigations include CT, octreotide scan, MRI and endoscopic ultrasonography.

Miscellaneous pNET

For VIPomas, glucagonomas, somatostatinomas and PPomas, the biochemical markers are VIP, glucagon, somatostatin and PP, respectively, and the clinical features are detailed in Table 15.6. These tumours are generally malignant and may present as large tumours with 70% having evidence of tumour spread at the time of diagnosis. Aggressive surgical removal of as much tumour as possible is often indicated to relieve the severe symptoms associated with excessive hormone secretion.

Multiple endocrine neoplasia type 1

Multiple endocrine neoplasia type 1 is characterised by hyperplasia and/or neoplasm of the parathyroid glands, enteropancreatic

15

NETs and pituitary adenomas. The gene for type 1 MEN has been localised to chromosome band 11q13 and is a tumour-suppressor gene that encodes menin, a nuclear protein. Some patients do not present with all these tumours, so it has been agreed that diagnosis is made when a patient presents with two of these concomitantly. To diagnose familial MEN-1 syndrome, a first-degree relative has to manifest at least one of the tumours previously mentioned. Hyperparathyroidism occurs in about 90% of patients, endocrine pancreatic tumours in 60% of patients; usually they are small and nonfunctional, and the most common hormonally active ones are insulinomas or gastrinomas. In contrast to sporadic insulinoma these are multiple in 90% of MEN-1 patients. Pituitary adenomas are present in 40% of patients, and in 60% of the patients skin manifestations can also be present. Biochemical screening for pancreatic NETs, in the presence of suspected MEN-1 syndrome, should include gastrin, insulin/pro-insulin, PP, glucagon and CgA, which together have a sensitivity of approximately 70% that can be increased if α- and β-HCG (human chorionic gonadotropin) subunits, VIP, postprandial gastrin, and PP measurements are added. It is recommended that carriers of MEN-1 mutation are screened biochemically every 1–3 years for hyperparathyroidism, prolactinoma, gastrinoma, insulinoma and other enteropancreatic tumours. MEN-2 is not associated with pancreatic endocrine tumours.

The spleen

Surgical anatomy

The spleen is a vascular organ lying in the left upper quadrant of the abdomen alongside the 9th, 10th and 11th ribs, and is usually impalpable. It weighs 75–150 g in the adult, is between 8 cm and 13 cm in length, and is ellipsoid in shape. The convex outer surface and superior pole lies against the diaphragm, the concave inner surface is related to the fundus of the stomach, the pancreatic tail and the upper pole of the right kidney, and its lower pole rests on the splenic flexure of the colon below. It has a fibrous capsule and, except at its hilum, is covered by peritoneum, which is reflected as supporting ligaments running to adjacent organs; the lienorenal, lienogastric and lienocolic ligaments (lieno-=spleen). The phrenicocolic ligament, which runs between the splenic flexure of the colon and the undersurface of the diaphragm, provides additional support.

Arterial inflow is primarily through the tortuous splenic artery arising from the coeliac axis, which carries 40% of the splanchnic blood flow into the spleen. Venous blood drains into the portal venous system via the splenic vein. The splenic vessels are closely related to, and may run within, the pancreas entering the spleen at the splenic hilum. The spleen has a secondary vascular inflow and outflow via the short gastric vessels that run within the lienogastric ligament to the upper part of the greater curvature of the stomach, which assume importance when the main splenic vessels are occluded through surgical division, radiological embolisation or spontaneous thrombosis.

Normally, the spleen is impalpable and cannot be percussed. When enlarged, it extends downwards and medially below the costal margin. It is then best palpated bimanually, with the patient lying on the right side with the left side turned slightly forward. The distinctive notch on the anteroinferior border of the spleen may then be felt. On percussion, an enlarged spleen causes dullness over the ninth rib in the midaxillary line. Splenomegaly is normally confirmed by abdominal ultrasound or CT.

Physiology

Circulatory filtration

The cut surface of the spleen reveals areas of red and white pulp surrounded by fibrous trabeculae. The red pulp is a loose honeycomb of reticular tissue that contains the splenic sinusoids, lined by macrophages, and blood vessels pass into the pulp along the trabeculae. As erythrocytes age, the normal lifespan being about 120 days, the cell membrane becomes less flexible and because erythrocytes are required to deform to pass through the sinusoids, senescent cells are trapped within the spleen and therefore removed from the circulating population of cells. Following phagocytosis iron is split from the haem portion, and stored as haemosiderin before being transported to the bone marrow bound to transferrin to be incorporated into a new population of erythrocytes.

Erythrocytes move in and out of the pulp tissue, so that 1% of the body's red cells and 20–30% of its platelets are sequestrated at any given moment. Unlike in some mammals, the spleen is not a site of significant blood pooling except in pathological conditions with splenomegaly, where the spleen may contain more than a litre of blood. Following splenectomy, there is an increased number of misshapen red cells in the peripheral blood, some containing nuclear remnants (Howell-Jolly bodies) and others containing clumps of iron (siderocytes).

Immunological function

The spleen is an important site for promoting both cell-mediated and humoral immunity. The spleen represents the largest aggregation (~25%) of lymphoid tissue in the body forming the white pulp, which consists of lymphoid follicles (Malpighian bodies) and lymphatic tissue, containing lymphocytes, macrophages and plasma cells, these cells having migrated from the bone marrow and 30–50% of them are thymus-dependent. Antigens entering the spleen are engulfed by macrophages, promoting antigen presentation, with subsequent antibody production in the germinal centres. Following splenectomy, immunological responses are impaired.

Haemopoiesis

In utero in the second and third trimester the spleen is an important source of erythrocyte and granulocyte production for the foetus. Although at birth this function usually ceases, in some disease processes with a high turnover of erythrocytes the spleen may continue to contribute to this process (extramedullary haemopoiesis).

Indications for splenectomy (nontraumatic)

Although the recommendation to remove the spleen often comes from the haematologist, the surgeon must be aware of the indications for splenectomy and the criteria that should be fulfilled before accepting a patient for operation. The common indications are outlined later (Table 15.7).

Table 15.7 Indications for splenectomy

Traumatic	Blunt penetrating trauma
	Iatrogenic intraoperative endoscopic trauma
Haematological	The purpuras
	Haemolytic anaemia
	Hypersplenism
	Proliferative disease
Miscellaneous	Distal pancreatectomy (for benign or malignant disease)
	Total radical gastrectomy
	Splenorenal shunt

The purpuras

Idiopathic thrombocytopenic purpura (ITP)

Of the two types of ITP, one affects children, and the other, adults. In children, the usual age for getting ITP is 2–4 years, may be post-viral and most recover without treatment. Most adults with ITP are young women. Immunoglobulin G (IgG) antibody develops against platelet membrane antigen, resulting in the premature destruction of platelets. The low platelet count is associated with reactive megakaryocytosis within the bone marrow. Epistaxis, bleeding from the gastrointestinal tract and other sites is associated with petechiae and ecchymoses. Platelet counts are below 50×10^9/L, and bleeding time is prolonged but clotting time is normal. The spleen is usually not overly enlarged, making it particularly suitable for laparoscopic removal.

Treatment is indicated in patients with platelet counts less than $20–30 \times 10^9$/L and when counts less than 50×10^9/L are associated with substantial mucous membrane bleeding (or risk factors for bleeding, such as hypertension, peptic ulcer disease, or the potential for substantial trauma to the body). Initial therapy with glucocorticoids, such as prednisone, is appropriate and may be augmented with intravenous immunoglobulin, and platelet transfusions but splenectomy is often appropriate with persistent thrombocytopenia ($<30 \times 10^9$/L after 4–6 weeks of medical treatment).

Secondary thrombocytopenia

Secondary thrombocytopenia may occur secondary to a number of conditions and comprises about 40% of all cases of thrombotic thrombocytopenic purpura (TTP). Predisposing factors include cancer, pregnancy, drugs (e.g., cyclosporine), HIV infection and bone marrow transplantation. Splenectomy is in general contraindicated in secondary purpuras, although it may be advised if hypersplenism is associated with symptomatic secondary thrombocytopenia.

Haemolytic anaemias

Hereditary spherocytosis

In this autosomal dominant disorder, red blood cells are spherical rather than biconcave, are fragile, and are destroyed when trapped within the splenic sinusoids. Excess haemolysis results in anaemia, jaundice and splenic enlargement. It is a disease of remissions and relapses, with 'haemolytic crises' requiring transfusion. Pigment gallstones occur in 30–60% of cases. Mild hereditary spherocytosis can be managed without folate supplements and does not require splenectomy. Moderately and severely affected individuals are likely to benefit from splenectomy, which

should be performed after the age of 6 years and with appropriate counselling about the infection risk. If gallstones are present, cholecystectomy is carried out simultaneously.

Acquired haemolytic anaemias

Excess haemolysis may occur following exposure to agents such as chemicals, drugs or infection, and with extensive burns, or it may be an immune phenomenon (e.g., *Mycoplasma pneumoniae* infection, systemic lupus erythematosus [SLE], chronic lymphatic leukaemia). In the latter, the red cells are coated with an autoantibody, which can be detected by agglutination when antihuman globulin is added to a suspension of the patient's erythrocytes (positive Coombs' test). Treatment consists of steroid therapy. Splenectomy is indicated if treatment fails from the outset or if there is a fall in the haemoglobin following the reduction or cessation of steroids.

Hypersplenism

This syndrome consists of splenomegaly and pancytopenia in the presence of an apparently normal bone marrow and the absence of an autoimmune disorder. There is sequestration and destruction of blood cells in the spleen, affecting predominantly white cells and platelets. Hypersplenism may complicate a number of inflammatory conditions (e.g., rheumatoid arthritis), infections (e.g., malaria), and myeloproliferative and lymphoproliferative disorders. In portal hypertension, splenic congestion frequently leads to splenomegaly and hypersplenism.

The enlarged spleen results in an expansion of the total blood volume to fill the increased vascular spaces of the enlarged spleen with pooling of cells and increased destruction within the sinusoids. This results in anaemia, leucopenia and thrombocytopenia, with reticulocytosis and leucoerythroblastosis in the marrow. Increased haemoglobin turnover results in increased amounts of urobilinogen in the urine. Splenectomy may be appropriate but the potential morbidity, the risks of late septic complications and the prognosis of the underlying cause of the hypersplenism require to be balanced with the potential alleviation of the pancytopenia.

Segmental portal hypertension (syn. sinistral portal hypertension, left-sided portal hypertension)

A localised form of portal hypertension associated with hypersplenism and oesophagogastric varices may follow occlusion of the splenic vein. Thrombosis may result from acute or chronic pancreatitis, or the vessel may become compromised by direct invasion from a carcinoma of the pancreas. Gastric varices are particularly prominent in this condition and often communicate directly with short gastric veins. Acute variceal haemorrhage in this situation is, however, relatively rare but may be best managed by splenectomy with ligation of the vessels on the greater curvature of the stomach, as endoscopic control can be difficult. Recurrent haemorrhage is unusual following surgery and the prognosis is favourable, given that there is often no associated liver disease.

Proliferative disorders

Myelofibrosis

It is recognised that this condition is due to an abnormal proliferation of mesenchymal elements in the bone marrow, spleen, liver and lymph nodes, and that extramedullary haemopoiesis occurs at many sites. Most patients present over the age of 50 years.

15

The spleen may be grossly enlarged and splenic infarcts may occur. Splenectomy decreases transfusion requirements and, by relieving the discomfort of a grossly enlarged spleen, also improves symptoms.

Lymphomas

In non-Hodgkin's lymphoma, splenectomy is only indicated in the rare event that a primary neoplasm is confined to the spleen or, in both myelo- and lymphoproliferative conditions, to reduce transfusion requirements when hypersplenism is a problem.

Other tumours

Of the other rare tumours, haemangiomas (capillary or cavernous) may reach sufficient size to cause splenic enlargement, with a consumptive coagulopathy and haemorrhagic tendency.

Miscellaneous conditions

Cysts of the spleen

Cysts of the spleen are uncommon and are usually single. *Congenital* cysts are due to an embryonic defect and result in a dermoid-like lesion. *Degenerative* cysts result from liquefaction of an infarct or haematoma. There may be a past history of minor trauma. The wall is fibrous and often calcified, and the cyst is filled with brownish fluid or paste-like material. Pancreatic pseudocysts may extend to involve the spleen and *parasitic* cysts may occur due to infection with *Echinococcus granulosus* (hydatid disease). Splenic cysts normally cause no symptoms and are often discovered by accident. Symptomatic cysts may present with left upper quadrant pain radiating to the back or left shoulder. The lesion may be recognised by CT or ultrasound scan, investigations that are usually sufficient to characterise the nature of the cyst. Intervention is not indicated for small congenital or degenerative cysts. Large symptomatic cysts are treated by partial or complete splenectomy.

Splenic infarct

Splenic infarct may present with acute onset of left upper quadrant pain in a patient with known hypersplenism. Asymptomatic infarcts may be observed in patients following a severe attack of pancreatitis or following a spleen-preserving distal pancreatectomy. These may resolve with the formation of a splenic cyst, but do not require surgical intervention.

Abscess of the spleen

A splenic abscess is rare. It should be suspected when progressive splenic enlargement is associated with bacteraemia and abscess formation at other sites. Image guided drainage may be appropriate in select cases but splenectomy is often required to achieve resolution.

Splenic artery aneurysm

This may occur primarily as a complication of atherosclerosis in elderly patients where the calcified wall of the aneurysm may be visible on x-ray or secondary to acute or chronic pancreatitis. The presence of a small, uncomplicated primary aneurysm is not necessarily an indication for intervention, particularly as they often affect elderly, frail patients. Bleeding can occur, however, and mesenteric angiography with embolisation is the treatment of choice. Bleeding is more common in secondary aneurysms, and again the treatment of choice is radiological if possible as surgery in an actively bleeding patient is associated with a high mortality rate.

Table 15.8 The American Association for the Surgery of Trauma (AAST) classification of splenic trauma

Grade	Injury	Description
I	Haematoma	Subcapsular, <10% of surface area
	Laceration	Capsular tear <1 cm parenchymal depth
II	Haematoma	Subcapsular, 10–50% of surface area, intraparenchymal, <5 cm in diameter
	Laceration	1–3 cm parenchymal depth that does not involve a trabecular vessel
III	Haematoma	Subcapsular, >50% of surface area, or expanding Ruptured subcapsular or parenchymal haematoma Intraparenchymal haematoma >5 cm or expanding
	Laceration	Laceration >3 cm in depth or involving trabecular vessels
IV	Laceration	Laceration involving segmental or hilar vessels producing major devascularisation (>25% of spleen)
V	Laceration	Massive disruption of spleen
	Vascular	Hilar vascular injury that devascularises spleen

Traumatic splenectomy

In the majority of situations that require an emergency splenectomy for trauma (Table 15.8), the potential for injury is relatively obvious through a history of blunt or penetrating trauma. Delayed presentation, an unusual mechanism (e.g., postcolonoscopy) or the absence of a history through intoxication make a high index of suspicion essential. In addition, in patients with splenic enlargement, the mechanism may be relatively trivial. The cardinal features are those of significant blood loss, and local signs of peritoneal irritation (peritonitis or left shoulder tip pain).

Patients that do not respond to initial resuscitation require an emergency laparotomy and usually a splenectomy along with a careful exploratory laparotomy to exclude injury to other structures. In the responding patient, cross-sectional imaging is advised.

Approximately 80% of splenic injuries may be managed conservatively, and of these the requirement for intervention is apparent within 72 hours in 95%. In the unstable patient, control of haemorrhage and restoration of circulating volume are paramount and consideration regarding organ preservation is of secondary importance. Unlike an elective splenectomy, a midline laparotomy is usually performed with packing of the left upper quadrant, which will normally control the splenic haemorrhage to allow the remainder of the abdomen to be examined. If examination of the spleen reveals bleeding from the splenic hilum, preservation is not appropriate and a splenectomy should be performed.

Splenic conservation

Because of the immunologic function of the spleen, interest over the last century has turned to salvage of the spleen rather than splenectomy. Minor lacerations may respond to topical haemostatic agents (Floseal, Baxter Healthcare, UK; or Surgicel or Evarrest, Johnson & Johnson, UK) coupled with enhanced haemostatic technology (argon diathermy, harmonic scalpel, Ethicon UK; or Ligasure, Covidien, UK) may allow haemorrhage to be controlled or a partial splenectomy to be performed. The role of interventional radiological embolisation of the splenic artery has been reported; however, it is dependent on the availability of appropriately skilled radiologists. As the majority of patients can be managed conservatively without embolisation, care needs to be taken that in striving to avoid laparotomy inappropriate delay in haemostasis does not occur in those with ongoing bleeding. In those who are being managed conservatively, awareness and ongoing careful observation are critical, as 'delayed rupture' of a subcapsular haematoma can occur.

Surgical decision-making regarding splenic preservation versus splenectomy also requires consideration of the patient's total injury burden and physiology. For example, the patient with blunt poly-trauma with competing priorities, such as a closed head injury, will not tolerate the haemodynamic compromise from a delayed bleed following an attempt at splenic preservation. A lower threshold for splenectomy is required in this scenario. Similarly, physiological instability including coagulopathy may necessitate splenectomy as part of a damage-control approach, even in the context of a spleen that was otherwise suitable for preservation.

Other indications for splenectomy

Removal of the spleen may be required as part of other surgical pro-cedures, such as distal pancreatectomy and radical gastrectomy for carcinoma and, less frequently, for proximal splenorenal shunt.

Effects of splenectomy

Following splenectomy changes occur in the blood cell composi-tion and immunological status of the patient. Absence of pitting leads to the presence of Howell-Jolly bodies and Pappenheimer granules. Occasionally erythroblasts and siderocytes are also seen. There is leucocytosis with an increase in platelet number. An increase in platelet adhesiveness is also seen, leading to an increased risk of thrombosis. The immunological defects seen after splenectomy include a poor response to immunisation with particulate antigens, decreased levels of phagocyte-promoting peptide, deficiency of serum IgM levels and decreased properdin levels.

Postsplenectomy immunisation

Loss of lymphoid tissue reduces immune activity and impairs the response to bacteraemia. The risk of overwhelming post-splenectomy sepsis is greatest when splenectomy is performed in childhood. The British Committee for Standards in Haematol-ogy recommends that all splenectomised patients should receive pneumococcal polysaccharide vaccine, *Haemophilus influenzae* type B vaccine, and meningococcal C conjugate vaccine. Lifelong prophylactic antibiotics are still recommended (oral phenoxymethylpenicillin or erythromycin). Elective sple-nectomy should be preceded by the administration of vaccines 2–3 weeks prior to surgery, but are still effective if given postoperatively.

15

16

Malcolm G. Dunlop

The small and large intestine

Chapter contents

Introduction 252

Surgical anatomy and physiology 252

Clinical assessment of the small and large intestine 253

Principles of operative intestinal surgery 254

Disorders of the appendix 255

Inflammatory bowel disease 255

Disorders of the small intestine 261

Small and large bowel obstruction 264

Non-neoplastic disorders of the large intestine 266

Intestinal stoma and fistula 272

Polyps and polyposis syndromes of the large intestine 272

Malignant tumours of the large intestine 275

Introduction

Any individual can reasonably expect to suffer gastrointestinal (GI) symptoms at least once a year. Most disorders are self-limiting, benign conditions but serious pathology can have enigmatic, or even, no symptoms until a late stage in the natural history of the disease. Infective diarrhoea most commonly affects the young; inflammatory conditions those in early and middle adulthood; cancer and diverticular disease in middle and old age. There are similarities in presenting symptoms despite varied underlying disorders and it is usually not possible to differentiate underlying causes from clinical assessment alone (see Box 16.1). Thus, self-resolving disorders, in which watchful waiting is appropriate, may be indistinguishable from those requiring timely investigation and active management. Investigation can be potentially harmful, since it frequently involves invasive investigations such as colonoscopy and radiation exposure. Careful history and examination, informed by knowledge of the hierarchy of likely age-related diagnoses is essential when assessing patients with intestinal problems.

16.1 Summary

Clinical assessment of a patient with gastrointestinal symptoms

- Gastrointestinal symptoms are very common
- Most symptoms are due to self-resolving illness
- Patient age is an important factor when considering the differential diagnoses
- Duration of symptoms is important in deciding the need for investigation
- Careful assessment of the nature and severity of symptoms is important and may indicate peritonitis, obstruction or severe inflammation
- Symptoms of self-resolving intestinal disorders that are managed conservatively often cannot be differentiated from major problems
- Investigation includes blood tests, stool culture, endoscopy, imaging and open or laparoscopic inspection.

Surgical anatomy and physiology

Anatomy and function of the small intestine

The small bowel extends from the pylorus to the ileocaecal valve and ranges in length from 3 to 7 metres. The jejunum comprises two-fifths of the small intestine and is of wider calibre than the ileum. The gut diameter narrows progressively from the duodeno-jejunal flexure to the ileocaecal valve. The small bowel mucosa is supported by a strong submucosa and comprises a single layer of columnar cells in a villiform structure that greatly increases the absorptive surface area. Columnar glandular epithelium is interspersed with mucus-secreting cells, Paneth cells and amine precursor uptake and decarboxylation (APUD) cells derived from the neural crest. Between the inner layer of circular muscle and the outer longitudinal layer runs Auerbach's myenteric plexus comprising vagal parasympathetic fibres and sympathetic fibres from the lesser and greater splanchnic nerves. This plexus controls orderly propulsive contractions of the muscular layers of the gut wall. The submucosal (Meissner's) neuronal plexus of autonomic nerves innervates the glandular cells in the epithelium. The sensation of visceral pain is mediated by the sympathetic nervous system, originating mainly from the thoracolumbar outflow and fed along the arterial supply to the gut.

The arterial supply to the small intestine is via the superior mesenteric artery, which runs in the root of the small bowel mesentery, supplying the bowel by a series of arterial arcades (Fig. 16.1). These midgut vessels communicate with the coeliac axis through the pancreaticoduodenal arcade, and with the inferior mesenteric artery by contributing to the colonic marginal artery through the left branch of the middle colic artery, which joins the ascending branch of the left colic artery. Venous blood drains via the superior mesenteric vein to the portal vein. Lymphoid aggregates in the submucosa (Peyer's patches) are more numerous in the ileum,

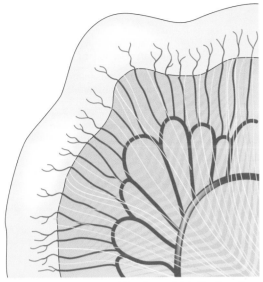

Fig. 16.1 Arterial arcades supplying the small intestine from the superior mesenteric artery.

and lymph drains to regional nodes in the root of the mesentery before passing to the cisterna chyli.

The main function of the small bowel is nutrient absorption (amino acids, short peptides, sugars, fats, minerals, vitamins and micronutrients). Its secretory and digestive functions supplement those of the upper gastrointestinal tract. The mucosa is thrown into circular folds (plicae semilunares) and is carpeted by fingerlike villi, giving an absorptive area of 200–500 m². Some 5–8 L of fluid enter the jejunum each day, of which only 1–2 L normally pass to the colon.

Anatomy and function of the large intestine and appendix

The main function of the large intestine is water absorption and to act as a reservoir until defaecation is appropriate. The large bowel mucosa consists of columnar epithelium interspersed with mucus-secreting goblet cells that secrete lubricating mucus. The villi are shorter than those of the small intestine, and crypts pass down to the muscularis mucosa, which is supported by a strong submucosa. The large bowel extends from the ileocaecal valve to the upper anal canal (approximately 1.6 metres). The caecum is a blind pouch at the most proximal part of the large bowel. The transverse and sigmoid colon are mobile because they have a mesentery, whereas ascending and descending colon are only partially peritonealised. The true rectum is demarcated by coalescence of the three taeniae coli of the sigmoid colon to form a continuous outer longitudinal muscular tube. The upper third of the rectum has peritoneal cover anteriorly and on both sides, the middle third is peritonealised only anteriorly and the lower third is normally wholly extraperitoneal.

The inferior and superior mesenteric arteries supply the colon via a marginal artery (Fig. 16.2) that allows collateral supply in the event of arterial occlusion, but is weakest at the splenic flexure. In contrast to the small bowel, each of the terminal arterial branches feeding the large bowel are end arteries which has implications for the risk of ischaemia. The superior rectal artery is the continuation of the inferior mesenteric artery, and with the middle and inferior rectal arteries (branches of the internal iliac arteries) supplies the rectum. The inferior mesenteric vein drains into the splenic vein. Lymph channels run along the course of the arterial supply (Fig. 16.2). Lymph from the rectum, sigmoid and descending colon drains to the superior rectal and inferior mesenteric nodes, whereas anal canal lymph drains to inguinal nodes. Knowledge of the lymphatic drainage has considerable relevance to the management of patients with rectal or anal cancers.

The appendix is lined by colonic epithelium but has no known function in humans. The submucosa contains prominent lymphoid follicles in childhood that regress in adolescence. In older patients, the lumen may be obliterated by fibrosis. The appendix projects from the medial wall of the caecum some 2 cm below the ileocaecal junction as the taeniae coli converge.

Clinical assessment of the small and large intestine

Clinical history taking

Painful contraction of the midgut (the duodenum distal to the ampulla of Vater, small bowel, right colon and right two-thirds of transverse colon; supplied by the superior mesenteric artery) secondary to obstruction or inflammation results in periumbilical colic due to referred pain related to its the embryological origin. Nausea, vomiting and pain are early and predominant features of many small bowel disorders, particularly obstruction. Disorders affecting the hindgut (the distal third of transverse colon to rectum; supplied by the inferior mesenteric artery) frequently present with poorly defined features including abdominal distension, colicky lower abdominal pain and altered bowel habit. Vomiting is a late feature of large bowel obstruction. Normal stool frequency ranges from one motion in 3 days to 3 motions/day. Hence, it is important to ascertain whether there has been any change in frequency from the patient's normal habit. Passage of blood or mucus per rectum is a common feature of large bowel disease. It is important to differentiate 'outlet type' bleeding (from the anal canal) from sinister blood loss, when the blood is mixed with the stool and there may be associated altered bowel habit or tenesmus (a painfully urgent but ineffectual attempt to pass stool). Outlet bleeding is typically bright red and may be present only on toilet paper or spattered in the pan, separate from the stool. There may be associated perianal pain, due to fissure or prolapsed piles. Blood originating from the distal bowel is usually bright red, whereas blood coming from the upper gastrointestinal tract is usually altered by gut bacteria and digestive enzymes, becoming black or tarry (melaena). Weight loss, malaise and anaemia are common nonspecific features of intestinal disease. A careful drug history is essential as many medicines can directly, or indirectly, cause GI upset.

Examination

The hands, fingernails, eyes, conjunctivae and oral mucous membrane should be inspected. Abdominal examination may reveal distension, a mass or visible peristalsis. In thin subjects, the caecum is often palpable, and the descending and sigmoid colon may be palpable when loaded with faeces. Hepatomegaly due to metastatic disease should be excluded. Abdominal auscultation is rarely of any value and has been shown to be nondiscriminatory. Digital rectal examination may detect a rectal tumour and may reveal blood or

16

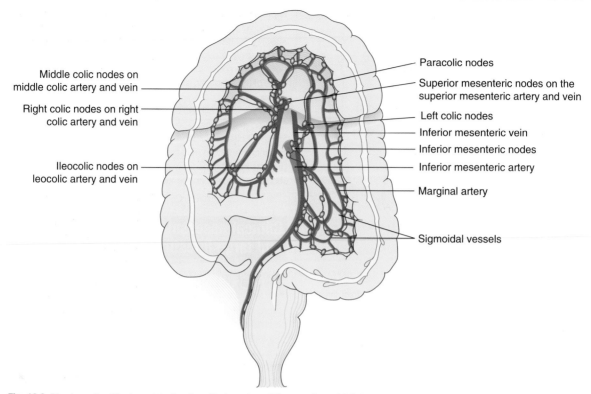

Middle colic nodes on middle colic artery and vein

Right colic nodes on right colic artery and vein

Ileocolic nodes on leocolic artery and vein

Paracolic nodes

Superior mesenteric nodes on the superior mesenteric artery and vein

Left colic nodes

Inferior mesenteric vein

Inferior mesenteric nodes

Inferior mesenteric artery

Marginal artery

Sigmoidal vessels

Fig. 16.2 Blood supply of the large intestine from the branches of the superior and inferior mesenteric arteries, with the lymphatic drainage of the colon and rectum.

mucus. In patients with lower GI symptoms, there is no rationale for checking the faeces for occult blood, as the sensitivity of the faecal occult blood (FOB) test is low. The more specific and sensitive faecal immunological testing (FIT) may have a place in stratifying symptomatic patients for investigation.

Investigation of the luminal gastrointestinal tract

Investigation of persisting diarrhoeal illnesses should include stool samples for faecal calprotectin (nonspecific test of intestinal inflammation), culture and testing for *Clostridium difficile* toxin. For recent foreign travel, hot stool should be assessed for cysts, ova and parasites. Imaging modalities for small bowel comprise plain radiography, magnetic resonance imaging (MRI) enteroclysis, computed tomography (CT), capsule video endoscopy, labelled white cell radionuclide scanning and labelled red cell radionuclide scanning. Barium follow-through and contrast small bowel enema have largely been superseded by MRI. Fibreoptic small bowel enteroscopy allows direct inspection of the proximal jejunum, whereas the terminal ileum can be inspected and biopsied at colonoscopy. Coeliac disease may be diagnosed by serum ELISA assays for autoantibodies, including antiendomysial IgA antigliadin or tissue transglutaminase (tTG) antibodies. Duodenal biopsy taken at endoscopy is the gold standard investigation and would reveal the characteristic subtotal villous atrophy of coeliac disease. Tests of absorptive capacity are rarely performed. Bacterial overgrowth can be assessed using the glucose breath test, ^{14}C-xylose and ^{14}C-glycocholate breath tests. Small bowel aspiration can be carried out by nasojejunal tube or at enteroscopy for bacterial culture.

Following digital rectal examination, direct inspection includes proctoscopy, rigid sigmoidoscopy, flexible sigmoidoscopy and colonoscopy. These techniques allow biopsy and snare removal of colorectal polyps using cauterising diathermy. Plain radiography is used extensively in the emergency situation. CT double contrast colonography has superseded double contrast barium enema. CT also has considerable utility in the assessment of the acute abdomen. CT of chest, abdomen and pelvis is routinely used in staging of colon and rectal cancer, along with MRI for rectal cancer. Positron emission tomography (PET) after administering a fluoride[18] labelled tracer (fluorodeoxyglucose) that is metabolised by tumours is reserved for staging of colorectal cancer when multi-organ resection is being considered. Colonic transit can be assessed in cases of suspected megacolon or slow-transit constipation by administering radioopaque markers or ingestion of radionucleotide (indium[111] or technicium[99]) labelled feed to assess large bowel transit time.

Principles of operative intestinal surgery

The nutritional function of the small bowel is crucial and so the principle of resectional surgery is to maximise residual bowel length. Conversely, loss of the large bowel can be tolerated with little impact on nutritional status, but water and salt depletion can occur, especially in hot climates. Specific nutritional deficits can follow resection.

Small intestinal anastomoses heal well due to their excellent blood supply and rich submucosal arteriolar plexus. The large intestine microcirculation consists of a series of small end-arteries. This feature, combined with the presence of faeces with a high density of bacterial colonisation, results in poor anastomotic healing and increased anastomotic leak rates compared with small intestine. There is a tendency towards formation of a stoma in the emergency setting due to the increased risk of anastomotic leakage but efforts are made to reconstitute large bowel continuity in both elective and emergency resectional surgery to avoid stomas.

Mechanical bowel preparation is no longer indicated for elective large bowel resections. Low-residue diet prior to surgery may have a place, whereas broad-spectrum antibiotic prophylaxis (e.g., gentamicin, amoxicillin and metronidazole) to cover coliforms and anaerobic bacteria is essential.

Disorders of the appendix

Appendicitis

Acute appendicitis remains the most common acute abdominal emergency in childhood, adolescence and early adult life (Chapter 12).

Appendiceal tumours

Tumours of the appendix

The appendix is the most common site for carcinoid tumours, which are neuroendocrine tumours (NETs), arising from the argentaffin cells of the APUD system and have an embryological origin from the neural crest. Tumours are typically yellow submucosal lesions located near the tip of the appendix and account for 85% of all tumours, being found in 0.5% of all appendices removed for appendicitis. Most are benign, but tumours >2 cm in diameter have a greater risk for mural infiltration and lymphatic spread to the mesenteric glands. It is rare for appendiceal carcinoid tumours to give rise to liver metastases and the carcinoid syndrome. Appendicectomy is sufficient treatment for most appendiceal carcinoid tumours, but right hemicolectomy is advised for tumours >2 cm, if it involves the caecum, or if the lymph nodes are affected.

Benign tumours include adenoma and cystadenoma. A mucocoele may arise due to chronic obstruction of the appendix base and luminal accumulation of mucin and may be confused on imaging with a tumour but is cured by appendicectomy.

Pseudomyxoma peritonei

This rare condition results from seeding of the peritoneal cavity with mucus-secreting cells from an appendiceal cystadenoma. It is important to differentiate the disorder from a true malignant mucus-secreting adenocarcinoma. In pseudomyxoma, the peritoneal tumour has a low mitotic rate but causes pressure symptoms owing to the amount of mucin produced. Median survival is 2.5 years and few patients are alive after 5 years. Surgical debulking is frequently necessary but rarely curative. The lesions are not responsive to conventional chemotherapy or radiotherapy. Extensive pseudomyxomas may be treated with radical cytoreductive resection with peritoneal stripping and intraoperative intraperitoneal hyperthermic chemoperfusion (HIPEC) using hot mitomycin C.

Adenocarcinoma of appendix

This rare, highly malignant neoplasm frequently presents with involved regional lymph nodes at diagnosis. The presentation may mimic acute appendicitis or appendix mass. Right hemicolectomy is the treatment of choice, even in cases where the diagnosis is only apparent at histological assessment of an appendicectomy specimen. Adjuvant chemotherapy may be considered when lymph nodes are involved. Adenocarcinoma often affects younger patients, and may arise in association with the autosomal dominant Lynch syndrome (see later).

16.2 Summary

Tumours of the appendix

- 85% of all appendiceal neoplasm are carcinoid tumours, the appendix being the most common site of carcinoid tumour in the gastrointestinal tract
- Carcinoid tumours are found in 0.5% of surgically removed appendices
- Carcinoids >2 cm have a greater risk of malignancy, but lymph node involvement is rare and metastases are extremely rare
- Appendix adenocarcinoma is rare and may be associated with hereditary nonpolyposis colorectal cancer (HNPCC)
- Mucin-secreting cystadenoma; if ruptured, may lead to pseudomyxoma peritonei
- Pseudomyxoma peritonei is a rare, unpredictable condition that causes pressure symptoms on intestine and other intraabdominal organs, and for which there is no curative therapy, but radical cytoreductive surgery with HIPEC has gained favour.

Inflammatory bowel disease

Crohn's disease and ulcerative colitis may be considered together due to similarities in clinical presentation and management (Table 16.1). Ulcerative colitis affects the colon and rectum exclusively, whereas Crohn's disease may affect any part of the gastrointestinal tract. Inflammation is restricted to the mucosa in ulcerative colitis but transmural inflammation is a hallmark of Crohn's disease. Surgery for ulcerative colitis can be curative, whereas Crohn's disease frequently follows a relapsing course, despite medical or surgical intervention.

Crohn's disease

Although originally described affecting the terminal ileum, any part of the gastrointestinal tract can be involved, from mouth to anus. In 50% of cases, both small and large bowel are involved, whereas in 25% of cases large bowel alone is affected. The incidence is increasing in developed countries and the annual incidence rate is 5–7 cases per 100,000 in the UK. Due to the life-long nature of the condition, the estimated UK prevalence is around 620,000 people. At the time of initial presentation, the clinical and histological features may be indistinguishable from those of ulcerative colitis, leading to the diagnostic category of IBDU (inflammatory bowel disease unclassified). The outcome from IBDU is worse and may follow a course eventually leading to overt evidence of Crohn's disease.

Cigarette smoking is the single most important risk factor, being associated with increased disease severity, likelihood of relapse and further need for surgical interventions. There is also evidence for the involvement of immunological factors and the gut bacterial flora in Crohn's disease pathogenesis. There is a substantial heritable contribution to disease aetiology, variously estimated at 20–50%.

Pathology

Macroscopically, Crohn's disease produces a cobblestone appearance, in which oedematous islands of mucosa are

16

Table 16.1 Clinical features of Crohn's disease and ulcerative colitis

	Crohn's disease	Ulcerative colitis
Incidence	5–7 per 100,000 and rising	10 per 100,000 and static
Extent	May involve entire gastrointestinal tract	Limited to large bowel
Rectal involvement	Variable	Almost invariable
Disease continuity	Discontinuous (skip lesions)	Continuous
Depth of inflammation	Transmural	Mucosal
Macroscopic appearance of mucosa	Cobblestone, discrete deep ulcers and fissures	Multiple small ulcers, pseudopolyps
Histological features	Transmural inflammation, granulomas (50%)	Crypt abscesses, submucosal chronic inflammatory cell infiltrate, crypt architectural distortion, goblet cell depletion, no granulomas
Presence of perianal disease	75% of cases with large bowel disease; 25% of cases with small bowel disease	25% of cases
Frequency of fistula	10–20% of cases	Uncommon
Colorectal cancer risk	Elevated risk (relative risk = 2.5) in colonic disease	25% risk over 30 years for pancolitis
Relationship with smoking	Increased risk, greater disease severity, increased risk of relapse and need for surgery	Protective, first attack may be preceded by smoking cessation within 6 months

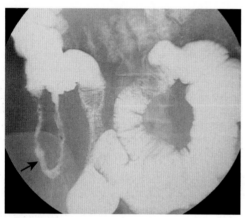

Fig. 16.3 Small bowel follow-through showing Crohn's disease strictures (*arrow* indicates long stricture).

separated by fissures that can extend through all coats of the bowel wall. Circumferential ulceration and associated fibrosis can result in multiple strictures of varying length. Multiple areas of inflammation are common with intervening normal bowel (skip lesions, Fig. 16.3). Full thickness involvement of the bowel wall leads to serosal inflammation, adhesion to neighbouring structures, and sinus or fistula formation. Microscopically, there are deep fissuring ulcers, oedema and inflammatory cell infiltrates with foci of lymphocytes and noncaseating granulomas in 50% of cases.

Clinical features

Crohn's disease is a chronic disorder with exacerbations, remissions and a varied clinical presentation. Continuous or episodic diarrhoea is associated with recurring abdominal pain and tenderness, lassitude and fever. There may be declining general health, malabsorption, weight loss and metabolic bone disease (osteoporosis or osteomalacia). Failure to thrive and to reach developmental milestones are common in affected children.

Examination may reveal malnutrition and there may be a palpable abdominal mass. Intestinal obstruction may be due to gross thickening of active disease occluding the lumen, stricturing of 'burnt out' disease, or adhesions from previous surgical intervention. Fistula formation occurs in 20% of patients with small *and* large bowel disease, but less in those with disease restricted to the large bowel. Fistulae may communicate with adjacent loops of bowel, other viscera (e.g., bladder, vagina) or the skin. Enterocutaneous fistulae may result from surgical intervention and commonly involve the anterior abdominal wall or perineum (Fig. 16.4). Abscesses can result from chronic bowel perforation, but free perforation is relatively uncommon because the inflamed segment usually adheres to surrounding structures. Although less common than in ulcerative colitis, toxic dilatation can complicate colonic disease. Fulminant Crohn's colitis with severe inflammation, mucosal oedema, deep linear ulcers and fibrosis is shown in Fig. 16.5.

There is an elevated risk of colorectal adenocarcinoma with long-standing Crohn's disease: 2.5-fold overall and 4.5-fold for colonic disease, with a 10-year cumulative risk following diagnosis of 2.9%. Lymphoma risk may also elevated, likely due to immunomodulatory therapy (e.g., thiopurines) and biological therapy (anti-TNF and antiintegrin). Evidence is limited that surveillance provides protection and many patients with long-standing colonic Crohn's eventually come to colectomy. Crohn's disease is also associated with ~30-fold excess risk of small bowel adenocarcinoma, but because that cancer is rare, the absolute risk only amounts to 0.2% at 10 years and 2.2% at 25 years after diagnosis.

Anorectal involvement is common (25% in small bowel Crohn's disease; 75% in large bowel disease), including abscess, fistula, fissures, ulceration, oedematous skin tags and anorectal stricturing. Anal fissures are often multiple and indolent, and extend to involve any part of the perineum, including the vagina or scrotum. Systemic manifestations include anterior uveitis, iritis,

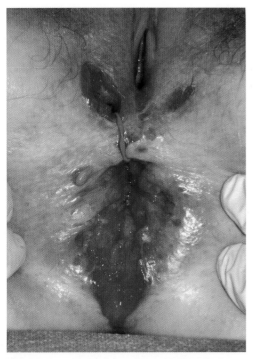

Fig. 16.4 Severe perianal Crohn's disease with fistulation.

Investigations

Assessment of nutritional status, including serial weight measurement, is essential. Anaemia may be due to iron deficiency from chronic blood loss and (rarely nowadays) malabsorption from short gut syndrome; a normocytic anaemia of chronic disease; macrocytic anaemia from vitamin B_{12} or folate malabsorption. Assays for circulating acute-phase proteins (C-reactive protein) is not a diagnostic test but is useful for monitoring disease activity. Until recently, the diagnosis was most frequently made on barium follow-through (Fig. 16.6): rose-thorn ulcers, long irregular terminal ileal stricture at the site of previous ileocaecal resection. Active disease produces radiological evidence of thickening, luminal narrowing and separation of bowel loops, and is often associated with mucosal ulceration, deep fissuring ulcers and cobblestone appearance. Skip lesions and fistula formation may be apparent. MRI enteroclysis (image enhanced by administering oral osmotically active agent, e.g., polyethylene glycol) is now the investigation of choice (Fig. 16.7) and has the advantage of limiting radiation exposure. Rectal examination, proctoscopy, sigmoidoscopy and colonoscopy determine disease extent, and biopsy of inflamed bowel is mandatory. Newer investigative techniques include video capsule endoscopy (Fig. 16.8), enteroscopy, and CT colonography. Double-contrast radiography still has a place for delineation of fistulous tracts.

16

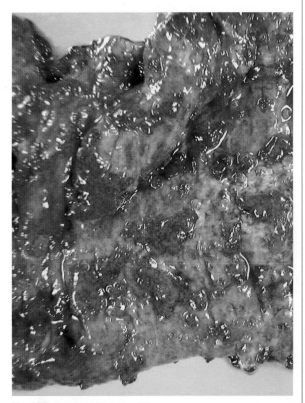

Fig. 16.5 Fulminant Crohn's colitis.

polyarthropathy, ankylosing spondylitis, liver disease (e.g., sclerosing cholangitis) and erythema nodosum. Terminal ileal involvement or ileocaecal resection may result in gallstone formation owing to poor absorption of bile salts.

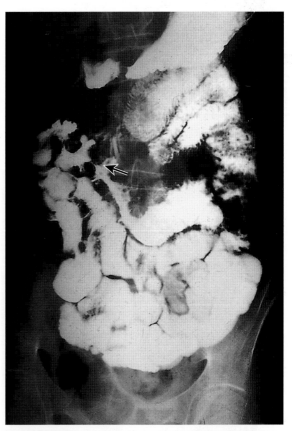

Fig. 16.6 Small bowel contrast enema in Crohn's disease, showing a long irregular stricture (*arrowed*) and typical rose-thorn ulceration.

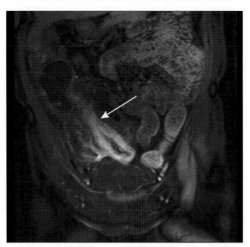

Fig. 16.7 Small bowel magnetic resonance imaging showing thickened strictured small bowel in Crohn's disease (arrow).

Management

Medical management

Attention to general nutritional state is crucial. Anaemia should be corrected by transfusion, iron and/or vitamin supplements, as appropriate. Oral protein and calorie supplements may be required and patients with short bowel syndrome may require parenteral nutrition. Bile salt diarrhoea secondary to previous terminal ileal resection may benefit from cholestyramine.

Corticosteroids may be used to induce remission (prednisolone 30–60 mg daily by mouth), but long-term therapy should be avoided. Some patients with colonic disease or relapsing terminal ileal disease may be maintained on 5-aminosalicylic acid agents (e.g., mesalazine, olsalazine), but there is no evidence that prophylactic maintenance therapy reduces relapse risk or need for further surgery. Immunosuppression using azathioprine or 6-mercaptopurine can be used in resistant cases to induce remission and for maintenance. There are concerns about complications of long-term immunosuppression: the agents are not generally continued beyond 2 years without review and are seldom used beyond 4 years. Monoclonal antibodies to tumour necrosis factor-α (TNF-α) (e.g., Infliximab) and humanised anti-TNF MAbs (Adalimumab) are now widely used. Newer biological agents are under development and those such as the gut-selective monoclonal antibody to alpha integrin (Vedolizumab) are widely used as second line therapy.

Surgical management

Many patients undergo surgery at some stage of their disease course and multiple operations are common. There are four main categories of indications for surgical management of Crohn's disease:

1. Onset of complications of luminal disease: fulminant colitis, life-threatening haemorrhage, obstruction, abscess/sepsis, perforation, fistulation.
2. Acute or chronic failure of medical management to control symptoms/disease activity, failure to thrive, complications of medical therapy.
3. Treatment or prophylaxis of malignancy.
4. Perianal disease: abscess, fistula, anorectal stricture (EBM 16.1).

EBM **16.1 Crohn's disease and ulcerative colitis**

'Colonoscopic surveillance may reduce colorectal cancer risk in longstanding inflammatory bowel disease.
Surgical resection is required in patients resistant to medical management, those with complicated disease such as abscess, fistulation and perforation, and those developing complications of medical therapy.'

Mowat C et al. Guidelines for the management of inflammatory bowel disease in adults. Gut. 2011;60:571–607. doi: 10.1136/gut.2010.224154.
Cairns SR et al. Guidelines for colorectal cancer screening and surveillance in moderate and high risk groups. Gut. 2010;59:666–89. http://gut.bmj.com/content/59/5/666.long
NICE Guideline. Colonoscopic surveillance for prevention of colorectal cancer in people with ulcerative colitis, Crohn's disease or adenomas. http://www.nice.org.uk/nicemedia/live/13415/53641/53641.pdf

---

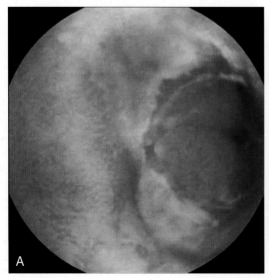
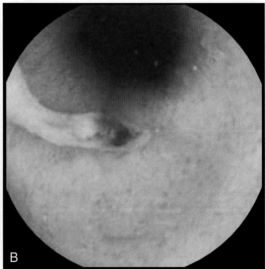

Fig. 16.8 Video capsule enteroscopy of Crohn's disease. **(A)** Extensive ulceration and stricturing. **(B)** A single deep ulcer.

Preservation of bowel length is the modern surgical maxim, limiting segmental bowel resection and using stricturoplasty (longitudinal enterotomy with transverse closure of strictures). Measured length of residual small bowel should be documented in patient records. Relapse is common following small bowel resection, but small bowel relapse occurs in less than 20% of patients with exclusively colonic disease. However, many patients with colonic disease eventually come to proctocolectomy and permanent ileostomy. In perianal Crohn's disease, loculated pus must be drained and radical surgery should be avoided. Simple fistulae may be laid open, but long-term Seton drainage is used for complex fistulae involving sphincter muscle. Complex reconstructions such as rectal advancement flaps should be avoided.

 16.3 Summary

Indications for surgery in Crohn's disease

Elective
- Chronic subacute obstruction due to fibrotic strictures, adhesions or refractory disease
- Symptomatic disease unresponsive to, or poorly controlled by, medical management
- Chronic relapsing disease on discontinuation of medical management and steroid dependency
- Complications of medical management (e.g., osteoporosis)
- Concerns about long-term immunosuppression, risk of malignancy and viral/atypical infections
- Perianal sepsis and fistula
- Enterocutaneous fistula
- Onset of malignancy, including colorectal adenocarcinoma and small bowel lymphoma
- Rarely, control of debilitating extracolonic manifestations such as iritis and sacroiliitis.

Emergency
- Fulminant colitis or acute small bowel relapse unresponsive to medical management
- Acute bowel obstruction
- Life-threatening haemorrhage
- Abscess or free perforation
- Perianal abscess.

Ulcerative colitis

The annual incidence of ulcerative colitis is ~10/100,000 population in Westernised countries but rare in developing countries. The aetiology is incompletely understood, but genetic, immunological and dietary factors all play a part. Any age group may be affected but peak incidence is in early adulthood. The disease may be contiguous, but almost universally affects the rectum and extends proximally (Table 16.1). In a minority, the rectum may be spared, and in untreated patients, this should raise suspicion about underlying Crohn's disease. There is an elevated risk of adenocarcinoma in ulcerative pancolitis. Although ulcerative colitis is primarily a disease of the large bowel, systemic manifestations (iritis, polyarthritis, sacroiliitis, hepatitis, erythema nodosum, pyoderma gangrenosum) can occur. Sclerosing cholangitis affects 2–5% of patients with ulcerative colitis and may necessitate liver transplantation.

Pathology

The characteristic feature is inflammation restricted to the mucosa and submucosa of the large bowel. In severe episodes, there may

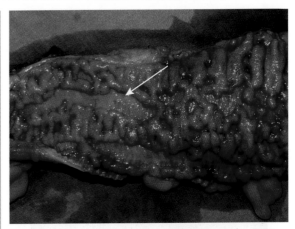
Fig. 16.9 Resected colonic specimen of fulminant ulcerative colitis showing denuded colonic epithelium (arrow).

be full-thickness involvement with inflammatory infiltrate. Abscesses develop at the base of the colonic crypts, which burst and unite to form crypt abscesses. These undermine the mucosa, resulting in ulceration (Fig. 16.9) and oedema of the intervening mucosa, with formation of inflammatory pseudopolyps. Histologically, there is also chronic inflammatory cell infiltrate, crypt architectural distortion and goblet cell depletion. Granulomas are absent but occasionally are present in severe cases, causing diagnostic difficulties. The thickened colon loses its haustrations and becomes rigid. Stricturing is rare and so its presence should raise the possibility of cancer or Crohn's disease.

Clinical features

Ulcerative colitis characteristically runs a relapsing/remitting course, although some patients may have a chronic continuous variant. The initial attack may be fulminant, and toxic dilatation with exacerbation of abdominal and systemic symptoms may occur at any time. Diarrhoea with the passage of mucus and blood is typical of relapse. Abdominal pain and tenderness may be present and intermittent pyrexia is common. Daily passage of 10–15 or more stools is not unusual in acute severe exacerbations. Incapacitating faecal urgency is the main symptom that degrades quality of life.

Careful rectal examination should be performed to detect anal complications such as fissure, fistula and haemorrhoids (present in 25% of cases); the rectal mucosa typically feels thick and boggy. Sigmoidoscopy and biopsy is essential and reveals red, granular mucosa with contact bleeding. In the early stages, sigmoidoscopy may only show loss of rectal mucosal vessels. As the disease progresses, severe ulceration leads to fulminant colitis, the complications of which include nutritional depletion, toxic dilatation, perforation and bleeding. During an exacerbation, the dilated colon may become paper-thin. Recent population-based studies have revealed that the mortality for all inpatient admissions for ulcerative colitis is ~15% at 3 years, emphasising the severity of the disorder.

Investigations

In the acute phase, stool cultures are essential to exclude supervening bacterial infection (especially *C. difficile*). Colonoscopy is the mainstay of diagnosis and assessment of disease extent/severity (Fig. 16.10). Abdominal CT should be reserved for

16

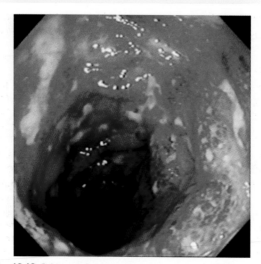

Fig. 16.10 Colonoscopic appearance of severe acute colitis.

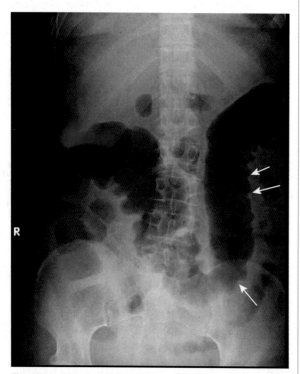

Fig. 16.11 Plain abdominal radiograph of fulminant colitis showing distension and mucosal oedema and thumbprinting (arrows).

suspected perforation, to minimise radiation exposure. Typical changes include loss of haustrations, fluffy granularity of the mucosa and pseudopolyps. Undermining ulcers may create a double contour to the edge of the colon. Widening of the retrorectal space, due to perirectal inflammation and reduced distensibility of the rectum, is common. In long-standing colitis, the bowel may become short and featureless, resembling a smooth tube ('leadpipe' colon). In an acute attack, plain films of the abdomen may reveal a dilated gas-filled colon in which pseudopolyps are evident ('thumb printing'). When toxic dilatation is suspected, daily plain x-rays are mandated (Fig. 16.11). 'Backwash ileitis' may produce a dilated and featureless terminal ileum in which the mucosa

appears granular and can lead to diagnostic difficulties with Crohn's disease.

Management

Medical

Repeated clinical and laboratory assessment is key during an acute exacerbation to identify those with a severe episode that requires escalation of therapy and/or surgical resection. Daily stool charting, temperature and pulse, along with C-reactive protein and albumin assays are essential. Various criteria are used to identify those with a severe episode and these include Truelove and Witt's score: stool frequency $>6\times/24$ h *AND* any of Hb <105 g/L, ESR (erythrocyte sedimentation rate) >30 mm/h, pulse >90 bpm, T $>37.5°$C.

Fluid and electrolyte replacement, correction of anaemia, nutritional support, intravenous corticosteroid therapy, and timely surgical intervention are the mainstay of treatment of an exacerbation. High-dose systemic steroids are needed during an acute relapse. In fulminant colitis, unresponsive to steroid therapy, it is now standard of care to escalate therapy to immunosuppression with cyclosporin A or biological therapy with anti-TNF agents (e.g., Infliximab). Topical steroids delivered by enema or suppository usually control mild attacks of proctocolitis. Long-term aminosalicylates, such as mesalazine or olsalazine, reduce the risk of relapse once a remission has been induced. Azathioprine is also used for maintenance therapy. Around 15% of all patients diagnosed with ulcerative colitis will eventually require surgery; 1 in 50 for mild proctitis, 1 in 20 for moderately severe colitis, and 1 in 2 for extensive disease.

Surgical

Indications for surgery in the emergency setting include fulminant colitis that fails to respond to aggressive medical therapy, perforation and toxic dilatation. The primary aim of monitoring is to operate before perforation occurs, when mortality increases dramatically. Patients presenting as an emergency are catabolic, malnourished, immunosuppressed, bacteraemic and septic. Hence, surgical reconstruction in the acute phase is inadvisable and management comprises colectomy and ileostomy as a 'first aid' operation. The rectum is closed over as a stump in the pelvis, or by bringing out the distal end as a mucous fistula. Completion proctectomy and the formation of an ileoanal pouch are undertaken ~6 months following the emergency operation to allow nutritional recovery. The residual rectum is removed because of the elevated rectal cancer risk over the remaining lifetime.

Indications for elective surgery include failure of medical management or repeated relapses on medical treatment. Failure to thrive, as reflected in retardation of growth and sexual development in children, or malnourishment and anaemia in adults, is a common indication for operation. The onset of biopsy-proven dysplasia or carcinoma in chronic disease necessitates surgical intervention.

Modern surgical practice comprises restorative proctocolectomy with retention of anal sphincters and reconstruction with an ileal pouch anastomosed to the upper anal canal to maintain the ability to defaecate. A temporary ileostomy may be required. Median stool frequency is 4–6 liquid or soft motions/day, but the debilitating faecal urgency associated with colitis is eliminated and the overall quality of life is excellent. Where pouch anal anastomosis is not possible, a Koch's continent ileostomy may be considered. Proctocolectomy and permanent end ileostomy still have an important place in management.

16.4 Summary

Indications for surgery in ulcerative colitis

Elective
- Symptomatic disease unresponsive to, or poorly controlled by, medical management
- Chronic relapsing disease on discontinuation of medical management and steroid dependency
- Complications of medical management
- Concerns about long-term immunosuppression, risk of malignancy and viral/atypical infections
- Severe dysplasia on surveillance biopsies of colorectal epithelium
- Onset of colorectal adenocarcinoma
- Rarely, control of debilitating extracolonic manifestations such as iritis and sacroiliitis.

Emergency
- Fulminant colitis unresponsive to maximal medical management
- Toxic megacolon
- Free perforation
- Life-threatening haemorrhage
- Acute complications of medical management.

Cancer surveillance in ulcerative colitis

Colorectal cancer risk in long-standing ulcerative colitis is a major factor contributing to surgical decision-making. Carcinoma is typically difficult to detect, is usually poorly differentiated and has a poor prognosis. Historical data indicate that 2% of patients develop cancer at 10 years, 8% at 20 years and 18% at 30 years (25% in patients with pancolitis). Early age at first onset (<15 years), pancolitis, a family history of colorectal cancer and associated primary sclerosing cholangitis (PSC) are strong cancer risk factors. However, recent evidence suggests that overall cancer risk may be lower, due to aggressive suppression of inflammation by newer agents. Nonetheless, 2-yearly colonoscopic surveillance with random colonic biopsies to detect dysplasia is mandated in chronic pancolitis (EBM 16.1). Dysplasia-associated lesion or mass (DALM) is a high-risk indicator of impending, or concurrent, cancer development. Cancer risk for patients with high-grade dysplasia or DALM is >60% in the next 2 years and prophylactic proctocolectomy is recommended. Even without dysplasia, patients with pan-ulcerative colitis may opt for prophylactic restorative proctocolectomy, rather than undergo life-long surveillance, especially when diagnosed in teenage years.

Disorders of the small intestine

Small bowel neoplasms

Small bowel tumours account for less than 5% of all gastrointestinal neoplasms.

Benign tumours

Solitary tumours include adenomatous polyps, hamartomas, lipomas and haemangiomas. Multiple hamartomas are found in Peutz–Jeghers syndrome. Benign tumours are rarely symptomatic and so the true incidence is unknown. Symptoms may arise as a result of intussusception or bleeding.

Malignant tumours

Malignant small intestinal tumours are rare and frequently diagnosed late because symptoms are nonspecific and so initial presentation may be at laparotomy for small bowel obstruction.

In symptomatic cases, imaging modalities include MRI enteroclysis, barium follow-through, CT, flexible enteroscopy and video capsule endoscopy.

Gastrointestinal stromal tumours (GIST)

GISTs are the most common form of mesenchymal tumour of the intestinal tract. The lesions are derived from smooth muscle of the gut tube; 50–60% arise in stomach, 20–30% in small bowel, 10% in rectum and 5% in oesophagus. There is a spectrum from benign to malignant assessed by mitotic figures and proliferation markers such a Ki67. Malignant lesions have a poor prognosis, tending to recur locally and metastasise. Expression of the oncogene p16/*c-Kit* differentiates malignant from benign characteristics. Malignant GISTs have a mutation in the *c-Kit* gene or the platelet-derived growth factor receptor alpha gene (PDGFRA). The resultant up-regulation of tyrosine kinase activity promotes tumour cell growth. New effective tyrosine kinase inhibitor anti-cancer agents (e.g., Imatinib mesylate) inhibit *Kit* or PDGFRA, and are one of the paradigm examples of 'precision medicine'.

Small bowel adenocarcinoma

The duodenum and upper jejunum are the most common sites of this rare tumour. Adenocarcinomas, which are usually poorly differentiated and are mucin-secreting, may be associated with HNPCC (Lynch syndrome). Resection of the affected segment is carried out, but palliative bypass may be all that is possible, as the disease often presents late.

Lymphoma

Small bowel is the most common site for lymphoma to arise in the intestine and may present as intermittent obstruction, bleeding or perforation. Coeliac disease is associated with an increased risk of various types of non-Hodgkin's lymphomas but particularly enteropathy-type T-cell lymphoma (ETTL). Antigliadin, anti-TTG and antiendomysial antibodies should be determined and a biopsy of adjacent normal small intestine or duodenum should always be assessed for villous atrophy in cases of lymphoma. Treatment is frequently surgical in the first instance because the diagnosis is made histologically after small bowel resection, but chemotherapy is required in most cases.

Carcinoid tumour

The small bowel is the second most common site for carcinoid tumour, after the appendix. Metastasis to lymph nodes is common at presentation, and obstruction and bleeding are the usual modes of presentation. Abdominal CT typically reveals a small bowel mass lesion with prominent calcification (Fig. 16.12). There may be features of the carcinoid syndrome with liver metastases. Urinary 5-HIAA (hydroxy-indole-acetic acid) and blood levels of chromogranin A should be assessed. The primary tumour should be resected where possible. Lesions are frequently multifocal and may require multiple resections.

Peutz–Jeghers syndrome

Peutz–Jeghers syndrome is an autosomal dominant inherited disorder with high penetrance, caused by mutations in the *STK11/LKB1* gene, located on the short arm of chromosome 19. Some cases are due to as yet unmapped genes. The clinical manifestations include gastrointestinal polyps and melanin pigmentation at mucocutaneous junctions, characteristically around the mouth and eyes. Occasionally there is pigmentation on the dorsum of the hands and feet. Affected individuals are at considerably elevated risk of colorectal, gastric, pancreatic, breast and ovarian

16

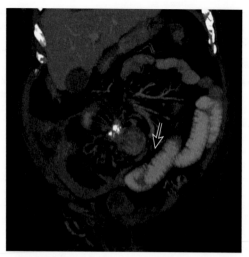

Fig. 16.12 Computed tomography showing small bowel carcinoid tumour with characteristic calcification and desmoplastic reaction. There is small bowel obstruction proximal to the lesion (*arrow*).

cancers. Small intestinal and gastric cancers occur in around 7% of patients and colorectal cancer in 10–20%.

Pathology

Polyps occur most commonly in the jejunum; they have a short pedicle with a lobulated surface resembling that of an adenomatous polyp or sometimes a villous tumour. On microscopy, the hamartomas consist of branches of muscularis mucosae covered by epithelium and lamina propria. There is a greatly increased (~30%) risk of colonic adenocarcinoma, but it is not clear whether this arises in a hamartoma or an adjacent area of normal epithelium.

Clinical features

Most cases present in childhood or adolescence. There are usually dark brown or bluish spots on the lips and inside the mouth. The face, palms, soles, arms and perianal region can also be affected, but patients without pigmentation have been described. The usual presentation is with abdominal pain or obstruction due to intussusception of a polyp, but rectal bleeding and iron-deficiency anaemia are also common. The diagnosis may be made in childhood or early adulthood on clinical grounds due to the association of abdominal colic and typical pigmentation. The investigation of choice in suspected Peutz–Jeghers syndrome is MRI enteroclysis (Fig. 16.13).

Management and surveillance

Laparotomy, enterotomy and polypectomy are often required because an emergency admission with obstruction is the frequent mode of presentation. On-table enteroscopy can reduce the number of enterotomies and allows inspection of the whole length of the gut from oesophagus to anus, with removal of all polyps. Combined upper and lower GI surveillance endoscopy biennially is recommended. MRI surveillance of the pancreas and intensive breast screening are also required due to the elevated cancer risk at these sites.

Meckel's diverticulum

This remnant of the vitello-intestinal duct is the most common congenital abnormality of the gastrointestinal tract, present in 2% of people. The diverticulum is ~5 cm long and arises from the anti-mesenteric border of the ileum some 50 cm from the ileocaecal valve (rule of 2: present in 2% of population, 2 inches long, 2 feet from ileocaecal junction). It is a true diverticulum and in 10% of cases its tip is connected to the umbilicus by a fibrous cord. Heterotopic mucosa is found in 50% of symptomatic diverticula; most often acid-secreting gastric mucosa although pancreatic tissue may be present. Only 5% of diverticula cause symptoms, most frequently in childhood or early adult life. Peptic ulceration distal to a Meckel's diverticulum is the most common cause of severe gastrointestinal bleeding in childhood. Intestinal obstruction may occur due to intussusception, or to a loop of bowel twisted around the band to the umbilicus (volvulus). Abdominal pain and tenderness, pyrexia and leucocytosis due to peptic inflammation may mimic acute appendicitis. Symptomatic Meckel's diverticulae

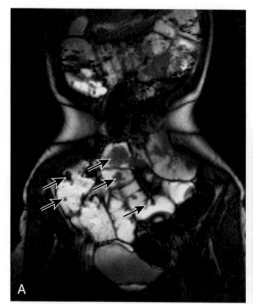

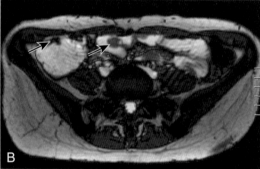

Fig. 16.13 Peutz–Jeghers syndrome. (A) Abdominal magnetic resonance imaging (MRI) (coronal view) showing multiple polypoid filling defects due to hamartomatous polyps (*arrowed*). (B) Cross-sectional MRI showing jejunal polyps.

should be excised. In patients with unexplained gastrointestinal bleeding, heterotopic mucosa within a Meckel's diverticulum can be detected by radionuclide scanning after injection of ^{99m}Tc-labelled sodium pertechnetate. Incidental Meckel's diverticulum found at laparotomy should generally be left alone.

Jejunal diverticulosis

Jejunal diverticulosis is an acquired disorder that is usually extensive along the length of the jejunum. There are multiple wide-mouthed sacs caused by herniation of mucosa into the mesentery at the site of vessel penetration of the gut wall. Jejunal diverticulosis may be first diagnosed at laparotomy for complicated disease, or incidentally on imaging studies (Fig. 16.14). Diverticulae may cause perforation, bleeding or an inflammatory mass. Malabsorption may occur due to bacterial over-colonisation. Occasionally, fish bones or nonsteroidal antiinflammatory drug (NSAID) tablets can become trapped in a diverticulum and cause local perforation. In symptomatic disease, the extensive nature of the disorder often necessitates a conservative approach with antibiotics and intravenous fluids. However, a bowel segment with complicated diverticulosis may require limited resection, leaving other affected areas in situ.

Radiation enteritis

External beam irradiation or radioactive implants can cause enteritis. The terminal ileum is the most commonly affected site within the small bowel. In the acute phase, oedema, inflammation and ulceration may produce watery diarrhoea, lower abdominal pain, tenesmus, mucus discharge and rectal bleeding. Subsequently, the bowel may thicken, with fibrosis and stricture which may require resection. The small bowel may fistulate to other loops, to large bowel or to the vagina. The involved segments require resection but anastomotic leakage rates are high because of the radiation damage.

Small bowel ischaemia

Small intestinal ischaemia is usually due to atheromatous occlusion with superadded thrombosis of the superior mesenteric artery. Predisposing factors include thrombophilia, hyperviscosity syndromes, dehydration, hypovolaemia or hypoperfusion of the gut resulting from trauma, cardiogenic shock, cardiac arrhythmia and septic shock. Arterial embolism can result from atrial fibrillation or recent myocardial infarction. In a third of patients dying from

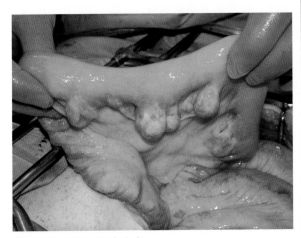

Fig. 16.14 Jejunal diverticulosis.

acute ischaemic necrosis of the midgut, there is no demonstrable occlusion of a major vessel, and in these cases low perfusion is responsible. Other causes include polycythaemia, sickle cell disease and disseminated intravascular coagulation. Arteritis should be suspected where there are other stigmata or a history of disseminated arteritis, such as preexisting renal failure. Impaired venous return from the gut can be due to hyperviscosity syndromes and prothrombotic tendency, but are also seen in the presence of malignancy and portal hypertension. Ischaemic necrosis may progress to necrosis of all bowel layers with gangrene and perforation.

Clinical features

Early diagnosis is often difficult as the symptoms and signs are nonspecific. There may be a preceding history of chronic or episodic abdominal pain associated with meals ('mesenteric angina'), diarrhoea and weight loss. Cardiac arrhythmias, notably atrial fibrillation, are often present on initial presentation. Abdominal pain is a predominant symptom and may be associated with vomiting. In a third of cases, there is watery or bloody diarrhoea. The pain varies in its location but is generally central, severe and constant in nature. Symptoms are out of proportion to signs. Abdominal tenderness, guarding and rigidity are late signs denoting gangrene and perforation, and cardiovascular collapse signifies hypovolaemia and sepsis.

Investigations and diagnosis

Clinical suspicion is essential in making a prompt diagnosis. Plain abdominal films may reveal calcified atheroma in the mesenteric arteries and aorta, and there may be dilated thickened gas-filled small bowel loops. Gas in the bowel wall or in the peritoneal cavity is a grave sign. Marked leucocytosis and hyperamylasaemia are common, but the finding of metabolic acidosis on blood gas analysis should raise strong suspicion of bowel ischaemia. Contrast enhanced CT is usually diagnostic and will show lack of gut enhancement. Formal arteriography is only occasionally helpful in practice because of the late presentation of most cases.

Management

Following vigorous resuscitation, gangrenous bowel requires resection, but this may be futile in elderly patients with extensive midgut involvement and a decision may be taken to limit intervention and keep the patient comfortable with palliative care. In some instances of acute occlusion, arterial flow can be restored by embolectomy or thrombectomy. A 'second-look' laparotomy 24 hours later may be useful. Massive resection is inevitable unless flow can be restored within 6 hours. Even if the patient survives, there may be substantial nutritional problems. The prognosis is poor (overall mortality 70–90%) and survival is restricted almost exclusively to patients in whom a defined vascular occlusion is treated early. Mesenteric venous occlusion has an equally bleak prognosis, and treatment is usually confined to resection of the gangrenous bowel and anticoagulation.

Chronic mesenteric ischaemia

Chronic mesenteric ischaemia results in repeated bouts of ill-defined colicky central abdominal pain, typically commencing 20–30 minutes after eating, leading to 'fear of food' and almost universally resulting in weight loss. Diagnosis is often elusive and is usually preceded by extensive investigation to exclude other conditions of the small or large bowel, such as Crohn's disease and malignancy. Mesenteric arteriography may be diagnostic but must be taken in the context of symptoms because atheromatous change in mesenteric vessels is common. Mesenteric revascularisation may be feasible in a minority of cases.

Small and large bowel obstruction

Obstruction refers to a mechanical impedance to the normal propulsive action through the intestine. The most common causes of small intestinal obstruction are adhesions (60%), obstructed hernia (20%) and malignancy (primary or secondary; 5–8%). In the large bowel, colorectal adenocarcinoma predominates (>70%), followed by stricturing diverticular disease (10%) and sigmoid volvulus (5%). The aetiology of large and small bowel obstruction can be systematically classified as intraluminal, intramural and extramural (Table 16.2). Treatment should be focused on the underlying cause of obstruction and surgery is required frequently.

The clinical presentation of bowel obstruction reflects the anatomical location of the lesion. The four symptoms of bowel obstruction are: abdominal pain, vomiting, distension and constipation. Depending on the level of obstruction, one or more symptom(s) will be prominent.

Proximal jejunal obstruction: very short history of anorexia, profuse vomiting, relatively severe upper abdominal pain and absent/minimal abdominal distension with limited, if any, change in bowel habit.

Distal small bowel obstruction: short history of colicky midgut (periumbilical) pain, distension, vomiting and recent absolute constipation.

Colonic obstruction presents more insidiously with poorly defined lower abdominal pain, weight loss, pronounced abdominal distension, history of altered bowel habit tending to constipation with little or no vomiting.

Initially the small bowel proximal to an obstruction contracts vigorously to overcome the mechanical impedance. However,

eventually peristalsis subsides and paralytic ileus ensues due to electrolyte imbalance and gross distension proximal to the obstruction. Patients with obstruction frequently present with profound dehydration due to a combination of vomiting, enforced fasting and 'third space' losses into the wall and lumen of the thickened intestine and peritoneal transudate. If the situation continues without decompression and resolution, there is progressive bacterial translocation into the portal circulation and the condition of the patient becomes increasingly toxic. Eventually bowel viability becomes compromised and may perforate. Features that indicate imminent perforation, strangulation or established peritonitis from perforation are: pyrexia, tachycardia, dehydration, hypotension, leucocytosis, peritonism on abdominal palpation and completely absent bowel sounds. It must be noted that none of these features reliably predict imminent perforation or strangulation.

Full clinical history and examination is essential, along with immediate instigation of intravenous fluid and electrolyte therapy. Digital rectal examination may reveal rectal or extrinsic malignancy, empty rectum or constipation. Hernial sites must be inspected carefully and any previous surgical abdominal scars noted. Abdominal x-ray will reveal distended small bowel or large bowel loops (Fig. 16.15) and may give an indication of the level of obstruction. Free gas under the diaphragm indicates perforation and mandates laparotomy. Grossly distended bowel loops or evidence of a closed loop obstruction also merit early surgical intervention. Increasingly CT is used to assess bowel obstruction, because it allows interpretation of the likely need for surgery, as well as identifying the underlying aetiology (Fig. 16.16). Right iliac fossa tenderness along with radiological evidence of caecal distension and distal colonic obstruction is a critical sign, indicating imminent caecal perforation and the need for urgent operation. The caecum perforates because it is anatomically the largest diameter. Since tension in the wall is directly proportional to the radius (law of Laplace), the tension is greatest in the caecal wall even though the intraluminal pressure is equal throughout the distended colon.

Closed loop obstruction in either small or large bowel is more likely to strangulate and perforate. Closed loop obstruction can occur in small bowel due to adhesions or malignant involvement of two parts of the small bowel. If the ileocaecal valve remains competent in colonic obstruction, this acts as one end of a closed loop and the risk of perforation is high, typically at the caecum as described previously.

Table 16.2 Causes of small and large bowel obstruction

	Small intestine	Large intestine
Intramural (intrinsic)	Crohn's disease Radiation stricture Tuberculosis Ischaemic stricture caecal carcinoma Primary tumour: lymphoma, adenocarcinoma, carcinoid tumour Intussusception secondary to: hypertrophy of Peyer's patches, Peutz–Jeghers polyp	Colorectal adenocarcinoma Diverticular stricture Sigmoid volvulus Radiation stricture (rectum/sigmoid) Ischaemic stricture Caecal volvulus Crohn's disease
Extrinsic	Postoperative adhesions Adhesions from previous inflammatory condition Congenital band Hernia Compression by tumour mass Volvulus	Rare owing to lumen diameter and retroperitoneal location Compression by tumour mass Massive inguinal hernia Incisional hernia
Intraluminal	Foreign body Gallstone ileus Worm infestation Bezoar	Faecal concretion (very rare)

Pseudoobstruction and nonmechanical gut functional disorder

Paralytic ileus

Paralytic ileus should not be confused with mechanical obstruction, although it is a sequela of the end stages of mechanical obstruction. The term refers to lack of propulsive contractions of both jejunum and ileum, although the ileus can be localised in some instances. It is common as a secondary feature of peritonitis due to any cause. It also may occur (1) after any surgical procedure due to handling of the bowel; (2) due to electrolyte abnormalities such as hypokalaemia, hyponatraemia, uraemia, diabetic ketoacidosis or; (3) secondary to drugs such as tricyclic antidepressant; lithium therapy, excessive opiate use. Management is conservative with bowel rest, nasogastric aspiration and fluid and electrolyte support. Treatment is otherwise focused on the underlying cause.

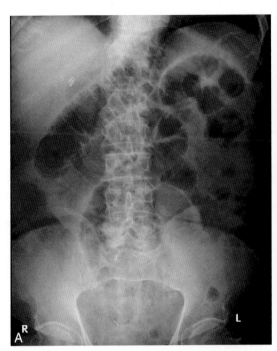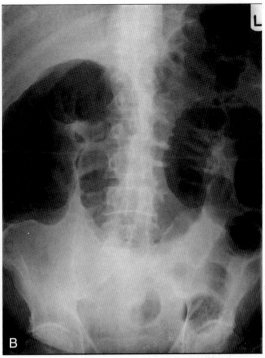

Fig. 16.15 Plain abdominal x-rays showing obstruction. **(A)** Small bowel obstruction. **(B)** Large bowel obstruction.

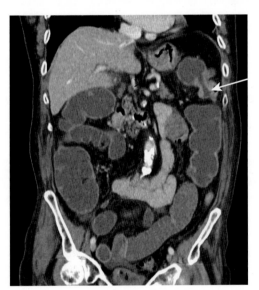

Fig. 16.16 Computed tomography showing large bowel obstruction caused by splenic flexure carcinoma (*arrowed*). Ileocaecal valve is incompetent resulting in small bowel dilatation.

Table 16.3 Causes of nonmechanical bowel dysfunction/ pseudoobstruction
Systemic/metabolic
• Hypokalaemia
• Hyponatraemia
• Hypocalcaemia
• Hypoxia
• Diabetic ketoacidosis
• Uraemia
• Dehydration
Drugs
• Tricyclic antidepressants
• Lithium therapy
• General anaesthesia
Miscellaneous
• Idiopathic
• Retroperitoneal malignancy (Ogilvie's Syndrome)
• Spinal trauma
• Retroperitoneal haematoma
• Brain injury
• Pelvic surgery
• Postoperative ileus
• General debility from any wasting illness
• Extra-abdominal sepsis
• Peritonitis

Pseudoobstruction

The underlying mechanism of pseudoobstruction is not fully understood (Table 16.3) but the pathogenesis involves autonomic imbalance resulting from decreased parasympathetic tone or excessive sympathetic output. It is essential to consider pseudoobstruction in patients who present with signs and symptoms of bowel obstruction.

The majority of cases of pseudoobstruction are due to large bowel dysfunction, although small bowel may be affected. It usually arises in the elderly and frail. Around 15% of all patients who present with signs and symptoms of large bowel obstruction in fact have pseudoobstruction. Operative mortality in patients with pseudoobstruction is >15% and so surgery should be avoided wherever possible. Blood electrolyte analysis is essential, along with imaging to exclude mechanical obstruction, using water-soluble rectal contrast with fluoroscopy and/or abdominal CT.

Management is conservative and involves stimulant enemas or colonoscopic deflation. Intravenous erythromycin can stimulate motility by binding to colonic motilin receptors, and is reserved for nonresolving cases. Intravenous neostigmine has been shown to be effective when other measures fail to resolve the pseudoobstruction. In a small minority of cases, colectomy with ileorectal anastomosis, or with ileostomy, may be required.

Common Disorders in Global Surgical Practice

Round worm infestation

Ascaris lumbricoides is one of the commonest nematode parasites affecting the human population worldwide. Fertilised eggs of *Ascaris* are present in faeces-contaminated soil and are ingested. Predominant symptoms are attributable to the presence of adult worms in the intestine: anaemia, malnutrition, failure to thrive, intestinal colic ('worm colic' in young children), intestinal obstruction due to a bolus of worms, and rarely perforation due to pressure necrosis of the wall of the intestine. Worms in the hepatobiliary tree can cause jaundice, cholangitis and acute pancreatitis.

Surgical complications of typhoid fever

Typhoid fever is caused by *Salmonella typhi* and *Salmonella paratyphi* A and B, which are gram-negative bacilli ingested when food or drink is contaminated due to poor sanitation. The incubation period for the ensuing febrile illness is 10–14 days. Bacteria localise in the ileal Peyer's patches. Blood culture is usually positive for *S. typhi* or *S. paratyphi* in the first week. Widal test for the presence of agglutinins to O and H antigens of *S. typhi* and *S. paratyphi*, respectively, is usually positive in the second week. Total leucocyte count, which is usually low and predominantly lymphocytic in typhoid fever, becomes elevated with neutrophilia in the presence of peritonitis. Haemorrhage can result from ileal, caecal or colonic ulcers. Typically in the third week of illness, ileal ulcers may perforate, usually on the antemesenteric aspect of the bowel. Perforation of colonic ulcers is uncommon. Urgent laparotomy after adequate fluid resuscitation is needed and perforations can be trimmed and closed or the segment resected if there are multiple perforations, with or without a stoma. Antibiotics should cover *Salmonella and* enteric organisms (ceftriaxone/ ciprofloxacin, gentamicin, metronidazole). Other surgical complications of typhoid fever include paralytic ileus, acute cholecystitis, acute osteomyelitis, acute pancreatitis, hepatic and splenic abscess and urinary tract infection.

Abdominal tuberculosis

Tuberculosis may arise after foreign travel or may reactivate in ethnic minorities. It is caused by the acid-fast bacillus *Mycobacterium tuberculosis* and less commonly *M. bovis*. The usual modes of spread by which the bacilli reach the abdomen are through ingestion of material contaminated by infected sputum or drinking contaminated milk. In tuberculous peritonitis, bacilli reach the peritoneum from intraabdominal lymph nodes or by haematogenous spread. Symptoms are nonspecific and include fever, anorexia, weight loss, night sweats and abdominal distension. Examination may reveal ascites; a transversely placed mass of 'rolled up' omentum in the upper abdomen may be palpable. The plastic form may present with acute or subacute intestinal obstruction

(Fig. 16.17). Miliary tubercles, yellowish white in colour and 2–5 mm in diameter, are seen in disseminated tuberculosis. Confirmation of diagnosis is best done by histopathological examination and peritoneal culture obtained at laparoscopy. In tuberculous lymphadenitis, the diagnosis may be made on CT or at laparotomy or laparoscopy for nonspecific symptoms. Small bowel mesenteric nodes (known previously as tabes mesenterica) are prominent and histologically the nodes exhibit caseation necrosis or calcification. Intestinal tuberculosis usually manifests in the distal small bowel and ileocaecal region. Initially an ulcerating course progresses to transversely orientated strictures in line with the lymphatics. After a diarrhoeal episode, patients may present with peritonitis due to perforation of a tubercular ulcer; however, fibrosis and stricture formation is more common and leads to intestinal obstruction. The differential diagnosis includes appendix mass, Crohn's disease, malignancy and amoeboma. Resection of the strictured segment usually provides a definitive diagnosis. A 'pulled up' caecum due to fibrosis of the mesentery is a classic feature on CT. Wherever possible antituberculosis therapy is preferable to surgical intervention to minimise loss of intestinal length.

Colonic amoebiasis and amoeboma

Entamoeba histolytica cyst forms are ingested in contaminated food and water. The trophozoites are released in the small bowel and travel to the large bowel, often remaining there without causing disease. If they invade the bowel wall they cause amoebic colitis; spread through the portal vein may cause abscesses in the liver (see Chapter 14), lung or brain. Clinical presentation is often a mild diarrhoeal illness, but amoebic dysentery can mimic ulcerative colitis and in severe cases may present as fulminant amoebic colitis with perforation. An 'amoeboma' (5% of cases) is a mass formed due to long-standing amoebic infection of the large bowel. The differential diagnosis includes malignancy, tuberculosis and Crohn's disease. Stool may show the presence of trophozoites. The lump rapidly resolves with antiamoebic therapy, which can be a helpful diagnostic test.

Non-neoplastic disorders of the large intestine

Colonic diverticular disease

Colonic diverticulosis is an acquired condition linked with low dietary fibre and stool bulk. It is extremely common in developed countries, present in more than 60% of people over age 70 years. The true population prevalence is unknown because estimates are derived from studies of incidental findings in people undergoing GI investigation for symptoms unrelated to the disease itself. In most cases, it is asymptomatic (diverticulosis) and asymptomatic disease can be classified as uncomplicated or complicated.

Although the whole colon can be affected, the sigmoid colon is by far the most commonly involved. The high intraluminal pressure at this site seems to relate to low residue in the diet. Muscular hypertrophy can be detected radiologically before diverticulae develop. Pulsion diverticulae, consisting only of herniated mucosa, emerge where feeding arteries pass through the circular muscle, between the mesenteric and antimesenteric taeniae. This relationship to feeding vessels has important clinical implications for bleeding risk. The true rectum is never affected due to differences in feeding vessels and because the outer longitudinal

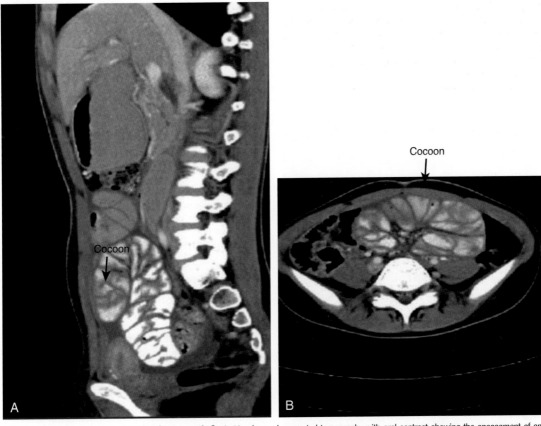

Fig. 16.17 Tubercular cocoon (*arrow* showing cocoon). Contrast enhanced computed tomography with oral contrast showing the encasement of small intestine in a central location in the abdomen. Note the large bowel relatively free on both flanks. (Courtesy Dr Bharat Agarwal, New Delhi).

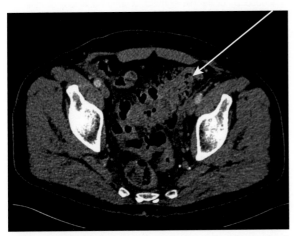

Fig. 16.18 Diverticular disease, computed tomography showing local perforation and collection (*arrow* showing localised collection with free air within it suggestive of bowel perforation).

smooth muscle tube encompasses the full circumference of the rectum.

Symptomatic diverticular disease often presents with intermittent lower abdominal/left iliac fossa pain, altered bowel habit, urgency of defaecation and episodic rectal bleeding. The sigmoid colon may be tender on examination. Abdominal CT (as CT colonography or plain abdominal CT) is the standard investigation (Fig. 16.18). This should involve intravenous, oral and rectal contrast to assess the overall extent of the disease, degree of surrounding inflammation, abscess formation and whether this communicates with the lumen. Colonoscopy reveals the ostia of diverticulae and will reveal any mucosal inflammation and fibrotic stricturing. Barium enema has now largely been abandoned for CT colonography as first investigation (Fig. 16.19).

In uncomplicated diverticular change, patients should be advised to take a high fibre diet, supplemented by bran or a bulk laxative such as methylcellulose. Stimulant laxatives and purgatives are best avoided. Antispasmodics (propantheline or mebeverine) may be useful if there is smooth muscle spasm and colicky pain. NSAIDs are associated with increased risk of complications and should be avoided. Surgical resection of the affected segment may be indicated for persistent symptoms, complications, or when carcinoma cannot be excluded by colonoscopy and/or radiology (EBM 16.2).

Congenital solitary diverticulum of the caecum is a rare condition that can arise from the medial wall close to the ileocaecal valve, extending upwards retroperitoneally. This may become obstructed by a faecolith and inflamed, producing a clinical picture indistinguishable from appendicitis.

Complicated diverticular disease

Although most diverticular disease is asymptomatic, complications are a frequent cause of emergency admission to surgical wards and are causally linked to inflammation (Table 16.4). Faeces inspissated in a diverticulum produce stasis and a local inflammatory response (diverticulitis). Infection may spread locally, resulting

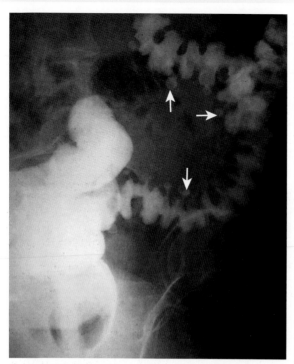

Fig. 16.19 Diverticular disease; barium contrast radiography.

EBM 16.2 Diverticular disease

'*Surgery is required for complicated diverticular disease (fistula, stenosis) and acute cases where abscess freely communicates with the lumen or there is failure to respond to antibiotics. Multiple episodes of diverticulitis is not in itself a requirement before surgery is indicated.*'

Fozard JBJ, Armitage NC, Schofield JB, Jones OM. Association of Coloproctology of Great Britain & Ireland Position Statement on Elective Resection for Diverticulitis. http://www.acpgbi.org.uk/assets/documents/Position_Statement_Elective_Resection_for_Diverticulis.pdf
Regenbogen SE et al. Surgery for diverticulitis in the 21st century: a systematic review. JAMA Surg. 2014;149:292–303. doi: 10.1001/jamasurg.2013.5477.
Jacobs DO. Clinical practice. Diverticulitis. N Engl J Med. 2007;357:2057–66. http://www.nejm.org/doi/full/10.1056/NEJMcp073228
Shaikh S, Krukowski ZH. Outcome of a conservative policy for managing acute sigmoid diverticulitis. Br J Surg. 2007;94:876–9.

in peridiverticulitis, and can result in a diverticular inflammatory mass or 'phlegmon'. Persistent infection may cause necrosis and the formation of a peridiverticular abscess. Septic complications are classified by Hinchey grade (Table 16.5). Patients presenting with established diverticular abscess are in a toxic condition and free perforation may result. Diverticulitis is also the underlying cause of diverticular bleeding as the feeding arteries are at the apex of each appendix.

Diverticulitis

Peridiverticulitis presents with pyrexia, leucocytosis, nausea and vomiting, and there is often a history of altered bowel habit. Pain and tenderness in the left iliac fossa are almost universal and a mass may be palpable. The initial diagnosis is primarily a clinical one, with the typical presentation being sufficient to treat the patient expectantly. The diagnosis is usually confirmed by CT.

Table 16.4 Complications of colonic diverticulae

Inflammation

- Peridiverticulitis
- Pericolic abscess
- Purulent peritonitis
- Faecal peritonitis
- Inflammatory mass
- Portal pyaemia

Obstruction

- Fibrotic stricture
- Adherent small bowel loops

Bleeding

- Massive lower gastrointestinal haemorrhage
- Chronic intermittent blood loss
- Anaemia

Fistula formation

- Colovesical fistula
- Colovaginal fistula
- Enterocolic fistula

Table 16.5 Hinchey classification of septic complications of diverticular disease

Hinchey grade I	Localised paracolic abscess
Hinchey grade II	Distant abscess (e.g., pelvic, subphrenic)
Hinchey grade III	Purulent peritonitis
Hinchey grade IV	Faecal peritonitis

Colonoscopy or flexible sigmoidoscopy and biopsy of inflamed segments are not usually necessary in the acute phase and best left until acute inflammation settles. CT colonography is the imaging modality of choice. Colonoscopy may be necessary if there is suspicion of malignancy on CT colonography.

Treatment comprises fasting or clear fluids by mouth, bed rest and intravenous fluids. The place of antibiotics remains controversial in uncomplicated flare up of clinical diverticulitis. If the patient shows signs of sepsis, broad-spectrum antibiotics are indicated, such as cephalosporins or gentamicin, along with metronidazole. If there is failure to improve within 36–48 hours, contrast-enhanced CT should be undertaken, preferably combined with rectal contrast to reveal any communication with abscess cavity or free perforation. The development of pericolic abscess usually necessitates surgical resection and peritoneal toilet, combined with surgical drainage of the abscess. There is no evidence to support percutaneous drainage of diverticular abscess but it is used by some in clinical practice. Such patients have a very high chance of ongoing sepsis and future surgery is almost certain due to chronic symptoms, even if the acute bout settles with antibiotics. Approximately one-third of all patients admitted with complicated acute diverticular disease require surgery during the index admission, while the remainder settle. Around 10% of these patients will eventually require surgical resection, preferably with primary anastomosis.

Perforation

Rupture of a pericolic abscess gives rise to purulent peritonitis, whereas free perforation of the bowel produces faecal peritonitis.

The patient is usually profoundly ill, with septic shock, dehydration, marked abdominal pain, tenderness and distension. Intravenous broad-spectrum antibiotics and vigorous preoperative resuscitation are essential, followed by resection of the affected bowel and peritoneal lavage. Specialist colorectal surgeons may elect to perform an anastomosis, given that only 30% of colostomies are subsequently closed. Hence, a second laparotomy may be avoided. If peritoneal contamination is severe and there is poor bowel perfusion of the gut, a colostomy may be preferable. The most common approach is to bring the end of the proximal colon through the abdominal wall and close the rectal stump (Hartmann's procedure). The distal end may be exteriorised as a mucous fistula. Continuity can be restored after 3 or more months, once the patient has recovered from the septic episode. Laparoscopic washout and drain replacement has gained much recent popularity, but is of unproven benefit and trials have been stopped due to concerns about safety. The mortality of perforated diverticular disease is 10–20%, but may be as high as 50% in the elderly with faecal peritonitis.

Stricture formation and obstruction

Long-standing diverticular disease may cause stricture formation and intestinal obstruction. Such strictures are often very difficult to distinguish from malignancy, particularly as the population most at risk of diverticular disease are the same demographic group as those at risk of cancer. Hence, resection may be necessary to rule out colorectal adenocarcinoma.

Fistula

Diverticular disease can give rise to fistulae to other viscera, particularly to the bladder or vagina. Colovesical fistula is more common in men because in women the uterus is interposed between bladder and sigmoid colon and prevents direct contact to some degree. The patient with a colovesical fistula usually complains of dysuria and the passage of cloudy urine, with bubbling on micturition ('pneumaturia'). The diagnosis may be confirmed by CT colonography with water-soluble rectal contrast but may not universally reveal the fistula. Cystoscopy is frequently performed. Many patients present to the urology service with chronic bladder instability and infections. Pelvic CT or MRI may reveal air in the bladder and show the fistulous tract itself. Treatment consists of resection of the affected segment, usually a sigmoid colectomy, with synchronous repair of the bladder.

Bleeding

Diverticular disease is the most common pathology responsible for major lower GI haemorrhage. It may present with persistent fresh rectal bleeding or massive haemorrhage. In the UK, the main differential diagnoses include colorectal cancer or adenomas, angiodysplasia (which frequently coexists with diverticular disease), haemorrhoids, inflammatory bowel disease and radiation proctitis, which may arise many years after prostate or cervical radiotherapy. Rare causes include amoebic colitis and typhoid ulcers in the ileum or colon. In the face of major lower GI haemorrhage, colonoscopy is not helpful in identifying the bleeding site, and in any case diveriticular disease is highly prevalent in UK populations. Hence, CT angiography is widely used, but bleeding is only visible if greater than 1 mL/min. Intraarterial angiography may be helpful and may allow embolisation of the bleeding vessel using gel foam. In some cases of unremitting torrential haemorrhage, operation has to be undertaken when a source of bleeding

has not been localised. On-table colonic lavage and colonoscopy will allow localisation of the affected bleeding segment and enabling the surgeon to perform a more localised resection. Rarely, in the face of life-threatening haemorrhage, a total colectomy and ileorectal anastomosis may be required.

Large intestinal ischaemia

The aetiology of ischaemia of the large bowel is similar to that of the small intestine. Atheroma at the origin of the inferior mesenteric artery results in relative insufficiency of the arterial supply from the marginal artery (Fig. 16.2). In rare cases where the inferior mesenteric artery is patent and an abdominal aortic aneurysm is present, colonic infarction may complicate aortic surgery if the inferior mesenteric artery is ligated. Untreated colonic ischaemia often progresses to gangrene and perforation. Some cases present with an acute bloody diarrhoeal illness known as ischaemic colitis, but others may declare symptoms from a chronic stricture.

Ischaemic colitis

In around 80% of cases, ischaemia of the large intestine is transient and is confined to the mucosa and submucosa. The patient presents with lower left-sided abdominal pain, nausea/vomiting and there may be bloody diarrhoea. Cardiovascular comorbidity should raise suspicion of the diagnosis. Examination reveals tenderness and voluntary guarding, often maximal in the lower left abdomen. There is usually a leucocytosis and pyrexia. Plain abdominal radiography may reveal a thickened segment of colon and thumb printing due to submucosal oedema, which may be evident on barium enema or CT (Fig. 16.20). Contrast studies should be carried out with water-soluble contrast because of the risk of perforation. The sigmoid colon is most often affected (Fig. 16.21). Ischaemic colitis is treated conservatively in the first instance unless abdominal signs reveal peritonitis, but symptoms should resolve after a few days of supportive therapy. Further assessment by colonoscopy is indicated once the acute episode has settled, to exclude diverticular disease and colorectal cancer. Biopsy features indicating ischaemic colitis comprise hyalinisation of lamina propria, withered crypts and relatively sharp demarcation from adjacent normal mucosa.

Gangrenous ischaemic colitis

The clinical presentation may initially be enigmatic, with severe pain but very little clinical signs. A profound lactic acidosis and leukocytosis should raise suspicion. In the late phases there is localised or generalised peritonitis. Without surgery, death is virtually certain, but given that operative mortality is over 50%, a considered decision on patient fitness and general state of premorbid health is required following consultation with the patient and family. Resection of the infarcted segment with formation of a colostomy or ileostomy is the rule, since anastomosis is not appropriate in the presence of poor blood supply.

Ischaemic stricture of the colon

Colicky abdominal pain, constipation and abdominal distension, following a history of an attack of bloody diarrhoea or a documented episode of ischaemic colitis, may suggest the diagnosis of ischaemic stricture. The patient may present with frank large bowel obstruction. Contrast CT or enema reveals a smooth narrowing of a segment of bowel, with a smooth appearance, lacking

16

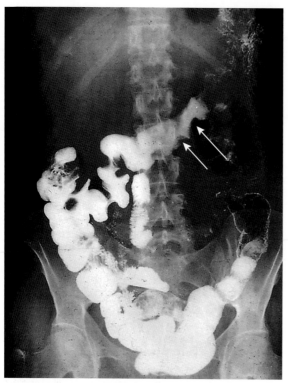

Fig. 16.20 Typical features of ischaemic colitis. Barium enema showing mucosal oedema and 'thumb printing' (arrows).

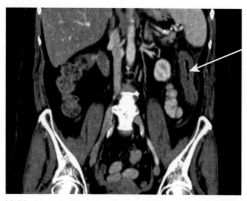

Fig. 16.21 Computed tomography showing gross mucosal thickening typically affecting the left side of the colon and sigmoid colon (*arrowed*).

the shouldering characteristic of malignancy (Fig. 16.22). Colonoscopy reveals a smooth, narrowed stricture with unremarkable biopsies, or occasionally histology may reveal evidence of chronic fibrosis. Symptomatic cases usually require resection, partly to exclude malignancy, although colonoscopic balloon dilatation may be attempted initially.

Irritable bowel syndrome

Although not discussed here, irritable bowel syndrome is a common functional bowel disease that is highly relevant to surgical practice because it presents with symptoms that are indistinguishable from structural bowel disease, such as inflammatory bowel disease, diverticular disease and cancer. Because of the

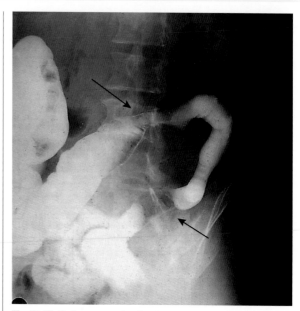

Fig. 16.22 Barium enema showing the smooth tapered appearance of a chronic benign stricture (between arrows).

lack of discriminatory clinical features, the diagnosis is largely one of exclusion by appropriate investigation.

Volvulus

Volvulus of the colon most commonly affects the sigmoid colon, and rarely the caecum, and is an important differential diagnosis of any cause of large bowel obstruction, such as cancer and diverticular disease. Sigmoid volvulus is due to a twist around a narrow origin in the sigmoid mesentery. It is an acquired condition and is the most common cause of large bowel obstruction in countries with a high level of dietary fibre; those affected are frequently young adults. By contrast in the UK, patients are usually elderly and chronic constipation is associated. The clinical presentation is of a bowel obstruction with lower abdominal pain, abdominal distension, nausea, vomiting and absolute constipation. Occasionally, the patient may present with sepsis owing to an established visceral perforation. Plain radiography reveals a characteristic Y-shaped shadow surrounded by a grossly distended colon arising out of the pelvis on a plain radiograph ('coffee bean' sign) (Fig. 16.23). Water-soluble contrast radiography or CT may show the characteristic 'beaking' at the site of the twist.

Sigmoid volvulus can be treated conservatively in the emergency situation by reduction and deflation, using rigid or flexible sigmoidoscopy and the placement of a large-bore tube into the sigmoid. Elective sigmoid colectomy following full bowel preparation is curative in the fit patient. In frail and demented patients or those with significant cardiac or other comorbidity, a conservative approach may be taken, but relapse is likely and frequent readmission the rule. Hence, surgery is the preferred option wherever possible (Fig. 16.24).

Caecal volvulus is a misnomer because it involves both the caecum and the small intestine, with the twist occurring around the longitudinal axis of the superior mesenteric artery. The presence of a congenital intraperitoneal caecum predisposes. It is usually suggested by plain radiography showing anticlockwise rotation of dilated small bowel loops around a grossly distended caecum. Caecal volvulus usually requires emergency laparotomy because

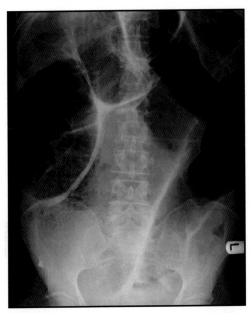

Fig. 16.23 Sigmoid volvulus. Plain abdominal radiograph showing characteristic 'coffee bean' sign.

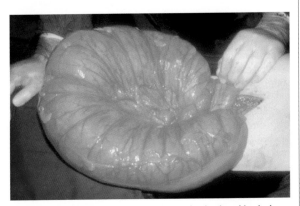

Fig. 16.24 Operative view of gross distension in sigmoid volvulus.

of the danger of compromise to the arterial supply of substantial lengths of the small bowel.

Angiodysplasia

Angiodysplasia frequently coexists with diverticular disease and is an important cause of massive lower gastrointestinal haemorrhage. The acquired submucosal arteriovenous malformations commonly affect the caecum and sigmoid colon, but any part of the large bowel can be involved. The diagnosis may be secured by visualisation of a bleeding point at colonoscopy. Bleeding angiodysplastic lesions can be treated by angiographic embolisation, by laser ablation at colonoscopy or injection sclerotherapy. Occasionally severe symptoms necessitate emergency laparotomy and resection.

Pseudomembranous colitis

Pseudomembranous colitis is due to *C. difficile* superinfection in the vast majority of cases. It is an important differential diagnosis of diverticulitis and inflammatory bowel disease (IBD). Stool should be screened for *C. difficile* in all patients with a flare up of IBD. The superinfection is almost always a healthcare-associated infection (HAI), associated with the use of oral broad-spectrum antibiotics. Typically patients present with an acute diarrhoeal illness, Left iliac fossa (LIF) pain and tenderness. Necrosis of the colorectal mucosa causes watery diarrhoea, toxaemia, shock and collapse. The stools are watery, green, foul smelling and blood stained, and often contain fragments of mucosal slough. A typical pseudomembrane may be visible on sigmoidoscopy but is not a prerequisite. Assays for the presence of *C. difficile* toxin in stool or blood, or colonic biopsy will confirm the diagnosis. The patient may be profoundly unwell, with dehydration and sepsis, and may require intensive resuscitation with intravenous fluid replacement. Treatment consists of oral metronidazole or vancomycin for 10 days. Severe cases may develop a toxic megacolon indistinguishable from that associated with inflammatory bowel disease, necessitating emergency colectomy and ileostomy. An ileorectal anastomosis can be performed at a later date when the patient is fully recovered.

Microscopic colitis

Rare subtypes of colitis include collagenous and lymphocytic colitis (collectively known as microscopic colitis), characterised by chronic diarrhoea, normal endoscopic and radiological findings, and typical findings on histological examination of colonic tissue. Microscopic colitis occurs more commonly in females; it can affect people of all ages but mean age is in the seventh decade. Collagenous colitis is characterised by macroscopically normal colonic mucosa overlying a typically thickened subepithelial collagen band on histological examination. Lymphocytic colitis is characterised by an increased number of lymphocytes in the submucosa but lacks the features of either ulcerative or Crohn's colitis. It can have a segmental distribution and so differentiation from Crohn's colitis is important. There is an association with coeliac disease and this should be excluded. There may be an association with a coexistent autoimmune disorder or the use of drugs such as NSAIDs. Treatment comprises avoidance of caffeine and other aggravating factors. 5-aminosalicylic acid agents may have a place in nonresponding cases. Antidiarrhoeal agents may be helpful. The disorder tends to resolve with such measures, but some resistant cases may benefit from topical steroid.

Hirschsprung's disease

Hirschsprung's disease affects 1 in 5000 live births and is due to the absence of ganglion cells in Auerbach's and Meissner's plexuses. It is an inherited disorder showing incomplete penetrance and variable expressivity. Mutations of the *RET* oncogene on chromosome 10 are responsible for most familial cases. *RET* mutations are also associated with multiple endocrine neoplasia (MEN) type II. In most cases, the distal 5–20 cm of large bowel is affected and presents in childhood, but presentation in adult life is also possible. Loss of peristalsis in the affected segment leads to large bowel obstruction with gross distension of the colon proximal to the aganglionic segment. The differential diagnosis in the neonate includes imperforate anus and meconium ileus, and in older children, megacolon acquired as a result of chronic constipation. Ischaemic colitis and, in children, necrotising enterocolitis have been reported due to superinfection with *Staphylococcus aureus*.

MRI in children and CT colonography in adults will reveal grossly dilated bowel above the narrowed aganglionic segment. Lack of ganglia is confirmed by full-thickness biopsy of the abnormal area.

16

In neonates, treatment consists of irrigation of the bowel with saline, followed by operation at about 6 weeks to bring ganglionated bowel down to the anal verge. In older children, a preliminary colostomy may be needed to allow bowel decompression. In the rare instance where the disease is not diagnosed until adulthood, the proximal colon is usually dysfunctional due to chronic megacolon and proctocolectomy with ileoanal pouch reconstruction may be preferable to anterior resection.

Acquired megacolon and idiopathic slow-transit constipation

Chronic constipation throughout life may result in megacolon. It may be associated with behavioural problems and difficulty with toilet training in childhood. The initial complaint is often faecal soiling, but a vicious cycle of constipation and anal fissure may ensue. In adults, defaecatory problems ranging from idiopathic slow-transit constipation to adult megacolon and megarectum may arise. Electrophysiological studies have shown changes reminiscent of Hirschsprung's disease affecting the whole of the large bowel, and there may be associated gastric motility dysfunction. Examination reveals gross faecal loading of the colon and rectum. Barium studies reveal a capacious and poorly contracting bowel with huge redundant loops. Transit studies following oral radioopaque markers or radioisotope labelled material typically show delayed transit.

Initial conservative management with aperients, bulk laxatives and regular enemas is successful in many cases, but faecal disimpaction under general anaesthesia may be required. Colectomy may be indicated in resistant cases but severe cases often involve neuropathy of the whole gut and surgery may not be curative.

Intestinal stoma and fistula

Stoma

Intestinal stomas have an important place in the management of intestinal disease. An ileostomy is formed by bringing out the ileum through the abdominal wall, usually through the rectus muscle in the right iliac fossa. Ileal bowel content is irritant to skin and a spout is fashioned to allow appliances to be fitted and so prevent skin contact with bowel content (Fig. 16.25). Ileostomy comprises either an 'end' stoma, or a 'loop' or 'defunctioning' stoma. A loop (defunctioning) ileostomy may be employed as an adjunct to resectional surgery when the disease process prevents

reanastomosis, or as a temporary measure to minimise the consequences of a leak from an anastomosis to the low rectum or anus. An end ileostomy may be established when the entire colon and rectum has been removed.

The colon can be also be formed into an end or loop colostomy, through the rectus muscle in the left iliac fossa. Transverse colostomy is seldom used in modern surgical practice. A colostomy does not require a spout, as faeces are not usually irritant to the skin. End colostomy is used as part of a Hartmann's procedure and is an integral part of an abdominoperineal resection for rectal cancer (see later). A loop colostomy of the sigmoid colon is used to divert faeces from a diseased anorectum, such as during the management of complex perianal fistula or faecal incontinence surgery. It may also be used as palliation for pelvic cancer or during radical radiotherapy for rectal cancer.

Given the requirement for formation of an abdominal wall defect, stomal and parastomal hernia is very common. Hence avoiding stomas is a key part of specialist colorectal surgical practice. Retraction and necrosis are serious early complications and require urgent surgical correction. Other complications include stenosis, bleeding from the skin–mucosa junction and prolapse.

Intestinal fistula

Fistula is defined as an abnormal communication between two epithelialised surfaces and can manifest between intestine and other parts of the gastrointestinal tract, skin, urinary tract or vagina. Intestinal fistulae may arise as part of a disease process (Crohn's, complicated diverticular disease or radiation enteritis) or as an iatrogenic complication, such as leak from a surgical anastomosis. Anastomotic leak may result in a cutaneous fistula, with bowel content appearing through the wound several days after intestinal surgery. The overall leak rate from colorectal surgery is around 5%, but around 10% for anastomoses involving the rectum. Anastomotic leak may present as a rectovaginal fistula, when defunctioning stoma with conservative management may be the best option but laparotomy and drainage of pus combined with taking down of the anastomosis with the formation of a stoma may be required. Radiation fistula typically present several years after the primary treatment, owing to the late development of endarteritis obliterans and chronic microvascular ischaemia. Malignant tumours of the upper and lower intestine can result in any combination of fistulation. Actinomycosis and tuberculosis are rare causes of cutaneous fistula. Treatment of disease-related fistula usually requires management of the primary problem.

Polyps and polyposis syndromes of the large intestine

The terms 'polyp' and 'tumour' are not synonymous. A polyp is a descriptive term referring to an excrescence of the mucosa and is not a pathological definition. The histological classification of colorectal polyps into four groups is shown in Table 16.6. Polyps may be identified by rigid sigmoidoscopy, flexible sigmoidoscopy, colonoscopy or CT colonography. Colonoscopy affords the opportunity for polypectomy and so enables histological assessment.

Colorectal adenoma

Neoplastic epithelial polyps are classified as tubular, tubulovillous or villous adenomas, depending on histological architecture. Such

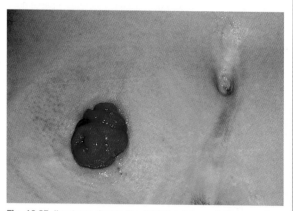

Fig. 16.25 Ileostomy sited in the right iliac fossa and demonstrating a spout.

Table 16.6 Classification of benign intestinal polyps

Type	Solitary	Multiple
Neoplastic hamartomatous	Adenoma (tubular, tubulovillous, villous) Juvenile polyp Peutz–Jeghers polyp	Familial adenomatous polyposis (FAP) Polymerase proof-reading associated polyposis (PPAP) Juvenile polyposis syndrome (JPS) Peutz–Jeghers syndrome (PJS) Cronkhite–Canada syndrome Cowden's disease
Inflammatory	Benign lymphoid polyp	Benign lymphoid polyposis Pseudopolyposis in ulcerative colitis
Hyperplastic	Hyperplastic Serrated adenoma	*MYH*-associated polyposis (MAP) Multiple hyperplastic polyposis

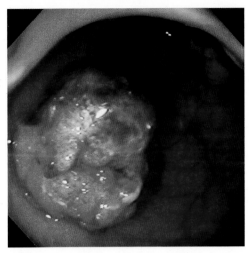

Fig. 16.26 Endoscopic appearance of a rectal adenomatous polyp.

classification has clinical relevance to cancer risk. Adenomas affect 40% of people over 50 years of age and 70% of those aged 65–69 years. Tubular adenomas account for 75% of all adenomas and are frequently pedunculated but may be sessile. Villous adenomas account for 10% and tubulovillous types for 15% of all adenomas. However, villous adenomas account for 60% of lesions larger than 2 cm. Villous adenomas are most commonly located in the rectum and may be large, carpeting the rectum. Around 50% of such tumours have a focus of carcinoma at presentation. Villous adenomas greater than 1 cm in diameter have an approximately 30% chance of malignancy, whereas the risk in a similar-sized tubular adenomas is around 10%. Multiple adenomas are common, with 24% of patients having at least two tumours.

Clinical features

The vast majority of polyps are asymptomatic, but symptoms include rectal bleeding or large bowel colic (especially when a large polyp intussuscepts). Occasionally, a rectal polyp may prolapse through the anus. Patients with giant villous adenoma of the rectum may present with severe watery diarrhoea due to excessive mucus loss, resulting in dehydration and profound hypokalaemia. Rectal adenomas may be palpable on rectal examination, but villous tumours are soft and can be missed. Distal polyps are detected readily by sigmoidoscopy, but there is a need for full colonoscopy in view of the risk of proximal synchronous lesions (Fig. 16.26).

Management

Colonoscopic polypectomy using an electrocautery snare prevents future risk of malignant conversion as well as enabling histological assessment (Fig. 16.27). Small adenomas can be biopsied and a current applied to destroy the entire polyp ('hot' biopsy). In many cases, polypectomy is the only treatment required, even when there is a malignant focus, if there are none of the following features: poor differentiation, stalk invasion at the resection margin, or invasion of submucosal lymphatics or microvasculature (Fig. 16.28). Surgical resection may be indicated if

16

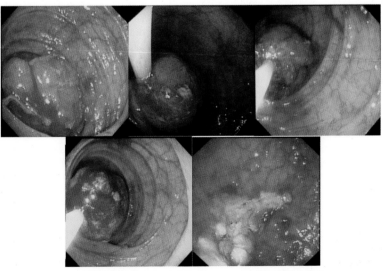

Fig. 16.27 Large adenoma of sigmoid colon resected endoscopically.

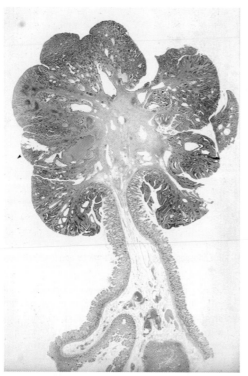

Fig. 16.28 Histological appearance of an adenomatous polyp, with malignant degeneration and early stalk invasion.

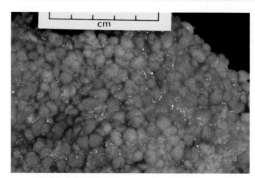

Fig. 16.29 Macroscopic features of dense polyposis due to familial adenomatous polyposis.

these histological features are noted, because there is a risk of bowel wall invasion or lymphatic spread. Polypectomy may be technically impossible or the risk of perforation too high (caecal lesions) and so bowel resection may be indicated for larger polyps. Transanal endoscopic microsurgery (TEM) allows resection of large rectal villous adenomas and repair of the rectal defect using an operating microscope. Advanced colonoscopic techniques such as lasering or submucosal resection are now well-established endoscopic techniques for larger lesions.

Follow-up colonoscopy is recommended after 6–12 months and 2–3 years. Long-term follow up is unnecessary once the colon has been cleared of any further polyps, unless the polyps fulfill high-risk criteria (>3 lesions and/or one >1 cm) or there were recurrent lesions at the 3-year screen.

Familial adenomatous polyposis (FAP)

FAP is caused by protein-truncating mutations in the *APC* gene (chromosome 5q22.2) and inherited as an autosomal dominant trait. It is one of the most common single-gene cancer predisposition disorders. APC has a critical role in colorectal carcinogenesis, because almost every sporadic colorectal cancer has a somatic defect in *APC* or another component of the Wnt signalling pathway. The annual incidence of FAP is 1 in 6670 live births and the population prevalence is 1 in 13,528. Around 25% of affected individuals have no family history of FAP, the disease arising in these sporadic cases as the result of a new germline mutation. There may be many hundreds or thousands of polyps (Fig. 16.29) but oligopolyposis is also possible. There are certain genotype–phenotype correlations. Adenomatous polyps usually develop during teenage years and early adulthood, with >90% chance of colorectal cancer by the third or fourth decade without

prophylactic colectomy. Because of effective surgical prophylaxis, FAP now accounts for less than 0.2% of all cases of colorectal cancer in the UK. The prevalence of colorectal cancer at diagnosis is 65% for symptomatic 'sporadic' cases and <5% for screened family members, emphasising the effectiveness of prophylaxis and surveillance.

Extracolonic features

Cystic gland polyps (not adenomas) are detected in 70% of FAP patients in the gastric fundus. Gastric antral and duodenal adenomas are apparent in over 90% of cases and malignant degeneration of periampullary adenoma is now the major cause of death: 7% of patients eventually develop periampullary cancer. Ileal adenomas also occur in FAP, but the risk of progression to malignancy appears to be very low. Craniofacial and long bone osteomas occur in the majority of FAP patients, and when these are a predominant feature, especially when associated with epidermoid cysts, the term Gardner's syndrome is widely used. However, Gardner's syndrome is simply a subgroup of FAP.

Intraabdominal desmoid tumours arise in around 10% of FAP cases. Although benign, these lesions expand and compress adjacent structures. Treatment with COX2 inhibitors (aspirin, sulindac, indomethacin) may induce regression or halt progression. The lesions express oestrogen receptor beta and so tamoxifen and or letrozole have been shown to be effective. Chemotherapy and radiotherapy may provide benefit in nonresectable cases with problematical symptoms or complications.

Epidermoid cysts arising in childhood should raise suspicions of FAP. Bilateral asymptomatic pigmented retinal lesions, known as congenital hypertrophy of the retinal pigment epithelium (CHRPE) are a feature of FAP. There is an increased risk of papillary thyroid carcinoma in women (160-fold excess risk <35years), but no increased risk in men. Other rare associations with FAP include hepatoblastoma, carcinoma of the gallbladder, bile duct and pancreas, and an increased risk of brain tumours.

Diagnosis and management

The diagnosis can be established by sigmoidoscopy and biopsy but mutation analysis is the mainstay of diagnosis in current practice. All FAP patients should be referred to a regional genetics service for registration and gene analysis. Presymptomatic detection of FAP allows prophylactic colectomy (EBM 16.3). There is no general consensus on the preferred surgical strategy, as both restorative proctocolectomy with ileoanal pouch formation and total colectomy with ileorectal anastomosis have advantages. The upper gastrointestinal tract should be screened for duodenal adenoma or carcinoma.

EBM 16.3 Colorectal adenomas

'Prophylactic surgical resection of the large bowel is indicated for familial adenomatous polyposis and MUTYH associated polyposis.'

Cairns SR et al; British Society of Gastroenterology; Association of Coloproctology for Great Britain and Ireland. Guidelines for colorectal cancer screening and surveillance in moderate and high risk groups. Gut. 2010;59:666–89. http://gut.bmj.com/content/59/5/666.long

Juvenile polyposis syndrome (JPS)

JPS is an autosomal dominant genetic disorder characterised by the development of multiple hamartomatous polyps throughout the gastrointestinal tract, usually around age 10 years. Juvenile polyps are usually classified as hamartomas, although some regard them as inflammatory, with blockage of crypts resulting in retention cysts. Single juvenile polyps occur in ~1% of the population, but juvenile polyposis is rare (~1:50,000). Estimates for gastrointestinal cancer risk range from 9% to 68%, but is probably ~50% lifetime risk of colorectal cancer. In JPS families, or individuals with a documented SMAD4 or BMPR1A mutation, colonoscopic surveillance is recommended 1–2-yearly from the age of 15–18 years. Surveillance intervals can be extended after the age of 35 years. Documented gene carriers or affected cases should, however, be kept under surveillance until the age of 70 years. Consideration should be given to prophylactic colectomy. Although it is essential that cases are recognised and managed appropriately, because of its rarity <0.1% of all cases of colorectal cancer are attributable to JPS.

Hyperplastic polyposis syndrome, MUTYH-associated polyposis (MAP) and polymerase proof-reading associated polyposis (PPAP)

Hyperplastic polyps are usually less than 5 mm in diameter and occur in increasing numbers with age, being present in some 75% of the population over the age of 40 years. Polyps tend to be pale, flat-topped, sessile plaques, found mainly in the rectum and often on the crest of mucosal folds. Histologically, the crypts are elongated, dilated and lined by columnar epithelium that has a sawtooth pattern. These polyps are often indistinguishable from adenomatous polyps, and are frequently removed because of the difficulties in differentiating them from adenomas. Some of the larger metaplastic polyps take on the features of a serrated adenoma and principally affect the caecum, where they are highly likely to progress to cancer. A subset of individuals with multiple hyperplastic polyps early in life has a substantially elevated cancer risk.

A gene involved in DNA base excision repair (MUTYH) has been shown to be responsible for colorectal hyperplastic polyposis in association with adenomatous polyps. The syndrome should be considered as a differential diagnosis of FAP, but with smaller numbers of adenomas. Mode of inheritance is autosomal recessive and colorectal cancer risk is very high. The management of documented homozygous MUTYH mutation carriers is controversial. Some advocate colonoscopic surveillance in the same manner as JPS but others cite the penetrance for colorectal cancer >90% and recommend prophylactic colectomy and ileorectal anastomosis.

PPAP is a recently described autosomal dominant oligopolyposis syndrome in which the adenomas may be indistinguishable from FAP. Somatic mutations in polymerase E1 and PolD1 genes are identified in 2–3% of all colorectal cancers, analogous to the situation with APC, although much less prevalent.

Other rare polyposis syndromes

Turcot's syndrome

Turcot's is an adenomatous colorectal polyposis syndrome associated with astrocytoma (also medulloblastoma or glioblastoma) of brain or spinal cord.

Cowden's disease

This is a rare gastrointestinal hamartomatous polyposis with an autosomal dominant pattern of inheritance. There is an increased risk of colorectal cancer, but benign and malignant disease of the breast and thyroid are the main risks. Periorbital warty tricholemmomas are pathognomonic in association with oral fibromas and keratoses of the hands and feet.

Cronkhite–Canada syndrome

This is a rare, nonheritable, syndrome comprising intestinal polyposis with alopecia, nail atrophy and brown macular hyperpigmentation. Histological examination shows cystic crypt dilatation similar to juvenile polyposis.

Miscellaneous colorectal polyps

Other differential diagnoses of colorectal polyps include benign lymphoid polyps; pseudopolyps in chronic ulcerative colitis; submucosal lipoma; lymphosarcoma; carcinoid tumour; leiomyoma. Neurofibromatosis rarely results in colonic polyps. Mucosal ganglioneuromatosis has been described in association with multiple adenomatous or juvenile polyps and in MEN type IIb.

Malignant tumours of the large intestine

Colorectal adenocarcinoma

Adenocarcinoma of the large bowel is the most common gastrointestinal malignancy. It is second only to lung cancer as a cause of cancer death in developed countries. There are ~45,000 new cases in the UK annually, accounting for around 15% and 12% of all cancer registration in males and females respectively. Lifetime risk is ~5%. It is the third ranked cancer overall after lung and prostate in males, and breast and lung in females. The male/female ratio for colon cancer is close to unity, whereas that for rectal cancer is 1.7:1. Incidence rates increase substantially with age. The rectum and sigmoid are particularly common sites for tumours (Fig. 16.30). However, in low-incidence countries, tumours are more evenly distributed. Around 3% of patients present with synchronous tumours and 3% develop metachronous tumours.

Aetiology

The aetiology is multifactorial, but there is a substantial environmental aetiological contribution, as evidenced by comparison of incidence between populations and observations that migrant populations take on the risk of the host population within a

16

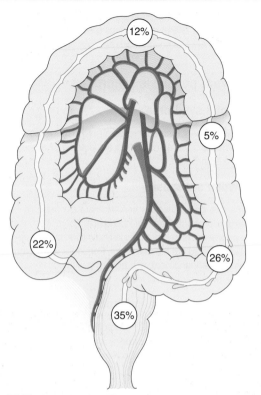

Fig. 16.30 Distribution of colorectal cancer in the large bowel in the UK.

EBM 16.4 Prevention and detection of colorectal adenocarcinoma

'Aspirin and non-steroidal anti-inflammatory drugs protect from colorectal neoplasia and are associated with reduced cancer mortality. Population screening by faecal occult blood test reduces mortality by 18% in those accepting screening. Population screening by 'once-only' flexible sigmoidoscopy may have a place in reducing colorectal cancer mortality.'

Rothwell PM et al. Effect of daily aspirin on long-term risk of death due to cancer: analysis of individual patient data from randomised trials. Lancet. 2011;377:31–41. Epub 2010 Dec 6. PubMed PMID: 21144578.
Hewitson P et al. Cochrane systematic review of colorectal cancer screening using the fecal occult blood test (hemoccult): an update. Am J Gastroenterol. 2008;103:1541–9. Epub 2008 May 13.
Atkin WS et al; UK Flexible Sigmoidoscopy Trial Investigators. Once-only flexible sigmoidoscopy screening in prevention of colorectal cancer: a multicentre randomised controlled trial. Lancet. 2010;375:1624–33. Epub 2010 Apr 27. PubMed PMID: 20430429.

generation. Risk factors include male gender (lifetime risk of males is 1.5 times that of females), increasing age, a strong family history of the disease and consuming a 'Westernised' diet.

Diet

Diet is a major environmental risk factor but no single dietary factor is solely responsible. Recently, dietary fibre has again gained favour as a protective factor. A high-fibre diet is associated with lower cancer rates in certain populations and within the UK population, whereas the consumption of a diet high in fat and red meat is associated with higher cancer rates. A high-energy diet is an associated risk factor. A low-fibre, high-fat diet appears to increase faecal pH, and this may enhance bile acid toxicity. Brassica vegetables, such as broccoli, contain antioxidants and other potential antineoplastic compounds. Dietary deficiency of calcium and vitamin D is associated with increased colorectal cancer risk. Despite strong supporting epidemiological evidence, intervention studies have not so far definitively shown that any dietary intervention reduces risk of colorectal adenoma or cancer, suggesting that a combination of risk factors is responsible.

Protective agents

Aspirin has been shown conclusively in case–control and cohort epidemiological studies and also recently in randomised trials to substantially reduce colorectal adenoma and cancer risk (variously 30–50% risk reduction). Other NSAIDs also appear to be protective. Dietary calcium supplements and vitamin D also are associated with a reduced risk. Hormone replacement therapy also seems to be protective (EBM 16.4).

Smoking, alcohol and exercise

Smoking and alcohol excess are risk factors for men but women appear not to be subject to the excess risk. An association between lack of physical exercise and colorectal cancer has been observed.

Inflammatory bowel disease

Colorectal cancer risk associated with IBD was discussed earlier.

Genetic susceptibility

Genetic susceptibility contributes 35% to the overall incidence of colorectal cancer. This genetic component ranges from an ill-defined increased risk in individuals with a positive family history, to well-defined autosomal dominant genetic traits in which the responsible genes have been identified and mutations characterised. Three broad categories of genetic susceptibility trait have been defined at the clinical and/or molecular level: autosomal dominant hereditary colorectal cancer susceptibility syndromes; recessive inheritance; common genetic inheritance.

Autosomal polyposis syndromes (FAP, PJS, JPS, PPAP) and the recessive disorder, MAP, were described earlier. HNPCC (Lynch syndrome) is the most common autosomal dominant cancer syndrome, accounting for 3–5% of all colorectal cancer cases. It is associated with small numbers of adenomas, but the lifetime risk of colorectal cancer is high (70% in males, 35% in females). There is also an elevated risk of other malignancies, including endometrial, gastric, ovarian, upper urinary tract and small intestinal. Lynch syndrome is of major clinical relevance because it is a relatively common definable genetic cause of colorectal cancer and gene carriers can be identified by DNA analysis of blood samples. Mutation analysis allows targeting of those at risk for colonoscopic screening and adenoma removal, and this has been shown to be an effective cancer control measure.

Inactivating mutations in one of the genes that participate in DNA mismatch repair is responsible: *MSH2*, *MLH1*, *MSH6* or *PMS2*. Around 90% of large dominant HNPCC families from research studies have identifiable mutations. In clinical genetics practice, however, only 30% of selected families have mutations in one of the genes responsible. Overall, causative mutations have been identified in ~3% of all colorectal cancer cases, but patients who develop colorectal cancer at an early age are more likely to have developed the disease because of an underlying DNA mismatch repair gene defect; 1 in 4 of patients aged <40 years and 1 in 20 aged <55 years at diagnosis of colorectal cancer carry a mutation, irrespective of family history.

Common genetic variance has been shown to contribute to colorectal cancer through genome-wide analysis. Over 40 common genetic variants have been identified with allele frequencies in the general population in the range 10–50%. Many of the variants are in genes encoding proteins participating in cellular growth such as SMAD and TGF signalling pathways. However, the colorectal cancer risk associated with these variants is low (typically RR 1.05–1.2) and so they currently cannot be used for individual risk prediction.

Clinical features of established colorectal cancer

Intestinal symptoms are extremely common in the general population but there are no specific symptoms that discriminate cancer from benign intestinal diseases or from symptoms common in healthy individuals. Presentation may include intermittent rectal bleeding, blood mixed with mucus, altered bowel habit, iron deficiency anaemia and colicky lower abdominal pain. Tenesmus occurs in over 50% of patients with low rectal cancers. Massive lower gastrointestinal haemorrhage is rare. Abdominal wall invasion may manifest as parietal pain and occasionally leads to abscess formation. Perianal or sciatic-type pain is an ominous sign suggesting locally advanced rectal cancer. Around 15% of all patients present with obstruction and 3% have a perforation at presentation, complications which are associated with poorer stage-specific prognosis.

A full history is essential, as clinical examination is often negative. There may be signs of anaemia, and abdominal examination may reveal hepatomegaly or an abdominal mass, especially in right-sided colon cancer. There may be signs of bowel obstruction. Digital rectal examination is mandatory to detect low cancers and to assess fixity and sphincter involvement. FOB testing will not alter the decision to investigate the symptomatic patient and so is a superfluous investigation.

Population screening for colorectal cancer

Early detection of colorectal cancer by population screening in asymptomatic individuals aged 50–75 years has been shown to result in ~20% improvement in survival. The most extensively studied screening test is the FOB test using guaiac-impregnated paper (Haemoccult) but sensitivity is only 50–60%. The predictive value is around 10% for cancer and 50% for adenomas >1 cm. Specificity is the main problem with the test, as it generates large numbers of people with positive slides but no cancer. A faecal immunological test for human haemoglobin (FIT) is being adopted by many national screening programmes due to an improved specificity/sensitivity profile. Population screening using colonoscopy is widespread in the USA, but is unlikely to be implemented in other countries due to cost implications. Once-only flexible sigmoidoscopy at age 50–55 years has recently been shown to reduce colorectal cancer mortality by detecting early rectosigmoid cancers and identifying individuals prone to develop adenomas. Other screening modalities are also under assessment, including cancer-specific stool DNA testing, but these approaches are many years away from formal clinical evaluation.

Investigations

Colonoscopy is the investigation of choice (Fig. 16.31). CT colonography (Fig. 16.32) is employed in the investigation of altered bowel habit. It has similar diagnostic accuracy to colonoscopy, although diagnostic biopsy and snaring of adenomas requires

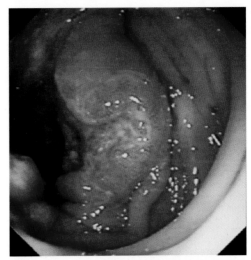

Fig. 16.31 Typical colonoscopic features of colorectal cancer.

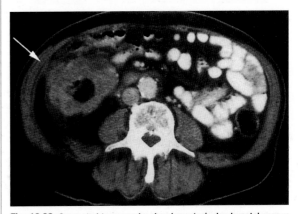

Fig. 16.32 Computed tomography showing a typical colorectal cancer with thickening, shouldering and mucosal ulceration.

subsequent colonoscopy. Barium enema (Fig. 16.33) is no longer used for diagnosis. Typical features of colorectal cancer are shouldering and mucosal destruction. In some instances diagnosis is only made at laparotomy for a perforated or obstructed viscus.

Preoperative staging

Staging is a central component of preoperative work-up, as it provides important information on prognosis, helps inform surgical strategy and indicates the need for adjuvant radiotherapy for rectal cancer and adjuvant postoperative chemotherapy. All patients with colon or rectal cancer should undergo CT of the chest, abdomen and pelvis (Fig. 16.34). Liver ultrasound and chest x-ray have now been almost totally superseded by CT. For rectal cancer, digital examination and rigid sigmoidoscopy should be undertaken to assess the degree of tumour fixity (examination under anaesthetic may be necessary). Pelvic MRI is essential to assess the degree of local invasion of rectal cancer. Endoanal ultrasound may also be useful for local staging of rectal cancer, but requires considerable experience and interpretational skill. In cases being considered for major debilitating surgery, ^{18}F-radio-labelled fluorodeoxyglucose (FDG) positron emission tomography in combination with CT (FDG-PET-CT) is indicated to detect unsuspected distant metastatic disease that may influence surgical strategy and planning.

16

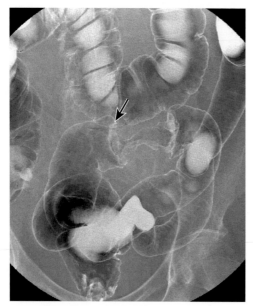

Fig. 16.33 Barium enema showing a malignant 'apple core' appearance in the sigmoid colon (arrowed), due to stenosing colorectal cancer.

Management of colorectal adenocarcinoma

Surgery

Elective colorectal resection with curative intent

The mainstay of treatment comprises resection of the primary tumour and locoregional nodes. This achieves cure in 75% of cases undergoing intended 'curative' resections. Excision of the colonic mesentery, ligation of the arterial supply at its origin, and excision of all accompanying lymph nodes achieve locoregional lymphadenectomy for the respective segment of bowel (Fig. 16.35). Resection offers cure for patients with localised disease; even for patients with lymph node metastases but no distant metastases, cure can be expected in 50% of cases with surgery alone. For rectal cancer, excision of the entire mesorectum can reduce local recurrence rates to <5%. Wherever possible, bowel continuity should be restored. In specialist hands, low rectal cancer should be treated by low anterior resection

and coloanal anastomosis. However, for low rectal cancer involving the sphincter muscle, it may be necessary to remove the anal sphincter as part of an abdominoperineal resection and fashion a permanent end colostomy. Laparoscopic colorectal resection is increasingly used and provides short-term benefits (less pain, shorter hospital stay). However, there is no definitive evidence of improved long-term outcomes over open surgery.

Rectal cancer can be excised peranally under direct vision or using transanal endoscopic microsurgery (TEM). TEM is particularly applicable to small low-lying T_1 or T_2 cancers (<3 cm) and major abdominal surgery may be avoided. However, careful staging is essential because the recurrence rate is 25–30% if there are incomplete excision margins or if the lesion was staged inaccurately. Pathology assessment may indicate the need to proceed to formal resection and mesorectal excision. Early polyp cancers removed by colonoscopic snare polypectomy may be treated without the need for formal transabdominal resection. However, where the pathology specimen of the snared polyp cancer shows poor differentiation or submucosal lymphatic or vascular invasion, or where the diathermised margin is involved, formal resection and regional lymphadenectomy are indicated. With the introduction of population colorectal cancer screening by faecal occult blood test (FOBT), this is becoming a more common scenario.

In the elective setting, the patient should be fasted having undergone full preoperative work-up to assess cardiac, respiratory and any other comorbidity; reversible risk factors for major surgery should have been addressed. Bowel preparation has been changed radically in recent years. Fluid diet is advised for 48 hours prior to surgery but mechanical bowel preparation is now avoided for the majority of resections and only a phosphate enema 2 hours prior to surgery is required for left-sided resections. Recent meta-analyses indicate that there is no benefit for mechanical bowel preparation (comprising polyethylene glycol, sodium picosulfate or phospho-soda), and it may even be harmful. However, bowel preparation does have a place for low rectal anastomoses, especially if a defunctioning ileostomy is planned. Antibiotic prophylaxis comprises perioperative broad-spectrum antibiotics (e.g., a third-generation cephalosporin, or gentamicin and amoxycillin, and metronidazole). Chemical thrombo-prophylaxis (low molecular weight fractionated heparin or calcium heparin), along with compression stockings and intraoperative intermittent pneumatic calf compression (EBM 16.5) is indicated as the risk of deep venous thrombosis and pulmonary embolism is high.

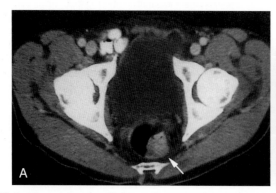
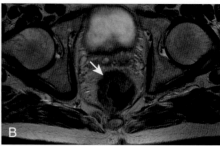

Fig. 16.34 **Rectal cancer imaging. (A)** Computed tomography features of early T_1 cancer (*arrowed*), restricted to the bowel wall. **(B)** Pelvic magnetic imaging resonance showing T_3 cancer, invading through the bowel wall and into the mesorectum (*arrowed*).

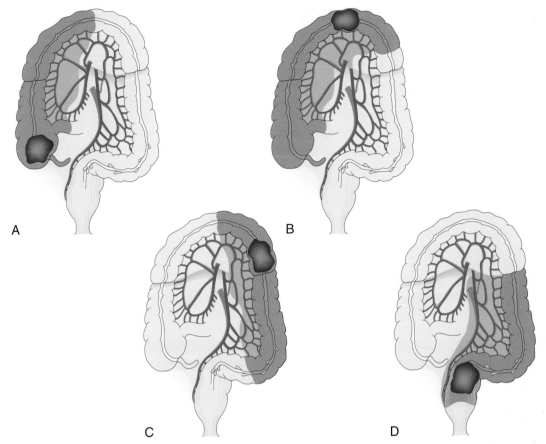

Fig. 16.35 Surgical resection for colorectal cancer arising at various locations within the large bowel. Radical tumour resection requires clearance of the primary tumour and also the arteries supplying that part of the colon. Lymphatic drainage follows the path of arterial supply, allowing a regional lymphadenectomy. **(A)** Excision of a right-sided tumour and the ileocaecal, right colic and right branch of middle colic arteries. **(B)** Tumours of transverse colon are usually treated by extended right hemicolectomy, again taking the feeding vessels at their origin from the superior mesenteric artery. **(C)** For left colonic lesions, the feeding vessels are taken. **(D)** Anterior resection is treated by high ligation of the inferior mesenteric artery.

EBM | **16.5 Preparation for surgery in patients with colorectal adenocarcinoma**

'Preoperative staging is required to guide surgery and pre-operative adjuvant radiotherapy.
Bowel preparation is not required for colorectal resection.
Compression stockings and heparin are required thromboprophylaxis for patients undergoing colorectal surgery.
Patient should be fasted prior to surgery.
Co-morbidity should be addressed wherever possible to limit perioperative mortality risk.
Perioperative antibiotic prophylaxis is essential and should cover coliform and anaerobic organisms.'

The Association of Coloproctology of Great Britain and Ireland. Guidelines for the Management of Colorectal Cancer 3rd ed; 2007. *http://www.acpgbi.org.uk/assets/documents/COLO_guides.pdf*

Güenaga KF, Matos D, Wille-Jørgensen P. Mechanical bowel preparation for elective colorectal surgery. Cochrane Database Syst Rev. 2011;(9):CD001544. DOI: 10.1002/14651858.CD001544.pub4

Scottish Intercollegiate Guideline Network. Prevention and management of venous thromboembolism. http://www.sign.ac.uk/pdf/sign122.pdf

Wille-Jørgensen P, Rasmussen MS, Andersen BR, Borly L. Heparins and mechanical methods for thromboprophylaxis in colorectal surgery. Cochrane Database Syst Rev. 2004;(1): CD001217. DOI: 10.1002/14651858.CD001217

Scottish Intercollegiate Guideline Network. Antibiotic prophylaxis in surgery. http://www.sign.ac.uk/pdf/sign104.pdf

Nelson RL, Glenny AM, Song F. Antimicrobial prophylaxis for colorectal surgery. Cochrane Database Syst Rev. 2009;(1):CD001181. DOI: 10.1002/14651858. CD001181.pub3.

Emergency colorectal resection

In cases of perforation or obstruction of colorectal cancer, there is a substantially increased risk of perioperative mortality. The patient should be resuscitated before laparotomy is undertaken. For obstructed right-sided colon cancer, right hemicolectomy is the operation of choice. An ileotransverse anastomosis can be safely performed, as the ileum has an excellent blood supply and the distal colon is not obstructed. Treatment of obstructed left colon cancer is best achieved by a one-stage resection with anastomosis whenever possible. Measures that may be employed to reduce the risk of anastomotic leakage in such cases include on-table colonic lavage to remove upstream faecal residue. Resection of the entire colon and ileorectal anastomosis avoids a colo-colic anastomosis and any synchronous tumour. Patients with faecal peritonitis secondary to perforation usually require resection with the creation of an end colostomy (Hartmann's procedure). If contamination is minimal, the surgeon may carry out a resection and primary anastomosis. As in the elective setting, surgery should be covered with perioperative antibiotics and deep venous thrombosis prophylaxis.

Pathology and staging

Macroscopically, colorectal cancer may be polypoidal, ulcerating or stenosing (Fig. 16.36). Two-thirds are ulcerating and a typical

16

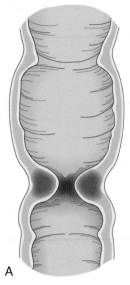
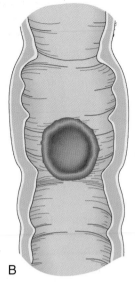
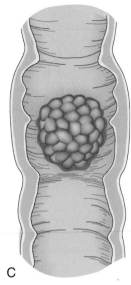

Fig. 16.36 Macroscopic characteristics of colorectal cancer. **(A)** Stenosing. **(B)** Ulcerating. **(C)** Polypoidal.

Table 16.7 Dukes' staging for colorectal cancer

Dukes' stage	Description	Proportion of colorectal cancers (%)
A	Spread into, but not beyond, muscularis propria	10
B	Spread through full thickness of bowel wall	30
C	Spread to involve lymph nodes	30
D[a]	Distant metastases	20

[a]There is formally no D stage in Dukes' staging; this is a misnomer, as Dukes' staging refers only to degree of local invasion and to lymphatic spread. However, the term is widely used in clinical practice.

Table 16.8 TNM staging of colorectal cancer

T (Tumour)

- T_x — Primary tumour cannot be assessed
- Tis — Carcinoma in situ
- T_1 — Cancer invades submucosa
- T_2 — Cancer invades into muscularis propria
- T_3 — Cancer invades through muscularis propria and into subserosa or adjacent nonperitonealised tissues
- T_4 — Cancer perforates the visceral peritoneum or directly invades adjacent organs

N (Node)

- N_x — The regional lymph nodes cannot be assessed
- N_0 — No regional lymph nodes involved
- N_1 — Metastases in 1–3 pericolic or perirectal lymph nodes
- N_2 — Metastases in 4 or more pericolic or perirectal lymph nodes
- N_3 — Metastases in lymph node along the course of a major named blood vessel

M (Metastases)

- M_x — The presence of distant metastases cannot be assessed
- M_0 — No distant metastases
- M_1 — Distant metastases

lesion has raised everted edges, a slough covered floor and indurated base. Tumours of the caecum tend to be large exophytic growths. Tumour differentiation may be classified as good, moderate or poor. Around 10–20% of tumours have mucinous histology and this tumour type has a poor prognosis. There is an increasing proportion of proximal tumours in the UK due to an ageing population and as right-sided colon cancer is more common in the elderly.

Colorectal cancer may spread by lymphatic invasion, via the portal blood to the liver and/or by transperitoneal seeding. Invasion of lymphatics results in regional lymph node involvement. Very low rectal tumours may also involve the inguinal nodes. Systemic metastases may occur in the later stages of the disease. Tumour staging systems include Dukes' and TNM staging (Tables 16.7 and 16.8). TNM stages can be grouped using the American Joint Committee on Cancer (AJCC) system (Table 16.9). Pathological staging has important implications for prognosis and also for directing clinical management (EBM 16.6). Staging information informs both predicted survival outcome and also decision-making on whether adjuvant chemotherapy is indicated.

Adjuvant therapy

Radiotherapy

Adjuvant preoperative radiotherapy has an important place in the management of rectal cancer, and so preoperative staging of rectal cancer is essential in order to plan optimal management. Radiotherapy has been shown to reduce local recurrence rates but there is no effect on overall survival (EBM 16.6). Many patients will be cured by surgery alone and so most UK specialist centres offer selective preoperative radiotherapy for those at increased risk of local recurrence, because there is significant morbidity associated with pelvic irradiation. Risk factors for recurrence include a low tumour, bulky fixed lesion, anterior lesion, evidence of T_3 or T_4 stage and/or involved lymph nodes

Table 16.9 American joint committee on cancer (AJCC) stage groupings and equivalence with Dukes' staging

AJCC	TNM		Dukes
I	$T_1N_0M_0$ or $T_2N_0M_0$	Spread into submucosa or just into muscularis propria. No lymph node or distant spread	A
IIA	$T_3N_0M_0$	Spread through bowel wall into outermost layers. No lymph node or distant spread	B
IIB	$T_4N_0M_0$	Spread through bowel wall into other tissues or organs. No lymph node or distant spread	B
IIIA	$T_{1-2}N_1M_0$	Spread into submucosa or just into muscularis propria. Spread to ≤ 3 nearby lymph nodes but no distant spread	C
IIIB	$T_{3-4}N_1M_0$	Spread through bowel wall into other tissues or organs. Spread to ≤ 3 nearby lymph nodes but no distant spread	C
IIIC	Any T N_2M_0	Any T stage and spread ≥ 4 lymph nodes but no distant spread	C
IV	Any T Any N M1	Any T and N stage but distant spread (e.g., liver, lung, peritoneum)	D[a]

[a]There is formally no D stage in Dukes' staging; this is a misnomer, as Dukes' staging refers only to degree of local invasion and to lymphatic spread. However, the term is widely used in clinical practice.

on imaging. Either a 5-day short-course regimen of 45 Gy daily or a long-course regimen of 52 Gy given weekly over 3 months is administered. The former is reserved for patients with operable but tethered tumours or very low or anterior tumours, or if extrarectal spread is evident. Fixed, inoperable tumours are best dealt with by radical radiotherapy over 3 months, and this may be combined with chemotherapy (capecitabine or 5-fluorouracil [5-FU]). Postoperative radiotherapy results in poor bowel function and may damage the small intestine, and hence the importance of preoperative staging to guide administration of radiotherapy before surgery whenever possible. Trials of radiotherapy alone for rectal cancer, without resection, have yet to establish the place of this approach.

Adjuvant chemotherapy

Systemic adjuvant chemotherapy using 5-FU alone or in combination with other agents has been shown to improve survival for Dukes' C colorectal cancer after surgical resection (EBM 16.6). Intravenous 5-FU regimens have largely been replaced by the less toxic oral agent capecitabine, targeting the same pathway through inhibition of thymidylate synthase. There is an overall 30% improvement in survival for patients with Dukes' C tumours who receive chemotherapy, equating with an 11% absolute improvement in survival for that group and a 6% overall improvement in survival for patients with colorectal cancer. In the UK, it is now routine practice to offer adjuvant chemotherapy (capecitabine with oxaliplatin as first line therapy) to all patients with stage C cancers who do not have significant comorbidity, particularly cardiovascular disease. Adjuvant chemotherapy for Dukes' B tumours is restricted to poor prognosis lesions (poor differentiation, venous or lymphatic invasion). Capecitabine (or 5-FU) chemotherapy is considered a conventional 'first line'

chemotherapeutic regimen for colorectal cancer. Other newer agents, such as cetuximab (monoclonal antibody to epidermal growth factor receptor) have been shown to be ineffective in tumours with Kras or Braf mutations. Hence, Kras/Braf mutation analysis is required to identify patients with tumours that might respond to cetuximab therapy. Other agents such as temozolomide, alone or in combination with other agents, are also used in relapsed disease. Although irinotecan (CPT-11) showed initial promise, many negative trials indicate the agent has a very limited place in the management of colorectal cancer.

EBM **16.6 Improving postoperative survival rates in colorectal adenocarcinoma**

'Improved surgical and anaesthetic management has had a major impact on overall survival. Preoperative adjuvant radiotherapy reduces local recurrence rates, but not overall survival.
Postoperative adjuvant chemotherapy improves survival by 30% for stage III tumours and 2% for stage II tumours. Postoperative intensive follow-up is associated with a 9% survival improvement by identifying those with surgically salvageable relapse.'

The Association of Coloproctology of Great Britain and Ireland. Guidelines for the Management of Colorectal Cancer, 3rd ed.; 2007. http://www.acpgbi.org.uk/assets/documents/COLO_guides.pdf
Scottish Intercollegiate Guideline Network (and update). Management of colorectal cancer. Guideline No 67. http://www.sign.ac.uk/guidelines/fulltext/67/index.html
Wong RKS et al. Pre-operative radiotherapy and curative surgery for the management of localised rectal carcinoma. Cochrane Database Syst Rev. 2007;(2):CD002102. DOI: 10.1002/14651858.CD002102.pub2
Midgley R, Kerr DJ. Adjuvant chemotherapy for stage II colorectal cancer: the time is right! Nat Clin Pract Oncol. 2005;2:364–9. Review. PubMed PMID: 16075796.
Gill S et al. Pooled analysis of fluorouracil-based adjuvant chemotherapy for stage II and III colon cancer: who benefits and by how much? J Clin Oncol. 2004;22:1797–806. Epub 2004 Apr 5. PubMed PMID: 15067028.

Palliative therapy

In addition to resection with curative intent, surgery can provide valuable palliation for patients with local disease relapse, hepatic or other distant metastases. This is achieved through improving symptoms or by averting distressing features of advanced local disease. In some instances, diversion of the faecal stream through a defunctioning colostomy or ileostomy may be all that is feasible. Wherever possible it is preferable to resect the tumour. Hence, the vast majority of patients undergo surgical resection, whether curative or palliative. In a small number of cases with poor functional status and/or extensive metastatic load and in whom surgical resection is relatively contraindicated, combined radiological and colonoscopic placement of an *intraluminal expanding stent* will palliate an obstructing colonic cancer.

Radiotherapy has an important role in palliation of locally advanced irresectable rectal cancer and can control pain, mucus discharge, disordered bowel habit, bleeding and faecal incontinence. It also has a value in palliation of rectal cancer recurrence and in alleviating bone pain from metastases. It may rarely be used to palliate locally invasive colonic cancer invading the abdominal wall, but this approach is restricted because the fields are difficult to define and damage to adjacent bowel is likely.

Palliative chemotherapy is used extensively to treat symptoms of disseminated disease, and to control disease progression and extend survival. This is especially the case with the introduction of oral capecitabine. Median life expectancy from diagnosis of unresectable hepatic metastases is approximately 12–14 months.

16

Prognosis

Overall 1-year and 5-survival is 75% and 57%, respectively, having improved by over 20% in both males and females in the last 10 years. The marked improvement in survival from colorectal cancer is due to a combination of earlier diagnosis across all stages, improved perioperative anaesthetic and surgical management, and improved adjuvant therapies, especially chemotherapy. However, overall prognosis is even better for patients who have no evidence of metastases on preoperative staging tests and who have undergone a resection with curative intent. This underscores the importance of preoperative staging when performing radical surgery. The 5-year survival by Dukes' stage is 90–95% for Dukes' stage A, 65–75% for Dukes' stage B and 40–50% for Dukes' stage C. Only a minority of patients with unresectable liver or lung metastases will survive to 5 years and most die within 2 years. Operative mortality is low (~3%) for elective resections but is 18% in patients requiring emergency surgery for complications such as obstruction and perforation, emphasising the importance of early detection and timely surgery. Patients with isolated hepatic metastases may be candidates for hepatic resection with a view to cure (see Chapter 14), and there is significant evidence for long-term survival benefit in selected patients.

16.5 Summary

Colorectal cancer

- Colorectal adenocarcinoma is the most common gastrointestinal malignancy, with 45,000 cases per annum in the UK
- It is second only to lung cancer as a cause of cancer death in developed countries, accounting for 15% of all cancers in males and 12% in females, with a 6% lifetime risk
- 2–3% of patients present with synchronous tumours, and a further ~3% develop metachronous tumours
- Risk factors include male gender, increasing age, family history of an affected relative, 'Westernised' diet, inflammatory bowel disease and preexisting adenomatous polyps
- Genes have been identified for a number of autosomal dominant colorectal cancer predisposition syndromes, accounting for ~3% of all cases
- Around 35% of the aetiology of colorectal cancer is attributable to genetic factors and a number of common genetic variants have recently been identified, offering future potential for genetic profiling
- Two-thirds of all large bowel cancers occur in the rectum and sigmoid colon, and the most common clinical features are alteration in bowel habit and the passage of blood per rectum
- Diagnosis involves CT colonography, colonoscopy and biopsy, Preoperative staging involves CT, MRI and PET-CT
- Surgery is the mainstay of treatment, involving radical local clearance combined with regional lymphadenectomy
- Adjuvant therapy options include preoperative radiotherapy for rectal cancer and postoperative chemotherapy
- Presymptomatic diagnosis may be achieved by population screening using faecal occult blood testing or by surveillance colonoscopy in high-risk groups
- Overall 5-year survival is 57%. Staging systems provide useful prognosis to guide therapy and inform patients of expected outcome.

Other malignant tumours of the large intestine

Squamous cancer of the large bowel

These poor-prognosis tumours are not metastatic anal carcinomas, but arise in the caecum and proximal colon from an area of squamous metaplasia in long-standing ulcerative colitis. In the absence of chronic inflammation, an adenosquamous pattern may be seen.

Carcinoid tumour of the large bowel

Large bowel carcinoid tumours are very rare, but benign lesions may be found incidentally during rectal examination as solitary, spherical, hard, sessile, yellowish submucosal nodules. Malignant carcinoid tumours of the colon are highly malignant and may give rise to the carcinoid syndrome if liver metastases are present (60% present with metastases at diagnosis).

Lymphoma

Primary lymphomas usually arise in the rectum or caecum but are occasionally multicentric. Secondary involvement of the large bowel in generalised nodal disease is more common. CT colonography shows a long rigid segment with intramural thickening. The diagnosis is established by endoscopic or operative biopsy. Primary lymphomas are treated by resection, followed by chemotherapy and radiotherapy. Secondary malignant lymphoma and malignant lymphomatous polyposis are treated by systemic chemotherapy and targeted radiotherapy.

Gastrointestinal stromal tumours (including leiomyosarcoma)

These tumours are rare in the large bowel and were discussed earlier with respect to the small bowel. They arise from the muscle of the bowel wall, most usually the rectum, and are usually diagnosed by digital examination or by sigmoidoscopy. There is a spectrum from benign to malignant and the tumours are often impossible to distinguish clinically; resection is therefore advisable. Metastases occur via the bloodstream to the liver and lungs.

Farhat Din

17

The anorectum

Chapter contents

Introduction 283

Applied surgical anatomy 283

Anorectal disorders 285

Miscellaneous benign perianal lumps 292

Anal cancer 293

Rectal prolapse 294

Anal incontinence 296

Pruritus ani 297

Pilonidal disease 297

Introduction

Anorectal complaints are extremely common; 2–3% of the population have anorectal symptoms at any given time. It is important to differentiate patients who merit specialist assessment from those who can be treated symptomatically in the first instance. Symptoms are often ignored or hidden by the patient from relatives and doctors. It is important that perianal symptoms are elicited without embarrassment and, because these overlap with conditions affecting the large bowel, a full gastrointestinal history is essential.

Applied surgical anatomy

The anus enables the passage of stool or flatus (when socially convenient) but is also essential in maintaining continence to gas, fluid and solid at almost all other times in healthy individuals.

Anal musculature and innervation

The anal canal is 3–4 cm long in males and slightly shorter in females. It consists of two concentric muscle layers known as the internal and external sphincters (Fig. 17.1). The internal sphincter is a condensation of the circular smooth muscle of the rectum and is a continuation of the circular muscle of the gastrointestinal (GI) tract. It is controlled by the autonomic nervous system with fibres from the pelvic sympathetic nerves, the lower lumbar ganglia and the preaortic/inferior mesenteric plexus. Parasympathetic fibres arise from the sacral plexus. The smooth muscle of the internal sphincter maintains tone and contributes to resting pressure within the anal canal, playing an important role in maintaining continence. The longitudinal muscle of the gut ends at the anus as a series of fibrous bands that radiate to the perianal skin, and is of little consequence to perianal disease. The striated muscle of the external sphincter is under voluntary control, being innervated bilaterally by the internal pudendal nerves and the fourth branch of the sacral plexus. The circular muscle tube of the external sphincter blends with the lower part of the levator ani, known as the puborectalis sling (Fig. 17.2). The puborectalis fibres of the levator ani originate from the posterior aspect of the pubic symphysis and pass posteriorly to join the external sphincter. The levator ani muscles themselves are also important in maintaining the relationship of the anus and rectum during defaecation.

Anal canal epithelium

The cell type of the anal canal epithelium determines why certain diseases, such as tumours and viral infections, affect only particular levels of the canal. The anal canal epithelium is specialised and contains three distinct zones. The external zone (from dentate line to anal verge) is keratinised, stratified squamous epithelium. The short modified anal transitional zone of nonkeratinised squamous epithelium lies immediately proximal to the dentate line, separated from the columnar epithelial of the anal canal but continuous with the rectal epithelium. The anal valves are crescentic mucosal folds that form a serrated or dentate line on the luminal aspect of the mid-anal canal (Fig. 17.3). The dentate line represents the line of fusion between the endoderm of the embryonic hindgut and the ectoderm of the anal pit. Thus, the epithelium is innervated by the autonomic nervous system and is insensate with respect to somatic sensation. The canal lining below the dentate line is innervated by the peripheral nervous system and pathology affecting this area, such as abscess, anal fissure or tumour, cause anal pain.

The composition of the epithelium of the anorectum determines the type of tumour that affects the region. Thus, squamous cell carcinoma of the anal canal arises from the epithelium below the dentate line or in the transitional zone of nonkeratinised

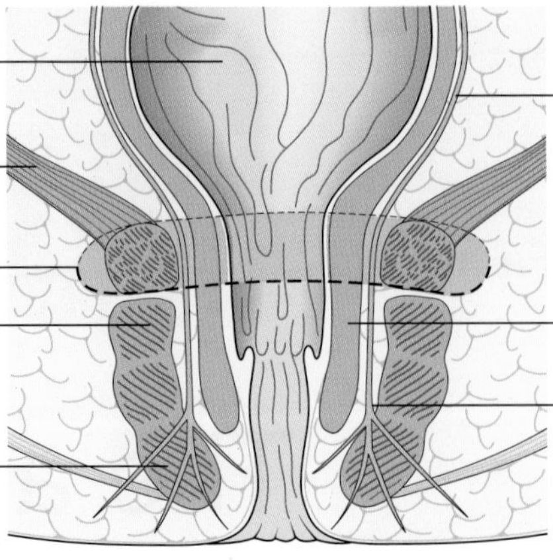
Rectum
Levator ani
Anorectal ring
Puborectalis
External sphincter
Longitudinal muscle of rectal wall
Internal sphincter
Longitudinal intersphincteric muscle

Fig. 17.1 Musculature of the anorectum.

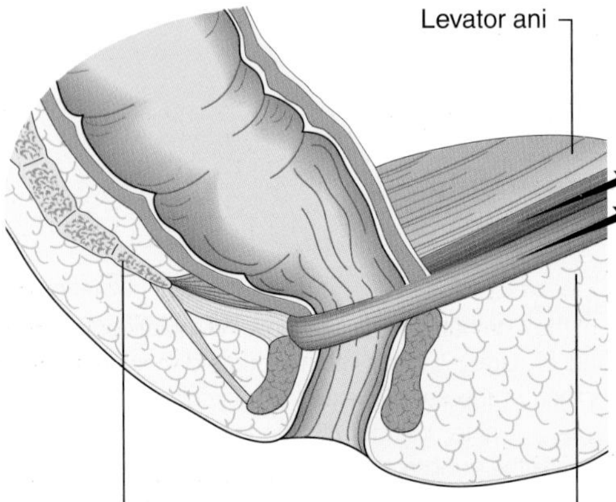
Levator ani
Coccyx
Puborectalis sling

Fig. 17.2 The puborectalis sling establishing the anorectal angle.

squamous epithelium. Because the canal above the anal transition zone contains columnar glandular epithelium, tumours of the upper anal canal are adenocarcinoma; they are best considered as a low rectal cancer and treated accordingly.

There are 4–8 specialised anal glands located within the substance of the internal sphincter or in the space between the internal and external sphincters at the level of the mid-anal canal; these glands have ducts that open directly on to the dentate line (Fig. 17.4). The ducts from these glands open into the mucosal folds at the dentate line. The function of the anal glands is mucus secretion which lubricates and protects the delicate anal transition zone epithelium. The glands are clinically relevant as they are the source of most perianal abscesses and fistula-in-ano.

The anal (haemorrhoidal) cushions

Although the internal and external sphincters, the puborectalis sling and anorectal angle play important roles in maintaining anal continence, fine control is aided by the submucosal anal 'cushions' above the dentate line. The anal cushions are specialised vascular structures comprising fibroconnective tissue containing arteriovenous communications, fed by the terminal branches of the superior rectal artery with inconstant anastomoses to the middle and inferior rectal arteries. There are usually three anal cushions corresponding to the three terminal branches of the artery (left, right posterior and right anterior, corresponding with the 3, 7 and 11 o'clock positions when the patient is in the lithotomy position). These positions determine the position of haemorrhoids, which are caused by distension and prolapse of the anal cushions. Haemorrhoids are not 'varicose veins' of the anal canal,

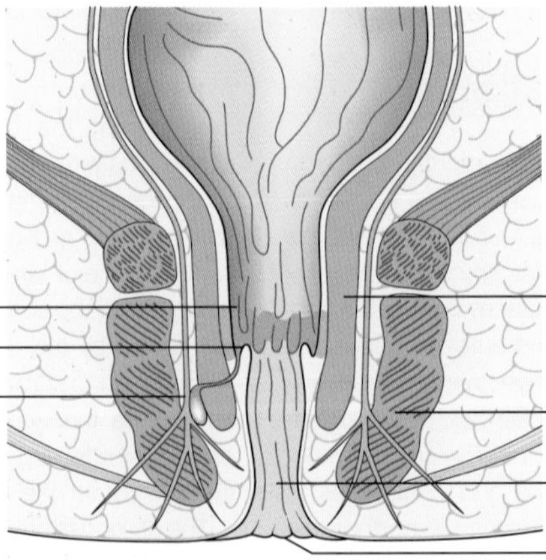
Anal transition line
Pectinate line
Anal gland and duct
Internal sphincter
External sphincter
'Pecten'
Anal verge

Fig. 17.3 The lining of the anorectal canal.

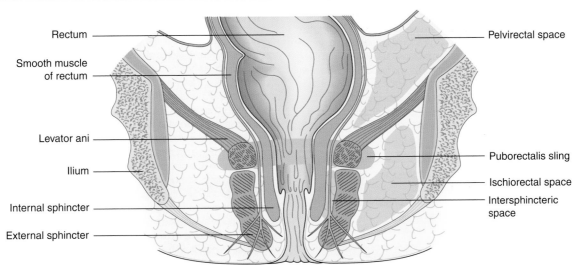

Rectum

Smooth muscle of rectum

Levator ani

Ilium

Internal sphincter

External sphincter

Pelvirectal space

Puborectalis sling

Ischiorectal space

Intersphincteric space

Fig. 17.4 Principal anorectal spaces in relation to the anal sphincters and rectum.

but prolapse of the specialised anal cushions; indeed, haemorrhoids are uncommon in patients with portal hypertension, despite the fact that the anal canal represents a potential portosystemic anastomosis.

17.1 Summary

Factors maintaining anal continence

- Intact anorectal and pelvic floor sensation
- Intact anal sphincters and levator ani
- Preservation of the anorectal angle
- The bulk provided by the anal haemorrhoidal 'cushions'.

Lymphatic drainage of the anal canal

Lymphatic drainage of the anus below the dentate line is to the inguinal lymph nodes. This contrasts with the lower rectum where lymphatic drainage passes superiorly through the mesorectum to follow the superior rectal artery and on to the inferior mesenteric and aortic chains. There are also some lymphatic channels that follow the course of the middle rectal arteries to drain to the nodes around the internal iliac arteries. This anatomical distinction between the lymphatic drainage of the anus and the rectum has important implications for the management of tumours of the rectum and anus. Anal cancer frequently metastasises to inguinal lymph nodes, whereas rectal cancer metastasises upwards to the mesorectum and onwards to the paraaortic chain. Thus, anal squamous cancer radiotherapy fields incorporate the inguinal nodes.

17.2 Summary

Causes of severe acute anal pain

- Perianal abscess
- Intersphincteric abscess
- Anal fissure
- Thrombosed haemorrhoids
- Perianal haematoma
- Anorectal cancer.

Anorectal disorders

Haemorrhoids

Haemorrhoids (colloquially known as piles) are very common; however, the aetiology remains obscure. Almost all haemorrhoids are primary, with only a tiny proportion due to other factors, such as a cancer in the distal rectum.

Definition

Haemorrhoids are enlarged, prolapsed anal cushions arising from arteriovenous communications within connective tissues

Pathogenesis

The pathophysiology involves degeneration of the supporting fibroelastic tissue and smooth muscle, with enlargement of anal cushions and protrusion at the 3, 7 and 11 o'clock positions. As the cushions prolapse, there is keratinisation and hypertrophy of the overlying anal transitional zone and eventually prolapse of the columnar epithelial component in later stages.

Risk factors

The underlying cause of the stretching of the fibroelastic support is unknown. Constipation and straining at stool are common features. These may be aggravated by a high anal sphincter pressure, with further entrapment of prolapsed piles. Haemorrhoids during pregnancy are very common and are probably due to hormonal effects inducing connective tissue laxity, combined with constipation and pressure from the baby's head. Sitting on the toilet for long periods, such as when reading, is also held to be an associated aetiological factor. However, as with other presumed aetiological factors, there is no real evidence for cause and effect.

Clinical features

Bleeding and prolapse are the cardinal features and may occur in isolation or together. The bleeding is typically intermittent 'outlet-type' bleeding, separate from the stool and evident in the pan or only on wiping. There may also be aching or dragging discomfort

17

on defaecation, and patients may self-reduce their piles to obtain relief after each bowel motion. Severe constant pain is unusual and in such cases other pathology should be suspected. In the later stages, haemorrhoids remain prolapsed at all times and there is staining of the underwear with mucus and faecal fluid. However, it is very unusual for patients to present with incontinence of solid faeces and a sphincter defect should be suspected in such cases. In cases of constant prolapse, there is often pruritus due to the discharge, with irritation of the perianal skin.

Classification

- *First-degree* piles are those that bleed, are visible on proctoscopy but do not prolapse.
- *Second-degree* piles are those that prolapse during defaecation but reduce spontaneously.
- *Third-degree* piles are prolapsed constantly but can be reduced manually (Fig. 17.5).
- *Fourth-degree* piles are irreducibly prolapsed.

Key point: Although staged according to the degree of prolapse, it is important to note that this classification is not necessarily proportional to symptoms and distress.

Acute presentation

Patients may present as an emergency with a complication of haemorrhoids.

1. *Thrombosis:* Prolapsing haemorrhoids may acutely thrombose and there is associated marked sphincter spasm. Thrombosed haemorrhoids are large, swollen and irreducible. They may be dark blue or even black due to necrosis and submucosal haemorrhage, and diagnosis is easily made on inspection. Acute pain and tenderness usually render rectal examination impossible.
2. *Major haemorrhage:* Haemorrhoids rarely cause massive lower GI haemorrhage but should be excluded in patients presenting with a major fresh rectal bleed resulting in significant hypovolaemia and anaemia.

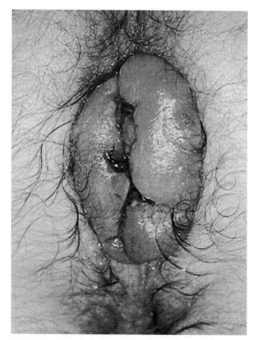

Fig. 17.5 Third-degree haemorrhoids.

History

Haemorrhoids may occur at the same time as more serious pathology. Because the symptoms of piles and colorectal cancer can be very similar, careful history is essential to guide clinical assessment and investigation. However, piles are very common and so it is important to avoid indiscriminate large bowel investigation for such a common complaint as rectal bleeding. 'Outlet-type' bleeding comprises fresh red blood, dripping in the pan, on wiping and separate from the bowel motion. If the bleeding is outlet type, there is no alteration in bowel habit and the patient is under 50 years of age, then the chance of rectal cancer is remote. In such cases, digital rectal examination, combined with proctoscopy and rigid sigmoidoscopy, should secure the diagnosis. If piles are confirmed, then management can be instigated without recourse to imaging the rest of the colon by colonoscopy. Notably, prescriptions for topical haemorrhoidal creams increase in the year before rectal cancer is diagnosed. Hence, if no demonstrable cause of rectal bleeding is identified on examination or in older patients (>50 years) with a change of bowel habit, further colonic investigation is essential.

Examination

Following abdominal examination in the supine position, perianal examination should be performed in the left lateral position with a chaperone (all patients). Inspection may reveal prolapsed piles, associated anal skin tags or evidence of perianal excoriation from scratching. Digital rectal examination is essential to assess sphincter tone and to exclude other anal conditions. First- or second-degree piles are rarely palpable, as they compress on pressure, and diagnosis is made by proctoscopy. The proctoscope should be gently inserted to the hilt and withdrawn; bulging haemorrhoids will be visible at right anterior, right posterior and left lateral positions. Rigid sigmoidoscopy should be performed to exclude other rectal pathology.

Management

Reassurance after appropriate evaluation is all that many patients require. Specific treatment is not required for most cases, as symptoms are minor and intermittent. A high-fibre diet with plenty of vegetables is commonly recommended, although there is no good evidence that this actually provides any benefit at all. However, if constipation is a feature, it does seem reasonable advice; in some cases, bulk laxatives or stool softeners may be indicated. Patients often self-medicate with proprietary ointments containing local anaesthetic. There is no good evidence from controlled trials that these are effective, but if patients find that they help, then it seems reasonable to advise their intermittent use.

Nonoperative approaches

Nonoperative haemorrhoid management approaches aim to cause fibrosis and shrinkage of the protruding haemorrhoidal cushion to prevent bleeding and prolapse. Current outpatient clinic approaches include application of small rubber bands to strangulate the pile (using a special Barron's bander) or heat application by infrared photocoagulation. Submucosal injection of a sclerosant (e.g., 5% phenol in almond oil) has largely been abandoned due to potential severe side-effects (intraprostatic injection). There is no strong evidence that any of these approaches is much better than doing nothing at all. In the long term, the symptoms of untreated piles tend to wax and wane, and symptom recurrence after any of these procedures is much the same as without any treatment. Rubber band ligation may be the most

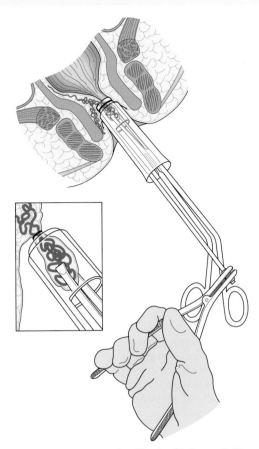

Fig. 17.6 Application of Barron's rubber band to haemorrhoids.

effective in the short term but does carry risks of bleeding and pain postprocedure (Fig. 17.6). Where there is a significant cutaneous component to the piles, any of the outpatient treatments is likely to be painful because of the cutaneous nerve supply, and is also unlikely to succeed. In these circumstances, the decision should be to do nothing but reassure the patient, or to offer an operation.

Operative approaches

Standard haemorrhoidectomy

The principle of haemorrhoidectomy involves total removal of the haemorrhoidal mass and securing of haemostasis of the feeding vessel. The wound can be left open (Milligan–Morgan) or can be closed (Ferguson), but there are rarely problems with healing or infection. In some cases, there are secondary haemorrhoids between the main right anterior, right posterior and left lateral positions, and these are also removed as part of the operation.

Stapled haemorrhoidectomy/haemorrhoidopexy/anopexy

This technique, using a circular stapler, aims to divide the mucosa and haemorrhoidal cushions above the dentate line to transect the feeding vessels and hitch-up the stretched supporting fibroelastic tissue, rather than whole haemorrhoidal mass excision in the standard haemorrhoidectomy. Stapled haemorrhoidopexy is now used extensively for symptomatic second-degree and the majority of third- and fourth-degree piles (EBM 17.1). With all surgical approaches to treating piles, it is important to consider that the haemorrhoidal cushions contribute to fine control of continence. Hence, an element of anal

EBM 17.1 Haemorrhoids

'Non-operative treatment is preferable wherever possible but surgery may be required for a small proportion of cases. Open haemorrhoidectomy is superior to stapled haemorrhoidectomy both in terms of symptom control and recurrence; rubber band ligation has similar efficacy to haemorrhoidectomy.'

Acheson AG, Scholefield JH. Management of haemorrhoids. BMJ. 2008;336:380–3.; Aly EH. Stapled haemorrhoidopexy: is it time to move on? Ann R Coll Surg Engl. 2015;97:490–3.; Hollingshead J, Phillips R. Haemorrhoids: modern diagnosis and treatment. Postgrad Med J. 2016;92:4–8.; Lumb KJ, Colquhoun PH, Malthaner R, Jayaraman S. Stapled versus conventional surgery for hemorrhoids. Cochrane Database Syst Rev. 2006;(4):CD005393.; Simillis C, Thoukididou S, Slesser A, et al. Systematic review and network meta-analysis comparing clinical outcomes and effectiveness of surgical treatments for haemorrhoids. Br J Surg. 2015;102:1603–18.

incontinence can be one of the long-term sequelae of any haemorrhoidopexy. Surgery should not be considered lightly. Staple line bleeding is the most important early complication requiring intervention to control bleeding vessels. Pain can occur if the staple line involves the sensitive anal mucosa. However, the instrument is expensive and open haemorrhoidectomy remains a good option when indicated.

Haemorrhoidal artery ligation operation (HALO)

This operation involves suture ligating the feeding blood vessels to the haemorrhoid with (or without) the aid of a Doppler ultrasound probe to identify the vessels. Although the haemorrhoidal mass is not excised, the operation may be combined with procedures aimed at reducing associated prolapsed tissue (rectoanal repair, mucopexy). A recent meta-analysis comparing clinical outcomes and effectiveness of surgical treatments for haemorrhoids revealed that traditional haemorrhoidectomy had greater complications and lengthier recovery, but less recurrences. HALO and stapled haemorrhoidectomies were associated with less pain and faster recovery, but higher recurrence rates. Emerging data suggest that the stapled technique is associated with serious complications perhaps heralding a retreat from this operation. As with any operation informed consent and discussion with the patient is essential.

 17.3 Summary

Haemorrhoids

Haemorrhoids are common and best treated conservatively
Classification:
• First-degree: visible in the lumen on proctoscopy but do not prolapse
• Second-degree: prolapse on defaecation but return spontaneously
• Third-degree: remain prolapsed but can be replaced digitally
• Fourth-degree: long-standing prolapse and cannot be replaced in the anal canal

Symptoms:
• Outlet-type bleeding, prolapse, mucous discharge, discomfort and thrombosis

Treatment:
• First-degree: advice on avoiding constipation and straining
• Second-degree: conservative management, banding, haemorrhoidectomy
• Third-degree: if symptomatic, haemorrhoidectomy
• Fourth-degree: thrombosed piles are usually treated conservatively in the first instance; interval haemorrhoidectomy may not be required.

Fissure-in-ano

Fissure-in-ano is common and usually affects people in their twenties and thirties, with a slight male preponderance. Fissures are most frequently observed in the posterior midline of the anal canal. Anterior fissures may occur in women following childbirth; they are rarely seen in males.

Definition

An anal fissure is a linear ulcer below the dentate line, often exposing the internal sphincter at its base, affecting the anal canal from the anal transition zone to the anal verge (Fig. 17.7). There is often minimal granulation tissue in the ulcer base. Failed attempts at healing may lead to a skin tag, or 'sentinel pile', at the lowermost extent of the fissure. At the proximal extent of the fissure there may be a hypertrophied anal papilla. Incomplete fissure healing, where mucosa bridges the fissure edges, may result in a low perianal fistula that can present years later.

Pathogenesis

A fissure develops when the anal mucosa is excessively stretched or traumatised. The pathophysiology involves ischaemia in the base of the ulcer, associated with marked anal spasm and a significantly raised resting anal pressure. Successive bowel motions provoke further trauma, pain and anal spasm, resulting in a vicious circle of pain and sphincter spasm leading to further anal mucosa trauma during defaecation. Fissures may be acute and settle spontaneously. Chronic anal fissure is defined as an ulcer that has been present for at least 6 weeks.

Aetiology

Most fissures are idiopathic. Recurrent, multiple or unusually extensive fissures affecting areas other than the midline should raise the suspicion of Crohn's disease, which can occasionally present with anal fissure as the sole initial complaint. Occasionally, anal fissure may be associated with ulcerative colitis. A fissure is an uncommon complication of haemorrhoidectomy and results from a nonhealing wound combined with anal spasm.

Paediatric

Fissure-in-ano is one of the commonest causes of constipation in infants and children. The associated pain leads to a behaviour pattern in which the child avoids defaecation. This results in stool retention and rectal stool bolus formation. The rectum becomes overdistended and the child becomes unaware of the need to pass stool. Overflow incontinence and soiling result.

Clinical features

History

The typical presentation is severe pain on defaecation in a young patient. Pain is the predominant symptom and may be burning, tearing or sharp in nature. It is usually painful to wipe the anus and pain may last a few hours after defaecation. There is often associated outlet-type rectal bleeding, with blood on the paper or dripping into the pan postdefaecation, or blood streaking of the stools. The amount of bleeding is usually minor and there may be some staining or mucous discharge in the underwear. There may be a history of constipation, which could be responsible for the tear, but is more likely secondary to the pain. A full history is important to exclude previous perianal surgery, perianal abscess, trauma during childbirth or symptoms consistent with Crohn's disease. It is important to remember that fissures can follow an acute attack of diarrhoea. It is important to document reproductive history for females, as surgery may have implications for future anal continence.

Examination

The diagnosis should be suspected from the history alone and is confirmed by gently parting the superficial part of the anal sphincter with the gloved fingers to reveal the characteristic linear ulcer. There may be an associated 'sentinel pile', which consists of heaped-up skin at the lowermost extent of the linear ulcer (Fig. 17.7). It is often too painful to perform a digital rectal examination or a proctoscopy, and so this is best left until after treatment is started. However, it is important to complete clinical assessment with rigid sigmoidoscopy at a later date.

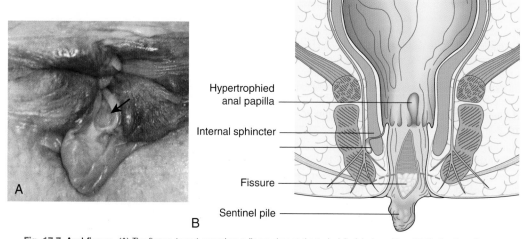

Hypertrophied anal papilla

Internal sphincter

Fissure

Sentinel pile

Fig. 17.7 Anal fissure. (A) The fissure (*arrow*) comprises a linear ulcer at the typical 6 o'clock position. **(B)** Explanatory diagram.

Management

Nonoperative

Many acute fissures resolve spontaneously and so treatment should be reserved for chronic symptoms with duration of 6 weeks or more. Having established that the fissure is primary, treatment is aimed at alleviating pain and anal spasm to break the vicious circle. The optimal approach is conservative in the first instance. Stool softeners may help, but rarely effect a cure as the sole treatment. Chemical sphincter relaxation is first-line treatment of choice using topical 0.5% diltiazem or nitrates (glyceryl trinitrate 0.2–0.5%) as a cream applied 12-hourly to the anal canal. Headaches can be a dose-limiting side-effect, especially with topical nitrates, but healing can be achieved in about 80% of acute fissures. Other means of reduction in sphincter tone include direct injection of the sphincter with botulinum toxin, which temporarily paralyses the sphincter. Anaesthetising the pain-sensitive anoderm using topical 5% lignocaine acts as an adjunct to the treatment, and provides immediate symptomatic relief.

Operative approach

Until the relatively recent advent of chemical sphincterotomy as first-line treatment, surgery was the only option. Surgery still has a major role in the management of patients who have fissures resistant to medical treatment, or who have recurrence. Anal stretching (Lord's procedure) has been abandoned, as it is associated with significant sphincter damage and incontinence (EBM 17.2). Lateral (internal) sphincterotomy (Notara's procedure) is the commonest operation for anal fissure and involves controlled division of the lower half of the internal sphincter, either to the level of the dentate line, or to the length of the fissure at the lateral position (3 o'clock or 9 o'clock with the patient in the lithotomy position). There is a small but appreciable risk of late anal incontinence following lateral sphincterotomy. This is usually only to gas, but occasionally faecal incontinence to liquid or solid can occur, particularly in women who have had birth-related anal sphincter damage. Hence, in women, it is more appropriate to avoid further sphincter muscle division, by using an anal advancement or rotation flap to cover the ulcerated fissure base and allow new, well-vascularised skin to heal the ulcer and reduce associated anal spasm. Any surgical intervention should also excise the sentinel pile.

EBM | 17.2 Anal fissure

'A step-wise hierarchical approach to treatment is optimal comprising medical therapy (diltiazem cream then botulinum toxin), internal sphincterotomy or anal advancement flap. Anal stretch is an outdated surgical treatment and is associated with a significant excess risk of faecal incontinence.'

Nelson RL, Thomas K, Morgan J, Jones A. Non surgical therapy for anal fissure. Cochrane Database Syst Rev. 2012;(2):CD003431.; Nelson RL, Chattopadhyay A, Brooks W, et al. Operative procedures for fissure in ano. Cochrane Database Syst Rev. 2011;(11):CD002199.

 17.4 Summary

Anal fissure

Pain on defaecation and outlet type bleeding are the cardinal symptoms
Typically affects younger age groups (18–30 years)
In older age groups, Crohn's disease or cancer should be suspected
Treatment
- Medical treatment is preferred in the first instance
- Stool softeners
- Chemical sphincterotomy (0.5% diltiazem or 0.4% glycerol trinitrate cream)
- Topical local anaesthetic (5% lignocaine)
- Botulinus toxin paralysis of anal sphincter
- Anal skin advancement flap (mainly reserved for females)
- Lateral internal anal sphincterotomy.

Perianal abscess

Perianal abscess is a nonspecific term encompassing abscesses in the perianal, intersphincteric, ischiorectal or pelvirectal spaces (Fig. 17.8). It is three times more common in men than women.

Predisposing factors

These include Crohn's disease and ulcerative colitis, and immunosuppressive disorders such as haematological disease, diabetes mellitus, chemotherapy and human immunodeficiency virus (HIV) infection.

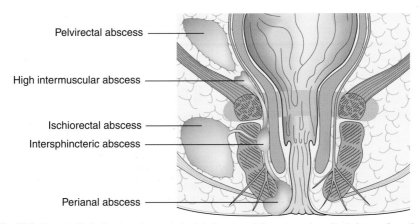

Pelvirectal abscess

High intermuscular abscess

Ischiorectal abscess
Intersphincteric abscess

Perianal abscess

Fig. 17.8 Spread of infection from the anal gland to the anorectal spaces and resultant abscess formation.

Pathogenesis

Most patients have no predisposing factors. Most abscesses are cryptoglandular, initiated by blockage of the anal gland ducts (see Fig. 17.3); followed by secondary infection with colonic organisms such as *Bacteroides*, *Streptococcus faecalis* and coliforms. The intersphincteric location of the anal glands (see Fig. 17.4) explains the routes that infection may take as pus tracks along the line of least resistance through the tissue spaces. Rarely, patients with established sepsis elsewhere may develop metastatic suppuration in the perianal region.

Clinical features

True perianal abscess

This is the most common type, in which pus tracks inferiorly to appear at the perianal margin between the internal and external sphincters (Fig. 17.8). Symptoms are usually of 2–3 days' duration and the abscess may have discharged spontaneously. Systemic upset is minimal and anal pain is the predominant presenting complaint.

Intersphincteric abscess

This occurs if the abscess remains localised within the intersphincteric space; the patient presents with acute anal pain and tenderness. There is usually no evidence of suppuration on inspection of the perianal region. Pain often prevents digital examination, and so general anaesthetic is required. The main differential diagnosis is acute anal fissure. Diagnosis is confirmed by demonstration of a localised pea-sized lump in the intersphincteric space.

Ischiorectal abscess

Infection may extend into the ischiorectal space resulting in ischiorectal abscess, which is a relatively uncommon but serious problem. Poorly controlled diabetes is a common underlying correlate and should be excluded in all cases. As the ischiorectal space is horseshoe-shaped with no fascial barriers within it, infection can track extensively, including posteriorly around the anus to the contralateral space. In such cases, the patient's condition is toxic and pyrexial with a large, painful, fluctuant, brawny swelling affecting both buttocks, due to large volumes of pus. Perianal pain, associated with difficulty sitting, is reported in the preceding days.

Supralevator abscess

Infection tracking proximally from the infected anal gland through the upper intersphincteric space may result in a high intersphincteric (high intermuscular) abscess or a pelvirectal abscess. As these spaces encircle the anorectum above the levator muscles, abscesses can be bilateral and often present with a major systemic upset. These are complex problems meriting specialist management. With high abscesses, it is also important to consider intraabdominal sepsis from Crohn's disease or a diverticular abscess.

Management

An established abscess will not respond to antibiotics alone and requires surgical drainage. Treatment of perianal abscess is usually straightforward and involves drainage of the pus under general anaesthetic. Most cases are adequately dealt with by incising and deroofing the abscess at the point of maximal fluctuance.

However, anatomical considerations are critical, as inappropriate incision of sphincter muscle can result in incontinence. Furthermore, drainage of pus through the wrong space will create a perianal fistula (see below). Pus should be sent for bacteriology to determine the causative organism(s). In uncomplicated cases, antibiotics have no place after drainage. Where there is extensive cellulitis, as is often the case with ischiorectal abscesses, parenteral antibiotics, such as broad-spectrum cephalosporins and metronidazole, should be administered. Parenteral antibiotics are mandatory for diabetic patients with perianal sepsis. Unusually complex perianal or recurrent sepsis should raise suspicion of Crohn's disease. Sigmoidoscopy and rectal biopsy should be undertaken and the abscess roof sent for histology.

17.5 Summary

Anorectal sepsis

- Most anorectal sepsis is cryptoglandular
- Perianal and ischiorectal abscesses are the most common anorectal abscesses
- Recurrent abscess should raise suspicion of fistula and Crohn's disease
- Abscesses require incision and drainage.

Fistula-in-ano

The underlying pathogenesis of the vast majority of cases of perianal abscess or anal fistula is anal gland duct obstruction. This results in stasis and anal gland infection (cryptoglandular infection). Abscess precedes all such cases of fistula, although the sepsis is often subclinical. Inappropriate surgical drainage of perianal abscess is responsible for a small but significant proportion of fistulae. Fig. 17.9 is a simplified diagram showing the classification of fistula-in-ano. A fistulous tract should be suspected in all patients with recurrent perianal abscess. Typically the patient presents repeatedly with an abscess that intermittently points and discharges pus on to the perianal skin. However, fistulae should not be routinely sought when draining straightforward perianal abscesses and inexpert probing may inadvertently induce a fistula.

In addition to cryptoglandular aetiology, perianal fistula may be due to Crohn's disease, anal trauma, inexpert surgical drainage and anorectal cancer. In populations with a high prevalence of tuberculosis (resource-poor nations, immunosuppressed individuals), fistulae can be tuberculous in origin, especially if there is evidence of tuberculosis elsewhere in the body. They are often complex. The external opening may have an undermined edge and a bluish tinge. Other rare causes include ulcerative colitis and actinomycosis. Around 10% of patients with small intestinal Crohn's disease, without colorectal involvement, have perianal disease. Crohn's should be excluded in those with recurrent perianal fistula or sepsis resistant to treatment.

Clinical features and assessment

Patients usually present with a chronically discharging opening in the perianal skin, associated with pruritus and perianal discomfort. It is essential to determine predisposing medical conditions or previous surgery. Investigation requires examination under anaesthetic (EUA) by a colorectal specialist when the fistula should be probed to trace the tract from external to the internal openings. Goodsall's Law is a rough rule of thumb as to the likely course of fistulous tracts. Thus, when the fistula opens on the perianal skin of the anterior anus, the tract usually passes radially directly to the anal canal. However, when the opening is posterior to a line drawn

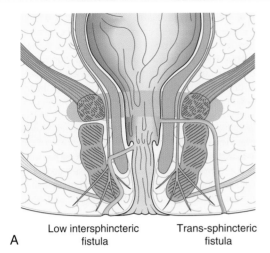

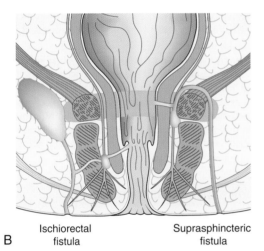

Fig. 17.9 Categories of fistula-in-ano. (A) Low intersphincteric and transsphinteric. (B) Ischiorectal and suprasphincteric.

A

Low intersphincteric fistula   Trans-sphincteric fistula

B

Ischiorectal fistula   Suprasphincteric fistula

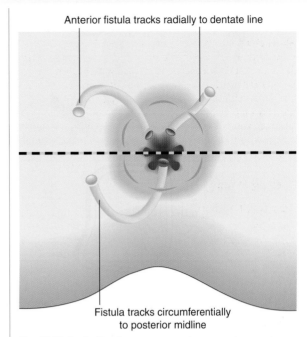

Anterior fistula tracks radially to dentate line

Fistula tracks circumferentially to posterior midline

Fig. 17.10 Goodsall's rule.

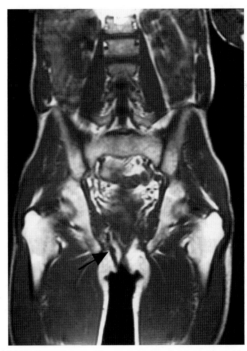

Fig. 17.11 Coronal magnetic resonance imaging scan of complex pelvirectal fistula (*arrow*).

between the 3 o'clock and 9 o'clock positions, the tract usually passes circumferentially backwards to enter the anal canal in the midline (6 o'clock position) (Fig. 17.10). It is essential to avoid inducing further fistulae by ill-advised probing of the region. It is important to determine whether the fistula is low or high, as the prognosis and treatment are different for each (Fig. 17.9). Most fistulae can be delineated and treated at EUA, but complex cases may merit magnetic resonance imaging (MRI) (Fig. 17.11). Endoanal ultrasound is useful, portable and relatively inexpensive. However, these modalities of investigation are rarely necessary and EUA can provide useful information. Further investigation to exclude Crohn's disease may be appropriate, involving colonoscopy, small bowel MRI or small bowel follow-through.

Management

Treatment is determined by the course of the fistula tract. Usually, low fistulae can simply be laid open and allowed to heal. However, where a significant proportion of the internal and/or external sphincter is involved, then laying open the tract will result in faecal incontinence. In such complex cases, the fistula tract can be probed and a seton passed along its length (Fig. 17.12) to allow the fistula to drain. Once it is drained, a tighter seton can be

applied that will gradually cut out through the sphincters, allowing them to heal behind the seton. Applying such a cutting seton maintains the ends of the sphincters together and minimises the risk of incontinence. Draining setons are not tightened, and these also cut through the sphincters if left in long enough. High fistulae may be treated by an anorectal advancement flap. This involves raising a flap of rectal wall and upper internal sphincter. The flap is advanced distally to close the internal opening. The

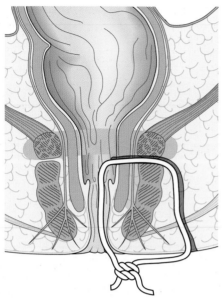

Fig. 17.12 A seton encircling a transsphincteric fistula. A seton is a piece of surgical thread, suture material or specialised tie that is passed through the fistula. It is tied in a loop to allow the fistula to drain (loose seton) and/or to cut slowly through the sphincter muscle, with the muscle healing behind the advancing seton (tight seton).

external opening and superficial part of the tract heals as there is no faecal stream to maintain the sepsis. Newer surgical procedures, such as the anal fistula plug and the LIFT procedure are still under evaluation. In some complex cases, a defunctioning colostomy may be necessary. All fistula tracts should be sent for histopathological examination and if clinically suspected, for mycobacterial staining and culture. Tuberculous fistula-in-ano will need antituberculosis therapy for at least 12 months.

 17.6 Summary

Fistula-in-ano

Aetiology
- Idiopathic (cryptoglandular) due to blockage of anal gland duct
- Crohn's disease
- Anorectal trauma
- Iatrogenic (surgical)
- Anorectal carcinoma

Rare causes
- Ulcerative colitis
- Tuberculosis
- Actinomycosis

Treatment
- Low fistulae should be laid open
- Complex high fistulae require repair and/or seton insertion.

Miscellaneous benign perianal lumps

Perianal haematoma

Perianal haematoma is a painful condition caused by subcutaneous haemorrhage and thrombus formation in the superficial space between the anoderm and the anal sphincter. A localised lump forms at the anal verge due to blood tracking subcutaneously from haemorrhoids after the passage of a hard bowel motion. It can also arise in patients with a bleeding diathesis or those on anticoagulants. The condition is readily treated by surgical drainage under local anaesthetic, with almost instantaneous relief. It would settle eventually without surgery, but perianal haematoma evacuation will prevent many days of pain.

Perianal haematoma is easily recognised as a well-circumscribed, bluish dome-shaped lump under the perianal skin. The main differential diagnosis is thrombosed haemorrhoids, and so it is essential to make an accurate diagnosis. Inappropriate incision of haemorrhoids will result in considerable bleeding. Perianal haematoma should be readily differentiated from perianal abscess by the colour and by the surrounding erythema and induration.

Anal warts

Anal warts cause discomfort, pain, pruritus ani and difficulty with perianal hygiene. Warts are also associated with an increased risk of squamous carcinoma as they are usually associated with human papillomavirus (HPV). The lesions may be very extensive or relatively sparse.

After viral infection and the development of an initial crop of warts, they may be spread extensively by scratching, which is provoked by the associated pruritus ani. Many cases resolve spontaneously, but those requiring treatment can usually be managed effectively by the application of podophyllin. More extensive cases may require surgical excision, and very extensive cases associated with dysplasia may require excision and skin grafting, combined with a temporary colostomy.

Fibroepithelial anal polyp

Fibroepithelial anal polyp is not a neoplasm, but hypertrophic epithelium arising on a stalk from the anal canal itself. Histologically, it comprises keratinised squamous epithelium supported by scarred, fibrotic subcutaneous tissue. The clinical history may suggest haemorrhoids as the main differential diagnosis, but this is easily discounted by digital examination and proctoscopy, which reveals the polyp on a stalk. The main differential diagnosis is of a prolapsing rectal adenomatous polyp on a long stalk. However, rectal polyps arise above the dentate line. Excision biopsy confirms the nature of the polyp.

Patients with a fibroepithelial polyp may present with a prolapsing anal lesion, discomfort on defaecation, or pruritus ani due to faecal-stained mucus irritating the delicate perianal skin. Anal polyps are usually associated with a history of perianal disease, including haemorrhoids or fissure-in-ano. Symptomatic polyps are excised under general anaesthetic.

Anal skin tags

Prolapse of haemorrhoids is usually followed by a degree of regression, and may leave irregular skin at the anal verge, known as anal skin tags. Haemorrhoids often present with minor anal skin tags, but it is important to stress that the tags themselves are not haemorrhoids. Although the anus may not look particularly tidy, there is no indication to operate unless the patient is having significant perianal hygiene or pruritus problems. Anal tags associated with haemorrhoids that merit surgery can be removed at the same time as haemorrhoidectomy.

Anal cancer

Anal cancer accounts for less than 1% of all new cases (UK) and is rare in comparison with colorectal cancer. There are around 1200 new cases annually in the UK. Most patients with anal cancer present in the sixth or seventh decade, but younger cases are well recognised, particularly in those with HIV and high risk activities.

Histological types

Over 85% of anal cancers are squamous arising from the keratinised squamous epithelium of the anal margin or from the nonkeratinised squamous epithelium of the anal transitional zone immediately above the dentate line. Around 5% of tumours are adenocarcinomas arising from the glandular epithelium of the upper anal canal or rarely from the intersphincteric space anal glands. These are distinct from low anorectal adenocarcinoma. Other rarer tumours include melanoma, lymphoma and sarcoma.

Risk factors

Human papilloma virus (HPV) infection causes the majority of anal carcinomas and is strongly associated with HPV types 16 and 18. Smoking is a risk factor and likely interacts with viral infection. Anogenital warts are also a risk factor, as is anoreceptive intercourse. HIV infection is also a predisposing factor, owing to immunosuppression and susceptibility to viral infection. Chronic immunosuppression associated with organ transplantation may also increase risk. The premalignant lesion, anal intraepithelial neoplasia (AIN), is probably the precursor of most anal carcinomas and is analogous to cervical intraepithelial neoplasia (CIN), the precursor lesion of cervical cancer. The level of AIN (1–3) is dependent on the degree of cytological atypia and the depth of that atypia in the epidermis. A high proportion of AIN 3 progresses to carcinoma and is shown in Fig. 17.13. It is important to perform a cervical smear in women with proven anal cancer. There is also an association with vulval intraepithelial neoplasia (VIN), which also has a common HPV aetiology. Screening for AIN using either anal cytology or high resolution anoscopy and biopsy may be undertaken in patient populations at high risk.

Clinical features and assessment

Anal cancer is frequently misdiagnosed in the early stages because of its rarity and because symptoms of benign anal conditions are highly prevalent. Anal verge tumours often present earlier than canal tumours because the patient becomes aware of a mass or irregular area at the anal margin. Early cancer may be confused with fissures, piles and warts. Anal tumours are readily accessible and detectable by careful clinical examination; anal pain/discomfort, bleeding or discharge into the underwear, and pruritus ani should be sought. Advanced tumours that have spread to the anal sphincters may present with incontinence. Clinical examination of anal cancer at the margin reveals an ulcerated discoid lesion at the anal verge (Fig. 17.14). Anal canal cancer may not be visible, although extensive lesions may protrude to the anal verge by direct spread. Examination under anaesthetic allows tumour biopsy and sigmoidoscopy. Biopsy is essential to confirm the diagnosis, but also to determine the tissue of origin, as the treatment for squamous carcinoma varies from that for adenocarcinoma.

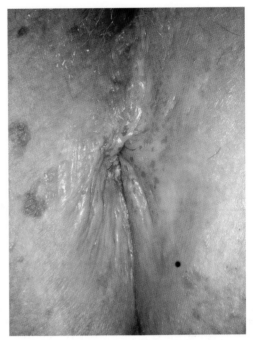

Fig. 17.13 The most severe degree of anal intraepithelial neoplasia (AIN 3), the precursor of most anal squamous cancer.

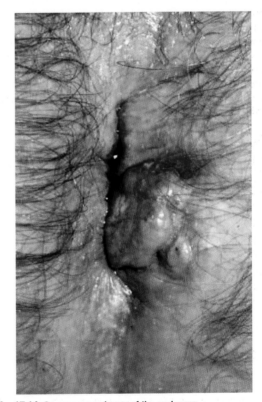

Fig. 17.14 Squamous carcinoma of the anal verge.

Staging

Staging is important for both prognosis and guiding treatment approaches (TNM staging in Table 17.1). The lymph nodes most commonly involved are the inguinal groups, particularly for anal

Table 17.1 TNM staging of anal cancer	
T (Tumour)	
• TX	Primary tumour cannot be assessed
• T0	No evidence of primary tumour
• T1	<2 cm
• T2	2–5 cm
• T3	>5 cm
• T4a	Invading vaginal mucosa
• T4b	Invading structures other than skin, or rectal or vaginal mucosa (i.e., local spread to muscle or bone)
N (node)	
• NX	Regional lymph nodes cannot be assessed
• N0	No regional lymph node metastasis
• N1	Metastasis in perirectal lymph node(s)
• N2	Metastasis in unilateral internal iliac and/or inguinal lymph node(s)
• N3	Metastasis in perirectal and inguinal lymph nodes and/or bilateral internal iliac and/or inguinal lymph nodes
M (Metastases)	
• MX	Distant metastasis cannot be assessed
• M0	No distant metastasis
• M1	Distant metastasis

verge cancers. Canal tumours may spread proximally to the mesorectal nodes or to the internal iliac nodes via the middle rectal lymph nodes. Lymphadenopathy alone is not sufficient to confirm lymph node spread because reactive changes due to infection are common. Hence, accessible nodes should be biopsied. Examination under anaesthetic is an important part of clinical staging, as the tumour is often painful and the anus too tender to examine. Computed tomography (CT) and MRI are essential; endoanal ultrasound may help but usually needs to be performed under anaesthetic.

Management

It is important to detect anal cancer at an early stage, as extensive local invasion and metastatic disease are associated with a poor outcome. Multidisciplinary treatment of anal cancer is essential, with surgeon and radiotherapist involved in assessment and treatment.

For early, well-circumscribed superficial (T_1N_0) carcinomas, wide surgical excision is the optimal treatment, and avoids chemoradiotherapy morbidity. However, for T_2, T_3 and T_4 tumours, treatment comprises radiotherapy to the anal canal and inguinal lymph nodes, combined with 5-fluorouracil (5-FU) (recently capecitabine is preferred) and mitomycin C (EBM 17.3). Newer

---

EBM 17.3 Anal cancer

'Combination chemoradiation is the primary treatment modality for anal canal and T2, T3 and T4 tumours. Abdominoperineal resection is reserved for salvage procedures in cases of relapse after chemoradiation.'

Anal Cancer. Position Statement of the Association of Coloproctology of Great Britain and Ireland. http://www.acpgbi.org.uk/assets/documents/Anal_Cancer_Position_Statement.pdf; Glynne-Jones R, Northover JM, Cervantes A; ESMO Guidelines Working Group. Anal cancer: ESMO Clinical Practice Guidelines for diagnosis, treatment and follow-up. Ann Oncol. 2010;21 Suppl 5:v87–92. PubMed PMID: 20555110.

---

radiotherapy regimens, combined with capecitabine and cisplatinum, are being introduced. The usual approach is external beam radiotherapy, but radioactive implants such as selectron wires are also used in selected cases. Surgery has a limited role in the primary treatment of these lesions but is important in the management of advanced disease. Surgery is reserved for radiotherapy treatment failures, when 'salvage' abdominoperineal excision of the anus and rectum may afford a cure in some cases and alleviate symptoms in others.

Modern multimodality approaches involving tailored surgery and chemoradiation have radically improved the morbidity of treatment by avoiding abdominoperineal resection and permanent colostomy for many patients; the 5-year survival rate is now around 65%.

  17.7 Summary

Anal carcinoma

- Anal carcinoma is associated with human papillomavirus (HPV) types 16 and 18
- Anal intraepithelial neoplasia (AIN) is a malignant precursor
- Local surgical excision is the treatment of choice for T1N0 lesions
- Chemoradiotherapy is treatment of choice for T2, T3 or T4 lesions
- Chemoradiotherapy is mandatory for those with involved lymph nodes
- Abdominoperineal resection is reserved for failures of chemoradiation.

Rectal prolapse

Rectal prolapse is a distressing condition that can affect both children and adults. The term rectal prolapse encompasses three types of abnormal protrusion of all, or part of, the rectal wall:

- *Full-thickness* rectal prolapse (procidentia) includes the mucosa and the muscular layers.
- *Mucosal* prolapse, as the name suggests, involves only the mucosal lining of the rectum.
- *Occult* rectal prolapse refers to rectal wall intussusception but without the prolapse protruding through the anus. This also refers to the much rarer condition of *solitary rectal ulcer syndrome* characterised by a full-thickness prolapse of the anterior rectal wall only. The terms occult rectal prolapse and solitary rectal ulcer syndrome are not synonymous.

Pathogenesis

The pathological process that results in rectal prolapse is incompletely understood. However, certain factors are clearly implicated in predisposing to the condition. Mucosal prolapse should not be confused with full-thickness prolapse. It is often associated with a degree of haemorrhoids, but whether these are causal or simply the result of a common aetiology is not understood. The majority of cases of full-thickness rectal prolapse occur in elderly women, with no obvious aetiological basis. Weight loss in the elderly with loss of fat supporting the rectum, combined with degeneration of collagen fibres and weakness of the musculature of the pelvic floor, results in loss of the anorectal angle and laxity of the rectal wall (see Fig. 17.2). In many cases, there is a deep rectovaginal pouch with a long loop of sigmoid colon that pushes down into the rectovaginal pouch and contributes to the prolapse. Occasionally, there is a clear history of obstetric injury but most patients are nulliparous.

Predisposing factors

Chronic constipation and straining at stool are the commonest aetiological factors in young adults, although spinal injury, psychiatric illness, multiple sclerosis and spinal tumour can predispose. In children, the lack of a sacral hollow, combined with constipation and excessive straining at stool, leads to evagination of the rectum and prolapse protrusion through the anus. In children with cystic fibrosis, excessive coughing increases intraabdominal pressure.

Clinical features and assessment

Patients present with an uncomfortable sensation of 'something coming down' the back passage. Initially, this is only on defaecation, but eventually the rectum remains constantly prolapsed and will not reduce spontaneously. The patient may be able to reduce the prolapse digitally. Constipation is usually an accompanying feature. There is often faecal incontinence and mucous discharge. Blood-stained mucus is common when the rectum remains prolapsed. The prolapse may become ulcerated and strangulated. In extreme cases, there may be associated uterine prolapse, alluding to the underlying aetiology relating to weakness of the entire pelvic floor.

Examination confirms the diagnosis in most cases. If the prolapse is not apparent, it will usually appear when the patient strains on a commode (Figure 17.15). Digital examination reveals a patulous anus, poor sphincter tone and evidence of a weak pelvic floor on straining. Rigid sigmoidoscopy will reveal cases of occult prolapse. If the history is short, consideration should be given to the presence of a spinal tumour, a spinal stenosis or a prolapsed intervertebral disc. In occult rectal prolapse, radiological assessment using a defaecating proctogram or dynamic MRI may secure the diagnosis. Conditions that might be mistaken for a rectal prolapse include large fourth-degree haemorrhoids, prolapsing rectal neoplasia, anal warts, skin tags and fibroepithelial anal polyp. On the basis of symptoms alone, the differential diagnosis of rectal prolapse includes rectal cancer and inflammatory bowel disease, which should be excluded by investigation.

Management

Childhood rectal prolapse

Rectal prolapse in children is usually treated effectively by maintaining a regular bowel habit with stool softeners, combined with digital reduction of the prolapse by the parents. The condition is self-limiting and surgery is rarely indicated.

Mucosal rectal prolapse

In adults, mucosal rectal prolapse can be treated by submucosal injection of sclerosant, by photocoagulation or by applying Barron's bands to the prolapsed area. In resistant cases, a limited excision of the area, similar to a haemorrhoidectomy, is effective. Stapled anorectal rectopexy has gained favour in some centres.

Full-thickness rectal prolapse

Surgery is the only effective treatment for established full-thickness rectal prolapse. However, none of the available surgical options is wholly satisfactory. The aim of surgery is to treat the prolapse and improve any associated incontinence. Operations for rectal prolapse can be undertaken employing perineal or abdominal approaches:

- *Perineal approaches* aim to fixate or excise the prolapse surgically from below. Delorme's procedure involves the excision of the mucosa lining the prolapse, with plication of the muscle tube. Perineal rectosigmoidectomy entails excision through the anus of the prolapsed rectum and lower part of the sigmoid. The latter may be combined with a repair of the pelvic floor (Altmeier procedure).
- *Abdominal approaches* aim to mobilise the rectum to the pelvic floor safe-guarding the pelvic nerves and blood vessels and to fix the rectum to the bony pelvis using sutures or foreign material (mesh). Increasingly these procedures are performed laparoscopically. Circumferential fixation aggravates constipation and has given way to posterior 120-degree fixation (Notara's mesh rectopexy). Recently, anterior (ventral) laparoscopic mesh rectopexy has gained acceptance and proponents claim better results. The abdominal approach may also include resection of the redundant sigmoid colon, particularly when constipation is a predominant feature, because rectal fixation usually aggravates the constipation. Injury to pelvic nerves in a male can lead to problems of impotence and therefore needs to be carried out after discussion and performed with meticulous care.

Solitary rectal ulcer syndrome

This rare condition is difficult to treat effectively because the main aetiology is behavioural and there may be a psychological overlay. The peak age-group affected is 20–40 years. The condition is associated with an introspective and anxious personality. Patients with this condition spend an inordinate amount of time attempting to defaecate. The diagnosis is confirmed by visualising the anterior ulcer in the low rectum. Biopsy shows the typical features of submucosal fibrosis, hypertrophy and reorientation of the muscularis mucosae and overlying ulceration. Management is conservative

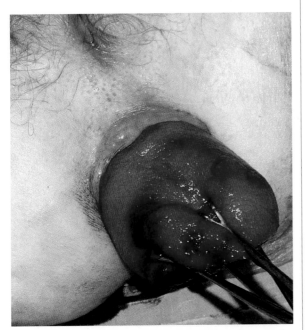
Fig. 17.15 Full-thickness rectal prolapse at operation prior to repair.

with stool softeners and psychology input. Biofeedback may help in suitable compliant patients. Various operations have been attempted including rectopexy and even low anterior resection. However, the results are usually poor and surgery should be avoided.

17.8 Summary

Rectal prolapse

- Rectal prolapse may occur at any age but is most common in the elderly
- Diagnosis is clinical
- Defaecating proctogram may be required to confirm the diagnosis in a minority
- Dynamic MRI delineates the extent of the entire pelvic floor problem
- Treatment is usually surgical: either perineal or transabdominal.

Anal incontinence

Anal incontinence is defined as the involuntary loss of faeces or flatus. Faecal incontinence is both distressing and socially disabling so patients are often reluctant to discuss the issue with relatives or medical professionals. Hence, the population prevalence of incontinence is probably underestimated but has been variously estimated at 2–5% in the general population and 10% of adult females.

Aetiology

There are a variety of specific aetiological factors (Table 17.2) but the majority of cases are 'idiopathic', most commonly affecting older parous women. Several factors are involved in maintaining

Table 17.2 Aetiology of anal incontinence

Trauma

- Obstetric sphincter injury (including episiotomy)
- Accidental trauma (e.g., road traffic accident, bicycle injury)
- Surgical trauma (injudicious fistula surgery, drainage of perianal abscess or haemorrhoidectomy)
- Perianal sepsis

Congenital

- Anorectal atresia (usually treated surgically in childhood)
- Spinal dysraphism (spina bifida)

Neurological

- Denervation of pelvic floor following childbirth
- Multiple sclerosis
- Low spinal or sacral tumour
- Spinal trauma
- Dementia

Miscellaneous

- Rectal prolapse
- Haemorrhoids
- Rectal cancer invading sphincter
- Perianal Crohn's disease
- Faecal impaction
- Relative incontinence due to intestinal hurry (e.g., inflammatory bowel disease)
- Psychiatric or behavioural disorders (including enopresis)

anal continence (see Summary 17.1) and these may be adversely affected by any combination of structural damage to the musculature, disruption of the nerve supply, and marked intestinal hurry with defaecatory urgency (such as in ulcerative colitis). Neurodegenerative disease is also a recognised aetiological factor. Perianal sepsis, or the surgery required to treat it, may result in structural damage to the sphincter complex.

The majority of patients are women with a history of obstetric problems, and the underlying mechanism of subsequent incontinence is complex. Although full-thickness obstetric tears are rare, significant sphincter defects have been observed to occur in 10–30% of women after vaginal delivery. Peripartum nerve injury secondary to a prolonged second stage of delivery and pressure effects from the baby's head or due to forceps can affect the internal pudendal nerves, eventually leading to denervation and atrophy of the striated muscle of the external sphincter, the puborectalis sling and the levator ani in later life. Most cases of incontinence involve a combination of sphincter muscle damage and the secondary effects of denervation.

Clinical features and assessment

History

A full history is essential, with particular reference to obstetric history and previous perianal operations. Incontinence should be graded using established scoring systems, such as the Cleveland Clinic Incontinence Score, which incorporate frequency and severity of episodes of incontinence to gas, liquid or solid stool. Such scores enable more objective assessment of any improvement or deterioration in incontinence. Co-existing disease should be documented and neurological symptoms sought. A defaecation history should be sought, including the degree of defaecatory urgency. A history of co-existing urinary incontinence is often present.

Examination

Digital examination to determine sphincter tone, the presence of previous scars and the state of the rectovaginal septum should be undertaken. Poor anal sensation suggests a neurogenic basis for the incontinence. Other anorectal causes of incontinence, as listed in Table 17.2, should be excluded by rigid sigmoidoscopy in all cases.

Investigation

Any cause of intestinal hurry (such as colonic cancer, inflammatory bowel disease or even infective diarrhoea) can render incontinent a patient who was previously coping with a more formed stool. Hence, colonoscopy is an essential part of assessment. Endoanal ultrasound scanning of the sphincters delineates the presence and extent of any sphincter defect. Anorectal physiology studies document resting and squeeze anal sphincter pressures, and also define whether there is a predominant neurogenic element. Where there is any concern from the history or clinical examination regarding a spinal lesion, MRI should be performed.

Conservative management

Any remedial causes of incontinence (Table 17.2) should be addressed appropriately. However, women with 'idiopathic' faecal incontinence constitute the majority of cases. In older women, who almost universally have a combination of sphincter and nerve damage, conservative measures should be instigated in the first instance. Dietary advice is important to avoid exacerbating factors in the diet, such as caffeine, spicy foods and excessive alcohol. Stool-bulking agents (e.g., Fybogel) should be combined with loperamide to reduce the propulsive activity of the GI tract and induce a degree of constipation. In cases with a predominant neurogenic basis, rectal irritability resulting in faecal urgency may respond to therapy with amitriptyline (25–50 mg at night). Conservative measures may be combined with regular emptying of the rectum using stimulant suppositories or enemas. In many cases, these measures dramatically improve quality of life even when minor degrees of incontinence persist.

Surgical management

Surgery is indicated only in a small minority of patients with idiopathic faecal incontinence. In a small subset of patients with a clear history of sphincter injury due to trauma or to surgical injury, overlapping sphincter repair is frequently highly successful. However, it is important to underline that overall the results of anterior sphincter repair are poor in the long term. Patients with evidence of denervation tend to have poor results. Complex total floor repairs have been performed with some success in a limited proportion of patients. Other surgical approaches include stimulated gracioloplasty (transferring the gracilis muscle on a proximal pedicle to wrap it subcutaneously around the anal canal). An electrical stimulator is implanted, which delivers an electrical signal to maintain the muscle in a tonic state by conversion of muscle fibres to slow-twitch type. This allows long-term tonic contraction of the gracilis muscle to maintain continence. The procedure has an acceptable level of success in around 50% of patients, but at a cost of major surgery and potentially major complications.

Implantable artificial anal sphincters have also been developed and these are placed to encircle the anorectum. Results from the use of the available devices are encouraging but, as with any foreign material, these are susceptible to infection and many have to be removed. Nevertheless, prosthetic devices have a place in the management of a small subset of patients with anal incontinence. Sacral nerve stimulation has been introduced with good effect. This involves insertion of an electrode through the S3 sacral foramina and inducing a low-voltage electrical stimulus. The underlying mechanism is poorly understood but in a substantial proportion of selected patients the effects are dramatic. Another surgical option for the patient with anal incontinence is the creation of a permanent colostomy. Although this might be seen as an admission of failure, a well-sited stoma and input from a stoma care specialist can transform a patient's life, from being afraid to leave the house to leading a virtually normal existence.

The management of anal incontinence remains imperfect, but it is clear that patients should be managed by specialist surgeons. This allows a full investigative work-up and bespoke management for individual patients. In a specialist setting, the management of anal incontinence can be highly successful. Improvements in obstetric practice are reducing the incidence in sphincter and nerve damage during childbirth. Unfortunately, progress in this area is hampered by the fact that patients present with anal incontinence many decades after the initial insult.

17.9 Summary

Faecal incontinence

- Faecal incontinence is most common in females
- Childbirth injury is a common aetiological factor
- Associated with neurological disorders, trauma and perianal sepsis or surgery

Treatment:

- Most respond well to conservative management
- Stool bulking, antidiarrhoeal agents such as loperamide
- Enemas may be required to maintain the rectum free of faeces
- Surgery reserved for debilitating incontinence after failed conservative management:
    - sphincter repair: excellent results for (rare) discrete sphincter injury, poor for majority
    - artificial sphincter implant
        - stimulated gracioloplasty
        - sacral nerve stimulation
        - colostomy may be only option in debilitating cases.

Pruritus ani

Perianal itching can range from a minor, short-lived episode to an all-consuming obsession. It is a particular nocturnal problem with some patients unconsciously scratching the perianal region, promoting further trauma and irritation. Itching may be secondary to anorectal disorders, including haemorrhoids, fistulae, fissures, faecal incontinence, anal carcinoma and rectal prolapse. Dermatological disorders such as psoriasis, dermatitis, lichen planus, anal warts and infections may predispose. Fungal infections (candida, tinea) should be considered, especially in diabetics. Worm infestation (*Enterobius vermicularis*, pinworm) is common in children.

Management

Underlying conditions, such as anal cancer, perianal fistula and haemorrhoids and fungal skin infections, should be treated and diabetes mellitus excluded. Idiopathic pruritus ani requires full explanation and support for the patient. The cycle of trauma to the delicate perianal skin, followed by irritation and scratching, should be explained. Advice on avoidance of scratching and a requirement for willpower is essential. Patients may need to wear cotton gloves in bed, to avoid nocturnal scratching. Perfumed soaps, antiseptics or lotions should be discouraged as should nylon undergarments to minimise sweating. Certain foods (e.g., spicy foods or alcohol) may also contribute. Overzealous perianal cleansing should be avoided. Gentle cleaning, followed by washing with mild soap is necessary, but trauma whilst drying must be avoided. 'Nappy rash' barrier cream may be helpful for some patients, but it is best to avoid relying on creams. Although it may take months to control, it is possible to improve idiopathic pruritus ani symptoms in nearly all cases, providing there is the necessary commitment from the patient.

Pilonidal disease

Pilonidal disease is characterised by chronic inflammation in one or more sinuses in the midline of the natal cleft that contain hair

17

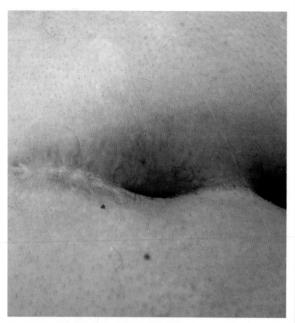

Fig. 17.16 Pilonidal sinus in the natal cleft.

and debris (Fig. 17.16). The name derives from the Greek terms 'pilus', meaning hair, and 'nidus', meaning nest. The superficial part of the midline sinus is lined with squamous epithelium, but the tracts are lined with granulation tissue due to chronic infection. Pilonidal disease can also affect the digital clefts in hairdressers.

Epidemiology

Perianal pilonidal disease is a common disorder with a population incidence of 20–30 per 100,000. It is more common in males than females, and affects around 2% of the population between the ages of 15 and 35 years. The disease is rare before puberty, when sex hormones act on hair follicles and sebaceous glands, and after the age of 40, suggesting that there is an aetiological relationship with age and skin character.

Pathogenesis

Pilonidal disease, although initially thought to be congenital, is an acquired condition. Hair follicle enlargement, secondary to repeated friction, allows the accumulation of extraneous hairs that are caught in the natal cleft. A foreign-body reaction occurs leading to a chronic discharging sinus that attracts other debris and hairs.

Risk factors

A sedentary occupation, particularly where sweating is common, is a predisposing factor. The condition was described in large numbers of American troops in the Vietnam war, owing to the use of Jeeps in the warm climate.

Clinical features

Many people have asymptomatic pilonidal sinuses and so it is important to treat the condition only if it is causing problems, in view of the high prevalence and the fact that it seldom presents after the fourth decade. Typical presentation comprises midline natal cleft pits discharging mucopurulent material which may smell mildly offensive and may be blood-stained. There is often tenderness on pressure and the patient may avoid long periods of sitting. When a sinus becomes infected and the pus is loculated, the disease presents as pilonidal abscess, with the abscess typically pointing just off the midline. However, there is invariably a communication with a midline sinus containing hair and granulation tissue. Occasionally, pilonidal sinus may present with extensive and complex branching sinus tracts. In these cases, it is important to consider perianal Crohn's disease, and careful examination of the anal canal is essential.

Management

Acute abscesses

Surgical drainage is indicated for established abscess and the incision should avoid the midline to minimise recurrence. Antibiotics have a place in the early stages of abscess formation and may avert the need for incision and drainage of an established abscess.

Chronic discharging disease

Nonoperative approach

Pilonidal disease treatment may be conservative or surgical. Conservative management comprises attention to natal cleft hygiene and hair removal by depilatory creams or by careful shaving. Hair removal from the sinus tract itself on a regular basis allows the sinus to drain and avoids the collection of hair and debris.

Operative procedures

Debilitating, chronically discharging sinus tracts merit surgery. There are a number of surgical options.

1. *Laying open and healing by secondary intention.* Tracts are laid open, granulation tissue removed with a curette and allowed to heal from the base.
2. *Excision and primary closure.* Following tract excision, the wounds are closed primarily with sutures. The wound is prone to break down and heal by second intention. Asymmetric (off midline) closure is associated with faster healing and less recurrence.

Recurrence is common, due partly to inadequate or inappropriate surgery in some cases, but mostly due to the fact that the underlying aetiology remains: namely, the natal cleft and a predisposed skin type. Recurrent disease can be treated using rotation flaps to replace the pitted skin with fresh skin from the buttock (Karydakis procedure). For complex recurrent disease, ablation of the natal cleft using a flap procedure (cleft closure) is highly effective but leaves a fairly large unsightly scar. The patient should keep the natal cleft hair-free postoperatively.

 17.10 Summary

Pilonidal disease

- Pilonidal disease is due to hair creating chronic inflammatory natal cleft sinuses
- Abscess should be drained
- Symptomatic tracts should be excised
- Recurrence is common and managed by natal cleft closure or other plastic surgery.

Section 3

Surgical specialties

Plastic surgery including common skin and subcutaneous lesions 301

The breast 326

Endocrine surgery 351

Vascular and endovascular surgery 375

Cardiothoracic surgery 409

Urological surgery 429

Neurosurgery 461

Transplantation surgery 487

Ear, nose and throat surgery 502

Orthopaedic surgery 528

Patrick Addison

Plastic surgery including common skin and subcutaneous lesions

Chapter contents

Introduction 301

Structure and function of the skin 301

Wounds 301

Burns 308

Skin and soft tissue lesions 315

Introduction

Reconstructive plastic surgery, as opposed to cosmetic surgery, is concerned with the restoration of form and function following trauma, ablative surgery, necrotising infection or congenital anomaly. The various techniques by which this is achieved are applicable throughout the body whether male or female, young or old, and the surgeon must therefore have an excellent knowledge of applied anatomy and reconstructive techniques. The 'reconstructive ladder' stratifies these increasingly complex and demanding procedures and is useful conceptually, although in practice it is often necessary to skip a step or even to take the elevator directly to the top of the ladder (Fig. 18.1). The specialty is highly varied and includes the surgical management of skin and soft tissue malignancy; soft tissue trauma; breast, trunk and perineal reconstruction; burns; soft tissue infection; hand surgery, brachial plexus and nerve compression; facial reanimation; cleft lip and palate and craniofacial deformity; and cosmetic surgery.

Structure and function of the skin

The outermost layer, or epidermis, is composed of keratinised, stratified squamous epithelium through which three appendages (hair follicles, sweat glands and sebaceous glands) pass from the underlying dermis and subcutaneous tissue (Fig. 18.2). These appendages can escape destruction in partial-thickness burns and are therefore a source of new epidermal cells for reconstitution of the epidermis. The basal layer of the epidermis generates keratin-producing cells (keratinocytes), which become flatter as they migrate towards the surface through substrata (spinosum, granulosum, lucidum and corneum), where they are shed. The basal layer also contains pigment cells (melanocytes) that produce melanin, which is passed to the keratinocytes and protects the basal layer from ultraviolet light and determines hair colour.

The dermis, which is bound to the epidermis through a basement membrane, is composed of three cell types (fibroblasts, macrophages and adipocytes), collagen, elastic fibres and an extracellular gel-like matrix. It supports the blood vessels, lymphatics, nerves and the epidermal appendages as well as pressure and temperature receptors. At the junction between the epidermis and the superficial papillary dermis, vascularised papillae push upwards to nourish the epidermis. Beneath this, the reticular dermis provides the strength and elasticity of the skin.

Sebaceous glands within the dermis secrete sebum into the hair follicles to lubricate the hair and skin. The coiled tubular sweat glands are of two types: eccrine glands exist throughout the entire skin surface and secrete salt and water, primarily for thermoregulation, whereas the apocrine glands, which are largely confined to the axilla and genital skin, secrete a more fatty odorous fluid that is a good medium for bacterial growth. Hidradenitis suppurativa is an infective process affecting the latter.

Wounds

A wound may be defined as disruption of normal tissue continuity and structure due to trauma or disease processes.

Types of wound

Wounds may be classified according to the mechanism of injury. *Trauma* caused by a sharp implement tends to produce 'incised' wounds whereas blunt trauma is associated with lacerations, abrasions, crush and degloving injuries. Special consideration should be given to *crush injuries* where the underlying tissue damage may exceed that apparent on the surface. Associated bleeding and oedema beneath the deep fascia can lead to

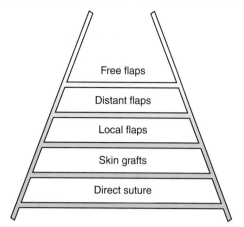

Fig. 18.1 The reconstructive ladder.

compartment syndrome with ensuing ischaemic necrosis of involved tissues. *Degloving injuries* result from shear forces, for example when a limb is compressed between rollers or beneath the wheel of a vehicle, which cause parallel tissue planes to separate. Due to the vascular anatomy in humans, such injuries can render large area of intact skin ischaemic. *Gunshot wounds* caused by low- or high-velocity projectiles can produce massive internal destruction due to cavitation, despite relatively minor skin wounds. In contrast, *burn wounds* caused by flame, hot fluids (scalds), chemicals, irradiation and electricity may involve large areas of skin with profound metabolic consequences. The management of burns is described in more detail later. Finally, natural disease processes such as neoplasia, vascular disorders and necrotising infections may also predispose to wounds.

Principles of wound healing

The essential features of wound healing are common to almost all soft tissues and result in the formation of a scar. 'Primary healing' is achieved when the wound edges are approximated shortly after injury. Epithelial cover is quickly achieved and healing produces a relatively fine scar. 'Delayed primary' healing refers to sharp debridement and direct closure of an old wound, whereas 'secondary healing' occurs when a wound is left to heal spontaneously usually resulting in excessive fibrosis and an unsightly scar (Fig. 18.3). Conceptually, there are three phases of wound healing mediated by several growth factors including fibroblast growth factor (FGF), vascular endothelial growth factor (VEGF), platelet-derived growth factor (PDGF), epidermal growth factor (EGF) and transforming growth factor beta (TGF-β) (Table 18.1).

Inflammatory phase (Days 1–6)

The initial phase begins with immediate vasoconstriction and coagulation followed by vasodilation and increased vascular permeability that is mediated by histamine, nitric oxide (NO) and serotonin produced by platelets and endothelial cells. Neutrophils (1–2 days), macrophages (2–4 days) and lymphocytes (5–7 days) coordinate the inflammatory and growth factor response.

Proliferative phase (Days 3–21)

Fibroblasts attracted to the wound by a process known as chemotaxis, arrive by day 3 and predominate by day 7. They produce the collagen necessary for scar formation and remodelling. Angiogenesis, the ingrowth of new blood vessels under the influence of VEGF and NO, occurs simultaneously and wound tensile strength increases steadily (Fig 18.4).

Maturation or remodelling phase (Weeks 3–52 +)

During weeks 3–5, the rate of collagen breakdown approaches and then temporarily surpasses its synthesis. Subsequently there is no net increase in collagen within the wound although it becomes more organised and better cross-linked. The type III collagen that predominates initially is gradually replaced by type I collagen, eventually restoring the normal ratio of 4:1, although skin and fascia usually recover only 80% of their original tensile strength.

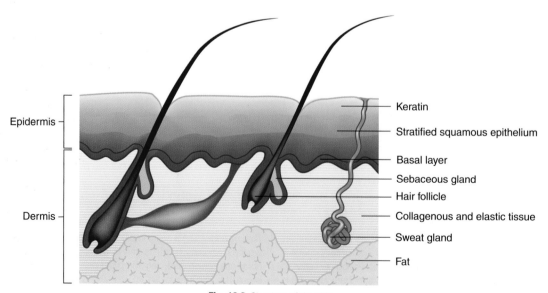

Fig. 18.2 Structure of the skin.

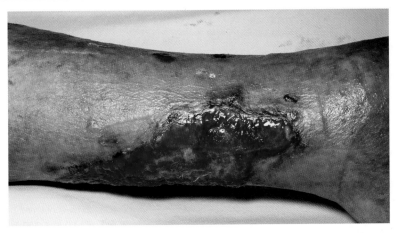

Fig. 18.3 Healing by secondary intention.

Table 18.1 Phases of wound healing

Inflammatory phase (days 1–6)

- Immediate vasoconstriction and coagulation
- Increased vascular permeability mediated by histamine, nitric oxide and serotonin
- Co-ordination of the inflammatory and growth factor response by neutrophils (1–2 days)
- Macrophages (2–4 days) and lymphocytes (5–7 days)

Proliferative phase (days 3–21)

- Fibroblast migration
- Capillary ingrowth (granulation tissue)
- Collagen synthesis with rapid gain in tensile strength
- Wound contraction

Remodelling or maturation phase (weeks 3–52+)

- Organisation of scar
- Gradual gain in tensile strength to 80% of normal

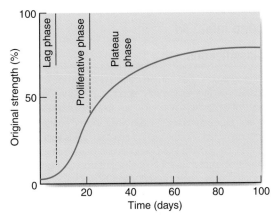

Fig. 18.4 Phases of wound healing.

Clinically, wound healing is considered to be complete once the surface of the wound has been reepithelialised. Epidermal cells from the wound edges and from within the skin appendages are mobilised to migrate across the wound surface, multiplying as they do so, until contact is made with the opposing wound edges. At this point contact inhibition is reestablished and the cells differentiate once more to form the normal epidermal layers. Concurrently, myofibroblasts scattered throughout the wound lead to wound contraction, especially in the absence of viable dermis.

Abnormal scarring

Hypertrophic scarring occurs in up to 15% of wounds and is more common following healing by secondary intent, in areas of tension or in the presence of infection and on flexor surfaces. It appears as raised, red and often itchy scars whose borders are by definition, confined to the original wound. Type III collagen and myofibroblasts predominate. Such scars tend to develop over the first 6 months and subsequently settle, although this may take 2 years or more. Resolution can be accelerated with regular massage, the application of topical silicone gel, steroid injections or pressure dressing. In some cases, surgical scar revision may be beneficial.

Keloid scars are similar to hypertrophic scars, except that they typically continue to enlarge beyond 6 months and expand outwith the original wound, appearing to invade the uninvolved adjacent skin. They most commonly occur across the upper chest, shoulders, and earlobes. Black or dark skinned individuals and those with a personal or family history of keloid formation or blood group A are particularly at risk. Such scars are notoriously difficult to treat and surgical intervention is the last resort. In addition to the treatment options described for hypertrophic scarring, intralesional 5-fluoururacil, interferon, bleomycin and botulinum toxin have been used successfully, as has low-dose external beam radiation and cryotherapy.

Unstable scars are prone to repeated cycles of ulceration and rehealing. They can develop where the dermis and subcutaneous tissue are thin, where the circulation is poor and pressure or shear forces are ever present. Genetic errors accumulate and Marjolin's ulcers, a form of squamous cell carcinoma, can develop. All chronic ulcers should therefore be biopsied to exclude such transformation.

18.1 Summary

Classification of wound healing

- Healing by primary intent is most efficient and rapid resulting in minimal scarring. It is achieved through early debridement and direct closure of a wound
- Healing by secondary intent occurs when a wound is left open. Healing is delayed and often results in hypertrophic scarring and contracture
- Delayed primary healing occurs when an old wound is debrided and closed. The wound will heal more rapidly and with better scarring.

Factors influencing wound healing

Many factors influence wound healing and consideration should be given to optimising these where possible.

Blood supply

Any local or systemic condition that compromises the ability of blood to deliver oxygen and nutrients whilst removing waste products from the wound, will adversely affect wound healing. This includes peripheral vascular disease, anaemia, cardiopulmonary disease, smoking and microvascular disease associated with diabetes, Raynaud's disease and scleroderma. Poor surgical technique that damages or applies excessive tension to the wound edges can also render tissue ischaemic. Such wounds are more prone to infection and frequently break down because arterial oxygen tension (Pao_2) is a key determinant of the rate of collagen synthesis. Similarly, wound healing in previously irradiated areas is often impaired due to injury to the circulation.

Infection

The risk of wound infection reflects patient age, the mechanism of wound formation, its location and exposure, the presence of intercurrent infection, steroid administration or other immunosuppression states, smoking, diabetes mellitus, severe malnutrition, and cardiovascular or respiratory disease. Microbial contamination can be minimised by careful skin preparation, aseptic technique and thorough wound debridement of devitalised tissue and foreign material. Poor hand hygiene before and after patient contact is perhaps the single greatest source of infection spread. The immune system provides natural defences against microbial invasion. Common infecting organisms include skin commensals as well as opportunistic organisms such as staphylococci, streptococci, coliforms and anaerobes. Pseudomonal infections are common in burns and chronic wounds.

When wound contamination is anticipated or the consequences of infection would be severe, prophylactic antibacterial treatment may be used topically or systemically. In acute traumatic wounds, tetanus prophylaxis is routinely considered, but antibiotics are not normally necessary if prompt treatment is undertaken.

Nutritional status

Protein, glucose and fatty acids are essential to wound healing and, in deficiency states, wound dehiscence and infection are common. Highly exudative wounds can contribute to total protein loss by up to 100 g each day. Healing problems should be anticipated if recent weight loss exceeds 20%.

Vitamin A is required for epithelial formation, cellular differentiation and normal functioning of the immune system, and supplements have been shown to mitigate the negative effects of steroids on wound healing. Vitamin C is essential for proline hydroxylation in collagen synthesis, and deficiency leads to reduced collagen production and tensile strength, immature fibroblast formation and capillary haemorrhage, all features of scurvy. Zinc is a cofactor for several important enzymes involved in healing. Although supplements of zinc and vitamins A and C are effective in patients with known deficiencies, they do not appear to improve healing in normal subjects.

Intercurrent disease

Healing may be affected by concurrent disease or its treatment. For example, cancer may be associated with severe malnutrition and marked impairment of healing. Diabetes mellitus impairs healing by promoting infection and by causing peripheral vascular insufficiency and neuropathy. Haemorrhagic diatheses increase the risk of haematoma formation and wound infection. Respiratory disease may lower arterial oxygen tension, and coughing can contribute to abdominal wound dehiscence. Treatments such as corticosteroids, immunosuppressive therapy, chemotherapy and radiotherapy each contribute to poor wound healing through various mechanisms including impaired cellular function and inflammatory response, impaired collagen synthesis and decreased resistance to infection.

Surgical technique

Tension-free primary wound closure and meticulous technique promote effective wound healing. Dead space should be avoided, as potential accumulation of blood and exudate encourages infection and increases tension on the wound. Drain placement can be helpful in the management of dead space but they should be removed as soon as possible and typically when the output falls below 40 mL/24 hours. Appropriate dressings are essential to protect the wound from infection, trauma and desiccation and to remove exudate whilst providing a favourable warm and moist environment.

Wound infection

Classification

All surgical procedures can be classified as 'clean', 'clean–contaminated' or 'contaminated', according to the likelihood of intraoperative contamination and subsequent wound infection.

- *Clean procedures* are those in which wound contamination is not expected and the wound infection rate is less than 1%.
- *Clean–contaminated procedures* are those in which no frank focus of infection is encountered, but where a significant risk of infection is present nevertheless. Bowel surgery is a classic example. Infection rates up to 5% may occur.
- *Contaminated procedures* are those in which gross contamination is already present or inevitable and the risk of wound infection is high. Examples include bowel perforations, trauma and drainage of an abscess.

Antibiotic prophylaxis may be considered for the first two, whereas contaminated wounds are very likely to require therapeutic antibiotics (for further details on perioperative antibiotic prophylaxis, see Chapter 4).

18.2 Summary

Factors affecting wound healing

Local factors
- Wound location and cause
- Presence of infection, contamination, foreign body, necrotic or devitalised tissue.

General factors
- Age
- Family history
- Genetic predisposition (progeria, cutis laxis, Ehlers-Danlos syndrome)
- Smoking.

Systemic disease:
- Malnutrition
- Diabetes mellitus
- Haemorrhagic diatheses
- Hypoxia states (e.g., cardiopulmonary and peripheral vascular disease)
- Corticosteroid therapy
- Immunosuppression
- Chemoradiotherapy.

Surgical factors:
- Meticulous tissue handling and haemostasis
- Minimal tension
- Accurate tissue apposition
- Appropriate suture materials and dressings.

Clinical features

Wound infection typically becomes evident 3–4 days after surgery, although it can be delayed if prophylactic antibiotics have been used. Earlier infections suggest significant contamination of the wound at the time of surgery or initial injury.

The clinical signs of infection include bright erythema radiating from the wound, associated with swelling and discharge that is often malodorous. On palpation there may be fluctulance indicative of an abscess, an infected haematoma or a seroma, whilst crepitus may be felt in the presence of gas-forming organisms. In deep-seated infection, there may be no signs on the skin surface although the patient may have wound tenderness, pyrexia and other signs of sepsis. Toxaemia, bacteraemia and septicaemia can complicate any wound infection, especially where there is a collection of pus.

Prevention

Careful preoperative planning and preparation, meticulous aseptic technique, tissue handling and debridement, and the prophylactic use of antibiotics in high-risk patients all help to reduce the risk of wound infection. In addition, severely contaminated wounds may be left open for subsequent inspection and closed days later; most blast and gunshot wounds are treated in this way.

Management

In the event of infection, a wound swab or specimen of pus is routinely sent for bacteriological culture and sensitivity determination. In urgent cases, Gram staining may be useful to indicate the class of bacteria involved. The area of erythema is 'mapped out' with an indelible marker so that any progression can be monitored. Whilst trivial superficial cellulitis can be managed expectantly, spreading cellulitis is an indication for intravenous antibiotic therapy, with surgical drainage of an abscess or debridement of necrotic tissue as required. Antibiotic therapy is usually initiated on an empirical basis and refined later, depending upon wound culture and antibiotic sensitivities.

18.3 Summary

Principles of management of contaminated traumatic wounds

- Contaminated wounds should be debrided under general anaesthesia: the margins must be cleansed or sharply excised, and grit, soil and foreign bodies removed. Devitalised tissue is formally excised until viable bleeding tissue is encountered
- Primary closure is best avoided if there has been gross contamination or when treatment has been delayed for many hours. In such circumstances, attempts at primary closure increase the risk of wound infection, especially with anaerobes
- Wounds may be suitable for delayed primary closure after 24–48 hours or later
- Appropriate protection against tetanus and the use of antibiotic prophylaxis should be considered.

Involvement of other structures

All wounds must be examined carefully to assess the skin viability and injury to deeper structures. Even small, apparently innocent wounds may conceal extensive damage to underlying muscle, tendons, nerves and blood vessels. Damage to most of these structures should be evident on examination of distal motor and sensory function and circulation. In some cases, appropriate radiological imaging may help to establish the extent of soft tissue and bony injuries.

Extensive injury or severe contamination usually necessitates inpatient exploration and repair under general anaesthesia. The wound and its margins are cleansed and all foreign material removed. Devitalised tissue is excised to a healthy bleeding wound edge (Fig. 18.5). Bleeding from the wound margin is not, however, a guarantee of its ultimate survival, as impaired venous drainage can lead to progressive necrosis, particularly after a crushing or degloving injury. If there is any doubt, the wound should not be closed primarily and a 'second-look' procedure undertaken after 48 hours. When closure is delayed, any granulation tissue is usually excised and secondary closure performed if possible. If not, skin grafts (see later) can be applied to the wound bed.

The frequency of subsequent dressing changes depends upon the risk of wound healing problems. If there is a high risk of infection or skin necrosis, a wound inspection should be carried out daily. If there is little concern, however, dressing change can be carried out on alternate days.

Devitalised skin flaps

When a traumatic injury causes skin to be undermined, this usually occurs at the level between the subcutaneous fat and underlying deep fascia, which may seriously compromise the circulation to the elevated flap. This commonly occurs in the pretibial lacerations so often seen in the elderly. Skin of dubious viability will appear pale initially, becoming purple in colour before finally changing to a more obvious dark purple-black with impending necrosis. In many cases where viability is initially uncertain, staged reassessment should be considered after patient resuscitation. Closing such a wound under tension risks exacerbating the ischaemia as ensuing tissue inflammation and oedema compromise the circulation further.

18

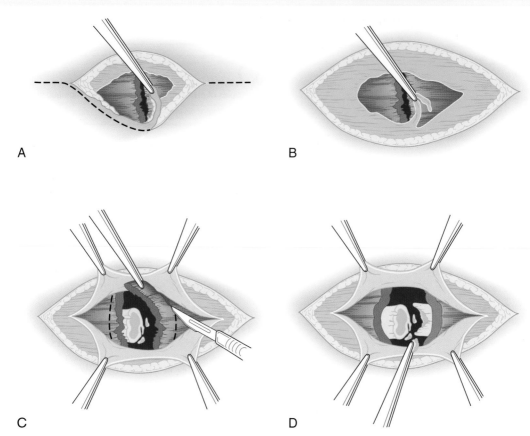

Fig. 18.5 Technique of wound debridement for a compound fracture. (A) Excision of skin edges. **(B)** Excision of fascial layer. **(C)** Excision of traumatised muscle. **(D)** Removal of small bone fragments.

Wounds with skin loss

Regardless of the cause, if significant amounts of skin and subcutaneous tissue have been lost, direct closure will not be possible. Smaller defects in less functionally or aesthetically important areas may be allowed to heal by secondary intention, especially in patients who are not fit for reconstructive surgery or where the necessary skills and resources are unavailable. For initial management of larger wounds, a vacuum-assisted closure (VAC) device can be employed to encourage granulation tissue formation and shrink the wound whilst providing protection and removing exudate. The device is contraindicated in the presence of infection, necrosis and neoplasia, but is often used to render a wound more graftable or to 'buy time' whilst complex reconstruction is planned. Nonetheless, it is often preferable to accelerate wound healing and reduce complications or scarring by 'importing' skin and other tissues from elsewhere in the body. This is done with either a 'graft', which by definition has no intrinsic circulation and therefore requires a vascularised recipient bed, or a 'flap', which by contrast incorporates its own vascular supply.

Skin grafts

These may be split- or full-thickness. The former include the epidermis and a thin layer of dermis and are harvested freehand using a specialised guarded blade (Watson Knife) or by means of a powered dermatome. Split-thickness grafts can be harvested from any region of the body although the thighs are commonly

used for ease of access and their acceptable donor site morbidity. The donor site heals by secondary intent with rapid reepithelialisation from epithelial appendages within the remaining dermis. After just 2–3 weeks the donor site can be reharvested once more if required. When it becomes necessary to cover very large wounds with limited availability of donor sites (in major burns for example), the graft can be 'meshed', permitting expansion of 1.5–6 times its original size.

Full-thickness skin grafts include the epidermis and all of the dermis, leaving a donor defect that must be closed directly or grafted. The graft size and donor sites are therefore limited: the neck, inner arm and groin are commonly used. The advantages of full-thickness grafts are that they exhibit less secondary contraction and generally produce a more aesthetic and robust scar; hence they are commonly used in reconstructive surgery of small defects of the face and hands.

All grafts require close contact with a well-vascularised wound for nourishment and survival. They will not 'take' on bone, cartilage or tendon denuded of periosteum, perichondrium or paratenon. In such cases, fresh tissue with an intrinsic blood supply must be brought into the wound.

Flaps

Flaps can be categorised by their components (skin, fascia, fat, muscle, bone or viscera such as bowel or omentum), their circulatory supply or 'pedicle' (random or named vessels, perforator vessels) and their congruity (local, distant or free). Thanks to the large variety of flap designs, they can be used to fill defects of any size, as well as to replace missing bone, muscle and nerve as required. The simplest flaps employ local skin, fat and fascia in various configurations (designs and methods of transfer), and are good alternatives to grafting for smaller defects such as those resulting from the excision of facial tumours (Fig. 18.6). Where no local option is suitable, a 'distant' flap may be brought to a wound whilst remaining attached temporarily to its original blood supply (Fig. 18.7). After 2–3 weeks the flap will have picked up a local blood supply and the original pedicle can be safely divided.

When local or distant flaps are not available or appropriate, the pedicle of almost any flap can be divided and anastomosed to a donor artery and vein adjacent to the wound (Fig. 18.8). These so-called 'free' flaps have almost completely replaced the need for complex staged reconstructions that were commonly used before the introduction of microsurgical techniques in the developed world (Fig. 18.9).

Major advances in our knowledge of the blood supply to the skin and underlying tissues have led to an explosion of new flap designs and compositions, which have revolutionised plastic

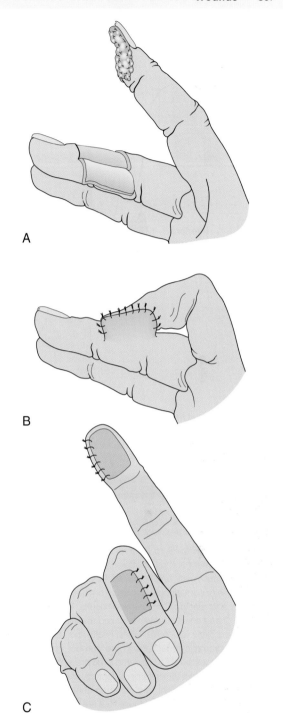

C

Fig. 18.7 Example of a pedicled (cross-finger) skin flap used to cover a defect on the tip of the index finger. **(A)** Raised. **(B)** Inset. **(C)** Divided.

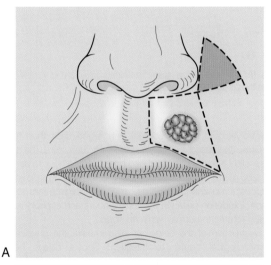

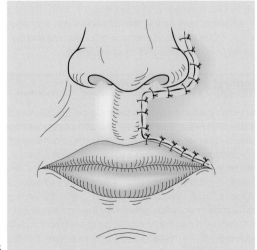

Fig. 18.6 Local skin flap used to repair a defect after the excision of a lip lesion. **(A)** Before surgery. **(B)** After surgery.

and reconstructive surgery. One example is the use of the deep inferior epigastric artery perforator (DIEP) flap for reconstruction of the breast following mastectomy. Another is the masseter muscle transfer used to restore the ability to smile for patients with a facial paralysis. The ability to join small blood vessels and nerves under the operating microscope now allows the surgeon to close defects and restore both form and function in a single operation (see also Chapter 26).

18

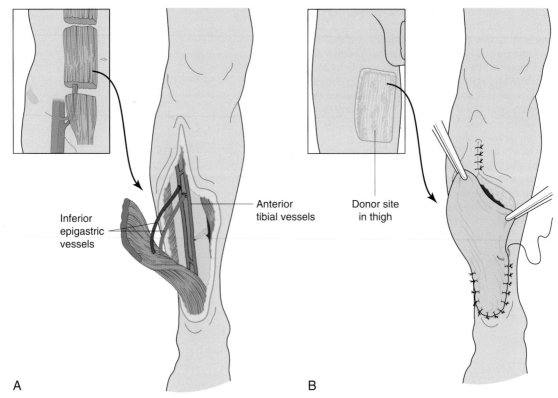

A   B

Fig. 18.8 Example of free tissue transfer based on inferior epigastric vessels. (A) Rectus abdominis muscle transferred to shin and its vessels (inferior epigastric vessels) anastomosed to anterior tibial vessels. **(B)** Muscle covered by split-skin graft.

Burns

Mechanisms

Burns range from trivial to life-threatening injuries that require extensive treatment and rehabilitation, with the prospect of permanent disfigurement and impaired function. The aetiologies include flame or contact burns, scalds from hot liquids or gasses, irradiation and electrical or chemical insults. Individuals at the extremes of age and those with impaired mental or physical abilities are particularly vulnerable. Whilst health and safety legislation has led to dramatic reductions in the number and severity of burns, most cases are still considered to be preventable. Industrial accidents account for the majority of electrical and chemical burns whilst alcohol and smoking are common contributing factors in many domestic burn injuries. House fires are often accompanied by smoke inhalation that injures the lung parenchyma and impairs tissue oxygenation. In every case, it is important to diagnose and treat concurrent preexisting comorbidities as well as other injuries that may have occurred at the time of the accident.

Local effects of burn injury

The local effects of a burn result from destruction of the tissues and the inflammatory response of the adjacent areas (Table 18.2). In its least severe form, the dermal inflammatory response consists of capillary dilation, as seen with the erythema of sunburn. With deeper burns, however, the damaged capillaries become permeable to protein, and an exudate forms with an electrolytic and protein content only slightly less than that of plasma. Increased capillary permeability can raise the typical insensible fluid loss of 15 mL/m^2 body surface/hour to as much as 200 mL/m^2 within the first few hours, resulting in blistering, hypovolaemia and oedema as lymphatic drainage fails to keep pace. Exudation peaks in the first 12 hours and capillary permeability returns to normal within 48 hours.

Destruction of the epidermis also impairs the physical and immunological barrier to infection. Sepsis delays healing, increases energy demands, and poses a threat to life, making early wound care and protection essential. With deeper burns, the epidermis and dermis are converted into a coagulum of necrotic tissue known as eschar which contracts and can compromise limb circulation and chest expansion.

General effects of burn injury

The systemic effects of a burn depend more upon its size than its depth. Large burns lead to water, salt and protein loss, hypovolaemia and increased catabolism. Circulating plasma volume falls as oedema accumulates, and fluid leaks from the wound surface. With large burns, the effect is compounded by a systemic increase in capillary permeability with widespread oedema. Red cell loss is small compared to plasma loss in the early period, and haemoconcentration, reflected by a rising haematocrit, is normally evident. If circulatory volume is not restored, hypovolaemic shock ensues. The metabolic rate increases such that in severe burns, some 7000 kcal may be expended daily, and consequent weight loss of 0.5 kg each day is not unusual unless steps are taken to prevent it.

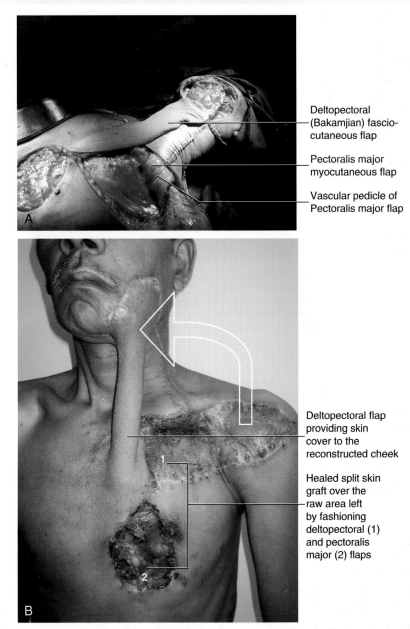

Deltopectoral (Bakamjian) fascio-cutaneous flap

Pectoralis major myocutaneous flap

Vascular pedicle of Pectoralis major flap

Deltopectoral flap providing skin cover to the reconstructed cheek

Healed split skin graft over the raw area left by fashioning deltopectoral (1) and pectoralis major (2) flaps

Fig. 18.9 Historical complex reconstruction of a patient with advanced oral carcinoma. (A) The pectoralis major myocutaneous flap provides muscle bulk to the cheek and the lining of the buccal cavity. The deltopectoral fascio-cutaneous flap provides skin cover to the cheek. **(B)** Postoperative photograph. Note the healed split-thickness skin grafts and the flaps. It should be noted that free flap reconstruction has superseded this type of procedure in many parts of the world.

Classification

Burns are classified according to the aetiology, the surface area affected and the burn depth: superficial, partial- or full-thickness (Fig. 18.10). In practice, many burns are of mixed depth.

Burn size

The approximate extent of any burn can be quickly calculated using a combination of three methods. Wallace's 'rule of nines' divides the body into areas that each represent approximately 9% of the total body surface area (TBSA) of an adult (Fig. 18.11). However, this technique is less useful in children because of the relatively large head size (about 20% of body surface at birth) and the relatively small limbs (legs are about 13%). In any case, burn injuries rarely conform to such neat patterns and another commonly employed technique is based on the assumption that the surface area of the patient's palm and closed fingers together constitute about 1% of their TBSA. Perhaps the most accurate and widely employed method is the Lund and Browder charts that provide a physical documentation of burn size and compensate for age (Fig. 18.12). Simple erythema usually subsides in a few hours and should not be included in overall burn size calculations. Hypovolaemic shock is more likely when more than 15% (10% in children) of the surface is burned.

Table 18.2 Effects of burn injury
Destruction of tissue
• Depth depends on temperature and contact time • Loss of barrier to infection • Insensible fluid loss from surface • Red cell destruction
Increased capillary permeability
• Oedema • Loss of circulating fluid volume • Hypovolaemic shock
Increased metabolic rate
• Cachexia • Immunological depression

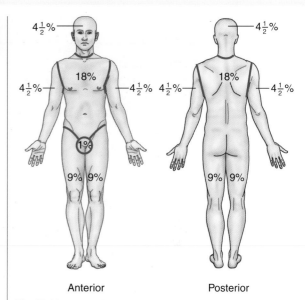

Anterior   Posterior

Fig. 18.11 Rule of nines for calculating surface areas of a burn.

Burn depth

The accurate assessment of burn depth is critical as it indicates the likelihood of spontaneous healing and therefore the need for grafting. Superficial burns are typically more painful with blistering and blanch on pressure, whereas the deeper burns may be dry, waxy and painless with no evidence of a dermal circulation. Burn depth is classically subdivided into three groups, superficial, partial and full thickness. In practice, many burns are of mixed depth (Fig. 18.13).

Superficial and superficial partial-thickness burns

Superficial and superficial partial-thickness burns affect the epidermis alone or epidermis and the superficial dermis, respectively. Reepithelialisation occurs from cells originating within the deeper epidermal appendages. Such wounds are therefore anticipated to heal spontaneously within 2–3 weeks and usually with excellent cosmetic outcomes. However, pain, swelling and fluid loss can be marked.

Deep partial-thickness burns

In deeper partial-thickness (also known as deep-dermal) burns, the epidermis and much of the dermis are destroyed. Restoration of the epidermis then depends on relatively few intact epithelial cells within the remaining appendages and those at the wound edges. Pain, swelling and fluid losses are again marked, but the burn takes longer than 3 weeks to heal and often leaves unsightly hypertrophic scars and contractures. Superimposed infection may delay healing further and can cause additional tissue destruction, effectively converting the injury to a full-thickness burn.

Full-thickness burns

Full-thickness burns destroy the epidermis and underlying dermis, including the epidermal appendages and therefore drastically limit the healing potential. The tissues undergo coagulative necrosis to form an eschar that if not debrided, begins to lift after 2–3 weeks. Without skin grafting, epidermal cover can only proceed from the inward migration of uninjured cells at the periphery of the burn, and by contraction of its base. Fibrosis, contracture and poor scars are inevitable in all but the smallest, ungrafted wounds.

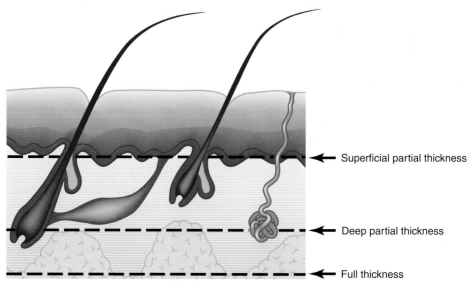

Superficial partial thickness

Deep partial thickness

Full thickness

Fig. 18.10 Depth of burn injury.

Name _____ Ward _____ Number _____ Date _____

Age _____

Lund and Browder Charts

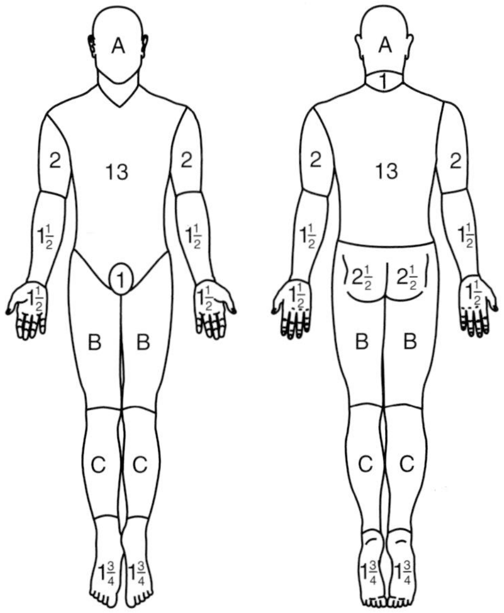

Ignore simple erythema.

▨ Superficial

▨ Deep

Region	%
Head	
Neck	
Ant. trunk	
Post. trunk	
Right arm	
Left arm	
Buttocks	
Genitalia	
Right leg	
Left leg	
Total burn	

Relative percentage of body surface area affected by age

Area	Age 0	1	5	10	15	Adult
A = 1/2 of head	9 1/2	8 1/2	6 1/2	5 1/2	4 1/2	3 1/2
B = 1/2 of thigh	2 3/4	3 1/4	4	4 1/2	4 1/2	4 3/4
C = 1/2 of one lower leg	2 1/2	2 1/2	2 3/4	3	3 1/4	3 1/2

Fig. 18.12 Lund and Browder charts for calculating percentage of the body surface area.

18

18.4 Summary

Consequences of burns

The morbidity and mortality of burns depend on the site, extent and depth of the burn and on the age and general condition of the patient

Early consequences
- Hypovolaemia (loss of protein, fluid and electrolytes)
- Metabolic derangements (hyponatraemia and hyperkalaemia, followed by risk of hypernatraemia and hypokalaemia)
- Sepsis
- Haemolysis with anaemia and need for transfusion
- Hypothermia

Short-term consequences
- Renal failure (due to hypovolaemia, haemoglobinuria and myoglobinuria)
- Respiratory failure (smoke inhalation, airway obstruction, acute respiratory distress syndrome) (ARDS)
- Catabolism and nutritional depletion
- Venous thrombosis
- Curling's ulcer and erosive gastritis

Long-term consequences
- Permanent disfigurement
- Prolonged hospitalisation
- Psychological disturbance
- Impaired mental and physical function.

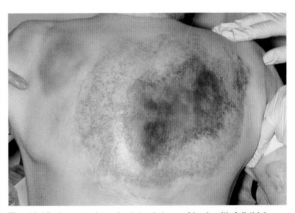

Fig. 18.13 An extensive mixed-depth burn of back with full-thickness burn evident centrally.

Determination of burn depth

There is no perfect method for the determination of burn depth and clinical experience is still essential despite newer technologies such as laser Doppler scanning. Even experienced surgeons may not be able to make an accurate initial assessment. Furthermore, burn depth may appear to evolve favourably or unfavourably depending upon local and systemic treatments.

Mechanism

Burn depth is proportional to the temperature of the causal agent and to the duration of contact. For example, scalds from liquids below 70–80°C usually produce partial-thickness injury, whereas scalds from boiling water or contact burns from an iron or radiator often produce full-thickness injury. All burns can be of mixed depth but flame burns in particular nearly always include areas of full-thickness skin loss. High-tension electrical burns are also almost always associated with full-thickness skin loss and can cause extensive injury to muscle, bone and nerve in deeper tissues.

Appearance

Erythema that blanches on pressure indicates that the epidermal damage is superficial, the dermal capillaries are intact and that the burn depth is superficial or partial-thickness. Likewise, blisters are accumulations of fluid superficial to the basal layer of the epidermis and are indicative of a viable dermal circulation and partial-thickness injury. A pale pink or white appearance frequently indicates deep partial- or full-thickness injury whilst a dry, pale and leathery eschar with visible thrombosed vessels denotes full-thickness destruction.

EBM **18.1 Burns**

'Mortality is roughly proportional to the size (% TBSA) and age of the patient.
Mortality ≈ (% BSA + age)/100
Large burns >15% in adults (>10% in children) require intravenous resuscitation.'

Strassle PD et al. Improved survival of patients with extensive burns: trends in patient characteristics and mortality among burn patients in a tertiary care burn facility, 2004–2013. J Burn Care Res. 2016. [Epub ahead of print]

Sensation

The intact cutaneous sensation evident in painful burns implies that the nerve endings have survived. As these lie at the same level as the epidermal appendages, these too are likely to be viable and reepithelialisation from such partial-thickness wounds will progress spontaneously.

Prognosis in burns

Patients at the extremes of age, with significant comorbidities or with alcohol, drug or nicotine addictions fare less well than healthy young adults following burn injury. Burn extent and depth also determine prognosis in terms of survival and scarring (EBM 18.1). Burns involving the face, neck, hands, feet or perineum are particularly liable to have cosmetic or functional implications and require inpatient management regardless of their size.

Associated respiratory injury

This is common in house fires and usually results from the inhalation of smoke from burning plastic and foam upholstery. Carbon monoxide (CO) preferentially binds to haemoglobin (Hb), displacing oxygen and therefore impairing tissue oxygenation. The half-life of CO–Hb is greatly reduced with the delivery of high flow oxygen (from 4–6 hours in room air to 75 minutes on 100% O_2). Cyanide is just one of many other commonly inhaled products of combustion that interferes with cellular mitochondrial metabolism. Despite supportive measures, respiratory injury in burn victims is frequently fatal.

Management

First aid

Safely extracting the victim from the source of injury and prompt irrigation and cooling of thermal or chemical burns is essential to minimise further damage. The ABDCE of resuscitation should be employed at the earliest opportunity and reevaluated regularly to save life or prevent prolonged suffering (Table 18.3). The burn itself should then be covered with a clean nonadhesive and preferably transparent covering such as clingfilm. The victim should be kept warm, but no other dressing should be applied to the wound until a burn surgeon has made an assessment.

Transfer to hospital

Patients with incipient hypovolaemia may take a surprisingly long time to decompensate, so it is essential that patients with significant burns are given fluid resuscitation, oxygen and analgesia as required, and transferred to hospital for specialist care as quickly as possible.

Adequate ventilation

The assessment and maintenance of an adequate airway remains the first priority. The absence of respiratory symptoms initially is no guarantee that the patient does not have an inhalational injury and attention should be given to the circumstances of the accident. Inhalational injury is suggested by dyspnoea, cough, hoarseness, cyanosis, coarse crepitations on auscultation, and the presence of soot particles around the nostrils, in the mouth or in the sputum. However, respiratory distress may not develop till several hours later. For this reason, endotracheal intubation is advisable whenever there is reasonable concern that smoke inhalation has occurred. Failure to do so can make intubation extremely difficult once airway swelling peaks.

Initial assessment and management

Once airway patency is secured, the time of injury, the type of burn and its depth and extent are established and treatment to date is documented. Intravenous fluid resuscitation is commenced for burns in excess of 15% in adults or 10% in children. Peripheral cannulation is usually straightforward but central cannulation may be required in shocked patients with vasoconstriction. Simultaneously, blood is withdrawn for cross-matching and for determination of blood count, haematocrit and renal function. Arterial blood gas analyses are performed and carboxyhaemoglobin levels measured if there is a possibility of smoke inhalation. Once an infusion has been established, the pulse rate, blood pressure and core/peripheral temperature difference are monitored. In patients undergoing fluid resuscitation, a urinary catheter is inserted to measure hourly urine output that is maintained above

---

Table 18.3 First aid for burns

- Arrest the burning process
- Remove victim to place of safety
- Ensure adequacy of airway
- Evaluate all injuries
- Avoid wound contamination with appropriate dressings (e.g., clingfilm)
- Transfer for definitive treatment as soon as possible.

Table 18.4 Hypovolaemic shock and burns

- Anticipate if total body surface area exceeds 15% (10% in children)
- Prevent by early, controlled intravenous fluid resuscitation
- Control pain with adequate intravenous administration of opiates
- Monitor patient's response to treatment and modify as required
- The formulae for fluid replacement only provide a guideline.

1 mL/kg per hour. Pain is relieved by appropriate analgesia, most often intravenous opiates.

In general, patients with burns involving more than 5% TBSA should be admitted to hospital, as should all those with significant full-thickness injury or burns in sites of important functional or cosmetic concern, including the face, hands and perineum. Patients in whom there are other significant injuries or a suspicion of non-accidental injury should also be admitted.

Prevention and treatment of burn shock

The aim of fluid resuscitation is to prevent hypovolaemic shock by prompt and adequate fluid replacement (Table 18.4). The need for fluid is greatest in the early hours, but excessive losses may persist for 36–48 hours. Various formulae are available to help calculate replacement volumes (EBM 18.2), but all should be considered as guidelines and the actual amounts of fluid given must be adjusted in the light of the patient's response to resuscitation.

Despite renal retention of sodium after injury, there is a tendency towards hyponatraemia in the first 2–3 days owing to the secre-

EBM 18.2 The Parkland formula is now widely used around the world.

'The fluid volume of crystalloid to be administered over the first 24 hours from the time of the initial burn is calculated as follows:

$$Volume = 4\,mL \times weight\,(kg) \times \%\,TBSA$$

Half of the total volume is given in the first 8 hours and the remainder over the next 16 hours. There is debate about introducing colloid, as purified protein solution (PPS) in the second 24 hours. Maintenance fluids must be calculated and administered in addition to the resuscitation volume indicated by the Parkland formula.'

Foster KN, Caruso DM. Fluid resuscitation in burn patients: current care and new frontiers. Crit Care Clin. 2016 Oct;32(4): xv–xvi.

tion of antidiuretic hormone and the sequestration of sodium in oedema fluid. As inflammatory oedema is reabsorbed, the serum sodium concentration returns to normal, and unless water intake is maintained, there is a danger of hypernatraemia. Tissue destruction releases large amounts of potassium into the extracellular fluid (ECF), but hyperkalaemia is largely prevented by increased renal excretion as part of the metabolic response to injury. After the first few days have passed, ongoing potassium losses can produce hypokalaemia in patients unable to eat and drink normally.

Oral intake

Although many burn patients are thirsty, paralytic ileus may occur during the first 48 hours in those with very large burns, so that giving oral fluids too soon can cause gastric distension, vomiting and aspiration. Most patients are able to drink normally after 48 hours and should be encouraged to do so.

Nutritional management

The increased energy expenditure following a severe burn can be reduced by nursing in a warm environment (30–32°C). A high calorie intake is impractical during the period of hypovolaemic shock, but is encouraged as soon as the patient can eat. The daily caloric intake in adults can be estimated as 20 kcal/kg body weight plus 70 kcal/% burn. It is particularly important to provide sufficient protein (1 g/kg body weight plus 3 g/% burn). In large burns, oral intake can usually be supplemented at 48 hours by enteral feeding using a fine-bore nasogastric tube and weight loss can be limited. Vitamin supplements and iron should also be provided. Enteral feeding helps to preserve gut integrity and minimise the risk of bacterial translocation, and is far preferable to parenteral nutrition in burned patients.

Blood transfusion

Blood transfusion is rarely indicated in the first 24 hours but may be needed thereafter in patients with large full-thickness burns. Continuing red cell destruction and bone marrow suppression in deep burns can necessitate repeated transfusion. Haemoglobin concentration and haematocrit should be monitored regularly.

Organ failure and burn shock

Organ failure and shock are discussed in more detail in Chapter 1.

Respiratory complications

Inhalation of smoke can cause direct heat damage to the upper airway, carbon monoxide poisoning and damage to the lung parenchyma from other chemicals, all of which predispose to infection and respiratory failure. Chest x-rays and blood gas analyses are repeated regularly in patients with ventilation problems. Arterial hypoxaemia and carbon monoxide poisoning require oxygen therapy, and may necessitate early endotracheal intubation and assisted ventilation. Patients with head and neck burns are best nursed head-up to encourage the dispersal of oedema. Continued observation is mandatory and physiotherapy is essential to clear bronchial secretions. Antibiotics should only be prescribed when chest infection is deemed likely to occur. Tracheostomy is occasionally unavoidable despite the problems associated with its management. Encircling eschar impairing chest or abdominal expansion must be incised (escharotomy) or excised.

Renal failure

Acute tubular necrosis may complicate extensive burns, especially in the elderly, those with preexisting renal disease and those who develop haemoglobinuria or myoglobinuria. These pigments appear in the urine after massive red cell destruction or extensive muscle damage (particularly after electrical injury), and can damage the tubules and obstruct urine flow by forming casts. Hourly urine output should be maintained at 30–50 mL in adults. Falling output reflects inadequate resuscitation or impending renal failure (acute tubular necrosis). Measurement of urine osmolality and the response to a test infusion will distinguish between them. Diuretics are used only if oliguria persists despite adequate fluid replacement, when 300 mg/kg of 15–20% mannitol may be infused following a test dose.

18

Sepsis

Septicaemia is a constant threat until skin cover has been fully restored. Wound colonisation amounts to a reservoir of infective organisms. Catheters, cannulae and tracheostomies are all potential sources of infection and they should be replaced regularly using aseptic technique. The incidence of septicaemia can be reduced with topical antibacterial agents and early excision and grafting. However, in large burns the risk remains high. Regular monitoring with blood cultures is advisable in some cases. Systemic antibiotics are not prescribed routinely because of the risk of promoting superinfection with multiresistant organisms. Their use is reserved for invasive infection, guided by positive blood cultures and sensitivities.

In full-thickness injury, thrombosis of cutaneous vessels impairs the normal resistance to infection. In large burns, cellular and humoral immune mechanisms are also depressed. Organisms readily colonise the burn wound and will multiply and invade surrounding tissues especially if necrosis is present. Commensal staphylococci remain the most common infecting organism and *Pseudomonas aeruginosa* is ever present in most burn units, whereas haemolytic streptococci are feared because of their ability to exacerbate burn depth, cause systemic illness and interfere with graft take.

Curling's ulcer and gastric erosions

Acute duodenal ulceration (Curling's ulcer) and multiple gastric erosions may follow major burns. Early resumption of enteral feeding reduces their incidence, and H_2-receptor antagonists such as omeprazole are prescribed prophylactically.

Initial cleansing and debridement

The wound is cleaned with a mild detergent containing antiseptic and saline, in an operating theatre or clean dressing room using aseptic technique. Loose devitalised tissues are removed and large blisters are deroofed. General anaesthesia may be necessary, but in many cases sufficient pain relief can be provided by intravenous opiates.

Dressings

Dressings are an essential part of wound management to protect the wound from contamination and promote a healing environment.

Exposure

Burns to the face and neck in particular are difficult to dress and may be exposed to the air. Evaporation of the protein-rich exudate leaves a dry, adherent crust. Alternatively the wound may be kept moist with the application of petroleum jelly.

Evaporative dressings

These basic yet comfortable dressings minimise contamination whilst allowing exudate to evaporate. The wound is covered by a layer of sterile nonadherent dressing such as paraffin gauze or Mepitel, a layer of cotton gauze swabs, a bulky layer of cotton wool or Gamgee and an outer crepe bandage. The dressing is reviewed daily but can be left in place for several days between changes, unless exudate soaks through to the outside.

Semi-occlusive and occlusive dressings

Hydrogel and hydrocolloid dressings absorb modest exudates but offer no particular advantages in acute management.

Polythene bags filled with sterile liquid paraffin provide excellent cover for hand burns when secured at the wrist, permitting mobility and ready access for physiotherapy and splinting.

Topical antibacterial agents

Silver sulfadiazine cream (Flamazine) and povidone-iodine (Betadine) impregnated dressings are valuable local antibacterial agents for large and small burns. In partial-thickness burns that are anticipated to heal spontaneously, Flamazine is a useful antimicrobial dressing. However, its use in the first 48 hours is discouraged because it can make interpretation of burn depth more difficult.

'Biological' dressings

Xenografts such as porcine skin and human allograft can be supplied freeze-dried and reconstituted for use as temporary 'biological' dressings, but they are expensive and of course are eventually rejected by the patient's immune system. 'Biobrane' is a biosynthetic dressing comprising a silicone layer bonded to a nylon mesh that is impregnated with porcine collagen. It is useful in the management of clean superficial and superficial partial-thickness burns. 'Transcyte' is similar to Biobrane but is impregnated with newborn human fibroblasts and is indicated for use in deeper partial-thickness burns. Both can also act as temporary dressings in excised burns awaiting autografting.

Relief of constriction (escharotomy)

The danger of progressive respiratory embarrassment from encircling and contracting eschar has been mentioned. Increasing oedema beneath circumferential eschar in the limbs may also imperil peripheral circulation. Relieving incisions (escharotomies) that avoid important superficial nerves and vessels are made across deep circumferential burns in the first few hours after injury. Because these incisions can bleed profusely, it is important to have cautery readily available.

Restoration of epidermal cover

Small full-thickness and deep-dermal burns may be suitable for primary excision and grafting, usually within 48–72 hours of injury. For larger burns, the necrotic layers of skin must be excised and the defect grafted. Tangential excision is used for deep-dermal burns in order to spare the viable deep dermis. The dead outer layers of skin are progressively shaved down to bleeding dermis and a split-skin graft is applied immediately. With full-thickness burns, it may be quicker and more successful to deeply excise necrotic skin and subcutaneous tissue before grafting. In the largest burns, however, there may be insufficient donor skin available for autografting. In these cases, grafting can be staged while donor sites recover or, where finances allow, the patient's own keratinocytes can be cultured over 2–3 weeks into sheets or a suspension for later application to the burn wound. In the meantime, excised burns can be covered with synthetic dermal substitutes such as Integra or Matriderm, which will become incorporated into the wound as a neodermis, helping to improve ultimate scar quality. Wound colonisation with haemolytic streptococci is a troublesome cause of graft failure and when such infection is present, grafting must be deferred until the patient has been successfully treated with appropriate topical and systemic antimicrobials.

Full-thickness grafts are rarely used for primary burn grafting but may be used in secondary reconstruction of cosmetically or functionally important areas such as the face, hands and genitalia.

Long-term functional and cosmetic outcomes

Wound closure is not the only end-point of burn management. Good cosmetic and functional outcomes are essential. To this end, skin grafts and donor sites must be kept soft and supple by regular massage and application of moisturising cream for many months. Splints and physiotherapy may be needed to mobilise joints and prevent joint contractures. Elastic pressure garments and silicone dressings may help to prevent the development of hypertrophic scars. In spite of this, secondary reconstructive procedures may be required over many years to release contractures or restore form and function. Psychological support is essential for patients having difficulty coming to terms with their disfigurement and physical limitations.

Skin and soft tissue lesions

Diagnosis

A thorough assessment of any lesion is necessary to determine its site, size, shape and consistency and whether or not it is attached to the skin or deeper structures such as muscle or nerve. Surface changes often indicate an epidermal origin, whereas the surface overlying dermal lesions appears normal. The colour of a skin lesion is also an important feature in its diagnosis.

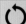

18.5 Summary

Key questions when examining skin swellings

- Is the swelling located in the skin or in the subcutaneous tissues?
- Is the swelling epidermal, dermal, subcutaneous or deep?
- Is the swelling pigmented?
- What is the size of the lesion?
- What is its shape: smooth and round or irregular and craggy?
- How firm is it: soft, fluctuant, firm or hard?
- Is there any associated ulceration or discharge?
- How long has it been present?
- Is it changing: increasing or decreasing or fluctuating in size?
- Are there any associated signs or symptoms: pain, pulsatility, nerve dysfunction?
- Is there any relevant personal or family history?

Infections

Skin infections and abscesses are relatively common and usually benign unless the patient is immunocompromised, diabetic or elderly. Commensal organisms such as *Staphylococcus aureus* are most commonly involved, whilst streptococci usually cause more aggressive and prolonged infections. A precipitating event should be sought and treated. Abscesses should be drained and cellulitis treated with appropriate empirical antibiotics that are modified once the results of culture and sensitivities are available.

Cellulitis

This is a nonsuppurative invasive infection commonly caused by β-hemolytic streptococci, staphylococci and *Clostridium* species. Lymphoedematous and immunosuppressed patients are particularly at risk. Often there is a history of a minor injury or bite that progresses to spreading erythema and inflammation, which should be carefully monitored. Tissue destruction and skin ulceration may also occur. Systemic signs including fever, tachycardia and an elevated white cell count, and erythrocyte sedimentation rate (ESR) may be seen. The signs of inflammation are classically present and the condition usually spreads due to enzymatic activity of the invading organisms. Systemic antibiotics and supportive therapy are required. Affected limbs should be elevated.

Necrotising fasciitis

This is a rapidly progressive necrotising infection affecting the subcutaneous tissue and deep fascia, which can occur de novo or as a complication following invasive procedures (Fig. 18.14). Like most infections, it is more prevalent in the immunocompromised patient. Group A β-haemolytic *Streptococcus* is frequently implicated, although the condition is usually polymicrobial including anaerobes and gram-negative aerobes. In the presence of organisms such as *Clostridium*, gas may accumulate under the subcutaneous tissue and may be visible on x-ray and palpable as crepitus. Fournier's gangrene is a form of necrotising fasciitis that is localised to the scrotum and perineal area and closely associated with diabetes, whereas infections that involve the abdominal wall are sometimes referred to as Meleney's gangrene.

These infections can be difficult to recognise in their early stages, but incredibly rapid progression and disproportionate pain are suggestive. The Laboratory Risk Indicator for Necrotising Fasciitis (LRINEC) score (incorporating measures of C-reactive protein (CRP), white blood cell count (WBC), haemoglobin, sodium, glucose and creatinine) may help support the diagnosis. Aggressive antimicrobial treatment is essential but urgent surgical debridement of all affected tissue is necessary and life saving.

18

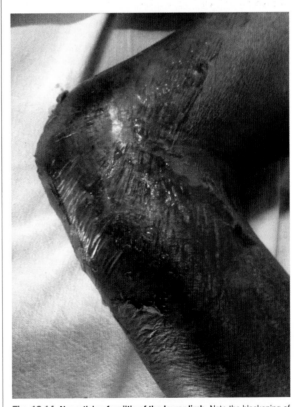

Fig. 18.14 Necrotising fasciitis of the lower limb. Note the blackening of the skin with exudation and partial sloughing of skin in places.

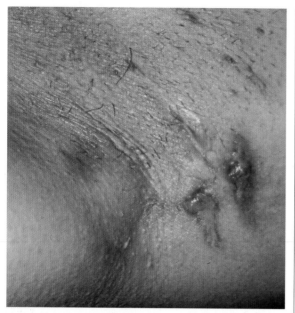

Fig. 18.15 **Hidradenitis suppurativa of the axilla.** Note the discharging sinuses and the surrounding cicatrisation.

Hidradenitis suppurativa

This is a chronic and cicatrising suppurative infection of the apocrine sweat glands that occurs commonly in females during their twenties and thirties. It often affects the axillary region, but also the perineum, groin and inframammary folds (Fig. 18.15). Patients, who are often obese and smoke, present with repeated episodes of painful swelling and discharge of pus from abscesses. There may be an association with Crohn's or other autoimmune diseases. Antianaerobic therapy (clindamycin, metronidazole) is often required, but lifestyle changes should be encouraged. If this fails, complete surgical excision may be needed to remove all subcutaneous tracts. Skin grafting or local flap reconstruction follows.

Cysts

Epidermoid cysts

Epidermoid cysts are common subcutaneous unilocular swellings arising from inflammation in a pilosebaceous unit, often in the head and neck, which are fixed to the overlying skin where a small central punctum is often visible (Fig. 18.16). On the scalp or scrotum they are known as 'pilar' or tricholemmal cysts. They have a thin wall of flattened epidermal cells and contain keratin and its breakdown products that appear cheesy-white and resemble sebum (hence the misnomer 'sebaceous cyst'). True sebaceous cysts arise from the sebaceous glands and are much less common. Treatment of an uncomplicated cyst is by simple excision. When infection occurs, excision should be deferred. An infected cyst may rupture spontaneously and the appearance can resemble a cutaneous malignancy (Fig. 18.17). In some cases, the inflammation destroys the cyst lining making excision unnecessary.

Dermoid cysts

Dermoid cysts arise from nests of epidermal cells that have been sequestered in the dermis during development or

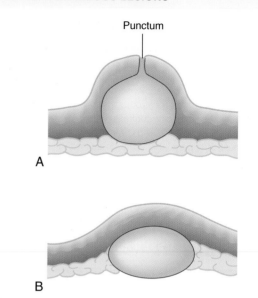

Fig. 18.16 **Types of cyst.** **(A)** Sebaceous (epidermoid). **(B)** Dermoid.

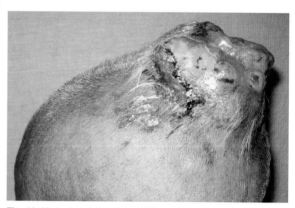

Fig. 18.17 **An infected cyst mimicking a cutaneous malignancy.**

implanted as a result of trauma (inclusion cysts) (Fig. 18.16). Congenital dermoid cysts are found at the sites of embryonic fusion, commonly at the root of the nose, the forehead, the occiput and in the midline of the neck. External angular dermoids lie adjacent to the lateral brow in the line of fusion of the maxilla and frontal bones and are the most common congenital dermoid cyst.

Implantation or inclusion cysts are found at any site of injury, notably the palmar surfaces of the hands and fingers. They are lined by squamous epithelium and contain sebum, degenerate cells and, in some cases, hair. Any troublesome cysts can be excised but care should be taken with congenital dermoids as they may extend deeply.

Tumours of the skin

Epidermal tumours are common and can arise from the basal cells, keratinocytes or melanocytes, whereas dermal tumours arising from connective tissue elements are relatively rare (Table 18.5). The skin may also be involved with metastatic tumour deposits from melanoma, breast cancer, oropharyngeal cancers and less commonly renal, lung, gastrointestinal and uterine cancers.

Table 18.5 Classification of skin tumours	
Epidermal neoplasms (common)	
From basal germinal cells:	**From melanocytes:**
Papilloma	Benign pigmented mole
Infective wart	Common mole
Seborrhoeic keratosis	Giant hairy mole
Papilloma	Blue naevus
Keratoacanthoma	Halo naevus
Premalignant keratosis	Malignant melanoma
Carcinoma in situ	Lentigo maligna melanoma
Epidermoid cancer	Superficial spreading
Basal cell carcinoma (rodent	melanoma
ulcer)	Nodular melanoma
Squamous cell carcinoma	Other forms of melanoma
Dermal neoplasms (rare)	
Benign	
Fibroma	
Neurofibroma	
Malignant	
Dermatofibrosarcoma protruberans	
Angiosarcoma	
Pleomorphic dermal sarcoma	

Benign lesions

Papillomas

Papillomas (or warts) are common sessile or pedunculated benign skin neoplasms that project from the skin surface.

Squamous cell papillomas (SCC) (viral warts)

These present as round or oval elevated, greyish-brown lesions with a filiform surface and keratinised projections that may be studded with spots of blood (Figs 18.18 and 18.19). They are common in children and immunosuppressed patients, often regressing spontaneously but may need to be treated with acetic acid, laser or cryotherapy. Plantar warts (verruca plantaris) become depressed into the sole and may be intensely painful and resistant to treatment (Fig. 18.20).

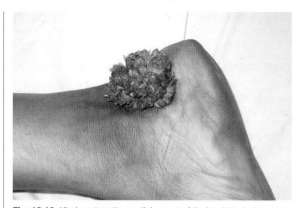

Fig. 18.19 Viral wart on the medial aspect of the leg. Note the keratinous projections from the surface.

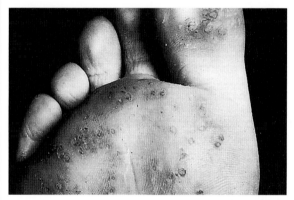

Fig. 18.20 Verruca plantaris (plantar warts). A plaque of closely grouped warts on the sole of the foot.

Seborrhoeic keratoses (senile warts)

These basal cell papillomas are common in the face and trunk in late middle age (Fig. 18.21). They present as yellowish-brown or dark, greasy plaques with a cracked irregular surface that

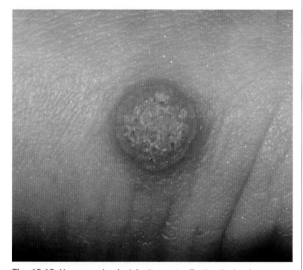

Fig. 18.18 Verruca vulgaris. Infective warts affecting the hand.

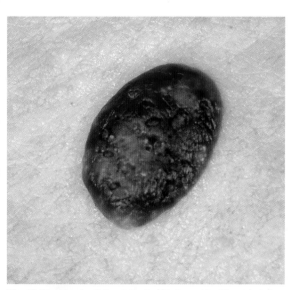

Fig. 18.21 Seborrhoeic keratosis (usually brownish, this example is unusually dark).

classically appears to be 'stuck on' to the skin surface. Parts of the lesion may fall off spontaneously but unsightly lesions may be treated by curettage or excision.

Fibro-epithelial polyps (acrochordon or skin tags)

These are typically small flesh-coloured lesions on a stalk of normal epithelium that appear around the neck, armpits, groins and eyelids. If necessary they can be easily excised.

Dermatofibroma

Also known as histiocytoma and sclerosing haemangioma, these are firm or hard, nodular lesions of the skin, which occur commonly over the hands and feet. They are thought to represent a stage between chronic inflammation and a benign neoplasm. They are brownish in colour and can have a rough surface. The lesions are freely mobile over deeper structures and are often itchy. Treatment is by surgical excision.

Keratoacanthoma (molluscum sebaceum)

These usually present as solitary lesions on the face, neck and hands of fair skinned individuals, most commonly in the sixth decade. They typically grow rapidly over 2–3 months from a small red papule to a large hemispherical nodule with a friable keratin core (Fig. 18.22). Growth ceases for a similar period of time before the lesion regresses spontaneously. The lesions do not metastasise, however they do resemble SCC both clinically and histologically, and for this reason simple excision is most often recommended.

Benign naevi (moles)

The total number of melanocytes in our skin is relatively fixed (approximately 800/mm^2), regardless of the colour of the individual, yet the amount of pigment produced varies greatly. Condensations of melanocytes form a naevus or mole that can be congenital or acquired (Fig. 18.23). The former are present at birth, tend to be larger and grow with the individual, often becoming darker, thicker and hairy with age. Congenital melanocytic naevi over 20 cm are known as giant hairy naevi and occur in around 0.002% of individuals, but are associated with a significant risk of malignant degeneration.

Normal

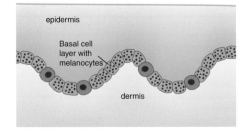

Junctional naevus

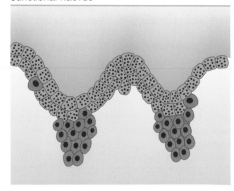

Dermal naevus

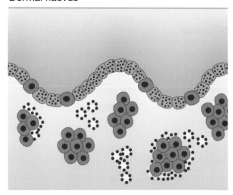

Compound naevus

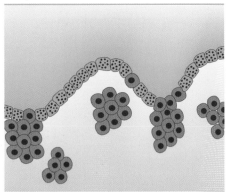

Fig. 18.23 Histopathological types of benign mole.

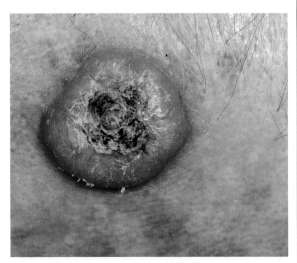

Fig. 18.22 Keratoacanthoma affecting the temple of an elderly man.

Acquired naevi are of three types: junctional, compound or intradermal depending upon the depth of the melanocytes within the skin. Their number is largely genetically driven but fair skin and sunburn are associated with increased incidence. Junctional naevi, which predominate in childhood, harbour cells at the junction between the epidermis and dermis. They are typically even coloured, mid to dark brown, flat and circular. Compound naevi are composed of cells within the dermis and epidermis. They tend to be similarly coloured but more elevated with a rougher surface and are hair bearing. The melanocytes of intradermal naevi are located in the dermis. Such lesions are typically paler or even skin coloured and more prominent than compound naevi. The vast majority of moles are asymptomatic and rarely undergo malignant transformation (1 in 100,000). Transformation is more likely in the presence of growth, deepening pigmentation, irregular shape or colour, ulceration, itch or bleeding. Any mole that develops these characteristics should be biopsied urgently.

Special types of naevi

Blue naevi are round, flat or elevated and have a blue hue from the relatively deep location of the melanocytes within the dermis. They tend to occur in older children but can develop at any age. Excision is only required for cosmetic reasons or when the diagnosis is in doubt.

Occasionally, the immune system targets a particular naevus giving rise to a *halo naevus* with a characteristic ring of depigmentation around the original naevus which itself fades and eventually disappears.

18.6 Summary

Epidermal neoplasms arising from melanocytes

- A mole is due to a condensation of melanocytes at particular levels in the skin
- Acquired naevi are common in childhood
- Migration of melanocytes into the dermis produces a dermal naevus, whereas migration to both dermis and epidermis produces a compound naevus
- Only 1 in 100,000 moles become malignant, so that the presence of a mole is not in itself an indication for removal. Active growth in childhood need not cause concern, but growth thereafter should cause concern
- Excision is indicated if a mole shows an increase in pigmentation, irregular colour or border, itching or bleeding, or if it looks different from the others—the 'ugly duck' sign.

Premalignant lesions

Actinic (solar) keratosis

This premalignant lesion is characterised by a scaly, erythematous macule or patch of skin that usually develops in the sun-exposed areas of elderly and fair skinned individuals, especially those with a history of excessive sun exposure (Fig. 18.24). They can expand slowly, becoming raised and crusty and may form hyperkeratotic horns or ulcers (Fig. 18.25). Although untreated lesions may regress, most persist or have a risk of developing into SCC in up to 20% of cases. Treatment options following diagnostic biopsy include cryotherapy or laser ablation, topical chemotherapy (5-fluoro-uracil, imiquimod, diclofenac), photodynamic therapy or surgical excision.

In situ or intraepidermal squamous cell carcinoma (Bowen's disease)

This is a localised patch of neoplastic cells that are confined to the epidermis. It appears as a flat, erythematous and scaly plaque that

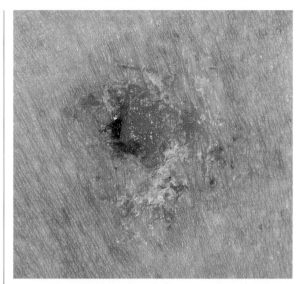

Fig. 18.24 Actinic keratosis.

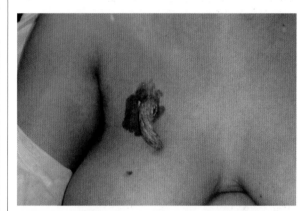

Fig. 18.25 A keratin horn in an elderly patient. The lesion was excised under local anaesthesia.

is well demarcated but irregularly shaped. It can occur anywhere on the skin but typically on sun-exposed areas, especially the legs. Prevalence is higher in females (60–80%). The lesions are slow growing and only 3–5% will progress to invasive disease that is usually manifest by thickening and rapid growth, more characteristic of an SCC. In situ SCC affecting the glans penis or vulva is known as erythroplasia of Queyrat and is associated with HPV infection. Treatment following targeted biopsy is as above for actinic keratosis, and the prognosis is similarly excellent.

Malignant lesions

Malignant skin lesions typically occur in later life following prolonged sun (UVA and UVB) exposure with episodes of sunburn especially in fair skinned individuals. Other risk factors include inherited disorders (albinism, XP), immunosuppression, infection (e.g., HIV, HPV), irradiation, chronic wounds, chemical exposure (arsenic, tar), family history and large numbers of moles, especially if atypical or dysplastic.

The most common forms of skin cancer are basal (90%) and squamous cell carcinomas (BCC/SCC) whilst malignant melanoma (MM) and malignant tumours of the adnexal structures are less common, but generally more aggressive with a worse prognosis.

Basal cell carcinoma (rodent ulcer)

This is the most common type of primary skin malignancy that typically presents on the head, neck (80%) and trunk. The lesions are slow growing and locally invasive but virtually never metastasise (Fig. 18.26). They classically present as firm nodules with pearlescence, telangiectatic, rolled borders and occasional central ulceration. Cystic degeneration results in increased prominence and translucence. Clinical subtypes include superficial, nodular, sclerosing (morphoeic), infiltrative, cystic and pigmented lesions. The infiltrative and sclerosing forms often have less distinct features and borders making full excision more difficult to achieve without employing Moh's micrographic surgery. Occasionally, the tumour is highly invasive and can burrow deeply, despite little apparent surface activity (Fig. 18.27). Some superficial lesions can be treated appropriately in a similar way to actinic keratosis and in situ SCC described above. Thicker lesions, however, necessitate formal excision (3–4 mm margin) and reconstruction, although radiotherapy can be very effective in patients who are not fit for surgery.

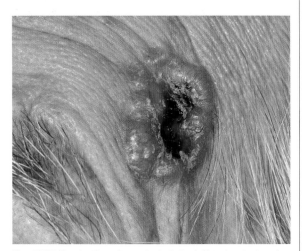

Fig. 18.26 Basal cell carcinoma (rodent ulcer). Note the raised pearly edge.

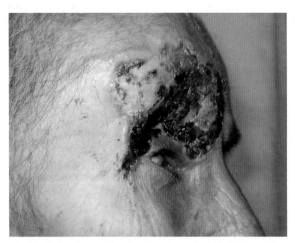

Fig. 18.27 An advanced basal cell carcinoma (rodent ulcer) near the inner canthus of eye. Note the destruction of the frontal bone.

Moh's surgery is also indicated for lesions that are recurrent or are adjacent to important structures that should be preserved if possible.

Squamous cell carcinoma

This is less common but more aggressive and faster growing than a BCC (Fig. 18.28). It arises from the stratum spinosum of the epidermis and may affect any area although is particularly common on exposed parts such as the ear, cheeks, lower lips and backs of the hands. It may develop from an area of epithelial hyperplasia or keratosis. The lesions appear as hard erythematous nodules, which proliferate and occasionally ulcerate. The regional lymph nodes can be involved early and should be examined at diagnosis and throughout follow-up. Treatment is by complete surgical excision (>4 mm margin) or radiotherapy if surgery is not possible. The role of sentinel lymph node biopsy is currently under review but positive nodal involvement necessitates formal regional lymphadenectomy with adjuvant radiotherapy in many cases.

Marjolin's ulcer

This represents malignant degeneration within a preexisting scar or chronic inflammatory lesion with an average latency period of around 30 years. The incidence is highest in old burn scars followed by osteomyelitic wounds; however, they also occur in areas of venous insufficiency and on pressure sores. The histological change is usually that of a well-differentiated SCC but other tumours are occasionally seen (Fig. 18.29). The lesions are typically slow to develop and metastasise late but are very aggressive thereafter. Treatment involves excision with wide (>4 mm) margins and appropriate reconstruction. Sentinel lymph node biopsy may also be undertaken but the role of radio/chemotherapy is less well established.

Malignant melanoma (MM)

This most aggressive form of skin cancer predominantly occurs in fair-skinned individuals and is rare in blacks in whom it typically occurs on the soles or palms (acral lentiginous type). Rarely, melanomas may arise on the mucosa, intestines or the eye. Whilst over-exposure to ultraviolet light (UVA and UVB), especially in

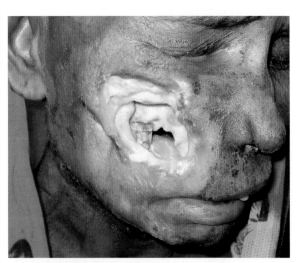

Fig. 18.28 An advanced squamous cell carcinoma of the cheek that has invaded into the maxilla and soft tissues of the cheek and formed an oro-cutaneous fistula.

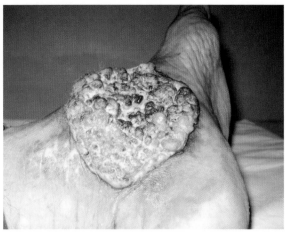

Fig. 18.29 A squamous cell carcinoma (Marjolin's ulcer) developing in a old scar. Note the everted edge characteristic of a squamous cell carcinoma.

childhood, is the major aetiological factor, the relationship is not as simple as widely thought. The incidence of MM is increasing globally and is highest in Australia and New Zealand (40/100,000 pa), then Europe and North America and much lower in Africa, Asia and South America. Malignant melanomas are more common in females, often on the legs, whilst on men they are more common on the trunk. About 25% of all MM are thought to arise from preexisting naevi. The lifetime risk of MM is increased in individuals with 100 or more common naevi or fewer atypical, dysplastic or giant naevi. Other risk factors include immunodeficiency, various genetic disorders including xeroderma pigmentosum and those with a personal or family history of MM and higher socioeconomic status. Five distinct clinicopathological subtypes are described.

Lentigo maligna (in situ melanoma/Hutchison's melanotic freckle)

One in ten melanomas arise from a melanotic or senile freckle. These occur most commonly on the face in old age, appearing as a light brown–red patch that grows slowly and darkens (Fig. 18.30). The well-defined edge of the lesion may appear serrated and the surface pigmentation is typically variable. This premalignant phase may last for 10–15 years following which the

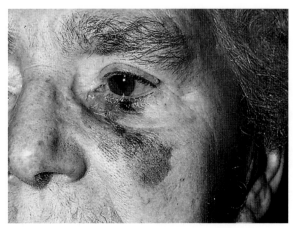

Fig. 18.30 Lentigo maligna (in situ melanoma) on the face of an elderly man.

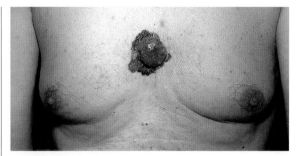

Fig. 18.31 Superficial spreading melanoma.

development of a thicker, darker papule within the lesion is suggestive of invasive, vertical growth, at which point the lesion is referred to as a lentigo maligna melanoma (LMM).

Superficial spreading melanoma (SSMM)

This is the most common type of malignant melanoma (Fig. 18.31). It most often occurs on the trunk in middle age. A preinvasive phase lasts for up to 2 years during which the malignant cells spread outwards (horizontal growth) in the epidermis. The surface is slightly raised, the outline is indistinct; pigmentation is patchy and there may be a range of colours. Invasion of the dermis (vertical growth) occurs when the lesion is still relatively small and produces an indurated nodule, which often ulcerates or bleeds. Once this phase has begun, metastatic spread is more likely.

Nodular melanoma

This elevated, deeply pigmented melanoma can occur at any site and at any age but is particularly common on the legs of females. In contrast to SSMM, nodular melanomas are vertically invasive from the outset and there is no prior intraepidermal spread and therefore no surrounding pigmented macule. The nodule grows and darkens progressively and the surface may ulcerate, itch and bleed readily. In time, satellite nodules may appear in adjacent skin.

Other types of malignant melanoma

Amelanotic melanomas are rare, pale pink lesions that can grow rapidly. The lack of pigment on clinical examination can lead to misdiagnosis although histological examination will demonstrate pigment in virtually every case. *Acral lentiginous melanoma* is seen on the soles and palms (Fig. 18.32). It resembles superficial spreading melanoma in its behaviour, although the thick skin of the affected regions may mask some of the features and late presentation is the norm. *Subungual melanomas* develop beneath a nail, typically the thumb or great toe, in the middle-aged and elderly. Pigmentation is not usually visible in the early stages and the lesion is often misdiagnosed as subungual haematoma. *Desmoplastic melanomas* are rare, aggressive, scar-like lesions accounting for 1% of all melanomas.

Spread of malignant melanoma

Malignant melanomas spread readily via the lymphatics and bloodstream and such spread can be unpredictable. In transit, metastases may develop in the lymphatics, forming painless dark nodules between the primary tumour and the regional nodal basin. Lymph node metastases most often present as firm enlargement of a node within the primary nodal basin from where the disease spreads to adjacent regional and central nodes.

18

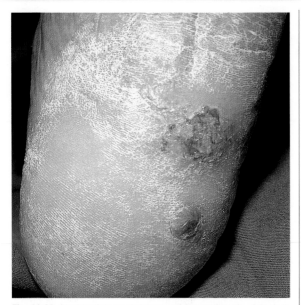

Fig. 18.32 Acral lentiginous melanoma arising on the sole of the foot.

Blood-borne metastases can occur at any site but are common in the brain, liver, lungs, skin and subcutaneous tissues. In about 5% of cases, metastases are present in the absence of a recognisable primary site.

18.7 Summary

Malignant melanoma

- Malignant melanoma is predominantly a disease of fair-skinned individuals
- Exposure to sunlight is the key aetiological factor
- The lesion is more common in females (legs) than males (trunk)
- 25% of all malignant melanomas arise from a preexisting naevus
- The essential feature of malignancy is invasion of the dermis by proliferating melanocytes (which show large nuclei, prominent nucleoli and frequent mitoses)
- Malignant melanoma spreads rapidly via the lymphatics and the bloodstream. 'In transit' metastases may develop in the lymphatics of the skin and subcutaneous tissues.

Management of malignant melanoma

Excision biopsy with a 2–3-mm margin down to, but not inclusive of the deep fascia, is essential to confirm the diagnosis and identify certain histological features that inform further clinical management. The Breslow thickness, defined as the vertical distance in millimetres from the granular layer of the epidermis to the deepest point of the tumour, is the most significant prognostic indicator and is used to determine the required secondary excision margins designed to reduce the chance of recurrence (EBM 18.3). For tumours less than 1 mm thick or when mitotic rate cannot be determined, Clark's level has more prognostic value than Breslow thickness (Fig. 18.33).

Tumours with a Breslow thickness of >1 mm or those with evidence of ulceration or a mitotic rate of $>1/mm^2$ are often candidates for sentinel lymph node biopsy (SLNB). This technique employs radioisotopes and blue dye injected around the primary tumour, which then migrates to and concentrates in the primary draining lymph nodes that are then easily identified and excised. This reduces the morbidity associated with a block dissection of the regional lymph nodes and allows the pathologist to concentrate their efforts on the two or three nodes that are most likely to be involved. However, if the sentinel nodes are involved or clinically enlarged nodes are present, regional completion or therapeutic lymphadenectomy is indicated. There is no role for elective (prophylactic) lymph node dissection in the absence of clinically involved nodes. The significance of micrometastases detected on SLNB remains under debate.

For metastatic disease confined to a single limb, isolated limb perfusion with cytotoxic drugs can be used in patients with recurrent disease or multiple in-transit lesions. The treatment of metastatic melanoma remains unsatisfactory; therefore the key to the successful management of malignant melanoma is early diagnosis and appropriate surgical excision (EBM 18.3), with appropriate reconstruction. Once disease is disseminated, systemic chemotherapy (dacarbazine, interferon, interleukin-2) has some benefit but more recently developed immunotherapies target the melanoma's ability to avoid innate immune responses and show great promise (PD-1, CTLA-4 inhibitors).

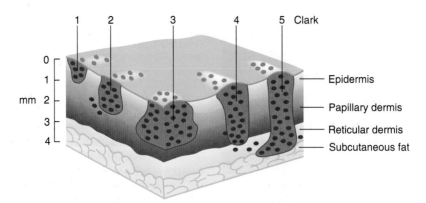

Fig. 18.33 Methods of grading malignant melanoma according to depth of invasion.

EBM | 18.3 Melanoma

'A superficial shave biopsy should not be carried out on suspicious pigmented lesions as it may prevent accurate assessment of Breslow thickness.

Excision margins for primary melanoma:

Melanoma in situ (0.5 mm)	Excision margin	5-year survival
Breslow thickness		
<1 mm	→ *1 cm*	*95–100%*
1–2 mm	→ *1–2 cm*	*85–96%*
2–4 mm	→ *2 cm*	*60–75%*
>4 mm	→ *2 cm*	*50%*

Elective lymph node dissection is not indicated in primary melanoma. Sentinel lymph node biopsy should be considered as a staging technique in appropriate patients, i.e. primary ≥1 mm, or <1 mm, if Clark level > 4, mitotic rate >0 per mm.'

National Institute for Health and Care Guidelines NG14 (July 2015). www.nice.org.uk

↻ | 18.8 Summary

Management of malignant melanoma

- The depth of the lesion is a key prognostic factor and is assessed by Breslow thickness and Clark's level
- Excision biopsy is essential to confirm the diagnosis and pathological features that inform prognosis and further management
- Once melanoma is confirmed, a wider excision with a 0.5–2-cm margin is performed
- Lymph node involvement or satellite deposits reduce 5-year survival rates from 70% to 30% and patients with distant metastases rarely survive for 5 years
- Block dissection of regional lymph nodes is no longer practised routinely but is indicated if the nodes are clinically involved or there is a positive sentinel lymph node biopsy.

Clinical and pathological staging

As for most cancers, staging has major prognostic and management implications. For melanoma, two overlapping staging systems are in common use. The TNM system describes the extent of the disease in terms of **T**umour size, lymph **N**ode involvement and **M**etastases (Table 18.6). In addition, five clinical stages are described (with several subgroups) by the American Joint Committee on Cancer (AJCC) (Table 18.7). Prognosis depends upon tumour size and mitotic rate, the presence of ulceration, evidence of vascular, perineural or lymphatic invasion and metastatic disease. The presence of tumour infiltrating lymphocytes and features of regression can also influence prognosis. Elevated levels of lactate dehydrogenase (LDH), thought to be released from melanomas that outgrow their blood supply, are associated with poorer prognosis in metastatic disease.

Vascular tumours

In recent years, much has been learnt about the aetiology, pathogenesis and treatment of vascular anomalies, whether predominantly capillary, venous, arteriovenous or lymphatic. They are broadly classified according to the presence of mitotic activity into vasoproliferative lesions (haemangiomas) and vascular malformations. The latter are subdivided into low flow (capillary, venous and lymphatic) or high flow (arteriovenous) malformations. Their pathophysiology and management are outwith the scope of this chapter.

Infantile haemangiomas (strawberry naevi)

These lesions occur in up to 10% of all newborns, making it the most common tumour of infancy. They commonly present at or shortly after birth especially in premature Caucasian females, as bright-red raised lesions with an irregular bosselated surface. Deep-seated lesions are more likely to present as a soft subcutaneous mass imparting a bluish hue to the overlying skin.

Table 18.6 TNM staging for melanoma

Primary (T)	Thickness	Ulceration status
Tis	N/A	N/A
T1	≤1.0 mm	a: no ulceration and <1 mitosis/mm^2 b: with ulceration and ≤1 mitosis/mm^2
T2	1.01–2.0 mm	a: no ulceration b: with ulceration
T3	2.01–4.0 mm	a: no ulceration b: with ulceration
T4	>4.0 mm	a: no ulceration b: with ulceration
Nodes (N)	**No. of metastatic nodes**	**Nodal metastatic mass**
N0	No evidence of lymph node metastasis	
N1	1 node	a: micrometastasis b: macrometastasis
N2	2–3 nodes	a: micrometastasis b: macrometastasis c: In transit metastases/satellites without metastatic nodes
N3	4 or more metastatic nodes, or matted nodes, or in-transit metastases/satellites and metastatic nodes	
Metastases (M)	**Site**	**Serum LDH**
M0	No evidence of metastasis to distant tissues or organs	
M1a	Distant skin, subcutaneous or nodal metastases	Normal
M1b	Lung metastases	Normal
M1c	All other visceral metastases Or any distant metastases	Normal Elevated

LDH, Lactate dehydrogenase.

18

Table 18.7 Prognosis in relation to the AJCC stage and depth of malignant melanoma

Clinical stage	5-year survival rate (%)
0 Melanoma	
I Primary lesion only	≈100%
Breslow depth (mm)	
1A <1 mm, no ulceration	
1B <1 mm with ulceration or 1–2 mm without ulceration	
II Primary lesion only	80% for men
Breslow (mm)	90% for women
2A 1–2 mm with ulceration or 2–4 mm without ulceration	
2B 2–4 mm with ulceration or >4 mm without ulceration	
2C >4 mm with ulceration	
III Metastatic disease	50% for men
3A, B or C depending upon the number and location of lymph node involvement, LDH level, satellite and in transit metastases	>50% for women
IV Distant metastatic disease	<5% for men
	<15% for women

LDH, Lactate dehydrogenase.

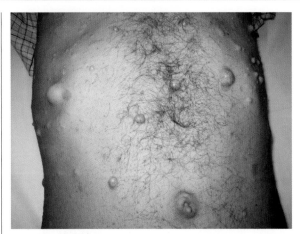

Fig. 18.34 Multiple neurofibromas in von Recklinghausen's disease (neurofibromatosis).

The skin is the most commonly affected organ, especially in the head and neck (60%), trunk (25%), and extremities (15%). The lesions typically proliferate for up to 6 months then remain static for 2–3 years, after which spontaneous involution occurs over several years, although large lesions may leave residual loose atrophic skin. Approximately 25% of cases present as multiple lesions and the presence of more than five should prompt investigation for cerebral and intraabdominal haemangiomas.

Despite the natural history of involution, perioral, aural or ocular lesions and those that are large or ulcerating may be treated with oral propranolol to accelerate involution. A rare complication can occur when platelets and fibrinogen are sequestrated by the lesion causing a consumption coagulopathy (Kasabach–Merritt syndrome).

Haemangiomas that are already fully developed at birth are either classified as rapidly involuting (RICH) or more commonly noninvoluting (NICH). The latter can be treated by surgical excision if required.

Tumours of nerves

Neurilemmoma (Schwannoma)

This is the most common neurogenic tumour and arises from the Schwann cells of the nerve sheath. They present as benign, encapsulated, solitary subcutaneous swellings that are somewhat mobile perpendicular to the nerve but fixed parallel to it. There may be symptoms due to nerve compression such as pain in the corresponding sensory distribution. Most neurilemmomas occur superficially in the neck or limbs of young and middle-aged adults. They grow slowly and are benign, though rare malignant degeneration to neurofibrosarcoma may occur. Most lesions are readily

excised, although neuropraxia is common and permanent nerve dysfunction can occur.

Neurofibroma

This is another form of benign nerve sheath tumour that can present in isolation but is more commonly associated with neurofibromatosis type 1 (NF-1, von Recklinghausen's disease), a genetic disease with an autosomal dominant inheritance pattern and incidence of 1 in 3000 (Fig. 18.34). The lesions typically appear during adolescence as numerous flesh-coloured, sessile or pedunculated nodules on or beneath the dermi. They can be painful and itchy and often cause significant cosmetic concern. In NF-1, there are also multiple lightly pigmented patches ('café au lait' spots). As well as the small discrete lesions, much larger 'plexiform' lesions can occur and invade through multiple tissue planes causing disfigurement and neurological symptoms, rendering complete excision extremely difficult. Unlike the dermal neurofibromas, plexiform fibroma has a 10% risk of malignant transformation to malignant peripheral nerve sheath tumour (MPNST). Surgery is the principle treatment for troublesome lesions although angiotensin-converting enzyme (ACE) inhibitors may have a role in suppressing tumour development.

Tumours of muscle and connective tissues

Lipoma

This is a very common, slow-growing and benign tumour of fat that forms a soft, mobile subcutaneous mass enclosed in a thin fibrous capsule. Most are asymptomatic. Small lesions can be managed conservatively but large (>5 cm) and deep-seated lipomas can rarely undergo sarcomatous change that is characterised by rapid growth. Therefore, large or symptomatic and deep lesions should be excised after appropriate imaging. Liposuction may be used where there is no suspicion of malignancy.

Sarcoma

Sarcomas are rare tumours arising from derivatives of the embryonal mesoderm including the dermis, blood vessels, bone, muscle and fat. They occur at any age. Some present primarily on the skin but the majority present as a deep-seated mass. Suspicious

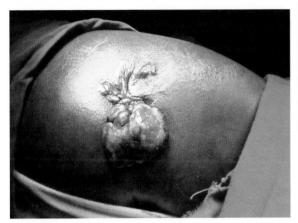

Fig. 18.35 Dermatofibrosarcoma protruberans (DFSP). Note the irregular multinodular surface and skin ulceration.

lesions should be investigated with magnetic resonance imaging (MRI) and in many cases core biopsy prior to formal wide excision (>2 cm margin) with selective adjuvant radio and chemotherapy. Excision and reconstruction of large tumours involving the skin, bone, muscle and nerve may be extremely complex. The prognosis depends upon the location of the primary lesion, the completeness of excision and the presence of metastatic disease as well as the degree of differentiation of the tumour cells and tumour grade (low, intermediate or high).

Dermatofibrosarcoma protruberans (DFSP)

This is a locally invasive sarcoma of the dermis arising from fibroblasts. It appears as a solitary firm, painless and reddish scar-like lesion measuring a few centimetres in diameter (Fig. 18.35). They usually arise on the trunk of adults over 30 years and grow slowly with indistinct margins and an irregular shape. Despite local invasion, metastases are rare (<5%). Moh's surgery may be indicated, especially in relatively common recurrent disease. The tyrosine kinase inhibitor, imatinib is promising for treatment of metastatic disease.

Dermal sarcoma

Despite features suggestive of malignancy, atypical fibroxanthoma (AFX) is a pleomorphic, often ulcerating, dermal neoplasm characterised by benign clinical behaviour. It affects sundamaged skin of elderly males, often on the scalp. The diagnosis is one of exclusion and histopathological distinction from the more aggressive pleomorphic dermal sarcoma, which can be difficult, although the latter often has features of necrosis and lymphovascular or perineural invasion.

Liposarcoma

Liposarcoma is the most common sarcoma of middle age. It may occur in any fatty tissue but is most common in the retroperitoneum and legs. Most liposarcomas grow relatively slowly and recurrence after excision may take a long time to develop.

Fibrosarcoma

This tumour arises from fibrous tissue at any site but is most common in the lower limbs of the middle aged. It forms a large, deep and firm mass often involving bone and representing approximately 10% of all musculoskeletal sarcoma and up to 5% of primary bone tumours.

Rhabdomyosarcoma

This greyish-pink, soft, fleshy lobulated or well-circumscribed tumour arises from striated muscle. It is more common in children under 5 years old and teenagers, and is the most common soft tissue malignancy in childhood. Common sites are the head and neck, genitourinary tract and the limbs. The lesions are highly malignant, and require treatment by radical excision and/or radiotherapy. Often neoadjuvant chemoradiotherapy is required to shrink the tumour prior to excision. Despite the aggressive nature of these tumours long-term survival is achieved in the majority of cases.

Angiosarcoma and Kaposi's sarcoma

Angiosarcomas are aggressive tumours arising form blood vessels of the skin, breast, liver and spleen. They occur in all ages but are rare in children. There is an association with long-standing lymphoedema and in patients having had previous radiotherapy for other tumours, with a latency of 15–20 years. The fact that the disease involves blood vessels probably explains why systemic spread has often occurred at the time of diagnosis and the disease has an extremely poor prognosis.

Kaposi's sarcoma is a form of angiosarcoma, which is often multifocal and associated with immunocompromised states. It was extremely rare in the West before the HIV epidemic. The AIDS-associated form is a rapidly progressive, extensive and painful disease. The lesions appear as brown macules and plaques and purple–red nodules. The legs are commonly sites, but the hands, ears and nose may also be involved. The disease has a poor prognosis.

18

19

J. Michael Dixon

The breast

Chapter contents

Anatomy and physiology 326

Assessment of a patient with breast disease 326

Benign breast conditions 331

Breast lumpiness and pain 331

Benign neoplasms 333

Breast infection 334

Breast cancer 335

Male breast 349

Anatomy and physiology

Overview

The breast is an appendage of skin and is a modified sweat gland. It is composed of glandular tissue, fibrous or supporting tissue, and fat. The functional unit of the breast is the terminal duct lobular unit, and any secretions produced in the terminal duct lobular unit drain towards the nipple into subareolar ducts. Although they are often described as being made up of segments, the glandular and ductal structures of the breast interweave to form a composite mass.

Anatomy

The breast lies between the skin and the pectoral fascia, to which it is loosely attached. It extends from the clavicle superiorly down onto the abdominal wall where it extends over the rectus abdominis, external oblique and serratus anterior muscles. The axillary tail of the breast runs between the pectoral and latissimus dorsi muscles to blend with the axillary fat. The breast is supplied by the lateral thoracic artery or the lateral thoracic branch of the axillary artery superolaterally, and by perforating branches of the internal mammary artery superomedially. The terminal duct lobular unit is lined, as are the draining ducts, with a single layer of columnar epithelial cells surrounded by myoepithelial cells. The major subareolar ducts in their terminal portion are lined by stratified squamous epithelium.

The main route of lymphatic spread of breast cancer is to the axillary nodes that are situated below the axillary vein. On average, there are 20 nodes below the axillary vein (Fig. 19.1). The nodes nearest the breast are usually affected first by breast cancer. In <5% of patients, higher nodes are involved without lower nodes being affected. Lymph also drains into the internal mammary nodes. Occasionally, the main route of lymph drainage of a cancer is to the interpectoral (Rotter's) nodes situated between the pectoralis major and minor muscles.

Congenital abnormalities

Only 1–5% of women and men have an extra or accessory nipple, and even less have accessory breasts. The most common site for an accessory nipple is between the normal breast and the umbilicus; the most common site for an accessory breast is the lower axilla. Some degree of breast asymmetry is normal, the left usually being the larger of the two. Surgery is indicated only if there is significant asymmetry.

Hormonal control of breast development and function

The life cycle of the breast consists of three main periods: development and early reproductive life, mature reproductive life and involution. Development occurs at puberty and involves proliferation of ducts and ductules associated with very rudimentary lobule formation. The breast then undergoes regular changes in relation to the menstrual cycle. By 30 years of age, involution is evident and continues to menopause and beyond. During involution, both the glandular and fibrous tissue atrophy and the shape of the breast changes.

Assessment of a patient with breast disease

In the UK, 1 in 4 women will attend a breast clinic at some time in their life, and 1 in 9 will develop breast cancer; whereas in India, rural women have a lifetime risk as low as 1 in 80, rising to 1 in 27 in urban areas. The most common breast symptoms are a breast lump or lumpiness, which may or may not be painful; pain alone; nipple discharge; nipple retraction; breast distortion; swelling and inflammation; or scaling or eczema of the nipple (Table 19.1).

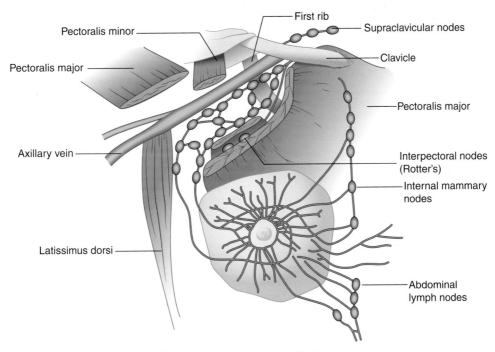

Fig. 19.1 Lymph node drainage of the breast.

Table 19.1 Symptoms and % of each symptom in patients attending a breast clinic	
Symptom	% of patients
Breast lump	36
Painful lump or lumpiness	33
Pain alone	17.5
Nipple discharge	5
Nipple retraction	3
Strong family history of breast cancer	3
Breast distortion	1
Swelling or inflammation	1
Scaling nipple (eczema)	0.5

History

The most important pointer to the diagnosis is the age of the patient. Breast cancer incidence increases with age, whereas benign conditions are much more common in young women. The duration of any symptom is important; breast cancers usually grow slowly, but cysts can appear overnight.

Clinical examination

In some cultures clinical examination may be difficult for a male doctor. The presence of a chaperone, a first-degree female relative, tact, good communication skills and a professional attitude will all aid in overcoming this barrier. The patient is asked to undress to the waist or expose the breasts adequately and sit facing the examiner. Inspection should take place in good light with the patient's arms by her side, above her head, and then pressing

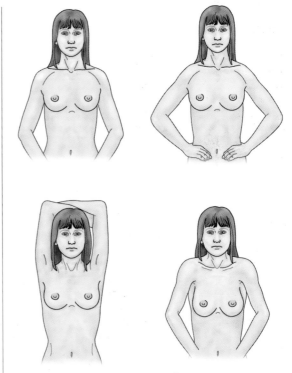

Fig. 19.2 Clinical inspection of the breast.

on her hips (Fig. 19.2). Skin dimpling or a change of contour is present in a high percentage of patients with breast cancer (Fig. 19.3). Breast palpation is performed with the patient lying flat with her arms above or under her head (Fig. 19.4). All the breast tissue is examined, using the fingertips (not the flat of the hand as is often described) to detect any abnormality. Any abnormal area

19

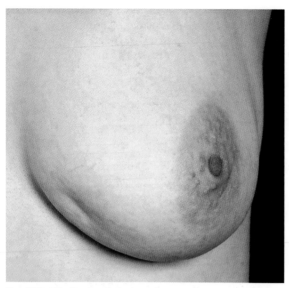

Fig. 19.3 Skin dimpling in the lower inner quadrant of the left breast associated with breast cancer.

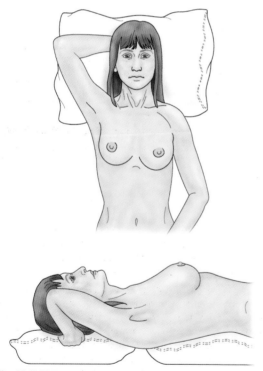

Fig. 19.4 Clinical examination of the breast.

should be examined in detail, again with the fingertips to determine the texture and outline of the mass. Deep fixation is assessed by asking the patient to tense the pectoralis major muscle; this is accomplished by asking her to press her hands on her hips. All palpable lesions should be measured with vernier callipers or a flat scale ruler, and the size and site (using the o'clock notation and relation to the areola) recorded in the hospital notes.

If the patient complains of nipple discharge, an attempt should be made to reproduce the discharge and to determine whether it arises from a single or multiple duct(s).

Assessment of regional nodes

Once the breasts have been palpated the nodal areas are checked (Fig. 19.5). Palpable axillary nodes can be identified in up to 30% of patients with no clinically significant breast disease and up to 20% of patients with breast cancer who have no palpable axillary nodes are found histologically to have metastatic disease in the axillary nodes. Ultrasound is better at assessing axillary nodes than clinical examination. The supraclavicular nodes are best examined from behind.

Imaging

Mammography

This requires compression of the breast between two plates and can be uncomfortable. Two views, a mediolateral oblique and a craniocaudal, are usually obtained. Mammography can visualise a mass or areas of increased density, areas of distortion and calcifications. Because the breasts are relatively radiodense in women under 40 years of age, mammography is of limited value in young women. In older women 10–15% of cancers are difficult to see on mammography because of persistently dense breasts. Any calcification can be biopsied using a stereotactic device attached to a mammography unit.

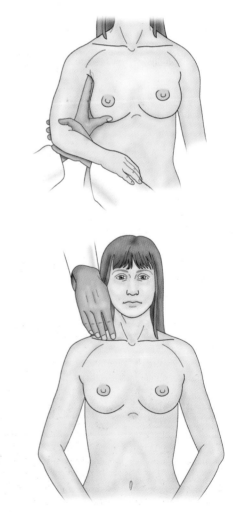

Fig. 19.5 Examination of the regional nodes.

Ultrasonography

High-frequency sound waves are beamed through the breast and reflections are detected and turned into images. Ultrasound can differentiate between solid and cystic lesions. Cysts show up as transparent objects (Fig. 19.6) and benign lesions tend to have well-demarcated edges (Fig. 19.7). In contrast, cancers usually have an 'irregular' indistinct outline and appear 'hypoechoic' because of their higher cellularity relative to the adjacent tissue (Fig. 19.8). They also absorb sound, producing a posterior acoustic shadow. Ultrasound is also used to assess axillary nodes in patients with

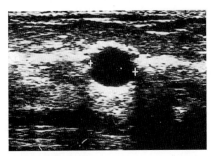

Fig. 19.6 Ultrasound of a cyst.

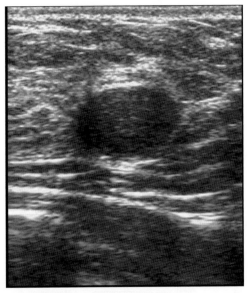

Fig. 19.7 Ultrasound of a fibroadenoma.

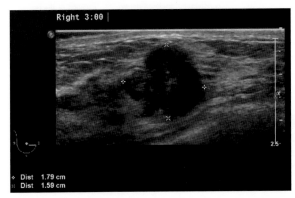

Fig. 19.8 Ultrasound of a cancer.

breast cancer. Where a node is enlarged and/or the cortex of a node is thickened, fine-needle aspiration cytology or core biopsy can be performed using ultrasound guidance to establish whether nodal metastases are present. Ultrasound is used commonly to localise small cancers immediately prior to surgery.

Magnetic resonance imaging (MRI)

MRI is an accurate way of imaging the breast. It has a high sensitivity for breast cancer and is of value in demonstrating the extent of both invasive and non-invasive disease. The indications are:

- Screening high risk young women who carry BRCA1 or BRCA2 gene mutations
- Assessing young women with dense breasts who have a lump or a cancer that is not well visualised on other imaging
- To identify a breast cancer in women with a malignant axillary node where there is no obvious primary cancer seen on mammography and ultrasound
- To assess response to chemotherapy or endocrine therapy
- To assess breast implants for leakage and rupture
- To assess treated breasts after surgery and radiotherapy.

(EBM 19.1)

EBM **19.1 Screening for breast cancer by MRI**

'MRI combined with mammography is more effective than mammography alone at screening women < 50 years who are at very high risk of breast cancer either because they carry a BRCA1 or BRCA2 mutation or because of their family history.'

MARIBS Study Group. Lancet. 2005;365:1769–78.

Core biopsy and fine needle aspiration (FNA) cytology

Core biopsy

Core biopsy offers several advantages over fine-needle aspiration cytology:

- It can differentiate invasive from in situ disease
- Cancer type and receptor status can be assessed
- It has an extremely low rate of false positives
- It has a very high sensitivity when image guided.

After injection of local anaesthetic several cores are removed from a mass or an area of microcalcification by means of a cutting needle technique (Fig. 19.9). Core biopsy can be performed using palpation to guide biopsy, although image-guidance using ultrasound is recommended for mass lesions and a stereotactic technique for calcifications. Vacuum-assisted core biopsy devices allow larger volumes of tissue to be removed and produce more reliable results in microcalcification biopsies.

Punch biopsy

Punch biopsy or core biopsy of any nipple ulceration or change can be used to diagnose Paget's disease of the nipple.

Fine-needle aspiration cytology

This is now rarely used to diagnose palpable breast lumps. If a lesion is a simple cyst on ultrasound, aspiration is indicated only for symptoms or reassurance. Any fluid aspirated should be discarded unless it is evenly blood stained, then it should be sent for

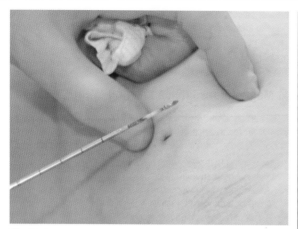

Fig. 19.9 Core biopsy being performed.

cytological analysis. Fine-needle aspiration (FNA) cytology cannot differentiate invasive from in situ cancer. It is used most frequently to sample lymph nodes that are abnormal on imaging in patients with breast cancer. FNA of nodes should be performed under image guidance with use of local anaesthesia.

Open biopsy

This should be performed only in patients who have been appropriately investigated by imaging and core biopsy. Removal of a lesion is indicated either if the lesion is benign and the patient requests removal or if core biopsy has not excluded malignancy. Removal of impalpable lesions requires localisation by a technique such as hooked wire insertion. Following excision, the specimen is x-rayed to confirm that the appropriate area has been removed.

Triple assessment

This is the combination of clinical examination, imaging (ultrasound ± mammography) and core biopsy or FNA cytology. All patients with a discrete localised mass or asymmetric nodularity should have triple assessment. The use of triple assessment minimises delay in diagnosis.

Accuracy of investigations

The sensitivity of clinical examination and mammography varies with age, and only two-thirds of cancers in women under 50 years of age are considered to be suspicious or definitely malignant on clinical examination or mammography (Table 19.2). Image-guided core biopsy is the most accurate and efficient of the various techniques used to diagnose breast masses.

Sentinel lymph node biopsy

Sentinel lymph node biopsy was first used in patients with breast cancer in the 1990s. The sentinel lymph node is the first lymph node that drains the breast and the most common node to be involved by metastasis. Sentinel node biopsy is performed in patients with invasive breast cancer who are clinically and/or on imaging believed to be node negative.

To identify the sentinel node(s), radioisotope ± blue dye is injected either under the nipple, into the skin over the cancer or around the cancer. Sentinel nodes are identified on scintigraphy with a hand-held gamma probe, or can be visualised (stained blue). A method using iron injections and a magnetometer that detects iron particles in the nodes is also available. There is rarely a single sentinel node and the average number of sentinel nodes removed at surgery is 2–3. When blue dye and radioisotope are combined, one or more sentinel nodes will be identified in approximately 97% of patients. The technique is 98% accurate in determining the presence or absence of involved nodes.

Removal of all axillary lymph nodes has been the standard in patients with any involved nodes, but axillary radiotherapy is an alternative treatment. If the sentinel nodes are negative, then no further axillary treatment is required. Sentinel lymph node biopsy has reduced the complications that were seen after axillary clearance such as lymphoedema, pain, numbness and infection. Recent studies from the USA have questioned the need to treat the axilla if only one or two sentinel nodes are involved in patients treated with breast-conserving surgery and whole breast radiotherapy.

Nipple discharge

There are a variety of causes for nipple discharge. Only spontaneous discharge requires investigation. Pressure applied deep to the nipple will usually elicit fluid for direct inspection. This allows assessment of the colour of the discharge and allows testing for the presence of blood. The presence of blood within a discharge increases the chances that cancer is present but has a poor sensitivity (<20% of women with a blood stained discharge will have cancer) and a low specificity for benign disease. The common causes, discharge type and their management are listed in Table 19.3.

Persistent (>2 times per week), troublesome discharge, is best treated by excision of the affected duct. Discharge from multiple ducts is managed by removal of all the ducts under the nipple. This operation renders the patient incapable of breast feeding and is best suited for those who have already completed their family.

Table 19.3 Causes and management of nipple discharge

Cause	Discharge characteristics	Management
Duct ectasia	Variable colour and consistency; multiple ducts	Reassurance Excision of ducts
Duct papilloma	Copious serous, bloody, single duct	Microdochectomy
Carcinoma in situ	Single duct, bloodstained, persistent, serous discharge	Image-guided biopsy or microdochectomy
Prolactinoma	Milky, multiple duct	Endocrine evaluation

Table 19.2 Sensitivity of investigations in the diagnosis of symptomatic breast disease in specialist clinics

	Clinical examination	Mammography	Ultrasonography	Core biopsy	Fine-needle aspiration cytology
Sensitivity for cancers	86%	86%	90%	98%	95%

Percentage of cancers detected by test as malignant or probably malignant (that is, complete sensitivity).

Benign breast conditions

Most benign conditions occur at particular times such as breast development, cyclical activity or involution, and are so common that they are best considered as aberrations rather than true disease (Table 19.4). Uncontrolled overgrowth of breast tissue is seen occasionally in adolescent girls, and is called virginal or juvenile hypertrophy, but it is not hypertrophy as there is an increase in the amount of stromal tissue rather than in the number of lobules or ducts.

Fibroadenoma

Fibroadenomas are a common cause of breast lumps, particularly in younger women. They were classified initially as benign tumours, but are best considered as aberrations rather than true neoplasms. Fibroadenomas develop from a whole lobule rather than from a single cell, and show hormonal dependence similar to that of normal breast tissue, lactating during pregnancy and involuting in the perimenopausal period. Fibroadenomas are most commonly seen immediately following breast development in the 15–25-year age group (Fig. 19.10). They are usually well-circumscribed, firm, smooth, mobile lumps, and can be multiple or bilateral. Although a small number of fibroadenomas increase

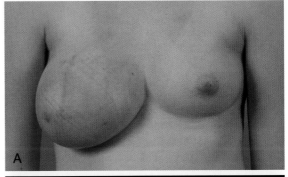

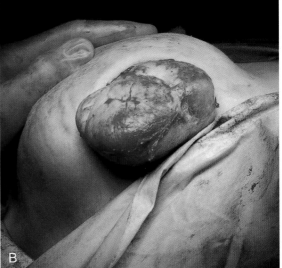

Fig. 19.11 (A) Juvenile fibroadenoma of the right breast. **(B)** Juvenile fibroadenoma being excised.

19

in size, most do not and over one-third become smaller or disappear within 2 years. Fibroadenomas have a characteristic appearance with easily visualised margins on ultrasound (Fig. 19.7). All discrete solid masses in patients over the age of 25 years should have a core biopsy. In younger women ultrasound alone is sufficient to establish the diagnosis of a fibroadenoma. Some institutions have a lower cut-off age and perform core biopsies on all solid lesions in patients over the age of 21 years, as cancers are sometimes seen in women aged 21–25 years. Large or giant fibroadenomas (>5 cm) are uncommon but are seen more often in women from certain African and Asian countries. Occasionally, a fibroadenoma in an adolescent girl undergoes rapid growth, a condition known as juvenile fibroadenoma (Fig. 19.11). Once a diagnosis of fibroadenoma has been established on core biopsy, options for management are reassurance with no follow-up or excision; fibroadenomas >4 cm in diameter are usually excised to ensure that a phyllodes tumour is not missed (see the section on Phyllodes tumours). Carcinoma arising in a fibroadenoma is extremely rare. Patients with simple fibroadenomas are not at increased risk of developing breast cancer.

Breast lumpiness and pain

Premenstrual nodularity or lumpiness and breast discomfort are common and considered part of the normal cyclical changes. Premenstrual pain that is severe and interferes with daily activities and

Table 19.4 Aberrations of normal breast development and involution (ANDI)		
Age (years)	**Normal process**	**Aberration**
<25	Breast development Stromal Lobular	Juvenile hypertrophy Fibroadenoma
25–40	Cyclical activity	Cyclical mastalgia Cyclical nodularity (diffuse or focal)
30–55	Involution Lobular Stromal Ductal	Palpable cysts Sclerosing lesions Duct ectasia

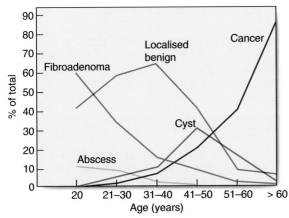

Fig. 19.10 Percentage of patients in 10-year age groups with a discrete breast lump who have common benign conditions and breast cancer.

decreases quality of life is a common reason for hospital referral. Reassurance and wearing a soft supporting bra 24 hours a day is the mainstay of treatment. Tamoxifen does not have a product licence for this condition but a dose of 10 mg improves premenstrual breast pain in 80% of patients. Agnus castus, a fruit extract, has also been shown in randomised studies to be somewhat effective in reducing breast pain.

Lumpiness or nodularity

This can be throughout the breast or localised. Diffuse bilateral nodularity is normal, particularly premenstrually and is not associated with any underlying pathological abnormality. Focal nodularity is a common cause for women seeking medical advice and is seen in women of all ages (Fig. 19.10). Patients with benign focal nodularity often report that the lump fluctuates in size in relation to the menstrual cycle. Breast cancer should be excluded by triple assessment in women with persistent localised asymmetric areas of nodularity as cancer in younger women can present as localised nodularity rather than a discrete lump.

Other lumps

A galactocoele is a cystic lesion that develops in lactating women and is full of milk. Most galactocoeles resolve upon cessation of breast feeding, but larger ones may require repeated aspiration.

Noncyclical breast pain

Noncyclical breast pain is much more common than cyclical pain and even cyclical pain can have its origins in the chest wall as when the breast swells premenstrually it increases breast volume and weight, pulling on the chest wall. Localised pain in the chest wall is a common reason for referral. The pain may appear to be in the breast but by examining the patient on her side and moving the breast away from the chest wall it is possible to demonstrate that the site of pain and discomfort is in the ribs or chest wall muscle (Fig. 19.12). Oral or topical nonsteroidal antiinflammatory agents (NSAIDs) can be effective in improving chest-wall pain.

Breast cysts

Approximately 7% of women in developed countries develop a palpable breast cyst at some time in their life. Cysts constitute 15% of all discrete breast masses. They are distended, involuted lobules and are most frequently seen in the perimenopausal period (Fig. 19.10). Clinically, they are smooth discrete lumps that can be painful and are sometimes visible. Mammographically, they have characteristic haloes and are easily diagnosed by ultrasonography (Fig. 19.6). Symptomatic palpable cysts are treated by aspiration and, provided the fluid is not blood-stained, it is discarded. All patients suspected as having a breast cyst should have an ultrasound, and if over the age of 40 should undergo mammography (Fig. 19.13). Patients with cysts do not have an increased risk of developing breast cancer.

Duct ectasia

The central subareolar ducts dilate and shorten with age; when symptomatic, this is known as duct ectasia. By the age of 70 years, 40% of women have dilated ducts, some of whom present with nipple discharge or nipple retraction. The discharge

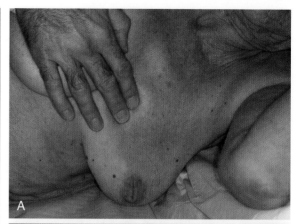

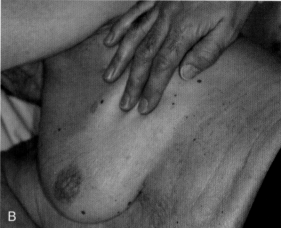

Fig. 19.12 Examination of chest wall underlying the breast to demonstrate whether the site of pain originates from the ribs medially (A) or chest wall muscle or ribs laterally (B).

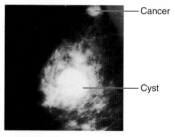

Cancer

Cyst

Fig. 19.13 Mammogram of a cyst and a cancer.

associated with duct ectasia is usually cheesy and the nipple retraction is classically slit-like (Fig. 19.14), in contrast to patients with breast cancer, where the whole nipple is pulled in (Fig. 19.15). Surgery is indicated if the discharge is troublesome or if the patient wishes the nipple to be everted.

Epithelial hyperplasia

An increase in the number of cells lining the terminal duct lobular unit is known as epithelial hyperplasia. If the hyperplastic cells also show cellular atypia, this condition is called atypical hyperplasia. Women with atypical hyperplasia have a significant increase (4–5 times) in their risk of developing breast cancer. The absolute risk of breast cancer development for a woman with atypical hyperplasia without a first-degree relative with breast cancer is

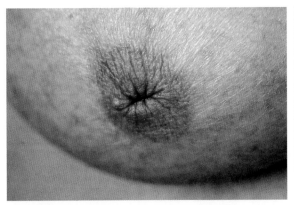

Fig. 19.14 Duct ectasia showing slit-like nipple retraction.

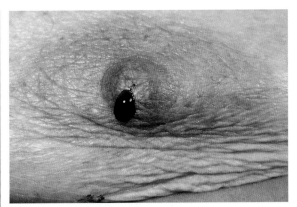

Fig. 19.16 Blood-stained nipple discharge.

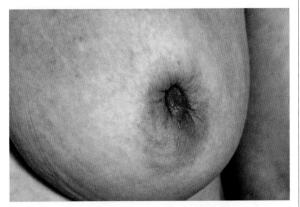

Fig. 19.15 Asymmetric nipple inversion in a patient with breast cancer.

8% at 10 years; and for women with a first-degree relative with breast cancer the risk is 20–25% at 15 years.

Benign neoplasms

Duct papilloma

These develop most commonly in the ducts under the nipple but can occur in any part of the ductal tree and can be single or multiple. They are very common and show minimal malignant potential. They can cause persistent and troublesome nipple discharge that can be either serous or frankly blood-stained (Fig. 19.16). Treatment involves removal of the discharging duct, removing the papilloma (if this is the cause) and allows exclusion of an underlying neoplasm.

Lipoma

These are soft, lobulated, radiolucent lesions and are common. They should be imaged to confirm the diagnosis. Biopsy is not required in most cases, as the diagnosis can be made by a combination of clinical examination and imaging.

Phyllodes tumour

These rare fibro-epithelial neoplasms are mostly benign, but a small percentage are malignant. They present as localised discrete masses that clinically feel like fibroadenomas, although they

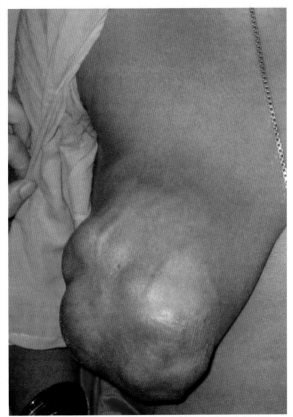

Fig. 19.17 'Cystosarcoma' phyllodes presenting with characteristic hard, mobile, bosselated lumps. Note the prominent veins on the chest wall.

tend to be larger (>4 cm) and appear bosselated, but despite their size they usually remain free from the overlying skin or underlying chest wall (Fig. 19.17). Up to 20% of benign phyllodes tumours recur locally following simple excision. In more malignant lesions it is the sarcomatous stromal element that recurs; approximately one-quarter of lesions metastasise, most commonly to lung. Treatment of such tumours, whether malignant or benign, is wide excision. If the lesion is large, mastectomy may be needed to ensure complete removal.

19

↻ **19.1 Summary**

Benign breast disease

- Is more common than breast cancer
- Can be difficult to differentiate from breast cancer
- Inappropriate treatment of benign conditions is associated with significant morbidity
- Many benign conditions occur in particular age groups
- The only benign condition associated with a significant increased risk of subsequent breast cancer is atypical hyperplasia.

Breast infection

Breast infection is less common than it used to be. It most frequently affects women aged 18–50 years. Infection can be divided into lactational and nonlactational. Infection can also affect the skin overlying the breast as a primary event or secondary to a lesion in the skin (such as an epidermoid cyst or an underlying condition such as hidradenitis suppurativa).

The principles of treating breast infection are:

- Give appropriate antibiotics early to reduce the incidence of abscess formation (Table 19.5).
- If an abscess is suspected, confirm pus is present by ultrasound before embarking on aspiration or surgical drainage.
- Exclude breast cancer using imaging and consider core biopsy in any inflammatory lesion that is solid and that does not settle despite adequate antibiotic treatment.

Most breast abscesses can be managed by repeated (ultrasound-guided) aspiration (Fig. 19.18), combined with oral antibiotics or incision and drainage under local anaesthesia. A sample of pus should be sent for bacteriological culture. Few abscesses require drainage under general anaesthesia. Simple drainage is preferred. Placement of a drain or packing the abscess cavity after incision and drainage is unnecessary and delays wound healing.

Lactating infection

Improvements in maternal and infant hygiene have reduced the incidence of infection associated with breastfeeding. When infection does occur, it usually develops within the first 6 weeks of breastfeeding. Presenting features are pain, swelling, tenderness and a cracked nipple or skin abrasion (Fig 19.19). *Staphylococcus aureus* is the most common organism, although *Staphylococcus epidermidis* and streptococci are occasionally implicated.

Table 19.5 Antibiotics most appropriate for treating breast infections[a]		
Type of infection	No allergy to penicillin	Allergy to penicillin
Lactating and skin-associated	Flucloxacillin (500 mg 6-hourly)	Clarithromycin (500 mg 12-hourly)
Nonlactating	Co-amoxiclav (375 mg 8-hourly)	Combination of clarithromycin (500 mg 12-hourly) with metronidazole (200 mg 8-hourly)

[a]Doses are for adults

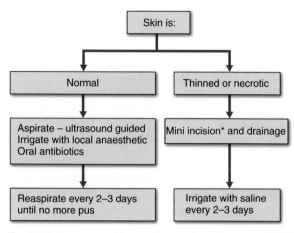

Fig. 19.18 Management of breast abscesses in relation to nature of overlying skin. *Through a small stab incision.

Skin is:
- Normal
  - Aspirate – ultrasound guided. Irrigate with local anaesthetic. Oral antibiotics
  - Reaspirate every 2–3 days until no more pus
- Thinned or necrotic
  - Mini incision* and drainage
  - Irrigate with saline every 2–3 days

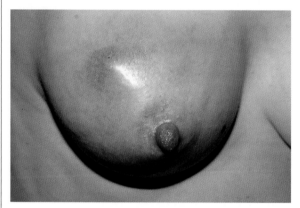

Fig. 19.19 Lactating breast abscess.

Drainage of milk from the affected segment is reduced, with the resultant stagnant milk becoming infected. Early infection should be treated with flucloxacillin or erythromycin. An established abscess should be treated by recurrent aspiration, or by incision and drainage. Women should be encouraged to breastfeed, as this promotes milk drainage from the affected segment.

Nonlactating infection

This can be separated into infections that occur centrally in the periareolar region and infection affecting the periphery of the breast.

Central (periareolar) infection

This is most commonly seen in young women (mean age 32 years). The underlying cause is periductal mastitis. Current evidence suggests that smoking is important in the aetiology of non-lactational infection, 90% of women with infection under the nipple are smokers. Substances in cigarette smoke either directly or indirectly damage the subareolar breast ducts, and the damaged tissue then becomes infected by either aerobic or anaerobic organisms. Clinical features include breast pain, erythema, swelling and tenderness. Nipple retraction may be present.

Treatment of periductal mastitis is with appropriate antibiotics (Table 19.5). Periareolar abscesses are managed by aspiration or incision and drainage (Fig. 19.20). Up to one-third of patients develop recurrence. Repeated episodes of periareolar infection require excision of the diseased duct(s).

Mammary duct fistula

This is a communication between the skin—usually at the areolar margin—and a major subareolar duct as a result of periductal mastitis (Fig. 19.21). Treatment is by excision of the fistula and diseased duct(s) under antibiotic cover.

Peripheral nonlactating abscesses

These are less common than periareolar abscesses and although some are associated with an underlying condition, such as diabetes, rheumatoid arthritis, steroid treatment or trauma, most develop without an obvious cause. Peripheral abscesses are treated by recurrent aspiration with antibiotics (Table 19.5), or incision and drainage under local anaesthesia.

Tubercular mastitis

This is sporadically seen in developing African and Asian countries. Females in the reproductive age group develop a painless lump that can simulate malignancy or a painful lump mimicking a breast abscess. A history of previous or concomitant tuberculosis (TB) may be present. FNAC and needle biopsy can provide definitive evidence of caseation in a background of epithelioid cell granulomas. Acid-fast bacilli are occasionally demonstrable. If TB

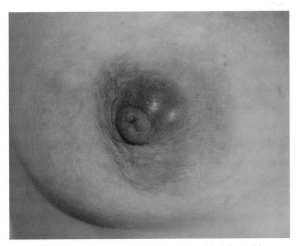

Fig. 19.20 Periareolar abscess secondary to periductal mastitis.

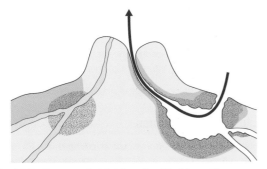

Fig. 19.21 Mammary duct fistula and periductal mastitis.

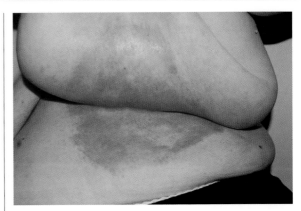

Fig. 19.22 Intertrigo under the breast.

is suspected, tissue should be sent for culture. A prolonged course of antitubercular treatment is preferred and provides complete resolution of disease.

19.2 Summary

Breast infection

- Antibiotics should be given early to reduce risk of abscess formation
- Hospital referral is indicated if infection does not settle rapidly on antibiotics
- If an abscess is suspected, this should be confirmed by ultrasound
- If the lesion is solid on ultrasound, a core biopsy should be performed to exclude an underlying inflammatory carcinoma
- Abscesses can be treated by aspiration or incision and drainage under local anaesthesia.

Skin-associated infection

Primary infection of the skin most commonly affects the lower half of the breast and can be recurrent in women who either are overweight or have large breasts. Intertrigo is infection related to chafing of the skin in the lower half of the breast and the abdominal wall (Fig 19.22). Treatment involves keeping the area as clean and dry as possible and avoiding all creams. Antifungal agents should not be used in this condition as there is no evidence that fungi are important in intertrigo.

Epidermoid, or so-called sebaceous cysts, are common in the skin of the breast and can become infected. Some recurrent infections in the skin of the lower part of the breast are due to hidradenitis suppurativa, which is more common in smokers. Abscesses associated with epidermoid cysts or hidradenitis usually require incision and drainage.

Breast cancer

Epidemiology

Over one and a half million new cases of breast cancer are diagnosed each year worldwide. It is the most common malignancy in women, comprising 18% of all female cancers. Known risk factors are shown in Table 19.6.

19

Table 19.6 Established and probable risk factors for breast cancer

Factor	Relative risk	High-risk group
Age	>10	Elderly
Geographical location	4–5	Developed country
Age at first full pregnancy	3	First child in early 40s
Previous benign disease	4–5	Atypical hyperplasia
Cancer in other breast	>4	Women treated for breast cancer
Weight	2	Body mass index >30 in postmenopausal women
Socioeconomic group	2	Social classes I and II
Alcohol consumption	1.3	Excessive intake
Exposure to ionising radiation	3	Abnormal exposure in young females after age 10
Oral contraceptives	1.24	Current use
Combined HRT	2.3	Use for ≥10 years
Family history	≥2	Breast cancer in first-degree relative

Risk factors for breast cancer

Age

The incidence of breast cancer increases with age, doubling every 10 years until menopause when the rate of increase slows dramatically (Fig. 19.23). Compared with lung cancer, the incidence of breast cancer is higher in young age groups.

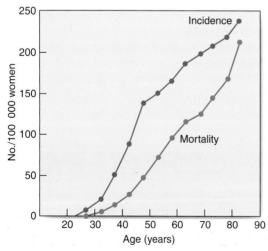

Fig. 19.23 Percentage of all deaths in women attributable to breast cancer.

Geographical variation

Incidence varies by up to a factor of four between different countries. Breast cancer rates around the world in premenopausal women are similar but there are striking differences after the age of 50 years, with a much higher incidence in Caucasian women from North America, Western Europe and Australia. Migrants who move from Japan, a low-risk area, to a high-risk area such as Hawaii show the same incidence of breast cancer as the local population in the host country within one or two generations. This indicates that environmental factors are important in the aetiology of breast cancer.

Menstrual and pregnancy factors

Women who start menstruating early in life, or who have a late menopause, have a slightly increased risk of developing breast cancer. Young age at first delivery protects against breast cancer. The risk of breast cancer in women who have their first child after the age of 30 years is twice that of women who have their first child before the age of 20 years. Breast cancer is more common in nulliparous women, who have a risk approximately 2.4 times that of women who have their first child before the age of 20 years. The highest risk is in women who have a first pregnancy over the age of 40 years. Breastfeeding has a small protective effect and although the effect of breastfeeding is small, in the developed world it can be substantial because women have four or more children and breastfeeding is continued for up to 2 years for each child.

Breast cancer in developing countries

In developing countries like India there has been an age shift and breast cancer is increasing in younger women in the 30–40 and 40–50 year age groups. Breast cancer is now the most common cancer in most areas of India and accounts for 25–32% of all female cancers. The types of breast cancer seen in India differ, with more HER2 positive or triple negative cancers (see later) and they also present at a later stage.

Radiation

A doubling of breast cancer risk was observed among teenage girls exposed to radiation during the Second World War. Women treated by mantle radiotherapy for Hodgkin's and non-Hodgkin's lymphoma during adolescence and teenage years are also at significant risk of developing early-onset breast cancer.

Benign disease

The only benign breast condition associated with a significantly increased risk of breast cancer is severe atypical hyperplasia diagnosed by core or open biopsy.

Diet

Although there is a correlation between the incidence of breast cancer and dietary fat intake in populations, the relationship is neither particularly strong nor consistent. A high alcohol intake does appear to increase breast cancer risk.

Exogenous hormones

Patients taking the oral contraceptive pill have a 1.24 times increased relative risk of breast cancer compared with that of the general population, but the risk is almost negligible with the newer preparations containing low doses of oestrogen. Hormone replacement therapy (HRT) increases breast cancer risk. Combined oestrogen and progestogen HRT is associated with a greater risk than preparations containing oestrogen alone.

Physical activity, weight and height

Numerous studies have shown that moderate physical activity reduces breast cancer risk by about 30%. Obesity doubles the risk of breast cancer in postmenopausal women, whereas in premenopausal women it may reduce risk. Some studies have shown that breast cancer risk increases very slightly with height; taller women having a greater risk.

Genetics

- Up to 5% of breast cancers in Western countries are due to inheritance of genetic abnormalities
- The abnormalities are mutations, insertions or deletions of the DNA that result in malfunction of the corresponding protein
- These genes are inherited as autosomal dominant genes with limited penetrance
- The abnormal genes can be transmitted through either sex and not all those individuals with an abnormal gene will develop cancer
- Many of the genes involved in breast and ovarian cancer are DNA repair genes.

High risk genes

BRCA1 and BRCA2 genes are thought to account for over three-quarters of highly penetrant genetic breast cancer. The vast majority of families that have members with both breast and ovarian cancer are linked to these two genes. The cumulative lifetime risk of developing breast cancer for BRCA1 mutation carriers is 60–85% for breast cancer and 40–60% for ovarian cancer, and 50–85% and 10–35%, respectively, for BRCA2. About 2 per 1000 women have a genetic mutation in BRCA1 or 2 that increases their risk of breast and/or ovarian cancer. In certain populations such as Ashkenazi Jews the incidence of mutations is higher and specific mutations are seen. Other cancers seen in families with mutations in BRCA1 or 2 include prostate cancer, fallopian tube cancer and pancreatic cancer.

Mutations in the p53 gene account for over 70% of cases of the Li Fraumeni syndrome characterised by soft tissue sarcomas, early-onset breast cancer, glioma, childhood adrenal cancer and other early onset malignancies.

Cowden's syndrome is caused by mutations in the phosphatase and tensin homolog (PTEN) gene and is associated with bilateral breast cancer, macrocephaly, multiple hamartomas and an increased risk of thyroid, endometrial, kidney and colon cancer. Women with Peutz–Jeghers syndrome caused by a mutation in the SKT11 gene have a 20–50% lifetime risk of breast cancer.

Other genes

A variety of other genes increase breast cancer risk by as much as two-fold. Mutations in these genes are generally rare and do not require any specific investigation or treatment.

Genetic testing

Testing for BRCA1 and 2 and the other high risk genes is available and based on family history. Pretest counselling is essential. Results are usually available in 6–8 weeks.

Management

High risk women have the following options:
- Bilateral risk reducing surgery: removal of as much breast tissue as possible ± nipple. This reduces risk by at least 95%. The uptake rate of this surgery is increasing as are the cosmetic results of surgery
- Regular screening: involves MRI in younger women and mammography ± MRI in older women
- Chemoprophylaxis: tamoxifen, raloxifene and the aromatase inhibitors given for 5 years reduce the rate of breast cancer development.

Types of breast cancer

Breast cancers are derived from epithelial cells that line the terminal duct lobular unit. Cancer cells that remain within the basement membrane of the lobule and the draining ducts are classified as in situ or noninvasive, and are termed invasive when cells invade outside the basement membrane into the surrounding adjacent tissue. Both in situ and invasive cancers have characteristic patterns by which they are classified.

The most commonly used classification of invasive cancers divides them into ductal and lobular types and is based on the belief that ductal carcinomas arise in ducts and lobular carcinomas in lobules. This is now known to be incorrect, as almost all cancers arise in the terminal duct lobular unit. The two types behave differently, so the classification remains in use.

Noninvasive cancer

Ductal carcinoma in situ (DCIS) is the most common form of noninvasive cancer, making up 3–4% of symptomatic and 17–25% of screen-detected cancers (Fig. 19.24). Screen-detected DCIS is most commonly associated with microcalcifications on mammography, which can be either localised or widespread (Fig. 19.25). Lobular carcinoma in situ (LCIS) (Fig. 19.26) and atypical lobular hyperplasia (ALH) have been combined into a single diagnostic condition called lobular intraepithelial neoplasia (LIN). This is usually an incidental finding and is treated by regular follow-up, as

19

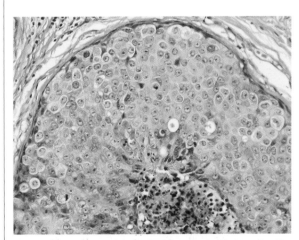

Fig. 19.24 Ductal carcinoma in situ. This is characterised by cells with irregularly shaped and often angular nuclei with variable amounts of chromatin. The cells themselves are variable in size and the necrosis seen in the lumen is a frequent finding.

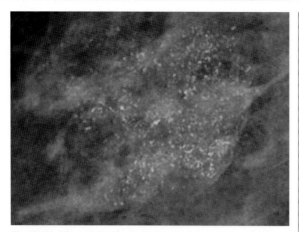

Fig. 19.25 Microcalcification in the breast characteristic of ductal carcinoma in situ.

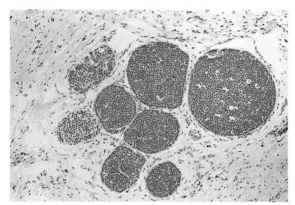

Fig. 19.26 Lobular carcinoma in situ (now called LIN). This is characterised by regular cells with regular round or oval nuclei. (Compare this with DCIS.)

these women are at significant risk of developing invasive cancer in either breast (Table 19.6).

Invasive cancer

The majority of invasive cancers are of no special type and are often referred to as ductal cancers. Certain invasive carcinomas show distinct patterns of growth and are classified as tumours of 'special type'; this includes lobular, tubular, cribriform, papillary, mucinous and medullary cancers. Invasive lobular cancer accounts for up to 10% of invasive cancers and is characterised by a diffuse pattern of spread that causes problems with clinical and mammographic detection. These tumours are often large at diagnosis. Tubular, cribriform and mucinous cancers are well differentiated and have a better than average prognosis. Mucinous cancers are rare circumscribed tumours characterised by tumour cells that produce mucin; these also have a good prognosis. Medullary cancers are circumscribed and soft, and consist of aggregates of high-grade pleomorphic cells surrounded by lymphoid cells, and this type of cancer is seen more often in BRCA1 carriers.

Breast cancers can be graded.

- Grade I have the best prognosis
- Grade II have an intermediate prognosis
- Grade III or high-grade cancers have a poorer prognosis than Grade 1 or 2 cancers.

The presence of tumour cells in lymphatics or blood vessels is associated with an increased risk of both local and systemic recurrence.

Hormone receptors

The hormones oestrogen and progesterone play important roles in breast cancer. Oestrogen receptors, called ERs after the American spelling (estrogen), are present in approximately 75% of breast cancers. ER is expressed in much greater amounts in cancer cells than in normal breast tissue. ER is a target for treatment, and depriving ER-positive cancer cells of oestrogen causes the cancer cells to stop growing and the tumour to shrink. The majority of cancers that express ER also have receptors for progesterone and these are called PRs. The presence of both ER and PR indicates the cancer is even more likely to benefit from removing oestrogen compared with a cancer which has neither ER nor PR (ER and PR negative), where there is no benefit from hormone treatment.

Growth factor receptors

Growth factors in cancer cells also control cancer growth rate. The most important group of growth factors are the human epidermal growth factor receptors (HER). There are four HER receptors, the most important of which is HER2. Between 15% and 20% of all cancers overexpress HER2 and are classed as HER2 positive. HER2 can be blocked with monoclonal antibodies; one is called trastuzumab, and a second antibody is known as pertuzumab. A drug called lapatinib is also effective in HER2 overexpressing cancers.

Testing for receptors

Currently all breast cancers have ER and HER2 measured. Some units check routinely for PR but others only check PR in ER-negative cancers. Most cancers have high levels of ER (ER rich). HER2 is reported as positive or negative but two tests are used in borderline cases and it can take 10–14 days to get a HER2 result.

Cancer types

Cancers are classified as hormone sensitive if they have high levels of ER ± PR. About 25–30% of cancers are hormone independent (ER− PR−). Cancers are considered to be triple negative if they are ER−, PR− and HER2−. Molecular classification of breast cancers recognises three main types of cancer. The first is the luminal or hormone-dependent cancers: Luminal A with high levels of ER and a low rate of proliferation, and Luminal B which has lower levels of ER and a higher rate of proliferation. The second type is the triple negative cancers (ER−, PR−, HER2−). Triple negative cancers are more common in BRCA1 gene mutation carriers and tend to have a worse outcome, although about half do respond very well to chemotherapy. The third group is HER2-positive cancers. These used to have a worse outlook than HER2-negative cancers before the widespread use of trastuzumab. The outcome in HER2-positive disease and HER2-negative cancers is now similar.

Screening for breast cancer

Randomised controlled trials have shown that screening by mammography can significantly reduce mortality from breast cancer

(EBM 19.2). Mortality is reduced by approximately 20% in women invited for screening, with the greatest benefit being seen in women aged over 50 years. This 20% reduction was considered in a review in 2012 to be a reasonable estimate of the impact of breast screening. The UK programme screens the 50–70 year age group, but the age range varies between countries.

<table>
<tr><td>EBM</td><td>19.2 Breast screening by mammography</td></tr>
</table>

'Mammography is at present the best screening tool available. Randomized controlled trials have shown screening by mammography reduces mortality from breast cancer by 20% in those invited for screening. For every 235 women invited for screening one breast cancer death will be prevented – this corresponds to screening 180 women to prevent one death as not all women are invited to attend. Between 11% and 19% of breast cancers diagnosed by breast screening represent over-diagnosis (this means that if left undiagnosed their cancers would not have become symptomatic within their lifetime). The consequence of this over-diagnosis is that women are turned into patients unnecessarily and will undergo surgery and other forms of cancer treatment that will adversely affect their quality of life and psychological well-being.'

Independent UK Panel on Breast Cancer Screening. Lancet. 2012;380:1778–86. Available online: http://www.cancerresearchuk.org/prod_consump/groups/cr_common/@nre/@pol/documents/generalcontent/breast-screening-report.pdf

The most appropriate interval between mammographic screens is yet to be determined. In the UK, screening takes place every 3 years but the rate of cancers diagnosed between the second and third years after the initial screen climbs rapidly, suggesting that this interval may be too long. Patients are currently screened by two-view mammography.

About two-thirds of screen-detected abnormalities are shown to be benign or normal on further mammographic or ultrasound imaging. Between 20% and 25% of all screen-detected breast cancers are noninvasive (DCIS) and the remainder are invasive. Compared with symptomatic cancers, screen-detected cancers are smaller and more likely to be noninvasive. The ability of screening to influence mortality from breast cancer (EBM 19.3) indicates that early diagnosis identifies cancers at an earlier stage of evolution, when metastatic spread is less likely to have occurred. Controversy has surrounded breast screening because overdiagnosis and overtreatment do occur. Women need to be informed of the pros and cons of breast screening so they can make an informed decision whether to attend.

<table>
<tr><td>EBM</td><td>19.3 Mortality rates in breast cancer</td></tr>
</table>

'Mortality rates from breast cancer are falling in all age groups and are approximately 2% per year. The major reason for the falls in mortality is a combination of earlier detection and better treatment.'

Mukhtar TK. J R Soc Med. 2013;106:234–42.; Weedon-Fekjaer. BMJ. 2014;348: g3701.

Mammographic features of breast cancer

Mammographically, a cancer most commonly appears as a dense opacity with an irregular outline from which spicules pass into the surrounding tissue (Fig. 19.27). Associated features include microcalcifications that can occur within or outside the lesion, skin tethering or thickening, distortion of the shape of the breast or overlying skin, and tenting or direct involvement of underlying muscle. Involved lymph nodes can also sometimes be seen (Fig. 19.28). Mammography is not always accurate in dense breasts. For this reason in the USA, ultrasound is advised in addition to mammography screening in women with dense breasts.

Staging of breast cancer

When invasive cancer is diagnosed, the extent of the disease should be assessed. The currently used tumour, nodes and metastases (TNM) system relies on clinical measurements and clinical assessment of lymph node status, both of which are inaccurate (Table 19.7). Breast cancer is also classed as being stage I–IV (Table 19.7). The imaging size is used when making

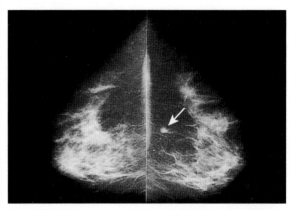

Fig. 19.27 Mammogram of a cancer detected at breast screening. A small lesion at the back of the left breast (*arrow*).

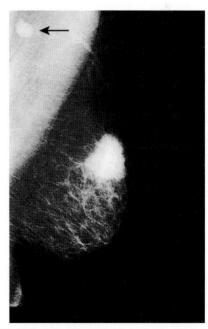

Fig. 19.28 Mammogram of a cancer (irregular dense mass) and involved axillary nodes (localised density in the axillary tail).

Table 19.7 TNM staging for breast cancer

T (Primary tumour)

T_X	Primary tumour cannot be assessed
T_0	No evidence of primary tumour
T_{1s}	Carcinoma in situ: intraductal carcinoma, lobular carcinoma in situ, or Paget's disease of the nipple with no associated tumour mass[a]
T_1	Tumour 2.0 cm or less in greatest dimension[b]
T_{1a}	0.5 cm or less in greatest dimension
T_{1b}	More than 0.5 cm but not more than 1.0 cm in greatest dimension
T_{1c}	More than 1.0 cm but not more than 2.0 cm in greatest dimension
T_2	Tumour more than 2.0 cm but not more than 5.0 cm in greatest dimension[b]
T_3	Tumour more than 5.0 cm in greatest dimension[b]
T_4	Tumour of any size with direct extension to chest wall or skin
T_{4a}	Extension to chest wall (includes ribs, intercostal muscles, serratus anterior only, *but not* pectoral fascia or muscle)
T_{4b}	Oedema (including orange peel appearance), ulceration of the skin of the breast or satellite nodules confined to the same breast
T_{4c}	Both of the above (T_{4a} and T_{4b})
T_{4d}	Inflammatory carcinoma[c]

N (Regional lymph nodes)

N_X	Cannot be assessed (e.g., previously removed)
N_0	No regional lymph node metastasis
N_1	Metastases to movable ipsilateral level I, II axillary lymph node(s)
N_2	Metastases in ipsilateral level I, II axillary lymph nodes that are clinically fixed or matted OR Metastases in clinically detected[c] ipsilateral internal mammary nodes in the *absence* of clinically evident axillary lymph node metastases
N_3	Metastases in ipsilateral infraclavicular (level III axillary) lymph node(s) with or without level I, II axillary lymph node involvement OR Metastases in ipsilateral internal mammary lymph node(s) with clinically evident axillary lymph node metastases OR Metastases in ipsilateral supraclavicular lymph node(s) with or without axillary or internal mammary lymph node involvement

M (Distant metastases)

M_X	Cannot be assessed
M_0	No distant metastasis
M_1	Distant metastasis present (includes metastasis to ipsilateral supraclavicular lymph nodes)

Staging based on TNM

Stage 0	T_{is} N_0 M_0
Stage I	T_1 N_0 M_0
Stage II	T_0 N_1 M_0, T_1 N_1 M_0, T_2 N_0 M_0, T_2 N_1 M_0, T_3 N_0 M_0
Stage IIIA	T_0 N_2 M_0, T_1 N_2 M_0, T_2 N_2 M_0, T_3 N_1 M_0, T_3 N_2 M_0
Stage IIIB	T_4 N_0 M_0, T_4 N_1 M_0, T_4 N_2 M_0
Stage IIIC	Any T N_3 M_0
Stage IV	Any T Any N M_1

[a]Paget's disease associated with tumour mass is classified according to the size of the tumour.
[b]Dimpling or tethering of the skin and nipple retraction or other skin changes may occur in T_1, T_2 or T_3 without changing the classification. They are only signs of underlying malignancy and occurs due to involvement of ligaments of Cooper.
[c]Inflammatory carcinoma of the breast: brawny induration of the skin of the breast with an erysipeloid edge usually without any palpable lump.

decisions on management, as it is more accurate than clinical measurement. Patients with small breast cancers (< 4 cm) have a low incidence of detectable metastatic disease and, unless they have specific symptoms, do not need investigations to search for systemic metastases. Patients with larger or more locally advanced breast cancers are more likely to have metastases and should be considered for CT of the chest, abdomen and pelvis (or liver ultrasound) and a bone scan. A simpler classification of breast cancer separates patients into three groups: operable, locally advanced and metastatic.

The curability of breast cancer

Almost half the women with operable breast cancer who are treated solely by local treatments (surgery, with or without radiotherapy) die from metastatic disease, indicating that cancer has spread by the time of presentation. Invasive breast cancers

spread via lymphatics and through the bloodstream. The most common site for spread is to the axillary lymph nodes. It was previously believed that spread through the blood stream took place only after lymph nodes were involved, but it is now appreciated that lymph nodes do not act as a filter and while the presence of nodal metastases usually means that the cancer has spread systemically, distant metastases are sometimes present in patients with negative axillary nodes. Metastasis can occur at any site, but the most commonly affected organs are the bony skeleton, lungs, liver, brain, ovaries and peritoneal cavity.

Prognosis of breast cancer

Factors related to prognosis include:

- Stage of the tumour at diagnosis: principally, its size and involvement of the axillary lymph nodes or the presence of any metastases (Fig. 19.29)

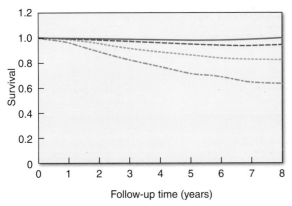

Fig. 19.29 Relation between number of involved axillary lymph nodes and survival after breast cancer. Patients treated between 2006–2012 (*blue*, N0, no nodes involved by pathology; *red*, N1, 1–3 nodes involved; *green*, N2, 4–9 nodes involved; *purple*, N3, ≥10 nodes involved by metastases).

- Biological factors that relate to tumour aggressiveness: these include histological grade, histological type, presence of lymphatic and/or vascular invasion, hormone receptor content and HER2 status
- Genomic indices that measure tumour proliferation, ER and HER2, or a panel of genes using messenger RNA from the cancer.

It is possible to combine prognostic factors. There are a number of online tools to help predict prognosis and determine the potential benefits of different treatments, e.g., Adjuvant! Online and Predict! These tools incorporate tumour size, nodal status, tumour grade, proliferation, patient age, general health status and the receptor status of the cancer. Mammaprint is a 70-gene profile and the Recurrence Score or Oncotype DX is a 21-gene panel. Both can be measured in paraffin-embedded breast cancer tissue. They are used to help determine prognosis and to predict whether chemotherapy is likely to benefit the patient.

Presentation of breast cancer

The most common presentation of cancer is with a breast lump or lumpiness, which is usually painless. Any discrete lump, no matter how small or mobile, may be malignant. The investigation of a breast lump is shown in Figure 19.30. Malignant lesions are usually firm and irregular and produce visible signs of breast asymmetry, such as flattening, dimpling or puckering of the over-lying skin. Retraction or alteration in nipple contour can also be features of malignancy. Approximately 50% of breast cancers are located in the upper outer quadrant of the breast. Diagnosis of breast lumps is a particular problem in young women, in whom the breasts are dense and lumpier and in whom cancer is rare. In this age group cancer commonly presents as lumpiness or asymmetric nodularity rather than a discrete lump. Some patients attend with features of locally advanced breast cancer such as skin ulceration, with direct infiltration of the skin by tumour or with oedema±erythema of the overlying skin (Fig. 19.31).

Breast pain alone is a rare presenting feature of breast cancer; 2.7% of patients with breast pain have cancer, whereas 4.6% of patients presenting with breast cancer have pain as their only

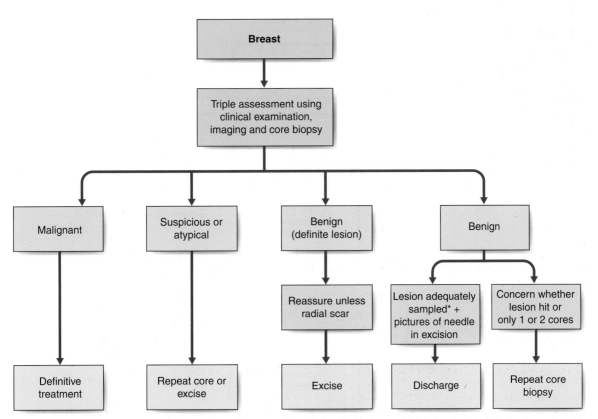

Fig. 19.30 Investigation of a breast mass. *A minimum of three cores is required, preferably image-guided, to be certain the lesion has been adequately sampled.

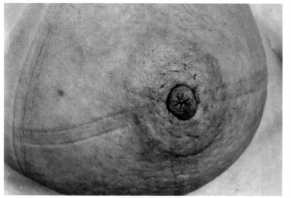

Fig. 19.31 Orange peel appearance of the skin around the nipple in a patient with inflammatory carcinoma.

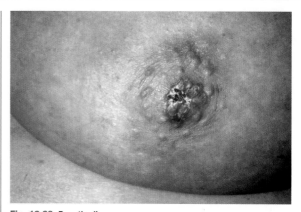

Fig. 19.33 Paget's disease.

symptom. Nipple discharge, which is either blood-stained or contains moderate or large amounts of blood on testing, can be a presenting feature of breast cancer. Investigation of patients who present with nipple discharge is shown in Figure 19.32.

Patients with breast cancer occasionally present with a dry scaling or red weeping appearance of the nipple known as Paget's disease; this signifies an underlying invasive or noninvasive cancer (Fig. 19.33) and should be differentiated from eczema (Fig. 19.34). Paget's disease always affects the nipple and only

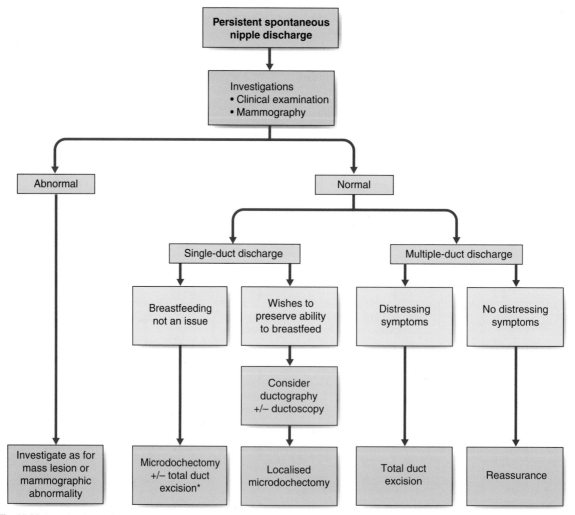

Fig. 19.32 Investigation of nipple discharge. *Some surgeons prefer total duct excision in women >45 years to reduce the incidence of further discharge from ducts (microdochectomy: removal of diseased duct).

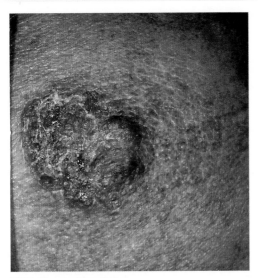
Fig. 19.34 Eczema of the nipple.

involves the areola as a secondary event, whereas eczema primarily involves the areola and only secondarily affects the nipple. Approximately 1–2% of patients with breast cancer have Paget's disease.

Patients can present initially with palpable axillary nodes or with signs or symptoms of distant metastatic disease: for example, an enlarged supraclavicular node, bone pain, a cough or breathlessness, lethargy and tiredness, jaundice, headaches, or a sudden onset of grand mal seizures. Fewer than 1 in 300 patients present with axillary nodal metastases without an obvious primary cancer in the breast. Up to 70% of these women have metastases from an occult breast cancer, most of which will be visible on mammography or MRI of the breast.

Management of operable breast cancer

In situ breast cancer

Localised DCIS can be treated by wide excision to clear surgical margins. Patients with small areas of low or intermediate grade DCIS that have been excised completely have a low rate of recurrence and may not require any follow up treatment. Patients with high grade DCIS have a much higher rate of recurrence or of invasive cancer development after wide excision alone and should be considered for postoperative radiotherapy, which significantly reduces the rate of recurrence. There is no evidence as yet that radiotherapy reduces the number of women dying from breast cancer. Tamoxifen reduces both the risk of recurrence and the rate of development of contralateral cancer in women with oestrogen receptor-positive DCIS, but because of side-effects its use for DCIS is not widespread. Larger areas of DCIS are usually treated by mastectomy, with or without immediate breast reconstruction.

Estimating risk of DCIS recurrence has until recently been based on the patient's age, extent, grade and margins. A new genomic-based DCIS prognostic index has been developed to

identify women at low and high risk of recurrence but is not yet in widespread use.

19.3 Summary

Ductal carcinoma in situ (DCIS)
- Localised disease is treated by wide local excision to clear margins
- All patients other than those at low risk of recurrence should be considered for adjuvant radiotherapy to the breast
- Tamoxifen reduces recurrence following wide excision, but is not in widespread use because of its side effects
- Large areas of DCIS are usually treated by mastectomy ± reconstruction.

Operable breast tumours

Operable breast tumours are those restricted to the breast alone or have mobile involved ipsilateral axillary lymph nodes (T_1, T_2, T_3, N_0, N_1, M_0). As only a minority of patients are cured by locoregional treatments alone, most women with operable breast cancer should be considered for systemic therapy after local therapy (EBM 19.4 and 19.5).

EBM 19.4 Breast conservation in operable cancers

'Breast-conserving surgery followed by radiotherapy is as effective as mastectomy for small operable breast cancer.'

Fisher B et al. N Engl J Med. 2002;347:1270–1.

EBM 19.5 Radiotherapy after surgery for invasive breast cancer

'Radiotherapy reduces local recurrence after breast conserving surgery for invasive breast cancer and reduces deaths from breast cancer.'

Early Breast Cancer Trialists' Collaborative Group. Lancet. 2005;366:2087–106.

Local therapy

There are currently two accepted methods of local therapy for operable breast cancer.

Breast-conserving surgery

This involves removing the cancer with a margin of macroscopically normal tissue. Breast conservation is only feasible when, once all the cancer or cancers have been excised, a good cosmetic outcome is achievable. Complete excision of all invasive and noninvasive cancer is necessary and if any invasive cancer or DCIS extends to a margin, then re-excision of that margin is usually recommended.

Axillary surgery in women with operable invasive breast cancer

Patients whose nodes appear normal on clinical examination and imaging should have a sentinel lymph node biopsy using a

19

radioactive isotope colloid ± blue dye. Patients with micrometastases ≤2 mm require no further axillary treatment. Patients with one or two involved sentinel lymph nodes may not require any further treatment to the axilla providing they are getting radiotherapy to the breast.

Patients with involved nodes proven on FNA or core biopsy, patients with involved sentinel nodes not having whole breast radiotherapy, and patients with >2 sentinel nodes should have the remaining nodes treated by surgery (axillary clearance or axillary dissection), or with radiotherapy. Patients with >4 axillary lymph nodes are at increased risk of recurrence after mastectomy and so are advised to have radiotherapy to the chest wall and the supraclavicular region.

Patients who have a good cosmetic result after breast-conserving surgery have low levels of anxiety and depression and better body image and self-esteem than those who have a poor result. The larger the volume of breast tissue excised, the poorer the cosmetic result. The aim of breast-conserving surgery is to remove the cancer in as small a volume of tissue as possible, and to obtain clear margins, classified as ≥1 mm in the UK and no ink on tumour in the US.

Radiotherapy

Wide excision should be followed by whole breast radiotherapy given over a period of 3–5 weeks. An additional boost is given to the tumour bed in women under 50 years of age or those with close margins. Studies comparing local radiotherapy with the tumour bed given intraoperatively using an intracavity balloon device or after operation using external beam are ongoing. Rates of local recurrence are higher for local radiotherapy than with whole breast radiotherapy. Long-term data are required before local radiotherapy is considered safe enough to use in routine practice.

19.4 Summary

Breast conservation

- Is suitable treatment for operable breast cancers in which there is no evidence of metastatic disease beyond the axillary nodes; excision must leave a reasonable cosmetic result
- Includes wide local excision of the cancer to clear histological margins, axillary surgery (sentinel node biopsy in patients without evident nodal involvement, or clearance of the axillary nodes in patients with proven nodal metastases) and whole-breast radiotherapy with an optional boost to the tumour bed.

Modified radical mastectomy

This is indicated in patients
- When breast conservation would produce an unacceptable cosmetic result (this includes some but not all central lesions directly underneath the nipple and most larger cancers). Breast-conserving surgery may be possible in these women if they have shrinkage following initial chemotherapy or hormone treatment
- When radiotherapy is not possible or when there is a wish to try and avoid radiotherapy
- Who elect to have a mastectomy
- Who have a localised invasive cancer but also a large area of surrounding DCIS.

Radical or so-called Halsted mastectomy, where all breast tissue with overlying skin including the nipple was removed along with part of the pectoralis major muscle in combination with complete axillary node clearance, is no longer used. The modified radical mastectomy preserves the pectoralis major and usually the pectoralis minor muscles and remains the most appropriate treatment for late-presenting breast cancers in developing countries. If reconstruction is being performed, a skin-sparing mastectomy can be performed. Mastectomy should be combined with some form of axillary surgery to assess involvement of lymph nodes. Radiotherapy to the chest wall is given after mastectomy to patients who are at high risk of local recurrence, i.e., those with involvement of multiple axillary lymph nodes, a grade III cancer, a cancer >5 cm in diameter (pathological measurement), or a tumour that involved the pectoral fascia or pectoral muscle or was close to any remaining skin.

19.5 Summary

Mastectomy

- For large operable breast cancers or patients with extensive noninvasive disease
- For women who have incomplete excision after one or more attempts at breast-conserving surgery and in some women with a central tumour
- Consists of removal of the whole breast together with sentinel node biopsy, or an axillary clearance
- Should be followed by chest-wall radiotherapy in women at high risk of local recurrence.

Systemic therapy

Systemic drug treatment can be given after surgery and/or radiotherapy (adjuvant), or before surgery and/or radiotherapy (neoadjuvant). The effectiveness of adjuvant treatment has been shown in clinical trials (EBM 19.6). Randomised studies comparing neoadjuvant therapy with adjuvant treatment have shown similar outcomes, with a higher rate of breast-conserving surgery in patients having initial treatment with chemotherapy or hormone therapy. Adjuvant systemic treatments include chemotherapy, hormone therapy and targeted treatments such as the anti-HER2 drug trastuzumab.

If neoadjuvant therapy is planned, core biopsy of the cancer and nodes (if involved) and marking of the cancer and the nodes with clips or a radioactive seed should be performed before starting treatment.

Adjuvant chemotherapy

- A combination of chemotherapy drugs is more effective than a single agent
- The optimal benefit appears to come from at least four cycles of postoperative chemotherapy
- The benefits of chemotherapy are greatest in women under the age of 50 years (Table 19.8); a smaller but still significant benefit is seen in older women
- Regimens that include anthracyclines are more effective than non-anthracycline-containing regimens
- Taxanes (taxol and taxotere) combined with an anthracycline appear more effective than anthracyclines alone

Table 19.8 Reduction in recurrence and mortality in polychemotherapy trials

Age	Reduction in annual odds of recurrence (% ± SD)	Reduction in annual odds of death (% ± SD)
<40	37 ± 7	27 ± 8
40–49	34 ± 5	27 ± 5
50–59	22 ± 4	14 ± 4
60–69	18 ± 4	8 ± 4
All ages	23 ± 8	15 ± 2

- Platinum agents are particularly effective in BRCA mutation carriers
- Chemotherapy is generally offered to all patients at significant risk of recurrence.

EBM 19.6 Adjuvant systemic treatment for breast cancer

'Adjuvant systemic treatment reduces the risk of relapse by 30–40%. In hormone receptor-positive breast cancer, reducing oestrogen levels or using an oestrogen antagonist reduces recurrence by 40–50% and improves survival in all ages. Chemotherapy reduces risk of recurrence by up to 40% and reduces deaths from breast cancer, the greatest benefit being in younger women and those with hormone receptor-negative cancer.'

Early Breast Cancer Trialists' Collaborative Group (EBCTCG). Lancet 2005;365:1687–717.

Adjuvant hormone therapy

Hormone therapy is only effective in patients with ER+ breast cancer and has its greatest benefit in women with ER rich breast cancers. Adjuvant hormonal treatments include oophorectomy, tamoxifen and the aromatase inhibitors letrozole, anastrozole and exemestane. Oophorectomy is only of benefit in women under 50 years of age with ER+ cancer. It can be achieved surgically, by radiation or by the administration of gonadotrophin-releasing hormone (GnRh) analogues such as goserelin. Tamoxifen is a partial oestrogen agonist taken orally in a dose of 20 mg once daily. At least 5 years of tamoxifen should be given. It reduces the risk of contralateral breast cancer by 40–50%. Tamoxifen is effective in both pre- and postmenopausal women. The aromatase inhibitors block the conversion of androgens to oestrogen in postmenopausal women and appear to be more effective than tamoxifen in postmenopausal women. Aromatase inhibitors combined with ovarian suppression or ablation appears to be better than ovarian suppression alone in younger premenopausal women with high risk ER+ cancers who regain regular menstrual cycles after chemotherapy. Aromatase inhibitors should be included as adjuvant therapy for most postmenopausal women with hormone receptor-positive breast cancer. Studies have shown that 10 years of hormone therapy is better than 5 years.

A summary of how hormone therapy and chemotherapy are used as adjuvant treatment is outlined in Table 19.9.

Table 19.9 Suggested adjuvant treatment for patients with breast cancer[a]

Risk group	Premenopausal	Postmenopausal
Very low-risk ER+	Nil or tamoxifen	Nil or tamoxifen
Low-risk ER+	Tamoxifen	Tamoxifen
Low-risk ER−	Chemotherapy or nil	Chemotherapy or nil
Moderate-risk ER+	Chemotherapy + tamoxifen[b]	Chemotherapy + AI[c]
Moderate-risk ER−	Chemotherapy	Chemotherapy
High-risk	Chemotherapy + tamoxifen + OS[d] (if ER+)	Chemotherapy + AI[c]

ER, oestrogen receptor.
[a]Patients whose tumours overexpress HER2 should also be considered for adjuvant trastuzumab.
[b]5 years of tamoxifen followed by 5 years on an aromatase inhibitor (AI).
[c]AI for 5 years.
[d]Ovarian suppression (OS): either luteinising hormone releasing hormone (LHRH) analogue or surgical oophorectomy.

Anti-HER2 therapy

Between 15% and 20% of cancers overexpress the oncogene HER2 and these cancers have a worse prognosis than those that are HER2-negative. A humanised monoclonal antibody (trastuzumab) has been shown to reduce the risk of cancer recurrence by up to 50% in women whose cancers overexpress HER2 (EBM 19.7).

EBM 19.7 Effect of trastuzumab on breast cancer

'Trastuzumab given to patients whose cancer over-expresses the oncogene HER2 reduces recurrence by up to 50%.'

Piccart-Gebhart MJ et al. N Engl J Med. 2005;353:1659–72.; Romond EH et al. N Engl J Med. 2005;353:1673–84.

Studies with pertuzumab (another monoclonal antibody), T-DM1 (a combination of trastuzumab and a chemotherapy drug called emtansine), and lapatinib (an oral HER2 targeted drug) are in progress.

Neoadjuvant therapy

Neoadjuvant or preoperative treatment should be considered in patients with large or locally advanced tumours that would otherwise require a mastectomy who may become suitable for breast-conserving surgery, or in patients with inoperable cancers that may become operable. It is used increasingly in Western countries. Pathological complete response rates to chemotherapy occur in 30–40% of patients with triple negative cancers, in up to 60% in HER2-positive cancers but in less than 10% in ER+ cancers.

19

19.6 Summary

Adjuvant therapy

Following surgery and/or radiotherapy for operable breast cancer, patients should receive adjuvant systemic therapy, which can be either hormonal therapy or chemotherapy.

Examples of hormonal therapy

- Premenopausal women: tamoxifen, goserelin, or goserelin + aromatase inhibitor
- Postmenopausal women: tamoxifen or aromatase inhibitors, or tamoxifen followed by an aromatase inhibitor.

Chemotherapy

- Commonly used regimens are AC, FEC, AT, ET[a].

Positive factors influencing the use of chemotherapy

- Young age (especially <50 years)
- Axillary node positivity
- Large tumour size
- Histological features
  Grade III
  Lymphatic/vascular invasion
- Negative oestrogen receptor.

[a]AC, Adriamycin cyclophosphamide; AT, adriamycin and a taxane; CET, epirubicin and a taxane; FEC, 5-fluorouracil, epirubicin and cyclophosphamide.

- Neoadjuvant hormonal therapy is being used increasingly in postmenopausal women with oestrogen receptor rich breast cancers.
- Randomised studies of neoadjuvant hormone treatment have shown that the aromatase inhibitor, letrozole, produces better responses than tamoxifen.

Breast cancer in pregnancy

Diagnosis during pregnancy occurs in 1–2% of breast cancers and develop in 1–3 of every 10,000 pregnancies. There is no evidence that breast cancer occurring during pregnancy is more aggressive, although up to 65% of patients have involved axillary nodes because diagnosis is often delayed. Treatment during pregnancy is usually by mastectomy, but breast-conserving surgery followed by radiotherapy after delivery is possible in small cancers. Radiotherapy is not given during pregnancy. Chemotherapy during pregnancy can be given but is associated with a small risk of foetal damage.

Pregnancy after treatment for breast cancer

Available data show no effect of pregnancy on the outcome of patients with breast cancer.

Complications of treatment

Haematoma and infection are the most common complications (<5%) after breast surgery. Removal of all the axillary nodes often damages the intercostobrachial nerve, resulting in numbness and paraesthesia down the upper inner aspect of the arm. Other nerves that can be damaged during axillary surgery include the long thoracic nerve (causes winging of the scapula), and the thoracodorsal nerve (results in atrophy of the latissimus dorsi muscle and prominence of the scapula). After axillary surgery about 5% of women develop a frozen shoulder. Up to 40% of women treated by a full axillary dissection develop lymphoedema. Even after a sentinel lymph node biopsy some women develop arm swelling. The treatment of lymphoedema involves massage, skin care, and wearing a supportive elasticated sleeve.

Radiotherapy

Following radiotherapy, the skin develops an erythematous reaction that can last for 3–4 weeks. Patients should avoid exposing the area to direct sunlight for several months. Following radiotherapy to the axilla, some patients develop fibrosis around the shoulder.

Chemotherapy

Hair loss or alopecia is the most common concern of patients before starting chemotherapy, but 80% report fatigue and lethargy as the most troublesome side effect. The occurrence of alopecia with some chemotherapy regimens may be reduced by scalp cooling. Nausea and vomiting can be controlled in most patients with appropriate antiemetic drugs. Trastuzumab, when combined with anthracycline-containing chemotherapy, can result in cardiac failure in a small but significant number of patients, so patients having this drug require cardiac monitoring.

Hormonal treatments

The side effects of hormonal treatments are greatest in premenopausal patients and include hot flushes, vaginal dryness or discharge and loss of libido. All these have a considerable impact on quality of life. Aromatase inhibitors cause fewer hot flushes than tamoxifen, but cause more muscular aches and pains, vaginal dryness and reduced bone density.

Psychological aspects

Most women who present with breast lumps are emotionally distressed. When breaking bad news, the first step should be to check the patient's understanding of what is wrong. Almost two-thirds of patients with breast cancer suspect that their lump is malignant. In patients with proven malignancy, the doctor's role is to confirm that their diagnosis is correct, pause to let this sink in, acknowledge their distress and establish what concerns are contributing to any distress. When a patient is unaware that she has cancer, the doctor should break the news more slowly. Breast care nurses help to ensure that the patient is fully informed about the nature of any disease and its treatment. They can provide advice on prostheses, and help recognise and support patients with significant psychiatric problems.

Up to 30% of women with breast cancer develop an anxiety state or depressive illness within a year of diagnosis, 3–4 times the rate of women without breast cancer. After mastectomy, 20–30% of patients develop persisting problems with body image and sexual difficulties. Breast-conserving surgery reduces problems with body image. Psychiatric morbidity is increased when radiotherapy or chemotherapy is used. Few patients mention psychological problems to their doctor because they think it is unacceptable to do so. Doctors can promote the disclosure of such problems by being empathetic and making educated guesses about how patients are feeling.

Breast reconstruction

There is evidence that patients benefit psychologically from immediate breast reconstruction. Options for reconstruction include the placement of an implant at the time of mastectomy, behind the pectoral muscle. The use of implants has increased because larger pockets can now be created by the use of decellularised collagen matrices or the use of a synthetic mesh that is sutured between the pectoralis major and the chest wall to create a sling or pocket into which an implant can be placed. Alternative options for breast reconstruction include myocutaneous flaps; the most commonly used are the latissimus dorsi myocutaneous flap with or without an implant (Fig. 19.35), and the rectus abdominis myocutaneous flap alone. Lipofilling or lipomodelling is now commonly used as part of breast reconstruction.

Follow-up

The aim of follow-up is to detect local recurrence at a stage when it is treatable, to support the patient psychologically and to discuss problems associated with adjuvant therapy. Patients should have an annual mammogram of one or both breasts. No investigations should be performed to detect asymptomatic metastases as there is no evidence that this influences survival.

Management of locally advanced breast cancer

Locally advanced breast cancer (LABC) is characterised by infiltration of the skin or chest wall by tumour or matted involved axillary nodes (Table 19.10). It has a variable natural history. The median survival was previously 2–2.5 years but this has improved dramatically with better systemic therapy. LABC can arise because of its position in the breast (for example, peripheral), neglect (some patients do not present to hospital for months or years after they notice a mass), or biological aggressiveness (Fig. 19.36). The latter includes inflammatory cancers characterised by erythema and/or widespread peau d'orange or orange peel appearance affecting the breast skin, due to oedema from obstruction of dermal lymphatics by tumour cells (Fig. 19.31). Inflammatory carcinomas are uncommon but they have the worst prognosis of all LABCs (Fig. 19.37).

Local and regional relapse was formerly a major problem in LABC and affected more than half of patients. Primary systemic therapy, followed by surgery and radiotherapy or radiotherapy alone, has improved local control. Systemic treatment consists

Table 19.10 Clinical features of locally advanced breast cancer
Skin
• Ulceration
• Satellite nodules
• Dermal infiltration
• Peau d'orange
• Erythema over tumour
Chest wall

• Tumour fixation to:
  ribs
  intercostal muscles
  serratus anterior

Axillary nodes
• Nodes fixed to one another or to other structures

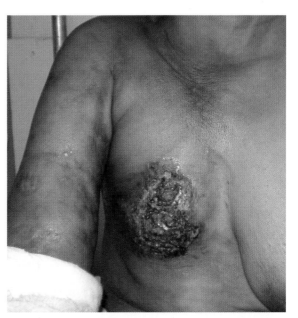

Fig. 19.36 Late presentation. This is common in certain countries such as India and this is an example of where the breast is destroyed with ulceration and evidence of 'cancer en cuirasse' (cutaneous metastatic breast carcinoma with lymphoedema of the chest wall and upper limb).

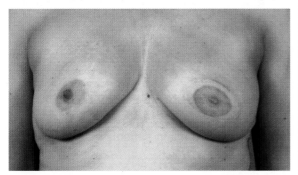

Fig. 19.35 A patient who had a left mastectomy and breast reconstruction with a latissimus dorsi reconstruction. The patient also had a nipple reconstruction with tattooing.

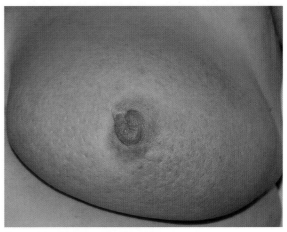

Fig. 19.37 Inflammatory breast cancer.

19

of either chemotherapy (inflammatory cancers, ER− tumours and rapidly progressive disease) or endocrine treatment (slow or indolent disease, ER+ cancers in women who are elderly or unfit). Following systemic therapy, the disease may become operable, at which point wide excision or mastectomy together with removal of any involved axillary nodes is followed by radiotherapy. In women whose disease remains inoperable following systemic treatment, radiotherapy is usually given. This can be followed by surgery in women in whom viable resectable cancer remains following radiotherapy.

 19.7 Summary

Locally advanced breast cancer

- Consider chemotherapy in patients who are young, have inflammatory cancers or have ER− disease
- Consider neoadjuvant endocrine therapy in the elderly or those who have ER+ cancers
- Radiotherapy can be given following primary chemotherapy, concurrently with hormonal therapy, or as an initial treatment
- Consider surgery if disease becomes operable following primary systemic therapy or after radiotherapy.

Management of metastatic or advanced breast cancer

The average period of survival after a diagnosis of metastatic disease varies widely between patients. Metastatic breast carcinoma can be present at diagnosis or may develop following treatment for an apparently localised breast cancer. The aim of treatment is to improve survival and produce effective symptom control with minimal side effects. There is no evidence that treating asymptomatic metastases improves overall survival, and chemotherapy is normally given only to symptomatic patients. Some patients with ER+ or HER2+ cancers survive over a decade with metastases.

Chemotherapy

A balance must be achieved between a high response rate and limiting side effects. The best palliation is obtained with regimens that produce the highest response rates. The most frequently used drugs in metastatic breast cancer are the anthracyclines (adriamycin and epirubicin) and the taxanes (taxol and taxotere). Overall response rates of metastatic disease to chemotherapy are approximately 40–60%, with a median time to relapse of 6–10 months. Subsequent courses have response rates of <25%.

Hormonal treatment

A variety of hormonal interventions are available for patients with ER+ metastatic breast cancer (Table 19.11). In premenopausal women these include oophorectomy (surgical, radiation- or drug-induced by GnRh analogues) combined with tamoxifen. Options in postmenopausal women include the aromatase inhibitors (anastrozole, letrozole and exemestane). The pure antioestrogen fulvestrant is used widely in the USA. Objective responses to hormonal treatments are seen in 50–60% of those with ER+ tumours. It is helpful to biopsy metastatic deposits, as cancers can change their ER and HER2 status. Response rates are 25% or less for second-line hormonal agents and 10–15% at most with third-line endocrine agents.

Table 19.11 Hormonal treatment of metastatic breast cancer

Premenopausal

- Ovarian suppression
- Gonadotrophin-releasing hormone analogues
- Oophorectomy
- Oestrogen receptor modulator: tamoxifen
- Ovarian suppression + tamoxifen[a]
- Ovarian suppression + an aromatase inhibitor

Postmenopausal

- Aromatase inhibitor[b,c]
- Tamoxifen
- Progestins, e.g., megestrol or medroxyprogesterone acetate
- Fulvestrant[d]

Note: These agents can be used in any order.
[a]There is evidence that combined ovarian suppression plus an antioestrogen is superior to single-agent treatment in premenopausal women.
[b]Letrozole or anastrozole are first-line agents in postmenopausal women.
[c]A steroidal aromatase inhibitor (e.g., exemestane) can have efficacy even if a tumour is resistant to the nonsteroidal aromatase inhibitors letrozole and anastrozole.
[d]Licensed in England, Wales and Northern Ireland, but not Scotland; continues to be evaluated in trials.

Anti-HER2 therapy

The humanised monoclonal antibody trastuzumab, raised against HER2, is very effective when combined with chemotherapy in patients with HER2 overexpressing cancer who have metastatic disease. The monoclonal antibody pertuzumab, a conjugate of trastuzumab and a chemotherapy drug maytansine, are also effective in metastatic HER2+ disease. Lapatinib an oral drug that blocks the HER2 pathways is also an option.

 19.8 Summary

Metastatic breast cancer

- The primary aim is to improve symptoms as well as improve the quantity and quality of life
- Consider hormone therapy if there is a long disease-free interval and the tumour is hormone receptor-positive
- Consider chemotherapy if there is a short disease-free interval, vital organs are affected and/or the tumour is oestrogen receptor-negative
- Treat HER2+ breast cancer with trastuzumab and consider combining it or sequencing with newer anti-HER2 agents.

Local treatments in metastatic breast cancer

The role of surgery in metastatic disease is to excise any fungating lesion that makes women in developing countries social outcasts. Simple 'toilet' mastectomy and basic skin cover with grafting can reduce suffering while systemic treatment is given for metastatic disease. Recurrence is common unless the cancer is controlled by systemic therapy. Radiotherapy is an option for local disease control and treatment can be modified to reduce the number of hospital visits.

Specific problems in patients with metastatic breast cancer

Bone disease

Three-quarters of patients who develop metastatic breast cancer have disease involving the bony skeleton. Bony metastases are more common in ER+ cancers particularly invasive lobular cancers. Treatment of localised pain includes radiotherapy and analgesics, including NSAIDs and opiates. Pathological fractures from bone metastases can be predicted by a sharp increase in pain over a few days or weeks. When x-rays show that fracture is likely, a combination of internal fixation by surgery and radiotherapy gives the best outcomes. Patients with widespread bony metastases should be treated with bisphosphonates (drugs that reduce osteoclast activity).

Hypercalcaemia

Up to 40% of patients with bony metastases develop hypercalcaemia. Symptoms include nausea, constipation, thirst, polyuria, personality change, muscle weakness and bone pain. Treatment is hydration with saline (about 3 L given over 24 hours) and the administration of intravenous bisphosphonates followed by a change in anticancer therapy.

Marrow infiltration

Immature cells in the peripheral blood (leucoerythroblastic blood film) suggest marrow infiltration. Chemotherapy is generally required, although hormones can be effective in oestrogen receptor rich disease. Chemotherapy is given initially in reduced doses with careful monitoring and adequate supportive care.

Spinal cord compression

Most often seen in patients with thoracic spinal metastases, it must be recognised early and treated promptly. Patients with isolated metastases causing cord compression and who are fit can be treated by surgery followed by postoperative radiotherapy and appropriate systemic therapy. In the remaining patients, treatment consists of steroids and radiotherapy.

Pleural effusion

Up to half of patients with metastatic breast cancer develop a malignant pleural effusion. Breathlessness is the most common symptom of a pleural effusion. Cytological examination of aspirated fluid reveals malignant cells in only 85% of such patients. Aspiration of the pleural effusion is ineffective treatment, as 97–100% of patients re-accumulate fluid. Tube drainage is better at controlling effusions. Instillation of bleomycin, tetracycline or talc to cause pleurodesis, and effective systemic treatment reduce recurrence. Lymphangitis (carcinoma in lung lymphatics) can also cause breathlessness.

Liver metastases

Right upper quadrant pain, general debility, tiredness, a feeling of nausea, lack of appetite, and the onset of jaundice are all symptoms suggestive of liver metastases. Chemotherapy is usually indicated, other than in postmenopausal patients with oestrogen receptor-rich tumours in whom aromatase inhibitors can be effective. Where jaundice is due to nodal disease at the porta hepatis, stenting of the common bile duct should be considered.

Brain metastases

These should be suspected in any patient with breast cancer who presents with focal neurological symptoms or signs, particularly if the cancer is HER2 positive. CT or MRI can detect even small volumes of disease. Treatment is high-dose corticosteroids (16 mg dexamethasone daily), followed by radiotherapy. The greatest benefits of radiotherapy are seen in patients whose neurological symptoms improve following steroid treatment, but the long-term results of treatment are disappointing. A small group of patients with solitary brain metastases, without evidence of involvement at other sites, are suitable for excision of the metastasis followed by postoperative radiotherapy and systemic treatment.

19.9 Summary

Metastatic disease: specific problems

- Bone metastases may require local radiotherapy, bisphosphonates or orthopaedic intervention, combined with a change of systemic hormonal therapy or chemotherapy
- Hypercalcaemia causes nausea, constipation, thirst, polyuria, weakness, pain and personality change, and is treated by rehydration followed by bisphosphonates
- Spinal cord compression should be treated by surgical decompression if feasible, or by steroids and radiotherapy
- Pleural effusions are best treated by tube drainage, followed by instillation of bleomycin, tetracycline or talc and a change of systemic therapy
- Discrete lung metastases may not cause acute symptoms but lymphangitis carcinomatosa can cause severe bronchospasm and dyspnoea, which may be relieved by steroids, bronchodilators and chemotherapy
- Liver metastases cause general debility, nausea and lack of appetite; they are usually treated by chemotherapy but hormone therapy with aromatase inhibitors is an option for postmenopausal women with ER rich cancers
- Brain metastases are treated initially with steroids, followed by radiation. Surgery is an option for isolated single metastases.

Miscellaneous tumours of the breast

Lymphoma of the breast is rare. Sarcomas are seen occasionally in the breast and include angiosarcomas (sarcoma of blood vessels); these may develop after previous radiotherapy to the breast.

Secondary tumours

Metastases from tumours elsewhere are seen in the breast and include cancers from the bronchus, thyroid, melanoma or the opposite breast.

Male breast

Gynaecomastia

Gynaecomastia (the growth of breast tissue in males to any extent in all ages) is benign and usually reversible. It occurs commonly at puberty and affects 30–60% of boys aged 10–16 years. In this age group it usually requires no treatment, as 80% resolve spontaneously within 2 years (Fig. 19.38). Embarrassment or persistent

19

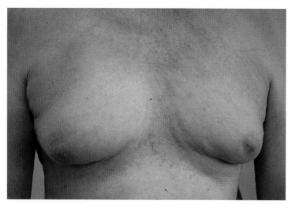

Fig. 19.38 Gynaecomastia in a male.

enlargement is an indication for surgery. Senescent gynaecomastia is also common and affects men aged 50–80 years, and in most cases is not associated with any endocrine abnormality. Drugs are common causes. Other causes include excess alcohol intake and a variety of conditions such as cirrhosis, hypogonadism and, rarely, testicular tumours. Gynaecomastia is usually easily diagnosed by imaging and biopsy is only indicated if there is suspicion that cancer could be present.

Male breast cancer

Less than 0.5% of all breast cancers occur in men and breast cancer comprises 0.7% of all male cancers. The peak incidence is 5–10 years later than in women. Klinefelter's syndrome and a strong family history are the only known risk factors. Young male breast cancers are seen in families with a BRCA2 gene mutation. The most common symptom is an eccentric breast mass often with retraction of the overlying skin. Direct involvement of the skin occurs more often in male than female breast cancer because of the smaller breast volume, and the disease is more likely to be advanced at diagnosis. Imaging and core biopsy will confirm the diagnosis. Treatment for localised breast cancer is by breast-conserving surgery or total mastectomy and the removal of sentinel or all the axillary nodes depending on whether the nodes are thought to be involved or not on preoperative imaging. Postoperative radiotherapy to the chest wall usually follows surgery. Adjuvant tamoxifen reduces recurrence in ER+ cancers. Adjuvant chemotherapy should be considered for fit patients with tumours that have nodal involvement or are oestrogen receptor-negative.

Sonia Wakelin

Endocrine surgery

Chapter contents

Introduction 351

Thyroid gland 351

Parathyroid glands 360

Pituitary gland 363

Adrenal gland 364

Other surgical endocrine syndromes 372

Introduction

In surgical endocrine disease, thyroid disorders are common, adrenal disease is uncommon and parathyroid disease is rare.

Thyroid gland

Surgical anatomy and development (see also Chapter 26)

The thyroid gland develops from the thyroglossal duct, which grows downwards from the pharynx through the developing hyoid bone. On the front of the trachea, the duct bifurcates and fuses with elements from the fourth branchial arch, from which the parafollicular (C) cells are derived.

The duct is normally obliterated in early foetal life but can persist in part to produce a thyroglossal cyst. The upper end of the duct is identified in adults as the foramen caecum at the junction of the anterior two-thirds and the posterior third of the tongue. Arrest of descent of the duct may result in an ectopic thyroid (e.g., lingual thyroid).

There are two pairs of parathyroid glands. The upper glands arise from the fourth branchial arch and are usually found at the back of the thyroid above the inferior thyroid artery. The lower glands arise from the third arch (in association with the thymus) and are less constant in position. They are usually found posterior to the lower pole of the thyroid lobes but can lie within the gland, some distance below it, in the upper mediastinum or within the thymus.

The lobes of the thyroid lie on the front and sides of the trachea and larynx at the level of the 5–7th cervical vertebrae (Fig. 20.1). They are connected by a narrow isthmus, which overlies the second and third tracheal rings. The thyroid normally weighs 15–30 g and is invested by the pretracheal fascia, which binds it to the larynx (oblique line of thyroid cartilage), cricoid cartilage (Berry's ligament) and trachea (Fig. 20.2). The strap muscles (sternohyoid and sternothyroid) lie in front of the pretracheal fascia and must be separated to gain access to the gland. It is difficult to feel the normal thyroid gland except at puberty and during pregnancy, when physiological enlargement occurs.

The superior thyroid artery runs down to the upper pole of the gland as a branch of the external carotid artery, whereas the inferior thyroid artery runs across to the lower pole from the thyrocervical trunk (a branch of the subclavian artery). As it nears the gland, the inferior thyroid artery divides into superior and inferior branches. The bifurcation is usually in front of the recurrent laryngeal nerve, but may be around it. Blood drains through superior, middle and inferior thyroid veins into the internal jugular and innominate veins. Lymphatics pass laterally to the deep cervical chain and downwards to pretracheal and mediastinal nodes. Two branches of the vagus nerve are closely associated with the thyroid gland (Table 20.1). The recurrent laryngeal nerve passes upwards in the groove between the oesophagus and trachea to enter the larynx and supply all of its intrinsic muscles except the cricothyroid. The superior laryngeal nerve, another branch of the vagus, runs with the superior thyroid vessels and the external branch supplies the cricothyroid muscles, which tense the vocal cords. The recurrent nerve also supplies sensation to the larynx below the vocal cords. The internal branch of the superior laryngeal nerve provides sensation above the cords. Normal sensory and motor function within the larynx is necessary for speech and coughing. Both nerves are at risk of damage during thyroid surgery and the consequences, if permanent, can be disabling.

Thyroid function

Histologically, the gland is a vascular organ made up of follicles containing colloid. The follicles are spheroids lined by cuboidal epithelium (thyrocytes). The parafollicular or C cells may be seen between follicles. The thyrocytes secrete triiodothyronine (T_3) and thyroxine (T_4). T_3 is the active hormone, and T_4 is converted to T_3 in the periphery.

T_3 and T_4 secretion is controlled by thyroid-stimulating hormone (TSH), which is secreted by the anterior pituitary

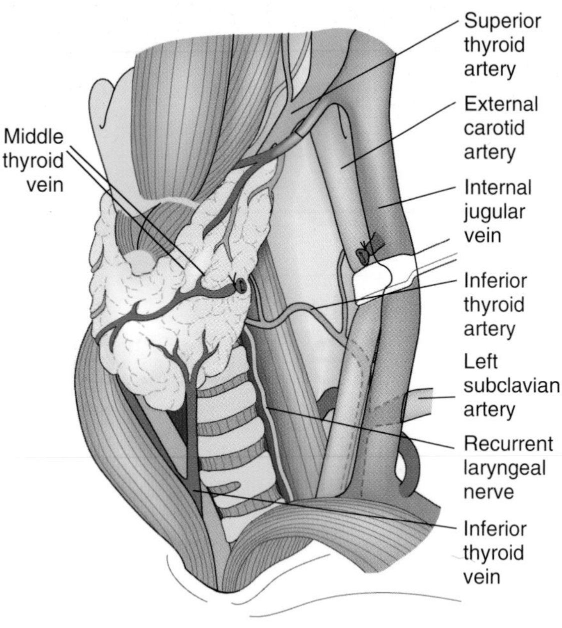

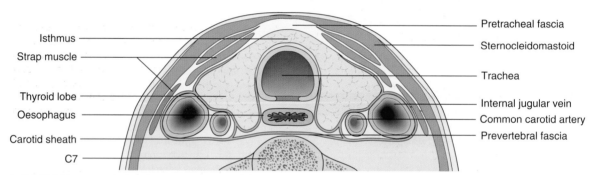

Fig. 20.1 Anatomy of the thyroid gland. The middle thyroid vein has been divided to allow forward rotation of the left lobe of the gland.

(Fig. 20.3). TSH release is controlled by thyrotropin-releasing hormone (TRH) from the hypothalamus. Circulating levels of T_3 and T_4 exert a negative-feedback effect on the hypothalamus and anterior pituitary. Calcitonin, which is released by the parafollicular cells following stimulation by ingested food, lowers the serum calcium but it is not an essential hormone and does not require replacement after total thyroidectomy.

Assessment of thyroid disease

Measurement of T_3, T_4 and TSH gives a biochemical estimation of thyroid function. TSH is totally suppressed in thyrotoxicosis and elevated in hypothyroidism. Pregnancy or oestrogen administration increases the level of thyroid-binding globulin, so that estimation of the ratio of free to bound hormone may be needed. TRH and TSH stimulation tests may be required to determine the site of failure of production of thyroid hormones.

The thyroid can be imaged by ultrasonography (Fig. 20.4) or radioisotope scanning (^{99m}Tc-sodium pertechnetate behaves like iodine and is 'trapped' by the gland). The practice of scanning is to differentiate between 'hot' (actively functioning), 'warm' (normally functioning) and 'cold' (nonfunctioning) thyroid nodules. It is of limited value in differentiating malignant from benign disease. The main value is in evaluating toxic nodular goitres to find out whether it is the nodule that is hyperfunctioning (will be treated

Fig. 20.2 Transverse section of the neck at the level of the seventh cervical vertebra to show the arrangement of the deep cervical fascia.

Table 20.1 Important nerves related to the thyroid gland				
Branches of vagus nerve	**Course**	**Muscles supplied**	**Sensory**	**Effect of permanent damage**
RLN	Passes upwards in groove between oesophagus and trachea	All intrinsic muscles of larynx except cricothyroid	Sensation to larynx below the vocal cords	**Unilateral division** • Vocal cord paralysed in the cadaveric position (midway between closed and open) • Voice is hoarse, weak and may be some stridor **Bilateral division** • Stridor and ineffective coughing • Laryngoplasty or permanent tracheostomy may be required
SLN	Runs with superior thyroid vessels	Cricothyroid (external branch of SLN)	Sensation to larynx above the vocal cords (internal branch of SLN)	• Inability to tense the vocal cord • Voice is weaker with change in pitch range • Anaesthesia of mucous membrane allows foreign bodies to enter larynx more easily
RLN, Recurrent laryngeal nerve; SLN, superior laryngeal nerve.				

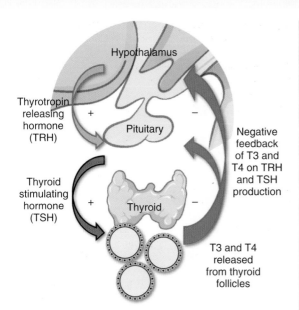

Fig. 20.3 Control of thyroid function.

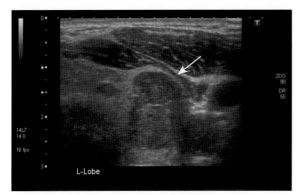

Fig. 20.4 Ultrasound demonstrating thyroid nodule.

by lobectomy) or is it the internodular tissue that is hyperfunctioning (will need subtotal thyroidectomy).

Magnetic resonance imaging (MRI) and computed tomography (CT) provide excellent means of determining the extent of goitre. Fine-needle aspiration cytology (FNAC) is used to determine the nature of thyroid nodules. Thyroid antibodies detected in significant titre may indicate autoimmune thyroid disease.

Enlargement of the thyroid gland (goitre)

Clinical features

Goitre is a visible or palpable enlargement of the thyroid (Fig. 20.5). The swelling appears in the lower part of the neck and retains the shape of the normal gland *(thyreos,* Greek for shield). The swelling characteristically moves upwards on swallowing because of the gland's attachment to the larynx and trachea. Patients may have a dry mouth, and when asking them to swallow, water should be provided.

'Physiological' enlargement

Transient enlargement may occur during puberty or pregnancy.

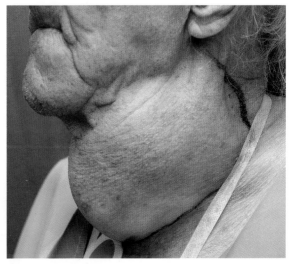

Fig. 20.5 Massive goitre.

Nontoxic nodular goitre

Aetiology

In the past, lack of iodine in the diet was a common cause of thyroid enlargement, but 'endemic goitres' in populations where iodine was deficient are now rare because table salt is iodised. However, nodular goitres still occur in iodine-sufficient populations and goitrogenous foods (e.g., brassica [cabbage] family), enzymatic defects in thyroid hormonogenesis and background radiation exposure may be responsible. It occurs more commonly in females.

Pathology

In a degenerative process called 'nodular hyperplasia', the gland initially enlarges diffusely as the follicles fill with colloid. Later, multiple nodules develop, some of which contain abundant colloid; others show hyperplastic changes or more commonly degenerative changes, with the formation of cysts, areas of old and new haemorrhage, and even calcification. The goitre varies greatly in size, from little more than normal to weighing several hundred grams. The whole gland may be involved, or the changes may be confined to one lobe.

Clinical features

Most multinodular goitres are asymptomatic. Others cause tracheal compression and dyspnoea, particularly when they extend behind the sternum (retrosternal goitre). Oesophageal compression can cause dysphagia. Rarely, bleeding into a nodule may cause pain and rapid enlargement and, for retrosternal goitre, respiratory distress. The thyroid is visibly enlarged and multiple nodules are usually palpable and mobile over the trachea. Sometimes only one nodule is palpable, giving the erroneous impression of a solitary nodule.

Investigations

In the case of retrosternal goitre, plain films of the thoracic inlet may reveal tracheal deviation (Fig. 20.6A) and CT may show tracheal compression (Fig. 20.6B). The presence of stridor indicates

20

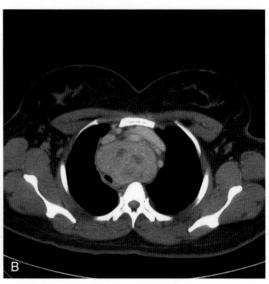

Fig. 20.6 Retrosternal goitre images showing marked tracheal deviation. **(A)** Plain x-ray. **(B)** CT scan.

compromise of the tracheal lumen. T_3, T_4 and TSH are usually normal, and that being the case isotope scans are not indicated.

Management

The administration of thyroxine rarely prevents further gland enlargement via the negative-feedback loop. Large goitres and those causing symptoms of compression require total or subtotal thyroidectomy. Some patients request surgery for cosmetic reasons. Patients usually choose total thyroidectomy with lifelong replacement therapy in preference to the high chance of recurrence and the need for reoperation with subtotal thyroidectomy.

Thyrotoxic goitre

Diffuse thyroid enlargement can result from stimulation by TSH or TSH-like proteins, resulting in increased production of T_3 and T_4 and thyrotoxicosis.

20.1 Summary

Goitres

- Physiological thyroid enlargement may occur during puberty or pregnancy
- Nontoxic nodular goitre can be associated with iodine deficiency and drug reactions; it is usually asymptomatic but can cause compression symptoms
- Thyrotoxic goitre results from stimulation of the gland by TSH or TSH-like proteins, resulting in excessive production of T_3 and T_4. About 25% of cases of thyrotoxicosis are due to a toxic multinodular goitre (a long-standing nontoxic goitre develops hyperactive nodule(s) that function independently of TSH levels)
- Thyroiditis can produce diffuse painful swelling that may be subacute (de Quervain's disease) or autoimmune (Hashimoto's disease). Riedel's thyroiditis is a very rare cause of painless thyroid swelling and tracheal compression
- A solitary thyroid nodule is often a conspicuous palpable nodule in a multinodular goitre. True solitary nodules may be adenomas, cysts or cancers, conditions that are distinguished by fine-needle aspiration cytology, ultrasonography, isotope scans and function tests
- Thyroid cancers can produce a goitre, particularly in the case of medullary carcinoma of the thyroid and lymphoma.

Thyroiditis

Subacute thyroiditis (de Quervain's disease)

This rare condition is associated with an influenza-like illness, during which there is painful diffuse swelling of the gland. Thyroid antibodies may appear in the serum. The disease may be viral in origin and usually resolves spontaneously.

Autoimmune thyroiditis (Hashimoto's disease)

Aetiology

This condition is believed to be due to the destruction of thyroid follicles by lymphocytes. Antibodies are detected in the serum against thyroglobulin, thyroid cell cytosol and microsomes. Histologically, there is marked lymphocytic infiltration around destroyed follicles.

Clinical features

The patient is usually euthyroid, but thyrotoxicosis can occur early. In the long term, the patient becomes hypothyroid as the gland is progressively destroyed. Postmenopausal women are most commonly affected (female/male ratio 10:1). The thyroid is diffusely enlarged and firm. A nodular form may be confused with multinodular goitre. Lymphoma may occur in a thyroid that has been affected by long-standing Hashimoto's disease.

Investigations

The diagnosis is made by demonstrating antithyroid antibodies, particularly to microsomal components of the follicle cells. Biopsy for cytology helps to confirm the diagnosis.

Management

Thyroidectomy is seldom needed and can be difficult because of the firm nature of the gland and inflammation of the surrounding structures. There is a higher than normal risk of damage to the recurrent laryngeal nerves or parathyroid glands.

Riedel's thyroiditis

In this very rare condition the thyroid is replaced by dense fibrous tissue, resulting in a firm painless swelling and tracheal compression. The cause is unknown. Surgery is reliably difficult but decompression of the trachea may be required.

Solitary thyroid nodules

Slow-growing and painless clinically 'solitary' nodules are common, although 50% really represent a clinically dominant nodule within part of a multinodular goitre. Amongst patients presenting with a thyroid nodule, the incidence of malignancy is approximately 10%. The others are benign adenomas or cysts. All patients with new thyroid nodules should be referred for investigation. Patients with concerning features (increasing size, family history of thyroid cancer, previous radiation exposure, patient over 65 years, unexplained hoarseness, cervical lymphadenopathy, stridor) should be referred urgently (EBM 20.1). Ultrasound is a very sensitive examination for thyroid nodules and allows identification of nodules suitable for FNAC. Isotope scans and thyroid function tests aid in the diagnosis (Fig. 20.7). Cysts can be aspirated and, provided that they do not refill and that the cytology is negative for neoplastic cells, they need not be removed. Very rarely, a cyst contains a carcinoma (often papillary) within its wall, and blood-stained aspirate or a residual swelling after aspiration should raise this possibility. A cytopathologist cannot distinguish between a follicular adenoma and follicular carcinoma; this can only be achieved on definitive histopathology by looking for capsular or vascular invasion. Diagnostic surgery is needed if aspiration reveals a follicular neoplasm. Intraoperative frozen section does not always provide a definitive diagnosis, but the demonstration of carcinoma by whatever means indicates that more extensive surgery may be needed (e.g., complete total thyroidectomy).

EBM | **20.1 Investigation and management of thyroid nodules**

'All patients with new thyroid nodules should be referred for investigation. Patients with concerning features (increasing size, family history of thyroid cancer, previous radiation exposure, patient over 65 years, unexplained hoarseness, cervical lymphadenopathy, stridor) require urgent referral.'*

'USS is the most sensitive first-line investigation in the management of thyroid nodules and is used to determine who needs FNAC. Specific USS signs give rise to a classification system that can be used to differentiate benign from malignant nodules (U1 Normal, U2 Benign, U3 Indeterminate, U4 Suspicious, U5 Malignant).'†

'Results from USS and FNAC, where suspicious for cancer, should be discussed in a specific MDT forum.'‡

*NICE Guidance – Improving Outcomes in Head and Neck Cancers https://www.nice.org.uk/guidance/csg6/resources/improving-outcomes-in-head-and-neck-cancers-update-773377597
†http://www.british-thyroid-association.org/Guidelines/
http://www.thyroid.org/professionals/ata-professional-guidelines/
‡NICE Guidance – Improving Outcomes in Head and Neck Cancers https://www.nice.org.uk/guidance/csg6/resources/improving-outcomes-in-head-and-neck-cancers-update-773377597

Other forms of neoplasia

All forms of thyroid cancer can produce goitre. Lymphoma and anaplastic tumours may cause diffuse thyroid swellings. Medullary and follicular tumours are often solitary swellings.

Hyperthyroidism

Thyrotoxicosis results from the overproduction of T_3 and T_4 and, because of the feedback mechanism, serum TSH levels are reduced or undetectable. High circulating levels of T_3 and T_4 increase the basal metabolic rate and potentiate the actions of the sympathetic nervous system. The clinical features of hyperthyroidism are outlined in Table 20.2. The three conditions that may produce thyrotoxicosis are:

1. Primary thyrotoxicosis (Graves' disease).
2. Toxic multinodular goitre.
3. Toxic adenoma.

Primary thyrotoxicosis (Graves' disease)

Pathophysiology

This condition accounts for 75% of cases. It is an autoimmune disease in which TSH receptors in the thyroid are stimulated by circulating thyroid receptor antibodies (TRAbs). The gland is uniformly hyperactive, very vascular and usually symmetrically enlarged. Histologically, there is marked epithelial proliferation, with papillary projections into follicles devoid of colloid. TRAbs can cross the placental barrier, so that neonatal thyrotoxicosis can occur.

Clinical features

The patient is usually a young female (female/male ratio 8:1) and the condition can be familial. The thyroid is usually moderately and diffusely enlarged and soft, and because of its vascularity a bruit may be audible.

In addition to the symptoms seen with hyperthyroidism of any cause, some clinical manifestations are more specific to Graves' disease. These include Graves' ophthalmopathy (Fig. 20.8) and pretibial myxoedema. In Graves' ophthalmopathy, inflammation of the extraocular muscles and connective tissue leads to proptosis (exophthalmos) and impaired function of the eye muscles. Pretibial myxoedema presents commonly as raised pigmented lesions typically on the shins.

Diagnosis

The diagnosis is usually obvious clinically, although in patients with anxiety, distinction from neurosis can be difficult. Raised T_3 and T_4 levels, coupled with low TSH levels, are confirmatory. The TSH response to intravenous injection of TRH is absent owing to atrophy of the TSH-producing cells of the pituitary.

Management

Antithyroid drugs

These drugs block the incorporation of iodine into tyrosine and so prevent the synthesis of T_3 and T_4. Carbimazole, given in full blocking doses (30–60 mg daily in four divided doses), can render the patient euthyroid within 4–6 weeks. However, up to 60% of patients will relapse within 2 years of stopping treatment.

Radioactive iodine

Many consider this to be the treatment of choice. As long as it is not used in pregnancy, the risks of genetic damage are minimal in both patients and their offspring. If ablative doses of iodine are used, patients require thyroxine replacement, but can lead an otherwise normal life with little risk of recurrence.

Surgery

Thyroidectomy is a highly successful form of treatment for many patients, especially younger ones. In experienced hands,

20

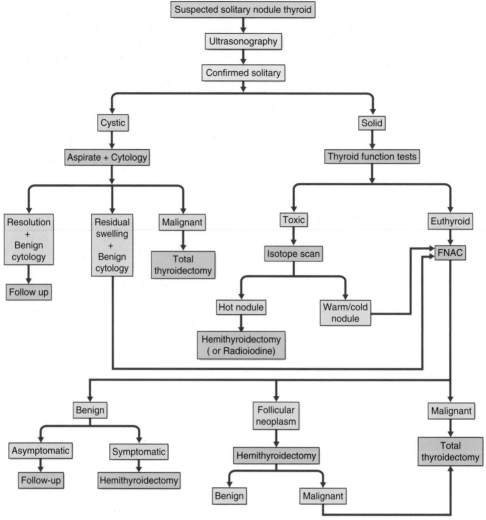

Fig. 20.7 Algorithm for the management of a patient with a suspected solitary thyroid nodule. *FNAC,* Fine-needle aspiration cytology.

Table 20.2 Symptoms of hyperthyroidism

System	Feature
Skin	Heat intolerance Skin moist and warm because of peripheral dilatation and excessive sweating
Cardiovascular	Cardiac output increased to meet metabolic demands Tachycardia even at rest Arrhythmias and palpitations; atrial fibrillation common
Gastrointestinal	Weight loss despite increased appetite Gastrointestinal motility increased
Eyes	Upper eyelid retraction and lid lag. The upper eyelids are retracted because the levator palpebrae superioris has some nonstriated muscle that is innervated by the sympathetic nervous system Exophthalmos common (Graves' disease)
Other	Fine tremor Hyperkinesia Anxiety and psychiatric disturbance may occur Menstrual irregularity Proximal myopathy Occasionally finger clubbing Pretibial myxoedema (Graves disease)

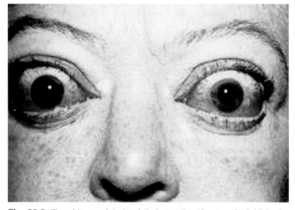

Fig. 20.8 **Thyroid-associated ophthalmopathy.** (Courtesy Prof. Michael Sheppard, University of Birmingham Medical School.)

operative mortality and morbidity are low. Patients are cured by surgery, total thyroidectomy being the operation of choice. Before surgery, patients must be rendered euthyroid with antithyroid drugs. Iodine has historically been given orally for 10 days before surgery to reduce vascularity, but the evidence base to support this is weak. It is thought to act by causing thyroid constipation, wherein the thyroid follicles swell with colloid and compress the interfollicular vessels. This in turn decreases the vascularity of the thyroid. β-Adrenergic blocking drugs can be used as an alternative means of countering the effects of thyrotoxicosis before operation. They block sympathetic overactivity and make the gland less vascular. Cardiac failure, obstructive airways disease and diabetes (where they may mask hypoglycaemic symptoms) are contraindications to the use of β-blockers. Propranolol is given in a dose of 40–80 mg every 6 hours, the aim being to reduce the pulse rate to below 80 beats per minute. Long-acting preparations may be preferred. The drug is continued on the morning of operation and for 7 days thereafter to avoid 'thyroid storm' or 'thyrotoxic crisis'. Excessive sweating or tachycardia after operation is an indication to increase the dose.

Toxic multinodular goitre and toxic adenoma

Pathophysiology

A toxic multinodular goitre is responsible for thyrotoxicosis in about 25% of patients. There is usually a long-standing nontoxic goitre in which one or more nodules become hyperactive and begin to hyperfunction independently of TSH levels. A single hyperfunctioning adenoma is a rare cause of thyrotoxicosis (1–2% of patients). The adenoma secretes thyroid hormones autonomously; TSH secretion and the remainder of the gland are suppressed.

Clinical features

Toxic multinodular goitre is more common in older women, and cardiac complications such as arrhythmias are particularly frequent due to the presence of an already compromised cardiovascular system. Eye signs are rare in these patients.

Diagnosis

In a toxic multinodular goitre, the isotope scan usually demonstrates multiple 'patchy' areas of increased uptake. In toxic adenoma, the nodule is 'hot' and the remainder of the gland is 'cold'.

Management

Treatment consists of removal of the hyperfunctioning glandular tissue by total thyroidectomy (multinodular goitre) or hemithyroidectomy (toxic adenoma), or, if surgery is contraindicated, radioiodine.

Malignant tumours of the thyroid

Thyroid cancer accounts for less than 1% of all forms of malignancy (Table 20.3). As with all thyroid disease, females are more often affected (female/male ratio 3:1). The two main types of thyroid carcinoma are papillary (50%) and follicular (30%), with the remainder comprising medullary carcinoma, anaplastic carcinoma and lymphoma (EBM 20.2). The incidence of thyroid cancer is increased by exposure to ionising radiation: for example, following the Chernobyl disaster. Other risk factors include rapid

EBM 20.2 Relevant websites and publications for the management of thyroid cancer

British Association of Endocrine and Thyroid Surgeons. www.baets.org.uk/Pages/guidelines/.php
    National thyroid cancer guidelines group of the British Thyroid Association. www.british-thyroid-association.org

Northern Cancer Network. Guidelines for management of thyroid cancer. Clin Oncol. 2000;12:373–91.

20

Table 20.3 **Thyroid cancers**		
Type	**Features**	**Prognosis**
Papillary (70%)	• Mostly affects <40 years of age • Lymph node spread common; may present first with lymphadenopathy (so-called lateral aberrant thyroid) • Commonly multifocal • Distant metastases rare • Focus of papillary carcinoma an incidental finding in 20% thyroids resected for other causes	Excellent 10-year survival: 90%
Follicular (20%)	• Affects patients typically 30–50 years • Haematogenous spread more common than lymph node spread. Common sites: lungs, bone, liver	More aggressive than papillary carcinoma. 10-year survival: 75%

Anaplastic	• Typically affects older patients
	• Aggressive tumour presents late
	• Local invasion may cause:
	  - *Stridor:* from either tracheal compression and/or recurrent laryngeal nerve involvement
	  - *Dysphagia:* involvement of the oesophagus
	  - *Horner's syndrome:* from invasion of cervical sympathetic nerves
	• Pulmonary metastases common
		Very poor prognosis;: most patients die within 1 year of diagnosis

Medullary	• Arises from parafollicular C cells • May occur sporadically or as part of MEN II (Sipple's syndrome). Exclude presence of concomitant phaeochromocytoma • Calcitonin levels elevated	10-year survival: 75%
Lymphoma (uncommon)	• Rare complication of autoimmune thyroiditis	10-year survival: 40%

growth of a thyroid lump, family history of thyroid cancer and thyroid cancer syndromes such as multiple endocrine neoplasia (MEN) II, familial adenomatous polyposis and Cowden's syndrome.

Papillary carcinoma

Clinical features

This tumour is most prevalent before the age of 40 years and presents as a slow-growing, solitary thyroid swelling. Enlarged lymph nodes are palpable in one-third of patients and may be the only finding in some patients with a microscopic primary (the so-called 'lateral aberrant thyroid'). Distant metastases are rare. In thyroid glands resected for nonmalignant causes, microscopic papillary carcinoma is discovered as an incidental finding in up to 20%. Histologically, complex papillary folds lined by several layers of cuboidal cells project into what appear to be cystic spaces. Psammoma bodies and nuclear inclusions with a resemblance to a comic-strip character (Orphan Annie) may be found. Lymph node spread is common in papillary carcinoma in comparison to follicular carcinoma.

Management

The disease is commonly multifocal, and thus total thyroidectomy is the optimal surgical procedure. Total thyroidectomy also has the advantage of facilitating early detection of metastases by using radioactive iodine scan, as no functional thyroid tissue is left in the body after surgery. Microscopic disease (<1 cm and unifocal) and tumours with favourable histology and <2 cm in size may be treated by hemithyroidectomy alone. Involved lymph nodes, usually identified by preoperative ultrasound scanning, are removed according to selective anatomical compartments, but routine prophylactic neck dissection is unnecessary. Thyroid-replacement therapy (T_3, 20 μg 6–8-hourly, or thyroxine 200–300 μg/day) is given with the intention of suppressing TSH. Widespread metastases are rare but may be amenable to radioactive iodine therapy. For this reason an isotope scan should be performed 4 weeks postoperatively to identify any iodine uptake in the neck or elsewhere. The disease has an excellent prognosis, with 10-year survival rates approaching 90%.

Follicular carcinoma

Clinical features

This disease typically presents as a solitary thyroid nodule in patients aged 30–50 years. Lymph node metastases are much less common than haematogenous spread, with deposits in the lungs, bone or liver (Fig. 20.9). Bony secondaries may be pulsatile. Histologically, malignant cells are arranged in solid masses with rudimentary acini. Vascular and capsular invasion characterise this neoplasm and distinguish it from a benign follicular adenoma. It is not possible to differentiate between adenoma and carcinoma preoperatively using FNAC, because only aspirated material and cells are seen.

Management

Treatment consists of total thyroidectomy with preservation of the parathyroids where the index of suspicion is high. Frequently, when a hemithyroidectomy has been done for a thyroid nodule that turns out to be a follicular carcinoma on biopsy, a completion thyroidectomy is preferred over radioactive ablation of the remaining gland. If a postoperative radioisotope scan (challenge scan) reveals increased uptake in the skeleton or neck, therapeutic doses of radioiodine are given. Prior to challenge scanning the short half-life hormone T_3 should be given, and once all treatment is completed T_4 is administered to suppress TSH secretion. Plasma thyroglobulin levels should be undetectable after a successful surgery and radioiodine therapy. Subsequent detection of thyroglobulin indicates recurrent disease. The disease is more aggressive than papillary carcinoma and the 10-year survival rate is 75%.

Anaplastic carcinoma

Clinical features

These rapidly growing, highly malignant tumours tend to occur in older patients. The tumours feel hard and are usually locally fixed at the time of presentation. Local invasion may involve the recurrent laryngeal nerve(s) and cause hoarseness, the

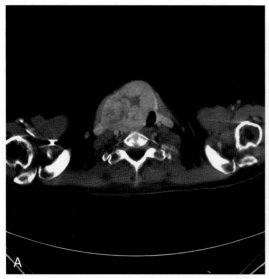 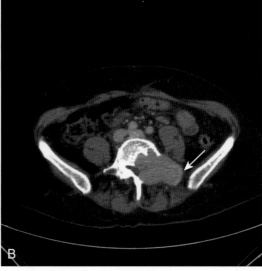

Fig. 20.9 Metastatic follicular cancer. (A) Primary tumour. **(B)** Bony metastases (*arrowed*).

trachea causing dyspnoea and stridor, and the oesophagus causing dysphagia. Invasion of the cervical sympathetic nerves may cause Horner's syndrome (contraction of the pupil, enophthalmos, narrowing of the palpebral fissure and loss of sweating on the face and neck). Pulmonary metastases are common.

Management

Resection is rarely curative in the early stages of the disease, but the main goal of surgery is to relieve tracheal compression and alter the manner of death to avoid asphyxiation. External beam radiotherapy may be of value but chemotherapy seldom is. Pre-operative chemoradiation may render more tumours operable but no treatment has been shown to prolong survival.

Medullary carcinoma

Clinical features

This tumour arises from the parafollicular C cells. There is hard enlargement of one or both thyroid lobes, and in more than 50% of patients the cervical lymph nodes are involved. The tumour may occur sporadically or as part of an inherited multiple endocrine neoplasia (MEN) syndrome type II (Sipple's syndrome). Calcitonin levels are elevated, and can be used to monitor progress and screen relatives. The gene causing the inherited form of this tumour is the *Ret* protooncogene, and the finding of a mutation allows the diagnosis to be made at any age. Prophylactic thyroidectomy for affected children is recommended at different ages depending on the specific mutation and level of risk associated with that mutation. This varies from 1 year of age for the 918 mutation through to 5 years of age for the most common 634 mutation, and in some families with good prognosis it may be delayed to 13 years of age.

Management

Treatment consists of total thyroidectomy and, if the calcitonin level is raised, dissection of the lymph nodes in the central compartment of the neck (levels 6 and 7). Medullary carcinoma in MEN IIb syndrome (918 mutation) is particularly aggressive, and those affected rarely live beyond 30–40 years of age. Other forms, for example pure inherited medullary thyroid cancer occurring without other endocrine tumours, can be very indolent. Preoperative CT of the neck and mediastinum is advised, and the exclusion of a phaeochromocytoma before neck surgery is mandatory.

Lymphoma

Primary lymphoma of the thyroid is a rare complication of autoimmune thyroiditis. It can also occur as a primary tumour that originates in an otherwise normal gland. It is amenable to treatment by radiotherapy and chemotherapy, and selective radiotherapy. Patients often require core biopsy of the gland to characterise the type of lymphoma. Thyroidectomy may be indicated if there is diagnostic doubt or in some cases of isolated thyroid involvement where it may be curative. CT is used to stage the disease fully.

Thyroidectomy

The following terminologies are used in relation to surgery of the thyroid gland based on the extent of the gland removed for different indications:

- *Lobectomy*: Removal of one lobe of the thyroid gland leaving behind the other lobe and isthmus; usually for solitary nodule
- *Hemithyroidectomy*: Removal of one lobe along with the isthmus; most common operation for a solitary thyroid nodule and toxic nodule
- *Subtotal thyroidectomy*: Removal of majority of both lobes leaving behind 6–8 g (equivalent to the size of a normal thyroid gland) of thyroid tissue on one or both sides; most common operation for multinodular goitre
- *Near-total thyroidectomy*: Removal of entire thyroid gland leaving behind 1–2 g of tissue usually on the nonaffected or least affected side of a malignant gland to preserve damage to the parathyroid glands and avoid injury to recurrent laryngeal nerve
- *Total thyroidectomy*: Removal of the total thyroid gland sparing the recurrent laryngeal nerves by identification and preservation of parathyroid glands by individual ligation of the branches of the inferior thyroid artery, keeping their blood supply intact as far as possible, or by reimplanting the parathyroids in the sternomastoid muscle to prevent postoperative hypoparathyroidism.

Technique

The gland is exposed through a transverse skin-crease incision placed 2–3 cm above the sternal notch. Subplatysmal skin flaps are raised. The deep cervical fascia is divided longitudinally in the midline and the strap muscles are separated. Each lobe is mobilised by dividing the vessels supplying the superior pole, the middle and inferior thyroid veins, and the inferior thyroid artery. A capsular dissection technique is used to divide the vessel branches close to the gland in order to preserve the recurrent and superior laryngeal nerves as well as the parathyroid glands. It is quick, easy and safe to do this using, for example, the harmonic scalpel or a vessel-sealing bipolar device in place of ligatures or clips. The recurrent laryngeal nerves should be identified so that they can be protected from injury. Generally, nothing less than a total lobectomy should be performed to avoid the need for reoperation on that side. The isthmus is usually removed along with a lobe (hemithyroidectomy). Care is taken to preserve the parathyroid glands. Haemostasis must be meticulous and drains are rarely necessary. The layers of the neck are reconstituted with continuous absorbable sutures and the skin with a subcuticular suture. Minimally invasive thyroidectomy via a small open incision or endoscopic technique can be performed for small goitres.

Complications

Haemorrhage

Early reactionary haemorrhage should not occur if meticulous haemostasis is achieved before closure. If bleeding does occur, it usually does so in the immediate postextubation period. If delayed bleeding is not recognised early, it can compress the internal jugular veins, leading to laryngeal oedema and asphyxia. The complication must therefore be recognised early and the wound re-explored in theatre. In patients who have stridor with critical airway oedema, small-bore intubation on the ward may be necessary prior to transfer to theatre. Opening the wound in the ward is rarely required.

Nerve damage

Two branches of the vagus nerve are closely associated with the thyroid gland and may be injured during surgery (Table 20.1) The external branch of the superior laryngeal nerve may be damaged while securing the superior thyroid pedicle, causing inability to tense the vocal cord and a weaker voice with noticeable pitch range changes. Anaesthesia of the mucous membrane of the upper larynx allows foreign bodies to enter the larynx more readily. It can be prevented by consciously ligating the superior polar vessels as close to the thyroid gland as possible, as the nerve travels away from the superior thyroid vessels as it approaches the thyroid gland.

Damage to the recurrent laryngeal nerve is more serious. Traction or bruising of this nerve causes temporary paralysis of a vocal cord in 1% of patients undergoing thyroidectomy, but recovery within 3 months is the rule. Division of the nerve paralyses the cord in the 'cadaveric' position (i.e., midway between the closed and open positions). The normal cord on the other side compensates by crossing the midline in phonation, but the voice is altered in timbre and is hoarse, weak and breathy. Some degree of stridor, especially on exertion, may be noted.

Bilateral nerve injury results in stridor and ineffective coughing when the endotracheal tube is withdrawn at the end of the operation. The tube is reinserted immediately and, if there is no early improvement, tracheostomy may be required. The paralysis is originally flaccid, but fibrosis draws the cords together and, even if tracheostomy has been avoided, increasing dyspnoea on exertion may be troublesome. Laryngoplasty may be needed to reconstitute the cords, but if this fails, permanent tracheostomy may be unavoidable.

Hypothyroidism

Thyroid function is monitored after unilateral lobectomy up to 1 year in case replacement therapy is needed (in one-third of patients). After total thyroidectomy, replacement therapy should commence the following day. The average replacement dose range for adults is 100–150 µg thyroxine daily, adjusted by changes of 25 µg according to clinical findings and thyroid function tests.

Hypoparathyroidism

Bruising or accidental removal of the parathyroid glands leads to hypoparathyroidism, manifest by hypocalcaemia and symptoms of increased neuromuscular excitability (Table 20.4).

Table 20.4 Signs and symptoms of hypoparathyroidism	
Symptoms	Paraesthesia affecting perioral region and hands and feet (early symptoms) Lethargy Stridor due to spasm of laryngeal muscles can be fatal
Clinical Signs	**Chvostek's sign** Twitching of the facial muscles on tapping of the facial (VII) nerve over the angle of the jaw Trousseau's sign Spasm of hand and forearm muscles after applying a tourniquet to occlude the pulse **Erb's sign** Hyperexcitability of the muscles on electrical stimulation *In extreme cases, tetany may develop*
ECG changes	Lengthened Q-T interval
Management	Acute hypoparathyroidism is treated with IV calcium gluconate (20 mL of a 10% solution diluted in 100 mL saline) until calcium levels rise For less severe hypoparathyroidism, calcium and vitamin D supplementation are prescribed according to serial blood calcium levels

Hypocalcaemic symptoms, or serum calcium less than 2.0 mmol/L, require calcium supplements. Severe hypoparathyroidism may require vitamin D therapy and correction of hypomagnesaemia as well. Serum calcium checks are required, with gradual withdrawal of supplements as the parathyroids recover. If supplementation is still necessary at 12 months, then the patient is likely to require lifelong treatment.

Scar complications

The scar can become hypertrophic or keloid, particularly when the incision has been placed low in the neck. Recurrent keloid formation is common after excision of the scar (with or without steroid infiltration), and reoperation is not advised lightly.

Patient information

A forewarned patient is much less aggrieved than one who learns about previously unmentioned complications on the first postoperative day. Full informed consent should be obtained by the surgeon who will carry out the procedure and should describe the potential complications with their own complication rates and information on how these compare with national averages. Explanations should be given in simple language and should be full and honest. Written advice may better inform the patient who may have accessed the Internet, which may not provide accurate and appropriate information.

Parathyroid glands

Surgical anatomy

The parathyroid glands receive a rich blood supply from the inferior thyroid artery, the branches of which are a valuable guide to their position. Histologically, the glands contain chief cells that secrete parathormone (PTH).

Calcium metabolism

Plasma calcium levels are kept constant in the range 2.25–2.6 mmol/L by regulating the amounts absorbed from the intestine, deposited in or withdrawn from bone, and excreted in the urine. PTH and vitamin D are the main regulators, with minimal modulation by calcitonin.

Hypercalcaemia and hypocalcaemia

Hypercalcaemia is a common biochemical abnormality and may be due to many causes other than excess PTH secretion (Table 20.5). Similarly, hypocalcaemia may be due to causes other than parathyroid removal or damage (Table 20.6).

Primary hyperparathyroidism

Pathology

In 90% of patients primary hyperparathyroidism is due to an adenoma, in 10% it results from hyperplasia (usually affecting all four glands), and in less than 1% it results from parathyroid carcinoma. Adenomas are normally small, spherical, brown nodules but can be ten-times larger than the normal gland. Most are single, but 20% of patients have multiple adenomas. Histologically, chief cells predominate. In hyperplasia, the gland is usually twice the normal weight, i.e., more than 70 mg.

Table 20.5 Causes of hypercalcaemia

Hyperparathyroidism

- Primary
- Secondary
- Tertiary

Increased calcium absorption

- Vitamin D excess
- Sarcoidosis
- Drugs (e.g., diuretics, lithium)

Excessive bone breakdown

- Metastatic disease (particularly breast cancer)
- Myeloma
- Immobilisation following multiple fractures

Ectopic secretion of parathyroid-like hormone

- Cancer of bronchus
- Cancer of breast

Table 20.6 Causes of hypocalcaemia

Hypoparathyroidism

- Thyroid surgery
- Parathyroid surgery

Hypoproteinaemia

- Nephrosis (excessive protein loss)
- Malnutrition (inadequate intake)
- Cirrhosis (deficient synthesis)
- Severe inflammation (e.g., burns, acute pancreatitis)

Vitamin D deficiency

- Pseudohypoparathyroidism

Table 20.7 Hyperparathyroidism

Pathology	Primary hyperparathyroidism • Adenoma (90%) • Hyperplasia (normally 4 gland; 10%) • Carcinoma (<1%) Secondary hyperparathyroidism • Usually renal disease • Occasionally malabsorption Tertiary hyperparathyroidism • Development of autonomous secretion in secondary hyperparathyroidism
Symptoms and Signs *'Bones, stones, groans and moans'*	Bones • Demineralisation and subperiosteal bone resorption • Cysts in long bones and jaw • Moth-eaten appearance to skull • Pathological fractures Renal stones • Nephrocalcinosis and calculi Gastrointestinal • Peptic ulcer • Pancreatitis • Nausea and vomiting (increase dehydration and increase serum calcium further leading to a vicious spiral of deterioration) Psychiatric • Psychosis and acute confusion (uncommon but indicate marked hypercalcaemia >3.5 mmol/L) Other • Lethargy and general weakness

Clinical features

Women are affected twice as often as men. The clinical features are outlined in Table 20.7. The disease usually presents in middle age. Increasingly, it is being diagnosed in asymptomatic patients found to have hypercalcaemia on routine biochemistry. If clinical manifestations occur, renal and bone effects predominate, including nephrocalcinosis (diffuse calcification) and urinary calculi. Polyuria is an early symptom of hyperparathyroidism.

Bone damage used to be common but is now rarely seen in high-income countries as the disease is diagnosed earlier. Gross demineralisation, subperiosteal bone resorption (seen typically in the middle and distal phalanges of the fingers), cysts in the long bones and jaw, and the moth-eaten appearance of the skull gave rise to the descriptive term 'osteitis fibrosa cystica'. Multiple pathological fractures were also once common. Significant bone disease is still a common manifestation in low-income countries where patients can be malnourished and present late in the disease course.

Other manifestations of hyperparathyroidism include peptic ulceration, acute and chronic pancreatitis, lethargy, muscle weakness, and psychotic symptoms. The clinical picture of florid hyperparathyroidism is often summarised as one of 'broken bones, renal stones, abdominal groans and psychic moans'. Rarely, patients present with a hypercalcaemic crisis characterised by marked hypercalcaemia (>3.5 mmol/L), mental confusion, nausea and vomiting. The vomiting increases preexisting dehydration, leading to higher levels of serum calcium, more confusion and prostration, more dehydration, and so on. Urgent expert attention is required to reverse this vicious downward spiral. The most pressing need is to correct the dehydration. The calcium may be further reduced by the use of bisphosphonates.

Diagnosis

If hyperparathyroidism is suspected, serum calcium and PTH levels must be measured on more than one occasion. PTH levels may be normal, but the detection of unsuppressed PTH values in a patient with hypercalcaemia supports the diagnosis of primary hyperparathyroidism. Other supportive findings include a low serum phosphate, hyperchloraemia (and an abnormal Cl/PO_4 ratio), and a raised 24-hour urinary calcium excretion. A low urinary calcium excretion should alert the clinician to the possibility of familial hypercalcaemic hypocalciuria, a disease of the renal tubules in which the parathyroids are normal. Alkaline phosphatase (skeletal) levels may be raised, even if there is no radiological evidence of bone disease.

Management

In symptomatic patients, the aim of treatment is to identify and remove all overactive parathyroid tissue. Preoperative imaging with ultrasound and sestamibi (MIBI) scans will allow selection of patients for a focused approach. Concordant scans permit a direct, targeted incision over the suspected adenoma, with or without frozen section confirmation and intraoperative PTH monitoring. The latter two intraoperative tests are not employed by all surgeons and rarely make a difference to the outcome of surgery enough to justify their expense. A minimally invasive video-assisted approach is favoured by some surgeons with equivalent outcomes. With discordant imaging or associated multinodular goitre and previous neck surgery, traditional cervicotomy and four-gland exploration will be required. If two or more glands are enlarged, they should be removed. If all four glands are thought to be hyperplastic, then all but a portion of the smallest gland should be removed. If exploration fails to identify an adenoma or hyperplasia, the incision is closed. Reoperation is considered after (re)confirming the diagnosis and attempting to localise the gland using CT, MRI or selective venous catheterisation (Fig. 20.10). Recurrent hyperparathyroidism is approached in the same way but repeating first ultrasound and MIBI scans.

With primary hyperparathyroidism being diagnosed increasingly in asymptomatic patients, the management of this condition has been the subject of much discussion (EBM 20.3). For those patients with serum calcium levels >1 mg/dL (>0.25 mM/L) above the upper limit of normal, or where end-organ disease (e.g., bone disease) or renal stone risk index is high, surgery remains the treatment of choice. In patients not keen on surgery or for whom surgery is not possible, medical management focuses on close monitoring of calcium levels, bone density and renal function. Treatments include measures to reduce calcium levels using calcimimetics (agents that increase the sensitivity of the calcium sensing receptor in the parathyroid gland to calcium) and bisphosphonates may be used to improve bone mineral density.

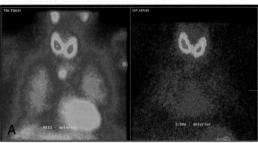

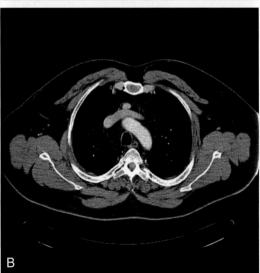

Fig. 20.10 Images of mediastinal parathyroid tissue. **(A)** MIBI scan. **(B)** Computed tomography scan. *MIBI,* Sestamibi

---

EBM 20.3 **Management of primary hyperparathyroidism**

'In symptomatic patients with primary hyperparathyroidism, the diagnosis and decision to operate are based on biochemical parameters and the patient's fitness for surgery. Parathyroid localisation using USS, MIBI and other imaging provide a roadmap to target the site of surgery.' *
'In asymptomatic patients, surgery may be indicated for:

- *Patients <50 years*
- *Serum calcium >1 mg/dL (>0.25 mmol/L) above the normal upper limit*
- *Evidence of end-organ disease, e.g.:*
  - *Impaired bone mineral density*
  - *24 hour urinary calcium >400 mg/day and increased stone risk*
  - *Reduced creatinine clearance*[†]

*Hindié et al. 2009 EANM parathyroid guidelines. Eur J Nucl Med Mol Imaging. 2009;36:1201.
[†]Bilezikian et al. Guidelines for the management of asymptomatic primary hyperparathyroidism: summary statement from the Fourth International Workshop. J Clin Endocrinol Metab 2014;99:3561.

Secondary and tertiary hyperparathyroidism

In secondary hyperparathyroidism, there is over-secretion of PTH in response to low plasma levels of ionised calcium, usually because of renal disease or malabsorption. This is an increasing problem in patients with chronic renal failure. It is managed initially by dietary phosphate restriction and by giving 1-α-hydroxyvitamin D_3 (alfacalcidol) to increase calcium absorption and provide negative feedback on the parathyroids.

Excessive PTH secretion in secondary hyperparathyroidism may become autonomous; it is then termed tertiary hyperparathyroidism. This may occur after renal transplantation. Total parathyroidectomy may be needed, with calcium and vitamin D replacement therapy, subtotal parathyroidectomy leaving half-equivalent of a normal gland in situ or autotransplantation of parathyroid tissue (equivalent in size to one normal gland) into an arm muscle (where it can be readily located if problems persist). Postoperatively, alfacalcidol and calcium are continued to heal bone disease and reduce the risk of recurrent hyperparathyroidism. Calcimimetics (e.g., cinacalcet) may also be used in patients with refractory hyperparathyroidism on dialysis if operative intervention is not possible.

Hypoparathyroidism

Hypoparathyroidism may occur temporarily after parathyroidectomy until the suppressed residual glands assume normal function. A fall in ionised calcium levels gives rise to the symptoms and signs outlined previously in Table 20.4. Acute hypoparathyroidism is treated with intravenous calcium gluconate (20 mL of a 10% solution given intravenously diluted in 100 mL of saline) 4-hourly until calcium levels rise. Oral calcium (effervescent calcium gluconate) and, if required, vitamin D (calcitriol) is prescribed according to serial blood calcium levels.

Parathyroidectomy

Patient information

To provide informed consent, it is important that patients understand several aspects of the glands and the disease, specifically:
- the variable position of the glands
- the function of the glands

- the results of hyperfunction: renal effects, bone disease and systemic effects
- that only one gland is likely to be diseased and overactive, and that this is very rarely malignant (<1%)
- that surgery will attempt to remove the abnormal gland but may fail to locate it because it is in an ectopic position
- that there may be a need for calcium and vitamin D supplements after surgery.

Pituitary gland

Surgical anatomy

The pituitary gland is small and weighs about 500 mg. It is enclosed within a bony shell, the sella turcica, which is sealed superiorly by a fold of dura mater, the diaphragma sellae. The pituitary stalk connects the pituitary to the hypothalamus. The pituitary has two parts: the anterior pituitary (adenohypophysis) and the posterior pituitary (neurohypophysis) (Fig. 20.11).

Anterior pituitary

The anterior pituitary develops from an epithelial outgrowth from the pharynx (Rathke's pouch). Some cells are thought to be of neural crest origin and belong to the amine and precursor uptake and decarboxylation (APUD) system. The anterior pituitary contains solid cords of secreting cells that used to be classified as acidophil, basophil or chromophobe on staining with haematoxylin and eosin. On the basis of immunofluorescence and other specific stains, these are now subdivided into cell types that secrete:

- Polypeptides: growth hormone (GH), prolactin (PRL) and adrenocorticotrophic hormone (ACTH)
- Glycoproteins: luteinising hormone (LH), follicle-stimulating hormone (FSH) and TSH.

The hypophysial stalk contains a portal venous system that connects capillaries in the median eminence of the hypothalamus with capillaries and sinusoids of the anterior pituitary. This system carries neurosecretory hormones that stimulate or inhibit specific endocrine cells in the pituitary. The most important messengers are GH-releasing and inhibiting factors, corticotrophin-releasing factor (CRF), gonadotrophin-releasing hormone (GnRH), TRH and prolactin-inhibiting factor (PIF). If the portal tract is divided, the secretion of all anterior pituitary hormones is suppressed, with the exception of PRL, the secretion of which is increased. A number of feedback loops ensure that the secretion of pituitary hormones is adjusted to need.

Tumours of the anterior pituitary

Pathophysiology

Functioning pituitary adenomas may result from overstimulation by hypothalamic factors. Initially small and confined within the gland (microadenomas), they grow slowly and can ultimately expand the sella turcica. Eccentric enlargement is common. Upward extension of the adenoma may stretch the diaphragm or herniate through it, to compress the optic chiasma and cause visual defects. It is therefore important that pituitary adenomas are detected before they enlarge the fossa or extend above it. CT with contrast enhancement and MRI (Fig. 20.12) are used to image the tumour. Three endocrine syndromes caused by anterior pituitary disorders have surgical relevance.

Acromegaly

Excess secretion of GH occurs most often in early adult life and results in overgrowth of the soft tissues of the hands, feet and face. This gives the patient 'large extremities' and a characteristically coarse face, with bulging supraorbital ridges and a protruding jaw (macrognathia). Endochondral ossification and periosteal new bone formation account for some of these changes. All viscera are enlarged and there is muscle hypertrophy, although muscle weakness and cardiac failure develop later. The skin is coarse and greasy, and acne is common. Headaches, sweating and carpal tunnel syndrome often develop. Glucose tolerance is impaired and galactorrhoea can occur in females. GH and somatomedin (insulin-like growth factor 1) levels are increased, and glucose or a meal does not suppress their secretion.

20

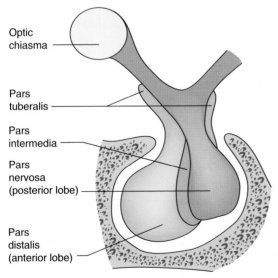

Optic chiasma

Pars tuberalis

Pars intermedia

Pars nervosa (posterior lobe)

Pars distalis (anterior lobe)

Fig. 20.11 Sagittal section through the pituitary gland.

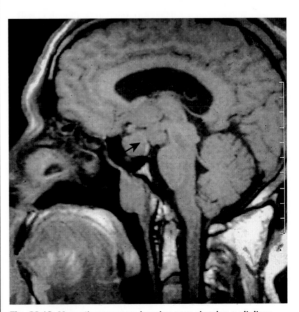

Fig. 20.12 Magnetic resonance imaging scan showing a pituitary tumour (*arrow*).

Treatment is directed at restoring GH levels to normal. For small adenomas, transsphenoidal removal is the treatment of choice. Somatostatin analogues, such as octreotide and lanreotide, offer an effective way of normalising GH levels and can be used to reduce the size of macroadenomas or to treat recurrent or residual tumour.

Hyperprolactinaemia

PRL is the most common hormone secreted by pituitary tumours. Hypersecretion results in galactorrhoea and amenorrhoea (owing to the suppression of gonadotrophin secretion) in young women, whereas in men gynaecomastia and impotence may occur. Basal levels of PRL are high, the nocturnal increase is absent, and the response to TRH is diminished. It is important to exclude other causes of hyperprolactinaemia, notably the administration of drugs such as metoclopramide.

Dopamine agonists, such as cabergoline and bromocriptine, are often used as first-line agents in the management of this condition because they reduce serum PRL levels and reduce the size of these adenomas. Surgery is reserved for refractory adenomas or for patients who cannot tolerate these agents.

Cushing's disease

This may be due to a functioning adenoma of ACTH-secreting cells. Only 15% of patients show expansion of the pituitary fossa. Removal of the microadenoma or its irradiation will relieve symptoms. Unsuccessful surgery may require bilateral adrenalectomy (removal of end organs) to terminate the syndrome of hypercortisolism, with its widespread destructive systemic effects.

Surgical hypophysectomy

The transsphenoidal approach is preferred for the removal of a small adenoma. An operating microscope is used to approach the gland through the sphenoidal or ethmoidal sinuses (Fig. 20.13). Diabetes insipidus is rare. By placing a free flap of muscle in the fossa, cerebrospinal fluid (CSF) rhinorrhoea is prevented. The transcranial approach is a major neurosurgical procedure that results in loss of the sense of smell and the development of diabetes insipidus. It is now reserved for the removal of large tumours with suprasellar extension, often in combination with a transsphenoidal approach. Following pituitary surgery careful monitoring of all pituitary hormones is required, as collateral damage can occur, leading to occult deficiencies (e.g., TSH, ACTH, LH and FSH).

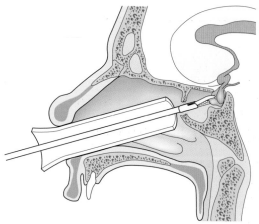

Fig. 20.13 Transsphenoidal removal of a pituitary adenoma.

20.2 Summary

Tumours of the anterior pituitary gland

- May be detected while still small (microadenoma) or after it has expanded, often with upward extension to compress the optic chiasma
- The three endocrine syndromes that have surgical importance are acromegaly, hyperprolactinaemia and Cushing's disease
- Acromegaly is due to excessive secretion of growth hormone (GH). Somatostatin analogues (or bromocriptine) can be used to normalise GH levels. Small adenomas are treated by removal; radiotherapy can be used for larger inoperable tumours
- Hyperprolactinaemia causes galactorrhoea and amenorrhoea in females, and impotence and gynaecomastia in men. Treatment is with dopamine agonists with surgery reserved for refractory cases
- Cushing's disease may result from a functioning adenoma of adrenocorticotrophic hormone-secreting cells, which is treated by removal or irradiation.

Radiation therapy

The pituitary is comparatively radioresistant and at least 100 Gy are needed to affect the function of a normal gland. Smaller doses (40–50 Gy) are used to treat acromegaly and Cushing's disease. A rotational technique avoids excessive irradiation of surrounding neural tissue. Larger doses can be delivered by the narrow focused beam of heavy particles that are generated by a cyclotron.

Replacement therapy

After total hypophysectomy, replacement therapy is required for life (hydrocortisone 20 mg each morning and 10 mg each evening). All episodes of stress or trauma, including hypophysectomy itself, require additional steroid to cover the stress response. An alert wrist band should be given to patients who are steroid dependent. Aldosterone secretion is unaffected and there is no need for mineralocorticoid replacement. TSH secretion is suppressed and thyroxine must be given. Diabetes insipidus is a common but often transient complication of pituitary surgery or the insertion of radioactive implants. Vasopressin, or an analogue, relieves polyuria.

Posterior pituitary

Pathophysiology

The neurohypophysis is part of a secretory and storage unit that includes the nerve cells of the supraoptic and paraventricular hypothalamic nuclei (Fig. 20.14). Fibres pass from these nuclei via the hypothalamohypophysial tract to the median eminence of the hypothalamus and posterior pituitary. The nerve cells secrete arginine vasopressin (antidiuretic hormone [ADH]) and oxytocin, both of which pass down the nerve fibres to be stored in vesicles in the pituitary. The close anatomical relationship of the anterior and posterior pituitary has functional significance in that oxytocin release during lactation is paralleled by increased TSH and PRL production, and the posterior pituitary may influence PRL secretion by dopamine release.

Adrenal gland

Surgical anatomy and development

Each adrenal gland weighs approximately 4 g and lies immediately above and medial to the kidneys. The right adrenal lies in

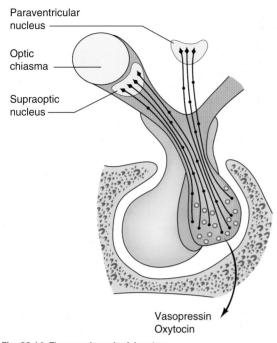

Paraventricular nucleus

Optic chiasma

Supraoptic nucleus

Vasopressin
Oxytocin

Fig. 20.14 The neurohypophysial system.

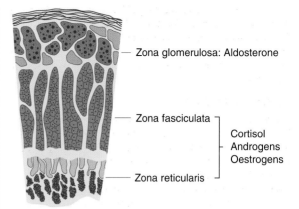

Zona glomerulosa: Aldosterone

Zona fasciculata ⎤
⎟ Cortisol
⎟ Androgens
Zona reticularis ⎦ Oestrogens

Fig. 20.16 Functional zones of the adrenal cortex.

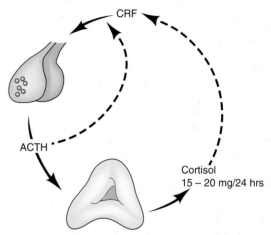

CRF

ACTH

Cortisol
15 – 20 mg/24 hrs

Fig. 20.17 Feedback loop in the control of cortisol secretion. *ACTH,* Adrenocorticotrophic hormone; *CRF,* corticotrophin-releasing factor.

close contact with the inferior vena cava, into which it drains by a short, wide vein that can be difficult to ligate at operation. The left adrenal vein drains into the left renal vein (Fig. 20.15). The glands are supplied by small vessels that arise from the aorta, and the renal and inferior phrenic arteries.

Each gland has an outer cortex and inner medulla. The cortex, like the gonads, is derived from mesoderm, whereas the medulla is derived from the chromaffin ectodermal cells of the neural crest. The cortex secretes corticosteroids. The medulla is part of the sympathetic nervous system. Its APUD cells secrete the catecholamines, adrenaline (epinephrine), noradrenaline (norepinephrine) and dopamine, and are supplied by preganglionic sympathetic nerves.

Adrenal cortex

Cortical function

Microscopically, the adrenal cortex has three zones (Fig. 20.16). The outer zona glomerulosa secretes the mineralocorticoid

aldosterone. The zona fasciculata and zona reticularis act as a functional unit and secrete glucocorticoids (cortisol and corticosterone) (Fig. 20.17), androgenic steroids (androstenedione, 11-hydroxy-androstenedione and testosterone), and the inactive androgen and oestrogen precursor dehydroepiandrosterone sulphate (DHA-S). Precursors of aldosterone (Fig. 20.18) are also synthesised by the fasciculata–reticularis zone, as are small amounts of progesterone and oestrogen. Only a fraction of the

20

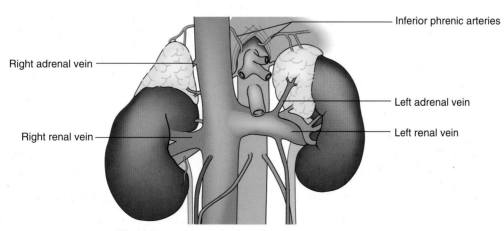

Right adrenal vein

Right renal vein

Inferior phrenic arteries

Left adrenal vein

Left renal vein

Fig. 20.15 Blood supply and venous drainage of the adrenal glands.

amount of hormone needed daily is stored in the cortex. The hormones are, therefore, secreted 'to order' and circulate either free (5%) or bound to α-globulin.

20.3 Summary

Adrenocortical hormones

- Cortisol secretion is controlled by pituitary adrenocorticotrophic hormone. Cortisol protects against stress, maintains blood pressure and aids recovery from injury/shock. Its metabolic activities include protein breakdown, increased gluconeogenesis, reduced glucose utilisation, and mobilisation/redistribution of fat and water
- In excess, cortisol has mineralocorticoid activity, can cause psychosis and has antiinflammatory effects (used in transplantation immunosuppression)
- Aldosterone secretion is controlled mainly by angiotensin levels (and thus by renin release from the juxtaglomerular apparatus during decreased renal perfusion)
- Aldosterone conserves sodium (by facilitating its exchange for potassium and hydrogen ions in the kidney) and is a major determinant of extracellular fluid conservation
- Androgenic steroids and dehydroepiandrosterone sulphate (DHA-S) are also secreted by the adrenal cortex. DHA-S is converted to testosterone and oestrogen in fat and liver, and this peripheral aromatisation is the main source of oestrogen in postmenopausal women.

Cushing's syndrome

This syndrome was first described by the American neurosurgeon, Harvey Cushing. It results from any prolonged and inappropriate exposure to cortisol, and has the following causes (Table 20.8 and Fig. 20.19):

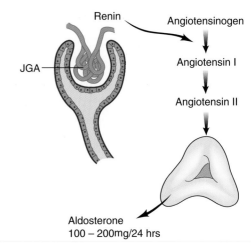

Fig. 20.18 Control of aldosterone secretion by the adrenal cortex. *JGA*, Juxtaglomerular apparatus.

- ***Tumours of the adrenal cortex (20%).*** Benign adenoma is the most common adrenal cause of Cushing's syndrome. It is almost invariably unilateral and is more common in females. Histologically, the tumour contains clear cells like those of the zona fasciculata, or compact cells like those of the zona reticularis. Autonomous cortisol secretion inhibits ACTH production, so that the contralateral gland becomes atrophic and ceases to function. Adrenal carcinoma is a rare cause of Cushing's syndrome that occurs more frequently in young adults and children. The tumour grows

Table 20.8 Cushing's syndrome

Causes	Features	Investigations
• Tumours of the adrenal cortex (20%) • Pituitary disease (Cushing's disease; 80%) • Ectopic ACTH production • Iatrogenic	Body habitus ('lemon on a stick' or 'tomato head, potato body and four matches as limbs'): • Truncal obesity • Buffalo hump • Moon face • Proximal muscle weakness Skin changes: • Thin skin • Purple striae • Capillary fragility • Purpura • Hirsutism • Acne Metabolic • Diabetes • Hypertension (mineralocorticoid activity) • Antiinflammatory effects Other • Loss of libido • Amenorrhoea • Cachexia • Psychosis	Exclude exogenous steroid use First-line investigations include one or more of the following: • Late-night salivary cortisol • Overnight 1-mg dexamethasone suppression test • 24-hour urinary free cortisol • 48-hour 2-mg dexamethasone suppression test The investigation of choice is performed at least twice to confirm the diagnosis Morning plasma ACTH • Suppressed ACTH indicates ACTH-independent Cushing's syndrome e.g., adrenal adenoma • Unsuppressed ACTH indicates ACTH-dependent Cushing's syndrome, either ACTH-secreting pituitary adenoma or ectopic ACTH production MRI can help demonstrate pituitary adenomas. Where a lesion is not seen inferior petrosal sinus sampling following CRH stimulation can aid in the diagnosis of pituitary lesions CT can help localise adrenal tumours and tumours responsible for ectopic ACTH secretion

ACTH, Adrenocorticotrophic hormone; CT, computed tomography; MRI, magnetic resonance imaging.

to a large size and has frequently metastasised by the time of presentation

- *Pituitary disease (80%).* Pituitary tumours causing Cushing's syndrome are usually basophil or sometimes chromophobe

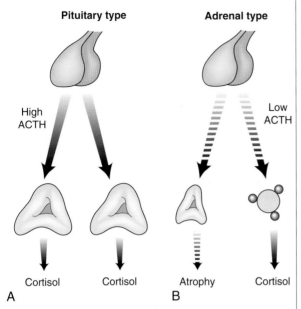

Pituitary type   **Adrenal type**

High ACTH   Low ACTH

Cortisol   Cortisol   Atrophy   Cortisol

A   B

Fig. 20.19 Types of Cushing's syndrome. (A) Overstimulation of the normal adrenal glands by excess ACTH. **(B)** Oversecretion of cortisol by a functioning tumour of the left adrenal gland, leading to suppression of function in the opposite gland. *ACTH,* Adrenocorticotrophic hormone.

adenomas of ACTH-secreting cells. They range from tiny 'microadenomas' to large and even invasive tumours. Because of the continued ACTH secretion, both adrenals become hyperplastic. When the syndrome is caused by a pituitary tumour, it is referred to as Cushing's disease
- *Ectopic ACTH production.* Inappropriate secretion of ACTH-like peptide by tumours of nonpituitary origin (e.g., pancreas, bronchus, thymus) is a rare cause
- *Iatrogenic.* Cushing's syndrome can be a major side effect of therapeutic steroid use. Adrenal atrophy occurs if the steroid dosage is supraphysiological (>20 mg equivalent of prednisone per day) and prolonged in duration.

Clinical features

Cushing's syndrome occurs most frequently in young women. The most striking feature is truncal obesity, a 'buffalo hump' (due to redistribution of water and fat) and 'mooning' of the face (Fig. 20.20). Cushing's original description was a 'tomato head, potato body and four matches as limbs'. As a result of protein loss, the skin becomes thin, with purple striae, dusky cyanosis and visible dermal vessels. Proximal muscle weakness is prominent. Other features include increased capillary fragility, purpura, osteoporosis, acne, loss of libido, hirsutism, diabetes, hypertension and amenorrhoea. The clinical signs develop insidiously over years and sometimes are only fully appreciated when the patients and their family review old photographs. The disease may run a fulminant course, particularly when due to an adrenal carcinoma or ectopic ACTH secretion. Electrolyte disturbances, cachexia, pigmentation, severe diabetes and psychosis are common in these patients.

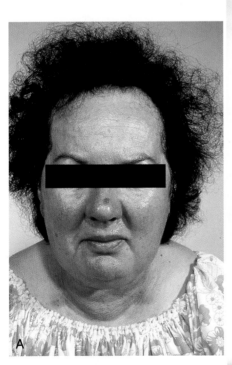
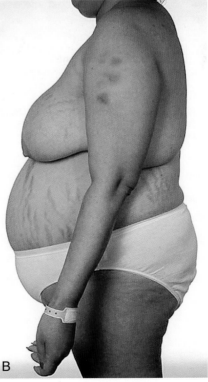

Fig. 20.20 Features of Cushing's syndrome. (A) Moon face and puffy eyes. (B) Papery skin with striae and a propensity to bruising, muscle wasting of limbs and centripetal obesity. (Courtesy Prof. Michael Sheppard, University of Birmingham Medical School.)

Investigations

Investigations to determine the cause of Cushing's syndrome are outlined in Table 20.8 and Fig. 20.21. Exogenous steroid use as a cause must be excluded. Proof of hypercortisolism is obtained by undertaking one of four highly sensitive first-line diagnostic tests: late-night salivary cortisol, overnight 1 mg dexamethasone suppression testing, 24-hour urinary-free cortisol or 48-hour 2 mg dexamethasone suppression testing. Whichever test is used as a first-line investigation, the test is repeated at least twice to confirm the result. A high morning plasma ACTH suggests a pituitary or ectopic source of cortisol. With a pituitary source, urinary cortisol excretion is suppressed by dexamethasone. In ectopic ACTH syndrome, the ACTH levels are often exceedingly high and there is an associated electrolyte disturbance. These patients may also have cancer cachexia. A suppressed morning plasma ACTH and the finding that urinary excretion of cortisol is not suppressed by high-dose dexamethasone suggests an adrenal source. MRI can help to identify lesions of the pituitary. In up to 40% of cases, MRI does not show a lesion but inferior petrosal sinus sampling in response to CRH may be helpful. CT is helpful in the identification of adrenal tumours (Fig. 20.22) and ectopic sources of ACTH.

Management

Adrenal adenoma

Adrenal adenomas are rarely bilateral and unilateral adrenalectomy is most commonly indicated. As the other adrenal is suppressed and atrophic, cortisone replacement is needed until the pituitary–adrenal axis recovers. This may take up to 2 years, and steroids must not be reduced or discontinued until a low-dose dexamethasone test shows normal function in the remaining gland.

Adrenal carcinoma

Adrenal carcinomas should be completely removed whenever possible; debulking may be helpful if chemotherapy is to be used.

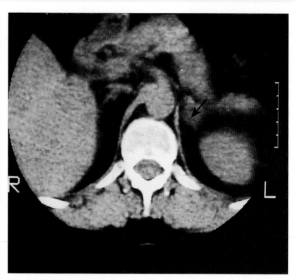

Fig. 20.22 Computed tomography scan of an adrenal tumour (*arrow*).

Patients often present late, with large tumours and lung metastases. Chemotherapy with mitotane may be tried, but this is a toxic drug and is often poorly tolerated. The therapeutic gain may be small.

Pituitary disease

The symptoms of bilateral adrenal hyperplasia due to pituitary hyperfunction can be relieved by bilateral adrenalectomy, but at the price of lifelong steroid therapy. Furthermore, adrenalectomy removes all feedback control, so that overproduction of ACTH and melanocyte-stimulating hormone (MSH) produces characteristic skin pigmentation, and continued growth of the

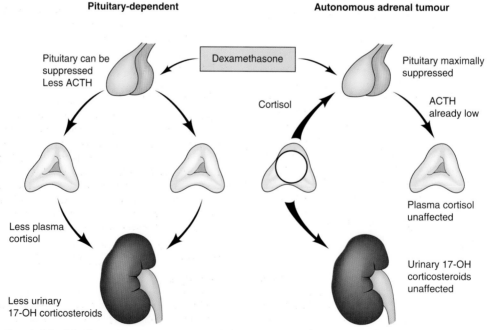

Fig. 20.21 The principle of the dexamethasone test in differentiating between adrenal and pituitary causes of excess cortisol secretion. *ACTH,* Adrenocorticotrophic hormone.

adenoma may compress the optic chiasma (Nelson's syndrome). Pituitary irradiation or surgery avoids the side effects of adrenalectomy, and microsurgical removal of the adenoma is now the treatment of choice.

Hyperaldosteronism

Primary hyperaldosteronism (Conn's syndrome)

This is usually due to a benign adenoma and is most common in young or middle-aged women. The adenoma is small, single, canary yellow on bisection and composed of cells of the glomerulosa type. Only rarely is the syndrome due to bilateral adrenal hyperplasia or multiple microadenomas. The high circulating levels of aldosterone suppress renin secretion, a helpful biochemical diagnostic observation.

Clinical features

Retention of sodium increases plasma volume and produces hypertension, often in association with headaches and visual disturbance (although serious retinopathy is uncommon). Potassium loss leads to worsening hypokalaemia, episodes of muscle weakness and nocturnal polyuria. Unrecognised, the syndrome progresses to severe hypokalaemic alkalosis, with periodic muscle paralysis, paraesthesia and tetany.

Diagnosis

Low serum potassium in a hypertensive patient should signal the possibility of hyperaldosteronism. Diagnosis then rests on the following:

- *Confirm hypokalaemia.* This may require repeated blood sampling without an occluding cuff; 24-hour urine collections usually show increased potassium excretion
- *Demonstrate hypersecretion of aldosterone.* Plasma and/or urinary aldosterone levels are measured at 4-hourly intervals to allow for diurnal variations. Giving the aldosterone antagonist spironolactone should reduce blood pressure and reverse hypokalaemia
- *Exclude secondary hyperaldosteronism.* Measurement of plasma renin is the critical investigation; renin levels are increased in secondary hyperaldosteronism but undetectable in the primary disease. Spironolactone causes further increases in renin levels in secondary hyperaldosteronism
- *Localise the adenoma.* If primary hyperaldosteronism is confirmed biochemically, attempts should then be made to localise the adenoma by CT or MRI. Failure to 'see' an adenoma may mean that there is no discrete tumour and that the patient has bilateral cortical hyperplasia. Plasma cortisol levels should always be measured to exclude Cushing's syndrome. Selective adrenal vein sampling to determine aldosterone levels is required to help localise small adenomas to one or other gland, and confirm which gland is hyperfunctioning.

Management

Primary hyperaldosteronism due to an adenoma is treated by removal of the affected gland after correcting the hypokalaemia with oral potassium and spironolactone. Hyperaldosteronism due to adrenal hyperplasia can be cured by bilateral adrenalectomy, but at such a high price that long-term drug treatment is preferable.

Secondary hyperaldosteronism

Hyperaldosteronism is most commonly secondary to excessive renin secretion (and stimulation of the zona glomerulosa by angiotensin) in chronic liver, renal or cardiac disease.

Adrenogenital syndrome (adrenal virilism)

Pathophysiology

This syndrome is due to one of a number of genetically determined enzyme defects that impair cortisol synthesis. The resultant increase in pituitary ACTH production causes adrenal hyperplasia and inappropriate adrenal androgen secretion.

Clinical features

The effects depend on the patient's sex and age. Female infants show enlargement of the clitoris and varying fusion of the labial folds. Later, other signs of virilism appear, leading to precocious heterosexual puberty. Young boys have precocious isosexual puberty. In both sexes, growth is at first rapid, but the epiphyses fuse early so that the final height is stunted. Excess muscle growth produces an 'infant Hercules' appearance. Milder forms of the disease may affect older girls and cause hirsutism and acne.

Management

The patient is given cortisol for replacement purposes and to suppress ACTH production. Surgical correction of the genital abnormality may be needed. Rarely, virilism is due to an adrenal tumour, which is usually large and malignant.

Adrenal feminisation

Exceptionally, a tumour of the adrenal cortex may secrete oestrogens. Such tumours are usually large and malignant. In the female, there is sexual precocity; in the male, there is feminisation, with gynaecomastia, decreased libido and testicular atrophy. Treatment consists of removing the tumour, although recurrence and metastatic spread are common.

Adrenal medulla

Pathophysiology

The adrenal medulla is not essential for life. There are other collections of chromaffin cells in paraganglia in the retroperitoneum, mediastinum and neck that release noradrenaline (norepinephrine). The normal adrenal medulla secretes catecholamines in the ratio 80% adrenaline to 20% noradrenaline. It also secretes the noradrenaline precursor dopamine. Small amounts of catecholamines are excreted in the urine in free and conjugated form. Larger amounts are excreted as metadrenaline, normetadrenaline and 3-methoxy-4-hydroxymandelic acid (VMA).

Phaeochromocytoma

Pathology

Phaeochromocytomas are tumours either of the adrenal medulla (80%), which secrete large amounts of adrenaline (epinephrine) and noradrenaline (norepinephrine), or of the extra-adrenal paraganglionic tissue (20%), which secrete only

20

noradrenaline. Virtually all (99%) arise within the abdomen; 10% are multiple and 10% are malignant. Benign tumours are usually chocolate brown and highly vascular. Associated conditions are medullary carcinoma of the thyroid (as part of MEN type II), von Hippel–Lindau disease (VHL) and neurofibromatosis. If it presents in pregnancy, phaeochromocytoma can be mistaken for hypertension of pregnancy, and may cause maternal and foetal mortality. Genetic testing for predisposition syndromes such as succinate dehydrogenase (SDH) B, C and D should be done in all patients under 50 years of age.

Clinical features

The median age for presentation of phaeochromocytomas is 40 years. Excess noradrenaline secretion causes hypertension; adrenaline excess has metabolic effects (e.g., diabetes and thyrotoxicosis). Paroxysmal hypertension is a very characteristic symptom due to the sudden release of catecholamines. It may be precipitated by abdominal pressure, exercise stress or postural change. During a paroxysm the blood pressure may rise to 200/100 mmHg, and there is headache, palpitation, sweating, extreme anxiety, chest and abdominal pain. Pallor, dilated pupils and tachycardia are prominent features. In some patients, persistent and severe hypertension develops at the age of 30–40 years, often in association with severe retinopathy, which can cause optic atrophy and blindness. Glycosuria is common. The skin may be mottled, with tingling of the extremities. Extra-adrenal phaeochromocytomas are also associated with persistent hypertension. On rare occasions, the tumour is in the bladder, and micturition may precipitate a syncopal attack. A few patients present with predominantly metabolic effects, such as those found in thyrotoxicosis. Occasionally, a phaeochromocytoma may cause sudden and unexplained death after trauma or during surgery, owing to severe hypertension causing a cerebrovascular accident or by precipitating a fatal arrhythmia.

Investigations

All young hypertensive patients (age <40 years) should be screened for a catecholamine-secreting tumour. Twenty-four-hour or overnight collections of urine should be analysed for metadrenaline and normetadrenaline levels. A CT or MRI may show the tumour. It may also be demonstrated by scintigraphy after giving radio-iodine-labelled metaiodobenzylguanidine (MIBG), a catecholamine precursor taken up by sites of synthesis (Fig. 20.23).

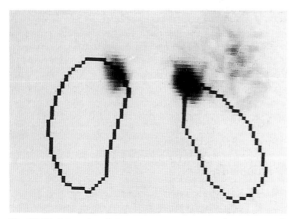

Fig. 20.23 Extra-adrenal phaeochromocytoma. Metaiodobenzylguanidine (MIBG) scan.

Management

Surgical removal of the tumour is the treatment of choice. The use of α- and β-blocking drugs has greatly reduced the risk of hypertensive crisis, tachycardia and arrhythmias during induction of anaesthesia or tumour handling. The patient should come to operation with blood pressure and pulse rate controlled. Adrenergic blockade also allows restoration of blood volume, so that sudden hypotension after removal of the tumour is unusual. To achieve blockade, an α-adrenergic receptor blocker such as phenoxybenzamine or doxazosin should be used, with incremental dose escalation according to response. A typical starting dose for doxazocin would be 1 mg 12-hourly, building up to 6 or 8 mg a day until hypertension is controlled and postural symptoms occur.

Once and only once α-blockade has been established, unopposed β effects, such as tachycardia, may become evident and are treated with a β-blocker such as propranolol. β-Blockade should not be instituted first, as this may allow unopposed α-agonist effects, which may make hypertension worse and precipitate heart failure.

Peroperatively, short-acting α- and β-blocking agents and sodium nitroprusside (which acts directly on vessels independent of adrenergic receptors and gives additional control of hypertension) should be available.

> ### 🔄 20.4 Summary
>
> **Phaeochromocytoma**
>
> - Usually benign tumours of the adrenal medulla (80%), but 20% arise in extra-adrenal paraganglionic tissue (see Fig. 20.24); 10% are multiple and 10% are malignant
> - May be associated with medullary carcinoma of the thyroid (MEN II), von Hippel–Lindau disease and neurofibromatosis
> - Usually presents clinically with hypertension, which is often paroxysmal, and with metabolic effects such as diabetes mellitus
> - All hypertensive patients <40 years old should be screened for phaeochromocytoma; overnight or 24-hour urinary and plasma metadrenaline and normetadrenaline levels are reliable methods of diagnosis
> - Location is best defined by CT and radiolabelled metaiodobenzylguanidine scanning
> - Treatment consists of adrenalectomy after careful preparation to control blood pressure and heart rate, and to re-expand blood volume (by α-adrenergic blockade with β-blockade).

Nonendocrine adrenal medullary tumours

Ganglioneuromas

These are benign, firm, well-encapsulated tumours of ganglion cells. They grow slowly, may become large and can cause diarrhoea. Surgical excision gives excellent results.

Neuroblastomas

These are highly malignant tumours arising from sympathetic nervous tissue. They are one of the most common malignant tumours of infancy and childhood, and metastasise widely. About 75% secrete catecholamines. Treatment by radical excision, radiotherapy and chemotherapy offers the only hope of cure, although spontaneous regression has been reported.

Adrenal 'incidentaloma'

The increasing use of imaging modalities such as CT or MRI has led to adrenal 'incidentalomas' being discovered in patients being investigated for other reasons (EBM 20.4). The vast majority of these will be benign (>80%). When discovered, it is important to determine whether there is cortical or medullary hyperfunction by the use of appropriate biochemical tests, as detailed earlier. If there is no hyperfunction and the swelling is <4.0 cm in diameter, further investigation and exploration are unwarranted. The lesion is likely to be a benign, nonfunctioning cortical adenoma. Endocrine hyperfunction, a swelling >4.0 cm or the suspicion of malignancy is an indication for further assessment and exploration.

EBM 20.4 **Adrenal 'incidentalomas'**

'All adrenal "incidentalomas" require radiological and biochemical evaluation to distinguish hyperfunctioning and possibly malignant lesions from benign lesions. Any suggestion of malignancy is an indication for surgical removal.'*
'Masses >4 cm warrant consideration of surgical removal since some will be adrenocortical carcinomas.'†
'Laparoscopic adrenalectomy is the surgical treatment of choice.'‡
'For benign lesions, further radiological assessment at 6–12 months is reasonable.'

*Kapoor et al. Guidelines for the management of the incidentally discovered adrenal mass. Can Urol Assoc J. 2011;5: 241.
†Grumbach et al. Management of the clinically inapparent adrenal mass ("incidentaloma"). Ann Intern Med. 2003;138:424.
‡Smith et al. Laparoscopic adrenalectomy: New gold standard. World J Surg. 1999;23:389.
Terzolo et al. AME position statement on adrenal incidentaloma. Eur J Endocrinol. 2011;164:851.

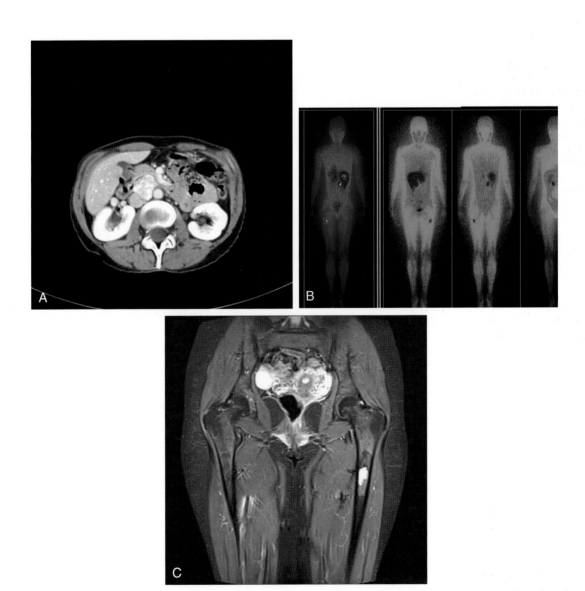

Fig. 20.24 Malignant paraganglioma. (A) Computed tomography scan abdomen showing primary. **(B)** Metaiodobenzylguanidine scan showing femoral metastases. **(C)** Magnetic resonance imaging showing femoral deposit.

Adrenalectomy

Indications

Indications for adrenalectomy include adrenal adenomas producing Cushing's syndrome, Conn's syndrome or excess catecholamines (phaeochromocytoma). Bilateral adrenalectomy may be needed for bilateral tumours, nodular hyperplasia producing Conn's or Cushing's syndrome, and if pituitary surgery fails to cure Cushing's disease.

Technique

The approach of choice is laparoscopically by the transperitoneal or posterior route. The exception to this is the known or suspected adrenal malignancy. If an open approach is required then the anterior transperitoneal route requires a large incision, inevitably causes ileus, and has a high incidence of wound and respiratory complications (especially in patients with Cushing's syndrome).

Large tumours that may be malignant are best approached through a flank incision, after removing a rib to allow access; if possible, the diaphragm, pleura and peritoneum are left intact.

The open posterior approach through the bed of the 11th or 12th rib is technically more difficult, but has low morbidity and patients return to normal activity more quickly. If pleura is breached in the course of adrenalectomy, it can be repaired on closing the wound, ensuring that the lung is fully inflated. There is no need for pleural or wound drains.

Adrenalectomy is best carried out using minimally invasive techniques. The usual route is anteriorly, beneath the costal margins, transperitoneally with reflection of liver on the right and spleen, pancreas and colon on the left. The adrenal vein can often be divided early in laparoscopic surgery, which, in phaeochromocytomas, prevents catecholamines from circulating, thereby reducing blood pressure swings following manipulation of the tumour. It is occasionally necessary to convert to an open procedure if bleeding is encountered or there are other technical or access problems. The posterior extraperitoneal approach is gaining popularity.

Replacement therapy

Corticosteroid replacement is needed for life after bilateral total adrenalectomy, but may not be needed permanently after unilateral adrenalectomy. Replacement is best achieved by a combination of oral hydrocortisone (30 mg daily in divided doses) and the mineralocorticoid fludrocortisone acetate (0.1 mg daily). If both adrenals are removed or the remaining adrenal is nonfunctional, the operation must be covered by commencing steroid replacement at the time of surgery. Adequacy of replacement is assessed by serum levels and by response to the dexamethasone test.

Doses of hydrocortisone are given intravenously until the patient can take oral steroid. It is important to note that blood pressure is the best early guide to adequacy of therapy. If hypotension occurs, 100 mg hydrocortisone is given immediately by intravenous injection, followed by 100 mg every 6–8 hours. All adrenalectomised patients must be warned to increase the dose of steroid if stress or infection occurs. Failure to anticipate the need for added steroid may precipitate an 'adrenal crisis', with acute hypotension and collapse. Such patients should carry a 'steroid card' giving details of dosage and possible complications, and should be able to recognise the symptoms of adrenal insufficiency (i.e., loss of appetite, nausea, cramps, muscle pains and malaise). If such symptoms occur, the patient should take an additional two tablets of hydrocortisone and seek urgent medical help.

Patient information

Although adrenal cortical function is vital for life, patients are unlikely to have heard of the adrenal glands. Adrenal tumours occur at a rate of about 1 per million population per annum, so patients may not have an awareness of cortisone or adrenaline. It is necessary to discuss the technicalities of surgery and the approach to be used, and to forewarn patients that a laparoscopic procedure may have to be converted to an open one. Complications should be minimal, but it is essential to mention blood loss and common complications as well as ones which, although rare, have a major impact on quality of life.

One of the most important features to describe will be any requirement for steroid-replacement therapy (necessary after bilateral adrenalectomy, unilateral adrenalectomy for an adenoma producing Cushing's syndrome, and after pituitary surgery) and the need for dosage increase at times of stress (e.g., other surgery) or intercurrent illness (e.g., pneumonia).

 20.5 Summary

Management of adrenal pathologies

- Hyperfunctioning benign adrenal masses should be removed surgically (phaeochromocytoma, cortisol secreting adenomas and Conn's syndrome). The laparoscopic approach is the preferred one
- Careful preoperative assessment to exclude multiple hormone secretions from a single or bilateral adrenal masses must be undertaken (e.g., a phaeochromocytoma that is also secreting cortisol)
- In primary hyperaldosteronism (Conn's syndrome) preoperative selective venous sampling from both adrenals should be considered to confirm the site of maximal secretion. It can be misleading to assume this will be the side with the mass lesion in it
- Incidentally found adrenal masses must be investigated for possible hypersecretion of all adrenal hormones prior to their removal or a decision to leave them in situ and follow-up
- Have a low threshold to remove nonfunctioning incidentalomas >3.5 cm in size, as the incidence of adrenocortical carcinomas increases significantly above this size
- Only biopsy an adrenal mass if you think it is due to a metastasis from a previous known malignancy. Always exclude a phaeochromocytoma before biopsy of any adrenal mass.

British Association of Endocrine and Thyroid Surgeons' Guidelines at www.BAETS.ORG.UK

Other surgical endocrine syndromes

Apudomas and multiple endocrine neoplasia

The APUD cell series

Distributed throughout the body (anterior pituitary, adrenal medulla, thyroid gland and intestine) are APUD cells that have in common the capacity to synthesise and store amines (e.g., ACTH, catecholamines, calcitonin, secretin, gastrin, cholecystokinin, enteroglucagon, somatostatin, vasoactive intestinal peptide). Hyperplasia and tumour of any APUD cell can produce specific endocrine syndromes.

Multiple endocrine neoplasia syndromes

In MEN syndromes, which are inherited as autosomal dominant traits of variable penetrance and expression, patients develop benign or malignant tumours in more than one endocrine gland (Table 20.9).

MEN type I

This is characterised by hyperplasia and/or adenomas of the parathyroid, pancreatic islets and anterior pituitary. There may also be nonfunctioning tumours of the thyroid, pituitary, adrenal cortex and soft tissues (lipomas), and functioning carcinoid tumours of the gut or lungs. The earliest biochemical sign in affected individuals is usually hypercalcaemia from hyperparathyroidism or hyperprolactinaemia from an asymptomatic pituitary tumour. Families are often uncovered when an index patient presents dramatically with small-bowel perforation or bleeding due to the Zollinger–Ellison syndrome, or with hypoglycaemia due to an insulinoma of the pancreas. Family members should be screened by measurement of fasting serum calcium and other hormonal markers such as PRL. Mutations in the MEN I gene on chromosome 11, encoding the tumour suppressor protein menin can be detected. A bracelet may be worn to alert medical attendants to the condition. Treatment is directed at the dominant clinical or biochemical feature. For example, pancreatic endocrine tumours are localised by endoscopic ultrasonography or CT and removed as necessary. Hypercalcaemia is treated by parathyroid surgery, where either all diseased glands are excised followed by calcium-replacement therapy, or by subtotal (three and a half glands) parathyroidectomy, when replacement therapy can be avoided but recurrence of the remnant to a hyperfunctioning state at some later date is inevitable.

MEN type II

This is characterised by medullary carcinoma of the thyroid, phaeochromocytoma and parathyroid hyperplasia. Genetic diagnosis, based on a mutation in *Ret* protooncogene chromosome 10, obviates the need for biochemical testing in family members. Unlike in MEN I, there is advantage in prophylactic surgery, with affected individuals undergoing total thyroidectomy at an age dictated by the mutation identified and the level of risk associated with that mutation. Kindred members not showing the mutation can be dismissed from follow-up and can be reassured that they will not pass on the genetic abnormality to their offspring. Phaeochromocytomas are diagnosed by annual screening using urinary metadrenaline and normetadrenaline levels, and localised by CT and MIBG scanning. Surgical treatment of the phaeochromocytoma must take precedence over the thyroid and parathyroid disease, as anaesthesia and surgery in patients with undiagnosed or untreated phaeochromocytoma can be life-threatening.

Carcinoid tumours and the carcinoid syndrome

Carcinoid tumours are most frequently found incidentally in the appendix of a patient undergoing appendicectomy for acute appendicitis, and account for 85% of all appendiceal tumours. They are usually less than 1 cm in diameter and are cured by appendicectomy, as metastases are exceptional in this situation. Carcinoid tumours larger than 2 cm in diameter are rare, but may have spread to lymph nodes and are best treated by right hemicolectomy. Liver metastases are extremely rare in patients with appendiceal carcinoids. Carcinoids occurring in the small intestine frequently spread to lymph nodes, and in 10% of cases there are liver metastases by the time the patient presents with obstructive symptoms or bleeding. Carcinoids in any site produce 5-hydroxytryptamine (5-HT) and other biologically active amines and peptides. In the case of gut carcinoids, these products are normally inactivated by the liver, but liver secondaries secrete these substances directly into the systemic circulation, giving rise to the carcinoid syndrome: periodic flushing, diarrhoea, bronchoconstriction, wheezing and distinctive red-purple discoloration of the face. Right-sided heart disease, notably pulmonary stenosis, may result and can prove fatal (Table 20.10).

20

Table 20.9 Multiple endocrine neoplasia syndromes

MEN type I	Characterised by hyperplasia or adenomas of the:
	• Parathyroid
	• Pancreatic islets
	• Anterior pituitary
	± Nonfunctioning tumours of:
	• Thyroid
	• Pituitary
	• Soft tissues (lipomas)
	± Functioning tumours:
	• Carcinoid of gut/lungs
	Variable presentation:
	• Hypercalcaemia from ↑ PTH
	• Hyperprolactinaemia
	• Small-bowel perforation or bleed due to Zollinger–Ellison syndrome
	• Hypoglycaemia due to insulinoma
MEN type II	Characterised by:
	• Medullary carcinoma of the thyroid
	• Phaeochromocytoma
	• Parathyroid hyperplasia

MEN, Multiple endocrine neoplasia; PTH, parathyroid hormone.

Table 20.10 Carcinoid tumours

Carcinoid tumours	*Appendiceal carcinoid tumours*	• Account for 85% of all appendiceal tumours • Usually <1 cm and cured by appendicectomy • >2 cm rare but may spread to lymph nodes and therefore require right hemicolectomy
	Small-intestine carcinoids	• Frequently spread to lymph nodes • In 10%, there are liver metastases by the time of presentation

Carcinoid syndrome		• Occurs when liver metastases secrete 5-hydroxytryptamine and other biologically active amines and peptides directly into the bloodstream
		• *Features:*
		  • Periodic flushing
		  • Diarrhoea
		  • Bronchoconstriction and wheezing
		  • Red–purple discolouration of the face
		  • Pulmonary stenosis and right-sided heart disease

The diagnosis of carcinoid syndrome is confirmed by detecting 5-hydroxyindoleacetic acid (a breakdown product of 5-HT) in the urine. If the primary tumour is causing symptoms, it should be removed surgically if possible (e.g., right hemicolectomy, small-bowel resection, lung resection). Hepatic metastases can be dealt with by resection, radiofrequency ablation or angiographic embolisation.

Somatostatin analogues or α-adrenergic antagonists may be useful in controlling symptoms. Chemotherapy (e.g., 5-fluorouracil) is sometimes effective, as is interferon, but side effects can be troublesome.

Hanafiah Harunarashid

21

Vascular and endovascular surgery

Chapter contents

Introduction 375

Pathophysiology of arterial disease 375

Chronic lower limb arterial disease 376

Arterial disease of the upper limb 386

Mesenteric artery disease 389

Acute limb ischaemia 389

Pathophysiology of venous disease 396

Venous thromboembolism 402

Other forms of venous thrombosis 404

Lymphoedema 405

Filariasis 406

Vascular access for haemodialysis 407

Introduction

The approach to vascular patients is multidisciplinary, and involves vascular surgeons, interventional radiologists, anaesthetists, angiologists, nurses, physiotherapists and occupational therapists. The increasing prevalence of elderly patients, diabetes and obesity is contributing to a rapid increase of vascular disease in the developing world, despite smoking reductions. The anatomy of the arterial and venous circulation is shown on Fig. 21.1

Pathophysiology of arterial disease

Pathophysiology of atherosclerosis (Fig. 21.2) is characterised by endothelial cell injury; subendothelial deposition of lipids and inflammatory cells; and smooth muscle cell migration and proliferation, all of which lead to plaque haemorrhage and rupture resulting in thrombosis and embolism.

Clinical features

The clinical manifestations of arterial disease depend upon the factors outlined in Box 21.1.

Mechanism of injury

The mechanism of injury has a major influence on the clinical presentation, prognosis and treatment of arterial disease (Fig. 21.3).

Haemodynamic mechanism

An atheromatous plaque must reduce the cross-sectional area of an artery by approximately 70% to cause an appreciable drop in blood flow at rest, a so-called critical stenosis. However, with exertion such as walking, a much lesser stenosis may become flow limiting. The pressure drop across a stenosis is proportional to the square of the velocity of the blood entering that stenosis, therefore blood velocity increases markedly on exercise. The clinical consequence is that the lesion only becomes symptomatic on exertion. This type of mechanism tends to have a relatively benign course; intermittent claudication (IC) due to superficial femoral artery stenosis is a common example.

Thrombosis

By the time a 'critical' stenosis occludes, the collateral supply may be so well developed that the event is clinically silent. However, acute thrombosis of the vessel can have severe consequences if a plaque that has been causing little or no haemodynamic impairment ruptures suddenly. Such an event can cause a myocardial infarction (coronary artery) or stroke (internal carotid artery) in a previously asymptomatic patient.

Atheroembolism

The effect that embolising plaque contents (predominantly cholesterol) or adherent thrombus (predominantly platelets) have upon the distal circulation depends upon the factors outlined above, as well as the embolic load. Perhaps the best-known example is atheroembolism from internal carotid artery plaque, which can cause small, discrete, and temporary areas of cerebral and retinal ischaemia that manifest clinically as a transient ischaemic attack (TIA) or amaurosis fugax. If the embolic load is high, however, these emboli may cause irreversible occlusion of major distal vessels, leading to stroke and retinal infarction (monocular blindness).

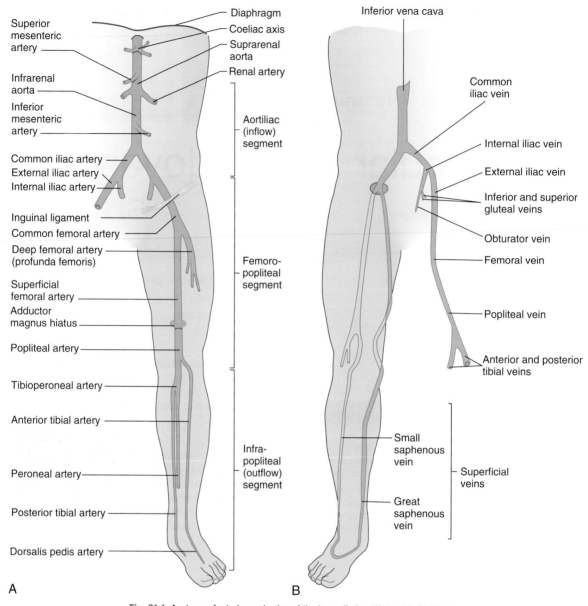

Fig. 21.1 Anatomy of arteries and veins of the lower limbs. **(A)** Arterial. **(B)** Venous.

Thromboembolism

The most common source of thromboembolism is the left atrium in association with atrial fibrillation (AF). The clinical consequences are usually dramatic, as the thrombus load is often large and tends to suddenly and completely occlude a large or medium-sized vessel that has previously been healthy, and around which there is therefore no collateral supply. This is an important cause of stroke and acute limb ischaemia.

Chronic lower limb arterial disease

Anatomy

The lower limb arterial tree comprises the aortoiliac segment above the inguinal ligament ('inflow'), the femoropopliteal segment and the infrapopliteal segment ('outflow')

Clinical features

Symptoms

Chronic lower limb ischaemia presents as two distinct clinical entities, IC and critical limb ischaemia (CLI), which have different epidemiologies, natural histories, treatments and prognoses.

Intermittent claudication

Epidemiology

IC affects up to 5% of people aged over 60 years. Provided patients comply with best medical treatment (BMT), only a small proportion (1–2%) of those affected by IC will deteriorate to a point where revascularisation or amputation are required. However, the annual mortality rate is 5–10% per year, which is 2–3-times higher than an age- and sex-matched nonclaudicant population. This is

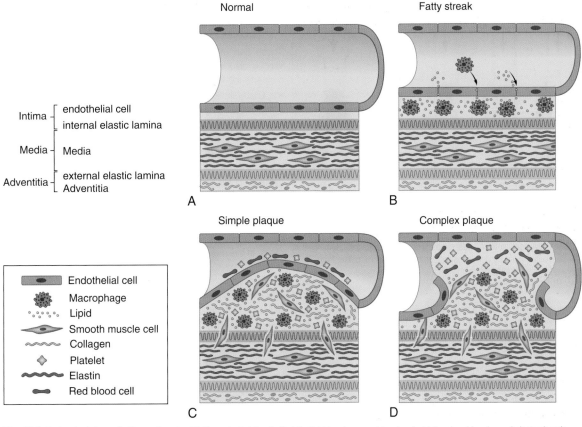

Fig. 21.2 Pathophysiology of atherosclerosis. (A) Normal arterial wall. Endothelial injury is caused by chemical injury (smoking, hypercholesterolaemia, hypertriglycerides, and diabetes) or physical injury or atheroma, where blood flow exerts shear stress on the arterial wall. Hypertension, which increases this stress, is an important predisposing factor for arterial disease. **(B)** Lipid deposition. Injury to the artery increases its permeability to lipids and inflammatory cells, which promotes deposition of lipids in the subendothelial layer. Leucocytes then adhere into the subendothelial space and digest lipids to become foam cells. Protease and free radicals liberate and further damage; cytokines attract more leucocytes and smooth muscle cells. **(C)** Smooth muscle cell proliferation. Through the internal elastic lamina, smooth muscle cells enter the media, where they proliferate, take on the characteristics of fibroblasts and produce collagen, raising the atheroma to occlude the lumen. **(D)** Complex plaque/plaque rupture. Proliferation forms an endothelial cap, which may rupture, ensuing further endothelial injury. This results in thrombosis and distal embolisation.

21

---

i | **Box 21.1 Factors determining clinical manifestations of arterial disease**

Anatomical site

- Coronary arteries: myocardial infarction
- Cerebral circulation: stroke, transient ischaemic attack, amaurosis fugax, vertebrobasilar insufficiency
- Renal arteries: hypertension, renal failure
- Mesenteric arteries: mesenteric angina, acute intestinal ischemia
- Limbs: intermittent claudication, chronic limb ischaemia, acute limb ischemia

Type of arterial supply

- End artery (only supply to tissue)
- Well collateralised (one of several arteries)
- For example, in a patient with a complete circle of Willis, occlusion of one internal carotid artery may be asymptomatic, whereas with an incomplete circle occlusion is more likely to cause a stroke

Speed of onset

- Slow development of atheroma may give chance for collateral development (e.g., profunda [deep] femoral artery collateralises around a diseased superficial femoral artery in patients with intermittent claudication).
- Sudden occlusion of a previously normal artery may cause severe ischemia (as there has been no time for collateral vessels to develop)

Mechanism of injury

- Haemodynamic mechanism: pressure drop across a stenosis is proportional to blood velocity. During walking, pressure drop is increased and is called critical stenosis (e.g., intermittent claudication)
- Thrombosis: rupture of plaque (myocardial infarction or stroke)
- Atheroembolism: embolic load. Small load = temporary (e.g., transient ischaemic attack), high load = irreversible (e.g., retinal infarct)
- Thromboembolism: most common source left atrium, thrombus load is high and often causes sudden occlusion (e.g., stroke or limb ischemia).

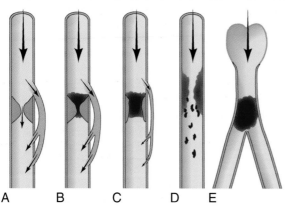

Fig. 21.3 Mechanisms of injury in atherosclerotic disease. (A) Critical stenosis compensated by collateral vessels, symptomatic on exercise. **(B)** Acute thrombosis of a critical stenosis, little change in symptoms due to collateral development. **(C)** Acute thrombosis of noncritical stenosis, symptoms are severe due to poorly developed collaterals. **(D)** Atheroembolism from ruptured plaque. **(E)** Thromboembolism from the heart; severe ischaemia because of lack of collateral supply.

because IC is a powerful marker of widespread atherosclerosis, and most of these patients succumb to myocardial infarction (MI), stroke and limb loss. The emphasis is, therefore, on the preservation of life.

Clinical features

Claudication pain is a muscular pain. Its characteristics are that:

- It is not present at rest
- It comes on walking a particular distance, which is known as the claudication distance

- It is quickly relieved by resting
- It is repetitive; the patient will develop the pain after walking the claudication distance.

These and other features distinguish it from neurogenic and venous claudication (Table 21.1). The site of claudication gives a clue to the likely site of arterial disease:

- Bilateral thigh and/or buttock: aortoiliac artery
- Unilateral thigh and/or buttock: iliac artery
- Calf: femoropopliteal artery
- Foot (instep): infrapopliteal tibial artery

In the lower limb, arterial disease most frequently affects the superficial femoral artery (SFA) (Fig. 21.4). IC is usually characterised by pain on walking in the muscles of one or both calves. Typically, the SFA first becomes narrowed at the adductor canal (Fig. 21.5A). Over the next few months or years, collateral vessels arising from the profunda femoral artery (PFA) enlarge so that they carry a higher proportion of the blood flow to the lower leg. As a result, in the majority of patients, symptoms gradually improve or even disappear. This phase of moderate claudication may remain apparently stable for several years. However, without BMT and a change in the patient's lifestyle, the atherosclerosis will progress to involve other segments, such as the PFA, iliac and tibial vessels (Fig. 21.5C). The IC will progress to become severe, requiring patients to stop every 50–100 m. As the disease progresses further in severity and extent, the scope for spontaneous improvement steadily diminishes and symptoms worsen to a point where CLI develops due to multilevel disease (Fig. 21.5D). Such patients will develop night/rest pain and are at risk of tissue loss (see later).

An understanding of this cyclical pattern of exacerbation and resolution in IC is important, as spontaneous improvement may mislead the patient into thinking that all is well and that there is no longer a need to comply with medical advice. In particular, they

Table 21.1 Differential diagnosis of claudication

	Arterial	Neurogenic	Venous
Pathology	Stenosis or occlusion of major lower limb arteries	Lumbar nerve roots or cauda equina compression (spinal stenosis)	Obstruction to the venous outflow of the leg due to iliofemoral venous occlusion secondary to deep venous thrombosis
Site of pain	Muscles: usually the calf but may affect thigh and buttock	Ill-defined; whole leg. Shooting in nature; may be associated with tingling and numbness	Whole leg. Bursting in nature
Laterality	Usually unilateral if femoro-popliteal, bilateral if aortoiliac disease	Often bilateral	Nearly always unilateral
Onset	Gradual onset after walking the 'claudication distance'	Often immediate upon walking or even on standing up	Gradual onset but may be present from the moment walking commences
Relieving features	On cessation of walking, the pain disappears completely in 1–2 minutes	On cessation of walking, the pain may gradually subside over 5–10 minutes. Often the patient has to sit down or lean against something to obtain relief	The subject usually needs to elevate the leg to obtain relief
Colour	Normal or pale	Normal	Cyanosed. Often visible varicose veins and venous skin changes
Temperature	Normal or cool	Normal	Normal or increased
Swelling	Absent	Absent	Always present
Pulses	Reduced or absent	Normal	Present, but may be difficult to feel because of swelling
Straight leg raising	Normal	Limited	Normal

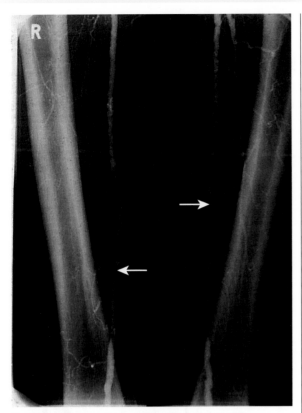

Fig. 21.4 Angiogram showing diffuse disease in both right and left superficial femoral arteries (*arrows*).

continue to smoke with impunity. Thrombotic occlusion of the SFA (Fig. 21.5B) may lead to a sudden deterioration in walking distance at any time.

Critical limb ischaemia

Whereas IC is usually due to single-level disease, CLI is caused by multiple lesions affecting different arterial segments down the leg (see Fig. 21.5). These patients usually have:

- Rest pain
- Tissue loss in the form of an ulcer or gangrene
- Low ankle/brachial pressure index (ABPI) (Fig.21.6).

Without revascularisation, such patients will often lose their limb, and sometimes their life, in a matter of months.

Rest pain

Rest pain occurs with the lower limb at rest; it is exacerbated by lying down or elevation of the foot. It is classically felt at night and is relieved by sleeping with feet hanging over the bed or sleeping on a chair. The patient may present with foot swelling due to gravitational oedema.

Examination findings

On examination, the chronically ischaemic limb is usually characterised by:

- Skin that is thin and dry
- Pallor, particularly on elevation. Upon dependency, the foot becomes bright red; this is known as dependent rubor or 'sunset foot', and is due to reactive hyperaemia (Buerger's test)

- Superficial veins that fill sluggishly in the horizontal position and empty upon minimal elevation (venous guttering)
- Nails that are brittle and crumbly
- Muscle wasting
- Reduced temperature
- Pulses that are weak or absent, and sometimes associated with thrills on palpation and bruits on auscultation.

Pulse status

All patients admitted to hospital must have their pulse status recorded. This includes superficial temporal, carotid, subclavian, brachial, radial, ulnar, femoral, popliteal, posterior tibial and dorsalis pedis. The pulses are recorded as normal, weak or absent. The presence of a thrill and/or bruit denotes turbulent flow. In the presence of effective collateralisation, especially in younger patients, pulses may sometimes be present at rest, despite significant proximal arterial disease.

Ankle/brachial pressure index

The severity of ischaemia in the leg can be simply estimated by determining the ratio between the ankle and brachial blood pressures. Pressures at both the posterior tibial and dorsalis pedis artery are measured, and the higher one is taken to calculate the index:

- Healthy person: 1
- Patient with IC: 0.5–0.9
- CLI: <0.5

Diabetic vascular disease

Approximately 40% of patients with CLI have diabetes, and such patients pose a number of unique problems for vascular specialists:

- Arteries are often calcified, which makes surgery and angioplasty technically difficult
- Calcification also leads to vessel incompressibility, which results in spuriously high ankle pressures and elevated ABPI measurements
- Reduced ability to fight infection
- Severe multisystem arterial disease (coronary, cerebral and peripheral), which increases the risks of intervention
- In the lower limbs, diabetic vascular disease has a predilection for the infrapopliteal vessels. Although vessels in the foot are often spared, the technical challenge of performing a satisfactory bypass or angioplasty to these small vessels is considerable
- Frequent coexisting neuropathy may lead to foot ulceration in its own right, but may also complicate peripheral ischaemia (see later).

The diabetic foot

This refers to the combination of ischaemia, neuropathy and immunocompromise that renders the feet of diabetic patients particularly susceptible to sepsis, ulceration and gangrene. Diabetic neuropathy affects the motor, sensory and autonomic nerves.

Sensory neuropathy

- Patient incapable of feeling pain
- It affects proprioception such that, when walking, pressure is applied at unusual sites
- This leads to ulcer formation and even joint destruction (Charcot's joint).

21

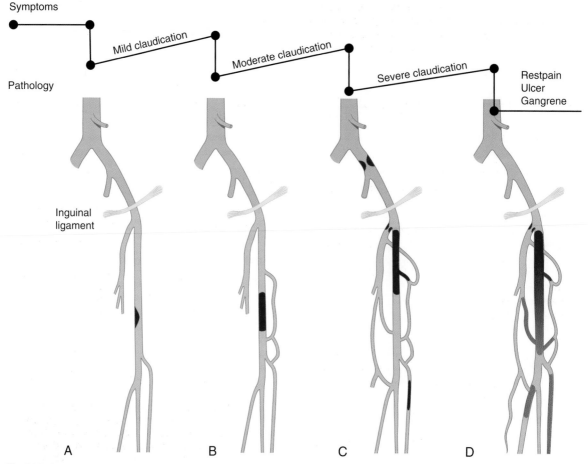

Fig. 21.5 **Symptoms and pathology in intermittent claudication.** (A) Superficial femoral artery (SFA) stenosis at adductor canal. (B) Occlusion of the SFA and development of a collateral circulation between the deep femoral (profunda femoris) artery (PFA) and the popliteal artery. (C) Iliac artery and PFA stenosis leading to worsening symptoms of intermittent claudication and further collateralisation. (D) Eventually critical limb ischaemia characterised by ischaemic rest pain and tissue loss develops due to multilevel disease affecting tibial arteries and collateral supply.

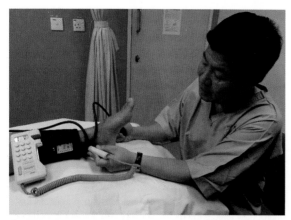

Fig. 21.6 Measurement of ankle/brachial pressure index (ABPI) using Doppler ultrasound.

Motor neuropathy

- The normal structure and function of the foot depends not only upon ligaments, but also upon the long and short flexors and extensors of the calf and foot

- The former are affected more than the latter by motor neuropathy, leading to weakness and atrophy
- The result is that the long extensors of the toes are unopposed and the toes become increasingly dorsiflexed
- This exposes the metatarsal heads to abnormal pressure, and they are a frequent site of callus formation and ulceration.

Autonomic neuropathy

- Dry foot deficient in the sweat that normally lubricates the skin and contains antibacterial substances
- The result is scaling and fissuring of the skin, and the creation of a portal of entry for bacteria
- Abnormal blood flow in the bones of the ankle and foot due to loss of autonomic control may also contribute to osteopenia and bony collapse (Charcot's foot).

Management

If the blood supply to the foot is adequate, dead tissue can be excised in the expectation that healing will occur, provided infection is controlled and the foot is protected from pressure (so-called off-loading). If there is ischaemia as well, the priority is to revascularise the foot, if possible. Sadly, many diabetic patients present late, with extensive tissue loss and 'unreconstructable' disease, which accounts for the very high amputation rate.

Management of lower limb ischaemia

Medical management

All patients with atherosclerotic vascular disease should be strongly urged to comply with BMT, which comprises:

- Cessation from smoking. This is by far the most important intervention and prognostic factor
- Control of hypertension
- Control of hypercholesterolaemia by statin despite the cholesterol level: usually with a lipid-lowering drug (statin)
- Prescription of antiplatelet agent: usually aspirin (75 mg daily), but clopidogrel (75 mg daily) is a more effective and safe alternative
- Regular exercise
- Control of obesity
- The identification and active treatment of patients with diabetes. This includes foot care
- Current clinical practice guidelines can be found at the following link: https://www.nice.org.uk/guidance/cg147/chapter/6-Related-NICE-guidance.

Compliance with BMT increases not only walking distance, but also affords very significant protection against cardiovascular events and improves the patient's quality of life and life expectancy. Unfortunately, many patients fail to comply and, in particular, continue to smoke. In patients undergoing intervention, BMT undoubtedly reduces the overall risks and increases the likely success of the procedure. Indications for intervention are:

- Disabling claudication pain
- CLI.

Intervention includes:

- Balloon angioplasty (BAP), with or without stenting
- Bypass surgery (BSX).

Endovascular management

BAP, with or without stenting, has been used successfully in the iliac, femoral, popliteal and crural arteries, and is usually performed under local anaesthesia (Fig. 21.7).

This is the treatment of choice for disease segments that are less than 10 cm long. The arterial lesion to be treated (stenosis or occlusion) is identified and crossed with a wire. A balloon is inserted and inflated. This enlarges the lumen by disrupting the atheromatous plaque. In patients with total occlusions and complex disease, metal stents may be deployed across the lesion to improve patency and reduce distal embolic complications. Sometimes these balloons and stents are coated with drugs that reduce the arterial scarring (neointimal hyperplasia) that follows such intervention and can lead to restenosis and reocclusion (drug-eluting balloons and stents). Endoluminal repair of the aortoiliac segment is the treatment of choice because of its high patency rates and low morbidity compared to open surgery. Infrainguinal BAP and, less commonly, stenting is also widely used in the management of CLI.

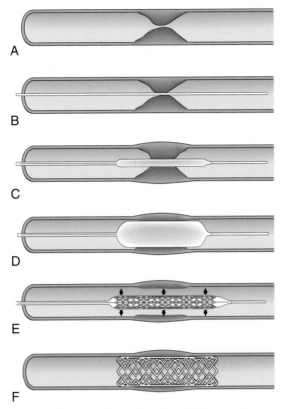

Fig. 21.7 Balloon angioplasty and stenting. (A) Critical arterial stenosis. **(B)** A guidewire is used to cross the lesion. **(C)** The guidewire is used to direct a balloon angioplasty catheter across the lesion. **(D)** The balloon is inflated. **(E)** A metal stent may be mounted on a catheter. The stent may be self-expanding or require expansion with a balloon. In many cases, the first manoeuvre is to cross the lesion with a stent and in this circumstance steps C and D may be omitted. **(F)** Metal stent holding open the stenosis.

Intermittent claudication

Endoluminal treatment (BAP, stent) should be used selectively in patients with IC because it may be associated with a 1–2% morbidity rate, rarely mortality, and many patients have a pattern of disease that is unsuitable for current endovascular technologies. There is controversy with regard to its role in the femoropopliteal and infrapopliteal segments because of a perceived lack of durability of benefit. In the future, this may be improved by the use of stents. By contrast, most vascular specialists believe that endoluminal therapy should be considered in patients with IC due to aortoiliac disease (absent or reduced femoral pulses) because they:

- Tend to be younger, so that their symptoms have a greater impact on their quality of life and livelihood
- Often have short-segment disease that is amenable to BAP, with or without a stent
- Often have (relatively) normal infrainguinal arteries, so that restoring flow in the aortoiliac segment effects a dramatic improvement in distal perfusion
- Tend to be more symptomatic, with shorter walking distances and bilateral symptoms

21

- May not achieve a satisfactory increase in walking distance with BMT alone, because the ability of the body to collateralise around aortoiliac disease is not as good as it is around femoropopliteal disease.

Furthermore, the long-term patency of BAP and stenting is optimal in high-flow, large-calibre vessels, leading to a durable clinical benefit in many patients.

Critical limb ischaemia

The role of BAP and stenting in CLI remains controversial and, with present technology, many such patients remain unsuitable for endovascular therapy. The only published randomised controlled trial to compare BAP and BSX reported that although BAP was safer and less expensive than BSX in the short term (12–18 months), BSX (with vein) offers a more durable and complete revascularisation in the longer term (3–5 years) (EBM 21.1). At the present time, CLI patients expected to only live 1–2 years and who do not have a suitable vein for the construction of a bypass are probably best treated by BAP where technically possible; all other CLI patients are probably best served by BSX. However, the role for endovascular therapy may increase in the future as technology improves.

> **EBM** **21.1 Bypass surgery (BSX) or balloon angioplasty (BAP) for severe limb ischaemia**
>
> 'For patients who survived for at least 2 years after randomization, a BSX-first revascularization strategy was associated with a significant increase in subsequent overall survival and a trend towards reduced amputation free survival. BAP was associated with a significantly higher early failure rate than BSX. Many BAP patients ultimately required surgery. BSX outcomes after failed BAP are significantly worse than for BSX performed as a first revascularization attempt. BSX with vein offers the best long term outcome but BAP appears superior to prosthetic BSX.'
>
> Basil Trial investigators and Participants. Final results of the BASIL trial (Bypass Versus Angioplasty in Severe Ischaemia of the Leg). J Vasc Surg. 2010;51:5S–17S.

Indications for arterial reconstruction

Intermittent claudication

Many surgeons are reluctant to perform infrainguinal BSX for IC because:

- The risk of limb loss is very low with BMT

- Those patients who fail to comply with BMT (fail to stop smoking) are those most likely to press for surgery because of ongoing symptoms. However, they are also those at greatest operative risk and those least likely to gain durable benefit from their bypass
- Surgery is associated with a significant risk of mortality and major morbidity, the size of that risk depending on the procedure and the patient but probably approaching 3–5% for infrainguinal bypass and 5–10% for aortobifemoral bypass
- As most patients have bilateral disease, even if they have unilateral symptoms, successful infrainguinal surgery on one side often reveals limiting IC symptoms on the other, requiring a second operation (the same for endoluminal treatment)
- Grafts have a finite patency, especially in those who fail to comply with BMT and, in particular, continue to smoke (the same for endoluminal treatment)
- As soon as a bypass graft is inserted, collaterals circumventing the original lesion shrink down. For this reason, when the graft occludes, usually suddenly, the patient is normally returned to a worse level of IC than before the operation. A previous claudicant may now have acute limb-threatening ischaemia, which then forces the surgeon or radiologist to re-intervene. Secondary interventions are technically more difficult, are associated with higher risk and a lower patency rate.

As with BAP and stenting, the balance of risks and benefits for open surgery is different in patients with aortoiliac disease. Although the risk of surgery is higher, the long-term patency rates of such grafts are excellent, and one operation deals with both legs. Whatever the treatment being considered, patients and their families must be made fully aware of the risks and benefits so that they can give fully informed consent. These discussions must always be carefully recorded.

Principles of arterial reconstruction

Endarterectomy

This involves the direct removal of atherosclerotic plaque and thrombus, and is a relatively uncommon operation in modern vascular surgical practice except at the carotid and femoral bifurcations (Fig. 21.8).

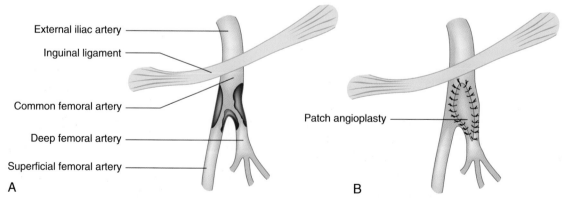

External iliac artery
Inguinal ligament
Common femoral artery
Deep femoral artery
Superficial femoral artery
A

Patch angioplasty
B

Fig. 21.8 Profundaplasty. (A) Focal atherosclerotic disease of the left common femoral artery is causing severe ischaemia because it is obstructing flow down the superficial and deep femoral (profunda femoris) arteries. **(B)** Local endarterectomy and closure of the profunda femoris using a vein or prosthetic patch (profundaplasty) restores normal flow to both vessels.

Bypass grafting

For a surgical bypass operation (Fig. 21.9) to be successful in the long term, three conditions must be fulfilled:

- There must be high-flow, high-pressure blood entering the graft (inflow)
- The conduit must be suitable
- The blood must have somewhere to go when it leaves the graft (outflow or run-off).

Two main types of conduit are available:

- Autogenous material, most commonly the ipsilateral great saphenous vein (GSV)
- Prosthetic material, most commonly expanded polytetrafluoroethylene (ePTFE) or Dacron.

The main advantage of vein is that it is lined by endothelium that is actively antithrombotic and profibrinolytic, and therefore much less liable to induce coagulation than even the most inert of man-made materials. This translates into much better long-term graft patency. Vein is also much more resistant to infection (see later) and less expensive. It is generally agreed that, wherever possible, vein from the leg or arm should be used for infrainguinal reconstruction.

In most bypass operations, the new conduit almost follows the course of the original artery, so-called anatomic bypass (Fig. 21.10). Various bypass operations, their indications and 'ideal' conduit are shown in Table 21.2.

Extraanatomic bypass

Where anatomic bypass is not possible and/or desirable, a so-called extraanatomic bypass can be inserted (Fig. 21.11).

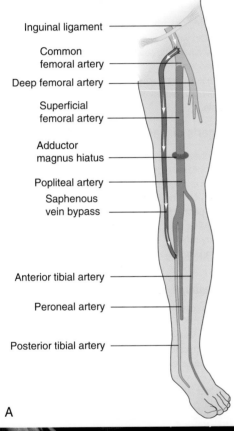

Inguinal ligament
Common femoral artery
Deep femoral artery
Superficial femoral artery
Adductor magnus hiatus
Popliteal artery
Saphenous vein bypass
Anterior tibial artery
Peroneal artery
Posterior tibial artery

A

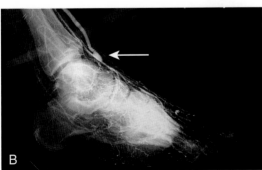

B

Fig. 21.9 Femorodistal bypass graft. (A) Diagram showing femoral to posterior tibial bypass graft. **(B)** On-table angiogram showing the distal end of the vein graft (*arrow*) anastomosed to the dorsalis pedis artery in the foot.

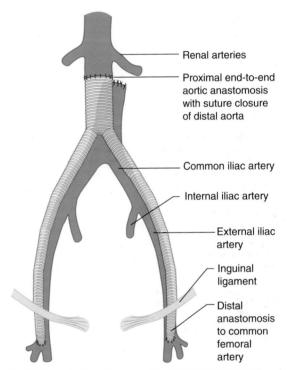

Renal arteries
Proximal end-to-end aortic anastomosis with suture closure of distal aorta
Common iliac artery
Internal iliac artery
External iliac artery
Inguinal ligament
Distal anastomosis to common femoral artery

Fig. 21.10 Anatomic aortic bypass. Reconstruction of an occluded aortoiliac segment by means of aortobifemoral bypass grafting.

Table 21.2 Types of bypass operation and preferred graft		
Bypass	**Indications**	**'Ideal' graft**
Aortobifemoral bypass	Aortoiliac disease	Dacron or PTFE bifurcated graft
Ileofemoral bypass	Isolated external iliac artery disease	PTFE graft
Femoropopliteal bypass above knee	Superficial femoral disease	Reversed GSV or PTFE graft
Femoropopliteal bypass below knee	SFA and popliteal artery disease	Reversed GSV graft
Femorodistal bypass	Popliteal and tibial arteries disease	In-situ GSV graft

GSV, Great saphenous vein; PTFE, polytetrafluoroethylene; SFA, superficial femoral artery.

21

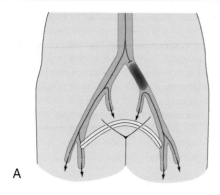

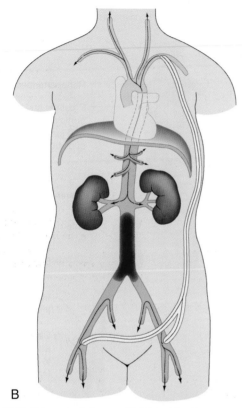

Fig. 21.11 Extraanatomic bypass. (A) Unilateral iliac disease may be treated by femoro-femoral crossover graft. **(B)** Bilateral aortoiliac disease may be treated with axillobifemoral bypass graft.

For example, if only one iliac artery is blocked, and the patient is unfit for abdominal surgery and unsuitable for endoluminal treatment, a femorofemoral crossover graft can be performed. If both iliac arteries are occluded, an axillobifemoral graft is employed. These extraanatomic grafts do not have as good long-term patency as anatomic aortoiliac reconstructions. However, they are lesser procedures, and so the preferred option in high-risk patients or those that have a limited life expectancy.

Complications of arterial reconstruction

Early morbidity and mortality associated with vascular surgery is related to the underlying cardiac disease that vascular patients invariably have. Meticulous perioperative care is essential for optimal results.

Long-term major complications include infection and graft occlusion, for which outcome is better when identified early.

Blockage of the graft

Serial ultrasound scans of grafts at regular intervals in the postoperative period, typically at 1, 3, 6, 12, 18 and 24 months, so-called graft surveillance, plays a role in early identification of a 'failing' graft before it has blocked. Despite not having strong evidence of benefit, it is generally believed that it is better to correct a 'failing' graft before it has blocked than to try to resurrect one that has already failed.

Infection of prosthetic grafts

This is largely due to the increasing prevalence of antibiotic-resistant organisms, including methicillin-resistant *Staphylococcus aureus* (MRSA). Measures to avoid graft infection include:

- Using vein wherever possible
- Perioperative antibiotic prophylaxis, use vancomycin for reoperations
- Strict aseptic technique in the operating theatre and ward
- Always using gloves and washing hands between examining patients.

Buerger's disease (thromboangiitis obliterans)

Buerger's disease is a nonatherosclerotic, idiopathic, recurrent, segmental, inflammatory, vasculopathy of medium- and small-sized arteries and veins of upper and lower extremities that is quite distinct from atherosclerosis. It is rare in Caucasians but more common in people from the South-East Asia, India, North Africa and the Middle East. Thromboangiitis obliterans refers to the inflammatory reaction of the arterial wall with involvement of the neighbouring vein and nerve, ultimately leading to thrombosis of the artery.

Clinical features

- Usually presents in young (20–40 years) male smokers
- Characteristically affects the peripheral arteries, but can also affect the veins commonly presenting as superficial thrombophlebitis
- Causes claudication in the feet, or rest pain in the fingers or toes
- Wrist and ankle pulses are usually absent, but branchial and popliteal pulses are palpable (Box 21.2).

Investigations

Arteriography typically shows segmental narrowing or occlusion of arteries with skip lesions with a corkscrew appearance in the affected limb, but relatively healthy vessels above that level.

Treatment

- BMT, especially smoking cessation
- Lumbar sympathectomy (surgical or chemical) provides relief from rest pain by causing vasodilatation in the skin vessels and abolition of pain carried through the sympathetic fibres. However, it is contraindicated in the presence of claudication, which may be worsened
- Prostaglandin infusions may be helpful
- Small-calibre vessel disease does not permit the use of any bypass or endovascular surgery

- Age younger than 45 years
- Current or recent history of tobacco use
- Presence of distal extremity ischemia (claudication, rest pain, ischaemic ulcers)
- Exclusion of autoimmune diseases, hypercoagulable states and diabetes mellitus
- Exclusion of a proximal source of embolisation by echocardiography and arteriography
- Consistent arteriographic findings in the clinically involved and noninvolved limbs.

- If amputation is required, it can often be limited to the digits at first. However, if the patient continues to smoke, then bilateral below-knee amputation is a frequent outcome.

Although the disease is uncommon in the UK, it is very important to consider and exclude in patients presenting with vascular symptoms in their legs and arms, especially if the symptoms are atypical and the patient is young (under 50 years of age). Failure to make the diagnosis often leads to avoidable limb loss and is a source of medicolegal activity.

Raynaud's phenomenon

Raynaud's phenomenon describes digital pallor due to vasospasm of the digital arteries, followed by cyanosis owing to the presence of deoxygenated blood, then rubor due to reactive hyperaemia upon restoration of flow, in response to cold and emotional stimuli (Table 21.3).

Amputation

Indications

Amputation should only be considered where arterial reconstruction is considered by a vascular surgeon to be inappropriate or impossible. In some cases, patients are admitted profoundly unwell and septic from spreading gangrene and immediate amputation may be the only means of saving the patient's life.

Table 21.3 Raynaud's phenomenon: disease and syndrome

	Primary (Raynaud's disease)	Secondary (Raynaud's Syndrome)
Age	15–30 years	Older people
Causes	Unknown; however, has family history	Connective tissue disease Vibration-induced injury Atherosclerosis
Aetiology	Reversible spasms	Fixed obstruction of the digital arteries
Progression	Self-limiting	Usually have fingertip ulceration and necrosis
Treatment	Avoid cold exposure Calcium channel blocker	Protect from cold and trauma If infected, antibiotics are warranted Vasoactive drugs have short-term benefits Sympathectomy Prostacyclin infusion

Some conditions that may require amputation are:
- Gangrene:, dry or wet
- Uncontrolled sepsis of the lower limb, which includes necrotising fasciitis
- Severe rest pain with no reconstruction option
- Paralysis with contractures
- Trauma.

Level of amputation

This is determined by local blood supply, the status of the joints, the patient's general health and his or her age. The broad principle is to amputate at the lowest level consistent with healing (Fig. 21.12). It is important to conserve the knee joint if at all possible, as the energy required to walk on a below-knee prosthesis is much less than that required to walk on an above-knee prosthesis. However, if the patient has other comorbidity or disability that would make walking with a prosthesis impossible, there is no point in attempting to conserve the knee joint at the expense of healing. A common situation is where a patient presents with a fixed flexion contracture of the knee. A below-knee amputation in such a patient is usually ill-advised because the contracture will prevent the patient from ever walking and will also result in the stump wound resting on the bed or chair, leading to poor healing and wound breakdown.

Surgical principles

A number of important principles must be observed if primary healing and satisfactory rehabilitation are to be achieved. The in-hospital mortality for major limb amputation may be as high as 20%, and can exceed 30% in the elderly undergoing above-knee amputation. The decision to amputate, the level of amputation and the procedure itself requires direct input from an experienced vascular surgeon. In some elderly patients, end-of-life care is more appropriate than amputation.

Rehabilitation and limb fitting

The speed of rehabilitation is variable:
- 1 week: patient should begin to bear weight on the other limb between parallel bars
- 10 days: walk with pneumatic walking aid
- 3 weeks: trial of temporary prosthesis, final fitting of the artificial limb must await shaping and firming of the stump.

Approximately 70% of below-knee amputees and 30% of above-knee amputees eventually walk, although many of these patients do not persist with their prosthesis. This is important to appreciate as due to the prolonged hospital admission, rehabilitation, home modifications and, in some cases, long-term care, amputation can be a much more expensive option than revascularisation leading to limb salvage.

Phantom pain

In some cases, patients will complain of feeling the amputated limb ('phantom limb') and may complain of pain in that 'limb'. It can be a serious problem, especially if pain has not been well controlled. With appropriate drug therapy such as gabapentin, reassurance and time, it usually settles but can take a long time to do so. There is some evidence that if the patient goes to theatre pain-free, the risk of phantom pain can be reduced. For this reason, some surgeons request epidural anaesthesia prior to surgery. Input from a pain specialist can be invaluable.

21

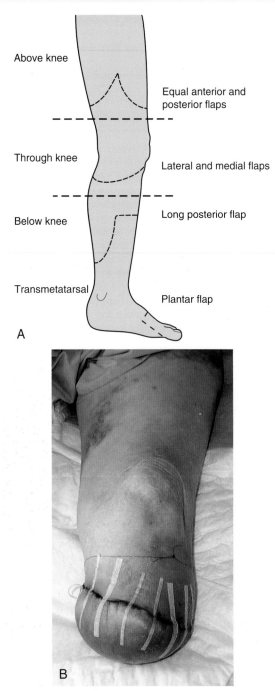

Fig. 21.12 Amputation. (A) Levels of amputation and types of flap used to close the residual defect. **(B)** Below-knee amputation.

Arterial disease of the upper limb

Overview

Occlusive arterial disease is about ten times more common in the leg than in the arm. Nevertheless, when the arm is affected, treatment can be difficult, and the loss of an arm (especially the dominant one) is even more devastating for the patient than loss of a leg.

Aetiology

Atherosclerosis rarely affects the upper limbs. Aetiologies to be considered when evaluating upper limb ischaemia are:

- Thoracic outlet obstruction
- Embolism
- Vasculitis
- Thromboangiitis obliterans.

The presentation and management principles are similar to that for the lower limb. The subclavian artery is the most common site of disease. This may lead to:

- *Arm claudication.* This is relatively unusual, even when the subclavian artery is completely occluded because of collateral supply, mainly from the vertebral artery
- *Atheroembolism to the hand.* Small emboli lodge in the vessels of the fingers and the hand, and lead to symptoms that are often mistaken for Raynaud's phenomenon, except that in this case the symptoms are unilateral (see later)
- *Subclavian steal.* If the block in the subclavian artery is proximal to the origin of the vertebral artery, then when the arm is used, blood is 'stolen' from the brain, with retrograde flow via the vertebral artery. This leads to vertebrobasilar ischaemia (VBI), characterised by dizziness, cortical blindness and/or collapse when the arm is used (Fig. 21.13).

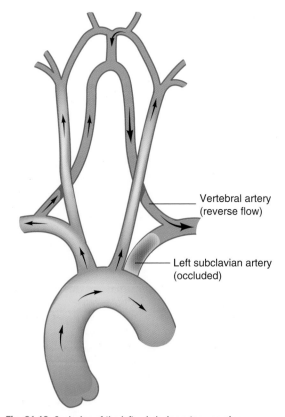

Vertebral artery (reverse flow)

Left subclavian artery (occluded)

Fig. 21.13 Occlusion of the left subclavian artery, causing 'subclavian steal'.

Management

Most subclavian artery disease can be treated by means of BAP and stenting, as the results are good and surgical access to the area is difficult. If surgery is required, then the usual operation is carotid-subclavian bypass.

Cerebrovascular disease

Definitions

Stroke

Stroke may be defined as an episode of focal neurological dysfunction lasting more than 24 hours, of presumed vascular aetiology.

Transient ischaemic attack

When such symptoms last for less than 24 hours, the episode is described as a TIA.

Amaurosis fugax

- Transient incomplete unilateral loss of vision, never synchronously bilateral (infinitely improbable that an embolus would enter both retinal arteries simultaneously)
- Described as a veil or curtain coming across the eye
- If bilateral loss of vision, usually due to occipital ischaemia secondary to vertebrobasillar insufficiency
- Nonsynchronous amaurosis fugax is possible in patients with bilateral carotid disease.

Carotid artery disease

Pathophysiology

Approximately 80% of strokes are ischaemic and about half of these are thought to be due to atheroembolism from the carotid bifurcation. The origin of the internal carotid artery is particularly prone to atheroma. The tighter the degree of stenosis, the more likely it is to cause symptoms. Atheroemboli entering the ophthalmic artery leads to amaurosis fugax or permanent monocular blindness on the same side (ipsilateral). If they enter the middle cerebral artery they may cause hemiparesis and hemisensory loss on the opposite side (contralateral). If the dominant hemisphere is affected there may also be dysphasia.

Assessment

The presence of a 'carotid' bruit bears no reliable relationship to the severity of underlying internal carotid artery disease and thus the risk of stroke. Such a bruit may arise from the external carotid artery or be transmitted from the heart. Furthermore, in the presence of a very tight internal carotid artery stenosis, flow may be so slow that no audible turbulence is present. It is important to exclude other causes of cerebral ischaemia and haemorrhage.

- Colour flow Doppler (duplex) ultrasound (CDU) is the initial investigation of choice for imaging the carotid arteries (Fig. 21.14)

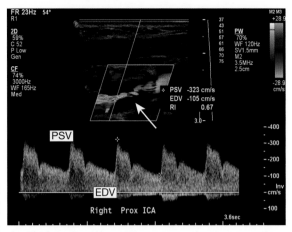

Fig. 21.14 Carotid ultrasound scan. The colour flow image shows the narrowing (*arrow*). By using Doppler ultrasound to measure the peak systolic velocity (PSV; about 300 cm/s in this case) and end-diastolic velocity (EDV; about 120 cm/s in this case) of the blood travelling through the stenosis it is possible to quantify the degree of narrowing. In this case the stenosis is estimated at greater than 70% and so further investigation with a view to surgery is warranted.

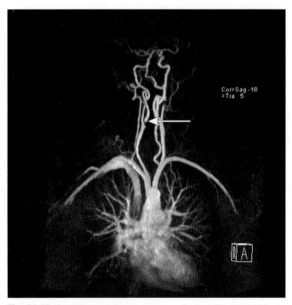

Fig. 21.15 Carotid magnetic resonance angiogram. The arterial blood to the brain from the origins of the great vessels from the aortic arch to the circle of Willis and cerebral arteries within the skull. The image confirms that there is a tight stenosis at the origin of the right internal carotid artery (*arrow*).

- Magnetic resonance angiography (MRA) or computed tomographic angiography (CTA) with perfusion scan provides excellent images and are increasingly used to plan treatment (Fig. 21.15)
- Intraarterial digital subtraction angiography (IA-DSA) is associated with a small risk of TIA/stroke as it is an invasive procedure. However, new evidence has emerged that DSA is playing a more important role, especially in the endovascular option of acute stroke treatment.

21

Management

Medical therapy

All patients should receive BMT.

Carotid endarterectomy

Patients with completed major stroke and little in the way of recovery are not candidates for carotid intervention; nor are those with an occluded internal carotid artery. However, carotid endarterectomy (CEA) combined with BMT is associated with a significant reduction in recurrent stroke, compared with BMT alone in patients with amaurosis, TIA and stroke with good recovery, provided that:

- There is a high degree of internal carotid artery stenosis (usually taken as a greater than 60–70% diameter reduction)
- The patient is expected to survive at least 2 years
- The intervention can be undertaken with a stroke and/or death rate of less than 3–5%
- The intervention can be performed soon after the index event. The exact timing remains controversial and is a matter of judgment for each patient but, in general, the sooner the better.

Patients who do not fulfil these criteria should, in most cases, be treated medically. The operation can be equally well performed under general or local anaesthetic (EBM 21.2).

The carotid bifurcation is dissected, heparin is given and the arteries are clamped. If this leads to cerebral ischaemia, a shunt is inserted. The plaque is shelled out (the endarterectomy) and the artery repaired with direct suture or a patch graft (patch angioplasty) (Fig. 21.16).

EBM **21.2 Carotid endarterectomy: general or local anaesthesia?**

'A definite difference in outcomes between general and local anaesthesia for carotid surgery has not been shown. The anaesthetist and surgeon, in consultation with the patient, should decide which anaesthetic technique to use on an individual basis.'

GALA Trial Collaborative Group. General anaesthesia versus local anaesthesia for carotid surgery (GALA): a multicentre randomised controlled trial. Lancet. 2008;372:2132–42.
Vaniyapong T, Chongruksut W, Rerkasem K. Local versus general anaesthesia for carotid endarterectomy. Cochrane Database Syst Rev. 2013;(12):CD000126. DOI: 10.1002/14651858.CD000126.pub4.

Carotid stenting

The role of carotid artery stenting (CAS) remains uncertain and controversial. While CAS avoids a neck wound and the risks of cranial nerve injury, and reduces the risk of perioperative myocardial infarction, there is a growing body of evidence to show that the short-term risks of clinical and subclinical brain injury are greater than with CEA. For these reasons, most vascular specialists believe that CAS should be reserved for patients where CEA is either not possible or desirable because of anatomic and clinical factors (e.g., recurrent stenosis after previous surgery or radiation arteritis) (EBM 21.3). However, all patients should have prompt access to all options to ensure maximal therapy. CAS may also be preferable to surgery of the common carotid and innominate arteries.

EBM **21.3 Carotid stenting**

'Completion of long-term follow-up is needed to establish the efficacy of carotid artery stenting compared with endarterectomy. In the meantime, carotid endarterectomy should remain the treatment of choice for patients suitable for surgery.'

International Carotid Stenting Study Investigators. Carotid artery stenting compared with endarterectomy in patients with symptomatic carotid stenosis: an interim analysis of a randomised controlled trial. Lancet. 2010;375:985–97.

Asymptomatic carotid disease

The evidence that undertaking CEA (or CAS) in addition to BMT confers clinical benefit in patients with asymptomatic ICA disease is weak. The risks of such people developing TIA/stroke are low (probably less than 10% at 5 years). So, even if one could halve that risk with intervention (relative risk reduction of 50%) the absolute risk reduction would be only 1% per year. This means the number of interventions needed to prevent one TIA or stroke is potentially quite large (perhaps 20–30 or more). By contrast, the number needed to treat for symptomatic disease is less than 10. CEA for asymptomatic carotid artery disease is, therefore, a highly cost-ineffective means of stroke reduction and a poor use of finite healthcare resources. Nevertheless, in many fee-for-service healthcare environments such as in the US, large numbers of CEA and CAS are still performed for asymptomatic carotid disease.

Vertebrobasilar disease

The vertebrobasilar system feeds the occipital cortex, cerebellum and brain stem. Patients with vertebrobasilar insufficiency may complain of (bilateral) cortical blindness, vertigo and loss of balance. Few patients have focal, discrete disease amenable to vascular or endovascular intervention, and the great majority receive BMT only.

Intravenous thrombolysis or mechanical thrombectomy

In acute stroke due to thromboembolic event, intravenous thrombolysis or mechanical thrombectomy (removing clot via endovascular route) has been increasingly used as a method of treatment in selected cases.

Renal artery disease

Pathophysiology

The most common cause is atherosclerosis:

- Underperfusion of the juxtaglomerular apparatus leads to an increase in renin and angiotensin, and the development of hypertension
- The disease may also lead to ischaemic necrosis of the renal parenchyma and progressive renal failure
- Fibromuscular hyperplasia: uncommon condition that mostly affects young and middle-aged women. Causes hypertension, but rarely renal failure.

Management

The indications of intervention remain controversial, especially since the ASTRAL trial results were published (EBM 21.4). Most patients

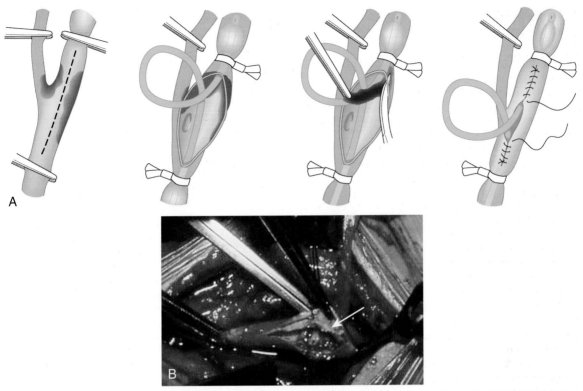

Fig. 21.16 Carotid endarterectomy. (A) Diagram showing carotid endarterectomy using a shunt in the internal carotid artery to maintain cerebral blood flow while the occluding plaque is removed and the artery repaired either by direct primary closure as shown here or, more usually, with a patch of vein or prosthetic material. **(B)** Operative photograph of plaque *(arrow)* being removed at carotid endarterectomy (no shunt being used in this case).

with renovascular disease are treated medically. Although the evidence for benefit is weak, primary stenting for atherosclerotic renal artery disease may be considered in selected patients to:

- Control hypertension that is refractory to medical therapy
- Preserve renal function.

Major complications (1–2%) include acute arterial occlusion, embolisation and rupture. BAP alone is effective for fibromuscular hyperplasia.

EBM 21.4 Intervention for renal artery disease

'Substantial risks but no evidence of a worthwhile clinical benefit from revascularization in patients with atherosclerotic renovascular disease was found.'

The ASTRAL investigators. Revascularization versus medical therapy for renal-artery stenosis. N Engl J Med. 2009;361:1953–62.

Mesenteric artery disease

Owing to rich collaterals, it is usually necessary for two of the three visceral vessels (coeliac axis, superior mesenteric artery [SMA] and inferior mesenteric artery) to be occluded or critically stenosed before symptoms or signs develop. Typically, the patient presents with severe central abdominal pain (mesenteric angina), sometimes with diarrhoea, 15–30 minutes after eating. Food avoidance and intolerance always leads to significant weight loss. The condition can mimic many much more common intraabdominal pathologies. Surgery is associated with significant morbidity

and mortality (5–10%), but long-term symptom relief is usually excellent. BAP and stenting are increasingly used, particularly in patients with high operative risk and in those who have limited life expectancy.

Acute mesenteric ischaemia is usually caused by occlusion of the SMA by embolus (usually from the heart in patients with AF) or acute thrombosis on top of preexisting atherosclerosis. There is usually sudden onset of excruciating abdominal pain, collapse, bloody diarrhoea and peritonitis. Symptoms are out of proportion to signs. Treatment comprises emergency SMA embolectomy (embolus) or SMA bypass (thrombosis), and resection of nonviable bowel. Unfortunately, extensive bowel necrosis is often already present at the time of surgery and mortality exceeds 50%. Endovascular techniques have little to offer, as the exclusion of bowel infarction requires laparotomy.

Acute limb ischaemia

Aetiology

Acute limb ischaemia is caused most frequently by acute thrombotic occlusion of a preexisting stenotic arterial segment (60%), thromboembolism (30%) and trauma, which may be iatrogenic. Distinguishing between thrombosis and embolism is important because investigation, treatment and prognosis are different (Table 21.4).

More than 70% of peripheral emboli are due to AF. Thrombosis in situ may arise from acute plaque rupture, hypovolaemia, increased blood coagulability (e.g., in association with sepsis) or 'pump failure' (e.g., heart attack; see later).

21

Table 21.4 Embolus versus thrombosis in situ

Clinical features	Embolus	Thrombosis
Severity	Complete ischaemia (no collaterals)	Incomplete ischaemia (collaterals)
Onset	Seconds or minutes	Hours or days
Limb	Leg 3:1 arm	Leg 10:1 arm
Multiple sites	Up to 15%	Rare
Embolic source	Present (usually AF)	Absent
Previous claudication	Absent	Present
Palpation of artery	Soft; tender	Hard/calcified
Bruits	Absent	Present
Contralateral leg pulses	Present	Absent
Diagnosis	Clinical	Angiography
Management	Embolectomy, warfarin	Medical, bypass, thrombolysis
Prognosis	Loss of life > loss of limb	Loss of limb > loss of life

AF, Atrial fibrillation.

Table 21.6 Symptoms and signs of acute limb ischaemia

Symptoms/ signs	Comment
Pain	May be absent in complete acute ischaemia; severe pain is also a feature of chronic ischaemia
Pallor	Also a feature of chronic ischaemia
Pulseless	Also a feature of chronic ischaemia
Perishing cold	Unreliable, as the ischaemic limb takes on the ambient temperature
Paraesthesia and paralysis	Loss of function is the most important feature of acute limb ischaemia and denotes a threatened limb that is likely to be lost unless it is revascularised within a few hours

inconsistently related to its severity, and should not be relied upon (Table 21.6)

Acute loss of limb function, of which vascular insufficiency is only one cause, must always be taken very seriously indeed; the patient should never be discharged until a diagnosis has been made. In the presence of ischaemia, pain on squeezing the calf indicates muscle infarction and impending irreversible ischaemia.

At first, acute complete ischaemia is associated with intense distal arterial spasm and the limb is 'marble' white. As the spasm relaxes over the next few hours and then fills with deoxygenated blood, mottling appears. This appears light blue or purple, has a fine reticular pattern, and on pressure, so-called nonfixed mottling. At this stage, the limb is still salvageable. As ischaemia progresses, blood coagulates in the skin, leading to mottling that is darker in colour, coarser in pattern and does not blanch. Finally, large patches of fixed staining progress to blistering and liquefaction (Fig. 21.17). Attempts at revascularisation at this late stage are futile and will lead to life-threatening reperfusion injury (see later).

Classification

Limb ischaemia is classified on the basis of onset and severity (Table 21.5). Incomplete acute ischaemia (usually due to thrombosis in situ) can often be treated medically, at least in the first instance. Complete ischaemia (usually due to embolus) will normally result in extensive irreversible tissue injury within 6 hours unless the limb is revascularised. Irreversible ischaemia mandates early amputation or, if the patient is elderly and unfit, end-of-life care.

Clinical features

Apart from those that indicate 'loss of function', namely paralysis (inability to wiggle toes/fingers) and paraesthesia (loss of light touch over the dorsum of the foot/hand), the so-called Ps of acute ischaemia, other features are nonspecific and/or

Table 21.5 Classification of limb ischaemia

Terminology	Definition/comment
Onset	
Acute	Ischaemia <14 days
Acute-on-chronic	Worsening symptoms and signs (<14 days)
Chronic	Ischaemia stable for >14 days
Severity (acute, acute-on-chronic)	
Incomplete	Limb not threatened
Complete	Limb threatened
Irreversible	Limb nonviable
Severity (chronic)	
Noncritical	Intermittent claudication
Subcritical	Night/rest pain
Critical	Tissue loss (ulceration ± gangrene)

Management

All suspected acutely ischaemic limbs must be discussed immediately with a vascular surgeon; a few hours can make the difference between amputation or death, and complete recovery of limb function.

- If there are no contraindications (e.g., trauma/suspected aortic dissection), an intravenous bolus of heparin (3000–5000 U) is administered to limit propagation of thrombus and protect the collateral circulation

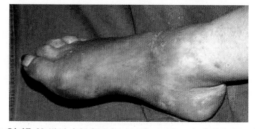

Fig. 21.17 Mottled right foot due to advanced acute limb ischaemia.

- If ischaemia is complete, the patient proceeds for embolectomy (preferably under local anaesthesia)
- If ischaemia is incomplete, preoperative imaging is obtained wherever possible, as simple embolectomy or thrombectomy is unlikely to be successful; a 'road-map' for distal bypass is helpful; and it is often possible, at least initially, to manage the patient medically depending on the results of imaging.

Acute embolus

Embolic occlusion of the brachial artery is not usually limb-threatening and, in an elderly patient, nonoperative treatment is reasonable. Younger patients should undergo embolectomy to prevent subsequent claudication, especially where the dominant arm is affected.

A leg affected by embolus is nearly always threatened and requires immediate surgical revascularisation. Femoral embolus is usually associated with profound ischaemia to the level of the upper thigh because the deep femoral artery is also affected. Acute embolic occlusion of the aortic bifurcation (saddle embolus) leads to absent femoral pulses and a patient who is 'marble' white or mottled to the waist. Such patients may also present with paraplegia due to ischaemia of the cauda equina, which may be irreversible. Embolectomy can be performed under local, regional or general anaesthesia (Fig. 21.18).

Postoperatively, the patient should continue on heparin. Warfarin reduces the risk of recurrent embolism but is associated with an annual risk of significant bleeding of 1–2%. The in-hospital mortality from cardiac death and/or recurrent embolism, particularly stroke, is 10–20%.

Thrombosis in situ

There is usually a reason why the limb affected by stable chronic ischaemia suddenly deteriorates due to thrombosis in situ on top of atherosclerosis. Causes include 'silent' or overt MI (drop in blood pressure); underlying, perhaps hitherto asymptomatic, malignancy (increase in thrombogenicity of the blood); septicaemia, particularly pneumococcal and meningococcal; and dehydration, which may be associated with widespread thrombosis. Many patients can be managed medically. If the limb remains threatened then it may be possible to clear thrombus by open surgical or endoluminal techniques, or

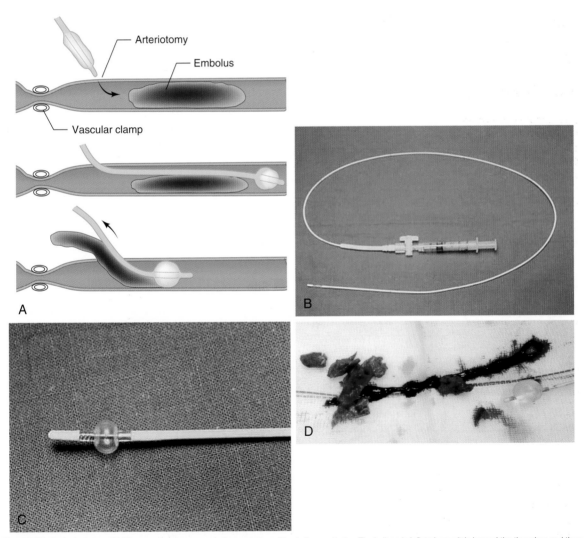

Fig. 21.18 Embolectomy. (A) Diagram showing removal of an embolus with a balloon catheter. The balloon is inflated once it is beyond the thrombus and then withdrawn. **(B)** Embolectomy catheter. **(C)** Tip of embolectomy catheter with balloon inflated. **(D)** Embolus postembolectomy, with a balloon catheter.

to dissolve the clot by thrombolysis or bypass of the affected segment. If urgent surgery is required, the in-hospital limb loss rate may approach 30%, with an in-hospital mortality rate of 10–20%.

Trauma

Acute traumatic limb ischaemia is frequently iatrogenic. The most common causes of noniatrogenic injury are limb fractures and dislocations, blunt injuries occurring in the course of road traffic accidents, and stab wounds. The presence of distal pulses emphatically does not exclude significant arterial injury, especially in otherwise young and fit trauma patients. Where there is any suspicion of major vascular injury, vascular imaging (e.g., MRA) should be performed immediately; operating 'blind' is to be avoided if at all possible.

Intraarterial drug administration

This leads to intense spasm and microvascular thrombosis. The leg is mottled and digital gangrene is common, but pedal pulses are often palpable. The mainstay of treatment is supportive care, hydration to minimise renal failure secondary to rhabdomyolysis, and full heparinisation. Vascular reconstruction is almost never indicated, but fasciotomy may be required to prevent compartment syndrome (see later). Limb loss rates are high.

Thoracic outlet syndrome

Pressure on the subclavian artery from a cervical rib or abnormal soft tissue band may lead to a poststenotic dilatation lined with thrombosis, predisposing to occlusion or embolisation. The distal circulation may be chronically obliterated and digital ischaemia advanced before the diagnosis is made. The diagnosis is confirmed on duplex scan and/or MRA. Treatment options include thrombolysis, thrombectomy/embolectomy, excision of the cervical rib and repair (replacement) of the aneurysmal segment.

Postischaemic syndrome

Reperfusion injury

Activated neutrophils, free radicals, enzymes, hydrogen ions, carbon dioxide, potassium and myoglobin released from reperfused tissue can lead to acute respiratory distress syndrome (ARDS), myocardial stunning, endotoxaemia and acute tubular necrosis, and, in turn, to multiple organ failure and death.

Compartment syndrome

- Endothelial cell injury during ischaemia leads to increased capillary permeability and oedema on reperfusion
- In the calf, where muscles are confined within tight fascial boundaries, the increase in interstitial tissue pressure can lead to continuing muscle necrosis despite apparently adequate arterial inflow: the so-called compartment syndrome
- There is swelling and pain on squeezing the calf muscle or moving the ankle or toes

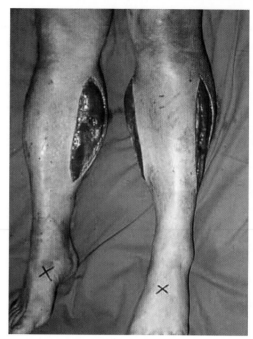

Fig. 21.19 Medial and lateral fasciotomy to decompress compartment syndrome in a patient who presented with bilateral acute limb ischaemia due to saddle embolus (the crosses marked on the skin indicate the position of palpable pulses).

- Palpable pedal pulses do not exclude compartment syndrome
- Management: prevention through expeditious revascularisation and a low threshold for fasciotomy to relieve the pressure (Fig. 21.19).

Aneurysmal disease

An aneurysm is defined as an abnormal focal dilatation of an endothelial-lined vascular structure (artery, vein, heart chamber). Arterial aneurysms are by far the most common. Aneurysms may be classified according to their site, underlying aetiology and morphology.

Site

Any artery can be affected. The most common site for aneurysmal disease requiring treatment is the infrarenal aorta; others include the popliteal, femoral and subclavian arteries.

Aetiology

Atherosclerotic

Most aneurysms are 'nonspecific' in aetiology; in the past they were termed *atherosclerotic*. However, it is now widely believed that aneurysmal disease is a distinct pathological process from occlusive arterial disease, although they share some of the same risk factors (smoking and hypertension) and may coexist in the same patient.

Mycotic

The term *mycotic*, meaning fungal, is a misnomer, because fungi do not cause aneurysms. The term is used nowadays to include all aneurysms that are believed to be infected. The infection can be primary or secondary to other pathology.

Arteries are generally resistant to infection, but two organisms, *Treponema pallidum* (syphilis) and *Salmonella*, have a particular ability to produce primary mycotic aneurysms. Septic emboli from heart valves affected by subacute bacterial endocarditis may also lodge in the distal vasculature and produce secondary mycotic aneurysms. 'Nonspecific' aneurysms and the layers of laminated thrombus within them may become infected secondary to bacteraemia from another site. Lastly, infection of prosthetic grafts can lead to infected anastomotic aneurysms.

Morphology

True aneurysms

All three layers of the arterial wall enclose a true aneurysm, which may be saccular or fusiform (Fig. 21.20).

False aneurysms

If the wall of an artery is damaged, the resulting surrounding haematoma can remain in continuity with the lumen, leading to a pulsatile swelling whose wall comprises compacted thrombus and surrounding connective tissue. Small aneurysms (1–2 cm in diameter) often thrombose spontaneously, but larger aneurysms tend to expand (especially if the patient is on aspirin, heparin or warfarin) and compress surrounding tissues. The most common site is the groin after common femoral artery instrumentation, and may cause femoral vein compression and deep venous thrombosis (DVT). Surgery is increasingly being replaced by ultrasound-guided thrombin injection. Where such aneurysms develop in less accessible sites, such as the aortoiliac segment, then the hole can be sealed using a covered stent introduced percutaneously or by blocking the artery (embolisation) usually via the femoral artery.

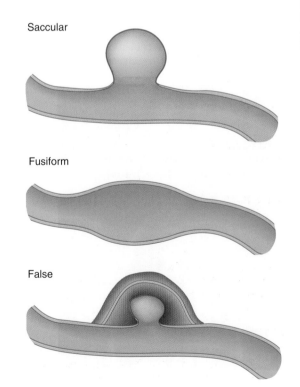

Saccular

Fusiform

False

Fig. 21.20 True and false aneurysms.

Abdominal aortic aneurysm

Epidemiology

Abdominal aortic aneurysm (AAA) is present in up to 5% of men aged over 70 years and is 2–3-times more common in men than in women of the same age. In about 70% of cases, only the infrarenal aortic segment is involved. In the remainder, the rest of the abdominal aorta, the thoracic aorta or a combination of both is involved.

Clinical features

An AAA may present in the following ways:
- Asymptomatic (60%). The AAA may be detected incidentally on routine physical examination, x-ray or, most commonly, abdominal ultrasound scan conducted for another reason. A large AAA can be difficult to palpate. Patients in whom an incidental finding of an AAA is made should be considered for treatment or surveillance
- Symptomatic (10%). AAA may cause pain in the central abdomen, back, loin, iliac fossa or groin. Thrombus within the aneurysm sac may be a source of emboli to the lower limbs. Much less commonly, the aneurysm may undergo thrombotic occlusion. AAA may also become inflamed and then compress surrounding structures such as the duodenum, ureter and the inferior vena cava (IVC)
- Rupture (30%). AAA may rupture, usually into the retroperitoneum, but sometimes into the peritoneal cavity or rarely into surrounding structures, most commonly the IVC, leading to an aorto-caval fistula.

Ultrasound screening for AAA results in a reduction in the number of deaths with asymptomatic AAAs that are not yet large enough to warrant surgical repair (Fig. 21.21; EBM 21.5). CTA will provide much more accurate information about the size and extent of the aneurysm, involvement of visceral arteries and the surrounding structures, and whether there is any other intraabdominal pathology. It is the standard preintervention investigation but is not suitable for surveillance because of the ionising radiation and cost (Fig. 21.22).

EBM	**21.5 Screening for abdominal aortic aneurysm (AAA)**
	'The mortality benefit of screening for AAA in men aged 64-73 years was maintained in the longer term and screening was cost effective.'
	Lindholt JS. Long-term benefit and cost–effectiveness analysis of screening for abdominal aortic aneurysms from a randomized controlled trial. Br J Surg 2010; 97: 826-834.

Asymptomatic AAA

The risks of open surgery generally outweigh the likelihood of rupture until an asymptomatic AAA has reached 5.5 cm in anteroposterior maximum diameter. It is, therefore, unusual in the UK for an AAA smaller than this to be operated upon in the absence of symptoms. Once a small AAA has been detected, the best way of following up the affected patient is by repeated ultrasound scans at regular intervals (depending on the size). Patients are encouraged strongly to comply with BMT, which affords the same benefits as it does in patients with occlusive

21

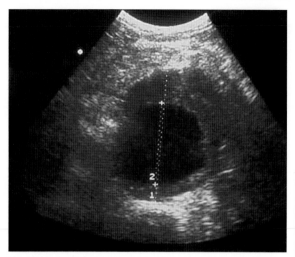

Fig. 21.21 Abdominal ultrasound showing a transverse section through a large abdominal aortic aneurysm. Measurement 1 shows the front to back (AP) diameter of the AAA from wall to wall while measurement 2 shows the diameter of the lumen through the thrombus lining the aneurysmal sac.

disease (which often coexists). Ultrasound is only accurate to about 0.5 cm and tends to underestimate AAA size. Thus, many specialists will arrange a CT scan when the AAA reaches 5.0 cm, along with other tests designed to assess fitness for surgery. Once the AAA reaches 5.5 cm, and assuming the clinical assessment and investigations indicate that the patient is fit for surgery, the surgeon will normally begin discussions with the patient with a view to open repair (OR) or endovascular aneurysm repair (EVAR).

Symptomatic AAA

All symptomatic AAAs should be considered for repair, not only to rid the patient of their symptoms, but also because pain often predates rupture. Distal embolisation is a definite indication for repair, even if the AAA is small, as limb loss is common if the AAA is left untreated.

Ruptured AAA

This is the most common emergency presentation of AAA. Patients survive rupture for the following reasons:

- The rupture is usually into the retroperitoneum, which tamponades (restricts the extent of) the leak
- There is intense vasoconstriction of nonessential circulatory beds
- The patient develops an intensely prothrombotic state
- The blood pressure drops, which helps to limit the blood loss.

Any medical intervention that upsets this delicate balance will convert a relatively stable, potentially salvageable patient into one unlikely to reach the operating theatre or to survive intervention. Specifically, large volumes of intravenous fluid (saline or plasma expander) increase the blood pressure, impair haemostasis and abolish vasoconstriction, and must therefore not be given. The only way of saving the patient is to either clamp and graft the aorta or insert a stent graft (EVAR; if necessary having controlled the bleeding through angioplasty balloon occlusion of the thoracic aorta); there must be absolutely no delay in getting the patient to a hospital where this can be done (Fig. 21.23).

Open AAA repair

OR entails replacing the aneurysmal segment with a prosthetic graft (Fig. 21.24). The 30-day major morbidity and mortality for this procedure is approximately 5–10% for elective asymptomatic AAA, 10–20% for emergency symptomatic AAA and up to 50% for ruptured AAA.

Endovascular aneurysm repair

EVAR involves placing a covered stent graft inside the aneurysm via a femoral arteriotomy, or percutaneously, under radiological guidance (Figs 21.25 and 21.26). The procedure can be performed under regional (epidural) or even local anaesthesia. Laparotomy and cross-clamping of the aorta are avoided. The patient

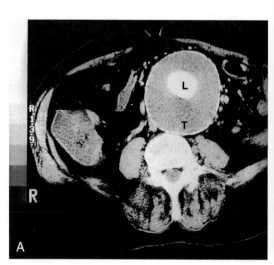

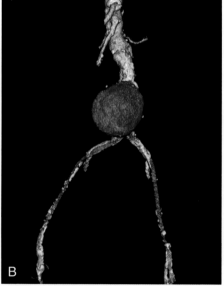

Fig. 21.22 Computed tomography in abdominal aortic aneurysm. (A) Transverse section. **(B)** Computed tomography angiography: 3D reconstruction. *L*, Lumen; *T*, thrombus.

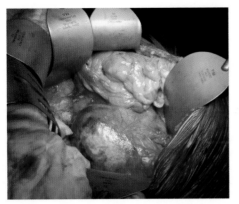

Fig. 21.23 Intraoperative photograph of repair of a ruptured abdominal aortic aneurysm.

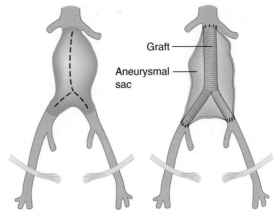

Fig. 21.24 Open repair of an abdominal aortic aneurysm. Diagram showing insertion of a 'trouser' bifurcation graft within the opened aneurysmal sac.

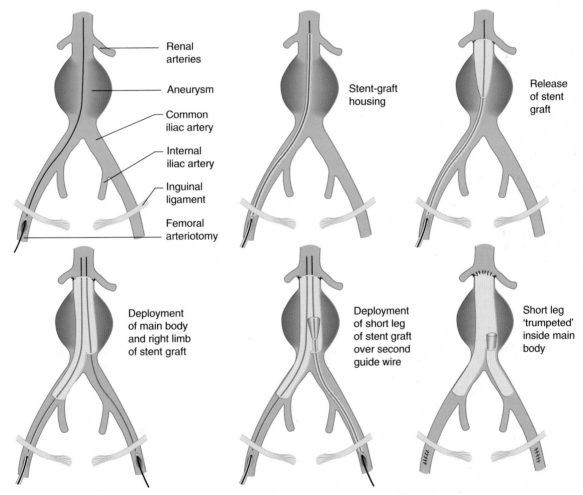

Fig. 21.25 Endovascular stent-graft repair of an abdominal aortic aneurysm. (A) A guidewire is passed through the aneurysm via an incision in the right common femoral artery. **(B)** A catheter containing the main body of the stent graft is passed over the guidewire and into position within the aneurysm. **(C)** The outer cover of the catheter is removed, allowing the upper part of the stent graft to spring open and become attached by hooks to the wall of the aorta just below the renal arteries. **(D)** The rest of the catheter is removed, allowing deployment of the main body of the graft and the right (long) limb within the common iliac artery. Note the short (left) limb of the graft. **(E)** Via an incision in the left common femoral artery a second guidewire is passed up through the short limb of the stent graft. A second catheter containing the rest of the stent graft is passed over the guidewire and into the main body of the stent graft. As before, retraction of the outer cover allows the top of the second limb of the stent graft to open within the short limb of the main body.
(F) Deployment is complete and the aneurysm sac completely excluded from the circulation. The femoral arteries are closed.

21

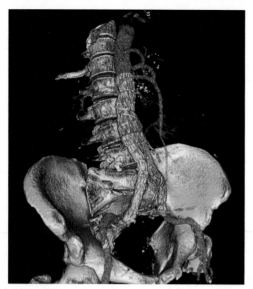

Fig. 21.26 3D computed tomography reconstruction of a stent graft deployed inside an abdominal aortic aneurysm. (Courtesy Mr Donald Adam.)

is often fit to go home within 48 hours, as opposed to the 7–10 days that are typical following OR. Patients also usually make a rapid return (4–6 weeks) to their preoperative functional status, whereas those who have undergone OR often take 4–6 months to feel as well as they did before their operation. Several trials have shown that EVAR is associated with a marked reduction in hospital mortality and morbidity, reduced hospital stay, and improved early postoperative quality of life (EBM 21.6). There are, however, downsides; the devices are expensive (£5000 or more); a significant proportion of AAAs are unsuitable for the procedure with present technology; and there are still questions over durability in that the secondary intervention rate following EVAR is much higher than it is following OR. In patients unfit for open surgery, the addition of EVAR to BMT is of no benefit when compared with BMT alone (EBM 21.6). With the development of newer devices, more anatomically challenging aneurysms can now be treated with EVAR.

Suprarenal aneurysms may be potentially treated with fenestrated grafts. The risk of pelvic and spinal ischaemia can be reduced with the use of iliac branching devices, which are used for aortoiliac aneurysms. With advancing technology, newer devices are being invented to reduce endoleaks.

Iliac aneurysms

In approximately 20% of patients, AAAs extend into one or both common iliac arteries, and about a third of these extend into the internal iliac artery; the external iliac artery is rarely affected. Isolated iliac aneurysms can also occur. The bifurcation of the aorta is at the level of the umbilicus, so that a pulsatile mass felt below that level is likely to be iliac in origin. Iliac aneurysms are most often treated in the course of AAA repair. Isolated iliac aneurysms should be considered for EVAR or surgical repair if they are causing symptoms, or have reached twice the normal diameter of the native artery.

Femoral aneurysms

There are three main types of femoral aneurysm: iatrogenic false aneurysm (see earlier), nonspecific aneurysm and anastomotic aneurysm. 'Nonspecific' aneurysms of the common femoral artery are found in 10% of patients with AAA and also as an isolated occurrence. Patients presenting with a femoral aneurysm should have an AAA excluded by ultrasound scan. In 50% of cases they are bilateral. They are frequently asymptomatic but may cause pain and compression of surrounding structures (femoral vein and nerve); rupture is uncommon. If large (>3 cm) or symptomatic, they should be considered for surgical repair. Anastomotic false aneurysms are increasingly being seen in patients who have previously undergone bypass grafting for occlusive aneurysmal disease. They may not present until many years after the original surgery, but once present, they usually grow inexorably and require repair. They are usually due to mechanical disruption of the anastomosis as a result of late suture failure or progressive disease of the femoral artery; less commonly, they are due to late graft infection.

Popliteal aneurysms

These are present in 20% of patients with AAA and their presence must be sought, if necessary with ultrasound, in all such patients. Around 50% are bilateral. If a patient presents with a popliteal aneurysm, there is a 50% chance that he or she also has an AAA, which again must be sought by ultrasound. The main complications of popliteal aneurysm are distal embolisation and acute thrombosis; the latter is associated with limb loss in up to 50% of cases because the calf vessels are often chronically occluded, which makes surgical bypass difficult. The best treatment is by exclusion of the aneurysm and bypass using the long saphenous vein. If a patient presents with acute ischaemia of the limb due to thrombosis, it is best treated by thrombolysis followed by exclusion and bypass. Rupture of popliteal aneurysms is extremely rare. Occasionally, they can compress the popliteal vein and present as a DVT.

Pathophysiology of venous disease

The lower limb venous system is divided into greater and lesser saphenous veins and their tributaries (see Fig. 21.1B). Some important landmarks of the venous systems are the perforators, namely the mid-thigh perforators and calf perforator. Perforators are communicating veins that perforate the fascia to connect the superficial and deep systems.

Physiology

Most venous disease arises as a result of incompetent valves, leading to reflux of blood or increased ambulatory venous pressure (the hydrostatic pressure exerted by the column of venous blood stretching from the ankle to the right atrium upon walking, see Fig. 21.27). This leads to symptoms and signs such as swelling, lipodermatosclerosis, ulceration and hyperpigmentation.

Varicose veins

Epidemiology

Varicose veins (VV) are so prevalent that they could almost be considered a variant of normal for a creature that spends its life on two as opposed to four legs. Their prevalence increases markedly with age and they are an almost universal finding in individuals over the age of 60 years.

Clinical features

The great majority of individuals with VV are asymptomatic, or at least they do not seek treatment. Those that do attend the surgical clinic do so because they are unhappy about the appearance of their leg(s), and/or they associate lower limb symptoms with their VV, and/or they are concerned about developing complications.

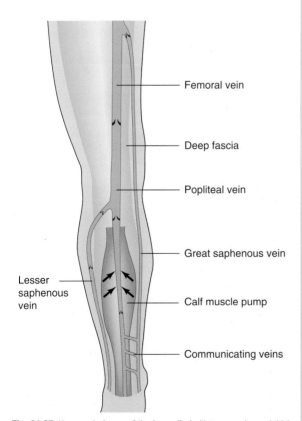

Fig. 21.27 Venous drainage of the lower limb. Note: upper leg and thigh perforators are not shown.

Femoral vein

Deep fascia

Popliteal vein

Great saphenous vein

Lesser saphenous vein

Calf muscle pump

Communicating veins

Cosmetic issues

Many patients, especially young women, seek treatment because they consider their veins to be unsightly. Possibly because they are unwilling to admit that cosmesis is the main issue, they frequently complain of various lower limb symptoms as well.

Symptoms

A wide variety of lower limb symptoms have been attributed to VV. Lower limb symptoms are present in about half of the adult population, and there is an inconsistent relationship between these symptoms, and the size and extent of VV on clinical examination and duplex ultrasound examination.

Complications

Only a proportion of patients with VV go on to develop the complications of chronic venous insufficiency (CVI): e.g., leg ulcers, haemorrhage and thrombophlebitis. There is ongoing controversy as to whether VV are a risk factor for DVT, but in young, otherwise healthy individuals, they are probably not. However, in the elderly, in whom VV are more likely to be associated with skin changes of CVI and in whom they may be a marker for coexistent deep venous disease, they probably are. At present, it is difficult to predict which patients will develop these complications and to know whether early VV surgery would prevent them, because the necessary longitudinal studies have never been done.

Indications for treatment

In correctly selected patients, it is clear that interventions for VV are associated with a marked improvement in health-related quality of life (HRQL) and symptom relief. In patients with uncomplicated VV, surgeons must use their own judgment and experience to determine whether the patient truly does have symptoms, whether those symptoms are of venous aetiology and, if so, whether they are likely to be relieved by intervention. Many VV interventions are performed in the private sector for purely cosmetic indications.

Aetiology

The true aetiology of VV remains unclear. The favoured hypothesis is that there is a structural defect in the vein wall, that may at least in part be inherited, which causes progressive dilatation in response to increased venous pressure consequent upon our bipedal posture and other factors. This leads to secondary incompetence of the valves (reflux), which in turn leads to more stress on the wall and more dilatation. These are sometimes termed *primary VV*. As in the deep venous system, thrombosis in the superficial veins (superficial thrombophlebitis) can destroy the valves leading to reflux. And, lastly, deep venous obstruction, usually due to DVT, can lead to the appearance of superficial varices that act as collateral pathways around that obstruction. These are sometimes termed *secondary VV*. Such secondary VV should not be removed, as that will result in a further reduction in the venous outflow of the leg, leading to worsening post-thrombotic syndrome characterised by pain and swelling, especially on walking (venous claudication).

Examination and investigation

The patient should be examined standing in a warm room; the whole leg is visualised from toes to groin with the lower abdomen also exposed. The distribution of VV may indicate whether they are great or lesser saphenous or both. Various percussion and

21

tourniquet-based tests, such as the Trendelenburg test, are highly inaccurate and should not be performed these days. Some surgeons use hand-held Doppler probes to help delineate patterns of reflux, but even in the best of hands the method lacks precision and accuracy. In reality, as duplex ultrasound machines become smaller, more portable, easier to use and cheaper, there is a move towards performing duplex examination in the clinic on all patients being considered for intervention.

Severe VV, especially in children, of atypical distribution or associated with skin discoloration, soft-tissue hypertrophy or limb overgrowth, should raise the suspicion of congenital arteriovenous malformations. Such patients should undergo MRI to assess the extent of the lesion and the arterial component.

Management

Conservative treatment: for uncomplicated varicose veins

The aim is to relieved tiredness and reduce swelling:

- Elastic support hose
- Weight reduction
- Regular exercise
- The avoidance of constricting garments
- Prolonged standing.

Surgery

Surgery aims to remove varices and intercept incompetent connections between deep and superficial veins so that further varices do not form. In patients with GSV disease, the Saphenofemoral Junction (SFJ) is ligated flush with the femoral vein (Fig. 21.28). Recurrence is very much less likely if the long saphenous vein (LSV) is stripped out from knee to groin. Care must be taken not to damage the saphenous nerve, which joins and runs with the GSV below the knee.

Endovenous treatment

Surgery is being increasingly replaced by a range of minimally invasive endovenous treatments that can be performed under local anaesthesia as a day case or even as an outpatient procedure. The techniques include:

- Radiofrequency ablation (RFA)
- Endovenous LASER ablation (EVLA)
- Ultrasound-guided foam sclerotherapy (UGFS) (Fig. 21.29).

Each of these techniques has pros and cons. However, performed correctly by appropriately trained clinicians, they appear to work at least as well as (often better than) surgery in many patients, and offer significant advantages in terms of less pain and a speedier return to normal activities.

Superficial thrombophlebitis

Inflammation and thrombosis of a previously normal superficial vein may result from trauma, from irritation due to an intravenous infusion or from the injection of noxious agents. Except when it arises from a septic puncture site, superficial thrombophlebitis

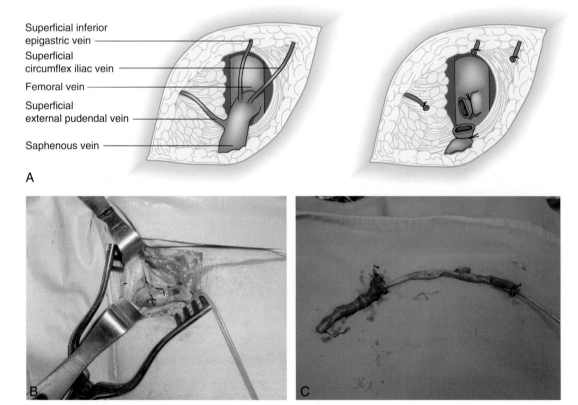

Fig. 21.28 **Saphenofemoral disconnection. (A)** Diagram showing ligation of the tributaries of the great saphenous vein. **(B)** Saphenofemoral junction with its tributaries ligated. **(C)** Great saphenous vein stripped.

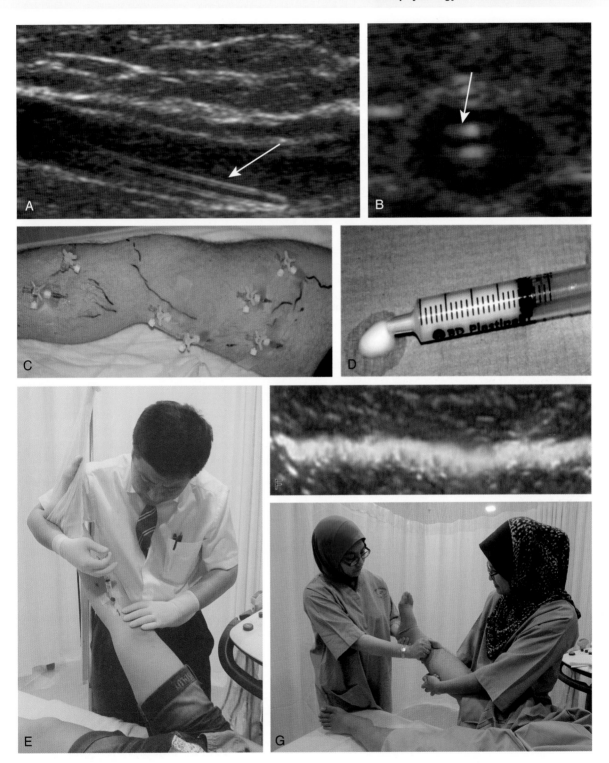

Fig. 21.29 Ultrasound-guided foam sclerotherapy. (A) Cannula (*arrow*) inserted into great saphenous vein under duplex ultrasound control (longitudinal view). **(B)** Tip of cannula in varicose vein (cross-sectional view). **(C)** Multiple cannulae inserted under local anaesthetic into a patient with recurrent great saphenous varicose veins that have previously been mapped using duplex ultrasound. **(D)** Foam made from 3% sodium tetradecyl sulphate (STS) sclerosant and a mixture of oxygen and carbon dioxide. **(E)** Injection of foam into great saphenous vein. The duplex ultrasound probe is used to check when foam reaches the saphenofemoral junction and that it does not enter the deep veins. **(F)** As soon as foam enters the great saphenous vein it goes into spasm. The foam destroys the endothelium leading to permanent occlusion. The bubbles in the foam make it extremely echogenic so it can be seen easily on ultrasound. **(G)** Once the varicose veins to be treated are full of foam compression bandaging and stocking is applied and worn for 5 days to keep the varicose veins closed.

is usually nonbacterial. When it arises spontaneously, it almost invariably occurs in VV. Redness and tenderness follow the line of the vein. Thrombosis may spread through communicating channels into the deep veins and give rise to DVT and pulmonary embolism (PE).

Treatment comprises analgesia, anti-inflammatory drugs, support stockings and exercise. Once the inflammation has settled, it is usually wise to remove the underlying VV, as recurrence is common. Propagation towards the deep veins usually requires heparin therapy, and rarely thrombectomy or vein ligation. Recurrent migrating superficial thrombophlebitis is occasionally seen in malignant disease (Trousseau's syndrome).

Chronic venous insufficiency

Pathophysiology

CVI may be defined as the presence of (usually irreversible) skin damage (such as eczema, lipodermatosclerosis) in the lower leg as a result of sustained ambulatory venous hypertension. This hypertension is due to failure of the mechanisms (see earlier) that normally lower venous pressure upon ambulation, namely:

- Venous reflux due to valvular incompetence (90%). This may affect the superficial veins, the deep veins or both, and may be due to primary valvular insufficiency (as in VV) or to postthrombotic damage
- Venous obstruction (10–20%). This is usually postthrombotic in nature and coexists with reflux.

CVI affects about 10% of the adult population and the lifetime risk of chronic venous ulceration (CVU) is around 1%.

Most patients with CVI and CVU (Fig. 21.30) are over 50 years of age and the incidence increases exponentially with advancing years. In 1992 it was estimated that the treatment of lower limb venous disease accounted for about 1–2% of healthcare spending in the UK (£400–600 million per annum at the time). The female-to-male ratio is about 3:1. Approximately 70% of all leg ulcers are venous in aetiology, and 20% are due to mixed arterial and venous disease. In many cases, the situation is aggravated by old age, poor social circumstances, obesity, trauma, immobility, osteoarthritis, rheumatoid arthritis, diabetes and neurological problems. It is usually possible to differentiate venous from arterial ulceration on clinical examination alone (Table 21.7).

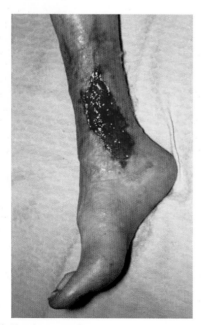

Fig. 21.30 Chronic venous ulcer.

Table 21.7 Differential diagnosis of leg ulceration

Clinical features	Arterial ulcer	Venous ulcer
Gender	Men > women	Women > men
Age	Usually presents >60 years	Typically develops at 40–60 years but patient may not present for medical attention until much older; multiple recurrences are the norm
Risk factors	Smoking, diabetes, hyperlipidaemia and hypertension	Previous DVT, thrombophilia, varicose veins
Past medical history	Most have a clear history of peripheral, coronary and cerebrovascular disease	More than 20% have a clear history of DVT; many more have a history suggestive of occult DVT, i.e., leg swelling after childbirth, hip/knee replacement or long bone fracture
Symptoms	Severe pain is present unless there is (diabetic) neuropathy; pain may be relieved by dependency	About a third have pain, but it is not usually severe and may be relieved on elevation
Site	Normal and abnormal (diabetics) pressure areas (malleoli, heel, metatarsal heads, 5th metatarsal base)	Medial (70%), lateral (20%) or both malleoli and gaiter area
Edge	Regular, 'punched-out', indolent	Irregular, with neoepithelium (whiter than mature skin)
Base	Deep, green (sloughy) or black (necrotic) with no granulation tissue; may involve tendon, bone and joint	Pink and granulating but may be covered in yellow-green slough
Surrounding skin	Features of severe limb ischaemia	Lipodermatosclerosis, varicose eczema, atrophy, blanched
Veins	Empty, 'guttering' on elevation	Full, usually varicose
Swelling	Usually absent	Often present

DVT, Deep venous thrombosis.

Assessment

The assessment and management of CVI and CVU should commerce as follows: the patient first, then the leg, and then the ulcer.

History

This should include history of the present and previous episodes of ulceration; previous thrombotic episodes; previous venous and nonvenous surgery to the leg, pelvis and abdomen; arterial symptoms; diabetes; autoimmune disease; other medical conditions; locomotor problems; current medications; and allergies.

Examination

This should include a description of the ulcer, concentrating on the features outlined in Table 21.5. Pulse status and ABPI should be recorded. Gait, particularly ankle mobility, which is vital for the proper functioning of the calf muscle pump, should be assessed.

Investigations

All patients must undergo duplex ultrasound to define the nature and distribution of superficial and deep venous disease, as this has an important bearing on both treatment and prognosis. In patients with absent pulses and/or a low ABPI, ultrasound can also provide valuable information about the pattern of arterial disease. Patients may require a full blood count, standard biochemistry, thyroid function tests, blood glucose determination, lipid profile and rheumatoid serology to exclude underlying systemic conditions. If there is any suspicion that the ulcer might be malignant, multiple biopsies of the base and margins should be performed without delay.

Management

All patients with a break in the skin below the knee that has not healed within 2 weeks should be referred urgently (within a week) to a vascular surgeon for a full clinical, haemodynamic and duplex ultrasound assessment, and consideration of surgical or endovenous treatment.

There is overwhelming evidence to indicate that the sooner an ulcer is diagnosed and appropriately treated, the more likely it is to heal and stay healed.

Medical therapy

Patients with leg ulcers often have multiple medical comorbidities, the treatment of which must be optimal if the chances of ulcer healing are to be maximised. There are no drugs that have been proven to increase ulcer healing or reduce recurrence. Most ulcers are colonised with bacteria (often mixed faecal organisms or pseudomonas, which explains the offensive smell) rather than infected, and antibiotics are usually contraindicated as they are ineffective and often select out resistant organisms. However, if the ulcer and surrounding skin are red and inflamed, or the ulcer is especially painful, then swabs should be taken. If β-haemolytic *Streptococcus* or *Staphylococcus aureus* is cultured, oral antibiotics guided by sensitivities are indicated. Topical antibiotics and antiseptics are contraindicated. The best way to treat heavy odorous colonisation is to wash the leg regularly in warm tap water (no soap or disinfectant should be added) as 'the solution to pollution is dilution'.

Dressings

Of the available types of dressing, none has been proven to increase ulcer healing. Leg ulcer patients are notorious for developing contact sensitivity to all manner of substances present in ointments and dressings. Thus, the least expensive, simplest and blandest forms of nonadherent dressings are to be recommended.

Compression therapy

Although it is still unclear exactly how compression therapy works, it continues to be the mainstay of treatment, and correctly applied, is highly effective in healing the majority of venous ulcers and preventing recurrence (Fig. 21.3A). To be maximally effective, compression should be:

- Elastic, as this achieves the best and most durable pressure profile
- Multilayer, as using many layers evens out the high–low pressure areas found under any bandage; the 'four-layer bandage' is a popular system
- Graduated, with the pressure greatest at the ankle (c. 30–40 mmHg) and least at the knee (c.15–20 mmHg).

It is vitally important to exclude arterial disease before compression is applied (Fig. 21.31B).

If pulses are not easily palpable, the ABPI should be measured (see earlier). Any patient with an ABPI of <0.8 should be referred to a vascular surgeon. Such patients will have to be treated with modified compression or undergo revascularisation to allow compression to be applied. Oedema is frequently present and significantly reduces the chances of healing. Even expertly applied graduated compression may fail to control severe oedema while the patient is still ambulant, and a period of bed rest for leg elevation may be required.

Elastic compression hosiery

Once the ulcer has healed with compression bandaging, compression stockings will reduce the chance of recurrence and should be prescribed to all patients for life (assuming the arterial circulation is adequate).

Surgical and endovenous therapy

Eradication of superficial venous reflux by means of surgery or endovenous treatment in addition to compression therapy definitely reduces CVU recurrence and probably increases CVU healing rates when compared with compression alone (EBM 21.7). Although many of these patients are elderly, unfit for and/or do not want surgery, nowadays most can be treated by endovenous methods. In particular, there is growing evidence that UGFS is not only as effective as surgery but also much less morbid. In patients with superficial and deep venous reflux, especially where the latter is postthrombotic in aetiology, the evidence that intervention for superficial reflux is beneficial is weaker. There is continuing controversy as to the benefit of ligating medial calf perforating veins either at open operation or endoscopically: so-called subfascial endoscopic perforator surgery (SEPS). The available data suggest that it adds little, if anything, to standard VV surgery in patients with isolated superficial venous reflux, and that it is as ineffective as VV surgery in patients with postthrombotic deep venous disease. Some surgeons believe that performing split-skin or 'pinch' grafting speeds up ulcer healing. This is only likely to be the case if the underlying venous abnormality has been corrected successfully. Patients with arterial disease may require angioplasty or BSX to relieve pain and allow compression therapy to be applied.

21

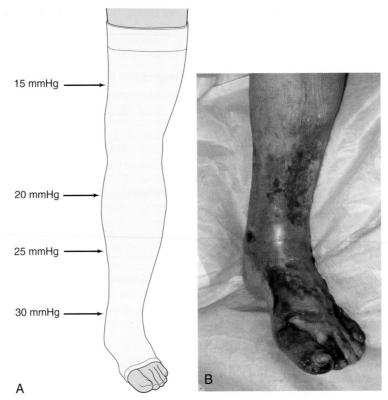

Fig. 21.31 Graduated elastic compression for venous ulcer. **(A)** Compression from the base of the toes to the tibial tuberosity usually suffices. **(B)** Extensive necrosis in a patient treated with compression for a venous ulcer in the presence of significant arterial disease. Above-knee amputation was required.

EBM **21.7 Surgery for chronic venous ulceration**

'Eradication of superficial venous reflux in patients with chronic venous ulceration reduces recurrence at 2 years by over 50%.'*
'Surgical correction of superficial venous reflux in addition to compression bandaging does not improve ulcer healing but reduces the recurrence of ulcers at four years and results in a greater proportion of ulcer free time.'[†]

*Barwell JR et al. Lancet 2004;363:1854–9.
[†]Gohel Manjit S et al. Long term results of compression therapy alone versus compression plus surgery in chronic venous ulceration (ESCHAR): Randomised Controlled Trial. BMJ. 2007;335:83.

Venous thromboembolism

Epidemiology

DVT is a common condition in medical and surgical patients, and PE is consistently cited as the most common cause of potentially preventable death in the surgical patient. DVT also renders the leg prone to CVI and ulceration (the so-called postphlebitic limb or syndrome).

Pathophysiology

DVT probably begins in the calf in most cases. Clot may extend into the popliteal, femoral or iliac veins, and even the IVC. In some cases, DVT originates in the pelvic veins. At first, the clot is free-floating within a column of flowing blood. The risk of PE is highest at this point. Later, when thrombus has completely occluded the vein and incited an inflammatory reaction in the vein wall, the clot becomes densely adherent and is unlikely to embolise. The classic text book features of DVT are due to this occlusion (leg swelling, dilated superficial veins) and thrombophlebitis (redness, pain and tenderness, heat).

The important point is that most surgical patients developing a clinically significant postoperative PE do so on about the 7th–10th day and nearly always have clinically normal legs. By the time a clinically apparent DVT has developed, the danger period for PE has largely passed; for this reason, thromboembolic prophylaxis must be considered in all patients undergoing open vascular or endovascular surgery.

Aetiology

Thrombogenesis (Virchow's triad):

- Venous stasis: immobility, obesity, pregnancy, paralysis, operation and trauma
- Intimal damage: external trauma to a vein, e.g., during a hip-replacement operation
- Hypercoagulability of the blood:
  - Congenital (primary): antithrombin, protein C and protein S deficiency, as well as factor V Leiden (activated protein C resistance [APCR]) in a young patient (<45 years), if there is a family history, or if thrombosis is recurrent or at an unusual site
  - Acquired (secondary): pregnancy, the puerperium, and malignancy.

In some individuals the left common iliac vein may be compressed between the right common iliac artery in front and the spine behind. This is known as *May–Thurner syndrome* and may be a cause of ileofemoral DVT.

Diagnosis

Clinical examination alone is unreliable at confirming or excluding the presence of DVT. This means that the diagnosis of DVT cannot be made on clinical grounds alone, and that some form of investigation is required. Colour duplex ultrasound imaging has largely replaced conventional venography in the diagnosis of DVT. It is noninvasive, avoids ionising radiation and contrast, and is as accurate as venography in most cases. At times of doubt, magnetic resonance (Fig. 21.32) or CT venography may be useful.

Venous gangrene

In certain circumstances, notably where there is underlying malignancy or severe sepsis, DVT may propagate to involve not only the main venous trunks, but also the venous collaterals and/or microcirculation (arterioles and venules). The former leads to an intensely swollen, cyanosed limb (phlegmasia caerulea dolens), whereas the latter can lead to obstruction of the arterial inflow and the development of a swollen white leg (phlegmasia alba dolens). The patient may then go on to develop venous gangrene.

Prevention

Rationale

Because of our inability to diagnose DVT easily in its early asymptomatic but dangerous phase, prevention is very important. The most important risk factors are a history of previous DVT or embolism, advanced age, malignant disease, obesity, and congenital or acquired thrombophilia. Identification of patients is important so that prophylaxis administered reduces the incidence of venous thromboembolism. For further guidance, see the National Institute of Clinical and Health Excellence (NICE), http://www.nice.org.uk/CG46.

General measures

Aspects of modern surgical care that help to reduce the likelihood of postoperative DVT include regional anaesthesia, accurate fluid replacement to avoid dehydration, effective pain control to facilitate early ambulation and, perhaps above all, the use of outpatient or day-case-based minimally invasive alternatives to traditional open surgery.

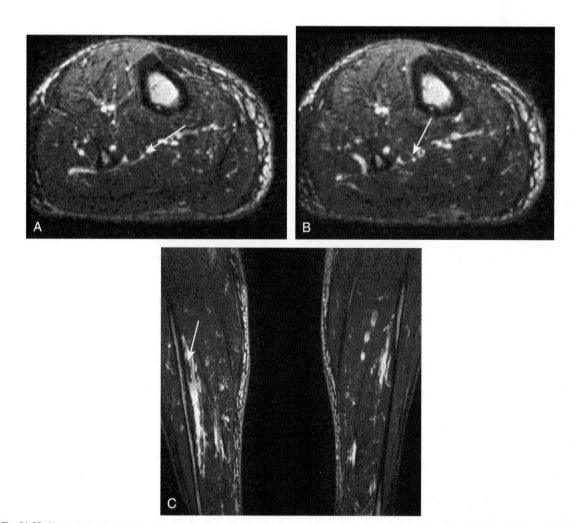

Fig. 21.32 Magnetic resonance venogram showing deep vein thrombosis (*arrows*). The clot appears as a black filling defect within the white blood inside the deep veins of the right calf.

Physical methods

Graduated compression (thromboembolic deterrent [TED]) stockings, which exert a pressure of about 20 mmHg at the ankle, augment flow in the deep veins and reduce the risk of thrombosis.

Pharmacological methods

Low-dose subcutaneous low-molecular-weight heparin (LMWH) protects against DVT and PE. The first dose may be given with the premedication (if an epidural is not being planned), and treatment is continued until the patient is fully ambulant. In 'high-risk' patients, it can be continued following discharge, and there is increasing evidence that this is of benefit in reducing venous thromboembolism and, probably therefore, postthrombotic syndrome.

Management

Overview

Before treatment is instituted, the diagnosis of DVT should normally have been established by means of ultrasound or magnetic resonance (computed tomography) venography. However, where the clinical suspicion of DVT and/or PE is high and there is no contraindication to heparin, the potential benefit of 'blind' treatment until the diagnosis is confirmed often outweighs the risk of withholding anticoagulation. The aims of treatment are to relieve the acute symptoms, protect against PE, and minimise the risk of recurrent thrombosis and postthrombotic sequelae to the limb.

Uncomplicated DVT

If thrombus is confined to the calf, the patient is fully mobile and other risk factors are reversible, then an elastic stocking and physical exercise may be all that is required. However, the 'surgical' patient does not usually fulfil these criteria postoperatively and there is a real risk of thrombus extension into the femoropopliteal segment. In these cases, specific treatment is indicated.

For most uncomplicated DVT, it is now clear that:

- Bed rest is unnecessary and the patient can be mobilised immediately, wearing an appropriately fitted compression stocking
- Low-molecular-weight heparin given by intermittent subcutaneous injection is more effective than unfractionated heparin given by infusion.

Thus, uncomplicated DVT is increasingly treated on an outpatient basis by protocol-driven, specialist nurse-run clinics.

Complicated DVT

In a proportion of patients, however, treatment is more complicated because of one or more of the following:

- The DVT is more extensive (iliofemoral, vena cava, phlegmasia)
- The DVT is recurrent
- The patient has had PE
- The patient has major irreversible congenital and/or acquired thrombophilia
- Heparinisation is contraindicated (heparin-induced thrombocytopenia, trauma—especially intracranial, recent haemorrhage).

Treatment must be tailored to the individual patient, and in selected instances it may be appropriate to use thrombolysis, insert a caval filter or consider thrombectomy. A high proportion of patients with extensive DVT have an underlying malignancy, and reasonable steps should be taken to ensure that this is diagnosed and appropriately treated in order, hopefully, to reduce the thrombotic risk.

Thrombolysis

Catheter-directed intraclot thrombolysis (CDT) using recombinant tissue plasminogen activator (rTPA) has been advocated as a means of rapidly clearing the iliofemoral segment in patients with extensive proximal DVT. It is hoped that CDT will reduce the incidence of PE and postphlebitic syndrome (by reducing venous pressure and preserving valves). Although the rate and extent of clot clearance is certainly greater with CDT than with heparin alone in the short term, it is not clear whether this results in improved patency and clinical outcome in the long term. CDT is also associated with a small risk of bleeding, which can be serious or even life threatening. The other potential role for CDT is in phlegmasia with venous gangrene. In this situation, not only is the rTPA given into the clot, it is also administered into the arterial circulation to try to clear the microcirculation. Again, although clots can be lysed in the short term, it is unclear whether this confers long-term benefit. Many of these patients have underlying malignancy and, unless the hypercoagulable state can be corrected, rethrombosis seems likely.

Surgical thrombectomy

In the UK, surgical thrombectomy to clear iliofemoral thrombus is very rarely performed nowadays. It is indicated in patients with iliofemoral thrombosis and impending venous gangrene.

Pharmacomechanical thrombectomy

There are now several catheter-based devices on the market that allow the thrombus to be isolated from the general venous circulation while being laced with thrombolytic (reducing systemic effects) and at the same time disrupted mechanically. Trials are ongoing to determine whether such pharmacomechanical thrombectomy (PMT) results in long-term benefits and if the cost is justified.

Venous stenting

If iliofemoral thrombus clearance reveals May–Thurner syndrome as the likely cause of DVT, then a stent may be placed to help keep the left iliac vein open in the long term.

Caval filters

The rationale behind inserting an IVC filter is that it will trap embolus that would otherwise have been destined for the lungs causing a PE. The use of IVC filters varies enormously around the world. In the UK, the accepted indications are in patients where:

- Anticoagulation is contraindicated or has had to be discontinued owing to a complication of therapy
- PE is still occurring despite adequate anticoagulation
- Compromised cardiovascular reserve means that even a small PE might have very serious clinical consequences.

Other forms of venous thrombosis

Superior vena cava thrombosis

Mediastinal tumours or enlarged lymph nodes (e.g., from breast or bronchial carcinoma) may obstruct the superior vena cava (SVC) and induce thrombosis. Central venous catheters (CVCs) for parenteral nutrition, pressure monitoring or haemodialysis may cause thrombosis of the SVC, or of the subclavian or axillary veins. The patient experiences an unpleasant bursting feeling in the head, neck and upper limbs. There is oedema, cyanosis and venous distension.

The obstruction is defined by CT or MR venography. In occlusion secondary to malignancy, percutaneous stenting,

Lymphoedema • 405

radiotherapy or chemotherapy may relieve malignant obstruction, and whilst the outlook remains poor, symptoms may be significantly relieved.

Subclavian and axillary vein thrombosis

Spontaneous axillary vein thrombosis is relatively common and usually occurs in otherwise healthy young adults following exercise, when it is termed *effort thrombosis*. There may be a previous history of intermittent venous obstruction in the limb due to a mechanical cause at the thoracic outlet. A cervical rib, abnormal muscle or ligamentous band at the inner border of the first rib, or a narrow interval between the clavicle and the first rib (the costoclavicular scissors) may constrict the vein and lead to thrombosis.

The patient complains of an uncomfortable, heavy, cyanosed arm with venous engorgement. Venous collaterals develop over the shoulder and anterior chest wall. Upper limb venous duplex scanning and/or venography define the occlusion. The arm should be elevated, e.g., in a towel suspended from a drip stand. Heparin therapy followed by oral anticoagulants is standard treatment. CDT and PMT can be very effective in early cases. Many surgeons believe that after the axillary thrombosis has been cleared, the thoracic outlet should be explored and the first rib or other obstructing element removed. Once the rib is out, stenting of any underlying venous stenosis may be of value.

Lymphoedema

Pathophysiology

The lymphatic system removes excess water and protein from the interstitial space. Lymph passes through lymph nodes before it re-enters the venous system, mainly through the thoracic duct. Failure of this mechanism leads to the accumulation of protein-rich oedema fluid in the tissues (lymphoedema) (Figs 21.33 and 21.34).

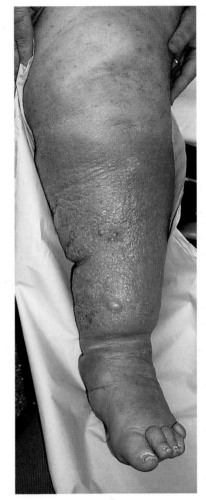

Fig. 21.34 Lymphoedema.

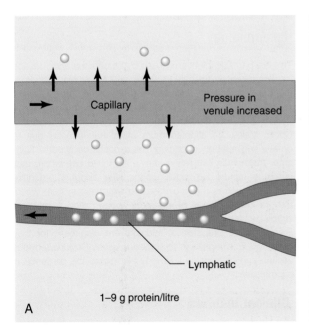

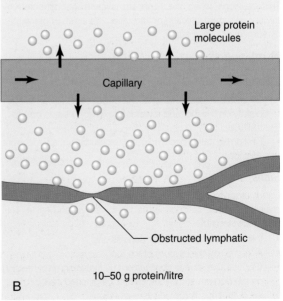

Fig. 21.33 **Types of oedema. (A)** Low-protein oedema due to abnormally high net fluid filtration. **(B)** High-protein oedema due to failure of lymphatics to remove interstitial protein.

Box 21.3 Differential diagnosis of the swollen limb

Nonvascular or lymphatic general disease states

- Cardiac, renal and liver failure
- Hyperthyroidism (myxoedema)
- Allergic disorders
- Immobility and lower limb dependency

Local disease processes

- Ruptured Baker's cyst
- Myositis ossificans
- Bony or soft tissue tumours
- Arthritis
- Haemarthrosis
- Calf muscle haematoma
- Achilles tendon rupture
- Other trauma
- Reflex sympathetic dystrophy

Gigantism

- Rare; all tissues are uniformly enlarged

Drugs

- Steroids

Obesity

- Lipodystrophy, lipodosis.

Lymphoedema must be differentiated from other causes of leg swelling (Box 21.3)

Primary lymphoedema

This often familial condition is estimated to affect 2% of the adult population and is caused by a developmental failure in which the lymphatics may be absent, hypoplastic, or varicose and dilated. It is usually categorised by the age of onset.

Secondary lymphoedema

This develops when the lymphatic system is obstructed by tumour, recurrent infection or infestation (filariasis), or obliterated by surgery or radiotherapy.

Clinical features

Symptoms

- Gradual painless swelling of one or both legs, commences distally on the foot and extends proximally, usually only to the knee
- First presentation because of acute cellulitis: usually recurrent episodes.

Signs

Unlike other types of oedema, lymphoedema characteristically involves the foot, as opposed to the lower calf and ankle. This is characterised by:

- Infilling of the submalleolar depressions
- A 'hump' on the dorsum of the foot
- 'Square' toes due to confinement by footwear; also, the skin on the dorsum of the toes cannot be pinched owing to subcutaneous fibrosis (Stemmer's sign)
- Pit easily initially, but with time fibrosis and dermal thickening prevent pitting.

Chronic eczema, fungal infection of the skin (dermatophytosis) and nails (onychomycosis), fissuring, verrucae, and papillae are frequently seen in advanced conditions. Frank ulceration is unusual.

Investigation

Lymphoedema is essentially a clinical diagnosis and most patients require no further investigation.

Management

Physical methods

- Feet elevation above the level of the hip, and avoid prolonged standing
- Intermittent pneumatic compression devices
- Graduated compression therapy, with pressure exceeding 50 mmHg at the ankle.

Drugs

Diuretics are of no value and are associated with side effects including electrolyte disturbance. No other drugs are of proven benefit.

Antibiotics

If there is evidence of infection, i.e., cellulitis, antibiotics should be administered based on the culture and sensitivity. Fungal infections should also be treated.

Surgery

Operations fall into two categories: bypass procedures and reduction procedures. They are only rarely performed.

Filariasis

Epidemiology

This is a parasitic infection caused by *Wuchereria bancrofti* and is transmitted by the bite of *Culex* and *Mansonia* species of mosquito. In 10% of patients the disease may be caused by the parasite *Brugia malayi*. Filariasis affects close to 100 million people worldwide in countries like India, South East Asia and China. Males are affected more often than females due to greater susceptibility to bites on the exposed body parts. Eggs enter the human circulation after a mosquito bite where they hatch to mature into adult worms after about 12 months. The adult worms then colonise the lymphatic system where they produce millions of immature larvae called microfilaria, which circulate in the blood with marked nocturnal periodicity. Blood smears prepared at midnight are diagnostic for their presence. Eosinophilia in the blood is usual. Chyluria, chylous ascites and hydrocoele fluid may also show the presence of microfilariae.

Clinical features

The adult worms cause lymphatic obstruction leading to lower limb oedema. Gradually, obstruction of the cutaneous

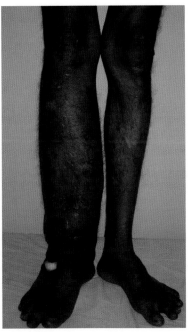

Fig. 21.35 Elephantiasis of the lower limb. Note that this oedema is nonpitting suggestive of chronic lymphoedema.

lymphatics leads to nonpitting oedema and marked thickening of skin, with an orange peel appearance. Repeated attacks of lymphangitis and cellulitis causes fibrosis, thereby aggravating the swelling further. Eventually, the thickening of the skin along with gross swelling resembles the elephant limb and thus the name 'elephantiasis' (Fig. 21.35). Blockage of lymphatics leading to secondary hydrocoele and scrotal oedema is not uncommon in endemic areas in the Indian subcontinent, as is chyluria and chylous ascites.

Treatment

Diethylcarbamazine is the drug of choice before chronic lymphoedema has set in. Intermittent pneumatic compression treatment and use of graduated compression stockings can reduce the oedema in the early stage. Elephantiasis does not respond to any conservative measure and has to be protected from repeated attacks of infection. Surgical excision has been abandoned due to failed results. Hydrocoele is treated by routine surgery with a course of medical therapy in proven cases.

Vascular access for haemodialysis

Ideal vascular access would have the following characteristics:
1. Reliable and repeatable access to the circulatory system
2. Sufficient flow rates
3. Long-term patency
4. Devoid of complications.

For acute haemodialysis, a CVC is the preferred route and provides high dialysis flow, but have high complication rates and are not suitable for chronic use. For long-term haemodialysis, an arteriovenous fistula (AVF) or graft (AVG) can provide a sufficiently high flow rate (>300 mL/min) to allow efficient dialysis.

Methods

See Table 21.8.

Access planning and preoperative assessment

The surgeon must consider numerous factors when planning dialysis access placement. One important factor is the diameter and quality of arterial inflow and venous outflow. This can be assessed by history and clinical examination, but many centres now routinely practice preoperative duplex ultrasound. Venography is reserved for cases with central venous stenosis or occlusion. One important factor to consider is the preservation of the venous real estate for subsequent access creation, hence the preference to create the AVF more distally.

Primary access

These are the commonly created access routes for haemodialysis. They can be performed under local anaesthetic as a day care procedure:
1. Snuff box AVF
2. Wrist radiocephalic fistula
3. Brachiocephalic fistula.

Secondary and tertiary access

When the cephalic vein is not available due to thrombosis or poor quality, the basilic vein can be used to create a fistula. However, this is not suitable for needling due to the depth and proximity to important structures, hence a secondary procedure is required to transpose the vein to a more superficial and safer site.

When an autologous AVF cannot be performed, a prosthetic graft (AVG) can be used. The most common is the non-ring-supported expanded polytetrafluoroethylene grafts. Lower limb access is less popular and reserved as the last option, as it has a very high complication rate.

Assessing a vascular access

A good access should have a strong thrill when palpated with an audible bruit. The distal pulses must be palpated, and evidence of swelling and venous hypertension must be recorded. The puncture sites must be inspected for aneurysms and infection. If there

Table 21.8 Methods of obtaining vascular access		
Method	Advantages	Disadvantages
1. Dialysis catheter	Immediate use Easy to insert	Infection rates high Short-term use Causes central vein stenosis
2. AV fistula	Suitable for long term Resistant to infection	Needs surgery to create Cannot be used immediately
3. AV grafts	Useful when small vasculature May cannulate early	Infection rates high Higher costs to maintain
AV, Arteriovenous.		

21

is central vein occlusion, there may be facial swellings and dilated veins on the trunks. Careful history and examination must be performed if there is a suspicion of steal syndrome.

A duplex ultrasound scan is performed to assess the diameter and flow rates when indicated. For central venous stenosis and occlusion, a formal fistulogram is needed.

Complications of vascular access

Failure to mature

About 10% of fistula remain patent but never achieve adequate flow for dialysis. This may be due to proximal arterial or a venous stenosis, which may be treatable by angioplasty or surgery. Otherwise a revision may be required.

Stenosis and thrombosis

Early thrombosis is usually due to technical error or inadequate assessment of both arterial inflow and venous outflow. Late failure may result from hypotension, dehydration and hypercoagulable states, traumatic needling, and juxta-anastomotic venous intimal hyperplasia. Treatment may involve angioplasty or surgery to bypass the stenotic segment. Thrombectomy alone without dealing with the underlying cause is doomed for failure.

Infection

Infection is the most common cause of hospitalisation among dialysis patients. It is most common in patients with a CVC or AVG, rather than those with an AVF. The most common organism is *Staphylococcus aureus*, which may lead to endocarditis and mycotic aneurysms. Local site infections may be controlled with antibiotics, although frequently removal of the infected catheter and grafts is needed.

Aneurysm and pseudoaneurysm

Occasionally the venous outflow becomes dilated, reaching aneurysmal proportions. This can be treated conservatively, although occasionally requires plication or ligation with a short jump graft bypass.

Pseudoaneurysm at the puncture sites may be due to poor puncture techniques or infections. Bleeding may occur and the fistula may need to be ligated. In AVGs, if it is sterile, local excision and interposition grafting may be possible.

Ischaemic steal syndrome (ISS)

The majority of the symptoms are mild and self-limiting, although in extreme cases patients may present with gangrene of the digits. Careful history taking is important; often patients present with numbness and pain at rest or during dialysis. Clinical examination may reveal a cool hand and an absent radial pulse, which promptly returns when the more proximal AVF is occluded. Duplex ultrasound will reveal reversal of flow. Treatment is by various procedures that reduce the flow though the AVF, but in severe cases a ligation may be necessary. The gold standard treatment to preserve access is the distal revascularisation and interval ligation (DRIL) procedure.

1. Haemorrhage

   Bleeding is often caused by traumatic cannulation, leading to a haematoma. Occasionally it is caused by infection, leading to torrential bleeding. This is treated by manual compression and subsequent ligation of the fistula

2. High-output congestive cardiac failure

   This is a rare complication, associated with fistula flow in excess of 1.5 L per minute. Treatment is by ligation of the AVF or flow reducing procedures such as plication or tapered grafts.

Robert R. Jeffrey

22

Cardiothoracic surgery

Chapter contents

Basic considerations 409

Acquired cardiac disease 411

Congenital cardiac disease 419

Thoracic surgery 421

Basic considerations

Pathophysiological assessment

Careful history and appropriate examination suggest the presence of possible cardiac pathology. The initial clinical assessment is then refined and specific investigations used to confirm and quantify any disease identified (Table 22.1).

Assessment of risk

As the risks of perioperative mortality and stroke are significantly higher with cardiac than with many other forms of surgery, a frank, informed discussion of these risks, recognising potential benefits of a successful operation, are essential elements of the preoperative consultation between the patient and surgeon.

Mortality

Risk stratification is important in cardiac surgery and Euroscore is a valuable tool for quantifying operative risk across all types of noncongenital cardiac surgery. Patient, condition and procedure-related factors contribute to a score that predicts 30-day mortality. Predicted operative mortality ranges from <1% for routine elective procedures to >50% for complex emergency operations.

Stroke

Stroke risk varies from 1% to over 10%, and is associated with preoperative risk factors including advanced age, history of prior embolic events, low cardiac output states, atrial arrhythmias, intracardiac thrombus, hypertension, diabetes, and severe atheromatous disease of the proximal aorta and carotids. Patients with evidence of peripheral vascular disease have a higher risk of stroke and those with high-grade symptomatic carotid disease may benefit from carotid endarterectomy prior to cardiac surgery (Chapter 21).

Specific aspects of surgical technique

Cardiopulmonary bypass

Modern cardiac and great vessel surgery became feasible with the development of cardiopulmonary bypass (CBP). Venous blood is drained via cannulae inserted into the right atrium or venae cavae and passes to a reservoir. It is then pumped through a heat exchanger coil so that its temperature can be varied and an oxygenator, which adds O_2 and removes CO_2, and filters it. Finally, the blood is returned to the arterial circulation via a cannula in the ascending aorta or other suitable artery (femoral, axillary) (Figs 22.1, 22.2 and 22.3). Full anticoagulation with intravenous heparin is required to prevent blood clotting in the bypass circuit. Roller or centrifugal pumps are used, as these minimise red cell trauma. Semipermeable membranes, or more commonly hollow fibres, form the blood–gas interface within the oxygenator. A trained perfusion technician controls the bypass machine.

CPB stimulates a systemic inflammatory response mediated by cytokine release, complement activation and white cell activation. These changes do not generally cause clinical problems but may be implicated in postbypass pulmonary, renal and cerebral dysfunction. Cerebral damage occurs in about 1% of cases due to intracerebral bleeding, embolisation of microbubbles or arterial debris, or inadequate cerebral perfusion. Subtle deterioration in cerebral function, as detected by psychological testing, is more frequent. Coagulopathy and haemolysis are associated with prolonged bypass.

Myocardial preservation

Cardioplegia

Cardioplegic arrest achieves a still bloodless heart. A cross-clamp is applied across the ascending aorta proximal to insertion of the arterial inflow cannula. This prevents blood flow into the coronary arteries. The heart is arrested by perfusing the coronary circulation with a cardioplegic solution, delivered either antegradely via the aortic root or coronary artery ostia utilising the native coronary arteries, or retrogradely via a catheter placed in the coronary sinus, which is accessed through the right atrium.

Table 22.1 Specific assessments of cardiac pathophysiological status

Investigation	Yield
ECG	
Resting	Rhythm; conduction abnormalities; atrial and ventricular hypertrophy; established ischaemic changes; evidence of previous myocardial infarction
Exercise	Exercise-induced ischaemic changes or arrhythmias
Chest x-ray	Cardiac enlargement; valvular calcification; evidence of pulmonary oedema (Kerley B lines, pleural effusion, interstitial marking, hilar flare); absent or enlarged cardiac or great vessel structures
Thallium isotope scan	Areas of low radio-uptake indicative of impaired myocardial perfusion
Echocardiography	
Precordial	Ventricular contractility; valvular stenoses, regurgitation or leaflet abnormalities; intracardiac morphology, including septal defects and intracardiac masses; pericardial effusion
Transoesophageal	Enhanced views of posterior cardiac structures (aortic and mitral valves, ascending aorta, great veins and posterior septae); posterior pericardial fluid collections
Cardiac catheterisation	
Chamber pressures	Assess left and right ventricular function via determination of left ventricular end-diastolic pressure; atrial pressures in valve disease; transvalvular gradients (Fig. 22.1)
Angiography	Coronary arterial anatomy; intracardiac anatomy; trans-septal flow
O_2 saturations	Intracardiac shunts
Cardiac output	Cardiac function and determination of secondary derived parameters, including peripheral and pulmonary vascular resistance

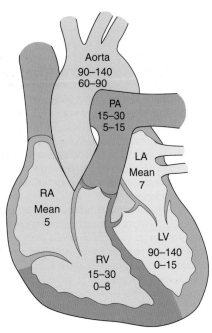

Fig. 22.1 Normal cardiac chambers. Normal pressures (mmHg) within cardiac chambers. *LA,* Left atrium; *LV,* left ventricle; *RA,* right atrium; *RV,* right ventricle; *PA,* pulmonary artery.

The essential component of a cardioplegic solution is a high potassium concentration (circa 18 mmol/L), which causes the heart to arrest in diastole. Cardioplegia is delivered as either a crystalloid solution or using the patient's own blood as a vehicle. Blood-based solutions are believed to contain abundant oxygen-derived free radical scavengers, and the blood's buffering characteristics may be helpful in reducing the deleterious effects of ischaemic metabolites generated by the arrested myocardium.

Cardioplegia solutions minimise myocardial energy requirements by abolishing the energy expenditure of contraction and by reducing basal cellular metabolism. This is enhanced with local tissue cooling, as cardioplegia is typically delivered at 4–6°C. Reducing core temperature on bypass to 26–34°C may further enhance cardiac cooling. Cardioplegia combined with mild systemic hypothermia (32°C) provides the surgeon with a safe period of cardiac arrest of up to 120 minutes, permitting surgery while minimising the risk of myocardial and critical organ damage.

Coronary artery bypass surgery (CABG) can be performed using a technique in which an aortic clamp is intermittently applied to cut coronary flow while the heart is electrically fibrillated so as to reduce movement. The resulting brief ischaemic episodes are tolerated. This cross-clamp fibrillation technique activates mechanisms within the myocardial cells that reduce damage caused by subsequent ischaemia (preconditioning).

In some circumstances, the surgeon may elect to leave the coronary arteries perfused while on bypass and to operate on a beating heart. Recently, there has been considerable interest in performing CABG on suitable patients without the use of CPB. Proponents of 'off-pump' surgery claim that the risks of artificial perfusion (particularly transient cognitive impairment) are avoided and that recovery may be quicker. Many surgeons, however, feel that the bloodless, still operative field resulting from cardioplegic arrest provides the optimum conditions for high-quality accurate anastomoses.

Postoperative care

Intensive care

Postoperatively, patients are usually ventilated for a few hours until they are fully rewarmed, have stable haemodynamics, satisfactory pulmonary gas exchange and normal acid–base status. Initial urine output is copious and potassium levels are, therefore, checked frequently and potassium is administered intravenously

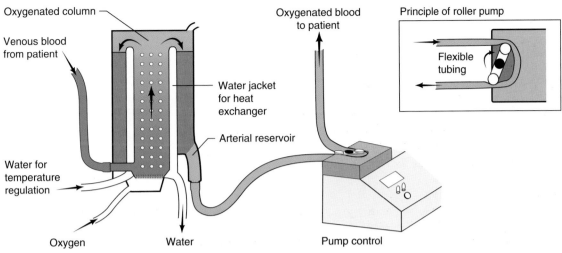

Oxygenated column

Venous blood from patient

Water jacket for heat exchanger

Arterial reservoir

Water for temperature regulation

Oxygen

Water

Oxygenated blood to patient

Principle of roller pump

Flexible tubing

Pump control

Fig. 22.2 Schematic of a bypass circuit.

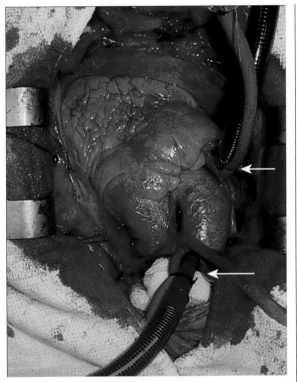

Fig. 22.3 Cannulation for cardiopulmonary bypass. *Upper arrow* from right atrium to pump. *Lower arrow* from pump to aorta.

to correct urinary losses. Invasive measurement of arterial and central venous pressure is standard. Pulmonary artery catheters may be used to measure pulmonary artery pressure, pulmonary artery capillary wedge pressure and cardiac output.

Complications

Other than death or stroke, established complications include:

- Bleeding: multifactorial causes including hypothermia, platelet dysfunction, CPB and pharmacological (aspirin, clopidogrel and other potent antiplatelet medication), hyperfibrinolysis, heparin excess, complement and leucocyte activation, and reduced coagulation factors

- Low cardiac output: inadequate perfusion, poor myocardial protection, previous poor left ventricular (LV) function, hypovolaemia, tamponade, etc.
- Arrhythmias: atrial fibrillation occurs in up to 40% after CABG
- Renal failure, hepatic failure, pulmonary failure
- Infection: wound, respiratory
- Short-term memory impairment, loss of concentration, intelligence, learning and dexterity.

Recovery time

Patients undergoing routine elective coronary or valve surgery will usually leave acute hospital care within 1 week. Those requiring more extensive surgery or emergency procedures may take longer to recover. Most patients will have undergone a median sternotomy (Fig. 22.4). This wound heals quickly and, as the sternal edges are approximated securely by wire or heavy sutures, chest discomfort eases rapidly. Leg vein donor sites may take longer to heal, particularly around the knee. By 2 weeks the patient should be able to walk a few hundred metres, and by 3 months should have returned to full activity, including work.

Acquired cardiac disease

Surgical intervention may be required in the management of:

- Ischaemic heart disease
- Cardiac valvular disease
- Aortic aneurysm
- Pericardial pathology
- Cardiac trauma.

Ischaemic heart disease

Surgery for ischaemic heart disease encompasses coronary artery disease (CAD) and its complications, which produce symptoms of heart failure, and include acute mitral regurgitation, post-infarction ventricular septal defect and LV aneurysm.

Coronary artery disease

Coronary artery atheroma (Chapter 21) results in narrowing of the vessels, and most patients will present for surgery because of angina, dyspnoea or previous myocardial infarction (MI).

22

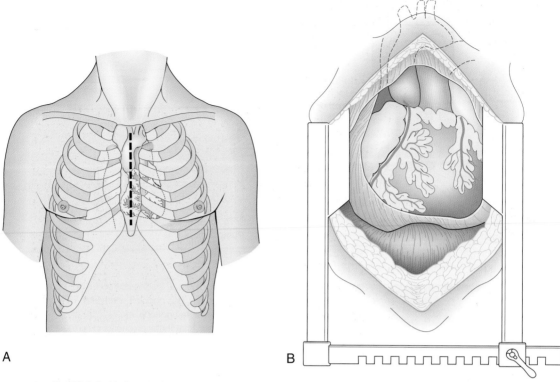

Fig. 22.4 Surgical approach to the heart. (A) Median sternotomy incision. **(B)** Right atrium and ascending aorta exposed.

Assessment

Exercise electrocardiography (ECG) is often used as an initial screening test for patients with suspected stable angina. Those with confirmed ischaemia then undergo coronary angiography and assessment of LV function with echocardiography. Computed tomography (CT) coronary angiography may be performed with the contrast medium delivered peripherally. Alternatively, contrast is injected into the coronary circulation (Fig. 22.5) via a catheter that is inserted through the arterial system. Previously, this was exclusively through the femoral artery but increased use is now made of the radial artery, which has benefits for day case-based procedures (Fig. 22.6). Images are obtained in several different planes so as to minimise the risk of missing eccentric lesions. Intervention is usually advised for stenoses that exceed a 70% reduction in vessel diameter. Such a reduction in internal diameter has a dramatic effect on flow as this is proportional to the fourth power of the radius (Poiseuille's law).

Indications

Elective surgery is indicated primarily for the control of angina that is refractory to medical treatment and is unsuitable for percutaneous intervention (PCI), usually with stent insertion. Historically, patients with three-vessel disease or left main stem disease have exhibited a high (circa 8% per year) risk of death from MI with medical therapy alone. Surgery improves long-term survival for such patients, particularly when LV function is also impaired. PCI has an important role in the management of patients with acute coronary syndrome ranging from ST elevation MI to unstable angina.

Some patients requiring other cardiac procedures may be shown to have significant coronary disease during cardiological

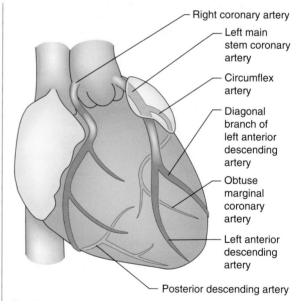

Right coronary artery
Left main stem coronary artery
Circumflex artery
Diagonal branch of left anterior descending artery
Obtuse marginal coronary artery
Left anterior descending artery
Posterior descending artery

Fig. 22.5 Coronary circulation.

assessment. In these cases, coronary surgery is performed with the other procedure to improve perioperative survival and prevent future ischaemic problems. Emergency coronary surgery is rare, and patients with incipient or established MI fare better with PCI and supportive medical therapy, as the mortality of surgery in this setting is much increased. Also, patients attending for noncardiac surgery who are demonstrated to have significant CAD may benefit from revascularisation.

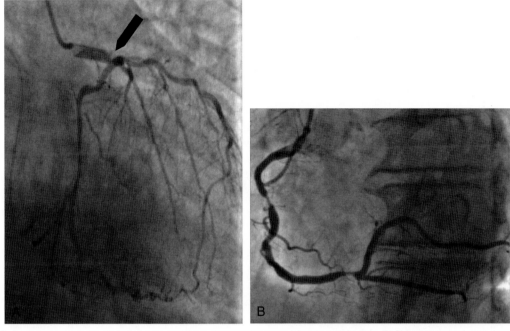

Fig. 22.6 Coronary angiography. (A) Left coronary angiogram demonstrating severe left main stem stenosis. **(B)** Right coronary angiogram demonstrating multiple stenoses.

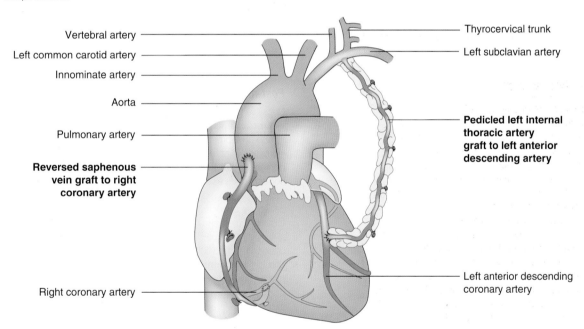

Fig. 22.7 Completed coronary bypass procedure with venous and left internal thoracic artery grafts in situ.

Coronary bypass

A CABG delivers blood to the distal coronary artery beyond a stenosis. If the distal artery is obliterated by atheroma, an endarterectomy procedure may be performed to restore the lumen. When first described, nearly all grafts comprised reversed segments of the long saphenous vein anastomosed proximally to the ascending aorta and distally to the coronary artery. Such grafts have patency rates of around 70% at 5 years and 40% at 10 years. Venous graft failure occurs as a result of intimal hyperplasia, which is thought to be, in part at least, a response to arterial pressure. The relatively high rate of vein graft failure stimulated interest in

arterial grafts and led to the almost universal use of the internal thoracic artery (ITA). This is usually employed as a pedicled graft when it remains attached at its origin from the subclavian artery, but it can also be used as a free graft in the same manner as a vein. ITA graft patency exceeds 95% at 5 years and 90% at 10 years. A common combination is to use the left ITA for the left anterior descending artery and vein grafts for the other vessels (Fig. 22.7).

The radial artery is a possible option as a free graft for use in people with poor-quality saphenous vein and critical proximal occlusion of more than 70% in the target vessel, and may be used together with ITA grafts to achieve 'total arterial revascularisation'. Occasionally, when there is a shortage of a good conduit (e.g., in a 'redo' operation), the surgeon may consider using the right gastroepiploic artery, the short saphenous vein or the cephalic vein. Prosthetic grafts occlude early and are not used.

Results

Uncomplicated coronary surgery carries a less than 3% risk of mortality and a 1–2% risk of stroke. Angina is relieved completely in about 70% of cases, is significantly improved in the remainder, and recurs with a frequency of about 10% per year. Successful revascularisation may also improve breathlessness if it is related to myocardial ischaemia, and survival is enhanced in patients with left main stem and triple-vessel disease. The use of arterial conduits is associated with better graft patency and improved survival. Although there is a trend in that direction for patients with multiple arterial grafts followed up beyond 10 years, the added benefit over one ITA graft placed to the left anterior descending coronary is small. This may reflect the progression of native coronary disease. Secondary prevention is mandatory in all patients with CAD and includes antiplatelet medication (aspirin) and cholesterol reduction (statin) (EBM 22.1).

 22.1 Summary

Coronary anatomy

- There are two coronary arteries (left and right), which have origin in the coronary sinuses: left or posterior sinus, right or anterior sinus.
- The left main coronary artery passes behind the pulmonary trunk and divides into two large branches: the left anterior interventricular artery or left anterior descending (LAD), which supplies the anterior left ventricle and anterior two-thirds of the interventricular septum, and the circumflex coronary, which supplies the posterior and lateral walls of the left ventricle.
- The right coronary artery passes down anteriorly in the right atrioventricular groove supplying the anterior right ventricle and acute marginal branches.
- Either the right or circumflex may terminate as the posterior descending artery, which supplies the inferior surface of both ventricles and the lower septum. This artery is then considered to be dominant.
- The right, LAD and circumflex are each considered to be a 'vessel system'. Disease within any one of these three vessels or its branches is termed *single-vessel disease*. Similarly, two- and three-vessel disease indicates involvement of two and three systems, respectively.

EBM 22.1 Coronary bypass surgery

'Revascularization to improve long term prognosis.
Patients with significant left main stem disease should undergo coronary artery bypass grafting.
Patients with triple vessel disease should be considered for coronary artery bypass grafting to improve prognosis, but where unsuitable be offered percutaneous coronary intervention.
Drug interventions to prevent new vascular events.
All patients with stable angina due to atherosclerotic disease should receive long term standard aspirin and statin therapy.'

SIGN. Management of stable angina. Scottish Intercollegiate Guideline 96; 2007.

Surgery for the complications of coronary artery disease

Mitral valve regurgitation

Chronic

Chronic ischaemia may cause regurgitation owing to papillary muscle fibrosis. Surgery may be indicated to repair or replace the valve as an elective procedure, usually concurrently with CABG. The operative mortality is around 8–11%.

Acute

Acute MI involving a papillary muscle may cause this to rupture, causing gross regurgitation. The patient is usually very unwell with pulmonary oedema due to MR and low cardiac output due to infarction, and often requires emergency ventilation. Emergency mitral valve replacement and CABG is associated with a mortality of 15–40%, mainly due to poor ventricular function and secondary multiorgan failure (EBM 22.2).

EBM 22.2 Valve replacement

- *Aortic valve replacement (AVR) is indicated for **symptomatic** patients with severe aortic stenosis (AS)*
- *AVR is indicated for patients with severe AS undergoing coronary artery bypass surgery (CABG) or surgery on the aorta or other heart valves*
- *AVR is indicated for **symptomatic** patients with severe aortic regurgitation (AR) irrespective of left ventricular (LV) systolic function*
- *AVR is indicated for asymptomatic patients with chronic severe AR and LV systolic dysfunction, or while undergoing CABG or surgery on the aorta or other heart valves*
- *Mitral valve (MV) surgery (repair if possible) is indicated in patients with symptomatic moderate or severe mitral stenosis*
- *MV surgery is recommended for the symptomatic patient with acute severe mitral regurgitation (MR)*
- *MV surgery is beneficial for patients with chronic severe MR.*

Class I recommendations from ACC/AHA 2006 Guidelines for the management of patients with valvular heart disease.

Post-myocardial infarction ventricular septal defect

Necrosis of the interventricular septum due to MI may lead to a ventricular septal defect. Blood flows from the high-pressure left to the low-pressure right ventricle (left-to-right 'shunt'). This increases right ventricular work and pulmonary blood flow, and decreases cardiac output. Typically, the patient complains of sudden, severe breathlessness 3–8 days after an MI and is noted to have developed a pansystolic murmur. The diagnosis is confirmed by echocardiography and coronary angiography is performed. Emergency repair is technically difficult due to the poor quality of the recently infarcted muscle to which the patch is attached. In addition, these patients have impaired cardiac function in the aftermath of an acute MI. Such patients will require mechanical support of their ventricle with an intra-aortic balloon pump. Surgical mortality ranges from 20% to 50%. Patients with minor shunts are managed medically and may be considered for surgery some weeks later to allow cardiac function to stabilise. The margins of the defect will have healed by fibrosis, making patch repair relatively straightforward with more acceptable operative mortality (<10%).

Left ventricular aneurysm

LV aneurysm complicates about 8% of MIs and occurs when a large LV free-wall MI scar becomes aneurysmal as a result of intraventricular pressure. A large aneurysm impairs cardiac contraction and increases myocardial work. Complications include clot formation within the aneurysm, which may embolise, and arrhythmias generated within the zone of ischaemic myocardium around the periphery of the aneurysm.

At operation, the aneurysm is excised, the clot removed and the resulting defect usually closed by direct suture, reinforced by buttressing strips of Teflon felt. Occasionally, a small patch repair is performed to preserve the shape of the LV. Surgery performed electively has a mortality of 6–10% with an increased risk of stroke.

Cardiac valvular disease

Valve disease may obstruct forward flow (stenosis) or permit reverse flow (incompetence/regurgitation), or both. The aortic and/or mitral valves are primarily affected; primary tricuspid pathology is rare and pulmonary valve disease is virtually unknown. Formerly, rheumatic fever following streptococcal infection was the most common aetiological factor. This remains the case in many developing countries, but is now rare in the Western world.

Assessment

Transthoracic echocardiography provides useful data on forward gradients using Doppler techniques and can quantify regurgitation. Transoesophageal echocardiography allows more detailed investigation of the valves and intracardiac anatomy. Coronary angiography is indicated in patients of middle age or older. LV angiography and aortic root angiography may allow the quantification of mitral and aortic regurgitation, but has been superseded by echocardiography, which is superior. A full catheterisation study should include measurement of cardiac output with chamber and pulmonary artery pressures. Pressure gradients and orifice areas may be deduced from echocardiography parameters.

Surgical management

Options include valve replacement or repair. Replacement utilises either a mechanical or a biological prosthesis. Mechanical valves have developed from the original ball-in-cage design through single disc designs to the current range of carbon bi-leaflet devices (Fig. 22.8). These should last indefinitely, but patients require lifelong warfarin to prevent thrombotic occlusion or embolism. Embolism risk is about 1–6% per year and is influenced by how closely the anticoagulant medication is controlled. Mechanical valves produce audible clicks.

Biological valves are derived from:

- Glutaraldehyde-preserved porcine aortic and mitral valves mounted on a frame (stent) (Fig. 22.9A)
- Glutaraldehyde-preserved bovine pericardium formed into a three-leaflet valve and mounted on a stent
- Glutaraldehyde-preserved porcine aortic unstented valves (Fig. 22.9B)
- Human aortic root homografts removed from cadaveric hearts and preserved in antibiotic solution (Fig. 22.9A).

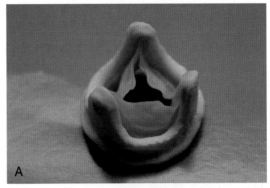
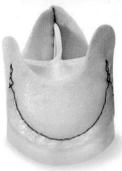

Fig. 22.9 Biological valve prostheses. (A) Stented. **(B)** Unstented.

Unstented valves and homografts offer the advantage of a larger effective orifice area minimising the residual pressure gradient. Warfarin is not required after 3 months with biological valves provided the patient remains in sinus rhythm. However, such valves deteriorate over time and after 15–20 years may need replacement with an increased operative risk. Unless there is a contraindication to anticoagulation, mechanical valves are commonly used in a younger age group (<60 years). In young women intending to have children it is usual to advise a biological valve, with the intention of replacing it with a mechanical device when the valve fails. This avoids problems with warfarin during pregnancy (placental separation, abortion and teratogenicity).

Repair is the preferred surgical option in regurgitation and is largely restricted to the mitral and tricuspid valves, but recently has also been applied to the aortic valve. It is superior to valve replacement, as the problems associated with a prosthesis are avoided. The techniques utilised for mitral incompetence include excision of portions of redundant leaflet, repositioning of the chordae and reduction in the size of the annulus (annuloplasty). Generally, only annuloplasty is applicable to the tricuspid valve. Rarely, isolated mitral stenosis without calcification may be found, in which case division of the fused leaflets under direct vision on bypass (commisurotomy) is performed.

Endocarditis

Abnormal native heart valves and artificial valves are prone to subacute bacterial endocarditis and prosthetic valve endocarditis, respectively. Antibiotic prophylaxis is contentious in patients with prostheses who undergo any surgical or dental procedure.

Patients with endocarditis require prolonged parenteral antibiotic therapy, which may be effective. However, surgery may be required if:

- The infection does not respond
- The patient presents with heart failure

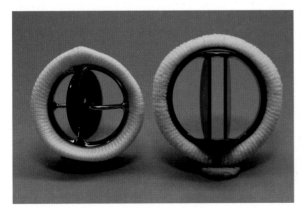

Fig. 22.8 Mechanical valve prostheses.

22

- There is evidence of dehiscence on echocardiogram
- There is evidence of increasing obstruction, regurgitation, or recurrent emboli
- The valve develops a significant paravalvular leak or annular abscess.

Surgery is a high-risk venture as the patient is systemically septic, the perivalvular tissues are of poor quality and the newly implanted prosthesis may itself become infected. Postoperative recovery is usually slow, with renal and ventilatory failure being common complications.

Aortic valve disease

Stenosis

Aortic stenosis is the most common indication for valvular surgery in the UK. Although rheumatic disease remains a common problem in underdeveloped countries, the most frequent aetiology in the Western world is calcific aortic stenosis, which develops in the older population, typically in patients over 70 years. The normal aortic valve has three cusps, but a congenital bicuspid valve calcifies at an earlier age (Fig. 22.10). Aortic stenosis causes LV hypertrophy, effort angina, episodes of arrhythmia with syncope or even sudden death, and LV failure.

Clinically, the patient has a slow rising pulse (pulsus parvus and tardus), a forceful apex beat and an ejection systolic murmur in the right upper parasternal area that may radiate to the root of the neck. Echocardiography will confirm a valvular gradient, which is considered severe aortic stenosis when this exceeds 60 mmHg. However, measurement of orifice area is independent of cardiac output and may be a more reliable measure. The onset of symptoms or LV dysfunction (ejection fraction <50%) should initiate referral for surgery. In the asymptomatic patient, a high transvalvular gradient (mean >40 mmHg), a low valve orifice area (<1 cm²), or an abnormal response to exercise (development of symptoms or asymptomatic hypotension) may indicate the need for surgery. Patients with cardiac failure have a low output and consequently a low gradient. In these cases, the decision to operate may be a difficult judgement, based on the absence of any other likely cause of poor LV function and echocardiographic evidence of severe aortic valve disease.

In some patients, e.g., the elderly, those with patent coronary grafts or significant other comorbidities, percutaneous replacement may be considered. TAVI (transcatheter aortic valve insertion) is the procedure where a biological valve on a holder is introduced percutaneously. Vascular access is achieved via the femoral artery or LV apex, or directly to the proximal aortic root via a right parasternal mini-thoracotomy.

Regurgitation

Native aortic regurgitation may be due to primary valve pathology (rheumatic fever, endocarditic valve destruction or, rarely, a bicuspid valve) or secondary to aortic root pathology with annular dilatation (see later). Prosthetic valve regurgitation can occur as a result of deterioration of a biological prosthesis, partial obstruction of a mechanical device, or paraprosthetic leakage. Chronic aortic regurgitation causes progressive LV dilatation and hypertrophy.

Clinically, there is a wide pulse pressure: collapsing pulse, lateral displacement of the apex beat and a diastolic murmur in the left parasternal area. Chronic aortic regurgitation is well tolerated and often asymptomatic. In severe cases, the patient may complain of dyspnoea and angina, and may exhibit features of congestive cardiac failure. Surgery is advised in symptomatic patients or if there is evidence of LV dysfunction (ejection fraction <50%) to forestall the onset of cardiac failure due to irreversible myocardial damage. The timing of surgery is determined by serial echocardiography measurements demonstrating LV dilatation.

Acute aortic regurgitation produces severe dyspnoea, with rapid onset of LV failure and pulmonary oedema. The patient may require emergency ventilation and urgent surgery.

Surgical outcomes

Elective aortic valve replacement is a relatively straightforward procedure, with a mortality of less than 3% and a stroke rate of 1%. The risk increases with age and comorbidities, and there is a several-fold increase in cases that have progressed to cardiac failure, and in emergency cases with acute severe regurgitation.

Mitral valve disease

Stenosis

Although the incidence of rheumatic valvular heart disease is declining, it is still the most common cause of mitral stenosis resulting in restriction of the flow of blood into the LV, which is consequently small and thin walled. Cardiac output is also reduced. The left atrium (LA) is dilated and left atrial and pulmonary artery pressures (PAP) are raised. Chronic pulmonary hypertension causes right ventricular hypertrophy and right atrial dilatation, and in advanced cases tricuspid incompetence may develop (see later).

Clinically, patients complain of shortness of breath on exertion and may experience palpitations. In severe cases the patient may have orthopnoea, paroxysmal nocturnal dyspnoea, haemoptysis, angina and fatigue. Thromboembolism may be a catastrophic complication. Chronic atrial fibrillation usually intervenes and the patient may be taking warfarin along with a diuretic for pulmonary congestion. Examination reveals a loud first heart sound, an opening snap after the second heart sound, and a harsh rumbling mid-diastolic murmur with presystolic accentuation. With the onset of pulmonary hypertension, there is a loud pulmonary component of

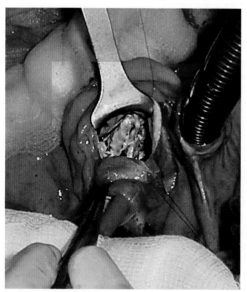

Fig. 22.10 Calcified aortic valve.

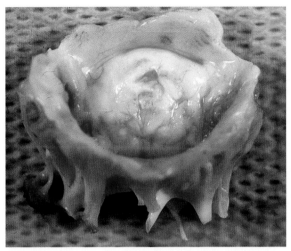

Fig. 22.11 Excised mitral valve showing the shortening and fusion of the papillary muscles and chordae tendinae in advanced mitral stenosis.

the second heart sound, a left parasternal heave due to right ventricular enlargement, a raised jugular venous pulse (JVP) and hepatomegaly. Chest x-ray shows straightening of the left heart border and evidence of left atrial enlargement.

Symptomatic patients with moderate or severe mitral stenosis (an echocardiographic calculated mitral valve area <1 cm^2) need surgery. Evidence of a LA thrombus, recurrent emboli or development of pulmonary hypertension (PAP >50 mmHg) are also indications for surgery. A percutaneous balloon mitral valvotomy is possible in patients with a pliable valve, with no evidence of a LA clot or mitral regurgitation. Conservative surgery with separation of the fused leaflets (commissurotomy) and reconstruction of the valve is possible in some younger patients. Usually, however, there is extensive leaflet calcification, with involvement of the subvalvular apparatus. There is shortening and thickening of the papillary muscles and chordae tendinae, tethering the leaflets to the tips of the papillary muscles (Fig. 22.11). Complex conservative surgery in experienced centres is possible but valve replacement is a practical option.

Rarely, patients with a mechanical mitral prosthesis may develop thrombotic occlusion of their valve secondary to inadequate control of anticoagulation or to fibrous tissue (pannus) ingrowth from the sewing ring. This acute emergency causes catastrophic pulmonary oedema and a severe reduction in cardiac output. Emergency salvage valve replacement or debridement is required.

Regurgitation

Chronic mitral regurgitation occurs with rheumatic disease, ischaemic papillary muscle dysfunction, myxomatous degeneration of the mitral valve, a variety of systemic connective tissue disorders and chronic paraprosthetic valvular leakage. Acute regurgitation is much less common and follows acute MI involving a papillary muscle, as noted above, but can also result from spontaneous rupture of a chorda tendina, sudden failure of a bioprosthetic valve leaflet or perforation of an infected native valve.

Chronic mitral regurgitation presents a volume load to the LV, which ejects blood preferentially backwards through the incompetent mitral valve to the pulmonary circulation. This situation is often well tolerated for years, with patients typically complaining of shortness of breath on exertion and of occasional episodes of palpitation.

Clinical examination is often relatively unremarkable, apart from a pansystolic murmur radiating from the lower left sternal edge to the axilla and leftward displacement of the apex beat. Surgery is indicated in symptomatic patients and where there is evidence of LV dysfunction, LV dilatation, or the new onset of atrial fibrillation or pulmonary hypertension. This process correlates with declining LV function consequent upon the continued volume overload.

Acute regurgitation causes pulmonary oedema and emergency surgery is necessary. Regurgitant mitral valves are frequently repaired but often prosthetic replacement is required.

Surgical outcomes

Elective mitral valve surgery for regurgitation is generally a low-risk procedure, with a mortality rate of 4–6% and a stroke rate of about 2%. The risk is much greater (10–15%) for patients with ischaemic regurgitation, owing to concomitant coronary disease and previous myocardial damage. Valve replacement for mitral stenosis carries a significant mortality (8–12%) due to established pulmonary hypertension, right ventricular failure and poor renal function. The stroke rate is increased to 3–4%. Emergency valve replacement for acute obstruction or regurgitation carries a mortality risk of approximately 20%.

Tricuspid valve disease

Stenosis is very rare. Tricuspid endocarditis is occasionally encountered in intravenous drug abusers. Tricuspid incompetence secondary to enlargement of the tricuspid annulus is the most common pathology and occurs when the right ventricle is dilated, as in advanced mitral valve disease. Typically, the patient will have the features of the underlying mitral valve disease, an elevated jugular venous pressure with 'v' waves, an enlarged pulsatile liver, peripheral oedema and, occasionally, ascites. Liver function tests are frequently deranged and clotting is impaired. The preferred surgical option is to restore the normal dimensions of the valve through annuloplasty. It is uncommon to replace the tricuspid valve, except in rare cases of organic stenosis. If replacement is performed, a biological prosthesis is preferable, as the risk of mechanical valve thrombosis is increased in this position.

Multiple and repeat valve procedures

Multiple-valve procedures typically comprise aortic and mitral valve replacement, or mitral replacement with tricuspid annuloplasty. Such operations attract a higher operative mortality (5–7%), as patients are often in poor general condition and may require prolonged periods of intensive care following surgery. Similarly, revisional valve surgery to replace a valve for a second time is technically more difficult and will involve a prolonged procedure against a background of impaired cardiac function or sepsis related to the defective prosthesis. Mortality is increased by two to three times the primary procedure risk, and intensive care unit stay is prolonged.

Aortic aneurysm

Tubulosaccular aneurysms

These are 'true' aneurysms that form either a fusiform (tubular) or a focal (saccular) type of swelling (Fig. 22.12). They are lined by

22

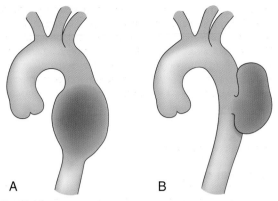

Fig. 22.12 Thoracic aortic aneurysm. **(A)** Tubular. **(B)** Saccular.

layered thrombus and most are due to medial degeneration secondary to smoking and hypertension (Chapter 21).

False 'aneurysms'

These result when bleeding from an aortic injury is contained within the mediastinum, so that the aneurysm wall is formed only by fibrous tissue and organised thrombus. There is usually a history of a road traffic accident or fall, which may have occurred many years previously.

Both true and false aneurysms may rupture and present as an acute emergency, with chest pain and catastrophic intrathoracic bleeding. However, they are often noted as incidental chest x-ray findings. Occasionally, an aneurysm may present with symptoms due to secondary pressure effects, such as dysphagia (oesophagus), stridor (left bronchus), chest wall pain (erosion of ribs), back pain (erosion of the vertebrae) or hoarseness (stretching of the left recurrent laryngeal nerve).

Aortic dissection

This is caused when blood enters into the wall of the aorta through a tear in the intima, creating a false lumen that spirals along the vessel within the medial layer but contained by the adventitia. The entry point is usually either just above the aortic valve or immediately beyond the left subclavian artery. However, the dissection process may extend along the entire length of the aorta

into the iliac vessels. The false lumen may rupture through the adventitia into the mediastinum or pleural cavity, causing massive and frequently fatal haemorrhage, or into the pericardium, causing fatal tamponade. The origins of aortic side branches, which are encountered by the false lumen, tend to be encircled and occluded. This process can lead to widespread ischaemic damage to the heart (coronaries), brain (branches of the aortic arch), spinal cord (spinal arteries), kidneys (renal arteries), abdominal viscera (coeliac and mesenteric arteries) and the limbs. A dissection that involves the aortic root (type A) tends to lift the aortic valve leaflets away from the wall, leading to regurgitation. Finally, a dissected aorta may dilate over months to years, causing a progressive aneurysmal process. Acute dissection is often fatal prior to arrival at hospital. There may be severe interscapular pain, collapse, shock, aortic incompetence, unequal peripheral pulses, features of a left haemothorax, stroke, paraplegia, abdominal discomfort and lower limb ischaemia.

Dissections that originate distal to the left subclavian (Fig. 22.13; type B), do not spread retrogradely to involve the aortic arch or ascending aorta, and are clinically stable are usually managed conservatively by control of blood pressure, as the results of medical and surgical treatment are not different. Endovascular stent placement via the femoral artery under radiological control has an emerging role in this difficult situation, and the decision to intervene on such patients is based on the development of rupture and organ/limb ischaemia.

In contrast, most patients with dissections that involve the ascending aorta or arch (type A) are offered emergency surgery to prevent rupture, stroke, MI and aortic valve incompetence. Surgery involves excising and replacing the portion of the aorta containing the entry point. This prevents more blood entering the false lumen and reapposes the layers of the aortic wall. Additional surgery to repair the aortic valve or to replace the aortic arch or descending aorta will be determined by individual circumstances.

Aortoannulo ectasia

This is characterised by a flask-shaped aneurysmal dilatation of the aortic root and ascending aorta. This expanding aneurysm may rupture, initiate a dissection and lead to severe aortic regurgitation, with all the potential sequelae of these conditions. Aortoannulo ectasia is frequently associated with connective tissue disorders, most commonly Marfan's disease.

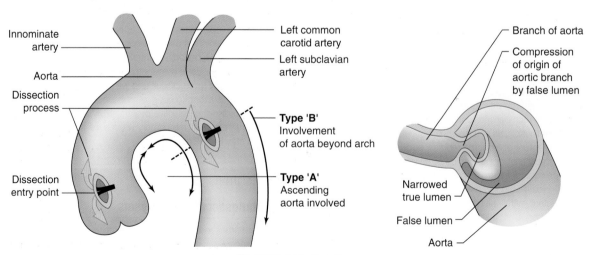

Fig. 22.13 Aortic dissection.

Assessment

A patient with an incidentally discovered aneurysm should be thoroughly investigated, including tests of respiratory function and coronary angiography with thoracic MRI and/or contrast CT to fully delineate the extent of the aneurysm. Aneurysms that extend from the chest into the abdomen (thoracoabdominal aneurysm) require further investigations to clarify the relationship of the aneurysm to the renal and visceral vessels. Larger aneurysms (5 cm on the ascending aorta and 6 cm on the descending aorta) are more likely to rupture, and serial investigation will confirm whether or not an aneurysm is enlarging. Based on these considerations, a decision can then be taken regarding the potential benefit of surgery. In patients presenting with acute rupture of an aneurysm, the diagnosis may have been made by one of the modalities described above or by transthoracic or transoesophageal echocardiography (Fig. 22.14). Surgery is recommended if patients are potentially salvageable and considered likely to benefit from operative intervention.

Surgery for aortic pathology

Lesions of the aortic root and ascending aorta are repaired on bypass via a median sternotomy. A woven Dacron tube graft is used to replace an ascending aortic aneurysm, but in aortoannulo ectasia a composite graft containing an aortic valve prosthesis is used to replace the whole aortic root. The coronary artery ostia are then attached as buttons onto side holes cut in the graft. Aneurysms involving the aortic arch require complex surgery. The patient is cooled to 16°C on bypass, the circulation arrested and the patient exsanguinated. Profound hypothermia protects against cerebral damage while the surgeon operates in a bloodless field. The brachiocephalic, left carotid and left subclavian arteries are anastomosed to the arch graft. Alternatively, antegrade cerebral perfusion is used during the repair of arch aneurysms, to prevent the cerebral complications of profound hypothermic arrest. Descending aortic aneurysms can often be repaired using a local shunt in order to deliver blood to the lower body. Clamps are applied to exclude the aneurysm, which is excised and replaced with a suitable length of graft. If a thoracoabdominal aneurysm is being repaired, the visceral arteries are also anastomosed to the graft. Interventional radiology with stent placement alone or in combination with open surgery (hybrid procedure) is increasingly being utilised.

Thoracic aortic aneurysm surgery is high risk. Elective procedures carry a 5–15% mortality risk and a substantial risk of stroke. Procedures involving the descending aorta carry an additional

5–10% risk of paraplegia, owing to interference with spinal arterial supply. Emergency thoracic aneurysm surgery is in most cases a desperate measure. Mortality rates vary between 10% and over 60%, depending upon the extent of surgery required, and the degree of preexisting and acquired comorbidities. It is not uncommon for the primary repair procedure to proceed satisfactorily only for the patient to die later from multiorgan failure and/or stroke.

Pericardial pathology

Pericardial effusion

In chronic pericardial effusion, the pericardial sac will stretch and the clinical effects of the accumulated fluid may be modest. In contrast, a rapidly evolving effusion will prevent the heart from filling in diastole (tamponade) and lead to a low stroke volume. In order to maintain cardiac output and blood pressure, there is a tachycardia and intense peripheral vasoconstriction. The raised intrapericardial pressure leads to elevation of atrial pressure, and hence the central venous pressure rises in order to maintain a filling gradient. A pericardial effusion can often be drained percutaneously through a catheter placed under echocardiographic guidance. This may help clarify the diagnosis, but surgical drainage is likely to be required in infection, malignancy with reasonable life expectancy, and in chronic effusions. Symptomatic chronic effusions may be drained into the left pleural cavity by creating a window in the left lateral pericardium using a minimal-access videothoracoscopic procedure (video-assisted thoracic surgery [VATS]). Acute and malignant effusions can be drained relatively simply into the peritoneal cavity via a short epigastric incision. Whichever approach is used, specimens of fluid and pericardium are sent for culture and histology.

Pericardial constriction

Chronic pericardial inflammation, often from tuberculosis, may heal by intense fibrosis and calcification (Fig. 22.15). This leads to chronic tamponade and investigations should include echocardiography, right heart catheterisation with record of chamber pressures, and CT or preferably MRI. Surgery is undertaken via a median sternotomy to remove the parietal pericardium and any fibrotic visceral pericardium, and can be performed without CPB. Such surgery is difficult and can be accompanied by significant blood loss. Results can occasionally be disappointing because the patient may have already developed irreversible hepatic cirrhosis and myocardial function is poor.

Cardiac trauma

Cardiac tamponade with penetrating trauma

This is a surgical emergency and the clinical diagnosis is made from an elevated JVP, hypotension and the site of the wound, which is commonly the result of an assault with a knife. Prompt anterior thoracotomy, relief of the bloody tamponade and digital control of the penetrating injury to the heart until suitable suture can be achieved may be life-saving. Major injuries to structures may require CPB.

Congenital cardiac disease

This may be classified as cyanotic or acyanotic, depending on the presence of central cyanosis. Those with cyanosis will have a

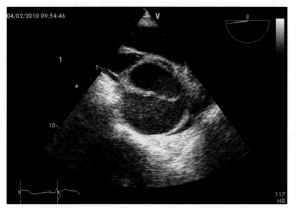
Fig. 22.14 Transoesophageal echocardiography of aortic dissection.

22

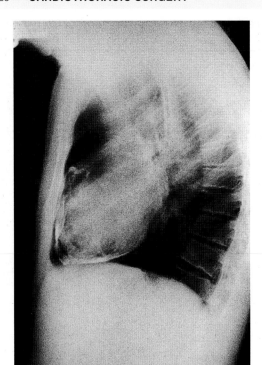

Fig. 22.15 Calcified constrictive pericardium.

right-to-left shunt, preventing complete oxygenation of systemic arterial blood. Some patients with high-flow left-to-right shunts develop severe pulmonary hypertension as a consequence of the massive pulmonary blood flow. This can result in pressures in the right heart chambers that are greater than those in the left heart and hence reversal of the shunt direction to right-to-left, causing cyanosis (Eisenmenger's syndrome). Primary repair is usually advised for congenital defects, but in some instances it may be helpful to delay definitive repair until the child is older, larger and fitter. In this situation, a temporising palliative procedure is performed. This is usually designed to augment or restrict pulmonary artery blood flow.

Atrial septal defect

This is the most common cardiac congenital abnormality, causing a left-to-right atrial shunt and hence an increase in right heart and pulmonary blood flow. Patients may be asymptomatic or may present with frequent chest infections. There is wide fixed splitting of the second heart sound and a pulmonary ejection systolic murmur. A diastolic flow murmur that does not change on inspiration is often present in the tricuspid area. ECG frequently demonstrates right ventricular hypertrophy and echocardiography is diagnostic.

Small defects are of little haemodynamic significance, but if the pulmonary-to-systemic flow ratio exceeds 2:1, closure is recommended and may be undertaken percutaneously or by open operation depending on the size and morphology of the defect. Three anatomical types exist, named after the developmental area giving rise to the defect: *ostium secundum defects* are the most common, *sinus venosus defects* arise in the upper atrium adjacent to the superior vena cava and *ostium primum defects* involve the anomalies of the mitral and tricuspid valves. Surgical repair in children carries a near 0% mortality, but adults presenting with pulmonary hypertension are at greater risk (2%).

Ventricular septal defect

Many ventricular septal defects close within the first year of life. Larger lesions cause a left-to-right shunt and pulmonary congestion. Defects may again be subdivided according to their embryological origins, but most (85%) occur in the perimembranous septum. Infants with large defects may present with frequent respiratory infections, but patients with small defects are often asymptomatic. A pansystolic murmur is audible, maximal at the left sternal edge. The second heart sound may be loud. Large shunts may cause a diastolic flow murmur in the mitral area. Biventricular hypertrophy is present on ECG and pulmonary plethora may be noted on chest x-ray. Echocardiography is diagnostic. Asymptomatic defects are observed, but early operation is preferred for larger defects to prevent irreversible pulmonary hypertension. Repair is undertaken using a patch, with a very low operative mortality of 1–2%.

Patent ductus arteriosus

If the ductus arteriosus fails to close after birth, pulmonary blood flow is abnormally high, producing pulmonary congestion and hypertension. Infants have retarded growth and a continuous 'machinery' murmur is audible over the precordium and back. The chest x-ray shows pulmonary congestion, and echocardiography can exclude concurrent intracardiac defect(s). In premature children, the duct may close with an indomethacin infusion (prostaglandin E_1 inhibition), but clipping or division at left thoracotomy is definitive. Endovascular closure is an option in older children. The operative mortality is low in older children (<1%) but high (25%) in preterm infants, who are generally very unwell.

Coarctation of the aorta

This condition is caused by a narrowing of the thoracic aorta, usually at the level of the ligamentum arteriosum. The lower body is perfused via extensive chest wall collaterals. Upper body hypertension develops and may lead to heart failure in infancy. Untreated adults develop hypertensive cerebrovascular and renal problems, and accelerated coronary atheroma. Most children and young adults are asymptomatic and present with high blood pressure or an abnormal chest x-ray. The femoral pulses may be impalpable or weak and delayed, and a systolic murmur may be audible over the back. Left ventricular hypertrophy (LVH) is seen on ECG and chest x-ray shows an enlarged heart, reduced aortic knuckle and characteristic rib 'notching', caused by enlarged and tortuous intercostal arteries eroding the ribs near the posterior angles (Fig. 22.16). Balloon angioplasty has been used to dilate some coarctations in infants, but surgical correction is usually required. At operation, the left subclavian artery may be used as an onlay patch. Older children and adults are usually managed with a resection and end-to-end anastomosis or a Dacron bypass graft. Surgical correction tends to reduce upper body hypertension in children. It is less effective in adults but pharmacological control of hypertension becomes more reliable. The operative risk is approximately 5%.

Tetralogy of Fallot

This most common cause of cyanotic congenital heart disease comprises a high ventricular septal defect, an aorta that overlies the interventricular septum, pulmonary valvular and subvalvular stenosis, and right ventricular hypertrophy. Right ventricular outflow obstruction causes cyanosis as a result of right-to-left shunting

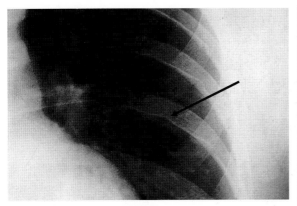

Fig. 22.16 Rib notching in coarctation.

across the ventricular septal defect. Clinical features depend upon the severity of the obstruction, particularly the subvalvular component. The child may become blue and faint during feeding or crying.

Right ventricular hypertrophy is evident on ECG and the pulmonary artery shadow is small on chest x-ray. Echocardiography is diagnostic. Correction entails closing the ventricular septal defect with a patch, resecting muscle bands contributing to right ventricular outflow obstruction, and enlarging the right ventricular outflow tract with a patch placed across the pulmonary valve annulus and along the pulmonary artery if necessary. In those not fit for this procedure or in those with very small pulmonary vessels, a shunt

is created in order to increase pulmonary blood flow and, hopefully, lead to further pulmonary arterial growth. Definitive correction may then be possible at a later stage. Operative mortality is approximately 5%.

Thoracic surgery

Assessment

This is concerned with confirming the diagnosis, determining in oncological cases whether resection is appropriate, and establishing that the patient is fit for the intended surgical procedure. The principal investigations are summarised in Table 22.2. History can be instructive in suggesting advanced malignant disease and in providing evidence of the patient's functional status.

Bronchogenic carcinoma

Aetiology, pathology and presentation

This usually presents from the fifth decade onwards and is the leading cause of cancer death in the UK for both men and women. The principal risk factor is cigarette smoking but other rare causes include exposure to various chemicals. The combination of asbestos exposure and cigarette smoking produces a many-fold increase in risk.

Table 22.2 Common thoracic surgical investigations

Investigation	Yield
ECG	
Resting	Rhythm; conduction abnormalities; atrial and ventricular hypertrophy; established ischaemic changes; evidence of previous myocardial infarction
Chest x-ray	
Posterior–anterior and lateral	Preliminary assessment of location of lesion; malignant involvement of phrenic nerve or ribs; presence of additional lesions or effusion; presence of pneumothorax or mediastinal air
Thoracic CT	Further refine radiological assessment of mass lesions as above; review mediastinum for enlarged nodes in bronchogenic carcinoma; inspect bronchi for dilatations in suspected bronchiectasis; determine areas of greatest disease in interstitial lung disease; locate intrathoracic collections; map out distribution of bullous/emphysematous lung disease
PET CT	Identify further disease elsewhere through metabolic uptake of ^{18}F-fluorodeoxyglucose not identified by conventional CT
Upper abdominal CT	Exclude or confirm liver abnormalities; identify adrenal metastases
Upper abdominal ultrasound	Determine probable nature of cystic hepatic lesions; provide guidance for biopsy of hepatic or adrenal lesions; review diaphragm motion in cases of suspected diaphragmatic rupture or phrenic nerve paralysis
MRI	Useful for assessing relationship of tumour to adjacent neural structures, e.g., detecting possible intraspinal extension of paravertebral neurogenic tumours or involvement of brachial plexus by superior sulcus (Pancoast) tumours
Isotope scans	
Bone	Search for skeletal metastases; review chest wall for possible direct invasion by carcinoma
Lung	Identify areas of low uptake indicative of impaired perfusion or ventilation
Pulmonary function tests	
FEV$_1$	Provides a measure of airway obstruction
FVC	Indicates presence of restriction of ventilation
CO transfer	Measures the diffusion capacity of the patient's lungs
Walking test	Measures distance walked by the patient in a set time period (4 minutes) and the perceived exercise level achieved as assessed by the final heart rate; useful as an indicator of functional status in patients with poor FEV$_1$, as they may not comply well with the methodology of formal respiratory testing and hence underachieve
Arterial blood gas	Useful in demonstrating patients with CO_2 retention who should be excluded from surgical consideration

CO, Carbon monoxide; CT, computed tomography; FEV$_1$, forced expiratory volume in one second; FVC, forced vital capacity; PET, positron emission tomography.

22

With the exception of alveolar cell carcinomas, which arise from cells lining the alveoli, primary lung cancers arise within the bronchial epithelium and are hence termed *bronchogenic carcinoma*. They are described as peripheral or central, according to their location within the lung (Figs 22.17, 22.18 and 22.19). Peripheral lesions may grow to 8 cm or more before causing local symptoms such as chest wall pain. Many are detected as incidental findings on a chest film taken for unrelated reasons, or for nonspecific symptoms such as weight loss. Central lesions tend to occlude the airways, causing varying degrees of pulmonary collapse and consolidation (Fig. 22.19). Nodal spread occurs to the intralobar, hilar and mediastinal nodes, and thence to the scalene nodes. Metastases occur in bone, brain, liver, adrenals and lung. Local direct spread may involve the chest wall, vertebrae, trachea, oesophagus and great vessels.

EBM   22.3 Surgery for lung cancer

- *Patients with Stage I and II non-small-cell lung cancer should be considered for curative surgery where possible*
- *Lung resection should be as limited as possible without compromising cancer clearance. Lobectomy is the procedure of choice for fit patients*
- *Every effort should be made to avoid a futile thoracotomy*
- *Systematic lymph node dissection is recommended as offering the best compromise between accuracy of staging and containment of morbidity.*

From SIGN management of patients with lung cancer. Scottish Intercollegiate Guideline 80. Quick reference guide.

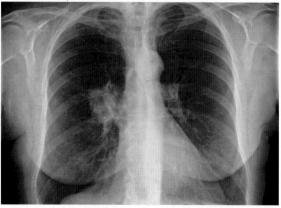

Fig. 22.17 Chest x-ray showing cancer in the right upper lobe.

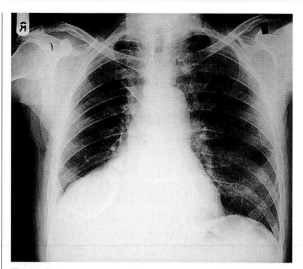

Fig. 22.19 Consolidation/collapse of the right middle and lower lobes associated with a central bronchogenic carcinoma.

The approximate frequencies of the various cell types are: squamous 35%, adenocarcinoma 35%, undifferentiated 10%, small cell 15% and rare cancers 5%.

Small-cell lung cancer is regarded as a systemic disease at presentation and patients are not usually referred for surgery but treated with chemotherapy and radiotherapy. All other varieties are resected if possible (EBM 22.3). Therefore, for surgical treatment purposes, bronchogenic carcinoma is categorised into small cell and non-small cell. However, cell type is important as recent advances in pathology and genetics have identified mutations that mark tumours that may be sensitive to some chemotherapeutic agents and allow tailoring of chemotherapy regimens to specific cell subtypes.

There may be no clinical features, but haemoptysis, pulmonary infection and weight loss are common presenting symptoms. Paraneoplastic syndromes are infrequent but well described, including ectopic hormone production (adrenocorticotrophic hormone, parathyroid hormone, antidiuretic hormone) and a painful periosteal reaction affecting the joints and long bones, termed *hypertrophic pulmonary osteoarthropathy*. Patients frequently have finger clubbing.

Assessment for pulmonary resection

Prior to referral to the surgeon, the diagnosis will often have been confirmed by sputum cytology, bronchoscopy or CT-guided

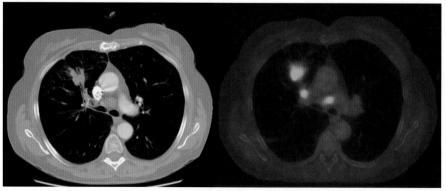

Fig. 22.18 PET CT images of right upper-lobe carcinoma with local nodal and subcarinal disease. Same patient as Fig. 22.17.

needle biopsy, but approximately 30% of cases will be undiagnosed at this stage. Assessment addresses two questions:

- Is the patient fit for pulmonary resection?
- Is the disease potentially curable?

Fitness for resection

Fitness is determined by cardiorespiratory assessment. A history of angina or MI does not preclude surgery, provided the symptoms are stable. However, patients with poor LV function and/or unstable angina are not suitable for pulmonary resection. Respiratory investigations, including the forced expiratory volume in one second (FEV_1) and carbon monoxide (CO) transfer data, will establish whether pulmonary reserve will be adequate following the intended resection. Patients with an $FEV_1 < 50\%$ predicted, prior to resection, are likely to be significantly breathless following surgery and may not be suitable candidates for surgical management. If the CO transfer value is low, implying poor alveolar gas exchange, the minimum FEV_1 figure would have to be revised upwards. However, resection of consolidated or collapsed lung does not affect residual respiratory capability.

Staging

Assessment of the potential for curative resection is determined by staging. Initial clinical assessment will normally filter out advanced disease and provide evidence of incurability because of local irresectability or disseminated disease (Table 22.3). Chest x-ray may reveal an elevated diaphragm, indicating phrenic nerve involvement, bone metastases or direct invasion of the rib cage. If an effusion is present, this should be aspirated; if malignant cells are noted on cytology, this would preclude resection.

Contrast-enhanced thoracic and upper abdominal CT will clarify the nature and position of the pulmonary mass, and should exclude other pulmonary lesions that might represent metastases or synchronous tumours. Mediastinal nodes <1 cm in long axis are generally considered to be benign, but surgical sampling is necessary to confirm this. Combined thoracic CT/positron emission tomography (PET CT) is helpful in both locating and

characterising mediastinal lymph nodes. A negative PET scan is highly accurate in predicting the absence of tumour involvement; a positive scan may indicate tumour but can also arise with inflammatory conditions, and, therefore, positive glands must be sampled by mediastinoscopy. The liver and adrenals are common sites for metastases. Suspicious areas can be sampled by ultrasound-guided biopsy. Further investigations, such as bone or brain scans, will depend upon clinical suspicion.

Surgical staging is concerned with further refining the intrathoracic assessment so as to ensure that thoracotomy will be associated with a reasonable chance of cure. In practical terms, this involves excluding those with involved mediastinal lymph nodes and, where possible, confirming the diagnosis and local operability. Techniques which are employed include:

- *Mediastinoscopy* is used to sample the paratracheal and subcarinal lymph nodes. A low anterior cervical incision is made just above the jugular notch and the mediastinoscope used to create a passage in the pretracheal region. The lymph nodes are dissected and biopsied
- *Mediastinotomy* is used mainly to assess lymph nodes within the concavity of the aortic arch or anterior to the aorta, as these areas cannot be reached at mediastinoscopy. Access is gained via a short left anterior second interspace incision
- *EUS*: under endoscopic ultrasound guidance, fine-needle aspiration of mediastinal nodes may be performed either transbronchially or transoesophageally
- *Videothoracoscopy* is a technique that allows the surgeon to inspect the pleural cavity, biopsy the primary lesion and sample the lower mediastinal and aortic arch lymph nodes. The extent of resection likely to be required can also be assessed in relation to the patient's lung function. Videothoracoscopy may also reveal unforeseen causes of irresectability, such as pleural seedlings.

Resection

Lung tumours are normally removed en bloc with the surrounding parenchyma and local draining lymphatics. This involves either lobectomy or pneumonectomy. Occasionally, in unfit patients, small cancers are excised within a wedge or segment of lung but the risk of local recurrence is greater in these lung-sparing cases. An area of anterior chest wall directly invaded by tumour can be excised and replaced with synthetic patch, provided it is lateral to the posterior rib angles. Following assessment and surgical resection, the final pathological Tumour, Node, Metastasis (TNM) stage (Table 22.4) is helpful in indicating prognosis and determining whether a patient might benefit from adjuvant therapy, usually within the setting of a trial. Patients who are found to have positive mediastinal nodes following resection are routinely referred for adjuvant radiotherapy to the mediastinum in view of the high risk of recurrence in that area. Postoperative chemotherapy may improve 5-year survival across all resected stages by approximately 5%. This form of adjuvant therapy is likely to become an increasingly common option for suitably fit patients. Operative mortality is about 2% for lobectomy and 6% for pneumonectomy.

Survival

Reported 5-year survival data are approximately 60% for stage I, 35% for stage II and <20% for stage IIIa disease. Relatively few patients (<20%) with non-small-cell bronchogenic carcinoma are suitable for resection at presentation. One strategy to address

Table 22.3 Clinical indicators of locally irresectable or incurable lung cancer

Clinical finding	Pathological implication
Local inoperability	
Horner's syndrome	Involvement of upper sympathetic chain
Hoarseness	Involvement of left recurrent laryngeal nerve
Upper-body venous congestion	Involvement of superior vena cava
Severe shoulder/inner arm pain	Involvement of brachial plexus (Pancoast tumour)
Disseminated disease	
Scalene node enlargement	Nodal spread out of operative field
Hepatomegaly	Hepatic metastases
Focal bone pain	Bone metastases
Skin deposits	Cutaneous metastases
Behavioural/balance disturbance	Cerebral/cerebellar metastases
Headache	

22

Table 22.4 TNM classification of lung cancer

Tumour	
T1a	<2 cm
T1b	2–3 cm
T2a	3–5 cm
T2b	5–7 cm or within 2 cm of main bronchus or partial lung collapse
T3	>7 cm, chest wall involvement, phrenic nerve involvement, whole-lung collapse or >1 tumour nodule in same lobe
T4	Direct involvement of mediastinum or tumour nodules >1 lobe
Nodes	
N0	No nodes
N1	Local node involvement
N2	Ipsilateral mediastinal nodes or subcarinal
N3	Contralateral mediastinal nodes or supraclavicular nodes
Metastases	
M0	No evidence of spread
M1a	Tumours in both lungs, malignant pericardial or pleural effusion
M1b	Distant metastases, e.g., bone, adrenal, brain
Staging of lung cancer	
Stage 1A	T1a or T1b N0M0
1B	T2a N0M0
Stage 2A	Any T1 or T2N1, T2b N0M0
2B	T2b N1M0 or T3N0M0
Stage 3A	Any T1 or T2N2M0, any T3N1 or N2, T4N0M0, T4N1M0
3B	Any TN3M0 or T4N2M0 or T4N3M0
Stage 4	Any T or N with M1a or M1b

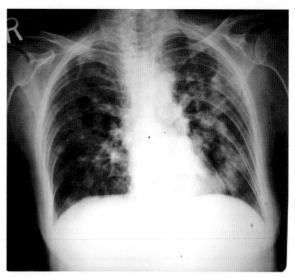

Fig. 22.20 Multiple pulmonary metastases.

this problem is the use of neoadjuvant preoperative induction chemotherapy to downstage tumours, although there are as yet no data to support the widespread use of this approach. The other obvious possibility for improving resection rates would be to detect lung cancers at an earlier stage. Previous mass chest x-ray screening studies did not appear to show an improvement in long-term survival, but there is currently renewed interest in screening high-risk individuals (smoking history, >50 years old) using CT as a more sensitive test.

Metastatic disease

Pulmonary metastases (Fig. 22.20) are the most common form of intrathoracic malignancy. A confirmatory diagnostic lung biopsy may be helpful for patients with no evident primary. A palliative pleurodesis in patients with associated pleural effusion can be achieved by instilling an irritant such as aluminium silicate powder (kaolin) into the pleural cavity.

Rarely, a solitary metastasis (e.g., renal carcinoma) or limited pulmonary metastases (e.g., in osteogenic sarcoma) may be found in patients without any other evidence of disseminated disease. Increasingly, patients with pulmonary metastases from colorectal cancer are considered for resection if there is evidence that intra-abdominal disease has been cleared and there is no increase in number or size of the metastases over a reasonable period.

Other lung tumours

These tend to present either as an incidental chest x-ray finding, in which case the concern is that they may in fact be malignant tumours, or as a cause of bronchial obstruction and infection. True benign lung tumours are rare and can arise from all tissue elements within the lung architecture. If the lesion can be shown to be benign by transthoracic biopsy, no treatment is required. Where there is doubt, local excision will be required. If a main bronchus is obstructed, lobectomy or sleeve resection will be necessary to remove the tumour and the damaged portion of lung. Carcinoid tumours arise from argentaffin-containing cells within the bronchial epithelium. They are divided on histological grounds into 'typical' tumours, which grow slowly locally, and 'atypical' tumours, which grow more quickly and can metastasise. Resection is by lobectomy or sleeve resection. As local recurrence may occur up to 15 years following resection, good local clearance is essential. Unlike abdominal carcinoids, thoracic carcinoids do not secrete vasoactive substances.

Mesothelioma

This causes progressive thickening of the parietal and visceral pleura, with subsequent encasement of the lung and the formation of a large pleural effusion. In the later stages, the growth penetrates the chest wall, causing pain, and involves the mediastinal structures and abdominal cavity. Metastatic spread is rare until an advanced stage is reached. Mesothelioma is strongly related to a history of asbestos exposure (e.g., boiler makers), but there is usually a latent period of 20–40 years before the onset of symptoms. The patient commonly presents with shortness of breath owing to a large pleural effusion. In many cases, the diagnosis is made by a percutaneous pleural biopsy but, if this is not successful, thoracoscopy or open pleural biopsy is useful. The main differential diagnosis is disseminated adenocarcinoma involving the pleural cavity. It can be difficult to distinguish these two pathologies on light microscopy, and diagnosis may be delayed while immunohistochemistry and electron microscopy studies are performed. Surgical resection by excision of the parietal pleura, lung, diaphragm and pericardium (pleuropneumonectomy) is not generally reported to offer a survival benefit, except possibly in very early lesions. Radiotherapy and chemotherapy have no curative value. Therapy is, therefore, usually directed towards controlling symptoms. If the lung re-expands after drainage of the effusion, kaolin may be instilled in order to promote pleurodesis and so prevent recurrence. Life expectancy varies from 1 to 4 years from initial presentation depending on age, the rate of tumour growth and the stage at presentation.

Mediastinum

Mass lesions

Benign and malignant masses may arise in the mediastinum. Some clue to the likely diagnosis is provided by the location of the lesion (Fig. 22.21) within the mediastinum. Anterior mediastinal masses include goitre, thymoma and lymph nodes, whereas posterior mediastinal masses include neurogenic tumours and enterogenous cysts. Where the diagnosis is in doubt, tissue

may be obtained by CT-guided needle biopsy. If this is either not feasible or is unsuccessful, a surgical biopsy can be obtained using mediastinotomy, mediastinoscopy or videothoracoscopy. The clinical features vary considerably, with some quite large masses being asymptomatic and identified on routine chest films. Nonspecific symptoms include vague chest pain, cough, weight loss, fever and general malaise. Other lesions may cause direct pressure effects, such as tracheal compression by a retrosternal thyroid goitre or oesophageal compression by malignant lymphadenopathy. Thymomas may be identified during the evaluation of patients with myasthenia gravis and resection of these may improve their neurological symptoms.

Wherever possible, primary mediastinal tumours are resected, although in many cases this is precluded because the growth involves the great vessels and mediastinal viscera. Benign cysts are usually resected or, less commonly, marsupialised in order to prevent pressure effects or the development of infection. Surgery is generally undertaken via a median sternotomy for anterior lesions or a thoracotomy for mid- and posterior lesions.

Video-assisted thoracic surgery

An increasing number of procedures are performed by VATS, which reduces the pain of long-access incisions on the chest wall and provides access by using conventional instruments aided by magnification of vision and lighting. This form of minimal-access surgery in the thorax does not need the use of any gas for creating space and can be aided by single-lung ventilation. Pulmonary resection is routinely performed and excision of mediastinal tumours such as thymomas, lung biopsies, mobilisation of the thoracic oesophagus as part of three-stage oesophagectomy for carcinoma, excision of the cervical sympathetic chain for hyperhidrosis are some of the other procedures that have become well established in expert hands.

Infection

Mediastinal infection is an uncommon but serious condition that is associated with a rapid onset of septicaemia and septic shock. It is almost always a consequence of oesophageal or pharyngeal leakage, which may follow perforation or breakdown of an oesophageal anastomosis (see Chapter 13).

Pneumothorax

Pneumothorax occurs when air enters the potential space between the visceral and parietal pleura through either an external chest wound or an internal air leak. External air entry occurs with a traumatic chest wall defect, and the resulting open pneumothorax is often associated with a 'sucking wound', where air moves in and out of a chest wound with respiration. Internal air leakage may follow oesophageal perforation or anastomotic breakdown, as air can enter the pleural cavity via the mouth.

However, the most common cause of pneumothorax is leakage of air from the lung, due either to a traumatic puncture wound or to spontaneous leakage from a large (bulla) or small (<1 cm, 'bleb') air sac on the lung surface. Occasionally, the pulmonary leak point may have a flap valve mechanism that allows air out of, but not back into, the lung, causing a rapid build-up of pressure within the pleural cavity (tension pneumothorax; Fig. 22.22). This can be fatal, as the high intrapleural pressure completely flattens the ipsilateral lung while deviating the mediastinum to the opposite side, impeding venous return.

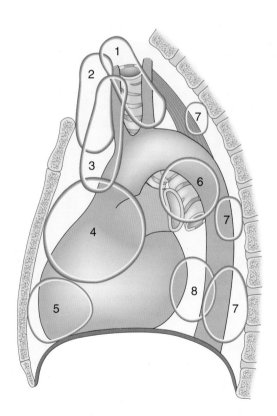

1 Goitre
2 Lymph node tumours, primary and metastases
3 Thymoma
4 Dermoid/teratoma
5 Pleuropericardial cyst
6 Bronchogenic cyst
7 Neurogenic tumour
8 Enterogenous cyst

Fig. 22.21 Topography of mediastinal lesions.

22

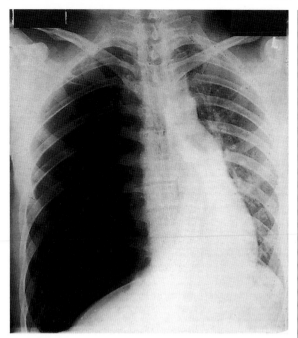

Fig. 22.22 Radiographic appearance of a right-sided tension pneumothorax. Note the mediastinal shift to opposite side.

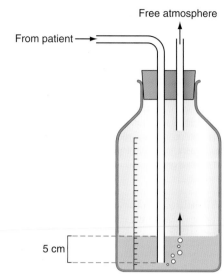

Fig. 22.23 **Underwater seal drain.** The water acts as a hydraulic valve. This allows air to escape from the pleural cavity with ease but the pressure required to cause reverse air flow is much greater, being increased by the ratio of the surface areas inside and outside the tube that enter the water.

Spontaneous pneumothorax is described as primary or secondary. Primary pneumothorax typically occurs in young (15–35 years) individuals with essentially normal lungs apart from a few apical bullae or blebs. Secondary pneumothorax develops in elderly patients (55–75 years) with a background of emphysema and chronic obstructive pulmonary disease. It is caused by rupture of a large bulla. Other common causes of secondary pneumothorax include iatrogenic (following subclavian vein catheterisation, pleural biopsy, tracheostomy, transbronchial biopsy etc.), pulmonary tuberulosis, bronchogenic carcinoma and lung abscesses.

Management

Initial management is aspiration or by insertion of a chest drain connected to an underwater seal into the pleural space (Fig. 22.23). This allows the lung to re-expand. In most cases of primary pneumothorax, air leakage stops within 48 hours or so, after which the drain can be removed. If the pneumothorax recurs or the air leakage does not stop, thoracoscopic surgery is indicated. The lung is inspected and any blebs or bullae are stapled. These are usually found at the apices of the upper or lower lobes (Fig. 22.24). Pleurodesis is then performed either by using an abrasion technique to scarify the parietal pleura or a pleural strip (pleurectomy), or by insufflation of kaolin. Bullectomy and abrasion or pleurectomy carry about an 8% risk of further recurrent pneumothorax. This is reduced to 1–2% with kaolin insufflation, but as this technique involves leaving foreign material in the chest of a young person, it is usually kept in reserve for recurrent pneumothorax or for patients with no obvious culprit bulla or bleb.

Secondary pneumothorax may not settle rapidly, owing to the poor quality of the underlying lung tissue. It typically occurs in individuals who are poor candidates for general anaesthesia and major thoracic surgery. It is customary, therefore, to wait for 1–2 weeks to see if the air leak will stop spontaneously. If not, videothoracoscopy is undertaken in better-risk patients to inspect

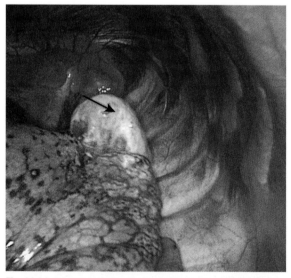

Fig. 22.24 Typical moderate-sized apical bulla seen at thoracotomy.

the lung for a leaking bulla, which can be closed by stapling. Alternatively, kaolin mixed with local anaesthetic can be introduced as a slurry via the intercostal drain. This option avoids general anaesthesia but results in significant pain. Either treatment is associated with an appreciable mortality of 2–5%, owing to respiratory and cardiovascular complications.

Emphysema

Emphysema is characterised by progressive loss of interalveolar septae. Large air spaces form throughout the lungs, which become grossly enlarged with severely affected areas that are neither ventilated nor perfused. This causes progressive loss of respiratory function, culminating in respiratory failure and death. Recurrent infection and pneumothorax are common.

This is typically a smoking-related disease affecting patients from the fourth or fifth decade onwards, with a tendency towards an upper lobar distribution. In less than 10% of cases, however, it can also result from a deficiency of α_1-antitrypsin, affecting younger patients from the third decade and having a lower lobar distribution. Medical treatment with bronchodilators and steroids may improve symptoms but transplantation is the only definitive cure. This is only an option for younger patients, and even in these individuals it should be postponed for as long as possible.

Lung volume-reduction surgery aims to improve lung function by excising portions of the worst-affected areas, typically the upper lobes. This removes the space-occupying effect of these nonfunctional areas and allows the overall lung volume to return towards normal, thereby improving diaphragmatic and chest wall function. The improvement in respiratory function is modest in absolute terms, being in the order of 0.5 L for FEV_1. However, patients eligible for this surgery typically have FEV_1 values of less than 1 L, so that the relative improvement and hence the perceived benefit can be significant. The procedure may be performed either as a videothoracoscopic operation or through a median sternotomy. The clinical improvement only lasts for a few years as lung function continues to fall, reflecting the progressive nature of emphysema. Case selection is important as the operative mortality is high (6–12%), reflecting the generally very poor condition of these patients.

Interstitial lung disease

This can arise from many causes and correct treatment depends on an accurate pathological diagnosis. Transbronchial biopsy can be effective in some instances, particularly sarcoidosis, but provides only a small tissue sample, which may not be diagnostic. It is usually preferable to use videothoracoscopic techniques to excise a wedge of affected lung. The patient is typically allowed home on the first postoperative day.

Pleuropulmonary infection

Empyema

This is a collection of pus within the pleural cavity. It commonly follows pneumonia due to secondary infection of a reactive parapneumonic effusion. In the initial phase, the infected fluid is thin and may be completely evacuated by a low intercostal drain. The empyema quickly becomes thick and loculated as a result of the deposition of fibrin, and at this stage formal surgical drainage is required. The collection is typically placed posteriorly towards the base of the pleural cavity and causes a D-shaped shadow on the chest film (Fig. 22.25). Drainage in this phase may be achieved by videothoracoscopic techniques or by excising a 2-cm segment of rib over the lowest part of the empyema and suctioning and curetting the cavity clean. As dense fibrosis surrounds an empyema, drainage creates a fixed cavity. In elderly or unfit patients, a simple open tube drain is left in situ for many months, during which the cavity gradually shrinks and finally obliterates. In younger patients, open formal thoracotomy with decortication allows the fibrous cavity to be excised and any cortex over the lung removed. This returns more lung function to the patient and avoids prolonged open drainage, so that recovery is more rapid.

Other causes of empyema include postsurgical bronchial or oesophageal suture line leakage, lung abscesses, oesophageal

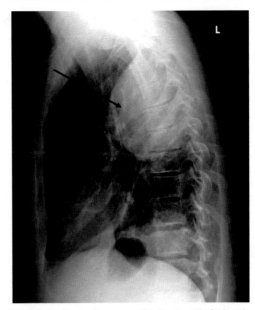

Fig. 22.25 Lateral x-ray of empyema. This film shows the D-shaped outline of a typical empyema with fluid level (arrow).

rupture or perforation, repeated aspiration of pleural effusion, secondary infection of a clotted haemothorax and, rarely, a subphrenic abscess.

Bronchiectasis

Dilatation of bronchi and bronchioles can follow childhood infections, e.g., measles or pertussis. The stagnant pools of secretions that collect are subject to continued infection, resulting in episodes of acute pulmonary infection or pneumonia and, more rarely, in haemoptysis. Management is by antibiotic therapy, physiotherapy and daily postural drainage. Evaluation by CT usually demonstrates that the condition is fairly widespread throughout the lungs, but occasionally one lobe may be particularly badly affected where the bronchiectasis is secondary to chronic bronchial obstruction by an inhaled object or tumour, or, more rarely, from external glandular compression as in tuberculosis. In this situation, lobectomy may result in a gratifying decrease in chronic sputum production and in the frequency of recurrent infection. Resection can be technically difficult, as dense vascular adhesions surround the affected lobe.

Pulmonary tuberculosis

Pulmonary tuberculosis is a disease of poverty, and globalisation has led to increased chances of spread of the disease. A large amount of money, energy and research has been put into its prevention and treatment. Besides being endemic in underdeveloped areas in the world, tuberculosis also affects people with weakened immune systems, those undergoing chemotherapy, and those with AIDS.

Initially, surgery was the only therapeutic option for pulmonary tuberculosis. Therapeutic lung collapse (by thoracoplasty, artificial pneumothorax, plombage and phrenic nerve division), together with rest was the preferred treatment prior to the availability of antitubercular therapy. Present indications for surgery in pulmonary tuberculosis include the complications of pulmonary tuberculosis: pneumothorax, empyema, bronchopleural fistula, bronchiectasis, massive haemoptysis, lung abscess and aspergilloma in a

22

tubercular cavity. Surgery may also be indicated in pulmonary tuberculosis if there is a solitary nodule and for multidrug-resistant tuberculosis (MDR-TB), especially if the focus of infection involves a localised area, i.e., a bronchopulmonary segment, or if there is a suspicion of malignancy.

Results of surgery are excellent, and in many cases lead to cure of the disease.

Chest wall deformities

Sternal protuberance (pectus carinatum) or retraction (pectus excavatum) may be obvious and corrected in childhood. Pectus excavatum can be associated with connective tissue disorders such as Marfan's syndrome, and with unilateral breast hypoplasia. There is often a mild degree of scoliosis present and patients characteristically stand with a hunched posture. Often, however, patients with these deformities present in their early teenage years. At this time, the deformity is exacerbated by accelerated growth and the individual becomes extremely sensitive about his or her appearance. Neither deformity is of physiological significance, and correction is only indicated when the patient's quality of life is clearly impaired because of appearance.

Correction involves major surgery. Open operation with resection of the costal cartilages from the third rib downwards bilaterally mobilises the sternum so that it can be repositioned. In addition, a steel bar is implanted behind the elevated sternum for excavatum cases so as to maintain the new sternal position. Alternatively the bar may be introduced with a minimally invasive technique through bilateral small incisions avoiding division of the costal cartilages (Nuss procedure). The patient and family must be advised that, as with all major thoracic surgery, this procedure can be associated with serious postoperative complications. Also, the sternum must be given time to fuse in the corrected position, and so contact or vigorous sports are not permitted for about 9 months after surgery. In general, if repair is to be undertaken, it is best delayed until the patient is at least 17 years old, as major growth has stopped by this time, thereby reducing the chance that further deformation could follow repair.

Cervical sympathectomy

This procedure involves removal of the lower half of the stellate (cervicothoracic ganglion) along with the second to fifth ganglia in the form of a chain. Conventionally performed by an open approach (axillary or transthoracic), this procedure is now performed by minimal access VATS. The indications for this operation include hyperhydrosis of the upper limbs, axilla and face characterised by excessive and unpredictable sweating, especially the palms, due to overactivity of the sympathetic system and troublesome Raynaud's phenomenon of the upper extremities.

Postoperative care

In the UK, despite the increasing application of VATS procedures, the majority of major thoracic surgery is performed through a lateral thoracotomy incision, which is inherently much more painful than a median sternotomy. Patients are not electively ventilated,

as this is not helpful to healing lung or to lung function. Patients undergoing major thoracic surgery are therefore usually cared for in a high-dependency unit (HDU) for the first 24–48 hours following surgery. The key objectives are to enable the patient to breathe effectively and to clear secretions properly.

Pain control

Pain management during the HDU phase is achieved normally by placement of an epidural catheter. It can have disadvantages related to increased fluid requirement, which may be detrimental to lung function, and marked pain increase when the epidural infusion is stopped. Many units prefer not to place an epidural catheter and to rely instead on a combination of patient-controlled morphine infusion supplemented by parenteral nonsteroidal analgesics and local intercostal nerve blocks. These can be conveniently given via a paravertebral catheter inserted at surgery.

Management of secretions

It is vital that patients cough and clear secretions. This requires humidification of oxygen to prevent the secretions becoming excessively viscous, effective pain control and considerable input from physiotherapy, since many patients have pre-existing impaired lung function. Excessive secretions may need to be removed by suction bronchoscopy under light general anaesthesia, and a minitracheostomy tube may be inserted via the cricothyroid membrane. In severe cases, ventilation and formal tracheostomy may be required.

Fluid management

Following major thoracic surgery, the pulmonary alveolar–capillary membrane becomes relatively leaky, so that fluid tends to accumulate within the pulmonary interstitial spaces. This decreases lung compliance and increases the work of breathing. A degree of postoperative fluid restriction for the first 48 hours ensures that the left atrial pressure is kept low, thereby decreasing pulmonary venous pressure and the transcapillary gradient.

Late management

All patients receive subcutaneous heparin as prophylaxis for deep venous thrombosis until fully mobile, because the risk of thrombosis is high in thoracic surgery and the consequences of pulmonary embolism are that much worse when lung has been resected. Drains are withdrawn when air leakage stops, and patients are mobilised as rapidly as possible. In an uneventful recovery, discharge home should occur about 6–9 days after major open resection, and after 1–5 days following a videothoracoscopic minimal-access procedure. The patient's age, general health and social circumstances will influence these estimates.

Cardiac and pulmonary transplantation

Transplantation for end-stage cardiac and pulmonary disease is discussed in Chapter 25.

Grant D. Stewart

23

Urological surgery

Chapter contents

Assessment 429

Upper urinary tract (kidney and ureter) 434

Infections of the kidney 438

Lower urinary tract (bladder, prostate and urethra) 441

Disorders of micturition: incontinence 452

External genitalia 454

Assessment

General points

Patients may present with symptoms clearly related to the urinary tract, but seemingly unrelated symptoms may also be due to a urological cause; backache from metastatic prostatic carcinoma, fever of unknown origin from renal carcinoma, lethargy and anaemia from obstructive renal failure.

Urinary tract symptoms

Pain

Afferent innervation of the urinary tract is rudimentary, and as such pain originating from these organs, though characteristic, may not easily be localised. Renal pain occurs in the angle between the 12th rib and the sacrospinalis muscles. Ureteric pain (or colic) typically radiates forwards and downwards towards the groin, testes or labia, following the dermatomes relating to the nerve roots from which the sympathetic innervation of the ureter originates (i.e., T10–L2). Acute bladder obstruction usually causes central lower abdominal pain. By contrast, chronic bladder obstruction may be virtually asymptomatic. Disease of the bladder and prostate causes ill-defined perineal or penile pains. A prostate that is grossly enlarged can cause rectal symptoms, including tenesmus.

Disorders of micturition

The history aims to distinguish between obstruction (e.g., poor stream), storage problems (e.g., urgency), infection (e.g., frequency, dysuria) and malignancy (e.g., dark, discoloured, or brown, pink or red urine). Frequency is recorded numerically: D/N 6/3 (by day, six times; by night, three times). Hesitancy, poor stream and dribbling are characteristic of bladder outflow obstruction (BOO).

Haematuria

Haematuria, or the presence of blood in the urine, is a very specific symptom of urinary tract disease. It may be nonvisible, where the urine appears clear on naked eye examination but contains red blood cells on microscopic examination. Visible haematuria is the condition in which the urine is red or brown in colour, and occurs when there is substantial bleeding in the urinary tract.

The haematuria may be intermittent in frequency with periods of clear urine in between, or it may be persistent. It may be present either throughout the act of micturition or only during a particular phase of micturition, providing a clue to the aetiology (Table 23.1).

Haematuria may be associated with pain or it may be painless. Conditions that may mimic haematuria are discoloration of urine due to certain drugs like phenazopyridine and rifampicin, or certain food items like beetroot. They are of no clinical significance other than that they may cause undue anxiety to the patient.

Dysuria

Dysuria or painful micturition is often described by the patient as a sensation of burning during micturition. It is usually localised to the urethra and is associated with acute inflammatory conditions of the lower urinary tract. The symptom may be associated with urinary frequency and urgency.

Frequency, nocturia, urgency

These symptoms are interrelated and are the result of inability of the bladder to hold urine. Frequency may be caused by an actual decrease in the capacity of the bladder (due to diseases causing fibrosis) or by a decrease in the functional capacity of the bladder (due to a large residual volume of urine). Acute inflammatory conditions also decrease the capacity of the bladder and lead to frequency and inability to postpone micturition (urgency).

Nocturia or night-time frequency may be a result of renal disorders leading to a decrease in the concentrating ability of the kidney, or due to excessive intake of fluids, caffeine or alcohol before bedtime.

Table 23.1 Sources of haematuria

Type of haematuria	Site of origin
Total/complete	At or above the level of bladder
Initial	Prostate, anterior urethra
Midstream	At or above the level of bladder
Terminal	Posterior urethra, bladder neck, trigone

Incontinence

True incontinence is when the passage of urine occurs without warning and without any precipitating factors (exstrophy of bladder, vesicovaginal fistula, ectopic ureteric orifices). Stress incontinence occurs with any increase in the intravesical pressure (straining, coughing, laughing) and leads to a loss of urine due to a weakness of the sphincter mechanism. Urge incontinence is associated with urgency and is seen in acute inflammatory conditions, patients with upper motor neuron injuries and in individuals with an overactive bladder. Overflow incontinence is seen in patients with chronic urinary retention, when urine dribbles out of the bladder due to an excessive rise in intravesical pressure.

Oliguria/anuria

Oliguria denotes decreased urinary output (<400 mL/day in adults; <6 mL/kg/day), while anuria is a complete absence of urine output. The causes are discussed in the section on acute renal failure.

Others

Rare presenting complaints include pneumaturia (air in urine), cloudy urine, chyluria (milky urine) and urethral discharge.

Examination

Examination should not be confined to the urinary system, as cardiological, neurological and gynaecological problems may be associated with urological symptoms and signs. Many urological patients are elderly and require an assessment of their fitness for further investigations and operative treatment. Furthermore, the patient's cardiovascular status may be relevant to subsequent treatment; for example, administration of oestrogens for carcinoma of the prostate.

With the patient relaxed, the kidney can be balloted between two hands, one placed posteriorly in the loin and the other one anteriorly; a sufficiently enlarged organ may be bimanually palpable when lifted with one hand placed behind the loin and compressed by the other hand pressing downwards (Fig. 23.1). The ureter cannot be palpated. An enlarged bladder rises centrally out of the pelvis, is dull to percussion and may be visible in thin patients. In men, the hernial orifices, cords, testes and epididymes are examined with the patient standing and lying. If the foreskin is uncircumcised, it must be confirmed that it retracts and that the glans and meatus are normal. In women, the vulva, urethra and vagina must also be examined. A speculum examination should be carried out if there is any suspicion of vaginal or cervical abnormality. A full pelvic bimanual examination, whether in males or females, is best carried out under general anaesthesia with a muscle relaxant. A rectal examination is mandatory, not only to examine the prostate but also to detect abnormalities of the anal margin (haemorrhoids, fissures) and lower rectum (carcinoma).

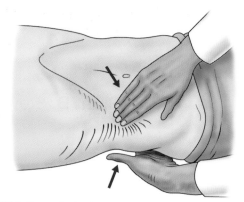

Fig. 23.1 Bimanual palpation of the right kidney.

Investigations

Urine

- Dipstick testing:
  - Proteinuria. In the absence of infection, urine is normally almost protein free. Proteinuria of more than 150 mg/24 hours mandates further investigation
  - Glycosuria suggests the presence of diabetes
  - Leucocytes and nitrites suggest urinary tract infection (UTI)
  - Specific gravity. A loss of concentrating ability of the kidney is seen in conditions affecting the renal medulla such as chronic renal failure, and presents as urine with a fixed low specific gravity (isosthenuria).
- Microscopy. May detect casts or tubular epithelial cells associated with renal parenchymal disease, crystals in patients with renal calculi, or ova in schistosomiasis
- Cytology and, more recently, urinary cellular markers are useful in the diagnosis and follow-up of bladder (and other urothelial) cancers
- Mid-stream specimen of urine (MSSU). The patient is asked to pass some urine into the toilet. Without interrupting the flow, the next part is directed into a special container, and the remainder into the toilet; collected samples are then sent for microbiological assessment.

Blood tests

Creatinine is a breakdown product of skeletal muscle and serum levels do not begin to rise until the glomerular filtration rate (GFR) is halved. Creatinine clearance can be used to estimate GFR. Patients with chronic renal disease often have disordered erythropoiesis, leading to normocytic, normochromic anaemia in addition to disordered calcium metabolism. The erythrocyte sedimentation rate (ESR) can be markedly raised in idiopathic retroperitoneal fibrosis, a cause of ureteric obstruction. Beta human chorionic gonadotrophin (β-HCG), α-fetoprotein (AFP) and prostate-specific antigen (PSA) are useful tumour markers.

Ultrasonography

Ultrasound (US) is a common first-line imaging approach (Fig. 23.2) providing information about the renal parenchyma but less about the collecting system and the ureters. It allows visualisation of other related organs, such as the liver, spleen and

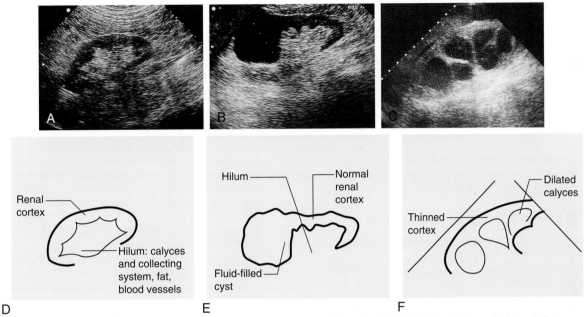

Fig. 23.2 **Renal ultrasound. (A)** Normal kidney. **(B)** A simple cyst occupies the upper pole of an otherwise normal kidney. **(C)** The renal pelvis and calyces are dilated by a chronic obstruction to urinary outflow. The thinness of the remaining renal cortex indicates chronicity. **(D–F)** The diagrams beneath show the anatomical features.

gynaecological organs, and is also helpful in evaluation of bladder, prostate, testis and epididymis.

Transrectal ultrasonography (TRUS) employs a high-frequency transducer via the rectum for evaluation of prostatic disease. The anatomical delineation is much better than with transabdominal US, as the prostate is in direct contact with the anterior wall of the rectum.

Plain x-ray film

A plain film, commonly called a KUB (kidney-ureter-bladder), is a simple imaging investigation for patients with urinary tract symptoms. It provides information about any calcification in the course of the urinary tract.

Intravenous urography

An intravenous urogram (IVU) involves injecting iodine-containing contrast material intravenously and taking serial x-rays (Fig. 23.3) to demonstrate the renal pelvis and calyces, the rate of kidney emptying, the calibre of the ureters, and the bladder outline. Once the bladder has filled, a 'postmicturition' film will demonstrate bladder emptying and the amount of residual urine.

Computed tomography (CT) scanning

The IVU has largely been superseded by the 'plain' computed tomography (CT) KUB, a noncontrast-enhanced CT, which has a higher specificity and sensitivity for the detection of renal and ureteric calculi. CT urography allows the ureters to be delineated by contrast, as in an IVU, but also allows other structures within the abdomen to be assessed. A CT urogram may be useful to detect other synchronous pathologies in the abdomen, and

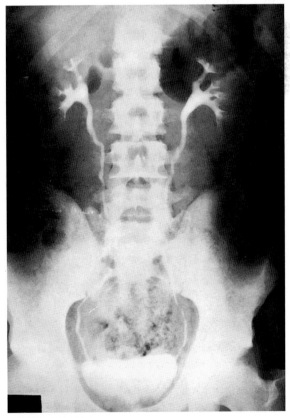

Fig. 23.3 Normal intravenous urogram.

to stage the extent of local and metastatic spread of any neoplastic lesion. CT has a distinct advantage in evaluation of the retroperitoneum.

Retrograde pyelography

This is a special investigation used to outline the collecting system and the ureters of use when evaluating the upper urinary tract in theatre. It is an invasive investigation, and carries the risk of introducing infection. The ureter on the side of interest is cannulated under cystoscopic vision in a retrograde fashion using a fine-calibre ureteric catheter. Radioopaque dye is then injected through the catheter under fluoroscopic screening to outline the collecting system (Fig. 23.4).

Special radiological investigations

Abnormalities of the renal vessels including assessment of active bleeding can be demonstrated by renal angiography. A micturating cystourethrogram (MCU) will outline the bladder, detect ureterovesical reflux, and examine the bladder neck and urethra (Fig. 23.5). The bladder is filled with contrast material (via a catheter) and emptying is then studied by x-ray screening (Fig. 23.5). An ascending or retrograde urethrogram, in which contrast medium is injected into the urethra, can be used to define strictures. When used in conjunction with a MCU, a descending urethrogram can also be obtained.

Nuclear imaging

Radiolabelled substances are used for two main purposes:

1. *Detecting bony metastases from carcinoma of the prostate (bone scan).* ^{99m}Tc-labelled methylene diphosphonate (MDP) is the most reliable method.
2. *Measurement of renal function (scintigraphic renography).* Occasionally 'how a kidney looks' does not correlate with 'how it behaves', e.g., hydronephrosis does not always mean the presence of obstruction. Nuclear scintigraphy allows assessment of obstruction to a kidney (e.g., from pelviureteric obstruction), differential kidney function (i.e., how much each kidney is contributing to overall function), assessment for nonfunctioning areas of renal parenchyma (e.g., scarring) and accurate assessment of GFR. Radiolabelled mercaptoacetyltriglycine (MAG-3) has largely superseded technetium-labelled diethylenetriamine pentaacetic acid (Tc-DTPA) for dynamic scanning (Fig. 23.6). It is secreted from the renal tubules and is used in the identification of obstructed kidneys and to assess differential function. Dimercaptosuccinic acid (DMSA) is concentrated in the renal tubules and static imaging can be carried out some 2–3 hours after injection. Parenchymal defects such as scars, haematomas, lacerations or ischaemia may be demonstrated. Differential renal function can be quantified by measuring the dimercaptosuccinic acid (DMSA) concentration/density in each kidney.

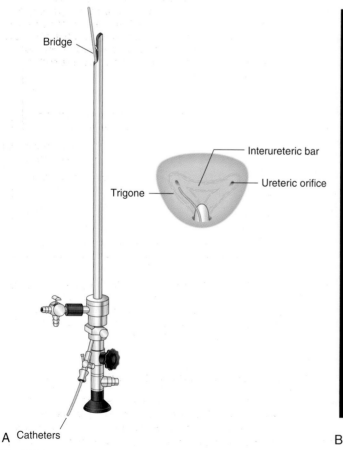

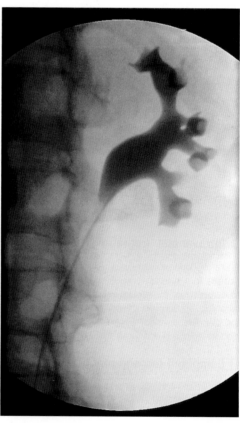

Fig. 23.4 Retrograde ureteropyelography. (A) Cystoscope and ureteric catheterisation. **(B)** The best views of the normal collecting system are shown by pyelography. A catheter has been passed into the left renal pelvis at cystoscopy. The anemone-like calyces are sharp-edged and normal.

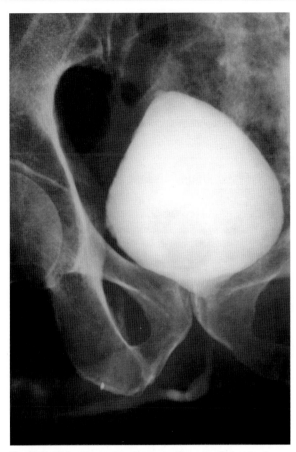

Fig. 23.5 Micturating cystourethrogram. Shows opacified and well-distended bladder, and a normal urethra in a male patient.

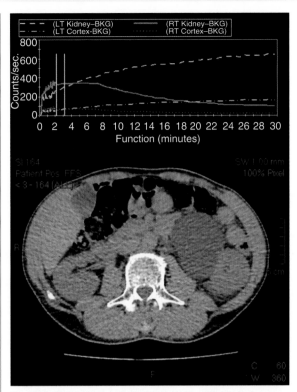

Fig. 23.6 MAG-3 (99mTc-labelled dimercaptoacetyltriglycine) scan (*left panel*) and accompanying computed tomography (*right panel*). The MAG-3 renogram curve demonstrates a normally draining right kidney (the curve started drops towards baseline after 7 minutes), whereas the curve for the left kidney continues to rise, despite the administration of a diuretic, suggesting an obstructed kidney. The computed tomography scan shows left-sided hydronephrosis, the patient was found to have a pelviureteric junction obstruction and treated with a pyeloplasty.

Urodynamic studies

The maximum urinary flow rate during micturition can be measured in the outpatient setting using a flow meter when the voided volume is at least 150 mL or the values may be misleadingly low. The norm in males is 15–30 mL/s and in females 20–40 mL/s; a flow rate of less than 10 mL/s is abnormal. The flow rate pattern can help to determine the cause of obstruction (Fig. 23.7). The residual volume of urine is assessed using US. More invasive urodynamics uses rectal and urethral pressure lines to indirectly assess detrusor pressure during filling of the bladder with contrast material or water. The cystometrogram provides a measure of bladder capacity, the capacity at which a desire to void occurs, and the detrusor pressures when the bladder is full and during maximum flow. Spontaneous detrusor contractions during bladder filling may indicate an unstable bladder, a cause of urgency and urge incontinence.

Semen analysis

Microscopic examination of the semen is a basic investigation in infertile males. The specimen is collected following a period of abstinence of at least 3 days and is examined within 2 hours. Normal semen has a volume of >1.5 mL and a sperm concentration of >15 million/mL. More than 40% of the sperm should be motile. The morphology, biochemistry and viability of the sperm may also be studied. In selected cases, immunological tests may help to determine the cause of infertility.

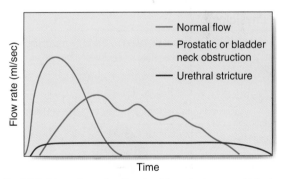

Fig. 23.7 Urinary flow rates. The normal flow rate shows a rapid rise to maximum high-peak flow. In a typical bladder outflow obstruction due to benign prostatic hyperplasia, there is a slow rise to poor maximum flow rate and prolonged variable flow. In a typical urethral stricture, there is prolonged flow with little variability, giving a plateau- or box-shaped curve.

Biochemical screening for stones

Recurrent urinary tract calculi should raise the suspicion of hyperparathyroidism, idiopathic hypercalciuria, hyperoxaluria, cystinuria, renal tubular acidosis or medullary sponge kidney. Serum calcium, phosphate, oxalate and uric acid should be measured. If more detailed investigation is required a 24-hour collection of urine for determination of calcium, phosphate, oxalate and uric acid excretion can be obtained. The composition of passed or removed stones should be analysed to determine their metabolic type.

Upper urinary tract (kidney and ureter)

Anatomy

The two kidneys lie retroperitoneally on the posterior abdominal wall. Each is approximately 12 cm long, 6 cm wide and 3 cm thick. The upper pole of the kidney lies on the diaphragm, which separates it from the pleura and the 11th and 12th ribs. Below this, it lies on the psoas, quadratus lumborum and transversus abdominis muscles from medial to lateral (Fig. 23.8). Anteriorly, the right kidney is covered by the liver, the second part of the duodenum and the ascending colon. The spleen, stomach, tail of pancreas, left colon and small bowel overlie the left kidney. The renal hilum lies medially and transmits from front to back over the renal vein, renal artery and renal pelvis. The ureter begins at the renal pelvis and runs for 25 cm to the bladder. The abdominal ureter lies on the medial edge of the psoas muscle, which separates it from the tips of the transverse processes. It then crosses the bifurcation of the common iliac artery, which separates it from the sacroiliac joint, to enter the pelvis. The pelvic ureter runs on the lateral pelvic wall to just in front of the ischial spine, when it then turns medially and forward to enter the bladder. In the male, it is crossed by the vas deferens. In the female, it lies close to the lateral fornix of the vagina and is crossed by the uterine vessels, where it is vulnerable to damage during hysterectomy. The section of ureter that lies within the bladder wall functions as a flap valve to prevent reflux. Stones tend to impact at the three points where the ureter narrows: namely, the pelviureteric junction (PUJ), the pelvic brim and the ureteric orifice.

Physiology

The healthy kidney produces between 0.3 and 17 mL of urine per minute, depending on the state of hydration, but on average produces 1 mL of urine per minute. This is transported down the ureter by 4–5 peristaltic waves per minute to reach the bladder.

Simple renal cysts

These are usually single and almost always asymptomatic. They are often found incidentally during ultrasonography and can usually be differentiated from carcinoma. Complex cysts containing multiple septa raise the suspicion of malignant change and need further evaluation by CT scanning.

Polycystic kidney disease

This is an autosomal dominant congenital anomaly affecting both kidneys, often leading to chronic renal failure in middle life. Despite their very large size, the cystic kidneys cause few symptoms. Infection or bleeding may occur in a cyst, causing pain or haematuria.

Horseshoe kidneys

The incidence is 1 in 400–800 live births, and is the most common fusion anomaly of the kidney. The fused mass usually has two collecting systems and two ureters. They are almost always malrotated with the pelves facing anteriorly, and also have an incomplete ascent, lying lower than the normal kidneys. They are usually asymptomatic and are discovered incidentally on imaging. Occasionally they may present with obstruction and resultant pain.

Other developmental anomalies

The common developmental anomalies seen are unilateral renal agenesis, renal ectopia, crossed renal ectopia and various degrees of duplication of the collecting system. All of these are compatible with a normal life, and are usually detected in adult life as incidental findings on imaging investigations.

Benign tumours

Oncocytomas are the commonest benign kidney tumour which can be difficult to differentiate from a kidney cancer on imaging. Angiomyolipomas, commonly associated with tuberous sclerosis, are characterised by a typical appearance on CT due to their high fat content. Treatment is observation, embolization or surgery and is dictated by symptoms and size.

Nephroblastomas

Epidemiology

Also known as Wilms' tumour, it usually occurs in children under 4 years of age, and is the most common childhood urological malignancy, with an incidence of 7 per million per year. Growth is rapid and there is early local spread, including invasion of the renal vein. Invasion of the renal pelvis occurs late, and so haematuria is seen in only 15% of cases. Distant metastases most commonly appear in the lungs, liver and bones. Tumours presenting in the first year of life have a better prognosis.

Clinical features

The cardinal sign is a large abdominal mass. Some of the unusual clinical features associated with a renal carcinoma in adults, such as fever or hypertension, may be present. Clinically it needs to be differentiated from neuroblastoma (Table 23.2).

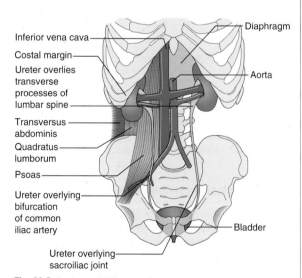

Inferior vena cava
Costal margin
Ureter overlies transverse processes of lumbar spine
Transversus abdominis
Quadratus lumborum
Psoas
Ureter overlying bifurcation of common iliac artery
Ureter overlying sacroiliac joint
Diaphragm
Aorta
Bladder

Fig. 23.8 Anatomy of kidneys and ureters.

Table 23.2 Childhood renal tumours

Feature	Nephroblastoma	Neuroblastoma
Frequency	7 per million children	1 per 8000-10,000 children
Age	Between 3 and 5 years of age	<2 years of age
Origin	Kidney	Adrenal, also extra-adrenal
Symptoms	Hypertension in 25–60%	Uncommon
Abdominal lump	Unilateral, never crosses midline	May cross midline
Radiologically	No change in renal axis	Outward and downward displacement of kidney; calcification common
Metastases at presentation	Uncommon	Bony metastases common
Tumour markers	Serum LDH may be raised	VMA may be raised
Treatment	Surgery mainstay, adjuvant chemotherapy for metastases	Chemotherapy, radiotherapy and surgery

LDH, lactate dehydrogenase; VMA, vanillylmandelic acid.

Investigations

CT of the abdomen and chest is essential for diagnosis and staging. The main differential diagnosis to consider is adrenal neuroblastoma, but other causes of a large kidney, such as hydronephrosis and cystic disease, must also be considered. The tumour is bilateral in 5–10% of cases.

Management

The diagnosis is confirmed by biopsy. Chemotherapy is followed by transabdominal nephrectomy with wide excision of the mass. Further chemotherapy with or without radiotherapy is administered dependent upon the histopathological features; the 5-year survival rate is in the region of 70–90%.

Renal cell carcinoma

Epidemiology

Renal cell carcinoma (RCC) arises from the renal tubules and is the most common malignant tumour of the kidney. The incidence is 16 cases per 100,000, being 1.6-fold more common in males. It is uncommon before the age of 40 years, but there is a sharp increase in incidence from 45 to 49 years and a peak incidence between 80 and 85 years of age. Invasion of the renal vein, often extending into the inferior vena cava, and occasionally into the right atrium, can occur. Direct spread into perinephric tissues is common, so that the whole fascial envelope and kidney should be removed en bloc. Lymphatic spread occurs to para-aortic nodes; blood-borne metastases (which may be solitary) are most common in the lungs (cannon ball metastases) but may develop anywhere.

Clinical features

The triad of pain, haematuria and a palpable mass occurs in only 15% of cases. Historically, 60% presented with haematuria, 40% with loin pain and 25% with a mass, but increasing access to US and CT has increased incidental diagnosis to ~50%. Patients may present with pyrexia of unknown origin, raised ESR, polycythaemia, disorders of coagulation, and abnormalities of plasma proteins and liver function tests, or with neuromyopathy due to secretion of renin, erythropoietin, parathormone and gonadotrophins; making RCC the 'great mimic'.

Investigations

The initial investigation is US or CT urogram, followed by a full staging CT of abdomen and chest (Fig. 23.9). In young RCC patients with a family history of the disease, genetic testing for a familial syndrome should be performed.

Pathology

There are numerous histological subtypes of RCC. The most common is clear cell RCC (85%), followed by papillary RCC (comprised of type 1 and type 2). Chromophobe and collecting duct RCC are less common. RCC may develop in a range of inherited syndromes, i.e., von Hippel–Lindau syndrome and Birt–Hogg–Dubé syndrome.

Tumour staging

Tumour, Node, Metastasis (TNM) staging is used (Table 23.3).

Management

Organ-confined RCC should be treated with curative intent, either by laparoscopic or open nephrectomy. Tumours (<7 cm) confined to one pole of the kidney are treated by partial nephrectomy (using an open, robot assisted or laparoscopic approach) with oncological results as good as with radical nephrectomy. Metastatic RCC is relatively radio- and chemo-resistant. Multitarget tyrosine kinase inhibitors (TKIs), which are antiangiogenic, provide a median 12 months progression-free survival benefit. It is unknown if there is a definite survival benefit by performing a cytoreductive nephrectomy prior to starting TKIs. Novel immunotherapeutic agents (T-cell checkpoint inhibitors) show promise in improving outcomes in metastatic RCC, they have a proven survival advantage in the 2nd line setting, further Phase III trials are awaited.

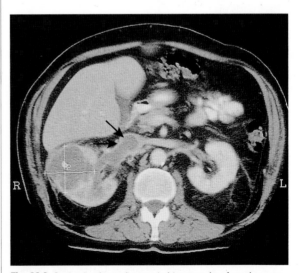

Fig. 23.9 Contrast-enhanced computed tomography of renal cancer. The right kidney is expanded by a low-density cancer that fails to take up the contrast. Tumour is seen extending into the renal vein and inferior vena cava (*arrow*).

Table 23.3 TNM-7 classification of kidney cancer

T (Tumour)

- T_0 — No evidence of primary tumour
- T_X — Primary tumour cannot be assessed
- T_1 — Tumour <7 cm in greatest dimension, limited to the kidney
  - T_{1a} — Tumour <4 cm in greatest dimension, limited to the kidney
  - T_{1b} — Tumour >4 cm but <7 cm in greatest dimension
- T_2 — Tumour >7 cm in greatest dimension, limited to the kidney
  - T_{2a} — Tumour >7 cm but <10 cm in greatest dimension
  - T_{2b} — Tumours >10 cm limited to the kidney
- T_3 — Tumour extends into major veins or perinephric tissues but not into the ipsilateral adrenal gland or beyond Gerota's fascia
  - T_{3a} — Tumour grossly extends into the renal vein or its segmental (muscle-containing) branches, or invades perirenal and/or renal sinus fat (peripelvic), but not beyond Gerota's fascia
  - T_{3b} — Tumour grossly extends into the IVC below the diaphragm
  - T_{3c} — Tumour grossly extends into IVC above the diaphragm or invades the wall of the IVC
- T_4 — Tumour invades beyond Gerota's fascia (including contiguous extension into the ipsilateral adrenal gland)

N (Nodes)

- N_0 — No regional lymph node metastasis
- N_X — Regional lymph nodes cannot be assessed
- N_1 — Regional lymph node metastasis

M (Metastases)

- M_0 — No distant metastasis detected
- M_X — Distant metastasis cannot be assessed
- M_1 — Distant metastasis

IVC, Inferior Vena cava.
Courtesy Sobin LH, Gospodariwicz M, Wittekind C (eds). TNM classification of malignant tumors. UICC International Union Against Cancer. 7th ed. Wiley-Blackwell, 2009: pp. 255–7 and 243–248, with permission.

23.1 Summary

Renal carcinoma

- Renal cell carcinoma is the most common malignant renal tumour and is 1.6 fold more common in males
- The carcinoma arises in the renal tubules. Renal cancer may involve the renal vein (with bloodstream dissemination), perinephric tissue and lymphatic spread
- The clinical presentation is varied. The triad of pain, haematuria and a mass may be late features, and early systemic effects include fever, polycythaemia, disordered coagulation and pyrexia of unknown origin
- The key investigation is CT of the chest and abdomen
- Treatment consists of radical nephrectomy; the tumour is not radiosensitive. The natural history of renal carcinoma is very variable and excision of solitary metastases may be worthwhile.

Upper urinary tract urothelial cell cancer

Epidemiology

Upper urinary tract urothelial cell cancer (UUTUCC) of the renal pelvis or ureter are rare tumours accounting for only 5–10% of urothelial cell carcinomas. They have a similar morphology to bladder carcinomas and nearly all UTUCs are urothelial in origin. UUTUCC is three times more common in males, with a peak incidence in patients aged 70–90 years. Patients with a carcinoma of the upper tract have a 30–50% risk of developing bladder carcinoma, whereas conversely, the risk of a patient with bladder carcinoma developing upper tract malignancy is only 1–4%. Smoking, exposure to dyes and solvents, and analgesic abuse have been identified as risk factors.

Clinical features

Visible haematuria is the most common symptom and is seen in 70–90% of patients. Flank pain and dysuria are other presenting symptoms.

Investigations

UUTUCC is usually identified as a mass or filling defect on CT urogram. Any suspicious filling defects require ureteroscopy and biopsy for pathological diagnosis. The extent of local and distant spread can be determined by CT of chest, abdomen and pelvis.

Management

The standard treatment for UUTUCC is radical (open or laparoscopic) nephroureterectomy along with a cuff of bladder as the disease can be multifocal within the ipsilateral collecting system. In frail patients or those with a single kidney, ureteroscopic laser fulguration of the UUTUCC may be adequate treatment, but requires close follow-up. In metastatic disease, chemotherapy is used if the patient has an adequate performance status.

Urinary tract calculi

Mechanism of stone formation

The ability of urine to keep compounds in solution and prevent calculus formation is a balance between forces keeping the solute in solution and those that promote crystal formation. Stones form when the amount of solute increases (e.g., hypercalciuria), the amount of solvent decreases (e.g., dehydration) or the concentration of inhibitors falls (e.g., decreased citrate excretion). Foreign bodies, anatomical abnormalities, and calculi can all act as a nidus for nucleation and promote further stone formation.

Types and causes of stone formation

The most common stone types are calcium oxalate (85%), uric acid (10%), mixed calcium phosphate calcium oxalate (10%), magnesium ammonium phosphate (5–15%) and cystine (1%). Calcium oxalate stones are commonly caused by hypercalciuria, hypercalcaemia, hyperoxaluria or hypocitraturia. Uric acid stones form due to increases in uric acid formation, either through gout or myeloproliferative disorders. Approximately 50% of patients with urate stones have gout but only 20% of patients with gout develop urate stones. Calcium phosphate stones are generally secondary to renal tubular acidosis. Magnesium ammonium phosphate (struvite) stones are usually due to UTI by pathogens that can break urea down into CO_2 and ammonia, thereby alkalinising the urine (e.g., *Proteus mirabilis*).

Radiolucent calculi

Uric acid, xanthine, indinavir, triamterene and matrix calculi are the common radiolucent varieties, and are not visualised on a plain film. A noncontrast CT KUB is the modality of choice for these, except indinavir calculi, which appear radiolucent even on a noncontrast CT.

Clinical features

Renal calculi cause flank pain, which may be colicky (arising from the renal pelvis) or a noncolicky dull ache (arising from renal capsule). Ureteric calculi cause colicky pain and the site of the stone in the ureter determines the site of the pain: upper ureteric calculi cause costovertebral angle or flank pain, mid-ureteric calculi cause pain radiating from 'loin to groin', and lower ureteric calculi cause pain radiating to the testicle in males and labia majora in females. Renal pain, renal colic and ureteric colic are characteristically unilateral. Vesical calculus may lead to suprapubic pain, recurrent UTIs, intermittent urinary stream or urgency. Any stone may also cause haematuria. However, a stone in the kidney may remain silent, even one large enough to fill the pelvis and calyces ('staghorn' calculus). Urethral calculi may be secondary (passing down from the bladder) or primary (due to a stricture or diverticulum in the urethra), and present with dysuria and pain radiating to the tip of penis.

Investigations

CT KUB provides all the necessary information on the position and size of the stone (Fig. 23.10). Ultrasonography is a noninvasive investigation that is easily available and provides a lot of information in renal and vesical calculus disease, without any radiation exposure (preferred in children, women of childbearing age and pregnant females).

Routine haematological and biochemical tests are needed to assess renal function and to exclude metabolic causes. Urine culture will determine if there is infection. If obstruction is acute, its relief is the prime clinical need; if it is chronic and has caused renal damage, the surgical approach depends on the function of the affected kidney. This is best determined by radioisotope methods.

Management

Symptomatic treatment should be instituted as soon as the diagnosis is confirmed. Intramuscular diclofenac, a nonsteroidal anti-inflammatory, is the most effective analgesic; pethidine is an alternative. The likelihood of spontaneous passage of a renal or ureteric calculus depends on the size of the stone and on its smoothness. A stone less than 5 mm in diameter should pass easily. The location of the stone in the ureter also determines the ease with which it will pass: small lower ureteric stones having a higher likelihood compared with larger upper or mid-ureteric calculus. Immediate treatment should be considered in cases of ongoing pain, renal obstruction or, more importantly, where there are signs of sepsis (infected obstructed kidney).

Extracorporeal shockwave lithotripsy (ESWL), the technique of focusing external shock waves to break up stones, has revolutionised the treatment of renal and ureteric stones. Stones visualised on x-ray or US can be treated by ESWL, especially those that are single and up to 2 cm in size. Other stones can be visualised directly by ureterorenoscopy (URS), and the stones broken up using a holmium laser or removed intact using a Dormia wire basket. Some stones in the kidney that are unlikely to pass, even if broken up, are best treated by direct puncture of the kidney, insertion of a sheath and removal under vision with a nephroscope with or without ultrasonic disaggregation (percutaneous nephrolithotomy). It is now very rare to perform open surgery to remove renal or ureteric stones. Even large staghorn calculi filling the entire renal collecting system can be treated by percutaneous nephrolithotomy (PCNL) with our without ESWL (multiple sessions may be required). In developing countries in Asia and Africa, where the expertise for the latest noninvasive techniques is not available, large kidney stones continue to be treated by conventional open surgery.

In patients with acute obstruction and sepsis (infected obstructed kidney) or renal impairment, decompression of the kidney either via insertion of a ureteric stent or percutaneous

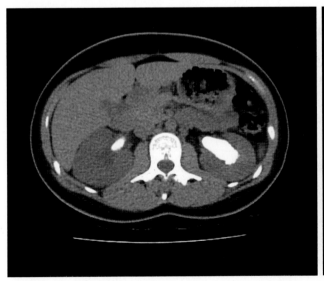
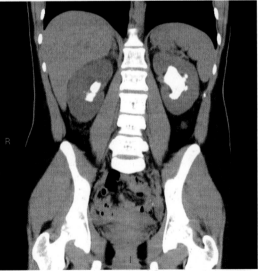

Fig. 23.10 Computed tomography kidney-ureter-bladder showing bilateral staghorn calculi. The patient was rendered stone free with bilateral percutaneous nephrolithotomies.

nephrostomy is required. Stones and infection within a kidney can be the cause of renal destruction and if the kidney contributes less than 15% of total renal function, then nephrectomy is recommended.

Vesical calculi can be treated endoscopically like ureteric calculi, using a stone-crushing device, pneumatic lithotrite or holmium laser. Alternatively, large stones can be dealt with through an open suprapubic cystolithotomy, or by suprapubic insertion of a nephroscope and the use of ultrasonic shattering.

Primary urethral calculi are treated along with the inciting cause. Secondary calculi impacted in the urethra may be removed intact endoscopically if small, or may have to be crushed and removed.

Infections of the kidney

Acute pyelonephritis

Acute pyelonephritis is a bacterial infection of the renal parenchyma and collecting system. The causative organisms are the same as for UTI (gram-negative enteric organisms), as most infections are ascending infections from the lower tracts. It classically presents as sudden onset of fever with chills and unilateral or bilateral flank pain. It may be associated with lower tract symptoms such as dysuria, frequency and urgency.

Diagnosis is by way of urine culture. Blood counts may show the presence of leucocytosis with predominance of neutrophils. Imaging modalities are seldom needed. US or CT may reveal the presence of an enlarged kidney on the affected side.

Management is aimed at treating the infection. Antibiotics are started empirically with clinical diagnosis, and may have to be revised once the culture and sensitivity reports are available. They should be continued for 2–3 weeks. Patients with sepsis may have to be hospitalised and administered intravenous antibiotics. Absence of response to treatment after 48–72 hours should alert the surgeon towards development of complications such as a renal abscess or the presence of associated urinary tract obstruction, which is an emergency and requires urgent decompression.

Chronic pyelonephritis

Chronic pyelonephritis denotes the process of scarring and atrophy of renal parenchyma, ultimately resulting in renal insufficiency. The most common association, especially in children, is with vesicoureteric reflux, hence it is often called reflux nephropathy.

The condition is usually silent and is discovered incidentally on investigating abnormal renal functions. Imaging may show a small contracted and scarred kidney that is poorly functioning.

Management is aimed at preventing further damage to the kidneys by recurrent UTIs. The damage that has already resulted is irreversible.

Renal and perinephric abscess

The aetiology and pathogenesis of renal abscesses has changed with the use of antibiotics. Whereas the haematogenous route was the most common route of infection in the past, currently most infections ascend from lower tracts. The haematogenous infections are mostly caused by gram-positive bacteria and are located in the subcapsular and cortical regions of the kidney. Ascending infections, on the other hand, are caused by gram-negative pathogens, and are located in the corticomedullary region. Perinephric abscesses usually result from extension of renal abscesses in the perinephric space. The bacteriology is therefore the same.

Patients usually present with fever associated with chills, flank pain, and systemic symptoms such as nausea and malaise. Blood counts may reveal neutrophilia and urinalysis pyuria and bacteriuria. Imaging studies are important in making a diagnosis, and CT is the modality of choice.

Management involves hospitalisation, antibiotic therapy and supportive treatment, followed by US- or CT-guided drainage. If percutaneous drainage fails to resolve the abscess, open surgical drainage may be needed.

Emphysematous pyelonephritis

Emphysematous pyelonephritis (EPN) is a severe necrotising infection of the renal parenchyma; it causes gas formation within the collecting system, renal parenchyma and/or perirenal tissues. It is common in diabetics, and the presentation is similar to that of acute pyelonephritis. However, the clinical course of EPN can be severe and life-threatening if not recognised and treated promptly.

Patients are usually unwell and typically present with fever, abdominal or flank pain, nausea and vomiting, and may be in septic shock. Radiological evaluation with CT diagnoses the problem.

Patients with EPN should be treated with aggressive medical management and, wherever needed, prompt surgical intervention. Initial resuscitation with fluids, control of diabetes, and administration of intravenous antibiotics empirically is important in stabilising the patient.

Percutaneous drainage combined with antibiotic therapy is useful in early cases associated with gas in the collecting system alone and when the patient is otherwise stable. It may also be useful in patients with compromised renal function. Nephrectomy is frequently the treatment of choice, especially when patients are sick, with evidence of gas in the renal parenchyma or if there is no access to percutaneous drainage.

The mortality rate associated with EPN was high before the advent of antibiotics; however, advances in imaging technology, control of diabetes, resuscitative management, and minimally invasive treatment have improved the outcome.

Genitourinary tuberculosis

Genitourinary tuberculosis is usually a secondary infection, the primary focus being somewhere else. Kidneys are the most frequently affected organ followed by bladder and ureter. *Mycobacterium tuberculosis* is the causative organism and the disease is still common in many developing countries and in the presence of HIV infection.

Pathogenesis

Haematogenous seeding of bacteria leads to involvement of the renal cortex in a susceptible individual. The infection is asymptomatic and slowly progressive. The focus slowly expands from the cortex and involves the calyces and the pelvis, resulting in (sterile) pyuria and bacteriuria. At a more advanced stage, caseous breakdown of the renal cortex and medulla occurs, resulting in formation of what is known as 'putty kidney'.

Involvement of the ureter and the bladder occurs, with the latter manifesting as urinary frequency. Ureteric involvement leads to progressive fibrosis and stricture formation, leading to back pressure changes. Ureteric fibrosis leads to straightening and shortening of the ureter, pulling the opening in the bladder, which therefore assumes a 'golf hole configuration'. Tuberculous cystitis leads to formation of tubercles, starting in the periureteric region, which may coalesce and ulcerate, leading to haematuria. Severe bladder involvement leads to fibrosis resulting in a small capacity contracted bladder (thimble bladder) and marked urinary frequency.

Passage of infected urine through the lower tracts may lead to involvement of prostate, seminal vesicles, epididymis and testes.

Clinical features

The symptoms of genitourinary tuberculosis are nonspecific. Early storage-type symptoms are due to involvement of the bladder. Renal involvement may lead to a dull ache in the flank. Occasionally there may be haematuria, but a more common finding is sterile pyuria. Clinical examination may reveal a thick and beaded vas deferens and a thickened epididymis.

Investigations and diagnosis

Urinalysis reveals the presence of pyuria without bacteria (sterile pyuria). Direct smears of the first morning-voided urine for acid-fast bacilli may provide an early diagnosis. Culture of first morning-voided urine for tuberculous bacteria is often positive.

An IVU is often normal in early disease. Advanced cases may reveal the presence of distorted calyces with partial obliteration and/or dilatation, or single/multiple ureteric strictures with proximal dilatation. In late stages, absence of visualisation of the kidney may occur due to complete ureteric obstruction or renal destruction (autonephrectomy).

Cystoscopic examination may reveal the presence and extent of vesical involvement and provide a biopsy specimen for confirmation of diagnosis.

Management

The primary treatment is medical. Standard antituberculous treatment for 12–18 months is effective. Shorter courses usually result in incomplete resolution and/or relapse. Complications like renal or perinephric abscess and nonfunctioning kidney may necessitate surgical intervention in the form of drainage or nephrectomy. A contracted bladder may need augmentation cystoplasty or cystectomy and urinary diversion.

Urinary tract obstruction

Obstruction may be classified according to cause (congenital or acquired), duration (acute or chronic), degree (partial or complete) and level (upper or lower urinary tract) (Table 23.4 and Fig. 23.11).

Pelviureteric junction obstruction

Narrowing of the junction between the renal pelvis and the ureter is a common cause of hydronephrosis. This condition can present at any age. It is likely to be congenital and can be bilateral.

Table 23.4 Cause of urinary tract obstruction

Variety	Unilateral	Bilateral
Upper tract		
Congenital	Unilateral pelviureteric junction obstruction Ureteric stricture Ectopic ureter Ureterocoele Unilateral vesicoureteric reflux Unilateral vesicoureteric junction obstruction	Bilateral pelviureteric junction obstruction Meatal stenosis Posterior urethral valves Bilateral ectopic ureters Ureterocoele Bilateral vesicoureteric reflux Bilateral vesicoureteric junction obstruction Neural tube defects
Acquired	Ureteric stricture Ureteric calculus Bladder tumour Local extension of ca prostate/ca cervix/ca rectum Retroperitoneal fibrosis Pregnancy	Ureteric stricture Bilateral ureteric calculi Bladder neck stenosis BPH Bladder calculus Bladder tumour Local extension of ca prostate/ca cervix/ca rectum Retroperitoneal fibrosis Urethral stricture Neurogenic bladder
Lower tract		
Congenital	Meatal stenosis Posterior urethral valves	
Acquired	BPH Bladder calculus Bladder tumour Urethral stricture Urethral calculus	

BPH, Benign prostatic hyperplasia; ca, cancer.

Clinical features

In its grossest form, PUJ obstruction may produce a large, painless mass in the loin and the volume of urine in the hydronephrotic sac may simulate free fluid in the peritoneal cavity. However, the more usual moderate hydronephrosis causes ill-defined renal pain or ache that may be exacerbated by drinking large volumes of liquid (Dietls' crisis). The patient may regard these symptoms as 'indigestion'. Rarely, there may be no symptoms.

Investigations

CT urogram provides sufficient information in many cases. The calibre of the ureter is normal. There are a few patients in whom there is doubt as to whether the dilatation of the pelvis and calyces is truly obstructive in nature. In these cases, a mercaptoacetyltriglycine (MAG-3) renogram is performed to provide information about drainage of the kidney and also an estimate of differential renal function.

Management

Laparoscopic, open or robotic assisted pyeloplasty is performed to remove the obstructing tissue and refashion the

23

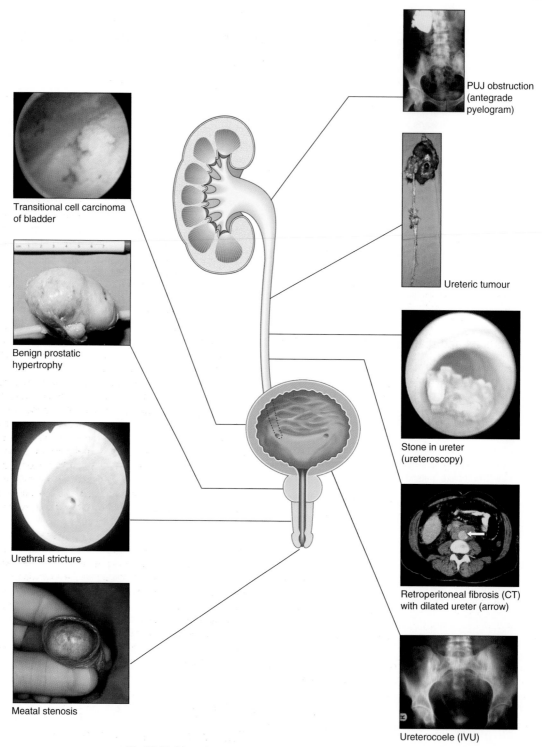

PUJ obstruction (antegrade pyelogram)

Ureteric tumour

Transitional cell carcinoma of bladder

Benign prostatic hypertrophy

Urethral stricture

Meatal stenosis

Stone in ureter (ureteroscopy)

Retroperitoneal fibrosis (CT) with dilated ureter (arrow)

Ureterocoele (IVU)

Fig. 23.11 Common causes of urinary tract obstruction with their sites.

PUJ so that the lower part of the renal pelvis drains freely into the ureter. The dismembered (Anderson–Hynes) pyeoloplasy (Fig. 23.12) is the gold-standard procedure. Not uncommonly, PUJ obstruction is due to an aberrant vessel supplying the lower pole of kidney crossing in front of it. This vessel can be preserved by bringing the newly formed PUJ anteriorly. It is not possible to predict the degree of recovery of renal function after the relief of obstruction, but a kidney contributing less than 15% of total renal function on a nuclear medicine scanning is usually removed.

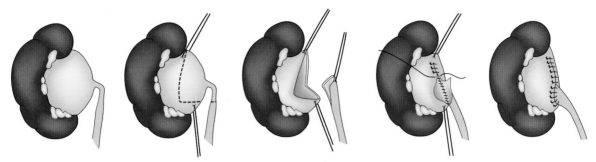

Fig. 23.12 Anderson–Hynes pyeloplasty.

23.2 Summary

Urinary tract obstruction

Common causes of obstruction of the lower outflow tract
- Benign prostatic hyperplasia
- Prostatic cancer
- Bladder cancer involving the bladder neck
- Bladder-neck obstruction (dyssynergia, infection, neurological disorders)
- Urethral obstruction (congenital posterior urethral valves, blocked urinary catheter, trauma, infection, stricture).

Common causes of obstruction of the upper urinary tract
- Renal and ureteric calculi (80% are calcium oxalate/phosphate stones)
- Pelviureteric junction obstruction (idiopathic hydronephrosis)
- Retroperitoneal fibrosis (idiopathic/malignant infiltration/radiotherapy)
- Urothelial cell cancer (with or without bleeding and clot)
- Congenital abnormalities (e.g., ectopic ureter, ureterocele)
- Infections (notably schistosomiasis and tuberculosis).

Renal trauma

Renal trauma may be blunt or penetrating, accounts for 10% of abdominal trauma and ranges from a contusion on/around the kidney to a shattered or avulsed kidney. Diagnosis is usually confirmed by CT, ideally with an angiographic phase to assess for vascular injury and a delayed phase to determine if there is a breach of the collecting system. The majority of patients with renal trauma can be managed conservatively, as the bleeding is tamponaded in the closed retroperitoneum, with close monitoring, bed rest and monitoring of the degree of visible haematuria. If active bleeding is identified on imaging and the patient is stable, radiological selective embolisation of the bleeding vessel can be utilised. However, if the patient is haemodynamically unstable, if surgery is being undertaken for other injuries or if there is avulsion of the kidney from the vascular pedicle, surgical management (usually a nephrectomy) should be undertaken.

Lower urinary tract (bladder, prostate and urethra)

Anatomy

The bladder is a muscular reservoir that receives urine via the ureters and expels it via the urethra. In children up to 4 years of age, it lies predominantly in the abdomen; in the adult it is a pelvic organ, well protected in the bony pelvis. Superiorly, the bladder is covered with peritoneum, which separates it from loops of small bowel, the sigmoid colon and, in the female, the body of the uterus. Posteriorly lie the rectum, the vas deferens and seminal vesicles in the male, and the vagina and supravaginal cervix in the female. Inferiorly, the neck of the bladder transmits the urethra and fuses with the prostate in the male and with the pelvic fascia in the female.

The bladder is composed of whorls of detrusor muscle, which in the male become circular at the bladder neck. They are richly supplied with sympathetic nerves that cause contraction during ejaculation, thereby preventing semen from entering the bladder (retrograde ejaculation). There is no such sphincter in the female. The bladder is lined with specialised waterproof epithelium, the urothelium. This is thrown into folds over most of the bladder, except the trigone where it is smooth.

The male urethra is 20 cm long; the prostatic urethra descends for 3 cm through the prostate gland, and the membranous urethra is 1–2 cm long and intimately associated with the main urethral sphincter, the rhabdosphincter. The spongy urethra is 15 cm long and is surrounded by the corpus spongiosus throughout its complete length, opening on the tip of the glans penis as the external meatus. The spongy urethra is further subdivided into the proximal bulbar urethra and the distal penile urethra. The female urethra is 3–4 cm long, descending through the pelvic floor surrounded by the urethral sphincter and embedded in the anterior vaginal wall to open between the clitoris and the vagina.

In the male, the prostate is pyramidal, with its base uppermost. It resembles the size and shape of a chestnut and surrounds the prostatic urethra. Traditionally described as having a median and two lateral lobes, it is better considered as being composed of a small central and a larger peripheral zone (Fig. 23.13). The prostate is surrounded by a venous plexus, which lies between its true and false capsule. Enucleation of the prostate gland in open prostatectomy leaves behind both the capsules since the plane of separation is between the enlarged adenoma and the compressed peripheral zone, which is prone to carcinoma.

Physiology

Neurological control of micturition

Detrusor contraction is mediated through cholinergic parasympathetic nerves arising from the nerve roots S2–S4, and relayed through ganglia lying predominantly within the detrusor. Sympathetic nerves arise from T10 to L2 and relay via the pelvic ganglia. Their exact role in the control of micturition is unclear. It is known that α-adrenergic receptors and their nerve terminals are found mainly in the smooth muscle of the bladder neck and proximal urethra. The α-receptors respond to noradrenaline (norepinephrine) by stimulating contraction, thereby maintaining closure of the bladder neck.

23

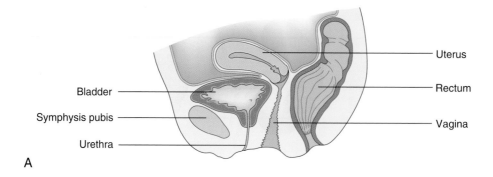

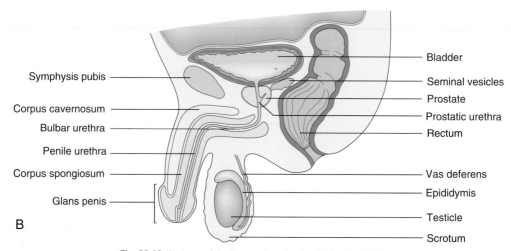

Fig. 23.13 Anatomy of the lower urinary tracts. (A) Female. (B) Male.

The distal sphincter mechanism is innervated from the sacral segments S2–S4 by somatic motor fibres that reach the sphincter either by the pelvic plexus or via the pudendal nerves. Afferent nerves are carried in both the parasympathetic and pudendal pathways, and transmit sensory impulses from the bladder, urethra and pelvic floor. These sensory impulses pass to the cerebral cortex and the micturition centre, where they produce reflex bladder relaxation and increased tone in the distal sphincter, so helping maintain continence. Cortical control is a basic part of the micturition cycle described below. The higher centres suppress detrusor contractions and their main function is to inhibit micturition until an appropriate time.

The micturition cycle

The micturition cycle has two phases.

Storage (or filling) phase

Due to the high compliance (elasticity) of the detrusor muscle, the bladder fills steadily without a rise in intravesical pressure. As urine volume increases, stretch receptors in the bladder wall are stimulated, resulting in reflex bladder relaxation and reflex increased sphincter tone. At three-quarters of bladder capacity, sensation produces a desire to void. Voluntary control is now exerted over the desire to void, which temporarily disappears. Compliance of the detrusor allows further increase in capacity until the next desire to void. Just how often this desire needs to be inhibited depends on many factors, not the least of which is finding a suitable place to void.

Emptying (or micturition) phase

The act of micturition is initiated first by voluntary and then by reflex relaxation of the pelvic floor and distal sphincter mechanisms, followed by reflex detrusor contraction. These actions are coordinated by the pontine micturition centre. Intravesical pressure remains greater than urethral pressure until the bladder is empty.

The normal control of micturition requires coordinated reflex activity of autonomic and somatic nerves, as described above. These responses depend on normal anatomical structures and normal innervation. There are thus two main types of disorders of micturition: structural and neurogenic. Examples are extensive carcinoma of the prostate that has damaged the sphincter mechanism (structural), and spinal cord injury that has damaged the innervation (neurogenic).

Lower urinary tract trauma

Bladder

Open injuries

The bladder may be damaged as a result of penetrating injury to the lower abdomen, or during pelvic surgery; damage to the urethra, rectum, vagina or uterus may also occur. Unrecognised damage during surgical procedures may lead to a wound fistula, a vesicovaginal fistula or a vesicocolic fistula.

Closed injuries

Intraperitoneal rupture typically occurs in a patient who has been drinking alcohol, has a full bladder and is assaulted and kicked in

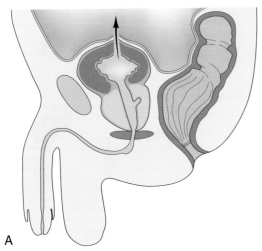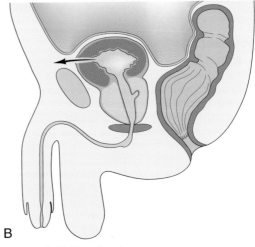

A   B

Fig. 23.14 Rupture of the bladder. (A) Intraperitoneal. **(B)** Extraperitoneal.

the abdomen. The dome of the bladder ruptures and urine extravasates into the peritoneum, causing intestinal ileus and abdominal distension. Extraperitoneal rupture is usually due to a major road traffic accident in which the pelvis has also been fractured, but may follow endoscopic resection of the prostate or a bladder tumour (Fig. 23.14).

Clinical features

The ileus and distension that occur with intraperitoneal rupture of the bladder are often detected late because of the circumstances surrounding the injury, although the patient may seek advice due to the inability to pass urine. Extraperitoneal extravasation of urine, due to major blunt trauma, adds to what already may be severe pelvic injuries. When the leak occurs following an endoscopic procedure, the patient subsequently complains of suprapubic pain with varying degrees of lower abdominal tenderness.

Investigations

Generally, the circumstances of the bladder injury establish the diagnosis. If confirmation of injury is required, water-soluble contrast is injected via a urethral catheter and the bladder examined on the x-ray screen (cystogram).

Management

Intraperitoneal rupture requires laparotomy and repair. Extraperitoneal rupture in the absence of other injuries tends to be managed conservatively with drainage of the bladder using a urethral catheter left in situ for 5–7 days. Occasionally, surgical exploration is required.

Urethra

Open injuries

Penetrating injuries resulting in damage to the anterior or posterior urethra are rare.

Closed injuries

Damage to the anterior urethra (penile and bulbar urethra) is typically due to falling astride a hard object, although a kick can cause a similar injury. The mechanism of injury to the posterior urethra (membranous and prostatic urethra) is similar to that of extraperitoneal rupture of the bladder. In the majority of cases, posterior urethral injuries are associated with a pelvic fracture. Both the posterior urethra and bladder are damaged in 10% of cases.

Clinical features

Anterior urethral injuries are usually located at the bulb, so that the patient presents with a perineal haematoma. If this becomes infected, there may be sloughing of the skin, urethra and even the scrotal tissues. If the patient has passed clear urine, the bladder and urethra are probably intact. If there is blood at the external meatus, urethral injury must be suspected. A distended bladder can occur because of spasm of the urethral sphincter or because of a torn posterior urethra.

Investigations

If physical signs suggest an anterior urethral injury, and the patient has passed clear urine, no further steps need be taken. If there is blood at the external meatus or the urine is blood-stained, a urethrogram using water-soluble contrast material may demonstrate extravasation (Fig. 23.15). *A catheter should never be passed in the emergency room.* If urine is blood-stained, retrograde urethrography may be carried out, but radiological distinction between a

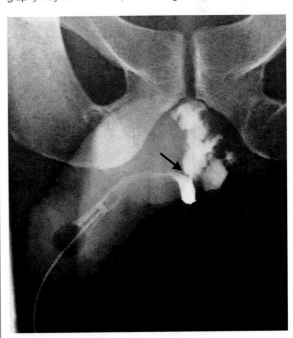

Fig. 23.15 Ascending ureterogram in urethral rupture. Contrast is seen extravasating at the site of the disrupted urethra (*arrow*).

23

rupture of the membranous urethra and an extraperitoneal bladder rupture may be difficult.

Management

All patients with an injury to the bulb of the urethra have a perineal haematoma. If the injury is only a contusion, this will resolve, but prophylactic antibiotics are indicated. A large haematoma may require drainage if the urethra has been lacerated. The extent of injury should be defined and the urethra repaired if possible. A urethral or suprapubic catheter drains the bladder. Treatment of a posterior urethral injury depends on the expertise available. It is quite acceptable to perform a suprapubic cystostomy and deal with the injury to the urethra at a later date. If laparotomy is necessary for other reasons, this may give an opportunity to pass a catheter. If the rupture is incomplete, the catheter will act as a splint. If the rupture is complete, the ends of the urethra can be approximated and splinted by the catheter. The late complications of these injuries are stricture and impotence. In the absence of investigations to visualise the exact site and extent of urethral injury, it is recommended that a suprapubic catheter is inserted and any attempt to introduce a urethral catheter is avoided. Urethral narrowing or stricture as a result of this is best managed by urethroplasty at specialist urology centres.

Bladder tumours

Pathology

The vast majority of bladder tumours arise from the urothelium or transitional cell lining, which it shares in continuum from the renal pelvis to the proximal urethra. The urothelium is exposed to chemical carcinogens excreted in the urine, such as naphthylamines and benzidine, which were extensively used in the chemical and dye industries in the past. The bladder is more susceptible to urinary carcinogens, as urine is stored in the bladder for relatively long periods of time.

Almost all bladder tumours are urothelial cell carcinomas (otherwise known as transitional cell carcinomas). Squamous carcinoma may occur in urothelium that has undergone metaplasia, usually due to chronic inflammation or irritation caused by a stone or schistosomiasis. An adenocarcinoma is a rarity but may occur in an urachal remnant in the dome of the bladder, or from local infiltration, e.g., bowel cancer. The prevalence of urothelial cell carcinoma of the bladder is 45 cases per 100,000, and it is three times more common in men than women. The appearance of a urothelial cell tumour ranges from a delicate papillary structure to a solid ulcerating mass. Papillary tumours are less aggressive superficial cancers, whereas those that ulcerate are much more aggressive.

Staging

Biopsy is essential to confirm the diagnosis (cell type), determine the degree of cell differentiation (grade), and assess the depth to which the tumour has penetrated the bladder wall (stage). The TNM system of tumour classification is applicable to bladder tumours. Assessment of the primary tumour (T) is of prime clinical importance and requires bimanual examination under anaesthesia to judge the degree of penetration through the bladder wall. This is especially important for T_2 and T_3 tumours (Fig. 23.16). Clinical examination, urography and CT are used to assess the involvement of regional and juxtaregional lymph nodes (N). Assessment of distant metastases (M) requires clinical examination and CT. Histopathological examination guides the choice of treatment. A transurethral resection of bladder tumour (TURBT)

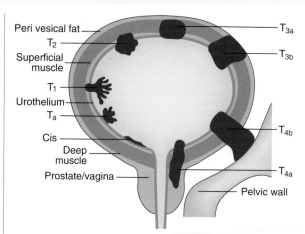

Fig. 23.16 T categories of bladder tumour. *Cis,* Carcinoma in situ.

with sampling of detrusor muscle is an essential treatment and staging modality which will determine if the cancer is superficial (CIS, pTa, pT1) or muscle invasive (pT2).

Clinical features

More than 80% of patients have haematuria, which is usually painless (Fig. 23.17). It should be assumed that such bleeding is from a tumour until proven otherwise. In women, symptoms of cystitis are so common that occasional bleeding may be thought to be part of an infective problem. Therefore, in cases of haematuria, an MSSU is mandatory with further investigation required if no growth is found. A tumour at the lower end of a ureter or a bladder tumour involving the ureteric orifice may cause obstructive symptoms. However, visible haematuria may be the only presenting symptom.

Investigations

Because upper tract tumours are much less common, they may be overlooked in the presence of an obvious bladder tumour. Both may occur together, and the whole of the urothelium must be examined using a CTU. Investigations for visible haematuria consist of local anaesthetic flexible cystoscopy and a CTU. Where a lesion is found within the bladder, cystourethroscopy and examination under anaesthesia are performed. With the patient relaxed under general anaesthesia, the bladder and tumour are examined bimanually to determine the depth of spread. The physical features of the tumour(s) are noted, the normal bladder mucosa is inspected and the tumour is fully resected if possible (TURBT), otherwise biopsies are taken from the tumour and any other suspicious areas.

Management

Superficial bladder tumours (T_a, T_1)

These lesions are treated by TURBT down to and including detrusor muscle. A single intravesical dose of intravesical chemotherapy (mitomycin C) reduces the risk of recurrence of superficial bladder cancer (EBM 23.1). A 6-week course of mitomycin C is also useful to treat multiple low-grade bladder tumours and to reduce recurrence. Regular check cystoscopies are required. Recurrences are mostly treated by repeat diathermy or resection, but, if they become very frequent and excessive, cystectomy may be advisable. Carcinoma in situ (Cis) may be present in mucosa that appears normal or in association with a proliferative tumour. Cis can also exist as a separate entity, when there may be only a generalised redness of the bladder mucosa. Cis should be considered in patients with ongoing

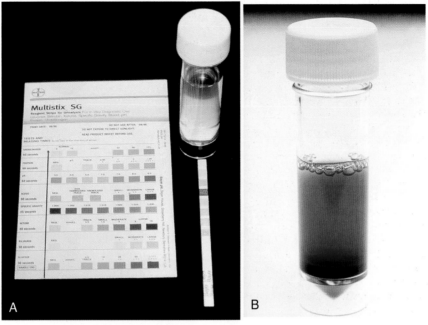

Fig. 23.17 Haematuria. (A) Non-visible (microscopic). **(B)** Visible (macroscopic).

storage urinary symptoms associated with pain or symptoms suggestive of ongoing UTI, in the absence of a positive urine culture. Untreated patients with Cis have a high risk of progression to invasive cancer. Cis responds well to intravesical bacillus Calmette–Guérin (BCG) treatment. However, if there is any doubt about the response, and especially if there is any pathological evidence of progression, cystectomy is warranted.

Invasive bladder tumour (T_2–T_4)

For patients under 70 years of age, radical cystectomy is recommended. In older patients, radiotherapy may be a better option. Unfortunately, this may not always cure the tumour and 'salvage' cystectomy may be needed. Cystectomy always necessitates urinary diversion. Where the urethra can be retained, it may be possible to construct a new bladder from colon or small bowel (orthotopic bladder replacement), so achieving continence. Alternatively, the urine is collected in an internal reservoir that is connected to the body surface via a continent conduit (ileum or appendix), through which the patient drains the urine at regular intervals with a catheter. In less favourable circumstances, an ileal conduit should be performed (Fig. 23.18). In some countries where an 'ostomy' is not acceptable, the ureters can be implanted into the sigmoid colon (ureterosigmoidostomy). However, renal infection and metabolic disturbances are potentially serious complications of this procedure. An invasive T_4 tumour, fixed to the pelvis or surrounding organs, is often unresectable and only palliative treatment can be given.

Prognosis

Outlook depends on tumour stage and grade. Superficial disease carries a much better prognosis with a 5-year survival of 70–90%. Muscle invasive disease has a 5-year survival of 10–60%.

Benign prostatic hyperplasia

Pathology

From about the age of 40 years, the prostate undergoes enlargement as the result of hyperplasia of periurethral tissue, which forms adenomas in the transitional zone of the prostate. Normal prostatic tissue is compressed to form a surrounding shell or capsule. There is considerable variation in the growth rates of the adenomas and in the proportions of stromal and epithelial tissue. Adenomas with an epithelial preponderance can grow to form large discrete masses weighing more than 100 g, and have a characteristic rubbery consistency, referred to as benign prostatic hyperplasia (BPH). Enlarging adenomas lengthen and obstruct the prostatic urethra, causing outflow obstruction and detrusor muscle hypertrophy. The muscle bands of the bladder form trabeculae, between which saccules

23

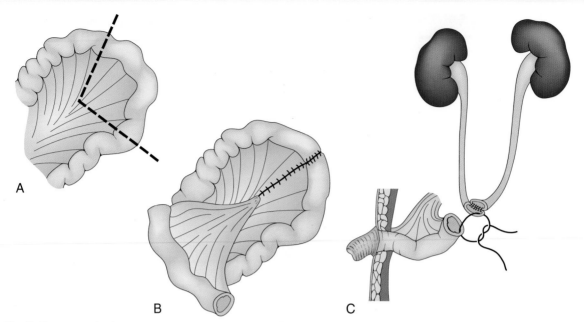

Fig. 23.18 Ileal conduit urinary diversion. (A, B) Isolation of segment of terminal ileum. **(C)** Fashioning of ureteroileal anastomosis. The stoma is made to protrude from the skin to minimise skin contact with urine and so reduce irritation.

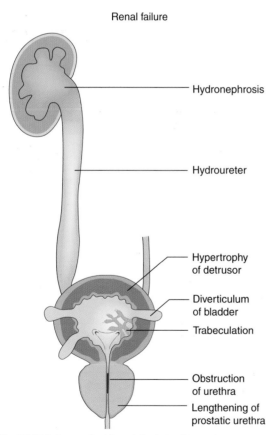

Renal failure

- Hydronephrosis
- Hydroureter
- Hypertrophy of detrusor
- Diverticulum of bladder
- Trabeculation
- Obstruction of urethra
- Lengthening of prostatic urethra

Fig. 23.19 Late sequelae of prostatic obstruction.

form diverticula (Fig. 23.19). Occasionally, a diverticulum may become quite large, even larger than the bladder. Bladder diverticula empty poorly and are liable to the main complications of urinary stasis: infection and stone formation.

With progressive inability to empty the bladder completely (chronic retention), the risk of urinary infection and stone formation increases. Eventually, the residual urine volume may exceed 1 L. In high-pressure chronic retention, progressive obstruction and dilatation of the ureters (hydroureter) and pelvicalyceal system (hydronephrosis) occurs, ultimately leading to obstructive renal failure.

Clinical features

Symptoms may be obstructive (poor flow, hesitancy, intermittent stream, straining to empty) or storage symptoms due to secondary detrusor overactivity (frequency, urgency and urge incontinence). Increasing frequency may deceive the patient into believing that an adequate amount of urine is passed, whereas the bladder has a small functional capacity and may be almost full all of the time (chronic retention). In high-pressure chronic retention frequency may progress to continual dribbling incontinence (especially nocturnally), leading over time to signs and symptoms of obstructive uraemia, including drowsiness, anorexia and personality changes.

Urinary infection, cold weather, anticholinergic drugs or excessive alcohol intake can provoke acute or acute-on-chronic retention. A bladder stone may result in obstructive symptoms during micturition, and may also cause bladder pain at the end of micturition. Examination reveals little except rubbery, symmetrical and smooth prostatic enlargement, with a median groove between the two lateral 'lobes'. Asymmetry or a hard consistency raises the suspicion of malignancy. In patients with chronic retention, the painless, enlarged bladder rises out of the pelvis, almost to the umbilicus. The overlying area will be dull on percussion.

Investigations

A good history and examination are paramount. A urinary frequency volume chart should be completed over 3 days. International Prostate Symptom Score (IPSS) (Table 23.5) provides

Table 23.5 International Prostate Symptom Score (IPSS)

	Not at all	Less than 1 time in 5	Less than half the time	About half the time	More than half the time	Almost always	**Your score**
Incomplete emptying Over the past month, how often have you had a sensation of not emptying your bladder completely after you finish urinating?	0	1	2	3	4	5	
Frequency Over the past month, how often have you had to urinate again less than two hours after you finished urinating?	0	1	2	3	4	5	
Intermittency Over the past month, how often have you found you stopped and started again several times when you urinated?	0	1	2	3	4	5	
Urgency Over the last month, how difficult have you found it to postpone urination?	0	1	2	3	4	5	
Weak stream Over the past month, how often have you had a weak urinary stream?	0	1	2	3	4	5	
Straining Over the past month, how often have you had to push or strain to begin urination?	0	1	2	3	4	5	

	None	1 time	2 times	3 times	4 times	5 times or more	**Your score**
Nocturia Over the past month, many times did you most typically get up to urinate from the time you went to bed until the time you got up in the morning?	0	1	2	3	4	5	
Total IPSS score							

	Delighted	Pleased	Mostly satisfied	Mixed – about equally satisfied and dissatisfied	Mostly dissatisfied	Unhappy	Terrible
Quality of life due to urinary symptoms							
If you were to spend the rest of your life with your urinary condition the way it is now, how would you feel about that?	0	1	2	3		4	5	6

Total score: 0-7 Mildly symptomatic; 8-19 moderately symptomatic; 20-35 severely symptomatic.

an objective measurement of symptoms and also helps in monitoring response to treatment. Other mandatory assessment includes blood for renal function, electrolytes and following counselling PSA. Prostate cancer can occur with normal PSA values (0–4 ng/mL), while BPH can cause elevated values, so careful interpretation is required (Table 23.6). If digital rectal examination (DRE) raises suspicion, TRUS-guided biopsy is indicated. Urine flow rate assessed by uroflowmetry and US assessment of postvoid residual will quantify a reduction in urinary stream and the need for intervention. In some patients, especially the elderly, neurological or pharmacological causes for changes in micturition must be considered. A pressure-flow urodynamic assessment may be necessary for equivocal symptoms or investigations.

Management

Patients can be divided into three treatment groups depending on the degree of bother of symptoms and the presence of complications, if any.

Table 23.6 Factors affecting the level of prostate-specific antigen

Causes of increase in PSA:

- Increase in age
- Acute retention of urine
- Urethral catheterisation
- Instrumentation of lower urinary tract
- Prostatitis
- Prostate cancer
- Large benign prostatic hyperplasia
- Prostatic biopsy

Cause of decrease in PSA

- Patient taking a 5-α reductase inhibitor (finasteride, dutasteride)

PSA, Prostate-specific antigen

Conservative management

In patients with mild symptoms (IPSS symptom score of 0–7) and no interference of daily activities, watchful waiting can be tried. The

23

prerequisite is absence of any complication arising due to BPH. Patients can be informed that a third of patients will have stable symptoms, a third will deteriorate and the remainder will show symptomatic improvement.

Medical management

Patients with moderate symptom scores (IPSS symptom score of 8–19) or those with a lower score opting for treatment are initially started on medical therapy. Availability of better drugs and improved understanding of the pathophysiology of the disease has resulted in a reduction in the need for surgery by almost half. The drugs used in treatment of BPH are of two broad categories:

- *α-blockers*. These act at the $α_1$ adrenoreceptors present in the bladder base and the prostatic capsule, and smooth muscle. Prostate-specific $α_{1a}$ blockers have been developed which have minimal systemic side effects that were common with the older nonselective agents. They include tamsulosin, doxazocin and alfuzosin, and act rapidly (three doses) by opening the bladder neck and relaxing the prostatic capsule. These agents are preferable in symptomatic patients with a smaller prostate
- *5α reductase inhibitors*. These drugs prevent the intraprostatic conversion of testosterone to its 9-times more active form, dihydrotestosterone, which is responsible for the growth and enlargement of the prostate. These drugs are therefore useful in large glands (>30 g) or in patients with a PSA >1.4 μg/L, causing the prostate to shrink. The commonly used agents are finasteride and dutasteride, but they take 4–6 months to have a full effect.

A combination of both classes of agents may be needed in patients who have severe symptoms, or those who do not improve on single-agent therapy.

Surgical management

Patients with severe symptoms (IPSS >19), those failing medical treatment, not able to tolerate the side effects of the drugs, not willing to try medical management or presenting with one of the complications of BPH are candidates for surgery. The absolute indications for surgery in a patient with BPH are: refractory urinary retention, recurrent UTI, recurrent haematuria, bladder stones, and/or diverticulae and high-pressure chronic urinary retention leading to renal insufficiency.

Acute retention

This condition usually requires emergency admission to hospital and intervention to relieve obstruction. If there is a history of bladder outflow obstruction, conservative measures aimed at encouraging micturition (a warm bath) only delay the inevitable requirement for catheterisation. A self-retaining Foley catheter is passed using strict asepsis and connected to a closed drainage system. If it is not possible to pass a urethral catheter, the bladder is drained directly by puncture with a suprapubic catheter. A specimen of urine is cultured and, if there is microbiological evidence of an infection, antibiotics are given. If the history of urinary symptoms is short, the catheter can be removed after 12 hours (known as *trial without catheter*), following which normal voiding may occur. This is more likely if the patient is given α-blockers (EBM 23.2). If retention recurs, then definitive treatment with endoscopic transurethral prostate resection is performed.

EBM 23.2 Benign prostatic hyperplasia: α-blockers in patients with acute urinary retention

'Alfuzosin 10 mg/day increases the likelihood of successful trial without catheter (TWOC) in men with a first episode of spontaneous urinary retention.'

McNeill SA et al. Urology. 2005;65:83–90.

Chronic retention

It is essential to determine whether the patient has any complications of obstruction, especially renal damage. If the patient is well, with no haematological or biochemical disturbance, there is no indication for preliminary bladder drainage and management may be planned in the usual way. Relief of high-pressure chronic obstruction is almost always followed by a diuresis, due partly to an osmotic (urea) diuresis and partly to renal tubular changes resulting from back pressure. Accurate intake/output fluid charts in addition to daily weights can detect these losses. The blood pressure, both lying and standing, should be monitored and intravenous fluid replacement may be necessary if there is a >20 mmHg postural drop in blood pressure. Medical therapy is contraindicated in patients who present with renal failure secondary to BPH; these patients should be managed either by long-term catheter or endoscopic transurethral prostate resection.

Endoscopy transurethral prostate resection

The gold-standard endoscopic management of bladder outlet obstruction due to prostatic enlargement is transurethral resection of the prostate (TURP). TURP entails removing the prostate piecemeal by electroresection using a resectoscope. The advantages are patient acceptance, short hospitalisation (2–3 days) and the precision of removal of the obstructing tissue. However, serious damage can be inflicted on the prostatic sphincter mechanism by inexpert use of the resectoscope. Prolonged resection can occasionally result in excessive absorption of glycine irrigating fluid and electrolyte imbalance (TURP syndrome). Favourable results are seen with laser prostatectomy, with improved haemostasis, reduced hospital stay, earlier catheter removal, and promising long-term follow-up data (EBM 23.3). The different types of laser prostatectomy are green-light laser prostatectomy and holmium laser ablation of the prostate (HoLAP), resection of the prostate (HoLRP), and enucleation of the prostate (HoLEP).

EBM 23.3 Management of benign prostatic hyperplasia with green-light laser prostatectomy

'The long-term (24 month) effectiveness and safety of green-light laser prostatectomy was similar to conventional TURP for the treatment of prostate enlargement.'

Thomas JA. Eur Urol. 2016;69:94–102.

Retrograde ejaculation is a common sequel to any operative procedure on the prostate and all patients should be advised preoperatively of this effect. Any associated bladder stone may be crushed with a lithotrite or intracorporeal lithotripsy using holmium or pneumatic energy. After endoscopic prostatectomy, the bladder must be allowed to drain freely via a urethral catheter while the prostatic bed heals and bleeding stops. After TURP, the catheter is normally removed on the second postoperative day. The main postoperative hazard is bleeding. If postoperative bleeding is excessive, clot may lead to obstruction (*clot retention*). This hazard can be minimised by continuous irrigation through a three-way urethral catheter.

Open prostatectomy

Open procedures are now rarely performed and are reserved for very large adenomas (>100 g) or patients with associated intravesical complications (stones or diverticulae). The various approaches for performing open prostatectomy are transvesical (Freyer's), retropubic (Millin's) and perineal (Young's). Apart from the length of hospitalisation (7–10 days) and the presence of an abdominal wound, enucleation of smaller adenomas may damage the external sphincter and cause incontinence. This is a particular problem with more fibrous glands and those that contain a focus of cancer.

Carcinoma of the prostate

Epidemiology

In the UK, this is the most common malignancy in males, with a prevalence of 105 cases per 100,000 population. It is the second most common cause of cancer death in men in the UK. The tumour is common in northern Europe and the USA (particularly in the black population), but rare in China and Japan. It rarely occurs before the age of 50 years but the incidence rises sharply from 50 to 54 years, peaking at 75–79 years of age. The mean age at presentation is approximately 70 years. The aetiology is unknown, but genetic, hormonal and possibly viral factors are implicated.

Pathology

Almost all malignant tumours of the prostate are carcinomas, with the most common being adenocarcinoma (>95%). If a prostate is examined by serial section, a small malignant focus is detected in almost all men over the age of 80 years. Thus, there is a very high prevalence of histological prostate cancer and many men will die *with* a cancer of the prostate, but not *from* prostate cancer. It is estimated that the prevalence of focal histological cancer in men aged 50–75 years is approximately 40%, whereas the prevalence of clinical prostate cancer is approximately 8%, one-quarter of whom will die from that cancer. The TNM system is used in classification (see Table 23.7). Metastatic spread to pelvic lymph nodes occurs early. One-third of clinically localised tumours at the time of presentation will have spread to regional nodes. Metastases to bone, mainly the lumbar spine and pelvis, occur in some 10–15% of patients.

The Gleason score is used to grade prostate adenocarcinoma. Cells are graded 1–5 depending upon their level of differentiation (grade 1 = most differentiated, grade 5 = least differentiated or most anaplastic). The pathologist uses the two most common malignant cell types to determine a Gleason score (most common type + second most common type = Gleason score). Therefore, Gleason scores range from 2 to 10 and are always expressed as an equation (e.g., 4+3=7); in practice the lowest Gleason score apportioned is 3+3=6.

Table 23.7 TNM classification of prostate cancer*

T (Tumour)
- T_0 — No evidence of primary tumour
- T_X — Primary tumour cannot be assessed
- T_1 — Tumour clinically inapparent and not palpable
  - T_{1a} — Incidental finding following TURP in <5% prostate chips
  - T_{1b} — Incidental finding following TURP in >5% prostate chips
  - T_{1c} — Prostate cancer detected by prostate biopsy
- T_2 — Tumour confined within the prostate
  - T_{2a} — Palpable nodule involving half of one lobe
  - T_{2b} — Palpable nodule involving one lobe
  - T_{2c} — Palpable nodule involving both lobes
- T_3 — Tumour extends through the prostatic capsule
  - T_{3a} — Extracapsular extension of prostate cancer
  - T_{3b} — Prostate cancer involving the seminal vesicles
- T_4 — Tumour is fixed or invades adjacent structures other than seminal vesicles: external sphincter, rectum, levator muscles, and/or pelvic wall

N (Nodes)
- N_0 — No regional lymph node metastasis
- N_X — Regional lymph nodes cannot be assessed
- N_1 — Regional lymph node metastasis

M (Metastases)
- M_0 — No distant metastasis detected
- M_X — Distant metastasis cannot be assessed
- M_{1a} — Metastasis to non-regional lymph nodes
- M_{1b} — Skeletal metastasis present
- M_{1c} — Metastasis to other sites

TURP, transurethral resection of the prostate.
*Sobin LH, Gospodariwicz M, Wittekind C (eds). TNM classification of malignant tumors. UICC International Union Against Cancer. 7th edn. Wiley-Blackwell, 2009 Dec; pp. 243–248.

Clinical features

In the 'PSA-era' most patients are asymptomatic. However, presentation of patients with localised prostate cancer can be similar to BPH. Occasionally, the tumour extends posteriorly around the rectum and causes alteration in bowel habit. Presenting symptoms and signs due to metastases are much less common, but include back pain, weight loss, anaemia and renal failure secondary to ureteric obstruction. On rectal examination, the prostate feels nodular and stony hard, but many irregular prostates, even those with nodules, are not malignant. Conversely, 50–60% of malignant prostates are not palpably abnormal on rectal examination.

Investigations

PSA is the serum marker used to aid detection of prostate cancer. A PSA of <4 ng/ml is generally regarded as normal, although there are age specific values that differ between regions. Metastatic disease is exceptional when the PSA level is <20 ng/ml, but levels >100 ng/ml almost always indicate distant bone metastases. PSA is the main test for monitoring response to treatment and disease progression. The diagnosis is confirmed by needle biopsy, usually performed under TRUS guidance. TRUS biopsy should be performed in men with elevated PSA or abnormal DRE. Histological examination of tissue removed at endoscopic resection for outflow obstruction may also reveal prostate cancer. Multiparametric prostate MRI is being increasingly used to evaluate the prostate for abnormal foci in men with a persistently elevated PSA with previous negative prostate biopsy. MRI is also useful to assess pelvic lymphadenopathy and evidence of locally advanced disease. A bone scan may be carried out at follow-up to localise and define the extent of metastases.

Management

Prostatic cancer is sensitive to endocrine influences (EBM 23.4) as testosterone is a trigger for moving prostate cells through the cell cycle, thereby stimulating mitosis. Management is best considered in three clinical groups, as follows.

EBM 23.4 **Hormone manipulation in prostate cancer**

'Reducing circulating testosterone levels (either by castration or by medication) results in a 70% initial response rate. Additional androgen blockade produces a small increase in survival but with poorer quality of life.'

Huggins C et al. Cancer Res. 1941;1:293–7.

Organ-confined disease

A patient with a small focus of well-differentiated carcinoma (Gleason score 3+3=6) may be managed by an active surveillance policy (close follow-up with DRE, PSA, MRI, repeat TRUS biopsy), as usually these patients remain unaffected by their prostate cancer for between 10 and 15 years. In patients with a life expectancy of >10 years and a less well-differentiated cell pattern (Gleason score 7 or more) there is an increased risk of progression. In these cases, treatment with curative intent by either radical prostatectomy or radiotherapy is suggested. The prostate can be removed laparoscopically, robotically or by the traditional open route. Radiotherapy can be performed by external beam radiotherapy (EBRT), intensity-modulated radiotherapy or by the insertion of radioactive seeds in the prostate (brachytherapy). There are no data to support one treatment over the other in terms of overall survival. However, each treatment modality has a different side effect and complication profile. Therefore, the choice of treatment tends to be based upon patient preference.

Locally advanced disease

This term refers to cases where the prostate cancer has invaded directly outside the prostate but has not metastasised. There is an evolving role for surgery as part of multimodality treatment in these patients; however, EBRT along with hormonal therapy is the standard of care. In patients not able to tolerate EBRT, hormone therapy alone or conservative symptomatic treatment can be considered.

Metastatic prostate cancer

20% of men with prostate cancer have metastatic disease at diagnosis. The basis of treatment in these cases is castration, either physically by androgen depletion (bilateral orchiectomy), or more commonly chemically by androgen suppression (gonadotrophin-releasing hormone analogues) and/or androgen receptor antagonists. A small number of patients fail to respond to endocrine treatment; a larger number respond for a year or two, but

then suffer disease progression known as castrate-resistant prostate cancer (CRPC). PSA levels are a useful marker of response, ideally falling to <0.01 ng/ml in well-controlled cases. Oestrogens are useful but are limited by their thromboembolic effects. Chemotherapy with taxanes has shown a marginal improvement in both symptoms and survival in patients with CRPC. Newer hormonal agents such as enzalutamide and abiraterone acetate also provide some survival benefit in CRPC. PSA is a very useful marker to determine response to treatment in addition to monitoring disease progression or recurrence. Bone-protective agents may be offered to patients with skeletal metastases (i.e., denosumab and zoledronic acid) to palliate bone pain, prevent loss of bone mass and reduce the risk of metastatic bone fractures. Radiotherapy is an effective treatment for localised bone pain.

Prognosis

The life expectancy of a patient with an incidental finding of focal carcinoma of the prostate is that of the normal population. With tumours localised to the prostate, a 15-year survival rate of 56–87% can be expected; if metastases are present, this falls to <10%.

 23.4 **Summary**

Prostatic cancer

- In the UK this is the most common cancer in men, and presents at a mean age of 70 years
- Prostate cancer is usually incidental (i.e., elevated PSA or found on histological examination), but may be clinically apparent (bladder outflow obstruction and a hard craggy prostate) or occult (metastatic disease)
- Metastatic spread may occur early; one-third of clinically confined cancers have spread to lymph nodes, and 20% of all new cases have bony spread (to lumbar spine and pelvis)
- Treatment of prostatic cancer varies:
  - *Well-differentiated, low-risk* cases. Life expectancy can be normal with an active surveillance policy. If the cancer contains undifferentiated cells, then either radical surgery or radiotherapy is considered
  - *Intermediate or high-risk localised cancer with no evidence of bony metastases*. Treated by either radical surgery, radiotherapy or brachytherapy
  - *Metastatic cancer*. Treated by androgen deprivation medically (gonadotrophin-releasing hormone analogues) or surgically (orchidectomy)
- Tumours localised to the prostate and amenable to radical curative treatment have a 10-year cancer specific survival of 95% or better.

Vesicoureteral reflux

Aetiology

Normal anatomical and physiological mechanisms prevent reflux of urine back into the ureters from the bladder whenever there is a rise in intravesical pressure. This protects the upper tracts against damage from the high pressures commonly seen in the lower urinary tracts. Any abnormality in this preventive mechanism may result in reflux. It may be unilateral or bilateral.

Pathology

Reflux causes dilatation of the upper tracts, the ureters, renal pelves and calyces. It may be associated with retrograde infection leading to pyelonephritis. All these factors ultimately lead to renal parenchymal damage, often referred to as reflux nephropathy.

Investigations

An IVU may show the sequelae of reflux in the form of hydroureteronephrosis. The modality of choice to document reflux is MCU or radionuclide scanning. A cystoscopic examination may reveal an abnormal ureteric opening (stadium, horseshoe or golf-hole type).

Management

Medical management is aimed at maintaining sterile urine and limiting the damage to the upper tracts. Primary reflux seen in children may correct on its own if it is not associated with any other abnormality. Careful follow-up is needed. Reflux secondary to other pathologies or in adults needs definitive surgical management in the form of vesicoureteroplasty.

Urethral obstruction

Pathology

Obstruction of the urethra may be congenital, due to a stricture or malignancy (Fig. 23.20). Foreign bodies, including urinary stones, may also be responsible. The complications include infection with periurethral abscess, fistulation and stone formation. Congenital valves in the posterior urethra occur only in boys. They lie at the level of the verumontanum and may cause gross obstructive changes in the bladder and upper urinary tracts at birth. Increasingly, this diagnosis is being established during pregnancy by US examination. If the diagnosis is established after birth, it is confirmed by micturating cystourethrography. Treatment consists of endoscopic fulguration of the valves. Urethral

diverticulum is a rare cause of obstruction. More commonly, it is secondary to obstruction and infection in women. Urethral trauma or infection may result in a stricture, the severity of which is related to both the site and the extent of the insult. A posterior urethral stricture following major trauma may be surrounded by dense fibrous tissue, whereas healthy tissues may surround a stricture of the bulb of the urethra. The former requires major reconstructive surgery, but urethral dilatation or incision can readily manage the latter. Rough inexpert use of any instrument (including a catheter) in the urethra can cause stricture formation. The principal organism responsible for inflammatory scarring and stricture of the urethra is *Neisseria gonorrhoeae*. Long-term use of a self-retaining catheter, although not necessarily associated with infection, can also cause an inflammatory reaction in the urethra.

Clinical features

The diagnosis should be considered if there is a history of urethral infection, instrumentation or trauma. The external meatus must always be examined and, if the foreskin is present, it should be retracted for full inspection. The urethra is palpated. It is still possible for a patient to pass urine, albeit with difficulty, in the presence of a urethral stone.

Investigations

Urinary flow rate will help differentiate urethral strictures from bladder neck and prostatic obstruction, the former giving a uniformly low and prolonged (box-like) pattern (see Fig. 23.7). Postmicturition US may exclude an increased residual volume. An ascending and descending urethrogram will adequately demonstrate the urethral anatomy. The final investigation to assess a urethral lesion is cystourethroscopy.

Management

Many simple strictures are easily treated by repeated dilatation with metal bougies, or may be incised under direct vision using a urethrotome. Most short strictures in the region of the bulb respond well, but recurrence is common (50%) and operative reconstruction (urethroplasty) may be required. Short strictures

23

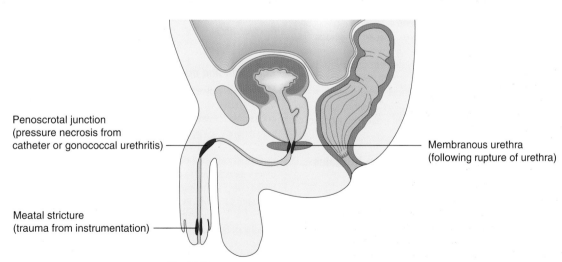

Penoscrotal junction
(pressure necrosis from
catheter or gonococcal urethritis)

Membranous urethra
(following rupture of urethra)

Meatal stricture
(trauma from instrumentation)

Fig. 23.20 Common sites and causes of urethral stricture.

can be excised and the healthy urethra reanastomosed. Longer strictures can be patched with full-thickness skin flaps or buccal mucosal grafts, to restore normal calibre.

Disorders of micturition: incontinence

Overview

Incontinence is defined as the involuntary leakage of urine. It may be due to problems in storage, resulting in urge and stress incontinence or continual incontinence with fistulae, or to problems in emptying, resulting in chronic retention with overflow incontinence. In stress incontinence, leakage occurs because passive bladder pressure exceeds normal urethral pressure. This may be because of poor pelvic floor support, because of a weak urethral sphincter or an element of both. In urge incontinence, leakage usually occurs because detrusor overactivity produces an increase in bladder pressure that overcomes the urethral sphincter. A hypersensitive bladder (sensory urgency) resulting from UTI or bladder stone may also drive urgency in the absence of overactive bladder contractions. Incontinence in these circumstances is less common. Stress incontinence and urge incontinence may coexist (mixed incontinence). All of the above terms, with the exception of a fistula, are descriptive only and do not accurately diagnose the underlying pathophysiology, which can only be determined by urodynamic testing.

Structural disorders

Clinical assessment

Abnormalities of function of the lower urinary tract are notoriously difficult to assess because there is frequently dual underlying pathology. Incontinence in an elderly man may be due to cerebral cortical degeneration, but could also be due to chronic outflow tract obstruction resulting from prostatic hyperplasia. The history is important but may be deceptive, and the exact character of the urinary abnormality must be determined so that structural causes can be separated from neurological ones. Details of drug treatment are noted since diuretics and drugs with anticholinergic side effects may tip the balance when there is already dysfunction. Urine is tested for glycosuria and infection. The range of more specific methods for assessing micturition, include radiology (cystourethrography), urodynamic studies (uroflowmetry, cystometrography and urethral pressure measurement) and direct inspection (cystourethroscopy and pelvic examination under anaesthesia). A full history and physical examination, with cystourethroscopy and bimanual examination, remain the basic initial investigation of structural disorders.

Structural causes of incontinence in males

Postprostatectomy

Disordered control of micturition occurs in 3–5% of patients after prostatectomy. In this operation, any inadvertent damage to the external sphincter can lead to difficulties with continence. Stress incontinence may occur, but as the damage to the sphincter is usually incomplete, it usually responds to physiotherapy. If not, insertion of an artificial urinary sphincter or male suburethral sling can be considered.

Chronic outflow obstruction

Changes within the bladder (detrusor hypertrophy) due to chronic obstruction commonly lead to secondary urgency and detrusor overactivity. Relief of obstruction alone is usually sufficient to correct the associated urgency and urge incontinence, but in about 10% of cases the instability is primary and antimuscarinics may be necessary. Chronic retention may also lead to overflow or dribbling incontinence. It must be emphasised that continence requires normal cortical control, and in an elderly patient this may be impaired. Possible abnormalities of both structure and innervation need to be considered in these patients.

Prostate cancer

The cancer may involve the external sphincter, preventing it from closing. Repeated transurethral resections for recurring obstruction may convert the posterior urethra into a rigid tube so that dribbling incontinence occurs. An indwelling catheter or condom incontinence appliance may be necessary.

Postmicturition dribble incontinence

This is very common, even in relatively young men, and is caused by a small amount of urine becoming trapped in the 'U-bend' of the bulbar urethra. This then leaks out passively when the patient moves. The condition is more pronounced if associated with a urethral diverticulum or urethral stricture. Milking of the urethra (from the perianal region towards the scrotum) will clear the last drops of urine from the bulbar urethra.

Chronic illness and debility

Especially in the elderly, incontinence may arise from poor tone in the periurethral striated muscle of the pelvic floor and from difficulty in getting to the toilet. This may be worsened by loss of cortical inhibition of micturition.

Structural causes of incontinence in females

Incontinence is more prevalent than generally suspected; approximately 14% of all women have been incontinent at some time, half of them within the last 2 months. This figure rises rapidly in older patients, and reaches 50–70% in geriatric units. Only a proportion of younger women seek advice, either because of embarrassment or because of stoical acceptance of some incontinence as being normal.

Childbirth and operations

Multiparous women commonly lose some of the tone in the pelvic floor muscles with each pregnancy. Symptoms may range from occasional stress incontinence to almost continual dribbling incontinence. Examination shows weakening of the pelvic floor muscles and anterior vaginal wall (cystocoele). It is important to distinguish stress incontinence from urge incontinence. The former responds well to pelvic floor exercises and to surgical procedures designed to support the bladder neck, but the latter should be treated by bladder retraining and drug therapy. Stress incontinence is characterised by an involuntary loss of urine during coughing, laughing, sneezing or any other activity that suddenly raises the intra-abdominal pressure. A cough, however, may stimulate involuntary detrusor contractions (cough-induced detrusor instability), which causes urge incontinence. This differential diagnosis can be made only by urodynamic assessment. In parts of the world where obstetric services are poor, prolonged labour may lead to a vesicovaginal fistula, which presents as continuous dribbling incontinence. The association with delivery is usually clear, but a small fistula may be missed. Investigation of dribbling incontinence must distinguish between urethral damage and a fistula. Treatment consists of closing the fistula through a vaginal or suprapubic approach.

Cystitis

Cystitis is common in women and, in addition to causing frequency, urgency and dysuria, sometimes causes sensory urge incontinence. Treatment of both the infection and the bladder spasm is required. Interstitial cystitis (painful bladder syndrome) is a chronic inflammatory condition that, in addition to causing frequency and dysuria, may also cause urgency and urge incontinence. Treatment can be challenging and centres on symptom control. Hydrostatic dilatation may be effective.

Ectopic ureter

Dribbling incontinence in a child should raise the suspicion of an ectopic ureter, in which the ureter from the upper pole opens outside the control of the urethral mechanism. The abnormal ureter must be reimplanted in the bladder.

Cervical cancer

Carcinoma of the cervix or its treatment by radiotherapy may cause vesicovaginal fistula and incontinence.

Neurogenic disorders

Clinical assessment

A full history, including an interview with relatives (especially in children), is required. Examination must include assessment of the plantar reflexes, and the sensation and tone of the anal canal. Glycosuria and urinary infection should be excluded. Urodynamic, radiological and electromyographic studies may all be required.

Aetiology of abnormal micturition

Impaired cortical control

Diseases affecting the frontal lobe can alter the pattern of micturition by increasing or decreasing its frequency, or by affecting the social awareness of incontinence. There may also be failure to inhibit initiation of micturition. The paracentral lobule controls the activity of skeletal muscle, so that lesions in this area may cause sustained pelvic and perineal muscular contraction. It must be remembered that a disorder of micturition may be accentuated by, or may even be due to, the physical inability to prepare for micturition such as poor mobility.

Emotional state

This may affect the postponement of micturition, giving rise to 'giggle' incontinence and possibly to enuresis in some patients. Incontinence with epilepsy is also due to a loss of inhibitory control. Excessive sensory stimuli, as with the pain of cystourethritis in women, may cause 'sensory urge incontinence'.

Drugs

Drugs, including alcohol, may alter cortical control of micturition. Sedatives can affect the postponement phase and precipitate incontinence, especially at night. The intoxicated patient may lack the mental alertness to maintain continence, or may continually suppress the desire to void, leading to prostatic congestion and retention.

Damage to the spinal cord

Two aspects of disease or injury to the spinal cord influence disordered micturition: namely, the level of the disease and the completeness of the damage.

Injury at or below the sacral outflow (S2, 3, 4) may be due to a fracture of the spine at the level of T12 and L1, which damages the conus medullaris, a central prolapsed intervertebral disc leading to cauda equina injury or spinal stenosis. The bladder distends without sensation, the external sphincter is weak and little detrusor contraction is seen upon urodynamic assessment. The patient develops retention with overflow, but emptying is possible with abdominal straining or hand pressure.

Injury between the sacral segment and the pontine micturition centres (upper motor neuron lesions) may be due to fractures of the spine; tumours that compress the cord; surgical removal of such a tumour; and diseases of the cord itself, such as multiple sclerosis, transverse myelitis and cervical cord stenosis. If these central connections are disrupted, the patient develops a reflex bladder with impaired or absent cortical control; that is, the bladder loses the coordination imposed by the pontine micturition centre. The detrusor becomes overactive and attempted voiding results in detrusor contraction occurring synchronously with that of the external sphincter (detrusor–sphincter dyssynergia). The net result is poor bladder emptying and the development of a thick, trabeculated bladder wall. The resultant high-pressure bladder will, over time, lead to renal impairment. Usually the central connections are not completely disrupted and there may be some sensation and some cortical inhibition.

Damage to pelvic nerves may occur in the course of surgery, especially when dissection involves the side walls of the pelvis, as in radical dissection of the rectum or the uterus. Similarly, aneurysm surgery may disrupt neural pathways in the pelvis. Diseases affecting the autonomic system, principally diabetes mellitus, also affect the control of micturition. With the loss of sensation and contraction, the bladder becomes atonic, prone to the complication of stasis infection. The external sphincter remains closed by uninhibited tonic contractions, but the internal sphincter is partly open as it, to some extent, depends on detrusor activity.

Primary failure of the detrusor has been described, but it is usually secondary to chronic overdistension. Atonic myogenic bladder is caused by prolonged outlet obstruction and is found in the late stages of bladder decompensation. The most common cause is silent prostatic obstruction, where progressive loss of the desire to void results in overflow incontinence. In women, conscious postponement can lead to a large atonic bladder.

Principles of management

More than one mechanism may account for disordered micturition and urodynamic assessment is mandatory in all patients with a suspected or proven neuropathic bladder.

Neurologically intact patients

Patients with congenital defects or fistulae should have these repaired surgically if possible. If the fistula is malignant or the surrounding tissues are poor because of radiation, urinary diversion is preferable. Stress incontinence should be treated initially with pelvic floor exercises. If it persists in males, it is best treated by the

23

insertion of an artificial urinary sphincter. In females, the urethra and bladder neck should be returned to their natural positions and supported by means of colposuspension or a pubovaginal sling. The injection of bulking agents at the bladder neck can improve continence, but remains under evaluation. Tension-free vaginal tapes (TVT) are the most effective surgical modality to treat stress incontinence. Urge incontinence should be treated initially by bladder retraining, supplemented by anticholinergic drugs. If this fails, excellent results can be obtained by intravesical injection of botulinum toxin type A via flexible cystoscopy. Alternatives are insertion of a sacral nerve stimulator device, a detrusor myectomy (which involves stripping off a substantial proportion of the detrusor muscle) or splitting the bladder in half and suturing a strip of small bowel to augment the bladder (clam ileocystoplasty). Patients with atonic bladders are best managed by regular intermittent self-catheterisation (ISC).

Neuropathic patients

These patients are prone to urinary infection and renal impairment, and preservation of renal function takes priority. The patient's overall condition is important, and those that are poorly motivated or immobile with poor cognition and hand function are best managed by suprapubic catheterisation or urinary diversion. Highly motivated patients should be treated in much the same way as the neurologically intact, although the results are often less successful.

23.5 Summary

Micturition

- Micturition requires parasympathetic innervation (S2–S4) of the detrusor, sympathetic innervation (T10–L2) of the bladder neck and proximal urethra, and somatic innervation (S2–S4) of the bladder, pelvic floor and urethra
- Structural causes of disordered micturition in the male include prostatic enlargement, prostatectomy (dribble, stress and urge incontinence) and chronic illness/debility
- Structural causes of disordered micturition in the female include childbirth, surgery, radiotherapy and cystitis (infection, chronic interstitial cystitis and urethral syndrome)
- Neurogenic causes of disordered micturition are:
  - Impaired cortical control
  - Alcohol abuse and drugs
  - Spinal cord damage (at/below T12–L1: flaccid bladder with overflow; above T12–L1; overactive bladder with incoordination of urinary sphincter, which results in poor bladder emptying)
  - Pelvic nerve damage (surgery, diabetic autonomic neuropathy)
  - Atonic myogenic bladder (prolonged outlet obstruction).

External genitalia

Anatomy

In the male, these comprise the penis, testicles and scrotum; in the female, the mons pubis, labia majora, labia minora and the clitoris (Fig. 23.21).

The penis consists of three cylinders of erectile tissue. The ventral corpus spongiosum is expanded proximally as the bulb and distally as the glans penis, and transmits the urethra. Two

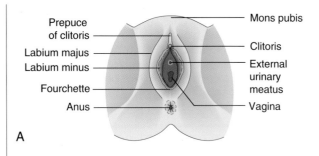

A

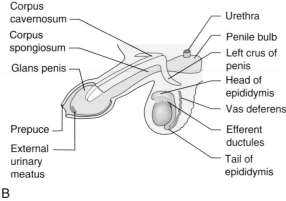

B

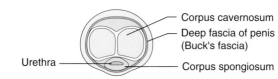

C

Fig. 23.21 Anatomy of the external genitalia. (A) Female. **(B)** Male. **(C)** Cross-section through the penis.

dorsolateral corpora cavernosa attach to each side of the inferior pubic arch as the crura. They form the body of the penis and become embedded in the glans.

The penile skin is hairless, free of fat, and extends over the glans as the prepuce or foreskin. Blood is supplied from the internal pudendal arteries. The scrotum is a thin rugose pouch of skin containing the two testicles. Each testicle is contained within a tough capsule (tunica albuginea) and has the epididymis attached to it posterior-laterally. This highly coiled tubular structure arises from the rete testis, where some 20 small tubules enter it. This head of epididymis is considerably larger than the lower tail, from which the vas deferens arises to traverse the spermatic cord and finally to open into the prostatic urethra as the ejaculatory duct. The testicle and epididymis are invaginated into the tunica vaginalis, which lies anteriorly, so providing a potential space where a hydrocoele may form. The testicular arteries supply the testes. Venous blood drains along the spermatic cord as the pampiniform plexus. The scrotum drains lymph to the inguinal lymph nodes, and the contents of the scrotum drain along the spermatic cord to nodes in the pelvis and abdomen.

In the female, the mons pubis is the fatty elevation over the pubis from which the labia run backwards, enclosing between them the vestibule into which open the vagina and urethra. The clitoris lies above the urethral opening and is a smaller replica of the penis, with the same erectile tissues.

Physiology

Parasympathetic stimulation leads to erection through the release of nitric oxide, with resultant vasodilatation of the arterioles, increased penile blood flow and passive closure of the venules. After sufficient stimulation, sperm from the epididymis and seminal fluid from the seminal vesicles are emptied into the prostatic urethra. Sympathetic stimulation is responsible for this emission, and also closes the bladder neck to prevent leakage of semen into the bladder. Ejaculation proper is due to rhythmic contraction of the bulbospongiosus muscles expelling the semen out through the urethra.

Circumcision

The foreskin is normally nonretractile for the first few months of life. By the end of the first year, half will retract, but it may be 3–4 years before >90% do so. Provided the parents are reassured, there is no reason, apart from religious grounds, to remove the foreskin within the first few years of life. In some children, the foreskin remains nonretractile and has to be treated by division of preputial adhesions or by circumcision. Otherwise, secretions collect under the foreskin, leading to infection (balanitis) and narrowing of the orifice (phimosis).

Severe phimosis may obstruct urinary flow, and if a poorly retracting foreskin remains retracted it can act as a tight band and cause engorgement and oedema of the glans (paraphimosis). This demands urgent treatment. It may be possible to compress the glans and draw the foreskin forwards, but if this fails, the tight band must be incised under general anaesthesia. Later, elective circumcision is advocated.

Congenital abnormalities of the penis

Hypospadias

Failure of the embryonic folds to fuse results in abnormal placing of the external urinary meatus on the ventral surface of the penis. The opening may be coronal, penile, scrotal or even perineal. The prepuce, which is in the form of a hood, should never be excised, as it is an important structure used in the reconstruction of the urethra. The corpus spongiosum may be scarred and fibrosed, leading to a ventral curvature or chordee of the penis. The aim of treatment is to correct the chordee by excising the fibrosis, and then to construct a new urethral opening in the normal position on the glans. This procedure should be ideally completed before the boy goes to school (Fig. 23.22).

Epispadias

In this condition the external urinary meatus opens on the dorsal surface of the penis. The extent of the malformation varies from an isolated penile abnormality to gross malformation of the bladder and urethra. The mucosa of the bladder and the ureteric orifices may be exposed and form the infraumbilical part of the abdominal wall (exstrophy). The urethra then lies opened out like a gutter. Other associated abnormalities include separation of the symphysis pubis and rectal prolapse. Reconstruction of these deformities is not always successful, and urinary incontinence may remain a major problem and require urinary diversion.

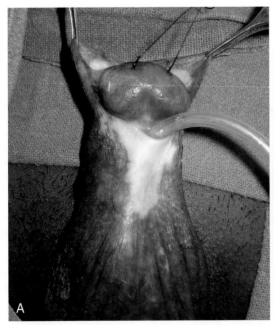
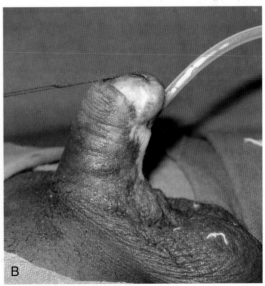

Fig. 23.22 Distal penile hypospadias. (A) Ventral and **(B)** lateral views. A silicone urethral catheter has been inserted through the urethral opening present on the ventrum of the distal third of the shaft of penis. The spatulated glans shows the vertically oriented urethral groove in the midline. The prepuce is hooded over the dorsum and is deficient ventrally. The edges of the prepuce are held with fine-tooth forceps on either side. Lateral view shows ventral curvature (chordee) distal to the urethral meatus. (Courtesy Dr Prabhat Shrivastava, Lok Nayak Hospital, New Delhi, India.)

23

Disorders of erection (impotence)

Impotence may be psychogenic, organic or drug-induced. Psychogenic problems, the most common cause, can usually be established from a careful history that includes details of sexual habits. Organic impotence is associated with cardiovascular disease, diabetes mellitus, neurogenic disorders, major pelvic injury or operations, vascular disease of the pelvic vessels (Leriche's syndrome), priapism and Peyronie's disease. Most of these conditions constitute irreversible impotence. Drug-induced impotence occurs with hormonal manipulation for prostatic cancer; some antihypertensive drugs may cause loss of erection or inability to ejaculate, and barbiturates, benzodiazepines, corticosteroids, phenothiazines and spironolactone may affect libido. Medical treatment is by oral sildenafil (Viagra), intracavernosal (self-)injection of papaverine or prostaglandin E. Vacuum suction devices or a prosthesis implanted into the corpora cavernosa are effective alternatives.

Priapism

This is a painful maintained erection unassociated with sexual desire. It is associated with intracavernosal self-injection for impotence (the most common cause), leukaemia, disorders of coagulation, renal dialysis and sickle-cell trait, and is believed to be due to venous sludging in the corpora cavernosa the corpus spongiosum and glans are unaffected.) Aspiration and intracavernosal injections of vasoconstrictors (phenylephrine) may be effective, especially in self-injection cases. If these fail, the creation of a venous shunt within 6–12 hours gives satisfactory results in up to 75% patients, and the patient can achieve normal erections subsequently. If treatment is delayed or incomplete, the erectile tissue is damaged and the patient will be impotent and require a penile prosthesis

Peyronie's disease

This is the occurrence of a hard fibrous plaque (or plaques) in the wall of a corpus cavernosum, causing curvature of the penis. The cause is obscure but is possibly related to trauma, leading to the formation of hard scar tissue. In addition to the deformity, the patient complains of pain during intercourse. Various treatments, including cortisone injections, vitamins and radiotherapy, have met with little success. Excision of the plaque and replacement by a dermal patch graft, or excision of a wedge of tissue on the convex (opposite) border of the penis, may be effective.

Carcinoma of the penis

This uncommon tumour has a prevalence of 1.5 cases per 100,000 and is generally attributed to poor hygiene associated with a nonretractile foreskin (Fig. 23.23). It occurs in males who were circumcised at birth and almost always occurs in the middle age. The cancer may be a papillary or an ulcerating squamous cell carcinoma. Local spread occurs early and the tumour may ulcerate and fungate. Lymphatic spread to inguinal lymph nodes is common; associated infection may also lead to lymphadenopathy. The patient may present with a purulent or blood-stained discharge. Unfortunately, many patients do not seek help until the lesion is advanced, some only when much of the penis is already destroyed and the inguinal lymph nodes are involved. The diagnosis must be confirmed by biopsy. Circumcision may cure early tumours confined to the prepuce. Early tumours confined to the glans may be treated by excision of the glans and skin grafting.

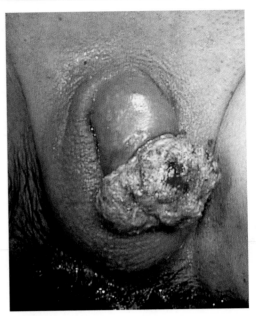

Fig. 23.23 Penile carcinoma.

Advanced tumours will require partial or total penile amputation, and often bilateral block dissection of the inguinal lymph nodes. Inoperable tumours are treated by chemotherapy and radiotherapy.

Inflammation of the penis

Inflammation of the glans penis (balanitis) usually also involves the prepuce (posthitis) and is common in children with poorly retractile foreskins. Circumcision usually cures recurrent nonspecific balanitis. Balanitis xerotica obliterans (BXO) is the local manifestation of lichen sclerosus et atrophicus of the glans and prepuce. It causes typical white scarring of the prepuce and glans, and may involve the urethral meatus and distal urethra. Meatal stenosis occurs as a result of recurrent infection, trauma or BXO. It may respond to removal of the inflammation (by circumcision) and meatal dilatation; alternatively, it may require meatotomy or meatoplasty.

Undescended testes (cryptorchidism)

Retractile testis

Normally, both testes are in the scrotum at birth or latest by 6 months of age. However, they may be excessively mobile and readily retract towards the external inguinal ring, even into the inguinal canal, especially when the patient is examined in a cold room due to an overactive cremasteric reflex. Such retractile testes may easily be misdiagnosed as being incompletely descended. The crucial clinical sign to differentiate a retractile testis from an undescended testis is the ability to bring the former down into the scrotal sac once the patient is relaxed. Since the testis remains in the scrotum most of the time, the development of the ipsilateral scrotum is also normal. Care must be taken to examine the baby in a warm room or after a bath.

Ectopic testis

An ectopic testis has developed normally, but after passing through the external inguinal ring it has strayed from its further path of normal descent into the scrotum. The common ectopic sites that the testis may lie in are the superficial inguinal pouch (most common), the perineum, the femoral triangle, and penile or prepubic sites (rare). The pathology may lie in abnormal distal attachment of gubernaculums, that (mis)guides the testis into the abnormal position.

True undescended testis

A true undescended testis is the one that is arrested at some point in the normal course of its descent between the kidney and the scrotum, and is hence hidden (cryptorchidism). The condition may be unilateral or bilateral, the former being more common. The incidence is about 3–4% at birth, half of which descend within the first month of life. The incidence of undescended testes is as high as 30% in premature infants. A few undescended testes may also complete their descent at puberty.

The aetiology is not clear and several hypotheses including defects of the gubernaculum, intrinsic testicular defects, and abnormalities of gonadotropin secretion or stimulation have been proposed.

The importance of identifying and treating the condition lies in the complications associated with this condition. Normally the temperature of the scrotum is about 1°C lower than the body temperature, which is important for the normal development of testis and for normal spermatogenesis. Exposure of testis to higher temperatures (as in abdominal cavity in undescended testes) leads to alteration in morphology as well as the function of the testes. This may occur as early as 1–2 years of life and therefore it is important to transpose the testes into the scrotum by the age of 1 year.

It has been theorised that some of these testes may have intrinsic defects, and may therefore not benefit from placement into the scrotum and will show abnormalities of function despite treatment.

Another important association of the undescended testes is a 30–40% higher incidence of malignancy, which affects not only the undescended testis but also its normally descended counterpart. This may suggest a role of testicular dysgenesis in the development of malignancy. Transposition of testes into the scrotum does not decrease the incidence of development of malignancy, but it nevertheless renders the organ amenable to clinical examination for an early detection of any abnormality.

Undescended testes are associated with an increased incidence of ipsilateral inguinal hernia and occasionally torsion.

Diagnosis is easy on clinical examination, as the affected hemiscrotum is empty and maldeveloped (cf. retractile testes). Localisation of the site may require the aid of radiological investigations, of which abdominal CT is the most accurate, examination under anaesthetic or laparoscopy.

Treatment is primarily surgical and consists of transposition of testis back into the scrotum, either laparoscopically or through an open approach. A staged procedure may be necessary in case the arrest is at a high level (Fowler–Stephens procedure). Care must be taken to preserve the vascular supply of the organ and to ensure that the transposition is tension free.

Torsion of the testis

Torsion of the spermatic cord is a urological emergency that develops due to rotation of the cord around itself, thereby resulting in strangulation of the blood supply to the testis. It is usually associated with anatomical abnormality of the tunica vaginalis or spermatic cord rendering the testis more prone to rotation.

The patient, usually a teenager, presents with sudden onset of testicular pain and swelling. There may be a history of minor trauma, or previous episodes of pain due to partial torsion. The initiating factor in most cases is a spasm of the cremaster, which inserts spirally into the cord, and therefore causes rotation of the testis. Due to the arrangement of the fibres of the cremaster, the direction of torsion is always constant, the anterior poles of the testes moving towards the midline. This is helpful when trying a manual detorsion of the organ.

On examination there is a red, swollen hemiscrotum that is usually too tender to palpate. It may be associated with nausea, vomiting and lower abdominal pain. The affected testis is retracted cranially (due to shortening of the cord by torsion), and lies horizontally in the scrotum when the patient is standing (due to abnormal investment of cord or tunica; Angell's sign). Elevation of the affected testicle may worsen the pain (Prehn's sign; cf. acute epididymo-orchitis). In a case of torsion, the cremasteric reflex is always absent.

Differential diagnosis includes acute epididymo-orchitis and trauma. A careful history and examination clinches the diagnosis. Acute epididymo-orchitis is rare in teenagers. The diagnosis is a clinical one, and no time should be wasted in performing radiological investigations.

Torsion of the testis is a surgical emergency; if the blood supply is not restored within 12 hours, the testis usually infarcts and must then be excised. If the patient is seen within the first 5–6 hours, manual detorsion may be attempted. The anterior pole of the affected testis is rotated outwards, away from the midline towards the ipsilateral thigh. If this fails urgent surgical exploration should be performed. If at operation the testis is found to be viable, it is sutured to the parietal tunica to prevent recurrence. As the underlying abnormality of the tunica is usually bilateral, the other testis must be fixed at the same time.

Testicular tumours

Pathology

Tumours of the testes are uncommon, with a prevalence of 5 cases per 100,000. They most commonly affect men between 20 and 40 years of age. Germ cell tumours make up 95% of testis cancers. Seminoma account for 60–70%, nonseminomatous germ cell tumours (NSGCTs) account for 25–35% and include teratoma, embryonal, choriocarcinoma and yolk sac tumours. Seminomas arise from seminiferous tubules and are of relatively low-grade malignancy. Metastases occur mainly via the lymphatics and may involve the lungs. NSGCTs arise from primitive germinal cells. They may contain cartilage, bone, muscle, fat and a variety of other tissues, and are classified according to the degree of differentiation. Well-differentiated tumours are the least aggressive; at the other extreme, trophoblastic teratoma is highly malignant. Occasionally, NSGCTs and seminoma occur in the same testis. A history of undescended testis increases the risk of malignancy in the ipsilateral testis. Orchidopexy does not reduce this risk but it does allow the testis to be moved into a position where it allows regular self-examination.

Clinical features

The most common presentation is the incidental discovery of a painless testicular lump. The history is often vague, however, and symptoms may be attributed to an injury, or there may be pain and swelling suggesting inflammation. The patient may have wrongly received treatment for 'acute epididymitis'. Very rarely, patients with teratoma may complain of gynaecomastia. Irrespective of the history, any new painless testicular lump in a young man must be regarded with suspicion. A hydrocoele in a young man also mandates investigation, as testicular tumours may be accompanied by blood-stained effusion in the tunica vaginalis.

23

Investigations

All suspicious scrotal lumps should be imaged by US, which provides a high degree of accuracy. As soon as a tumour is suspected, and before orchiectomy, serum levels of AFP, β-HCG and lactate dehydrogenase (LDH) should be determined. The levels of these 'tumour markers' are increased in extensive disease. Accurate staging is based on CT of the lungs, liver and retroperitoneal area, and an assessment of renal and pulmonary function.

Management

Through an inguinal incision the spermatic cord is divided at the internal ring; only then is the testis removed. Radiotherapy is the adjuvant treatment of choice for early-stage seminoma, as this tumour is very radiosensitive, although close surveillance will avoid unnecessary radiotherapy in 80%. The management of a NSGCT depends on the stage of the disease. Early disease confined to the testes may be managed without further treatment after orchidectomy, provided that there is close surveillance for at least 2 years; tumour progression is treated by chemotherapy. More advanced cancers are managed initially by chemotherapy, usually with a combination of bleomycin, etoposide and cisplatin. Retroperitoneal lymph node dissection (RPLND) is now only performed for stage I NSGCTs (to prevent recurrence), or for residual or recurrent nodal masses. AFP, β-HCG and LDH each offer a valuable means of monitoring response to treatment and detecting recurrent disease. These markers should be monitored in all patients with testicular tumours for at least 2 years after they are considered to be tumour free. CT is used to follow the response of enlarged lymph nodes to treatment.

Prognosis

The 5-year survival rate for patients with seminoma is 90–95%. The more variable prognosis of teratomas depends on tumour type, stage and volume. With more favourable tumours the 5-year survival rate may be as high as 95%, but in more advanced cases 60–70% is more usual.

23.6 Summary

Testicular tumours

- In the UK, there are about 2200 new cases of testicular tumour per year and the 20–40-year age group is predominantly affected
- Germ cell tumours account for 95% of all testicular tumours
- Seminomas arise from the seminiferous tubules, are of relatively low-grade malignancy, spread mainly via the lymphatic system and are very sensitive to radiotherapy
- Nonseminomatous germ cell tumours arise from germinal cells, their differentiation reflects their aggressiveness (well-differentiated tumours being the least aggressive) and they are not radiosensitive
- Treatment consists of radical orchiectomy (with division of the spermatic cord at the level of the deep inguinal ring). Radiotherapy is used if the tumour proves to be a seminoma, whereas chemotherapy (bleomycin, etoposide and cisplatin) is used for teratomas that are advanced or recurrent
- Seminomas have a 5-year survival rate of 90–95%, whereas teratomas have a more varied prognosis (60–95% 5-year survival rate).

Epididymo-orchitis

Acute epididymo-orchitis is usually the appropriate term, as both testis and epididymides are involved in the acute inflammatory reaction. The spermatic cord is also often thickened (funiculitis). After infection has subsided, the epididymis alone may remain thickened and irregular, so that chronic epididymitis may be diagnosed. Apparent involvement of the testis alone may be a feature of viral infections such as mumps orchitis. The usual cause of epididymo-orchitis is bacterial spread, either from infected urine or from gonococcal urethritis. The affected side of the scrotum is swollen, inflamed and very tender. In all cases, the urine or urethral discharge must be cultured. In the absence of a bacterial cause, a viral aetiology is likely. Treatment consists of antibiotics, analgesia, bed rest and a scrotal support. The choice of antibiotic depends on the results of culture and sensitivity determination of the organism responsible. If there is any doubt about the diagnosis, the testis should be explored. Abscess formation is now rare, but if signs of localisation or fluctuation develop, the pus should be drained. Infertility is an important late complication of epididymo-orchitis.

Tubercular epididymo-orchitis

In adults, this is usually secondary to urinary tuberculosis, wherein a retrograde infection of the prostate leads in turn to involvement of vas deferens, epididymis and testis. It is usually a slow process, which is painless. On examination the vas deferens is thickened and beaded, and the epididymis is enlarged, nontender and irregularly thickened (craggy). Rarely an epididymal abscess may rupture through the scrotal skin and may form a chronic sinus, which is pathognomonic of tuberculosis. Involvement of testis is rare and is usually secondary to tubercular epididymitis.

Involvement of epididymis and vas may lead to luminal obstruction due to scarring, and may result in infertility if bilateral. Treatment is medical with antitubercular drugs for 12–18 months.

Hydrocoele

This is a common condition, especially in older men, in which fluid collects in the tunica vaginalis, resulting in an enlarged but painless scrotum. Hydrocoele may be classified as vaginal, infantile, congenital or encysted hydrocoele of the cord, depending upon the anatomical region of the processus and tunica vaginalis in which the fluid collects (Fig. 23.24).

The inconvenience of its size usually leads the patient to seek advice. The cause of most hydrocoeles is unknown (idiopathic). The fluid is straw-coloured and protein-rich. In some patients, a hydrocoele develops as a reaction to epididymo-orchitis. Rarely, it may develop with a malignant testis (secondary hydrocoele) and the fluid may then be blood-stained. Another secondary hydrocoele seen only in tropical countries is filarial hydrocoele (Table 23.8).

On examination, a normal spermatic cord can be palpated above a smooth oval swelling. Typically, an idiopathic hydrocoele transilluminates (Fig. 23.25), although this may be difficult to elicit in long-standing cases owing to fibrosis and thickening of its wall. It is important to seek this physical sign and also to examine the neck of the scrotum carefully to exclude an inguinal hernia as the cause of the swelling. It may be possible to palpate the testis and confirm that it is normal, but this is unusual as it lies behind and is enveloped by the hydrocoele. If there is any doubt about the diagnosis, then an ultrasound should be performed. Injury to the scrotum may result in a swelling that resembles a hydrocoele but does not transilluminate because the tunica has filled with blood (haematocoele). Aspiration alone does not cure an idiopathic hydrocoele and the tunica soon refills. It is possible to obliterate the sac by injecting a sclerosant after aspiration, but surgical treatment is the most definitive treatment.

Opening and eversion of the tunica sac (Jaboulay's procedure) is the most commonly performed operation. The results are good,

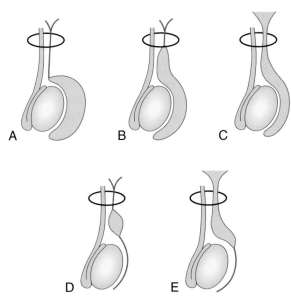

Fig. 23.24 Types of hydrocoeles. (A) Vaginal (most common), where the fluid collects in between the two layers of tunica vaginalis. **(B)** Infantile, where the hydrocoele sac extends from the scrotum up into the inguinal canal up to the deep ring. **(C)** Congenital, where there is a persistent communication between the hydrocoele sac and the peritoneal cavity across the deep ring. **(D)** Encysted hydrocoele of the cord, where a small part of the communication between the peritoneal cavity and the tunica remains unobliterated as a cyst in the inguinal canal. **(E)** Funicular, where the sac remains in communication with the peritoneal cavity but gets obliterated at the superficial ring or at the neck of the scrotum.

Table 23.8 Classification of hydrocoeles		
Feature	Primary hydrocoele	Secondary hydrocoele
Cause	Idiopathic	Trauma, infection, malignancy
Rate of development	Slow	Rapid
Size	Large	Small
Appearance	Tense	Lax
Testis	Not palpable	May be palpable
Primary abnormality	Defective absorption	Excessive secretion
Fluid	Clear/amber coloured	May be clear, purulent or blood stained

and it is believed that the secretory surface that faces outwards after the surgery secretes fluid that is absorbed by the scrotal lymphatics and passes to the inguinal channels, providing an alternate route for drainage. Small hydrocoeles with a thin small sac are best dealt with by plication of the sac (Lord's procedure).

Hydrocoele is a common abnormality in children. It is due to failure of closure of the processus vaginalis after descent of the testis. This patent processus vaginalis (PPV) allows fluid to drain into the scrotum around the testis. Most congenital hydrocoeles of this sort resolve before the first birthday. Those that persist require surgical treatment comprising ligation of the PPV through a small groin incision.

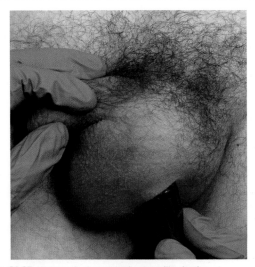

Fig. 23.25 Hydrocoele demonstrating transillumination.

Cyst of the epididymis

Cysts in the epididymis arise from diverticula of the vasa efferentia. The distinction between a cyst of the epididymis and a hydrocoele is easy. Epididymal cysts are almost always multiple and, therefore, nodular on palpation; they are located above and behind the testis, which is palpably separate from the cysts, and always transilluminate brightly. A solitary epididymal cyst may even resemble a testis, so giving rise to fables of three testes and the term 'pawnbroker's sign'. Sometimes the fluid within an epididymal cyst is opalescent and contains sperm (spermatocoele). Usually the fluid is clear. It is best to leave these cysts alone unless increasing size warrants excision. Careful dissection is needed to remove the cyst completely. Often several other little cysts are present which, if not removed, will eventually increase in size and produce a so-called *recurrence*. If all the cysts are removed, the pathway for sperm will almost certainly be damaged. Bilateral operations can result in sterility.

Varicocoele

The veins of the pampiniform plexus are dilated and tortuous, producing a swelling in the line of the spermatic cord that resembles a 'bag of worms' (Fig. 23.26). It is more common on the left side, possibly because the right-angled drainage of the left testicular vein into the renal vein renders it more liable to stasis.

The main symptom is that of a dragging sensation in the scrotum, and a feeling of heaviness. Varicocoele may also be associated with infertility or subfertility. The pampiniform plexus acts as a countercurrent mechanism that helps in heat exchange and keeps the temperature of scrotum about 1°C lower than body temperature, which is crucial for normal spermatogenesis. An interference with this mechanism, as in varicocoele, causes stasis of blood and leads to an elevation of the scrotal temperature, thereby interfering with spermatogenesis and/or sperm function.

Treatment involves ligation of the spermatic vein, which may be done surgically (open or laparoscopically). The advantage of the laparoscopic approach is that bilateral disease can be managed simultaneously. Alternatively, the feeding veins can be obliterated radiologically by means of coil embolisation.

23

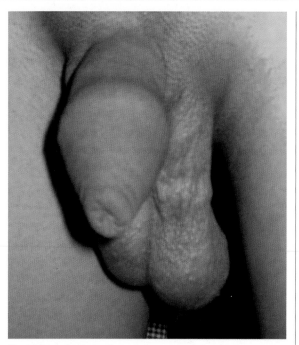

Fig. 23.26 Left-sided varicocoele in a young male. Note the 'bag of worms' appearance and a smaller testis.

The level at which the testicular veins are ligated vary and may be described as high approach (Palomo's), mid- or inguinal approach, and low or scrotal approach. High approach has the advantage of fewer veins as the tributaries of the pampiniform plexus join to form one or two veins at the level of deep ring. The presenting symptom also dictates the approach adopted. If symptomatic and fertility is not an issue, a high approach is preferred. On the other hand, if the surgery is to be performed for infertility, a low or scrotal approach is preferred. Use of optical magnification (operating microscope/loupes) ensures that the testicular lymphatics are spared, all the tributaries of the pampiniform plexus are ligated and the vas deferens is not damaged (micro-varicocoelectomy).

Lynn Myles
Paul M. Brennan

24

Neurosurgery

Chapter contents

Introduction 461

Surgical anatomy and physiology 461

Blood supply 462

Intracranial pressure 462

Investigations 465

Cerebrovascular disease 465

Neurotrauma 470

Intracranial infections 473

Intracranial tumours 475

Spinal dysraphism 480

Hydrocephalus 481

Malformations of the skull 482

Functional neurosurgery 483

Vertebral column 483

Peripheral nerve lesions 486

Introduction

The scope of neurosurgical operations continues to evolve with advances in such domains as imaging, anaesthesia, instrumentation, microsurgery, endoscopy and frameless image guidance, all of which contribute to reduced operative mortality and morbidity. There are many areas of continuing controversy and much of neurosurgery still lacks a quality evidence base to guide management. The results of randomised controlled trials (RCTs) have usually led to significant improvements in practice and a softening of entrenched opinion (see the EBM boxes throughout this chapter). There are many other areas, such as the management of low-grade and malignant gliomas, where evidence from RCTs is urgently required to improve patient outcomes.

Surgical anatomy and physiology

Anatomy and physiology is key to localising and treating pathology relevant to neurosurgery.

The skull

The skull has two main parts, a base and the calvaria. The calvaria comprises the frontal bone, the paired parietal and temporal bones, and the occipital bone. The frontal and parietal bones are joined by the coronal suture, the parietal bones by the sagittal (midline) suture, and the parietal and occipital bones by the squamosal sutures. These sutures are closed by about 18 months, and thereafter the brain is enclosed in a rigid container. The skull base comprises the orbital roof, cribriform plates and sphenoid bones (anterior cranial fossa); sphenoid wings and petrous temporal bone (middle

cranial fossa); and the squamous occipital bones, the clivus and petrous temporal regions (posterior cranial fossa). Holes in the skull base, known as foramina, permit transit of blood vessels, spinal cord and cranial nerves. The largest, called the foramen magnum, is at the base of the posterior cranial fossa through which the medulla projects inferiorly towards the spinal cord.

The spine

The bony axial spinal skeleton comprises 7 cervical, 12 thoracic and 5 lumbar vertebrae, as well as the sacrum and coccyx. Although vertebral structure varies between regions, the vertebrae basically comprise a body, pedicles, lamina and a posterior spine. The bony spinal canal is formed by the body (anteriorly), the pedicles (laterally) and the lamina (posteriorly). The canal contains the spinal dura, the spinal cord and, inferiorly, the cauda equina. The vertebral bodies are joined by fibroelastic discs and articulate via facet joints.

The brain

The brain is a gelatinous structure that in adults weighs about 1.4 kg. It comprises the paired cerebral hemispheres, the brain stem and the cerebellum. Primary fissures divide the brain into lobes (frontal, parietal, occipital, temporal and limbic). The temporal lobe is separated from the frontal and parietal lobes by the sylvian fissure, and the rolandic (central) sulcus separates the frontal from the parietal lobes. Some important brain functions can be localised to specific cortical regions, such as motor cortex (precentral gyrus), somatosensory cortex (postcentral gyrus) and speech/language (Broca's and Wernike's area). Commissural fibres, the largest of which is the corpus callosum, connect the cerebral hemispheres. Cortical grey matter lies on the surface of the brain and comprises laminae of neurons that project into the white matter (tracts). Important deep cortical nuclear regions include the basal ganglia, thalamus and hypothalamus. The brain stem comprises the midbrain, pons and medulla. The cerebellum attaches to the back of the pons and is responsible for movement, coordination, balance and posture.

The meninges and cerebrospinal fluid

The brain and spinal cord are encased by the meninges. The outer layer, the dura, is the most robust. The two inner layers are much finer: a spider's web-like tissue, the arachnoid, and a very thin layer over the surface of the brain called the pia. The pia and arachnoid layers bound the cerebrospinal fluid (CSF) space. CSF is made of fluid secreted from the choroid plexus and extracellular fluid from the brain that passes across the ependyma. The paired lateral ventricles, lined by ependyma, are the large CSF-containing spaces within the hemispheres. They communicate via the foramen of Monro with the third ventricle, which in turn communicates via the cerebral aqueduct with the fourth ventricle in the pons and medulla. Outflow foramina (Luschka and Magendie) connect with the basal and spinal subarachnoid spaces. There are several large CSF cisterns around the base of the brain (e.g., cisterna magna, cerebellopontine cistern). CSF flows over the hemisphere to be reabsorbed in the arachnoid granulations.

The cranial cavity is subdivided by thick folds of dura; the falx cerebri separates the two cerebral hemispheres and the tentorium cerebelli separates the middle from the posterior cranial fossa.

The cranial nerves

The 12 paired cranial nuclei arise from the base of the brain. The olfactory nerve (cranial nerve; CN I) transmits the sense of smell via the olfactory bulbs and tracts to the rhinencephalon in the temporal lobes. Vision is conveyed from the retina by the optic nerves (CN II) that connect through the optic tracts to the lateral geniculate body of the thalamus, whose fibres project to the occipital lobe. The oculomotor (CN III) and trochlear (CN IV) nerves project from the midbrain and along with CN VI control ocular motility. The trigeminal nerve (CN V) provides sensation to the face, as well as innervating the muscles of mastication. The abducens nerve (CN VI) controls abduction (lateral movement) of the eye. The facial nerve (CN VII) arises from the pontomedullary junction and controls the facial musculature, conveys taste from the anterior two-thirds of the tongue, and is secretomotor to the lacrimal and submandibular glands. The vestibulo-cochlear nerve (CN VIII) conveys hearing from the cochlea and balance from the labyrinth. Nerves IX (glossopharyngeal), X (vagus), XI (accessory) and XII (hypoglossal) project from the medulla to innervate the tongue, pharynx, larynx, bronchus and intestines.

The spinal cord

The spinal cord consists of central grey matter (neuron cell bodies) and white matter (axonal tracts), and gives off 8 cervical, 12 thoracic, 5 lumbar and 4 sacral paired spinal roots. Each root is actually formed from a ventral and a dorsal rootlet arising directly from the spinal cord. The dorsal root contains sensory fibres carrying information from the peripheral nervous system, whose cell bodies reside in the dorsal root ganglion, a small bulge on the

back of the dorsal rootlet. The ventral root carries motor fibres whose cell bodies are located in the spinal cord grey matter. The spinal cord is enlarged in the lower cervical region and at the thoracolumbar region (conus), and terminates in the adult at about L1–L2 level. Below the level of the conus is the cauda equina, a collection of the peripheral nerves that innervate the lower limbs, bladder, bowels and genitalia. The sympathetic division of the autonomic nervous system emerges from the thoracic and lumbar spinal cord. The parasympathetic division begins in selected cranial nerves and the sacral spinal cord.

Blood supply

The brain requires a large cerebral blood flow (CBF; 800 mL/min, 16% of cardiac output) to satisfy its oxygen and glucose requirements. The cell body-rich cortex receives about 50 mL/100 g/min, and the white matter about 20 mL/100 g/min. The blood supply to the brain is broadly divided into anterior and posterior circulations that communicate with each other, and across the midline, through the circle of Willis (Fig. 24.1). In some circumstances, occlusion of a major artery can be compensated for provided that collateral flow through the circle of Willis is adequate.

Anterior circulation

The major vessels supplying the anterior circulation of the brain are the paired internal carotid arteries. These arise from the common carotid artery, then pass through the skull base, along the middle fossa, and through the cavernous sinus before dividing into the anterior and middle cerebral arteries. Smaller but important branches include the posterior communicating artery, which interconnects the anterior and posterior circulations, the anterior choroidal arteries, and fine perforating vessels to the inferior part of the brain. The anterior cerebral arteries supply large parts of the frontal and medial parts of the parietal lobes. The middle cerebral artery supplies the posterior frontal region and most of the temporal and parietal regions.

Posterior circulation

The posterior cerebral circulation arises from paired vertebral arteries that pass through the cervical foramina, enter the skull and join to form a single midline basilar artery. This divides terminally into the paired posterior cerebral arteries that supply the brain stem, cerebellum, occipital lobes and inferior parts of the temporal lobes. Many of these are 'end-arteries', so occlusion often leads to a well-defined stroke syndrome, such as lateral medullary syndrome.

Intracranial pressure

Once the skull's sutures fuse, the brain is enclosed within a rigid bony container. Intracranial pressure (ICP) therefore depends on the relative volumes of intracranial blood, CSF and brain parenchyma; if one constituent increases then another must decrease, or else the ICP will increase; this is the essence of the Munro–Kellie doctrine. ICP fluctuates in response to normal variation in intrathoracic pressure (e.g., increased by coughing, defaecation) and cardiac pulsation. These transient increases do no harm. In a normal supine adult, ICP is the same as the CSF pressure obtained at lumbar puncture (LP; 5–15 cm H_2O, 4–10 mmHg). Symptoms of raised ICP may include headache,

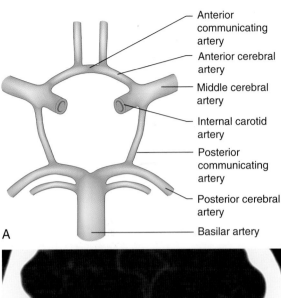

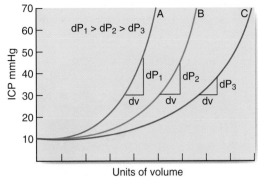

Fig. 24.2 The effects of a mass lesion on intracranial pressure. Generally, intracranial pressure (ICP) increases exponentially with the mass lesion. However, the shape of the pressure–volume curves varies depending on the brain. Thus, curve A would represent a mass lesion in a young healthy brain (limited compensation), curve B the brain of a middle-aged patient, and curve C a patient with brain atrophy who is thus able to compensate for a large intracranial mass lesion before ICP rises.

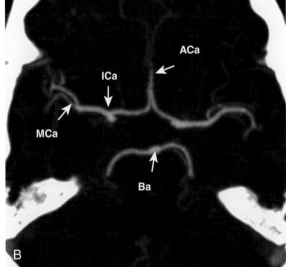

Fig. 24.1 Circle of Willis. (A) Diagram outlining the major arteries. **(B)** View on a CT angiogram. The basilar artery bifurcation, carotid bifurcation, anterior cerebral arteries and middle cerebral arteries can all be clearly seen. *ACa,* Anterior cerebral artery; *Ba,* basilar artery; *ICa,* carotid bifurcation; *MCa,* middle cerebral artery.

vomiting and visual disturbance (blurring of vision). Papilloedema may be apparent on examination. Neurological deficits may facilitate localisation of a causative lesion. If the raised ICP is chronic then there may be few clinical signs or symptoms. A rapid increase in ICP may precipitate acute reduction in conscious level.

In patients with intracranial mass lesions (tumour, haemorrhage), oedema or CSF obstruction, the extra volume is at first compensated for by a reduction in cerebral blood volume and CSF volume. A critical point is reached where no further compensation is possible. Any additional volume (e.g., increasing haematoma) leads to an exponential rise in ICP (Fig. 24.2). The rate of increase in the volume of intracranial mass is crucial (Fig. 24.2). With more chronic, slow-growing lesions such as some brain tumours, abscesses or congenital abnormalities, extraordinary degrees of compensation can actually occur. In some situations, even massive lesions can lead to minimal symptoms and signs, despite brain herniation (see later).

The consequence of changes in ICP can be understood in terms of the effect on cerebral perfusion pressure (CPP). CPP is the difference between mean arterial pressure (MAP; pushing blood into the brain) and ICP (effectively resisting blood flow into the brain) ($CPP = MAP - ICP$). So, if ICP increases, CPP will reduce unless the MAP increases. Simply speaking, a reduction in CPP will reduce CBF unless the heart rate increases. There is, however, also a system of vascular autoregulation to maintain optimal CBF (60–140 mmHg) over a range of CPP. For example, as MAP increases, the cerebral blood vessels vasoconstrict, reducing blood flow, and vice versa. Blood vessel diameter is also controlled by arteriolar carbon dioxide concentration (Pa_{CO_2}); increased Pa_{CO_2} causes vasodilation and increased CBF. Other compounds, such as nitric oxide and endothelin, also regulate local CBF. These different physiological mechanisms work in parallel to compensate for initial changes in ICP.

However, if there is a severe and sustained elevation of ICP the compensatory mechanisms become ineffective and cerebral perfusion may be focally or generally compromised, leading to cerebral ischaemia and infarction. The ability of blood vessels to autoregulate can also be impaired by brain injury itself. A CPP of >60 mmHg is generally required to sustain adequate cerebral perfusion, although children and young adults can tolerate lower levels.

Brain herniation syndromes

Generalised or localised increases in ICP can lead to marked displacement (herniation) of intracranial structures causing blood vessel compression, further compromising brain perfusion.

Subfalcine (cingulate gyral) herniation

A parasagittal lesion can cause the ipsilateral cingulate gyrus to herniate beneath the free edge of the falx (Fig. 24.3A). Anterior cerebral artery compression may cause medial hemispheric infarction, but otherwise the principal clinical effect is deteriorating conscious level.

Transtentorial (uncal) herniation

With large lesions, the medial part of the ipsilateral temporal lobe is pushed down through the tentorial notch to become wedged between the tentorial edge and the midbrain (Fig. 24.3B). The opposite cerebral peduncle is also pushed against the sharp tentorial edge. The aqueduct is compressed, obstructing CSF flow. Venous obstruction leads to midbrain haemorrhage. The clinical features of an uncal herniation are that the

24

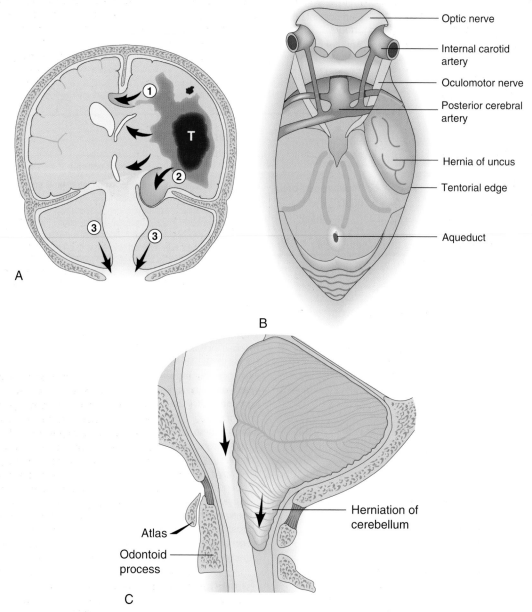

Fig. 24.3 Herniation syndromes. (A) Coronal diagram of the dynamics of an intracranial mass lesion. T causes mass effect that compresses the midline and the ventricles (*unnumbered arrows*), provoking subfalcine or cingulated herniation (*arrow 1*), and transtentorial herniation (*arrow 2*). If the mass effect is uncontrolled, tonsillar herniation may also occur (*arrows 3*). **(B)** Transtentorial herniation in the axial plane. **(C)** Foraminal herniation. T, Tumour.

- Glasgow Coma Score (GCS) falls and the motor component may become asymmetrical
- Ipsilateral pupil dilates and becomes nonreactive to light
- Blood pressure rises, the pulse slows, the respiratory rate falls (Cushing's response)
- The patient becomes apnoeic.

Foraminal (tonsillar) herniation

With posterior cranial fossa masses the cerebellar tonsils and medulla are displaced downwards through the foramen magnum (Fig. 24.3A and C). Cerebellar impaction leads to compression of the medulla, leading to a dramatic decrease in the GCS, bilateral extensor responses (decerebration) and bilateral fixed dilated pupils. A Cushing's response and sudden respiratory arrest can follow; this is called 'coning.' This can also occur following removal of CSF during LP in patients with raised ICP due to a posterior fossa mass, so in general LP must not be performed in patients suspected of having raised ICP caused by a mass lesion.

False localising signs

In a patient with a neurological deficit, the clinical history and examination aim to establish an anatomical localisation of the lesion and then generate a list of possible differential diagnoses. Thus, a patient with left hemiparesis may have a lesion in the right motor cortex, right corona radiata, right internal capsule, right crus cerebri, left half of medulla after the motor decussation or in the left half of the cervical cord. However, very occasionally the anatomy can be misleading in terms of localising the pathology.

Although a patient with a right frontoparietal extradural haematoma will usually have left hemiparesis, if there is also a transtentorial herniation then the right uncus displaces the midbrain against the tentorium, resulting in compression of the left crus cerebri, which can produce a right hemiparesis (paresis ipsilateral to the lesion is popularly referred to as *Kernohan's notch*). The clinician may therefore falsely localise the lesion to the left hemisphere. This is not common. In this situation, the dilated right pupil from right CN III compression is of true localising value and helps clinch the diagnosis.

The abducens nerve (CN VI) has a long course ascending from the pons to the cavernous sinus. Raised ICP can result in brain shift that stretches the 6th cranial nerve, falsely localising the anatomical site of the lesion to the pons.

24.1 Summary

Intracranial pressure

- The skull is rigid, so any increase in volume may increase intracranial pressure (ICP)
- Cerebral perfusion pressure = mean arterial pressure − intracranial pressure
- The principal symptoms of chronic raised ICP are headache, vomiting and visual disturbance (blurring of vision). Papilloedema may be apparent
- Reduced cerebral perfusion pressure can result in reduced blood flow, leading progressively to decreased Glasgow Coma Score, herniation syndromes, bradycardia, hypertension, respiratory abnormalities (e.g., apnoea) and death.

Investigations

Plain x-ray

There is rarely a role for plain x-rays in the acute assessment of raised ICP where computed tomography/magnetic resonance imaging (CT/MRI) is available. If CT/MRI demonstrates intracranial metastases then a plain chest x-ray may identify the primary lesion. Where CT/MRI is unavailable, 'normal' intracranial calcification, for example of the pineal gland or choroid plexus, may allow brain displacement to be inferred. Abnormal calcification can also develop in certain cysts and tumours. Plain x-rays of the skull and spine may also reveal evidence of bony erosion from metastatic tumour spread.

Computed tomography

CT does not image brain tissue as well as MRI, but images are acquired more rapidly. CT will demonstrate the cause of raised ICP in most patients, and spiral CT can also image the craniofacial skeleton (if traumatic injury) and blood vessels (CT angiography, or CT-A; may be useful in trauma or subarachnoid haemorrhage [SAH]).

Magnetic resonance imaging

MRI provides detailed information about the brain parenchyma and mass lesions (because of the relative water contents of the different tissues), but images bony structures less well than CT. As well as standard T1 and T2 sequences, additional MRI sequences permit further discrimination between possible differential diagnoses of mass lesions, e.g., Fluid-attenuated inversion recovery (FLAIR), or magnetic resonance spectroscopy. Diffusion tensor imaging localises white matter tracts. The function of brain tissues can also be evaluated, since active areas of the brain will have increased blood flow and oxygen consumption (functional MRI). With both CT and MRI, an intravenous enhancing agent can be administered (iodine-based compounds with CT and gadolinium-based for MRI). These compounds are normally excluded from the brain parenchyma by the blood–brain barrier (BBB), but breakdown of BBB integrity occurs with neoplastic, inflammatory or ischaemic processes. MRI is limited by certain conditions (e.g., cardiac pacemakers), but most modern neurosurgical implants will be MRI compatible.

CT and MR angiography

Both MRI and CT can be used to perform noninvasive angiography (magnetic resonance angiography, CT-A). These techniques are in some situations replacing conventional intraarterial digital subtraction angiography (IA-DSA), but digital subtraction angiography remains the gold standard. Angiography usually requires administration of a contrast agent, but Time of Flight MRI provides angiographic images without need for contrast.

Cerebrovascular disease

The management of patients with stroke will depend on its cause and clinical consequences. Most forms of embolic and ischaemic stroke are dealt with by medical neurologists, or stroke physicians. Occlusive disease affecting the extracranial vessels, a common cause of stroke and transient ischaemic attack (TIA), is usually managed by vascular surgeons (Chapter 25). Transient ischaemic attacks are associated with a high risk of major stroke within 5 years unless treatment is instituted (e.g., by carotid endarterectomy or aspirin therapy). The most common cause of large primary intracerebral haemorrhage (ICH) is small-vessel disease rather than large-vessel aneurysms. The optimal management strategy for these patients is uncertain, with no increased benefit or harm from surgical intervention. When SAH has occurred the priority is to determine whether there is an underlying aneurysm that has bled.

Brain tissue metabolism is vitally dependent on a consistent delivery of oxygen and glucose substrates for energy. If there is cessation of substrate delivery, the brain tissue will either die (if CBF is below a threshold of 12–15 mL/100 g/min) or stop functioning (if CBF is between 15 and 25 mL/100 g/min). These ischaemic thresholds are very important in terms of the extent of stroke (i.e., the amount of tissue that will die) and the penumbra (i.e., tissue that is damaged but still able to recover from these acute events). Urgent thrombolysis in ischaemic stroke with intravenous fibrinolytic therapy may improve prognosis if administered within 3-4 hours of onset of symptoms. Decompressive craniectomy can also save life (but with risk of significant morbidity) in selected cases if raised ICP due to ischaemic brain swelling is a problem, most commonly secondary to a middle cerebral artery infarction.

Subarachnoid haemorrhage

Spontaneous SAH affects 100 persons per million per year and most frequently (70%) results from the rupture of an intracranial 'berry' aneurysm. Other causes include small vessel rupture, arteriovenous malformation (AVM), cavernoma, tumour, infection and

24

Table 24.1 World Federation of Neurosurgical Societies grading system for subarachnoid haemorrhage

WFNS grade	Glasgow Coma Score	Focal neurological deficits
1	15	No
2	14–13	No
3	14–13	Yes
4	12–7	–
5	6–3	–

trauma. Typically, the patient complains of a sudden onset of severe headache that rapidly peaks in intensity (within 1 minute). Patients often describe it as like being 'hit on the head with a hammer' or as 'the worst headache they have ever had'. There is usually associated neck stiffness and photophobia. A positive Kernig's sign denotes meningism. In some cases, a small 'herald' bleed a few days earlier may have gone unnoticed. Nausea and vomiting are common. Conscious level is variably affected, ranging from mild disorientation to coma to rapid death.

Grading of SAH depends on the coma score of the patient at time of presentation. The most widely used system is the World Federation of Neurosurgical Societies' (WFNS) grading, graded 1–5 (Table 24.1). Sudden death is not uncommon when an aneurysm ruptures into the brain substance rather than the subarachnoid space. However, when the syndrome is of a grade 1 haemorrhage, a high degree of suspicion for SAH is required. SAH can mimic atypical migraines, thunderclap headache, coital cephalgia, pituitary apoplexy and meningitic-like syndromes. Focal signs depend upon the vessel affected. An unrecognised aneurysmal bleed may recur acutely and be devastating.

Saccular intracranial aneurysms

Risk factors include smoking, hypertension, polycystic disease of the kidney and female gender. The median age of affected patients is 55 years, although familial aneurysms may rupture earlier. Most aneurysms (85%) affect the anterior circulation and 15% of patients have more than one. The majority have no symptoms until rupture occurs, although a few may suffer compressive symptoms (e.g., oculomotor nerve [CN III] palsy from a posterior communicating artery aneurysm). Ectatic aneurysms may cause symptoms by embolic phenomena. Many intracranial aneurysms are now discovered as incidental findings when the brain is imaged for other reasons but are normally managed by interventional radiology because of the potential devastating consequences of SAH.

Investigations

The standard investigation is CT, which characteristically demonstrates blood in the CSF basal cisterns in the acute phase (Fig. 24.4). CSF blood is gradually broken down, so the CT detection rate falls after the first 72 hours. If the diagnosis is in doubt, then a LP should be performed, but only in patients whose clinical condition is good and in whom CT has excluded an intracranial mass lesion or midline shift. If this is performed early, the CSF will be uniformly blood-stained; later (after approximately 12 hours) it will contain haem pigments that will be apparent on naked-eye inspection (xanthochromia) or can be detected by spectrophotometry.

Next, a search must be made for the site of the bleeding. Conventionally, carotid or vertebral angiography has been

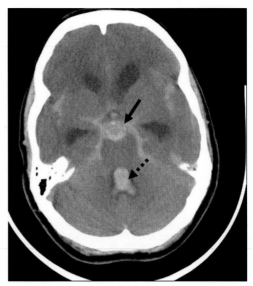

Fig. 24.4 Axial computed tomography of a patient following subarachnoid haemorrhage. Blood is seen in the basal cisterns as a white lesion (*solid arrow*), and also in the fourth ventricle (*broken arrow*). There is early enlargement of all ventricles. (Courtesy Dr R. Gibson.)

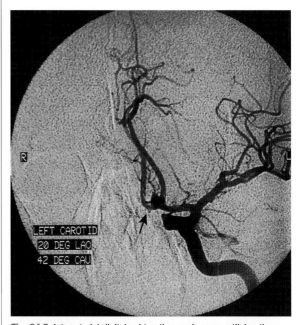

Fig. 24.5 Intraarterial digital subtraction angiogram outlining the cerebral vasculature and showing an aneurysm of the anterior communicating artery (*arrow*).

performed (Fig. 24.5). However, CT and MR angiography are equally good at revealing aneurysms greater than 5 mm and are noninvasive, thus associated with less morbidity. Missing the diagnosis of a ruptured aneurysm can be serious (if it rebleeds), so there is a tendency to perform angiography in patients in whom the diagnosis is equivocal. For that reason, a source of bleeding will be identified in only 70% of angiograms. In 30% of cases, no source is found despite a repeat angiogram after 3 months. Many of these patients will be diagnosed with a condition called *perimesencephalic SAH*, which is of unknown aetiology.

Management of aneurysmal SAH

The medical management of SAH includes intravenous fluids, the calcium antagonist nimodipine, analgesia and antiemetics. Patients in coma will usually be intubated and managed in a neurointensive care unit. Clinical deterioration may occur because of rebleeding, vasospasm, hydrocephalus, seizures, metabolic abnormalities and infections.

Rebleeding is a major cause of morbidity and mortality following aneurysm rupture. Rebleeding rates are maximum in the first 24 hours and subsequently fall off over the next few weeks, reaching a rate of 4% per annum. Thus, the initial focus of treatment is to prevent rebleeding. Until recently, standard management was occlusion of the aneurysm from the cerebral circulation by surgically clipping its neck (Fig. 24.6 and EBM 24.1). However, it is now standard to place detachable coils within the aneurysm via a catheter passed from the femoral artery into the cerebral circulation (Fig. 24.7). The coils unwind in the aneurysm and induce thrombosis. Coiling is a less invasive procedure than open surgery, and a prospective RCT

demonstrated that when an aneurysm can be treated by surgery or coiling, the latter is safer (EBM 24.2). Improvements in coil, stent and basket technology mean most aneurysms can now be coiled.

Even when an aneurysm has been successfully excluded by means of coiling or surgery, the patient can still suffer stroke. Patients may exhibit signs of focal or global cerebral ischaemia known as *delayed cerebral deficit*, 4–14 days following a SAH. This has been attributed primarily to vasospasm. It can be ameliorated by the prophylactic use of nimodipine, which has significantly decreased the risk of stroke (to 23%) and death (to 22%) (EBM 24.3). Clinical practice also includes induced hypertension (often using inotropes) and plasma volume loading (to keep up CPP), as well as haemodilution (to reduce blood viscosity in the hope of increasing flow). This 'triple therapy' has its own problems, such as precipitating cardiac failure.

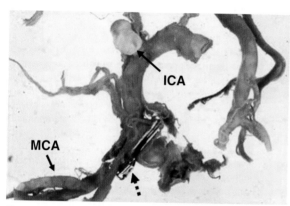

Fig. 24.6 Cerebral arteries at postmortem showing a surgical clip (*broken arrow*) on a ruptured middle cerebral artery aneurysm. There is also a nonruptured carotid bifurcation aneurysm (arrow). *ICA,* Internal carotid artery; *MCA,* middle cerebral artery.

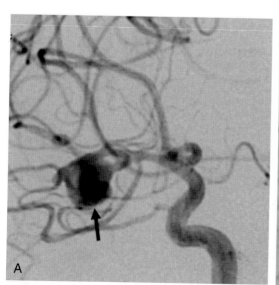
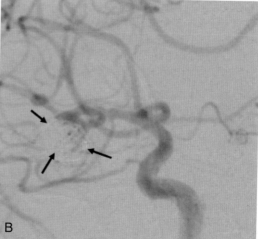

Fig. 24.7 Middle cerebral artery aneurysm. **(A)** Digital subtraction angiogram showing the aneurysm (*arrow*). **(B)** Its occlusion from the cerebral circulation after coiling (*arrows*).

The outcome following aneurysmal SAH is dependent upon the condition of the patient on admission and the CSF blood load (the more blood, the worse the outcome). About 90% of patients admitted in good condition (WFNS grade 1) enjoy a complete recovery. By contrast, about 50% of those admitted in coma (grade 5) die or are severely disabled. The outcome of intermediate patients is unpredictable. Hypotension and fever also predict poorer outcome.

Primary intracerebral haemorrhage

Primary ICH is becoming an increasing problem as the population of many developed countries ages. It is four times more common than SAH and, in about 30% of cases, is associated with amyloid angiopathy. Most cases are caused by hypertensive rupture of small arterioles, resulting in haematomas located in the putamen, cerebellum, thalamus, cerebral lobes and pons. Many haemorrhages are small and deep; others may be very large and cause death by raising ICP and provoking uncal or tonsillar herniation syndromes. Other causes of primary ICH include the rupture of a saccular aneurysm or AVM. The onset is usually abrupt, with many patients developing a flaccid hemiparesis or brain stem-cerebellar syndrome. One-third of patients die within a few weeks and many of those who survive are permanently disabled. The results of a recent prospective multicentre international RCT of surgery for ICH (STICH) have demonstrated that there are no significant differences in outcome with medical or surgical management of spontaneous, nonaneurysmal, supratentorial ICH (EBM 24.4).

EBM	24.4 Surgical evacuation of intracerebral haemorrhage

'Surgical evacuation of intracerebral haemorrhage is not superior to medical management (the STICH trial).'

Mendelow AD, et al. Lancet. 2005;365: 387–397 and Lancet. 2013;382:397–408.

Arteriovenous malformations

Cerebral AVMs are congenital vascular anomalies characterised by one or more feeding arteries, a cluster of abnormal capillaries forming the nidus, and a few draining veins either into the superficial or deep venous systems. This leads to gross dilatation of the draining cerebral veins, as well as ectasia and occasionally aneurysmal dilatation of the feeding artery. AVMs usually present with seizures or haemorrhage, while high-flow AVMs can 'steal' blood away from normal brain, leading to cerebral ischaemia. Rupture of an AVM typically causes an ICH rather than a SAH. As the haematoma is under less pressure, the overall prognosis is better than for aneurysmal SAH. The diagnosis is confirmed on CT or MRI and angiography (Fig. 24.8). If the AVM can be excised, then the risk of further haemorrhage is removed, and the incidence and frequency of seizures is considerably reduced. Sometimes, however, the AVM is large and in an important (eloquent) or inaccessible location. In these cases, endovascular 'glueing' or stereotactic radiosurgical treatment may be appropriate. The latter is a focused form of x-ray therapy that leads to fibrosis over a 2-year period.

Direct arteriovenous communications (fistulae) are usually located within the dura, either near a dural venous sinus in the brain or on a dural root sleeve in the spine. Cranial dural AVFs (Fig. 24.9) typically occur in the setting of dural venous sinus thrombosis secondary to trauma or infection followed by opening up of several normal arteriovenous connections in the dural sinus walls and a transmission of arterial pressure into leptomeningeal vessels, resulting in venous oedema and intracranial hypertension. Spinal dural AVFs commonly located in the thoracolumbar spine lead to venous hypertension in the spinal cord with progressive spastic paraparesis. Multiple tortuous vessels in the subarachnoid space on MRI representing normal dilated veins point towards the diagnosis. This can be confirmed with a spinal angiogram that detects the abnormal AV fistula along one or two roots (Fig. 24.10). Treatment is usually occlusion of the fistula by interventional neuroradiology or disconnection with open surgery.

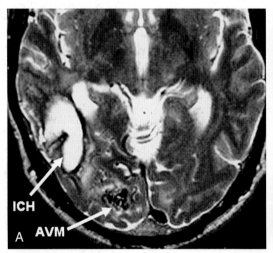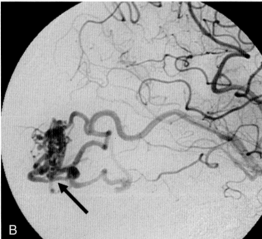

Fig. 24.8 Arteriovenous malformation. (A) Magnetic resonance scan showing an AVM that has bled, causing an ICH. **(B)** Angiogram of the same AVM (*arrow*). *AVM,* Arteriovenous malformation; *ICH,* intracerebral haematoma.

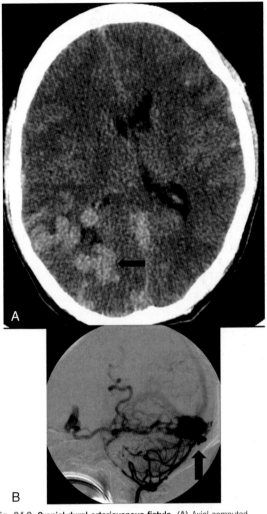

Fig. 24.9 Cranial dural arteriovenous fistula. (A) Axial computed tomography showing a left parieto-occipital haematoma (*arrow*). **(B)** The vertebral angiogram shows extradural feeding vessels entering the torcula (*arrow*).

Fig. 24.10 Spinal dural arteriovenous fistula. (A) Angiogram showing a fistulous connection (*vertical arrow*) between a radicular artery and vein. The tortuous subarachnoid veins are dilated secondary to the back pressure (*horizontal arrow*). **(B, C)** Sagittal and coronal magnetic resonance images reveal the dilated veins in the subarachnoid space dorsal to the thoracic cord (*white arrows*). Symptoms in these patients are caused by venous hypertension.

Cavernomas

These are well-circumscribed collections of small vascular channels (usually capillaries). Patients typically present with headaches, focal neurological deficits or epilepsy, owing to small, recurrent focal haemorrhages. The haemorrhages cause a clinical syndrome less dramatic than that associated with SAH or AVM rupture. CT and angiography often miss these lesions, but they have a characteristic hypointense rim on T2-weighed MRIs representing hemosiderin, described as a 'popcorn' appearance on MRI and may be much more common than was previously appreciated (Fig. 24.11). Those causing epilepsy or recurrent haemorrhage may be excised, unless they are in an eloquent and/or inaccessible place (e.g., brain stem). The risk of rebleeding from cavernomas and AVMs is poorly documented but is in the region of 4% per year.

24.2 Summary

Vascular disorders and the central nervous system

- Occlusive vascular disease most often originates from blockage of extracranial vessels by atherosclerosis. Intracranial occlusion can be thrombotic or embolic
- Patients with subarachnoid haemorrhage from an aneurysm should be considered for either clipping or coiling of the aneurysm to avoid recurrent bleeding
- 70% of subarachnoid haemorrhages result from aneurysm rupture. Intracerebral bleeding is frequently associated with hypertension and amyloid angiopathy
- Delayed ischaemic deficit should be managed aggressively with triple therapy.

24

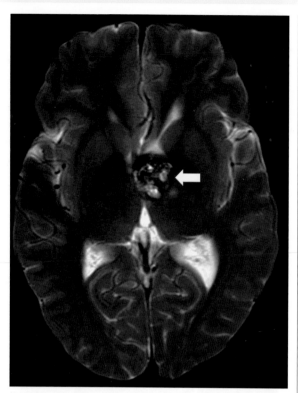

Fig. 24.11 Thalamic cavernoma. T2-weighted axial magnetic resonance image displaying a hypointense rim caused by hemosiderin.

Neurotrauma

Head injury comprises a large proportion of emergency neurosurgical practice. Severity can range from a minor concussive injury through to severe craniocerebral trauma associated with high-velocity motor vehicle accidents. The head injury may be associated with scalp or face injury, and may be penetrating (open) or nonpenetrating (closed). Management aims to minimise secondary brain injury. The primary brain injury results from the trauma. It may be diffuse or focal and of varying severity, and is essentially irreversible. Secondary brain injury occurs after the primary trauma as a result of hypotension, ischaemia, hypoxia, pyrexia, infection and raised ICP. Secondary brain damage can have a devastating effect even in patients with relatively minor injuries and can often be prevented.

Assessment

Glasgow Coma Score

The GCS is a measure of conscious level that facilitates objective management of head-injured patients (www.glasgowcomascale.org; Fig. 24.12). It is used internationally and records the best verbal, motor and eye opening responses to stimulus. The obtainable score ranges between 3 and 15. Changes in GCS over time are more informative than the reading at a single time point. The verbal component of the GCS can be modified for assessment in children. The best postresuscitation GCS is used to classify severity of head injury. Mild injury is GCS 15–13; moderate 12–9; and less than 8 is classified as severe. Coma is defined as a GCS of 8 or less.

Neurological examination

Routine assessment includes pupil size and reaction; a search for CSF leaks from nose, mouth and ears; a survey of the scalp for penetrating injuries; signs of a basal skull fracture (Battle's sign, raccoon eyes); and an assessment of the maxillofacial skeleton. Peripheral neurological examination will give a guide to focal brain injury, spinal injury or peripheral nerve injury.

Other systems

Patients with head injury often have extracranial injuries. Head injury alone does not cause hypovolaemic shock, except rarely in young children from scalp bleeding. Management of systemic complications such as chest injury or intraabdominal haemorrhage is a priority, since these can lead to hypoxia, cerebral ischaemia and hypoxia, and thus secondary brain damage.

Management

As with all injured patients, management commences with Airway, Breathing and Circulation assessment and management. The neck should be immobilised until a cervical spine injury has been excluded. The GCS should be documented on arrival and following resuscitation, and the findings of a neurological survey recorded. Patients may be under the effects of alcohol and other drugs that affect conscious level. If in doubt, assume that depressed consciousness is due to brain injury. Continued monitoring of conscious level over time by means of GCS is a key aspect of management, and sedatives must be avoided.

In general, patients with a GCS of 8 or less are intubated and ventilated to prevent hypoxia and aspiration pneumonitis, and to allow moderate hyperventilation, which reduces the Pa_{CO_2} to 30–35 mmHg. This lowers ICP through cerebral vasoconstriction. Following resuscitation, stabilisation and prioritisation of injuries, a head CT is performed to detect intracranial haematoma, brain contusions (bruises), depressed bone fragments, intracranial air and associated maxillofacial fractures. Mass lesions such as extradural or subdural haematomas and haemorrhagic contusions may cause brain swelling and shift, and are often surgically evacuated. Indications for clot evacuation include >5-mm midline shift, significant impairment of GCS, or protracted headache or vomiting. Compound cranial wounds need to be surgically explored, dead tissue and foreign bodies removed, and depressed bone fragments elevated. Depending on the age of the wound, bone fragments may be cleaned and replaced or discarded.

Brain injury evolves over several days and the principal aim of management is to limit secondary damage. ICP is often severely elevated following neurotrauma because of oedema, haematoma, contusions, engorgement of the brain vasculature, hydrocephalus or even infection. A sustained ICP that exceeds 25 mmHg is associated with a poorer outcome. Severely brain-injured patients are kept sedated and ventilated, and their ICP measured with a 'bolt' (pressure transducer). Hyperventilation, mannitol or hypertonic saline are used to reduce ICP, and the systemic blood pressure may be raised using fluids and inotropes. A CPP of more than 60 mmHg is generally required to sustain adequate cerebral perfusion. Many neurotrauma patients require rehabilitation. There is no evidence for administering steroids (EBM 24.5).

GLASGOW COMA SCALE : Do it this way

Institute of Neurological Sciences NHS Greater Glasgow and Clyde

GCS at 40 | EYES VERBAL MOTOR

CHECK

For factors Interfering with communication, ability to respond and other injuries

OBSERVE

Eye opening , content of speech and movements of right and left sides

STIMULATE

Sound: spoken or shouted request
Physical Pressure on finger tip, trapezius or supraorbital notch

RATE

Assign according to highest response observed

Eye opening

Criterion	Observed	Rating	Score
Open before stimulus	✔	Spontaneous	4
After spoken or shouted request	✔	To sound	3
After finger tip stimulus	✔	To pressure	2
No opening at any time, no interfering factor	✔	None	1
Closed by local factor	✔	Non testable	NT

Verbal response

Criterion	Observed	Rating	Score
Correctly gives name, place and date	✔	Orientated	5
Not orientated but communication coherently	✔	Confused	4
Intelligible single words	✔	Words	3
Only moans / groans	✔	Sounds	2
No audible response, no interfering factor	✔	None	1
Factor interfering with communication	✔	Non testable	NT

Best motor response

Criterion	Observed	Rating	Score
Obey 2-part request	✔	Obeys commands	6
Brings hand above clavicle to stimulus on head neck	✔	Localising	5
Bends arm at elbow rapidly but features not predominantly abnormal	✔	Normal flexion	4
Bends arm at elbow, features clearly predominantly abnormal	✔	Abnormal flexion	3
Extends arm at elbow	✔	Extension	2
No movement in arms / legs, no interfering factor	✔	None	1
Paralysed or other limiting factor	✔	Non testable	NT

24

Sites For Physical Stimulation

Finger tip pressure   Trapezius Pinch   Supraorbital notch

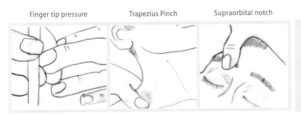

Features of Flexion Responses

Modified with permission from Van Der Naalt 2004 Ned Tijdschr Geneeskd

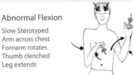

Abnormal Flexion
Slow Steretoyped
Arm across chest
Forearm rotates
Thumb clenched
Leg extends

Normal flexion
Rapid
Variable
Arm away from body

For further information and video demonstration visit www.glasgowcomascale.org
Graphic design by Margaret Frej based on layout and illustrations from Medical Illustration M I • 268093
(c) Sir Graham Teasdale 2015

Fig. 24.12 The Glasgow Coma Scale (GCS) assessment aid. (© Sir Graham Teasdale 2015, with permission.)

Skull fracture

The presence of a skull fracture is an important pointer to the likelihood of significant primary and/or secondary brain injury, especially if accompanied by a depressed GCS. However, the absence of a fracture does not exclude life-threatening brain injury, particularly in young children. A patient without a fracture who has a GCS of 15 has a risk of intracranial haematoma of 1:6000. If a fracture is present, this figure rises to 1:30; if the GCS is 14 or less, the figure is 1:4. CT is the investigation of choice after head injury, and certainly should be performed if there is a skull fracture.

Extradural haematoma

This is usually the result of a skull fracture with tearing of a meningeal vessel (Fig. 24.13). It is most common in the middle fossa after a temporal fracture and middle meningeal artery or vein tear. The primary brain injury is often minimal, with a typical 'lucid' interval followed by rapid deterioration as the haematoma enlarges. The haematoma has a classic biconvex or lenticular appearance on CT. The prognosis after treatment is usually good.

Subdural haematoma

This is more common than extradural haematoma and results from laceration of vessels (especially small cerebral veins) on the brain surface, or 'bursting' of the brain. CT shows a haematoma that is concave on its inner surface and whose extent is not limited between the cranial sutures, unlike extradural haematomas (Fig. 24.13B). Morbidity and mortality are often high, because of the severity of the primary brain injury.

An increasingly common problem in the ageing population is chronic subdural haematoma (CSDH). The initial acute bleed, which can occur apparently spontaneously or after relatively very minor head trauma, is rarely symptomatic. Patients with cerebral atrophy, or who are on antiplatelets or anticoagulants, are at greater risk of CSDH. The acute haematoma dissolves and the CSDH collection varies in viscosity from dissolving clot to blood-stained fluid. As the acute haematoma dissolves it draws in water, increasing in size. This process can evolve slowly, so there may be significant midline shift with few signs and symptoms. CSDHs can mimic most neurological syndromes in their presentation. Treatment involves drainage of the subdural collection through burr holes or minicraniotomy. Evidence from an RCT suggests that placement of a drain in the subdural space for 24-48 hours after surgery significantly reduces CSDH recurrence (EBM. 24.6). Patients with mild symptoms may be offered a short course of steroids (without surgery) for symptom management; there is not yet any quality evidence for this strategy, but clinical trials are ongoing.

Intracerebral haematoma and contusions

Trauma can cause focal intracerebral haematoma or, more commonly, foci of contusions or small areas of brain bruising. Such lesions can cause cognitive and focal deficits in the longer term, but acutely can be associated with severe pericontusional brain oedema and raised ICP. The STICH trauma trial was designed to investigate whether there was any benefit to surgical removal of traumatic intracerebral haematomas. The study was halted because of slow recruitment, so the hypothesis remains untested.

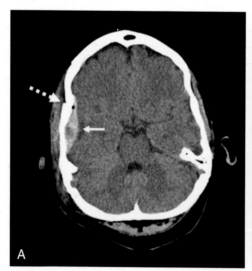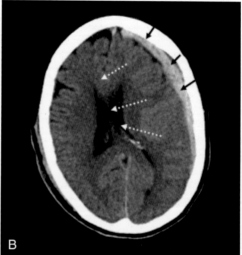

Fig. 24.13 Extradural and subdural haematoma. (A) Axial computed tomography (CT) scan showing an acute extradural haematoma. The extradural clot is lens-shaped (*solid arrow*), and is associated with a skull fracture and a small amount of intracranial air (*broken arrow*). **(A)** Axial CT scan showing a subdural haematoma. The subdural clot (*black arrows*) is compressing the brain and causing significant midline shift and subfalcine herniation (*white arrows*).

Diffuse axonal injury

This type of injury is caused by rotational head movements. It is common after high-speed motor vehicle accidents. The GCS is usually low. Paradoxically, the CT may appear normal, or there may be only small punctate brain contusions. The ICP may be normal, at least initially. However, because of the diffuse nature of the brain injury, severe neurological deficits are common. Treatment is supportive and it may be some time before the prognosis is known.

 24.3 Summary

Head injury

- Grading (Glasgow Coma Score [GCS]): minor, GCS 13–15; moderate, GCS 8–12; severe, GCS <8
- Injuries include extradural haematoma, subdural haematoma, intracerebral haematoma, cerebral contusions or diffuse axonal injury
- Avoidance of hypotension, hypoxia, hypercapnia, pyrexia and intracranial pressure >25 mmHg minimises secondary brain damage.

Traumatic spinal injury

Injury to the spinal cord may result from sports injuries, following accidents with or without severe craniocerebral neurotrauma, or after relatively minor falls in the elderly. The important factors are whether there is spinal axis instability, and whether there has been spinal cord or nerve root injury. Neural injury is almost invariably a consequence of the former, but many cases of spinal axis injury are not associated with neural injury. This is particularly the case for odontoid fractures and pedicular fractures of C2, and many burst lumbar fractures. Prompt recognition of unstable bony injury is required to avoid a devastating spinal cord injury.

Cervical spine trauma may produce subluxation of the cervical vertebra (often C5 on C6), a crush fracture of a cervical vertebral body, or hyperextension or hyperflexion injury in a patient with a narrow cervical spinal canal. The resulting neural injury may cause quadriparesis or a complete cord transection syndrome. A common pattern of injury in the elderly is a central cord syndrome, in which the segmental grey matter is contused but the fibre tracts are relatively spared. This produces weakness in the upper limbs, but relative sparing of the lower limbs.

Management consists of prompt recognition of the injury. Investigations usually consist of spinal x-rays and CT. MRI is useful if there are neurological deficits. With cord transection, there may be hypotension and bradycardia (due to loss of peripheral sympathetic tone), areflexia, hypotonicity and paresis. Sensory examination provides a clue to the level of spinal injury. The spine is then immobilised and, if necessary, spinal realignment is obtained with traction. Some fractures may be managed in a hard cervical collar or thoracolumbar brace. Other fractures require surgical stabilisation. Neurorehabilitation is important. There is no evidence to support the administration of steroids.

Intracranial infections

Infection of the central nervous system and its meninges acquires surgical importance if it produces a mass (abscess or oedema), hydrocephalus or osteomyelitis, or if it occurs as a result of a breach in, or absence of, the coverings of the brain. Infections may affect the scalp, cranium, meninges, or the brain itself (Fig. 24.14). Intracranial infections are relatively uncommon in

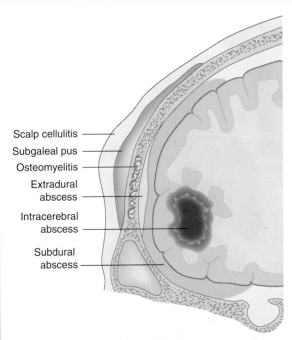

Fig. 24.14 Types of bacterial cranial infection.

Labels: Scalp cellulitis / Subgaleal pus / Osteomyelitis / Extradural abscess / Intracerebral abscess / Subdural abscess

immunocompetent patients, but immunocompromised patients, particularly those affected with HIV, can acquire a range of opportunistic organisms, e.g., toxoplasmosis and tuberculosis.

Bacterial infections

The brain is relatively resistant to infection but abscesses or subdural empyema (SDE) may form. Initially, there is cerebritis (encephalitis), following which the brain necroses to form pus surrounded by a tough glial capsule. There may be an obvious source of concurrent or contiguous infection (e.g., SDE complicating frontal sinusitis, temporal lobe and cerebellar abscesses complicating suppurative otitis media and mastoiditis [Fig. 24.15], brain abscess via haematogenous spread in patients with bronchiectasis), but in many patients the infection appears to arise de novo. Epidural infections and osteomyelitis of the skull can rarely occur after trauma with inadequate wound debridement. Brain abscess and SDE usually present in a subacute or acute manner with headache, seizures and focal neurological deficit. Meningism and pyrexia are common with SDE but can be absent with brain abscess.

Treatment is an emergency. As well as loculations of pus, the major problems are severe perilesional brain oedema and the propensity to venous sinus thrombophlebitis. CT permits the rapid diagnosis and localisation of pus and greatly facilitates surgical drainage. MRI may allow differentiation between an abscess or glioma, but should not delay treatment; if in doubt treat as an abscess. Abscesses may be excised or can be aspirated stereotactically; abscesses may need to be aspirated multiple times. Pus is sent for Gram staining, culture and sensitivity, and high-dose intravenous antibiotics are necessary. Anaerobic streptococci are the most common organisms. Infections due to middle-ear disease may be mixed. Dexamethasone can be used to reduce brain oedema, but cautiously, since it is immunosuppressive. Cranial melioidosis is a rare condition caused by *Burkholderia pseudomallei*. It can present with osteomyelitis, epidural empyema or cerebral abscesses, and requires prolonged treatment with ceftazidime and oral co-trimoxazole. If the abscesses are multiple they can mimic

24

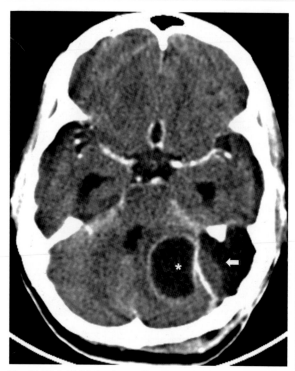

Fig. 24.15 Axial CT showing an otogenic cerebellar pyogenic abscess (*asterisk*) having arisen from a chronic suppurative otitis media and mastoiditis with an epidural abscess (*arrow*).

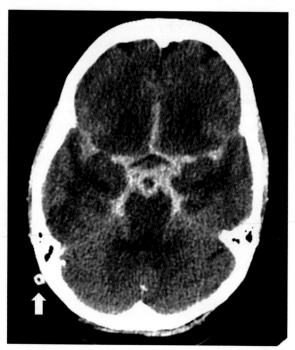

Fig. 24.16 Contrast brain computed tomography scan showing thick basal exudates in a patient with tuberculous meningitis. These exudates obstructed the flow of cerebrospinal fluid, causing a communicating hydrocephalus for which the patient underwent a ventriculoperitoneal shunt (*arrow*). In such patients an associated arteritis may result in cerebral infarcts.

metastatic neoplasia radiologically. Mortality from brain abscess and SDE has fallen considerably owing to earlier diagnosis, but patients frequently have significant neurological sequelae. There is a high incidence (50–60%) of postinfective seizures, so anticonvulsants are prescribed routinely and are often required indefinitely.

Tuberculous meningitis

Thick exudates fill the basal cisterns in chronic tuberculous meningitis, entrapping cranial nerves and causing secondary vascular inflammation. Patients usually present with hydrocephalus, cranial nerve palsies or strokes from vasculitis. Brain imaging detects contrast enhancement of the basal cisterns, hydrocephalus and small infarcts (Fig. 24.16). Emergency external ventricular drainage or ventriculoperitoneal (VP) shunting can be life-saving and provides CSF for analysis. Lumbar CSF analysis can be dangerous given the risk of uncal herniation in the presence of hydrocephalus. Antituberculous medication for 18 months is recommended.

Tuberculomas

This is a parenchymal manifestation of tuberculosis characterised by a conglomeration of granulomas containing giant cells and caseous necrosis, up to 4–5 cm in size (Fig. 24.17). These may present with raised ICP, focal neurological deficits or seizures. Brain imaging demonstrates a ring-enhancing lesion, but histopathological confirmation is recommended with stereotactic or open biopsy, followed by 18 months of antituberculous therapy.

Neurocysticercosis

This is the most common parasitic CNS infection in the world affecting about 50 million people, predominantly subsistence farming communities in Africa, Asia and Latin America. Faecal contamination of food by eggs of the pork tapeworm, *Taenia solium*, results in the larvae forming cysts in muscles and in the CNS. In the CNS, cysticercosis may manifest as solitary or multiple cerebral cysticercal granulomata, resulting in seizures or intraventricular cysts causing obstructive hydrocephalus. In endemic areas, if a patient presents with a seizure and brain imaging reveals a solitary lesion smaller than 2 cm, with absence of focal neurological deficits and raised ICP, the most likely diagnosis will be cysticercosis rather than tuberculosis (Fig. 24.18). In such patients, the administration of anticonvulsants alone followed by repeat imaging after 6 months is sufficient as these lesions usually resolve spontaneously and do not require excision or treatment with albendazole. Should hydrocephalus be caused by an intraventricular cyst, endoscopic removal of the cyst can be curative.

Postsurgical infection

Wound infections occur after less than 1% of craniotomies, usually caused by *Staphylococcus*. Most settle with antibiotics. Once the bone flap is colonised and a nidus of osteomyelitis has developed, craniectomy (removal of the bone flap) is usually required in addition to antibiotic therapy; cranioplasty (e.g., with acrylic) can be performed 12 months later. Infection of the brain itself following surgery is extremely rare, even following implantation of prosthetic material.

Meningitis

Although most forms of meningitis are medically treated, some require neurosurgery. For example, a dural tear following a skull-base fracture can result in egress of CSF into the paranasal sinuses (cranionasal fistula) or mastoid air cells. From there, the

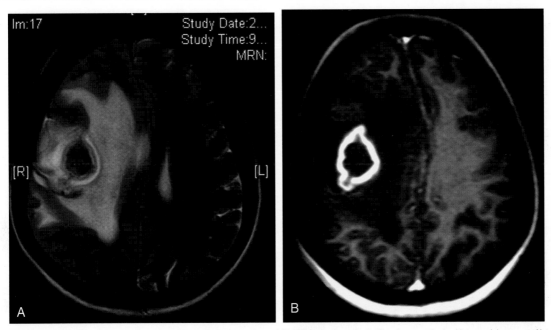

Fig. 24.17 Cerebral tuberculoma. T2-weighted **(A)** and gadolinium enhanced (B) MRI brain of a patient with seizures and raised intracranial pressure. Note the extensive white matter oedema in (A) and the peripheral enhancement of the lesion with central necrosis in **(B)**. The lesion was excised and the histopathology revealed granulomatous inflammation typical of a tuberculoma.

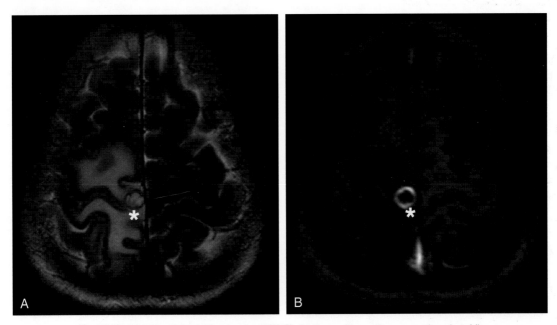

Fig. 24.18 Axial T2-weighted (A) and contrast MRI **(B)** showing a solitary cysticercus granuloma (*asterisk*).

CSF can pass through the Eustachian tube into the nasopharynx (cranioaural fistula). Under these circumstances, pneumococcal infection can occur, either early or extremely late following injury. Early treatment of post-CSF fistula meningitis is important and failure to recognise the disorder can result in death. However, there is not clear evidence that prophylactic antibiotics reduce the incidence of meningitis in post-traumatic CSF fistula. If the CSF leak continues, then the site of leakage needs to be surgically repaired.

Intracranial tumours

Tumours of the skull

These tumours are uncommon. The differential diagnosis includes osteomas, meningiomas with hyperostosis, metastatic malignancy, fibrous dysplasia (Fig. 24.19), histiocytosis and Paget's disease. Most are painless. Diagnosis may require CT, MRI and systemic investigations.

24

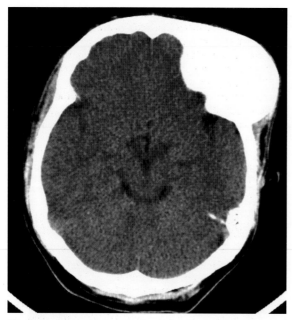

Fig. 24.19 Axial brain computed tomography scan showing fibrous dysplasia skull.

Gliomas

Gliomas are the most common (60%) primary intracranial tumour presenting clinically. They are named because the constituent cells resemble the brain's supporting cells known as glia and are thought to arise from cells with stem-like characteristics, so-called glioma stem-like cells. Gliomas include glioblastoma, astrocytoma, oligodendroglioma and ependymoma. Tumour cells infiltrate among normal brain cells and are graded using a WHO four-point scale based on features such as vascular endothelial proliferation, nuclear pleomorphism and mitotic rate.

- *Grade I tumours* (e.g., pilocytic astrocytoma, dysembryoplastic neuroepithelial, ganglioglioma) are on the borderline between hamartomas and extremely low-grade tumours. They are often cured by surgery
- *Grade II tumours* (astrocytoma, oligodendroglioma and ependymoma) have variable intrinsic malignancy and survival periods are usually long (median 8.5 years after surgery, radiotherapy and chemotherapy). Often transform into higher grade lesions
- *Grade III tumours* are anaplastic (e.g., anaplastic astrocytoma, anaplastic oligodendroglioma) and frequently have median survival periods of approximately 3 years after multimodality treatment (Fig. 24.20). As with grade II tumours, oligodendrogliomas tend to be more responsive to therapies than astrocytomas
- *Grade IV tumours* are highly malignant and comprise glioblastoma and gliosarcomas
  - Despite surgery, adjuvant radiotherapy and chemotherapy, median survival for patients with a glioblastoma is 14 months. Younger age and better function predict improved outcome.

Meningiomas

These arise from arachnoid cap cells of the dura (Fig. 24.21) and account for 20% of all primary intracranial tumours; many are not

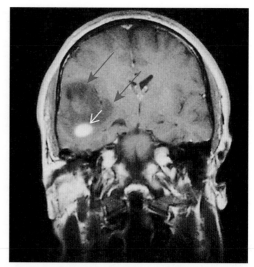

Fig. 24.20 Coronal magnetic resonance scan showing a right temporal mass lesion of low signal intensity (*red arrows*), with an oval-shaped region of gadolinium enhancement (*white arrow*). The latter suggests malignancy. This tumour was an anaplastic astrocytoma.

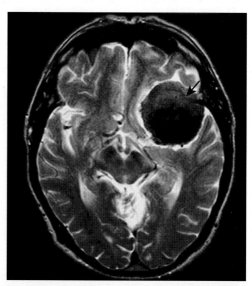

Fig. 24.21 Axial magnetic resonance image showing a large sphenoid wing meningioma (*arrow*). There is no associated brain oedema. This tumour caused troublesome seizures.

clinically apparent (and remain so), so the real incidence is much higher. Meningiomas are commonly located over the skull convexity, skull base or sagittal sinus region. They may compress the adjacent brain, causing functional deficits, and can precipitate seizures. They are generally slow growing (90% are WHO grade I tumours) but may spread widely over the dura ('en plaque' tumours). They can invade the skull to form a palpable mass. Treatment is excision and prognosis usually good. Recurrences are more common with grade II (atypical) or grade III (anaplastic) tumours, or with subtotal excision of grade I tumours, and may be treated with repeat surgery or radiotherapy.

Schwannomas

Cranial nerve tumours account for 10% of intracranial tumours. They usually affect the vestibulo-cochlear nerves (called *vestibular*

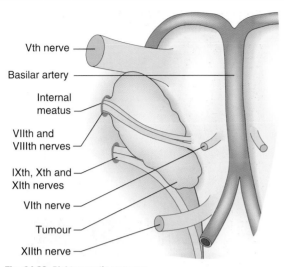

Fig. 24.22 Right acoustic neuroma.

schwannomas), where the tumour grows within, expands and erodes the internal auditory meatus (Fig. 24.22). The VII and VIII cranial nerves become stretched over its surface as it grows into the cerebellopontine angle. Early VIII cranial nerve symptoms include progressive nerve deafness, tinnitus and vertigo. Larger tumours affect the trigeminal nerve, leading to diminished facial sensation, and to the pons and cerebellum, leading to ataxia and nystagmus. Displacement of the fourth ventricle and aqueduct may lead to hydrocephalus. Patients may be misdiagnosed with Ménière's disease and tumours can reach a large size before diagnosis. Treatment options include excision, stereotactic radiosurgery or observation, depending on the symptoms, size and growth over time.

Pituitary tumours

These account for 10% of all intracranial tumours. Microadenomas (<10 mm in size) are generally functional tumours, so typically are diagnosed when small. They may hypersecrete adrenocorticotropin hormone (Cushing's disease), growth hormone (acromegaly), prolactin (amenorrhea–galactorrhoea syndrome or decreased libido in men) or a mixture of hormones. Nonfunctional adenomas are usually macroadenomas when diagnosed (>10 mm) and present with local pressure on the visual apparatus (e.g., distortion of the optic chiasma leading to bitemporal hemianopia), or occasionally pituitary hypofunction (Fig. 24.23). Growth hormone-secreting tumours may cause visual symptoms if diagnosis is delayed. Prolactinomas respond well to cabergoline, a dopamine agonist, so rarely require surgery. Growth hormone tumours may respond to octreotide or require surgery. Other tumours require transsphenoidal or endoscopic surgery. Recurrence is treated with repeat surgery or radiotherapy.

Craniopharyngiomas

These tumours are thought to arise from remnants of Rathke's pouch or the craniopharyngeal duct, either from proliferation of neuroectodermal cell rests or metaplasia of residual squamous epithelium. They are usually suprasellar in location and typically present with growth retardation, hypopituitarism, visual disturbances and diabetes insipidus. Brain CT and MRI show solid, cystic or mixed tumours, frequently with calcification (Fig. 24.24). Attempts at total surgical excision may impair hypothalamic function, resulting, for example, in diabetes insipidus and obesity. Tumour recurrence may be treated with further surgery or radiotherapy. Stereotactic aspiration and placement of catheters into cysts followed by radiotherapy are other options.

Brain metastasis

Metastatic tumours are present at postmortem in 20% of patients dying of cancer, and in 50% they are multiple (Fig. 24.25). The most common primary lesions are lung, breast, kidney, melanoma and colon. Brain metastases may be the presenting feature or appear only late in the course of a previously diagnosed primary cancer. Prostate cancer classically spreads to the cranium rather than the brain parenchyma. Gliomas rarely spread beyond the CNS.

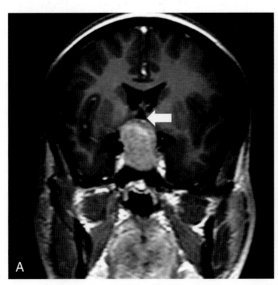
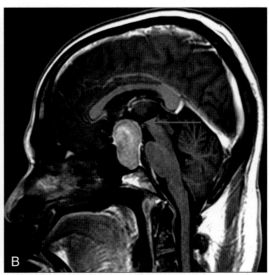

Fig. 24.23 Coronal (A) and sagittal (B) magnetic resonance image showing a pituitary macroadenoma indenting the floor of the third ventricle (*arrow*).

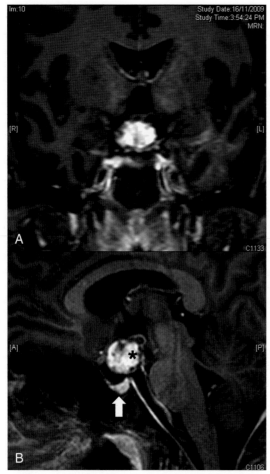

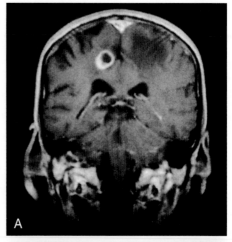

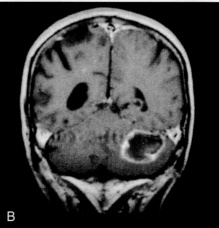

Fig 24.24 Coronal (A) and sagittal (A) magnetic resonance image showing a solid craniopharyngioma in the suprasellar cistern with the pituitary gland (*arrow*) inferior to the mass. * craniopharyngioma.

Fig. 24.25 Coronal magnetic resonance image scans showing two gadolinium-enhancing lesions in the brain. (A) The smaller lesion is in the cingulate region of the cerebral hemisphere. (B) The larger lesion is in the cerebellum. Both have low signal intensity centres, suggesting necrosis. The multiplicity of the lesions is highly suggestive of metastatic neoplasia. This magnetic resonance image appearance can also be seen with multiple brain abscesses.

Clinical features of intracranial tumours

Symptoms of raised ICP

Raised ICP may result from the tumour itself, surrounding peritumoral oedema, or obstruction to CSF flow. This classically results in morning headache aggravated by bending or straining. With large lesions there may be psychomotor slowing; the patient does everything normally but does it slowly and apathetically. This is a generalised sign of brain hypofunction.

Focal neurological deficit

A focal deficit is any sign or symptom indicating focal neuronal hypofunction. The most common is hemiparesis due to dysfunction of the motor cortex. Dysphasia occurs in about 50% of dominant hemispheric brain tumours and may be receptive, expressive or mixed. Visual field defects, dyslexia, dysgraphia and dyspraxia are also common.

Seizures

These may be generalised, partial or focal, and the precise nature of the seizures will often reflect the anatomical position of the lesion. Seizures are more common with lower grade tumours and meningiomas. They may respond well to anticonvulsant therapy and tumour excision.

Personality disintegration

There may be behavioural disturbances, cognitive decline and problems with insight, judgement, memory and planning abilities. The patient usually has no insight into this progressive decline and may be referred initially to a psychiatrist.

Diagnosis

MRI before and after contrast agent administration usually clarifies the location and pathology of tumours. In most malignant tumours there is a neovascular capillary bed, so the tumours enhance heterogeneously with contrast (see Fig. 24.20). Low-grade tumours are less likely to enhance. Meningiomas have a meningothelial cell origin, so do not have a BBB and therefore enhance avidly and uniformly. With the better resolution of MRI, apparently solitary lesions on CT are frequently found to be multifocal. Anaplastic and malignant tumours often have peritumoral brain oedema. This fluid occurs in the interstitial white matter because the neoplastic endothelium does not having the integrity of the normal BBB. Meningiomas and metastases can also be associated with oedema.

Management

The management principles of surgical neurooncology generally rely on:

- Obtaining tissue diagnosis
- Surgery to relieve signs and symptoms where possible
- Adjunctive radiotherapy and chemotherapy if appropriate
- Providing support services for the patient and family.

If peritumoral brain oedema is present it may be responsible for the symptoms, rather than the tumour itself. Oral or intravenous dexamethasone can dramatically reduce symptoms and signs over 12–24 hours. How steroids work in patients with brain tumours is not well understood, but their preoperative use has markedly reduced surgical morbidity and mortality. Surgical options include biopsy, or craniotomy for tumour resection or debulking. The choice of procedure is influenced by neuroradiological findings (i.e., the likely tumour pathology), the patient's age, symptomatology and functional status, as well as the accessibility and multiplicity of the tumour. To reduce risk from surgery on lesions adjacent to eloquent brain, the operation may be performed awake to allow real-time neurological assessment. Neurophysiology also allows intraoperative assessment of motor and sensory function, speech and language. Intraoperative localisation techniques include ultrasound, image guidance and intraoperative MRI.

If the lesion is a meningioma, then a total excision is generally planned, provided the tumour can be safely reached. Similarly, if a posterior fossa lesion looks like a vestibular schwannoma, complete excision may be the treatment of choice. A single brain metastasis may be removed if it is symptomatic and the patient's systemic disease otherwise controlled.

A diagnosis may be obtained from stereotactic or image-guided frameless biopsy if the tumour cannot safely be removed. CT or MRI images are used to either generate coordinates for a stereotactic frame affixed to the patient's head, or for frameless computer image-directed biopsy system, e.g., Stealth or Brain-Lab. A 2.5-cm incision is made in the scalp and a burr hole is drilled. The frame/frameless system guides the biopsy needle to the chosen tumour target. Accuracy is to within 1 mm and the tumour diagnostic rate is around 98%. Morbidity is generally very low (around 5%) and the 30-day mortality is less than 2%. Much of the mortality is related to the primary disease process rather than direct complications of the surgery.

Surgical excision of the lesion will reduce mass effect and may improve seizure control or restore brain function lost from compression of eloquent brain by the tumour. If the preoperative neuroradiology suggests a malignant glioma, then the extent of resection correlates with outcome. The reduced mass effect lowers steroid requirements and improves tolerance to radiotherapy. Total excision of gliomas is not possible because tumour cells invade into the brain. Extensive surgery risks brain injury. In a multicentre randomised study, temozolomide, an alkylating agent, when administered concomitantly with and after radiotherapy, optimised survival in patients with malignant gliomas (EBM 24.7). Temozolomide is most effective in patients whose tumour has a particular genetic profile called *MGMT methylation*.

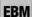

EBM | **24.7 Radiotherapy with concomitant temozolomide for malignant gliomas**

'The addition of temozolomide to radiotherapy for newly diagnosed glioblastoma resulted in a clinically meaningful and statistically significant survival benefit with minimal additional toxicity.'

Stupp R et al. N Engl J Med. 2005;352:987–96.

Outcome for all primary intracranial tumours depends largely on tumour type. After surgical resection for malignant glioma 30-day mortality is 5% and neurological morbidity 10%. Complications include iatrogenic neurological deficits, cavity and extradural haematomas, and superficial wound infections. Recurrence of meningiomas relates to the WHO grade and extent of resection. Outcome following surgical excision of brain metastases depends on the state of the primary disease, as well as the locality and multiplicity of intracranial disease. Excision plus radiotherapy of a solitary metastasis can give a median survival of 10–12 months.

 24.4 Summary

Tumours affecting the skull and its contents

- Tumours Involving the skull include osteomas and metastatic deposits
- The most common metastatic tumours are lung and breast
- Primary cerebral tumours can arise from the supporting cells of the brain (gliomas), from the ventricular walls (ependymomas) and from the fourth ventricle roof (medulloblastomas).
- Meningiomas usually grow slowly and are treated surgically if symptomatic
- Pituitary tumours may be functional, can cause pressure effects and apart from prolactinomas are best removed surgically
- Vestibular schwannomas develop near the internal auditory meatus and involve the VII and VIII cranial nerves, to cause deafness, tinnitus, vertigo and facial weakness. Involvement of the V nerve may cause loss of facial sensation.

Paediatric neurooncology

CNS tumours are the second most common childhood tumour after leukaemia. The UK incidence is 15 per million of the paediatric population. In children under the age of 2 years, the most common are teratomas, astrocytomas of embryonal tumours (formerly known as primitive neuroectodermal tumours). These can occur anywhere in the neuraxis. Between the ages of 2 and 15 years, tumours most commonly occur in the posterior fossa, and are usually medulloblastomas (a type of embryonal tumour) (Fig. 24.26), astrocytomas or ependymomas.

There may be an insidious onset of symptoms, such as lethargy, nausea, vomiting or progressive ataxia with posterior fossa tumours. Symptoms of raised ICP (headache, drowsiness, nausea and vomiting) from hydrocephalus or mass effect of the tumour itself may also precipitate admission. Children with posterior fossa tumours may present with a torticollis, which is persistent and not related to trauma. General surgeons may be asked to see a child because of persistent vomiting and weight loss, with no other symptoms or signs. Suprasellar tumours, such as craniopharyngioma, may present with visual failure, hydrocephalus or endocrine dysfunction. Brain stem gliomas may present with cranial nerve deficits (Fig. 24.27).

Information that a previously well child has lost ground or fallen behind his or her peers should be taken seriously. A clumsy child may have ataxia. Endocrine dysfunction may present as short

24

stature, obesity or cachexia. Optic atrophy or papilloedema should be excluded, as visual problems are difficult to diagnose in small children. Hemispheric neoplasms may present with hemiparesis. Spinal cord tumours are rare, but may present with back pain, scoliosis, limb weakness or bladder dysfunction. Children may present in coma, because of a catastrophic bleed into a tumour or the rapid onset of obstructive hydrocephalus. The investigation of choice is MRI, but a CT with contrast will often make the diagnosis, especially in an emergency. Even where a cranial lesion is found, MRI should include the spine to exclude drop metastases.

Treatment consists of surgery, chemotherapy and radiotherapy. Maximal safe surgical excision remains the mainstay of most treatment. It is usually not curative by itself for malignant tumours (e.g., embryonal tumours, ependymoma, malignant astrocytoma), but may be curative for benign tumours (e.g., pilocytic astrocytoma, pineocytoma). Many tumours (e.g., embryonal tumours and ependymoma) are radiosensitive, so radiotherapy is used after surgery in older children. However, radiotherapy risks damaging the developing brain and should not be used in children under 3 years of age. Between 3 and 8 years of age, radiotherapy may still cause loss of IQ and other neurodevelopmental delays, but to a lesser extent. Some childhood tumours are chemosensitive (e.g., germinomas), but most are not. Chemotherapy may still be used as adjunctive treatment or for recurrent disease. For example, chemotherapy after radiotherapy in embryonal tumours improves prognosis and is now standard practice. In children older than 3 years at presentation, with no CSF seeding or metastatic disease, and with gross total tumour excision, 5-year survival is 70%. Pilocytic astrocytomas of the cerebellum do well with complete surgical excision alone, and 90% 10-year survival is the norm.

Spinal dysraphism

This is a congenital abnormality of the spinal axis, with or without abnormalities of the spinal cord, meninges and nerves. It results from failure of the neural tube to close (Fig. 24.28). Closure begins in the mid-dorsal region and extends cranially and caudally. Thus, thoracic defects are rare. Cervical defects are uncommon. The lumbar/lumbosacral region is most affected. Maternal folate supplementation and prenatal screening (serum α-fetoprotein) at 16 weeks gestation have reduced the incidence. There are two categories of dysraphism: open and closed.

Fig. 24.26 Sagittal magnetic resonance image of a medulloblastoma. The tumour (*arrow*) can be seen filling the fourth ventricle between the pons anteriorly and the cerebellum posteriorly. There is associated obstructive hydrocephalus due to blockage of cerebrospinal fluid flow through the fourth ventricle.

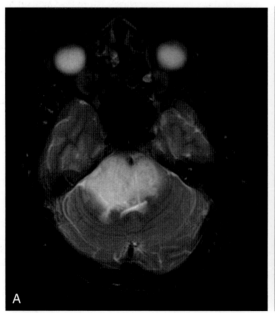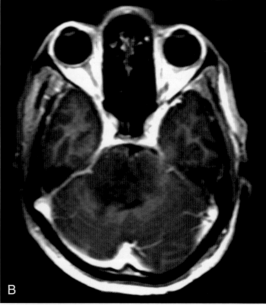

Fig. 24.27 Brainstem glioma. (A) T2-weighted axial magnetic resonance brain showing a diffuse expansion of the pons with displacement of the fourth ventricle posteriorly. There is no contrast enhancement of the mass. **(B)** Such nonenhancing lesions in children along with MR spectroscopic findings are highly suggestive of brainstem gliomas and patients are often referred directly for radiotherapy without histopathological confirmation.

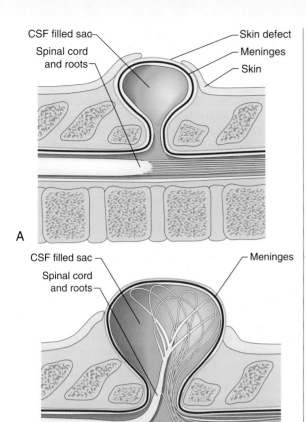

Fig. 24.28 **Spinal dysraphism.** **(A)** Simple meningocoele.
(B) Meningomyelocoele. CSF, Cerebrospinal fluid.

Open spinal dysraphism

This is known as classic spina bifida aperta or myelomeningo-coele. The child has an obvious open spinal defect and lower motor neuron signs below the level of the lesion, with numbness, weakness and a neuropathic bladder. Open defects require closure immediately after birth. These children often develop hydrocephalus following surgical closure of the spinal lesion and require VP shunting. Around 90% of these children have an associated abnormality of the hindbrain known as a Chiari II malformation, which may cause respiratory or feeding difficulties. They may develop scoliosis as they grow. These children require lifelong follow-up in a multidisciplinary clinic, where the renal tract, neurological status and orthopaedic deformities can be regularly reviewed.

Closed spinal dysraphism

This is also known as spina bifida occulta and includes lesions such as lipomyelomeningocoele, meningocoele, tight filum termi-nale syndrome, sinus tracts and intradural dermoids, split cord malformations, and caudal agenesis. It may be apparent at birth from characteristic overlying skin lesions including midline lumbar lipomas, hairy patches, dimples and sinuses. However, diagnosis

may be noted only when neurological symptoms develop later in childhood (often following minor trauma or a growth spurt), including leg pain and/or recurrent urinary tract infections. Late neurological deterioration and/or bladder dysfunction are due to tethering of the developing spinal cord at the level of the lesion. Treatment is surgical untethering, but symptoms may not improve. Other defects include splitting of the cord by a bony projection from the posterior vertebral body surface (diastemato-myelia), which can be removed, or the presence of intracord lipo-mas, which are often diffuse and multiple. Safe removal of these lipomas can be difficult. In severe cases, one foot may be smaller than the other. Dural sinus tracts to the skin surface may lead to meningitis. In general, affected individuals do not develop hydro-cephalus and there is no association with Chiari malformation. Low-lying sacral dimples, within the natal cleft, are more benign and rarely signify serious intradural pathology; if in doubt MRI is helpful.

Hydrocephalus

Aetiology and clinical features

Hydrocephalus is the accumulation of CSF within the ventricles or over the surface of the brain. This usually results from reduced CSF drainage secondary to obstruction of normal CSF flow ('non-communicating' or 'obstructive' hydrocephalus), or reduced reabsorption at the arachnoid granulations ('communicating' hydro-cephalus). It is rarely due to CSF overproduction, e.g., because of a choroid plexus papilloma (Fig. 24.29). Obstruction may be congen-ital, as in aqueduct stenosis (Fig. 24.30), or acquired, e.g., as a result of tumour or arachnoidal adhesions secondary to meningitis. In obstructive hydrocephalus the ventricular system distal to the obstruction will not be dilated. In communicating hydrocephalus, the ventricular system is patent and all ventricles are dilated. This may result from fibrosis following meningitis, subarachnoid or intra-ventricular haemorrhage, or from sagittal sinus thrombosis.

Congenital hydrocephalus usually presents at birth or in early infancy. The cranial sutures may start to open and the fontanelle will be tense and bulging. The veins of the scalp and the bridge of the nose may be dilated. As the hydrocephalus worsens, the eyes may become downcast (sunsetting). The child may be floppy and develop apnoeic spells and episodes of bradycardia. After closure of the fontanelles children have symptoms of raised ICP (head-ache, vomiting and drowsiness). The eyes may develop a squint secondary to VI cranial nerve palsy. Papilloedema may be present

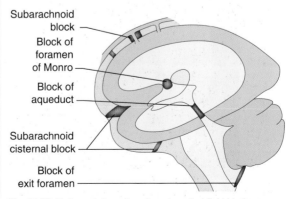

Fig. 24.29 **Hydrocephalus: sites of cerebrospinal fluid blockage.**

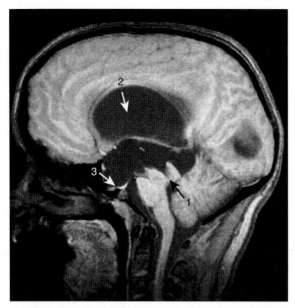

Fig. 24.30 Magnetic resonance image of aqueduct stenosis (*arrow 1*). This is an example of an obstructive hydrocephalus. There is gross ventricular enlargement (*arrow 2*) and herniation of the floor of the third ventricle into the interpeduncular cistern (*arrow 3*).

and, if severe or chronic, may lead to blindness. In adults, chronic hydrocephalus may cause the 'normal pressure hydrocephalus' syndrome of gait ataxia, incontinence and cognitive decline. Diagnosis is often difficult in the elderly because 'normal' brain atrophy causes ex vacuo dilatation of the ventricles, mimicking hydrocephalus. The differential diagnosis includes cognitive decline secondary to Alzheimer-like pathology or cerebrovascular disease, and urinary disturbances related to prostate problems.

Management and prognosis

Pressure can be relieved by bypassing the block to CSF drainage. In some cases this can be done in a minimally invasive way by endoscopic third ventriculostomy. Here an endoscope is passed into the lateral ventricle and through the foramen of Munro into the third ventricle. A small hole is formed in the floor of the third ventricle to permit CSF flow into the basal cisterns. If endoscopic third ventriculostomy is not possible or is unsuccessful, a VP shunt is required (Fig. 24.31). Here a catheter is inserted into the lateral ventricle that drains CSF through a valve (that sits on the skull under the scalp and drains at a fixed pressure) into the peritoneal cavity; shunts can also drain into the pleural space, right atrium or superior sagittal sinus. Insertion or removal of a VP shunt has a 1–2% risk of intraventricular bleeding. Early infection can occur, usually with skin commensal organisms such as *Staphylococcus epidermidis*. Shunts can also become infected months or years after insertion. Shunt blockage or malfunction can result in a rapid return of symptoms, which is a medical emergency. Infected, blocked or malfunctioning shunts have to be replaced, if necessary once the infection is treated. Shunts can also over drain. In a baby, overdrainage can result in premature closure of the cranial sutures and microcephaly. Overdrainage in older children and adults may also be symptomatic, with low-pressure headache and vomiting, or subdural haemorrhage.

The long-term prognosis depends on the underlying cause of hydrocephalus. If simple aqueduct stenosis is treated early, the prognosis is good for normal IQ and neurological function. Repeated episodes of raised ICP or ventriculitis can lead to reduced IQ and neurological deficit.

Malformations of the skull

Abnormalities of the scalp and skull often worry parents. The common problems are moulding at the time of birth, which is self-limiting, and scalp haematomas caused by ventouse extractions. These usually resolve spontaneously. Subgaleal haematomas in infants, often related to underlying skull fractures, can be extensive and can cause the haemoglobin to drop significantly. Growing skull fractures are peculiar to infancy and are caused when a fracture is associated with an underlying dural tear. The CSF pulsations cause the edges of the bone at the fracture site to absorb, and the child may present some months later with a palpable skull defect in the line of the fracture. The treatment is dural repair. Repair of the bony defect is not always required.

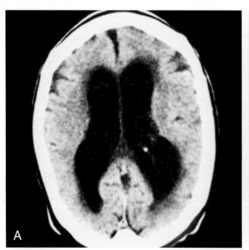

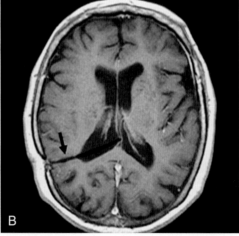

Fig. 24.31 **Hydrocephalus. (A)** CT showing adult hydrocephalus. **(B)** Magnetic resonance image after operation (ventriculoperitoneal shunt, *arrow*). There has been dramatic resolution of the hydrocephalus.

Craniosynostosis

Craniosynostosis is the premature closure or absence of a cranial suture. In normal development several intramembranous ossification centres occur in the skull vault and form plates of bone. Sutures form where these plates of bone meet and this is where further bone growth occurs. Overall, bone growth is driven by the expanding brain. The brain reaches 85% of its adult size by 2 years of age, and grows slowly after this time. Each suture fuses at a different age, but premature fusion leads to asymmetrical skull growth. Fusion of a single suture is associated with certain typical head shapes, depending on the affected suture (Fig. 24.32); e.g., scaphocephaly and plagiocephaly (premature fusion of the sagittal and coronal sutures, respectively). Plagiocephaly may more rarely be caused by fusion of the lambdoid suture. However, most plagiocephaly results from head moulding when a baby sleeps on its back. This usually resolves when the child starts to sit and walk; there is little if any evidence of benefit from fitted helmets.

Sometimes, more than one suture can be affected. This can be syndromal, e.g., Crouzon's or Apert's syndrome, which are associated with characteristic craniofacial deformities. Craniosynostosis may also lead to a reduction in cranial and orbital volumes, causing raised ICP, proptosis and visual loss. Surgery can be undertaken to remodel the skull into a more acceptable shape, or to increase the cranial and orbital volumes through an orbitofrontal advancement.

Cranial dermal sinuses and angular dermoids

Dermal sinuses are midline tracts lined with squamous epithelium that may communicate with the intracranial cavity and may predispose to meningitis. They are also found in the spine. In the head, most are found in the occipital region; 70–80% are associated with inclusion dermoids and 80% extend subdurally. In the face, because of the complex embryology, dermoids can be found at the tip of the nose and the lateral aspect of the eye.

Functional neurosurgery

Functional neurosurgery aims to modify brain function in the treatment of movement disorders, intractable epilepsy and certain psychiatric disorders.

Movement disorders

Stereotactic surgery for movement disorders such as tremor (Parkinson's disease, essential tremor), dystonia, chorea and tics involves selecting a central nervous system target for either ablation or stimulation. The latter is thought safer and therefore preferred. Neural transplantation is being evaluated and involves the implantation of neural tissues (often foetal or stem cells) into specific brain regions in the hope that they produce missing neurosecretory products. The target nucleus or subnucleus for each disorder is dependent upon an understanding of neuroanatomy and neurophysiology, e.g., the subthalamic nucleus to treat tremor in Parkinson's disease.

Epilepsy

Seizure disorders helped by neurosurgery are those that are intractable to medical therapies, have a focal onset of the seizure disorder and have a structural disorder of the brain that relates to the seizure focus. Consideration of surgery does not need to wait for failure of medical therapy though. The most common indication for neurosurgery is in patients with refractory complex partial seizures, usually known as *temporal lobe epilepsy*. Many of these patients have a hamartoma, a low-grade neoplasm or a condition termed *hippocampal sclerosis*. Resection of the involved temporal tissues and hippocampus can lead to seizure resolution in about 70% of cases. Success rates for surgery in nontemporal epilepsy are lower. However, chronic refractory childhood epilepsy associated with hemispheric dysgenesis may improve with resection of the anatomically and physiologically abnormal hemispheric tissues. Dramatic improvements in both motor and developmental milestones can also occur. Vagal nerve stimulators and deep-brain stimulators may also have a role for some refractory epilepsy.

Vertebral column

Spinal degenerative disease

Aetiology and clinical features

Degenerative changes in the lumbar and cervical intervertebral discs may be acute or chronic. Thoracic problems are less common because the rib cage limits movement at these levels. In response to acute trauma, or more chronic 'disc degeneration', the nucleus pulposus may protrude (herniate) through a tear in the annulus fibrosus (Fig. 24.33). Posterolateral protrusion usually compresses the adjacent nerve root, causing a radicular pain referred to as *sciatica* (lumbar) or *brachialgia* (cervical), with or

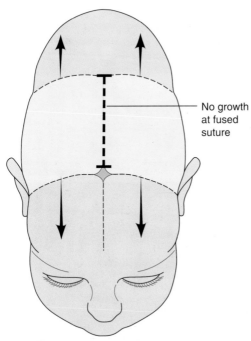

No growth at fused suture

Fig. 24.32 Sagittal suture craniosynostosis. The sagittal suture is prematurely fused (broken line). Growth normally occurs perpendicular to the suture line. In this case, the skull cannot widen, as there is no growth at the fused suture, which may be palpable as a ridge in the midline. There is compensatory growth at the coronal and lambdoid sutures, leading to an elongated head shape (scaphocephaly), with bulging of the forehead (frontal bossing) in severe cases.

24

without neurological deficit. Pain may be exacerbated by coughing or sneezing. With lumbar disc prolapse there is usually loss of normal lumbar lordosis, and a scoliosis may develop that is concave to the affected side. Straight leg raising is limited by exacerbation of the radicular pain. There may be paravertebral muscle spasm. Tendon jerks and muscle power are diminished according to the site of the lesion. The affected cervical or lumbar level is predictable by the symptomatic dermatome. A L5/S1 prolapse

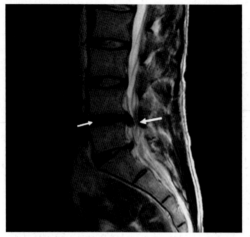

Fig. 24.33 Sagittal magnetic resonance image scan of the lumbar spine showing bulging and herniation of the L4/5 disc (*arrows*).

affects the S1 nerve root and produces pain down the back of the thigh, the lateral side of the calf and the lateral border of the foot. There is sensory loss in the latter region. The ankle jerk may be diminished or absent and, as plantar flexion of the ankle is weak, the patient may have difficulty standing on tiptoe. With an L4/L5 disc prolapse, the L5 root is compressed. Pain radiates down the posterior thigh, the lateral calf and dorsum of the foot into the great toe. There may be accompanying sensory loss; the ankle jerk is normal but ankle dorsiflexion is weak.

A surgical emergency occurs if the disc prolapses or herniates directly into the spinal canal (Fig. 24.34). In the cervical region, this will cause a progressive myelopathy, with numb, clumsy hands and spasticity. In the lumbar region, it is usually associated with severe pain in both lower limbs, loss of foot function, urinary retention, and numbness up the back of the legs and around the genitalia, anus and buttocks (saddle anaesthesia). A rectal examination should be performed to assess anal tone. These features, known as a *cauda equina syndrome*, may be unilateral if the disc prolapse is asymmetrical: Urgent advice from a spinal surgeon should be sought.

Chronic disc degeneration is associated with loss of 'disc space' height. This places abnormal strain on the intervertebral (apophyseal) joints, leading to osteophyte formation and narrowing of the intervertebral foramina. This condition is known as *spondylosis*; it may lead to nerve root (lateral recess stenosis), cord (spondylitic myelopathy) or cauda equina (lumbar canal stenosis) compression. These may result in a radiculopathic (i.e., a specific nerve root syndrome), myelopathic or lumbar claudication-type syndrome, with or without low-back or neck pain.

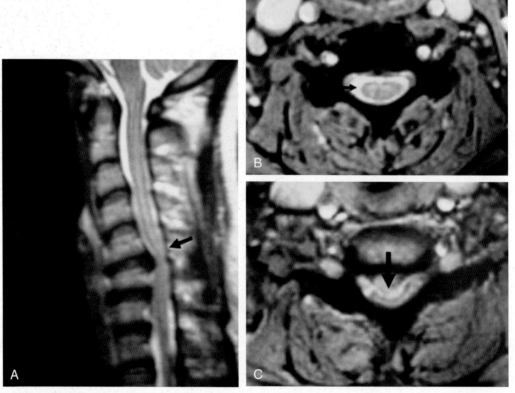

Fig. 24.34 Magnetic resonance image of the cervical spine. (A) The sagittal image shows severe spinal cord compression by a central disc prolapse (*arrow*). (B) Axial image showing the spinal canal, cord and cerebrospinal fluid (*arrow*) at a normal level. (C) Axial image at the level of compression. The posterior disc herniation (*arrow*) is easily seen.

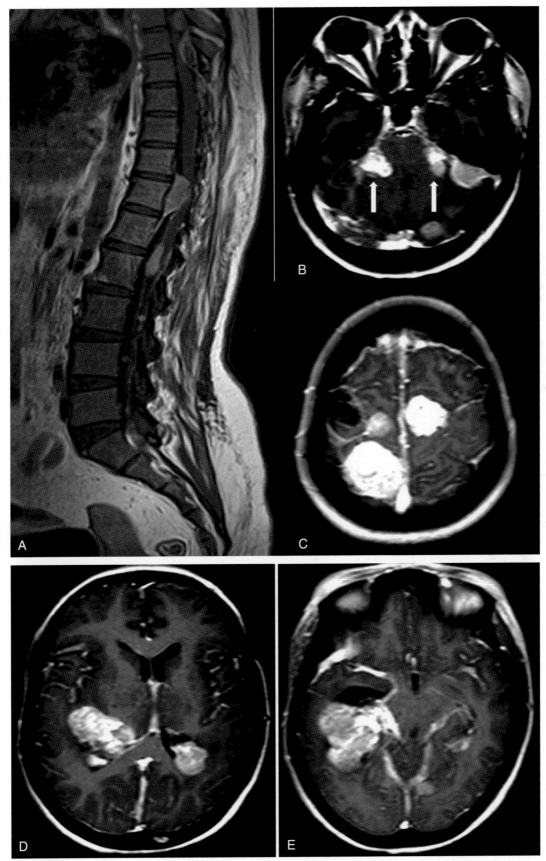

Fig. 24.35 Brain and lumbosacral magnetic resonance images of neurofibromatosis type 2. (A) Multiple spinal neurofibromata. **(B)** Bilateral vestibular schwannomas (*arrows*). **(C)** Multiple convexity meningiomas and bilateral lateral intraventricular meningiomas. **(D** and **E)** Imaging of the entire neuraxis is warranted in such patients.

Management

Ninety percent of acute radicular (sciatic) pain settles with conservative treatment (analgesia, physiotherapy and acupuncture) within 3 months. Persistent symptoms may prompt surgical decompression. The investigation of choice is spinal MRI. Flexion and extension x-rays may occasionally be useful if there is a spondylolisthesis (abnormal movement of one vertebra on another) contributing to the clinical syndrome. X-rays are not indicated in uncomplicated cases of back pain or sciatica. In some cases, metastatic tumours, neurofibromas, and spinal ependymomas or meningiomas are the cause of pain or neurological disability (Fig. 24.35).

The type of surgery is determined by the clinical syndrome and radiological investigations. A microdiscectomy may be performed for a simple posterolateral lumbar disc prolapse, causing a sciatica pain. A posterior foraminotomy or anterior cervical discectomy, with or without fusion and plating, may be performed for a cervical disc prolapse. For multiple-level lumbar or cervical spinal canal stenosis a laminectomy may be required. For lumbar spondylolisthesis associated with canal stenosis or radicular signs, decompression and fusion with pedicle screws for stabilisation may be necessary. Results depend on many parameters.

 24.5 Summary

Acute lumbar disc prolapse

- Most common in the fourth and fifth decades, and men most often affected
- The annulus fibrosus ruptures, allowing protrusion of the central nucleus pulposus. Prolapse most commonly occurs posterolaterally, compressing the spinal nerve(s) as it leaves the spinal canal. Less commonly, posterior disc ruptures can compress the cauda equina
- The most common levels for disc prolapse are L4–5 and L5–S1
- Most cases settle without surgery. Those with persistence of symptoms beyond 8 weeks should be considered for removal of the prolapsed material
- Cauda equina syndrome (severe back pain, urinary retention and weakness bilaterally below the knees) necessitates urgent surgical decompression.

Peripheral nerve lesions

Lesions of the peripheral nerves can be classified as traumatic, compressive, metabolic, inflammatory, autoimmune, neoplastic and genetic. Neurosurgeons will see mainly compressive lesions, some trauma and the occasional nerve tumour. The common compressive neuropathies are carpal tunnel syndrome, ulnar nerve compression at the elbow and meralgia paraesthetica.

Carpal tunnel syndrome

- Symptoms of pain and numbness in the distribution of the median nerve in the hand

- More common in patients with diabetes, hypothyroidism, acromegaly, pregnancy
- May be intermittent, usually worst at night, may be provoked by wrist flexion
- May be relieved by shaking hand while holding it in a dependent position.

The symptoms are often characteristic and the history can be key to diagnosis. The differential diagnosis includes cervical radiculopathy. On examination there are usually no signs, but there may be wasting of the thenar eminence, weakness of the abductor pollicis brevis, and diminished or altered sensation in the median nerve distribution. Tapping over the nerve in the carpal tunnel may elicit paraesthesia in the median nerve distribution (Tinel's sign). Phalen's test involves acutely flexing the wrist and holding it in this position. This may precipitate paraesthesia or numbness. This is abnormal if it occurs within 1 minute. Diagnosis can be confirmed with electrophysiology to measure nerve conduction velocity and distal motor latency. Treatment depends on symptom severity. Splinting the wrist or steroid injection into the carpal tunnel relieves a third of cases. The transverse carpal ligament can also be divided surgically, usually under local anaesthetic; risks include injury to the motor branch of the median nerve.

Ulnar nerve compression at the elbow

This is usually due to acute or chronic trauma, osteoarthritis or rheumatoid arthritis. The nerve may suffer repeated dislocation over the medial epicondyle on flexion of the elbow. Sometimes, the nerve may be compressed by the aponeurosis between the two heads of flexor carpi ulnaris. There is pain in the forearm and wasting of the small muscles of the hand, leading in the worst cases to an ulnar 'claw' hand. There may be reduced sensation in the ulnar distribution of the hand. The diagnosis may be made clinically, but electrophysiology is recommended to confirm the diagnosis. Treatment consists of surgically releasing and decompressing the nerve.

Meralgia paraesthetica

This is numbness and painful paraesthesia in the lateral thigh caused by compression or injury of the L2/3 sensory lateral cutaneous nerve. The nerve emerges from the lateral border of the psoas muscle just above the iliac crest and crosses the iliacus to pass beneath or through the inguinal ligament, 1 cm medial to the anterior superior iliac spine, into the thigh. Seat belts, pregnancy, trauma and postsurgical scar tissue can cause compression. Ten percent of patients have diabetes. Diagnosis can be confirmed by injecting local anaesthetic into the inguinal region 1 cm medial to the anterior superior iliac spine. Treatment includes weight loss, removal of constricting clothes and belts, nonsteroidal anti-inflammatory drugs, ice packs, and corticosteroid injection. Most cases settle within 2 years. Surgical decompression is reserved for those that do not, but is unsatisfactory.

Lorna Marson
John Forsythe

25

Transplantation surgery

Chapter contents

Introduction 487

Transplant immunology 487

Organ donation 491

Renal transplantation 494

Liver transplantation 496

Pancreas transplantation 498

Pancreatic islet transplantation 499

Heart and lung transplantation 499

Summary 501

Introduction

For many patients, the optimal treatment of end-stage renal failure (ESRF) is kidney transplantation because it improves quality of life and confers survival benefits (EBM 25.1). Liver, heart and lung transplantation can be truly life-saving, as there are few alternatives. The two main obstacles to transplantation are overcoming the recipient's immune response and a shortage of donor organs.

> **EBM** 25.1 **Transplantation versus dialysis in renal failure**
>
> 'Recent studies have demonstrated a significant survival benefit for renal transplantation compared with dialysis for virtually all ages. In addition, long-term dialysis is a major risk factor for graft loss, with best outcomes occurring in those patients transplanted early in the course of end-stage renal failure.'
>
> Wolfe RA, et al. N Engl J Med. 1999;341:1725–30.; Oniscu GC, Brown H, Forsythe JL. J Am Soc Nephrol. 2005;16:1859–65.; Meier-Kriesche HU, Kaplan B. Transplantation 2002;74:1377–81.

Transplant immunology

The basis of transplant immunology is the host's recognition of foreign tissue and its subsequent response. The major histocompatibility complex (MHC) encodes the predominant transplant antigens responsible for acute rejection, and these are identical to serologically defined human leucocyte antigens (HLA).

The recipient's immune response to the donor organ

Early events

Inflammation is at the centre of the rejection process and is activated through early events around the time of transplantation. Ischaemia–reperfusion injury (IRI) occurs as an inevitable consequence of the transplant process and contributes to the patient's subsequent course, evidenced by:

i)   Superior outcome following living donor transplantation, despite more significant MHC mismatching, and

ii) Adverse impact of prolonged cold ischaemia on graft outcome.

Indeed, the severity of inflammatory injury modulates the subsequent alloimmune response, generating a 'danger signal', which primes the immune response to the transplanted organ.

IRI impacts upon outcome, and may result in:

*   Delayed primary graft function
*   Increased acute rejection rates
*   Reduced long-term graft survival (EBM 25.2).

The afferent arm of the immune response

The immune response to the transplanted organ can be divided into afferent and efferent arms: the afferent arm includes presentation of donor antigen to recipient T cells, T-cell receptor binding and costimulation, and leads to T-cell activation. The efferent arm describes the sequence of events that occurs as a result of T-cell activation.

Afferent arm

Antigen presentation

Donor MHC antigens are recognised as foreign (allorecognition) by recipient T cells following presentation upon donor (direct) or recipient (indirect) antigen-presenting cells (Fig. 25.1).

EBM	**25.2 Impact of delayed graft function on long term outcome**
	'Delayed graft function, defined as the requirement for dialysis during the first week following transplantation is associated with: <ul><li>*41% increased risk of graft loss at 3 years*</li><li>*Higher serum creatinine at 3.5 years*</li><li>*38% relative increased risk of acute rejection,*</li></ul> *Compared with patients that have primary function'*
	Yarlagadda SG, Coca SG, Formica RN Jr, Poggio ED, Parikh CR. Association between delayed graft function and allograft and patient survival: a systematic review and meta-analysis. Nephrol Dial Transplant. 2009; 24:1039–47.

T-cell receptor binding and costimulation

MHC antigen binding to the T-cell receptor in the presence of costimulatory molecules can result in a number of possible outcomes, depending on the costimulatory stimulus, and these include T-cell proliferation, apoptosis (programmed cell death) or anergy (lack of response to antigen or antibody).

T-cell activation

Following their clonal expansion, T cells differentiate into helper (CD4+) and effector (CD8+) cells that secrete cytokines and kill target cells. Engagement of CD4+ T (helper) cells plays a central role in initiating and amplifying the rejection response.

B-cell activation

Traditionally seen as purely antibody-producing cells, it is clear that B cells contribute to the alloimmune response in a variety of additional ways: as antigen-presenting cells, and through cytokine production. Complex interactions between CD4+ T cells and B cells also lead to the production of donor specific antibodies, which play a crucial role in antibody-mediated rejection.

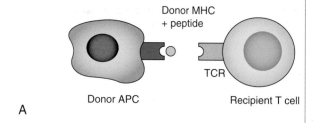

A

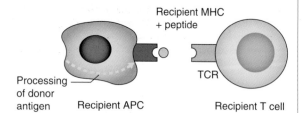

B

Fig. 25.1 Antigen presentation. (A) Direct. **(B)** Indirect. *APC,* Antigen-presenting cell; *MHC,* major histocompatibility complex; *TCR,* T-cell receptor.

Efferent arm

Donor organ damage can be mediated via cellular or antibody-mediated (humoral) mechanisms. The latter depends on B-lymphocyte maturation and the production of complement-activating antibodies. The former, also known as *delayed-type hypersensitivity* (DTH), involves cytotoxic T cells, natural killer (NK) cells, macrophages and neutrophils.

Patterns of allograft rejection

Hyperacute rejection

- Results from the presence of preformed cytotoxic antibodies directed against donor HLA or AB antigens
- Avoidable through blood group and tissue matching
- Apparent following removal of the vascular clamps as the donor organ becomes swollen and discoloured
- Leads to graft destruction within 24 hours.

Acute rejection

- Occurs in up to 50% of grafts, usually in the first 6 months
- Diagnosed on renal transplant biopsy and classified according to Banff 07 diagnostic criteria (Table 25.1)
- Cell-mediated rejection is the more common type; primarily involving T cells, it is treated with high-dose intravenous methylprednisolone
- Antibody-mediated rejection is characterised by specific histological findings along with elevated serum donor specific antibody. Treatment is more challenging, and usually involves plasma exchange and intravenous immunoglobulin.

Chronic allograft damage

- Occurs after 6 months and often leads to a progressive decline in, and eventual loss of, organ function

Table 25.1 Banff 07 diagnostic criteria for renal allograft biopsies
1. Normal

2. AMR
  a. Acute AMR
    i. ATN-like- CD4+, minimal inflammation
    ii. Capillary margination and/or thromboses, CD4+
    iii. Arterial-v3, CD4+
  b. Chronic active AMR. Glomerular double contours and/or peritubular capillary basement membrane multilayering and/or interstitial fibrosis/tubular atrophy and/or fibrous intimal thickening in arteries, CD4+

3. Borderline changes: suspicious for T-cell-mediated rejection, no intimal arteritis, foci of tubulitis

4. T-cell-mediated rejection
  a. Acute T-cell-mediated rejection
  b. Chronic active T-cell-mediated rejection
  c. Chronic allograft arteriopathy

5. IF/TA, no evidence of specific aetiology
Grade:
    I. Mild IF/TA (<25% cortical area)
    II. Moderate IF/TA (26–50%)
    III. Severe (>50%)

6. Other: changes not considered to be due to rejection.
AMR, Antibody-mediated rejection, ATN, acute tubular necrosis; IF/TA, interstitial fibrosis/tubular atrophy.

- Multifactorial aetiology: immune-mediated injury, IRI, toxicity from immunosuppressive agents and viral infections
- Characterised histologically by cellular atrophy and fibrosis, there are currently no therapeutic strategies to combat it.

Testing for histocompatibility

To minimise the risk of rejection, tests are undertaken by histocompatibility scientists to optimise the match between donor and recipient.

Tissue typing

- Prior to adding patients to the transplant waiting list, potential recipients are typed for class I (HLA-A, B and Cw) and class II (HLA-DR, DQ and DP) HLA antigens; this is known as *tissue typing*
- The majority of allocation schemes for kidney transplantation internationally place a high priority on donor and recipient HLA matching, as the better match the kidney is to the recipient, the better the outcome
- Newer technologies allow identification of specific antibodies produced by the recipient in response to pregnancies, previous transplants and blood transfusions, and this allows more thorough tissue matching.

Cross-match

A cross-match is undertaken in some transplant patients immediately prior to renal transplantation to ensure that there is no reactivity between donor and recipient cells.

Common cross-match techniques are:

- Complement-dependent cytotoxicity cross-match (CDC-XM), which, when positive in the presence of IgG antibodies, is likely to result in rapid rejection of the transplanted kidney
- Flow cytometry cross-match (FC-XM) is a more sensitive test, which, if positive, may represent an increased risk of rejection
- Virtual crossmatch: in patients with a known antibody profile who are at low immunological risk, it is possible to predict a negative crossmatch, and thus to proceed without waiting for the tests to be performed. This saves approximately 4 hours of cold ischaemia.

Immunosuppression

The challenge is to minimise the risk of graft rejection with as few side effects as possible. Various strategies are adopted: induction therapy, maintenance immunosuppression and treatment of rejection. The mechanisms of action of the common immunosuppressive drugs are outlined in Fig. 25.2.

Immunosuppressive drugs

Corticosteroids

- Play an important role in induction and maintenance, and are the first-line treatment for acute rejection
- Side effects of steroids are numerous and are responsible for many of the long-term complications of immunosuppressive therapy (Table 25.2)
- Several groups have explored reduction of the steroid load through various strategies:
  a) Steroid withdrawal, undertaken some time after transplantation
  b) Steroid avoidance, in which steroids are stopped a few days postoperatively
  c) Steroid free

Whilst the benefits of reduced steroid use have been observed in these studies, steroid free and steroid withdrawal are associated with an increased incidence of biopsy-proven acute rejection at 12 months posttransplant.

Antiproliferative agents

Azathioprine

- Prodrug of 6-mercaptopurine, it exerts its action by directly inhibiting purine synthesis
- Single daily dose of 1–3 mg/kg/day
- Side effects of azathioprine include severe myelosuppression, resulting in neutropenia and gastrointestinal symptoms.

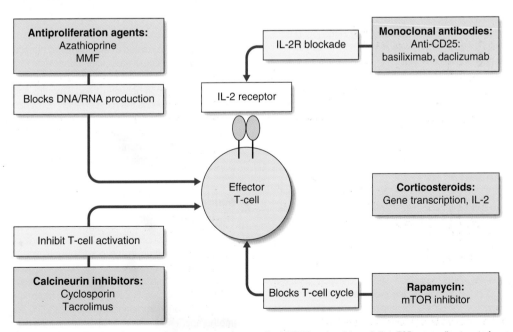

Fig. 25.2 Mechanisms of action of common immunosuppressive agents. *MMF,* Mycophenolate mofetil; *mTOR,* mammalian target of rapamycin.

Table 25.2 Side effects of corticosteroids

- Hypertension
- Diabetes mellitus
- Osteoporosis
- Peptic ulceration
- Cushingoid features
- Pancreatitis
- Poor wound healing
- Psychiatric disorders

Mycophenolate mofetil (MMF)

- Prodrug for mycophenolic acid (MPA), which prevents lymphocyte activation through inhibiting DNA formation
- Has replaced azathioprine in many renal transplant patients, following the publication of several randomised trials that demonstrated reduced treatment failure at 6 months post-kidney transplant
- Side effects include gastrointestinal disturbances, leucopenia, thrombocytopenia and anaemia.

Calcineurin inhibitors

Cyclosporin (CYA)

- Inhibits the production of key cytokines for early T-cell activation, such as interleukin-2
- Led to dramatic improvements in short- and long-term outcomes in transplantation when introduced in the 1980s
- Side effects include nephrotoxicity, hypertension, hyperlipidaemia and hyperglycaemia.

Tacrolimus

- Led to significantly improved 1-year outcome in liver and renal transplant patients compared with cyclosporin (EBM 25.3)
- Is now the mainstay of many immunosuppressive regimens
- Side effects include nephrotoxicity, neurotoxicity, diabetes and alopecia
- The ELITE symphony study compared low-dose cyclosporin, low-dose tacrolimus, low-dose sirolimus and standard-dose tacrolimus, and demonstrated superiority in the low-dose tacrolimus group in terms of acute rejection, renal function and allograft survival at 1 year.

EBM	25.3 Tacrolimus versus cyclosporin in renal and liver transplant patients

'Treatment with the calcineurin inhibitor, tacrolimus, reduces acute and steroid-resistant rejection rates when compared with cyclosporin following renal transplantation, and results in better long-term function. In liver transplant patients, tacrolimus is the agent of choice, with improved outcomes in patient and graft survival.'

Margreiter R, European Tacrolimus vs Ciclosporin Microemulsion Renal Transplantation Study Group. Lancet. 2002;359:741–6.; O'Grady JG et al. Lancet 2002;360:1119–25.

Sirolimus

Sirolimus inhibits T-cell activation and proliferation and early evidence supported its use for the prevention of acute cellular rejection. However, increasing concern about synergistic nephrotoxicity with the calcineurin inhibitors and other side effects such as impaired wound healing and increased incidence of lymphoceles, has limited its use.

Antibody therapies

Antibody therapies may be used as induction therapy or for treatment of acute rejection:

- Induction therapy, given at the time of transplantation, provides immediate immunosuppression after transplantation
- Treatment for steroid-resistant rejection.

Antibody therapies may be depleting or nondepleting:

- Depleting antibodies: target cells are removed from the peripheral blood, including rabbit antithymocyte globulin (ATG) and alemtuzumab. They may be used as induction therapy, or to treat steroid-resistant rejection.

Nondepleting antibodies: in which the function of the target cells is affected, e.g., the interleukin-2 receptor antibody, basiliximab. This is used as induction therapy, reducing acute rejection rates, with few side effects.

New therapies

- Belatacept: acts through T-cell costimulatory blockade, and has been introduced in clinical trials with the aim of reducing requirement for calcineurin inhibitors
- Bortezomib: acts as a proteasome inhibitor, thus inhibiting the production of antibody-producing plasma cells. It is used in antibody-incompatible transplants, to reduce the level of circulating donor-specific antibody, and in cases of refractory antibody-mediated rejection
- Eculuzimab: understanding the key role of complement in mediating antibody damage has led to the development of the complement inhibitors such as the monoclonal antibody, eculuzimab. It has been used to prevent antibody-mediated rejection, and to reduce the risk of recurrent atypical haemolytic uraemic syndrome (aHUS) posttransplant.

General risks of immunosuppression

Infection

The risk of infection is related to the dose of immunosuppression and is therefore greatest early after transplantation. Bacterial infections are most common during the first month. Viral infections are most common between 1 and 6 months and, of these, cytomegalovirus (CMV) is the most clinically relevant. The risk of CMV disease is reduced using antiviral agents such as valganciclovir prophylactically. Opportunistic infections with protozoa and fungi are also important, and most patients receive up to 6 months' co-trimoxazole prophylaxis against *Pneumocystis jirovecii*.

Malignancy

The risk of developing skin cancer is particularly high, with squamous cell carcinoma being 20 times more common in transplant patients than in the normal population. Posttransplant lymphoproliferative disorders (PTLDs) are usually related to infection with Epstein–Barr virus and are associated with a high risk of developing B-cell lymphoma. Treatment of PTLD involves reduction in immunosuppression and, in some cases, chemotherapy.

25.1 Summary

The immune response

- The immune response to a transplanted organ is largely mediated by T cells, and these are the target for immunosuppressive therapy
- Acute rejection is seen in up to 50% of grafts and episodes are treated with high-dose steroids
- Chronic allograft damage has a multifactorial aetiology and results in significant graft loss over the months and years following transplantation.

Organ donation

The shortage of organs for transplantation remains a major challenge, with demand consistently outstripping supply over many years (Fig. 25.3A). Such shortage has led to significant changes in practice over the last decade, with an increasing number of patients undergoing transplants from living donors, and from marginal or extended criteria deceased donors (Fig. 25.3B).

Deceased donation

The identification and selection of potential donors and the subsequent approach to the family has been the focus of much attention. Legislation around organ donation varies internationally, with some countries favouring an 'opt out' policy, which presumes consent for organ donation. The organisation of organ donation and close working between organ donation and critical care experts are key.

Few absolute contraindications for organ donation exist; those that do are directed against the avoidance of disease transmission from donor to recipient (Table 25.3). The most common deceased donation occurs after diagnosis of brain death (DBD), the criteria for this are shown in Table 25.4

Donation after circulatory death

Recent years have seen the expansion of donation after circulatory death (DCD) programmes and this has resulted in increased numbers of deceased donors. Donors after circulatory death are categorised according to the Maastricht criteria (Table 25.5). The majority of such donors in the UK are category III donors, with successful outcomes for renal, liver, pancreas and lung transplant patients.

- Renal transplantation following DCD is associated with increased rates of delayed graft function (DGF) because of longer warm ischaemic periods, but the long-term outcome is comparable to DBD, as long as cold storage time is kept to a minimum (EBM 25.4)

EBM 25.4 Outcomes following transplantation with kidneys from donors following circulatory death

'Kidneys from controlled cardiac-death donors provide good graft survival and function up to 5 years in first time recipients and equivalent to kidneys from brain death donors.'

'Circulatory death donors tolerate cold storage less well that do brain-death kidneys'.

Summers et al. Lancet. 2010:376:1303–11.; Summers et al. Lancet, 2013:381:727–34.

- An increasing number of liver transplants are being performed following DCD. With careful donor selection, primary nonfunction rates are comparable to DBD, but there is a higher risk of biliary complication
- Recently a small number of cardiac transplants have been performed using DCD donors.

Extended criteria donors (ECD)

The critical shortage of organs for transplantation has led to consideration of donors who would have been previously declined.

Extended criteria donors are defined as:

- Donors over the age of 60 years
- Donors aged 50–59 years plus two of the following: cerebrovascular accident as the cause of death, pre-existing hypertension or terminal serum creatinine greater than 1.5 mg/dL.

The long-term outcome of transplants performed from ECD is poorer than standard-criteria donors, and the potential risks to the recipient must be weighed against the benefits. The risks of ECD organs are general and organ specific:

- In liver transplantation, the risk of primary nonfunction is increased in donors with severe fatty liver disease (steatosis)
- In kidney transplantation, there is in an increased risk of delayed graft function.

Systemic risks from donors exist due to the possible transmission of infection, such as hepatitis B, C or HIV, and malignancy. Pre-donation screening minimises the risk of transmission of blood-borne viral diseases.

Organ preservation

Restricting the time between an organ retrieval and cessation of its blood supply to reperfusion in the recipient is acknowledged as important to final outcome, particularly in ECD. For many years, preservation of the organ was carried out by simple cold storage with the organ placed in sterile plastic bags and surrounded by ice. Recent research has examined the benefits of hypothermic machine perfusion and normothermic perfusion. The latter can either be in the donor (where the donor's own blood is recirculated to the organs that are going to be retrieved with regulation of oxygenation, temperature and pressure), or after simple cold storage (where the organ is perfused for a short period on a machine, prior to transplant). There is evidence that some of these techniques may be capable of resuscitating and monitoring the organ prior to transplantation, with the hope that this will lead to improved outcomes.

Living donation

There has been an increase in the number of transplants being performed from living donors. These are mainly kidney transplants but increasing numbers of living donor liver transplants are being performed.

Living donor kidney transplantation

Donor selection

Each potential donor must go through a rigorous assessment process, always bearing in mind that the major operation they are planning to undergo will have no direct benefit to the individual, and so great care must be taken to minimise risk. The assessment is outlined in Table 25.6, and evidence of significant comorbidity

25

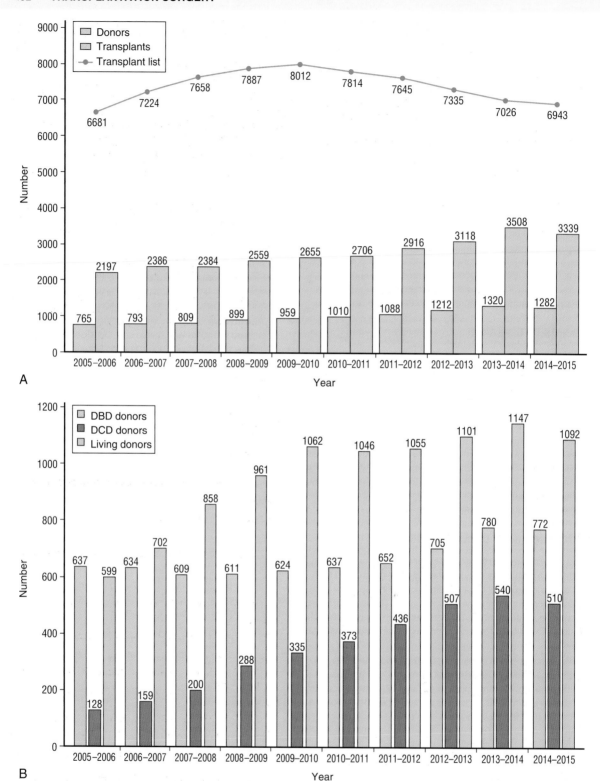

Fig. 25.3 (A) Number of deceased donors and transplants in the UK, 1 April 2005 to 31 March 2015, and patients on the waiting lists at 31 March each year (Organ Donation and Transplantation (ODT) statistics). **(B)** Number of deceased and living donors in the UK, 1 April 2005 to 31 March 2015 (ODT statistics). (Courtesy NHS Blood and Transplant. Transplant Activity in the UK, 2014–2015, with permission.)

should halt the work-up. Uncontrolled hypertension or diabetes should be considered absolute contraindications to living dona-tion, because of the risk of deterioration in donor renal function following nephrectomy.

Operative approaches

Laparoscopic surgery has revolutionised living donor kidney transplantation, making the operation more acceptable to the donor when compared with the traditional flank approach.

Table 25.3 Donor contraindications to organ donation

General contraindications

- HIV disease (not HIV infection; no AIDS-defining illness)
- Disseminated cancer (above and below the diaphragm)
- Melanoma (except local melanoma treated >5 years before donation)
- Treated cancer within 3 years of donation (except nonmelanoma skin cancer and in situ cervical cancer)
- nvCJD and other neurodegenerative diseases associated with infectious agents

Organ-specific donor contraindications

Liver
- Acute hepatitis (AST >1000 IU/L)
- Cirrhosis
- Portal vein thrombosis

Kidney
- CKD (stage 3B and below, eGFR <45)
- Long-term dialysis (i.e., not acute relating to acute illness)
- Any history of renal malignancy
- Previous kidney transplant, >6 months previously

Pancreas
- Insulin-dependent diabetes (excluding ICU-associated insulin requirement)
- Any history of pancreatic malignancy

AST, aspartate transaminase CKD, chronic kidney disease; eGFR, estimated glomerular filtration rate; ICU, intensive care unit; nvCJD, new-variant Creutzfeldt–Jakob disease.

Table 25.4 Criteria for diagnosis of brainstem death

Preconditions

- Ventilated and in a coma
- Known diagnosis for coma
- Sufficient length of time on ventilator to determine severity of brain injury
- Optimisation of condition, to reverse injury
- Interval of 6–24 hours from latest intervention and testing

Exclusions

- Drug or alcohol intoxication require a delay appropriate to half-life of drug
- Time for clearance of neuromuscular-blocking agents
- Primary hypothermia, metabolic and endocrine disturbances
- Coma of unknown aetiology

Investigation

Absent brainstem reflexes
- No papillary response to light
- Absent corneal reflexes
- Absent vestibulocochlear reflexes: caloric tests
- No motor response in cranial nerve distribution
- No gag reflex

Apnoea testing
- No attempt to breathe despite arterial $P_{CO_2} > 6.65$ kPa following preoxygenation with 100% oxygen

P_{CO_2}, Partial pressure of carbon dioxide.

Table 25.5 Maastricht criteria for donation after circulatory death

Category 1: Dead on arrival at hospital. The moment of sudden death must be witnessed and the time documented

Category 2: Unsuccessful resuscitation. Usually in the Accident and Emergency department

Category 3: Awaiting cardiac arrest. Patients in whom cardiac arrest is inevitable, but they do not fulfil criteria for brainstem death testing

Category 4: Cardiac arrest in a brainstem dead individual

Category 5: Unexpected death in a patient in ITU or critical care unit

Table 25.6 Assessment of the potential living kidney donor

History

- General health: obesity, hypertension, diabetes
- Cardiovascular risk: past medical history, family history, smoking, obesity
- History of thromboembolic events or bleeding disorders
- Respiratory risk (for anaesthetic): past medical history of asthma, chronic obstructive pulmonary disease, smoking
- Risk of renal disease: family history, particularly if disease in recipient is familial; past history of renal infections, haematuria
- Psychiatric history

Examination

- General
- Cardiovascular
- Respiratory
- Abdominal

Investigations

Immunology
- Blood group; HLA type; T- and B-cell flow cytometric crossmatching

Haematology
- Full blood count; coagulation studies

Biochemistry
- Urea and electrolytes; creatinine clearance; liver function tests; blood glucose

Urinalysis
- Protein; blood; sugar; culture sensitivity and microscopy

Cardiovascular
- Serial blood pressure measurements; electrocardiogram

Microbiology screen
- Hepatitis B and C; HIV; cytomegalovirus infection; Epstein–Barr virus; syphilis; *Toxoplasma*

Radiology
- Chest x-ray; isotope glomerular filtration rate; renal ultrasound; angiogram/spiral computerised tomography/magnetic resonance angiography

25

- Hand-assisted technique, with the ability to use a hand for retraction or to rapidly control intraoperative haemorrhage
- Open techniques include the traditional flank approach, which may be rib sparing or rib dividing, or performed via a mini-incision.

Procedure-related morbidity and mortality

The mortality of donor nephrectomy is low, estimated at 1 in 3000 for all surgical approaches. Life expectancy for living donors is

- Main benefits are improved cosmesis and shorter recovery time
- Hospital stay can be reduced by several days.

There are various technical options:
- Total laparoscopic surgery through a transperitoneal or retroperitoneal approach

probably higher than the general population due to bias in the selection process, although more recent data suggest a higher risk of ESRF in the long term. The risk of major complications such as pneumothorax, vascular or splenic injury is approximately 5%, and is 15% for all complications.

Living donation for liver transplantation

The surgical principle of living donation for liver transplantation (LDLT) is based upon the remarkable ability of the liver to regenerate to its full size and function, and due to a paucity of cadaveric liver availability for patients awaiting liver transplant. This property permits removal of a portion of an adult liver for transplantation into a child or small adult recipient. Mortality in the donor is approximately 0.5% and risk of significant complications around 20%. Although this procedure has been accepted in a number of countries around the world, the extra risks both for donor and recipient make any decision to proceed a very difficult one. In countries where a deceased donor programme has not been established, LDLT has successfully filled the void. Large series have been reported from Japan, Hong Kong, Taiwan and Korea with promising results. In India, where the waiting list for a liver transplant is in the thousands, LDLT has led to successful outcomes in 1500 cases. With experience and expertise increasing, more than 600 procedures are now being done annually in about five high-volume centres in the country.

25.2 Summary

Organ donation

- Shortage of organs for donation remains a significant challenge to the transplant community
- Strategies aimed at increasing use of organs for donation include use of marginal donors and donors without a heart beat
- Well-established programmes for living donor kidney transplants exist within the UK, with an increasing drive to establish living donor liver transplantation.

Renal transplantation

Indications and patient assessment

Absolute contraindications to renal transplantation:
- Active infection
- Malignancy.

Relative contraindications:
- Advanced age
- Severe cardiovascular disease
- Likelihood of noncompliance with immunosuppressive therapy
- High likelihood of the underlying disease causing problems in the transplanted kidney (e.g., diabetes mellitus, glomerulosclerosis, amyloidosis and hypertension).

Potential recipients undergo rigorous medical (Table 25.7), psychological and social evaluation. An important component of this is the education of the patient and family about the benefits and risks of transplantation and of immunosuppression, so that fully informed written consent can be obtained. Following full assessment and investigation, recipients can be listed on the national transplant waiting list.

Table 25.7 Assessment of the potential recipient for renal transplantation

General assessment

- History, clinical examination

Blood tests

- Haematology: full blood count, clotting screen
- Biochemistry: urea and electrolytes, liver function tests
- Virology: HIV, hepatitis B and C
- Immunology: ABO and HLA typing

Urinalysis and culture

- 24-hour urine collection for creatinine clearance

Other tests

- ECG, chest x-ray

Cardiovascular assessment

- Patients >45 years, history of diabetes or of cardiovascular disease: exercise tolerance test, stress echocardiogram or stress radionuclide scan; if abnormal, proceed to coronary angiography

Gastrointestinal assessment

- Abnormal liver function tests, history of peptic ulcer disease: liver ultrasound scan, upper GI endoscopy

Assessment for infection

- Active bacterial infection: contraindication to transplantation
- Viral infections: cytomegalovirus status

Urological assessment

- Urine culture and renal ultrasound; if positive, require assessment of bladder emptying, e.g., postmicturition ultrasound, cystoscopy

Immunological assessment

- Blood group: for ABO compatibility
- HLA typing, anti-HLA antibodies: for HLA matching and organ allocation

ECG, Electrocardiogram; GI, gastrointestinal; HLA, human leukocyte antigen.

The operative procedure

Back-table preparation

Final preparation of the donor kidney is undertaken at the recipient centre. This involves careful dissection of the donor renal artery and vein, removal of perinephric fat, and careful inspection of the kidney to ensure that there is no damage to the renal capsule, to the vessels or donor ureter. It is imperative to identify any damage at this stage, and prior to reperfusion, when haemorrhage can ensue.

Recipient operation

- A Rutherford Morris incision is made in the iliac fossa, and the iliac vessels are exposed by retroperitoneal dissection
- Lymphatics overlying the iliac vessels must be ligated and divided with care, to avoid the development of a postoperative lymphocoele
- The venous anastomosis is performed between donor renal vein and recipient external iliac vein
- The arterial anastomosis may be performed onto the recipient's internal or external iliac artery, depending on the calibre of the donor renal artery and the positioning of the arteries (Fig. 25.4)

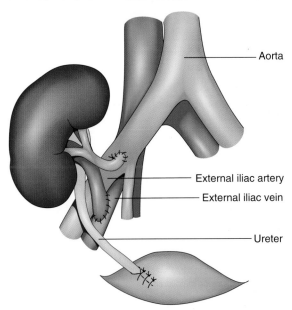

Aorta

External iliac artery

External iliac vein

Ureter

Fig. 25.4 Renal transplantation. The renal transplant is placed retroperitoneally on to the iliac vessels with the ureteric anastomosis as shown.

- The kidney is reperfused, and the ureteric anastomosis performed between donor ureter and recipient bladder, over a double J stent. Insertion of the ureteric stent has been shown to reduce the risk of early ureteric complications such as urinary leak.

Postoperative management

- The patient should be managed in a high-dependency unit by experienced nursing staff
- Primary function is expected in a transplant from a living donor, and if this is not the case, rapid and thorough investigation into the cause of delay is necessary, whereas a kidney from a DCD or ECD has a high likelihood of delayed graft function
  - Rigorous assessment and maintenance of fluids are essential. A brisk diuresis is common, and careful assessment and maintenance of volume status, blood pressure and serum electrolytes is crucial to optimise renal function
  - DGF is defined as the need for dialysis in the first postoperative week and occurs in up to 50% of all cadaveric transplants.

Management of delayed graft function

If the patient is well-filled, with a central venous pressure of around 8–10 mmHg, and there is no evidence of postoperative haemorrhage, an ultrasound scan is performed to exclude urinary leakage or obstruction, inadequate renal blood flow or the presence of a perinephric haematoma. If DGF is expected, the patient's fluids are carefully managed over the next few days. The patient is reassured that this is a common feature after transplantation. If the kidney is still not functioning at day 5, a renal biopsy is performed to check that there is no evidence of rejection, expecting evidence of acute tubular necrosis.

Complications

Early complications following renal transplantation may be general complications of major surgery, technical or immunological. The main immunological complications have been dealt with elsewhere in the chapter.

Technical complications:

- Acute renal artery thrombosis is rare (approximately 1%)
- Venous thrombosis (approximately 6%).

Both must be recognised rapidly, using Doppler ultrasound, and require that the patient is returned to theatre immediately if there is to be any chance of salvaging the transplant.

- Late vascular complications include renal artery stenosis, which occurs in about 3–5% of patients and usually presents several months posttransplantation with hypertension, and deteriorating graft function. The diagnosis is confirmed by angiography and the treatment of choice is angioplasty
- Urinary leaks occur less commonly now that ureteric stenting is adopted more widely: they present with falling urine output and increasing pain. They may be managed conservatively with prolonged urinary catheterisation, but may require surgical intervention
- Urinary tract obstruction can occur early or late. The diagnosis is confirmed by a percutaneous antegrade nephrostogram, during which a nephrostomy tube may be placed for temporary decompression. Subsequent percutaneous dilatation and insertion of a double J stent will often treat the stricture, with open surgery reserved for cases in which percutaneous management has failed
- Fluid collections (lymphocoeles) around the transplant are a common finding on ultrasound scan but are only relevant if they become symptomatic or cause urinary obstruction. Percutaneous drainage gives temporary symptomatic relief. Definitive management involves drainage of the lymphocele into the peritoneal cavity and this fenestration can be performed laparoscopically.

Outcome

The 1-year renal graft survival is approximately 90% and patient survival exceeds this. However, there remains a 2–5% perioperative mortality, as many renal patients have severe comorbidity. The 5-year graft survival is approximately 70%, and at this time graft losses are commonly due to chronic allograft damage or to cardiovascular death in a patient with a functioning graft.

Recent developments in renal transplantation

The significant benefits that arise from living donor renal transplantation and the ongoing shortage of organs for donation have led to an expansion in renal transplant programmes to perform higher risk transplants. In the UK, the kidney sharing scheme has developed considerably since its inception in 2006. This programme exists for donor–recipient pairs who are unable to directly donate due to incompatibility, be it due to blood group or HLA incompatibility. Pairs are entered into the national programme to determine whether a paired exchange transplant is possible. These transplants can then be undertaken in two

25

transplant centres simultaneously, with the kidneys being transported between centres. An additional resource that enhances the scheme significantly is the incorporation of nondirected altruistic donors, who offer an additional kidney into the matching scheme.

An alternative option for patients with incompatible donors is to undergo a blood group or antibody-incompatible transplant. Although these are associated with increased risk of rejection and infection, their outcome is superior to remaining on dialysis, but inferior to compatible transplants, supporting entry into a kidney-sharing scheme as the first option for such patients. Recipients undergo a period of desensitisation, usually involving treatment with the anti-CD20 antibody rituximab, and several rounds of plasma exchange with intravenous immunoglobulin G (IV Ig).

25.3 Summary

Renal transplantation

- Renal transplant is the optimal treatment for patients with end-stage renal failure, improving quality of life and survival compared with dialysis
- Renal transplantation is associated with a 90% 1-year and 70% 5-year graft survival
- Chronic allograft damage remains a significant cause of late graft loss.

Liver transplantation

Indications and patient assessment

The most effective therapy for end-stage liver failure is liver transplantation. Patients with chronic liver failure who show signs of hepatic decompensation despite optimal medical management, those with primary hepatocellular carcinoma or patients with acute liver failure should be referred to specialist liver transplant units.

Signs of decompensation in chronic liver failure include:

- Oesophageal varices
- Ascites
- Encephalopathy
- Infection, including spontaneous bacterial peritonitis.

All of these may be combined with poor synthetic liver function, as demonstrated by hypoalbuminaemia, hyperbilirubinaemia and prolonged clotting times. Indications for liver transplant are shown in Table 25.8.

A multidisciplinary team comprising surgeons, hepatologists, specialist anaesthetists and, where the patient demonstrates addictive behaviour, a specialist psychiatrist, must undertake patient assessment. In general, patients should be expected to have at least a 50% chance of surviving 5 years posttransplantation. The criteria to decide whether someone with fulminant liver failure should receive a liver transplant is detailed in Table 25.9. To help assess priority for organ allocation, the Model for End Stage Liver Disease (MELD) was developed in the USA. This was originally developed to assess the prognosis of cirrhotic patients who underwent treatment for portal hypertension. It has also been shown to predict short-term outcome in patients awaiting liver transplantation and therefore is used both in the US and, sometimes with modification, in other countries for identifying those patients most in need of liver transplant. The United Kingdom Model for End-Stage

Table 25.8 Indications for liver transplant

Common indications in adults

- Alcoholic liver disease
- Hepatitis C and B
- Primary biliary cirrhosis
- Primary sclerosing cholangitis
- Hepatocellular carcinoma
- Autoimmune hepatitis
- Nonalcoholic steatohepatitis (fatty liver)
- Cryptogenic cirrhosis
- Acute liver failure, e.g., paracetamol toxicity, drug reaction or virus

Rarer indications in adults

- Haemochromatosis
- Wilson's disease
- Alpha 1-antitripsin deficiency
- Budd–Chiari syndrome
- Polycystic disease
- Metabolic diseases (such as hyperoxaluria)

Common indications in children

- Biliary atresia
- Metabolic disorders including alpha 1-antytripsin deficiency
- Wilson's disease
- Crigler–Najjar type 1

Table 25.9 Criteria for liver transplantation in acute liver failure

Paracetamol toxicity

- pH <7.3
- Prothrombin time >100 seconds and creatinine >300 µmol/L in patients with encephalopathy

Nonparacetamol toxicity

- Prothrombin time >100 seconds (with encephalopathy)
- Any three of the following:
  Age 40 years
  Non-A/non-B hepatitis
  Drug reaction or halothane hepatitis
  Jaundice for >7 days prior to encephalopathy
  Prothrombin time >50 seconds
  Serum bilirubin >300 µmol/L

Table 25.10 Equation for determining United Kingdom Model for End Stage Liver Disease (UKELD) score

The UKELD score is calculated from the patient's INR, serum creatinine, serum bilirubin and serum sodium, according to the formula:

$5.395 \times \ln INR +$
$1.485 \times \ln creatinine +$
$3.13 \times \ln bilirubin$
$-81.565 \times \ln Na$
$+435$

INR, International normalised ratio; UKELD, United Kingdom Model for End-Stage Liver Disease.

Liver Disease (UKELD) is now used to assess severity of liver disease and allocate organs within the UK (Table 25.10). A patient requires a UKELD score ≥49 in order to meet listing criteria.

The operative procedure

Back-table preparation

The liver is examined carefully for any damage or underlying abnormality. The hepatic artery, portal vein and inferior vena cava are all prepared for anastomosis.

Recipient operation

- 'Mercedes-Benz' incision or through a midline incision, which is curved to the right following the line of the costal margin (Fig. 25.5)
- Hepatectomy is performed, leaving the inferior vena cava intact
- The liver is implanted by:
  - Anastomosis of donor to recipient inferior vena cava, using a 'piggyback procedure' and accomplished by performing a side-to-side anastomosis between the two venae cavae
  - Portal venous and hepatic arterial anastomoses (Fig. 25.6)
  - The liver is reperfused with recipient blood and haemostasis carried out carefully
  - The donor gallbladder is removed and an end-to-end common bile duct to common bile duct anastomosis performed unless there is a specific indication to perform a Roux-en-Y hepaticojejunostomy (retransplantation or primary sclerosing cholangitis in the recipient).

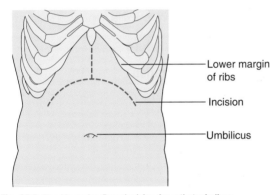

Fig. 25.5 The Mercedes-Benz incision for orthotopic liver transplantation.

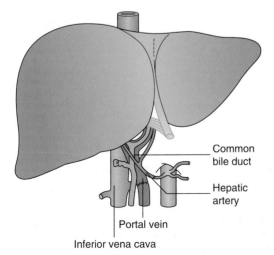

Fig. 25.6 Vascular and biliary anastomoses of a liver transplant.

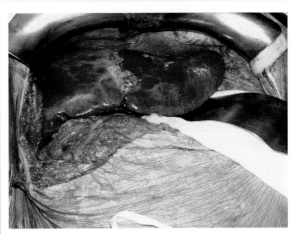

Fig. 25.7 Liver transplant postperfusion.

Fig. 25.7 shows a well-perfused liver following completion of the anastomoses.

Living donor liver transplant

No more than 65% of a healthy donor liver can be removed (right or left lobe can be removed) and the recipient should obtain at least 0.8% GRWR (graft-to-recipient weight ratio). Hepatic artery, portal vein, hepatic vein and biliary duct anastomoses are performed. The donor's remnant liver lobe regenerates to full volume and is functionally back to normal in 6 weeks.

Postoperative management and complications

- The patient is managed in an intensive care setting. Evidence of a functioning graft is based on the blood biochemistry of the recipient with falling blood lactate levels and return of clotting and blood glucose towards normal
- Primary nonfunction can occur in approximately 2% of patients who require urgent transplantation
- Re-exploration can be indicated, and there should be a low threshold for this
- Vessel thrombosis, most commonly in the hepatic artery, can be detected on colour Doppler and confirmed by computed tomography angiography. Suspicion of this serious complication necessitates re-exploration and it is possible that the patient may need a second transplant
- Rejection in the liver is much less common than with other organs for reasons which are not completely clear. Diagnosis of rejection is often made around day 7 with rising transaminases in the liver function tests. Biopsy may be performed to confirm the diagnosis and the rejection can be treated with daily boluses of methylprednisolone given over 3 days. It is rare, with modern immunosuppression, for acute rejection to cause complete failure of the graft.

Outcome

Many large, single-centre studies and information from registry data show that the 1-year survival for elective first liver transplant in adults is around 90%. The European liver transplant registry report an overall 5-year survival rate after adult liver transplantation

25

of 71%, but the most recent figures from the UK show a 5-year survival rate of 82%. Patients with acute liver failure fare less well, with approximately 70% surviving at 1 year. The vast majority of recipients report a very good quality of life but there remains the need, in most patients, to take immunosuppression in the long-term. In common with the recipients of other transplant organs, patients can experience nephrotoxicity and other side effects from immunosuppressive medication. However, without the liver transplant procedure, the outcome would have been certain death and so this procedure remains one of the miracles of modern medicine.

25.4 Summary

Liver transplantation

- Liver transplantation is a potentially life-saving treatment for patients with acute or chronic liver failure
- Patients must undergo rigorous medical and psychosocial assessment prior to being listed for this major operation
- Outcome for patients following liver transplantation is excellent.

Pancreas transplantation

Transplantation of the pancreas offers the only treatment that reliably offers insulin independence and normal glucose metabolism for patients with type 1 diabetes mellitus.

Indications and patient assessment

Patients undergo pancreas transplant in three distinct clinical settings:

- Simultaneous pancreas–kidney (SPK)
- Pancreas after kidney (PAK) and
- Pancreas transplant alone (PTA).

SPK transplant is the most common, and will be considered in more detail here.

There is little doubt that diabetic patients with renal failure should be offered a kidney transplant if they are fit enough. The potential benefits of dual transplant and insulin independence include:

- Improved quality of life

- Halting of the progress of diabetic complications
- Improved life expectancy.

However, this comes with significantly increased risk in terms of perioperative morbidity and mortality, with the potential for the pancreas transplant to affect adversely the outcome of the renal transplant. Thus, careful recipient selection is essential: cardiovascular comorbidity is the most important factor leading to postoperative mortality, and may not be apparent in the history.

Generally accepted indications for SPK transplant are:

- Inadequate glucose control by medical management alone
- Hypoglycaemic unawareness
- 'Brittle diabetes', where extremely high or low blood glucose levels are precipitated by minor dietary modifications.

Contraindications are:

- Systemic sepsis
- Malignancy
- Significant medical comorbidity
- Significant aortoiliac disease is a relative contraindication
- Insulin resistance. This should be suspected in obese patients, those with late-onset diabetes or those requiring high insulin doses.

Thorough assessment of these patients is essential as the majority have ESRF.

It is important to counsel patients and relatives that a pancreas transplant is a major undertaking and one that is life-enhancing rather than life-saving, as in the case of a liver transplant. Most patients will require a simultaneous renal transplant and the results for such combined transplants are better than for solitary pancreas.

The operative procedure

Back-table preparation

- The pancreas is retrieved en bloc with the spleen, and this is carefully excised on the back table, paying careful attention to the ligation and division of vessels
- The 'C' of duodenum is carefully reduced and the ends both stapled and oversewn to avoid leakage
- A Y graft (arterial conduit) is formed using donor iliac vessels onto the donor splenic and superior mesenteric vessels (Fig. 25.8)

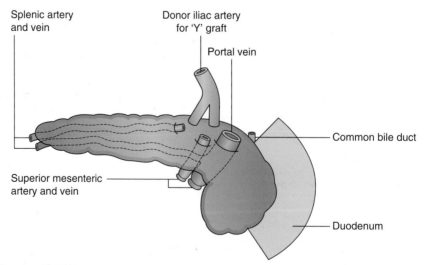

Fig. 25.8 Back-table preparation of the pancreas graft. Showing arterial Y graft using donor iliac vessels onto superior mesenteric and splenic arteries to create a single arterial conduit for anastomosis.

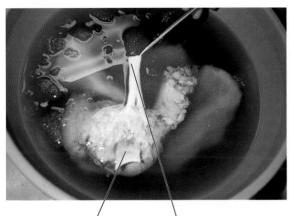

Portal vein Y graft from donor iliac vessels, anastomosed to recipient splenic and superior mesenteric arteries

Fig. 25.9 Pancreas graft showing interposition Y graft prior to implantation.

- Fig. 25.9 illustrates a pancreas graft just before implantation and shows the vascular reconstruction performed on the back table.

Recipient operation

- The pancreas is usually implanted first due to the ischaemic intolerance of the pancreas relative to the kidney. It is implanted intraperitoneally on the right side
- The venous anastomosis is performed between donor portal vein and the distal inferior vena cava
- The arterial conduit constructed on the back table is anastomosed to the recipient common iliac artery.

Reperfusion of the pancreas usually results in some haemorrhage, which has to be controlled with suture ligation of the small pericapsular vessels.

- Drainage of the exocrine secretions is achieved by an entero-enterostomy between donor duodenum and recipient small bowel.

Postoperative management and complications

Patients are often managed in the intensive care unit postoperatively, where close monitoring and early identification of postoperative complications are likely to improve early outcome.

Pancreas transplantation is associated with a higher incidence and a greater range of complications than kidney transplant due to a requirement for greater immunosuppression in a high-risk diabetic population with impaired infection resistance, poor healing and high levels of comorbidity. Between one-fifth and one-quarter of patients require relaparotomy in the early postoperative period. Complications of pancreas transplant are outlined in Table 25.11. Risk factors for complications include increasing donor age, prolonged preservation time, and donor and recipient obesity.

Rejection of a pancreas transplant alone is difficult to diagnose, with no reliable early markers. In SPK transplants, the diagnosis of rejection relies on monitoring renal function and undertaking renal biopsy when indicated. Acute rejection of the pancreas affects exocrine function first and gives rise to an inflammatory response,

Table 25.11 Complications of pancreas transplantation

Infective complications
Systemic infection (opportunistic infections)
Local infections (peritonitis, localised collections, fistulae)
Vascular complications
Haemorrhage: early or late
Thrombosis: arterial or venous thrombosis
Allograft pancreatitis
Ischaemia–reperfusion injury
Reflux pancreatitis

which may well be masked by the immunosuppressive regimen. Dysfunction of islets occurs as a late sign of rejection, which may then be less amenable to treatment.

Outcome

There has been considerable improvement in the 1-year patient and graft survival following pancreas transplantation over the last decade, with 95% patient survival, 92% kidney graft survival and 82% of pancreas graft survival. There is 89% patient survival at 5 years and there is also increasing evidence to suggest that pancreas transplantation has a favourable influence on diabetic complications and survival prospects.

 25.5 Summary

Pancreas transplantation

- Combined kidney and pancreas transplantation is an excellent treatment for a carefully selected group of patients with type 1 diabetes mellitus
- Patients must undergo rigorous medical evaluation prior to being listed, as they have complicated diabetic disease
- Pancreas rejection is difficult to diagnose and this may lead to delay in initiating therapy for such episodes
- Despite this, combined kidney–pancreas transplant is associated with a 5-year survival of 70%.

Pancreatic islet transplantation

Transplantation of islets alone offers an attractive alternative to whole-pancreas transplantation and is associated with less serious morbidity. Indications for islet cell transplantation differ from those of solid-pancreas transplant, and the primary indication is severe hypoglycaemic unawareness. It leads to long-term insulin independence in a small number of patients, and renders glucose control more predictable with less hypoglycaemic unawareness. Isolated islets from two pancreata are infused into the portal venous system, under sedation.

Heart and lung transplantation

Indications and patient assessment

Heart

Heart transplantation is undertaken to prolong life and improve its quality.

25

The main indications are:

- Coronary-related heart failure (38%)
- Cardiomyopathies (45%)
- Other indications such as valvular disease, adult congenital abnormalities and miscellaneous diagnoses account for the rest.

Potential candidates for heart transplant are patients with advanced heart failure who are on maximal medical therapy, including vasodilators, digoxin, diuretics and β-blockers. Patients should be considered if they have increasing medication requirements, frequent hospitalisations or overall deterioration in clinical status.

Contraindications to heart transplant include factors that:

- Increase perioperative mortality, such as irreversible pulmonary hypertension, active sepsis, severe obesity
- Affect long-term prognosis, such as age >65 years, severe renal impairment, active or recent malignancy, other major comorbidity
- Impair compliance, such as active mental illness, recent drug abuse refractory to treatment.

Lung

The lung has been the most challenging of the human organs to be transplanted in clinical practice. Lungs may be transplanted singly or sequentially as a bilateral lung transplant. Indications include:

- Chronic obstructive pulmonary disease (35%)
- Cystic fibrosis (15%)
- Pulmonary fibrosis (16%).

Bilateral lung transplantation is indicated when all native lung must be removed, e.g., when it is a significant source of sepsis, as in cystic fibrosis. Single lung transplantation is an attractive option for the treatment of lung failure, as it can be performed with reduced risk of acute lung injury and without the requirement for cardiopulmonary bypass.

The operative procedure

Heart

Cold ischaemic time must be kept to a minimum, such that the recipient operation may be commenced once the donor heart has been visualised and assessed for suitability. Through a midline sternotomy, cardiopulmonary bypass is established, the patient cooled to 32°C, and the heart removed. The donor heart is prepared for implantation. Donor and recipient atria are anastomosed, followed by the aortic anastomosis. Heart reperfusion is a critical time. The heart usually starts to beat and, if ventricular fibrillation occurs, the heart is promptly defibrillated. Reperfusion is followed by the pulmonary arterial, inferior and superior vena caval anastomoses. Once the implantation is complete the body temperature is brought back to 37°C. Cardioversion and temporary pacing may be required.

Lung

Lung transplantation similarly requires a short cold ischaemic time. For a single lung transplant, a lateral thoracotomy is performed and the native lung is excised with ligation of inferior and superior pulmonary veins and pulmonary artery. The bronchus is divided and the native organ removed. The pericardium is then incised, and the pulmonary veins and artery are mobilised for subsequent anastomoses.

Implantation starts with the bronchial anastomosis, followed by the left atrial and pulmonary arterial anastomoses. Ventilation of the new lung commences.

Postoperative management and complications

Heart

The principles of early postoperative management of heart transplant recipients are to:

- Maintain graft function
- Recognise and manage right ventricular impairment
- Establish adequate immunosuppression
- Prevent and treat early infections
- Allow the recovery of other organs, such as the kidneys.

Most patients have impaired myocardial function requiring inotropic support for the first 24–48 hours. Some patients develop ventricular dysfunction, which requires supportive management with inotropes.

Routine endocardial biopsies are taken from the right ventricle of heart transplant recipients using x-ray screening and right internal jugular venous access. If rejection is confirmed, augmentation of immunosuppression is carried out. Rejection can also cause rapidly progressive coronary artery disease, with thickening and narrowing of the coronary arteries. Because the donor heart is denervated, the patient will not experience angina, and therefore coronary angiography is performed annually from 2 years onwards.

Common causes of 30-day mortality following heart transplant are:

- Graft failure (41%)
- Non-CMV infection (14%)
- Multiorgan failure (14%).

Beyond 5 years, cardiac allograft vasculopathy and late graft failure are the most common causes of death. Malignancies are increasingly common after 10 years.

Lungs

Apical and basal chest drains are placed perioperatively and patients are managed in the intensive care unit.

Infection is a major cause of postoperative morbidity in lung transplant patients. Antibiotic prophylaxis with flucloxacillin and metronidazole is commenced and adjusted as microbiological results from donor and recipient samples become available.

Postoperative acute lung injury, occurring as a result of reperfusion injury, causes problems with ventilation, requiring meticulous supportive management of fluids, optimisation of ventilation and microbiology input. Another life-threatening complication of lung transplantation is dehiscence of the tracheal or bronchial anastomosis, with prolonged air leak and mediastinitis.

Transbronchial biopsies are performed regularly in the weeks and months posttransplant to diagnose rejection, which can be treated in the standard fashion.

Combined heart and lung transplant

Combined heart and lung transplant was the most common form of lung transplant, but its use has declined significantly over the last 15 years. Indications for the combined procedure are now confined to pulmonary hypertension without congenital heart disease. The operation is performed via a median sternotomy, and requires cardiopulmonary bypass. The results are similar to lung transplantation, with survival at 1 and 5 years of 60% and 40%, respectively.

Outcome

Survival following heart transplant is approximately 65% at 5 years, 50% at 10 years and 30% at 15 years. The success of cardiac transplantation, as is the case with other solid-organ transplants, has raised expectations that cannot be fulfilled, with the shortage of organs for donation and high death rates on cardiac transplant waiting lists. The 5-year survival of lung transplant recipients is close to 50%, and 25% after a decade.

Summary

Solid-organ transplantation provides excellent treatment for patients with end-stage organ failure, with 1-year graft survival exceeding 80% for most organs. The advantage of transplantation must be weighed against the price of immunosuppression and it is important that potential recipients are fully counselled. One of the greatest challenges facing transplantation is the shortage of organs for donation and this chapter has described specific strategies aimed at combating this: namely, use of extended criteria donors, living donors and donors after circulatory death.

25.6 Summary

Heart–lung transplantation

- Ischaemic heart disease and cardiomyopathy are the most common indications for heart transplantation
- Both heart and lung transplantation require short cold ischaemic times in comparison with intraabdominal organs
- Outcomes following heart and lung transplantation are similar to those seen following transplantation of intraabdominal organs.

25

Ear, nose and throat surgery

Chapter contents

Ear 502

Nose 507

Paranasal sinuses 509

Nasopharynx 510

Oral cavity 510

Oropharynx 515

Hypopharynx 516

Larynx 517

Neck 519

Ear

Anatomy

External ear

The pinna (Fig. 26.1) is made of fibroelastic cartilage. The external auditory meatus has an outer cartilage portion; the inner part is formed by the tympanic bone (Fig. 26.2). It is lined by squamous epithelium and contains ceruminous glands that produce wax. There is very little subcutaneous tissue, and soft tissue swelling is very painful.

Middle ear

The vibrating tympanic membrane is conical and attached to the margin of the bony ear canal peripherally, and to the handle of the malleus, the most lateral of the three ossicles, centrally (Fig. 26.2). The head of the malleus is attached to the body of the incus in the space superior to the middle ear known as *the attic*. The long process of the incus attaches to the head of the stapes. The stapes is joined to the oval window margin by the annular ligament. The middle ear is lined by simple cuboidal epithelium containing some mucus-secreting cells. The middle-ear space is connected to the nasopharynx by the Eustachian tube, which maintains the middle ear at atmospheric pressure.

The inner ear

The inner ear membrane encloses a labyrinth filled by a fluid called *endolymph*. This is surrounded by a bony labyrinth, the otic capsule, which is filled with perilymph. The cochlea, the hearing component of the inner ear, is a tube linking the oval and round windows, coiled up like a shell. The vestibular (balance) portion of the inner ear consists of three semicircular canals, together with their vestibule, which contains the saccule and utricle, medial to

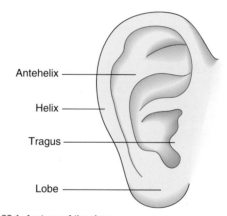

Fig. 26.1 Anatomy of the pinna.

Antehelix

Helix

Tragus

Lobe

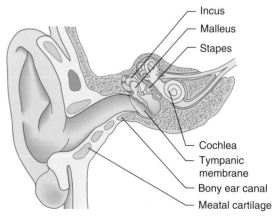

Fig. 26.2 Anatomy of the ear.

Incus

Malleus

Stapes

Cochlea

Tympanic membrane

Bony ear canal

Meatal cartilage

the stapes footplate. The cochlear and vestibular nerves combine in the internal auditory meatus and pass medially to the brainstem. The facial nerve enters the temporal bone through the internal auditory meatus and passes laterally to the geniculate ganglion, where it turns posteriorly (the first genu). It passes through the middle ear above the oval window and turns inferiorly (the second genu) to exit at the stylomastoid foramen.

Physiology

The pinna funnels sound into the ear canal. The tympanic membrane lever mechanism, the ossicular lever mechanism and the large size of the drum relative to the stapes footplate act as an impedance-matching transformer. Vibrations in air are thus transferred to the cochlear fluids without excessive loss of energy. The cochlea converts these endolymph vibrations into electrical impulses in the auditory nerve by stimulation of hair cells in the organ of Corti. The maximum response to high frequencies occurs in the basal turn of the cochlea. Low frequencies maximally stimulate the apex. Auditory neurons connect via the brainstem to the auditory cortex, where again different groups of cells are stimulated by nerve impulses coded for different frequencies. The hair cells in the ampullae of the semicircular canals are stimulated by angular acceleration. The saccule and utricle are stimulated by linear acceleration. Information from the labyrinths, eyes and limbs is processed in the brainstem. Connections from the vestibular nuclei pass to the cortex and the cerebellum.

Assessment

Clinical features

Disorders of the external or middle ear can impair sound transmission to the inner ear and cause conductive deafness. Sensorineural deafness results from lesions of the cochlea or its nerve. Deafness is often associated with a noise in the ear (tinnitus). Ear pain (otalgia) may be due to ear disease but may also be referred from other sites (Table 26.1). Ear-related disorders of balance usually cause a sensation of movement (vertigo), most often

Table 26.1 **Causes of referred otalgia**
Pharynx and larynx
• Tonsillitis
• Tonsillectomy
• Tumours
• Glossopharyngeal neuralgia
Mouth
• Dental disease
• Tumour
Temporomandibular joints
• Temporomandibular joint dysfunction/atypical facial pain
• Arthritis
Neck
• Cervical spondylosis
• Tumour
Paranasal sinuses
• Maxillary sinusitis

rotation. 'Unsteadiness', however, typically has a nonotological cause. Patients with ear disease occasionally fall to the ground but never lose consciousness.

Examination

The ear canal and tympanic membrane are inspected with an otoscope, a rigid telescope or a microscope. Microscopy can assist in wax or discharge removal. Tuning fork tests differentiate between conductive and sensorineural hearing loss (Rinne's test). In health or sensorineural deafness, a tuning fork is heard better via the ear canal (air conduction) than via the mastoid process (bone conduction). In conductive hearing loss, the tuning fork is heard better by bone conduction. When hearing is symmetrical, a tuning fork placed in the centre of the forehead is heard equally well in both ears (Weber's test). If a conductive hearing loss is present in one ear, the tuning fork is heard better in the deaf ear (confirmed by occluding one ear and applying the fork to your own head). Conversely, in unilateral sensorineural deafness, the sound is louder in the good ear.

Audiometry

Hearing by air conduction can be assessed by pure tone audiometry, in which sounds of known pitch and loudness are presented to each ear in turn via headphones. Bone conduction (cochlear function) can be separately tested by applying sounds to the mastoid process. A contralateral masking tone is needed if each cochlea is to be tested separately. The difference between the air and bone conduction gives the level of conductive hearing loss (Figs 26.3 and 26.4). The patient's ability to hear speech can be tested by presenting lists of words via headphones. Middle-ear function (compliance) can be assessed by tympanometry. The amount of sound from a probe reflected back from the drum is measured while the pressure in the ear canal is made to vary. The compliance is maximal when the pressure in the ear canal equals the pressure in the middle ear, because at this point the drum is maximally mobile. Tympanometry is most often used to confirm the presence of fluid in the middle ear.

26

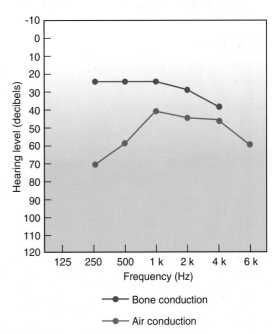

Fig. 26.3 **Audiogram showing conductive deafness.**

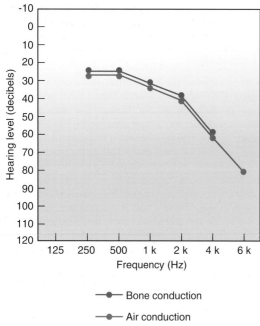

Fig. 26.4 **Audiogram showing sensorineural deafness.**

Temporal bone imaging

In patients with unilateral sensorineural hearing loss, magnetic resonance imaging (MRI) is used to detect an acoustic neuroma (Fig. 26.5). MRI also demonstrates the presence of normal fluid in the cochlea before attempting cochlear implantation. Computed tomography (CT) can be used to demonstrate temporal bone anatomy, congenital abnormalities, fractures or unusual pathology.

Diseases of the pinna

Bat ears

Bat ears are a developmental abnormality resulting in absence of the antihelical fold (see Fig. 26.1). This produces prominent ears that cause embarrassment. The abnormality can be corrected surgically.

Trauma

Trauma to the ear may result in a haematoma, which strips the perichondrium off the underlying cartilage. Secondary infection may lead to loss of cartilage, resulting in a 'cauliflower ear'. Haematomas should therefore be drained under strict aseptic conditions.

Tumours

Basal cell and squamous carcinomas may occur on the pinna and require excision (Fig. 26.6).

Diseases of the external auditory meatus

Wax

Wax (cerumen) is normally found in the ear canal. The ear canal has a migratory epithelium that carries wax to the opening of the external auditory meatus. Wax seldom causes deafness, unless it becomes packed against the eardrum. Sodium bicarbonate ear drops should be used regularly by those with a tendency to build up excess cerumen.

Otitis externa

This is a very common inflammatory condition of the ear canal skin. Secondary infection with bacteria or, less frequently, fungi may occur. It is managed by cleaning the ear, followed by local

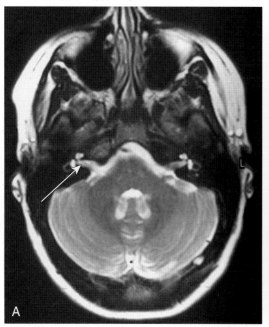
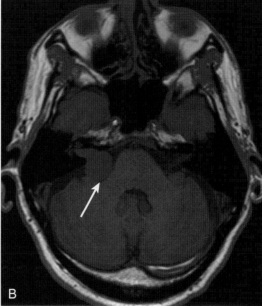

Fig. 26.5 **Magnetic resonance imaging of the cerebellopontine angle. (A)** Normal magnetic resonance image (MRI) scan of cerebellopontine angle. **(B)** MRI showing a acoustic neuroma. *Thin arrow,* internal auditory meatus (IAM); *thick arrow,* lesion compressing cerebellum.

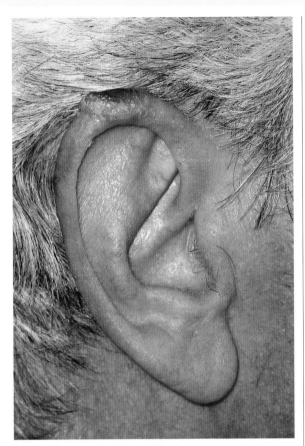

Fig. 26.6 Squamous carcinoma of the pinna.

treatment with eardrops, sprays or ointment containing a steroid, with or without antiseptic, or a weak acid solution (which controls the typical causative anaerobic organisms). Antibiotic preparations should be avoided. They cause contact sensitivity and predispose to fungal superinfection. Vaseline-coated plugs eradicate entry of water and irritant detergent (shampoo) or swimming pool water. The head and hair should not be cleaned under a shower spray but in a basin. Excessive hairwashing should be avoided. Cotton bud use must also be avoided.

Uncommonly, chronic otitis externa causes stenosis of the ear canal. Malignant otitis external is an aggressive variant usually seen in older people, particularly those with diabetes mellitus. It can culminate in skull base erosion and death if not adequately treated by prolonged intravenous antibiotic therapy.

Tumours

Squamous carcinoma of the ear canal occurs uncommonly and is treated by a combination of surgery and radiotherapy.

Diseases of the middle ear

Acute suppurative otitis media

This bacterial infection of the middle ear space is usually caused by *Streptococcus pneumoniae* or *Haemophilus influenzae*, most commonly occurring in young children (3 years of age and under). Children present with a combination of ear pain (otalgia), fever and malaise. On examination, dilated blood vessels are seen on the drum surface in the early stages. The drum then becomes red

and begins to bulge. Perforation with discharge frequently occurs, usually followed by spontaneous healing. Antibiotic therapy remains controversial: the majority of cases resolve spontaneously in a few days but antibiotics may play a part in those under 2 years of age with more severe signs (EBM 26.1). Antibiotics are also useful in high-risk patients (e.g., immunosuppression) as they shorten the episodes and reduce the rate of infective complications such as mastoiditis, facial palsy or meningitis.

EBM 26.1 Otitis media in children

- *In acute otitis media (AOM) antibiotics are most useful in children <2 years old with bilateral AOM, or with both AOM and otorrhoea. Most other children with mild disease in high-income countries can be offered an expectant observational approach*
- *In otitis media with effusion (OME) adenoid removal may decrease the risk of repeated surgery in children older than 4 years.*

Venekamp et al. Antibiotics for acute otitis media in children. Cochrane Database System Rev. 2015,6:CD000219.
Mikals et al. Adenoidectomy as an adjuvant to primary tympanostomy tube placement: a systematic review and meta-analysis. JAMA Otolaryngol Head Neck Surg. 2014;140:95–101.
For further information: www.cochrane.org

Otitis media with effusion, or 'glue ear'

In this condition, fluid accumulates in the middle-ear space, usually in children. A minority of adult cases are caused by nasopharyngeal tumours and systemic disease. Childhood otitis media with effusion (OME) causes hearing loss and may interfere with the acquisition of language and performance at school. Virtually all cases resolve spontaneously, but this may take as long as 10 years. Initial management involves documentation of the presence of effusion and the degree of hearing loss during a period of watchful waiting. If the effusions persist, hearing may be improved by drainage of the effusion (myringotomy) and insertion of a ventilation tube (Fig. 26.7). In children, removal of the adenoids may add benefit (EBM 26.2). Spontaneous resolution may also occur in adults, but often effusions persist. Ventilation tubes can be of value in adults. Some cases are better managed with a hearing aid.

Chronic suppurative otitis media

This causes aural discharge and deafness.

Tubotympanic or mucosal disease

This is characterised by the presence of a perforation of the tympanic membrane, which typically discharges. Swimming and other activities that involve water entering the ear may exacerbate the discharge. The hearing loss is worse when the ossicles are eroded, most commonly the incus long process. Discharge can be controlled by cleaning the ear and introducing eardrops, which should be used for a maximum of 2 weeks to minimise the risks of ototoxicity. Surgery is indicated to prevent discharge, improve hearing or allow the patient to swim. The operation to repair a perforation is called a *myringoplasty*. Defects of the ossicular chain can be repaired by removing the incus and repositioning it to bridge the gap between the malleus and stapes, or by using a prosthesis (ossiculoplasty).

Atticoantral or squamous disease

A cholesteatoma forms as a retracted area of the drum in which keratin accumulates. The drum tissue at the periphery of the cholesteatoma produces a number of chemical mediators that

26

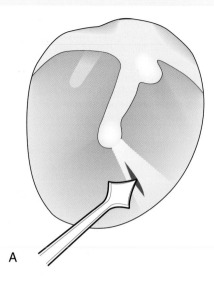

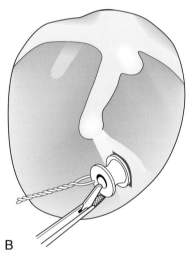

Fig. 26.7 Surgical treatment of otitis media with effusion.
(A) Myringotomy. **(B)** Grommet insertion.

stimulate osteoclast activity. Hence, the cholesteatoma can erode surrounding bone and cause complications such as disruption of the ossicular chain, facial palsy, meningitis and brain abscess. Surgical treatment (mastoidectomy) is mandatory to eliminate the disease in all but the very elderly and those who are medically unfit.

 26.1 Summary

Otitis media

- Acute otitis media is very common under the age of 3 years
- The child typically awakes crying at night with a painful ear. A red, inflamed, bulging drum on otoscopy is diagnostic
- Pain relief is important
- Otitis media with effusion (glue ear) occurs transiently in many children. Most resolve spontaneously. Bilateral persistent hearing loss may demand surgery (adenoidectomy, or insertion of a grommet)
- Chronic otitis media involves the middle ear and mastoid mucosa. There is tympanic membrane perforation, hearing loss and a mucopurulent discharge. Inactive ears require closure of the perforation (myringoplasty) and ossicular chain reconstruction. Cholesteatoma may require surgical removal of the posterior canal wall to open the attic or mastoid cavity and prevent complications.

Otosclerosis

This is a condition in which the stapes becomes fixed by new bone formation. It is more common in females and sometimes runs in families. The hearing loss can be managed with a hearing aid.

It can also be treated by an operation called a *stapedectomy*, in which the stapes is replaced by a piston attached to the incus. This produces excellent hearing improvement in the majority of patients, but a minority suffer from surgically induced, permanent inner ear damage.

Diseases of the inner ear

Deafness

Deafness is most commonly due to changes in the cochlea (Table 26.2). Ageing produces a gradual bilateral deterioration in hearing acuity (presbycusis). Unilateral hearing loss occurs in acoustic neuroma (see Fig. 26.5b). Most cases of inner-ear deafness are managed with a hearing aid, but in cases of profound deafness, hearing may be restored by a cochlear implant. This consists of a series of electrodes surgically introduced into the cochlea. An external speech processor converts sound into electrical energy, which stimulates the cochlear nerve.

Vertigo

In some cases, balance disorders may arise from abnormalities of the vestibular portion of the inner ear.

Benign paroxysmal positional vertigo is very common in middle age and is due to debris floating in the posterior semicircular canal, which stimulates the ampulla hair cells, producing vertigo. Episodes are triggered when the affected ear is down-most, as when the patient turns over in bed. Debris can be displaced therapeutically from the posterior canal by positioning the head so that it floats out of the canal into the vestibule (Epley's particle repositioning manoeuvre). If this fails, division of the ampullary (singular) nerve or occlusion of the posterior semicircular canal is beneficial.

Vestibular neuronitis causes severe vertigo that can last as long as several weeks. The hearing remains normal. It is due to severe temporary reduction of vestibular function in the affected ear. Patients are managed by bed rest and vestibular sedatives, such as prochlorperazine.

Abnormal fluctuations of fluid pressure within the inner ear (endolymphatic hydrops) produce a combination of fluctuating deafness, tinnitus and vertigo known as *Ménière's disease*. This uncommon condition is initially treated medically, using either a vasodilator agent (e.g., betahistine) or a diuretic. If medical treatment fails, the vestibular portion of the labyrinth may be destroyed by a middle-ear injection of gentamicin. Procedures of last resort

---

Table 26.2 Causes of sensorineural hearing loss

- Chronic noise exposure:
  - Heavy industry and agriculture
  - Playing in rock bands
  - Shooting
- Blast injuries
- Temporal bone fractures
- Inherited
- Manifestation of systemic disease
- Ototoxicity: aminoglycosides and cytotoxic agents such as cisplatinum
- Viral infections such as mumps and rubella.

are surgical destruction of the labyrinth or section of the vestibular nerve.

Disorders of the facial nerve

Upper motor neurone (central) causes of facial palsy, such as stroke, do not involve the forehead, which has bilateral central representation. Lower motor neurone facial palsy may result from temporal bone fractures or surgical trauma. A divided nerve may be repaired by end-to-end anastomosis or a cable graft derived from a sensory nerve of the right size, such as the sural nerve. Bell's palsy, an idiopathic (lower motor neurone) facial palsy, usually improves spontaneously. There is some evidence that it is caused by viral infection and steroid therapy given soon after the onset is beneficial. Herpes zoster infection of the geniculate ganglion causes facial palsy, often associated with deafness and vertigo (Ramsay–Hunt syndrome). Vesicles may be seen on the palate and on the tympanic membrane. Antiviral treatment appears helpful for Ramsay–Hunt syndrome, but evidence is less convincing in Bell's palsy (EBM 26.2). Malignant tumours in the parotid area of the neck can also cause lower motor neurone facial palsy.

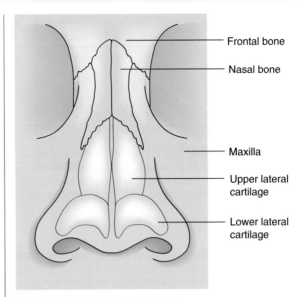

Fig. 26.8 Anatomy of the nasal skeleton.

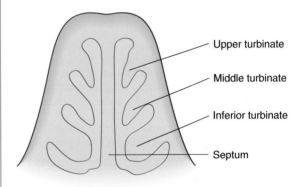

Fig. 26.9 Anatomy of the nasal cavity.

EBM 26.2 Antivirals alongside Steroids in Bell's palsy

- Low-quality evidence from randomised controlled trials shows a benefit from the combination of antivirals with corticosteroids compared to corticosteroids alone for the treatment of Bell's palsy of various degrees of severity
- Corticosteroids alone were more effective than antivirals alone
- There was no benefit from antivirals alone over placebo
- Moderate-quality evidence indicated that the combination of antivirals and corticosteroids reduced sequelae of Bell's palsy compared with corticosteroids alone.

Gagyor et al. Antiviral treatment for Bell's palsy (idiopathic facial paralysis). Cochrane Database Syst Rev. 2015;(11):CD001869.
Further information: Baugh et al. Clinical practice guideline: Bell's palsy. Otolaryngol Head Neck Surg. 2013;149(3 Suppl):S1–S27.

Nose

Anatomy

The nasal skeleton consists of two nasal bones superiorly and two pairs of cartilages inferiorly (Fig. 26.8). The nasal cavity is divided in two by a partition composed of cartilage anteriorly and bone posteriorly (the nasal septum). Three turbinate bones protrude from the lateral wall of the nose (Fig. 26.9). Between the inferior and middle turbinates is the middle meatus of the nose. Most of the paranasal sinuses open into this area under cover of a soft tissue flap known as the *uncinate process*. Obstruction of the sinus ostia can cause sinus pain and may lead to sinus infection. Above the superior turbinate is olfactory epithelium. The anterior portion of the nasal septum is called *Little's area*. It carries prominent veins. Nose bleeds most often arise here.

Physiology

The functions of the nose are to filter, warm and moisten inspired air. Olfaction is important in its own right and as an adjunct to taste.

Assessment

Clinical features

Nasal obstruction is a common symptom with a number of causes. Sneezing and rhinorrhoea are generally due to chronic rhinitis. Purulent nasal discharge and facial pain occur in sinusitis. Loss of smell may be due either to nasal blockage that prevents odours reaching the olfactory epithelium or to damage of the olfactory nerves. Smell is an important part of taste and reduced taste is therefore usually also reported by patients with anosmia.

Examination

The nasal cavity can be inspected using a nasal speculum or an otoscope. More detailed examination, particularly of the posterior part of the nose, is carried out with a rigid telescope.

Imaging

Imaging is not required if nasendoscopy is normal. Images are useful preoperatively to give the surgeon a guide as to individual variations, especially in the areas of potential surgical hazard: orbital wall, floor of the anterior cranial fossa (skull base). CT is

26

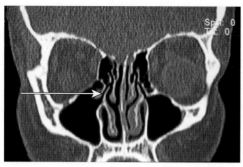

Fig. 26.10 Coronal computed tomography of sinuses. The narrow maxillary ostia and uncinate processes are seen on this cut (*arrow*), lateral to the middle turbinate.

the best means of imaging the paranasal sinuses and the middle meatus of the nose, where the sinus ostia are situated (Fig. 26.10). The sinuses can also be visualised by MRI, but the bony anatomy is not shown and mucosal disease is exaggerated.

Diseases of the nose

Trauma

This may result in fracture and displacement of the nasal bones. If the fracture is not reduced within 14 days, it is usually fixed and hard to mobilise. There may also be displacement and fracture of the septal cartilage and bone (deviated nasal septum; Fig. 26.11). Corrective septoplasty surgery requires a post-trauma interval of 3 months to allow for soft tissue repair before surgery. Bleeding into the septum causes a septal haematoma,

resulting in severe nasal obstruction. This should be drained under aseptic conditions, to prevent a septal abscess and collapse of the bridge.

Chronic rhinitis

Some cases are due to allergy to aeroallergens (pollen or dust). Otherwise, it seems to be a reaction to environmental conditions such as temperature and humidity. It may be seasonal (usually summer) or perennial. Patients complain of nasal blockage that often switches from side to side, sneezing and rhinorrhoea. Most cases are best managed medically with a steroid nasal spray. In severe cases with nasal obstruction, reduction of the inferior or middle turbinates may provide relief.

Nasal polyps

Oedematous paranasal sinus mucosa extrudes through sinus ostia to produce nasal polyps. Most are multiple swellings from the ethmoid sinuses. Rarely, there is a single posterior protrusion from the maxillary sinus (antrochoanal polyp). Unilateral disease is usually defined by a prebiopsy CT (Fig. 26.12). Temporary improvement in the resulting nasal obstruction can be produced by topical or systemic steroids. Most polyps eventually recur following excision. Thus, many patients opt for periodic courses of oral steroid therapy, and only resort to surgery for uncontrollably severe symptoms. Endoscopic clearance is facilitated by use of the microdebrider.

Epistaxis

Nose bleeds may be associated with a number of disease processes (Table 26.3). They are common in healthy children and young adults. Bleeding usually arises from Little's area and can be controlled by squeezing the nose (Fig. 26.13). In the elderly, more severe bleeding from further back in the nose may occur. In these cases, a nasal pack may be required to arrest the bleeding. Bleeding may be associated with the use of nonsteroidal anti-inflammatory drugs (NSAIDs) or other antithrombotic therapy in this group. Severe bleeding not controlled by a pack can be arrested by clipping either the sphenopalatine, anterior ethmoid or maxillary artery.

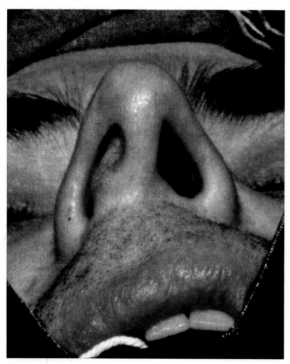

Fig. 26.11 Deviated nasal septum.

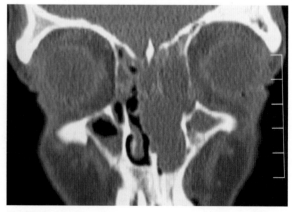

Fig. 26.12 Coronal computed tomography showing gross unilateral (left) nasal 'polyp'.

Table 26.3 Diseases associated with epistaxis

Bleeding disorders

- Excess alcohol consumption
- Iatrogenic (warfarin, clopidogrel, novel oral anticoagulants, aspirin)
- Haemophilia
- Thrombocytopenia
- von Willebrand's disease

Systemic disease

- Liver disease
- Renal disease
- Hypertension
- Hereditary haemorrhagic telangiectasia

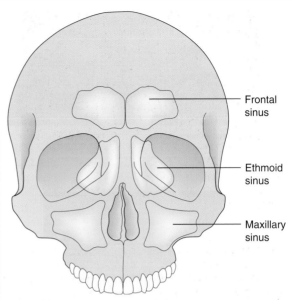

Fig. 26.14 Anatomy of the paranasal sinuses.

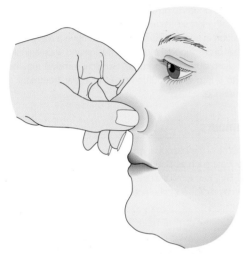

Fig. 26.13 Stopping epistaxis by squeezing the nose.

26.2 Summary

Epistaxis

- Epistaxis in young patients usually arises from a small blood vessel in Little's area; in older individuals, it arises from an arteriosclerotic vessel located more posteriorly
- Pressure on Little's area by compressing the anterior septum usually stops the bleeding. Topical 1:1000 adrenaline (epinephrine) on cotton wool may help
- Bleeding more posteriorly may require balloon compression or packing
- Consider coagulation defects including alcohol and nonsteroidal analgesics
- Persistent epistaxis may require embolisation or ligation of the sphenopalatine branch(es) of the maxillary artery.

Paranasal sinuses

Anatomy

The paranasal sinuses are air-filled cavities that open into the nasal cavity, mostly into the middle meatus of the nose. The maxillary sinuses occupy the cheeks (Fig. 26.14). The ethmoid labyrinth consists of a number of air cells lying between the orbit and the lateral wall of the nose. The frontal sinus is an ethmoid air cell that has migrated into the frontal bone, and it is connected to the middle meatus of the nose via the frontonasal duct. The sphenoid sinus is posterior to the ethmoid labyrinth, inferior to the pituitary fossa.

Diseases of the paranasal sinuses

Sinusitis

Any sinus may become infected. The most commonly involved is the maxillary sinus. Pain arising from the maxillary sinus is felt in the cheek, that from the ethmoid labyrinth is felt over the nasal bridge, and frontal sinus pain is felt in the forehead. Sphenoid sinus pain is said to be maximal at the vertex. Acute sinusitis is most commonly caused by *Strep. pneumoniae* or *H. influenzae*, and typically follows an upper respiratory infection. Gram-negative organisms may cause sinusitis related to a dental abscess. In some parts of the world, fungal infection is not uncommon.

Acute sinusitis is usually managed medically. Chronic sinusitis may result from failure of resolution of acute infection or may arise insidiously. Surgical treatment is frequently required and includes enlargement of the natural ostium of the maxillary sinus, often with clearance of infected ethmoid cells. Frontal and sphenoid sinusitis are much less common. Infection may spread from the sinuses, usually the ethmoid or frontal sinuses, to involve other areas such as the cranial cavity or orbit (Fig. 26.15).

Tumours

The most common malignant neoplasm found in the paranasal sinuses is squamous carcinoma. Adenocarcinomas are seen in workers in the furniture industry. The most common sites of origin are the maxillary and ethmoid sinuses. Unfortunately, the disease has often spread beyond the primary site at presentation

26

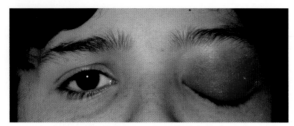

Fig. 26.15 Orbital cellulitis.

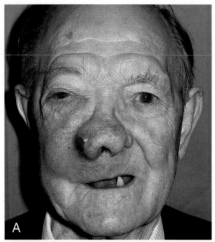

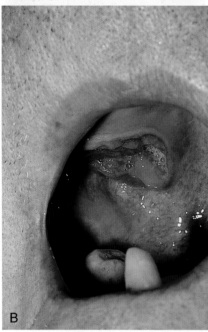

Fig. 26.16 **Spread of sinus cancer. (A)** There is evidence of spread into the cheek and orbit, with displacement of the eye. **(B)** There is ulceration of the hard palate, indicating spread into the mouth.

(Fig. 26.16). These relatively uncommon tumours are managed by a combination of surgery and radiotherapy, or by local surgery and topical chemotherapy.

Nasopharynx

Anatomy

The nasopharynx lies posterior to the nasal cavity and superior to the oropharynx. The skull base lies superiorly and the Eustachian tubes open into its lateral walls.

Diseases of the nasopharynx

Adenoids

The adenoids consist of B-cell predominant lymphoid tissue and in young children they occupy a significant proportion of the space within the nasopharynx. They increase in size until the age of 5 years and then become relatively smaller as the nasopharynx continues to grow. Few adults have significant amounts of residual adenoid tissue. Adenoid hypertrophy causes nasal obstruction in some children. They also have a role in the pathogenesis of childhood middle ear effusion and, increasingly in the West, sleep apnoea syndrome. Surgical removal may be indicated to improve the outcomes of glue ear treatment and in sleep apnoea.

Tumours

Carcinoma of the nasopharynx is very common in certain areas of the Far East such as South China. It is linked to the Epstein–Barr virus (EBV), rare familial clusters and heavy alcohol intake. Treatment is by radio- and chemotherapy.

> ↻ 26.3 Summary
>
> **Nasopharyngeal cancer presentations**
>
> - Painless cervical lymphadenopathy (75% of patients, often bilateral and posterior). Polymerase chain reaction evidence of Epstein–Barr virus material in nodal biopsy material is highly suggestive
> - Nasal obstruction or epistaxis
> - Diminished hearing, tinnitus or recurrent otitis media
> - Cranial nerve dysfunction (usually II–VI or IX–XII).

Male adolescents may rarely develop a benign but locally invasive angiofibroma of the nasopharynx. Juvenile nasopharyngeal angiofibroma presents with obstruction and epistaxis, and is treated by embolisation plus surgical excision. Endoscopic resection has lower intraoperative blood loss without increase in recurrence rate compared with open approaches.

Oral cavity

Anatomy

The oral cavity is bounded by the lips anteriorly. It extends posteriorly to the junction of the anterior two-thirds and posterior one-third of the tongue. Superiorly is the hard palate. Laterally is the buccal mucosa, which forms the inner lining of the cheek. The ducts of the submandibular salivary glands open anteriorly into the floor of mouth under cover of the tongue. The parotid ducts open just opposite the second upper molar teeth.

Diseases of the mouth

Stomatitis and gingivitis

Inflammation of the oral mucosa and gums is often associated with poor oral hygiene. It may also be a manifestation of a systemic disorder, such as anaemia. *Candida* is a common opportunist infection. It is characterised by white spots on the mucous membrane. Removal of the white material causes bleeding. Infection of the floor of the mouth may develop secondary to dental sepsis (Ludwig's angina). Pain, swelling, dysphagia, trismus and even acute airway obstruction may occur. Vincent's angina is the name given to an acute gingivitis (formerly known as *trench mouth*).

Mouth ulcers

Aphthous ulcers are the most common type. These have a punched-out appearance and are painful. They may have an immunogenetic origin. A minority relate to food allergy, smoking cessation, stress, or deficiency of iron, folate or vitamin B_{12}. Their spontaneous resolution is accelerated by steroid pellets. Oral ulceration is also a feature of drug reactions, lichen planus, Behçet's disease, pemphigus, mucous membrane pemphigoid or infections (HIV, herpes and other viruses, tuberculosis or syphilis).

Retention cysts

Mucous retention cysts may occur anywhere in the oral cavity. Those inferior to the tongue are called *ranulas*. Occasionally, a large ranula may push its way through the mylohyoid muscle to present in the upper neck (plunging ranula). They result from blockage of the openings of mucous and minor salivary glands. This may clear spontaneously, but otherwise excision may be required.

Leukoplakia

Leukoplakia (white patch) develops on the oral mucosa as a response to chronic irritation—e.g., by a rough tooth, tobacco or alcohol (especially brown spirits)—causing hyperkeratosis

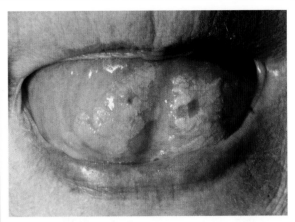

Fig. 26.17 Leukoplakia of the tongue.

(Fig. 26.17). This may progress to dysplasia and cellular atypia, and is therefore a premalignant condition. Removal of both the patches and the causative factors can prevent progression.

Tumours

Over 95% of oral cavity tumours present as ulcers or masses. Beware the nonhealing ulcer. The anterior two-thirds of tongue and the floor of mouth are the most common sites. Carcinogenesis involves irritants like cigarette smoking and alcohol, and overexpression of oncogenes. In South Asia, chewing tobacco along with betel leaves, betel nuts and slaked lime (*paan* or *khaini*), which is retained in the oral cavity for long periods of time, is a major risk factor. Human papillomavirus (HPV) plays a lesser role than in the oropharynx. The *p53* suppressor gene is important in smokers with oral cancer. Lip cancer is regarded as a separate entity as it behaves like a skin cancer.

Assessment

Othopantomograms (Fig. 26.18) may complement cross-sectional imaging (Figs 26.19 and 26.20). Positron emission

26

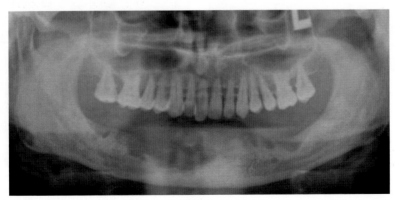

Fig. 26.18 Orthopantomogram showing mandibular involvement by carcinoma of the lower alveolus.

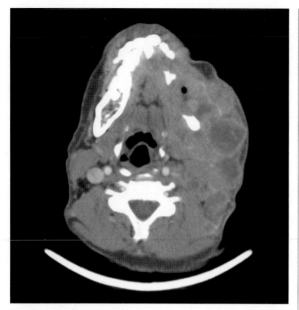

Fig. 26.19 Computed tomography showing mandibular involvement in carcinoma of left lower alveolus.

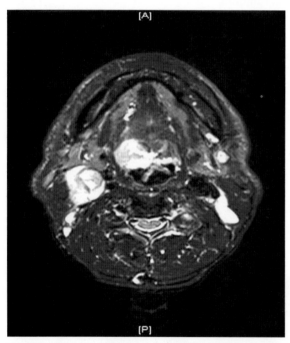

Fig. 26.20 Magnetic resonance image showing carcinoma of base of tongue with bilateral nodal metastases.

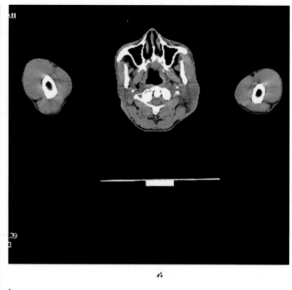

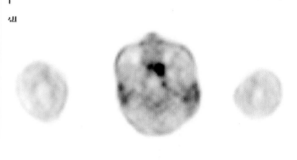

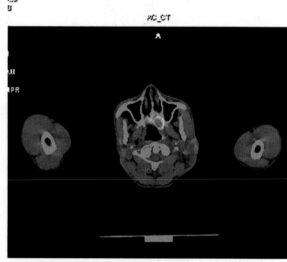

Fig. 26.21 PET-CT scan image showing an abnormal fluorine-18 fluorodeoxyglucose uptake in left soft palate region. Corresponding CT images show mild soft tissue thickening.

tomography co-registered with CT (PET-CT) is increasingly the gold standard for initial and follow-up assessment (Fig. 26.21).

Initial spread is to cervical lymph nodes (Table 26.4). Different intraoral sites have different considerations, as outlined in the following summaries. Early lesions respond equally well to radiotherapy or surgery.

Table 26.4 Causes of cervical lymphadenopathy

Infective bacterial

- Pyogenic infection in drainage area (e.g., streptococcal tonsillitis)
- Tuberculosis
- Brucellosis

Viral

- Infectious mononucleosis
- Cytomegalovirus
- HIV

Protozoal

- Toxoplasmosis

Neoplasms

- Lymphoma
- Metastatic squamous carcinoma
- Other metastatic tumours

Systemic disease

- Collagen diseases
- Sarcoidosis
- Amyloidosis

 26.4 Summary

Carcinoma of the lip

- The lower lip is more commonly affected (Fig. 26.22)
- Often a history of recurrent blistering (cheilitis)
- May be preceded by leukoplakia
- May present as a nodule, fissure or indurated area
- Very slow-growing tumour, but may spread if neglected (Fig. 26.23)
- The upper lip drains first to the buccal and parotid node
- The lower lip drains to submandibular nodes, then to upper deep cervical nodes
- The central portion of the lower lip drains first to the submental nodes
- Treatment is either surgical or radiation therapy; combined modality if advanced
- If more than two-thirds of the lip resected, use a radial free forearm flap for repair.

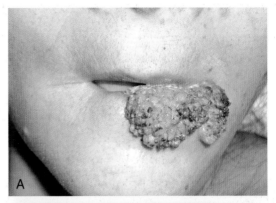

Fig. 26.23 (A) Carcinoma of the lower lip. **(B)** Carcinoma of the lip involving the adjoining skin of the cheek.

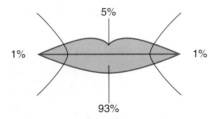

Fig. 26.22 Carcinoma of the lip: site-wise incidence.

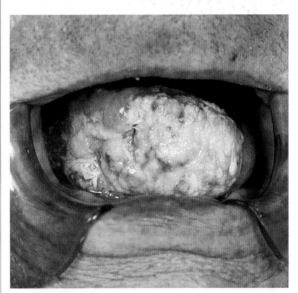

Fig. 26.24 Carcinoma of the tongue.

Carcinoma of the tongue

Clinically and anatomically, the tongue is divided into the anterior two-thirds or the oral tongue, and the posterior one-third, which lies in the oropharynx. The anterior lateral border is the most common source of oral cancer due to dental trauma. Tumours of the tongue (Fig. 26.24) are aggressive, with high metastatic potential. Nodal metastasis is related to poor differentiation, depth of invasion, involvement of extrinsic muscles of the tongue, tumour thickness >4 mm, lymphovascular invasion and perineural invasion. Anterior two-thirds of the tongue lesions require at least wide local excision with selective neck dissection of levels I–IV.

26

26.5 Summary

Carcinoma of the tongue

- The jugulodigastric node (level II) is the primary drainage
- 'Skip' metastases up to level IV are not uncommon
- Incidence of neck metastases is directly proportional to T stage: 15–75%
- 25% of patients occult nodal disease; 25% bilateral nodes
- Adjuvant radiation therapy for adverse prognostic factors
- Locally advanced disease requires composite resection
- Minimum of 5-mm histopathologically tumour-free margin
- Postexcision defects less than one-third of the tongue can be closed primarily or left to granulate. Larger defects need composite reconstruction.

26.6 Summary

Carcinoma of the buccal mucosa

- More common in developing countries (tobacco chewing; Fig. 26.25).
- Left buccal mucosa is more commonly involved
- Dental occlusal line prone to repeated trauma
- Frequently exophytic, painless
- Trismus may be due to masseteric spasm or pterygoid involvement
- Lymph drains initially to parotid, submental and submandibular nodes, then to deep cervical nodes
- Mandibular resection or partial maxillectomy may be required
- Reconstruction may require free microvascular tissue transfer with or without bone.

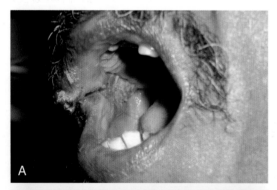

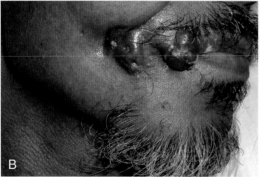

Fig. 26.25 **(A)** Carcinoma of the right buccal mucosa. **(B)** The same patient with involvement of the cheek. The tumour also infiltrated the masticator muscles.

Retromolar trigone

The retromolar trigone is the area of the mucosa overlying the ascending ramus of the mandible from the posterior surface of the last molar tooth to the apex superiorly. Tumours here are extensive, and often involve the posterior floor of mouth and the maxillary tuberosity. Lymph from the buccal mucosa drains into the parotid, submental, and submandibular lymph nodes, and from there to the upper deep cervical nodes. Involvement of the pterygoid muscles is a relative contraindication to operation.

26.7 Summary

Carcinoma of the alveolus

- Note history of loose tooth, bleeding on brushing the teeth, change in denture fit (Fig. 26.26)
- Trismus and altered lower lip sensation: inferior alveoli nerve involvement
- Primary lymph drainage to submental and submandibular triangle
- Treated by composite resection and free tissue reconstruction
- Osseointegrated dental implants are important in rehabilitation.

Floor of the mouth

It is a horseshoe-shaped space extending from the inner surface of the lower alveolar ridge undersurface of the tongue. Its posterior boundary is the base of the anterior pillar of the tonsil. The space is divided into two sides by the frenulum of the tongue. The floor of the mouth contains the openings of the submandibular and sublingual salivary gland ducts.

26.8 Summary

Carcinoma of the floor of the mouth

- Often presents with local infiltration even when relatively small in size (Fig. 26.27)
- Lymph drainage to the submental and submandibular triangle
- May require composite resection, including adjacent tongue and the mandible
- Small soft tissue defects may be closed by nasolabial flaps
- Floor of mouth muscle resection may impact speech and swallowing postoperatively.

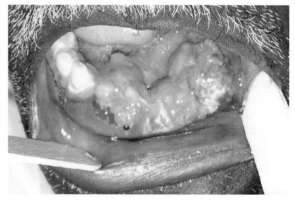

Fig. 26.26 Carcinoma of the lower alveolus.

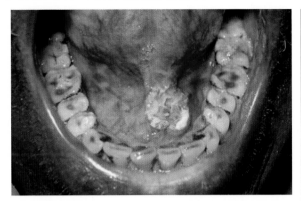

Fig. 26.27 Carcinoma of the floor of the mouth.

The hard palate

The hard palate is a concave semicircular area that extends from the inner surface of the superior alveolar ridge to the posterior edge of the palatine bone. It is lined with mucoperiosteum. Mucous glands can give rise to adenocarcinoma or minor salivary gland tumours.

 26.9 Summary

Carcinoma of the hard palate

- Lymph drainage is to retropharyngeal then deep cervical nodes
- Treatment may involve partial maxillectomy
- Dental obturators are required to prevent nasal regurgitation of food.

Oropharynx

Anatomy

The oropharynx lies posterior to the oral cavity between the nasopharynx superiorly and the hypopharynx and larynx inferiorly. At the junction of the mouth and oropharynx are the tonsils, which consist of lymphoid tissue. Together with the adenoids (see earlier) and the lingual tonsil in the base of the tongue, they form a ring of lymphoid tissue. This ring is important in the development of immunity during early infancy, but subsequently can be removed without ill effect. The pharynx itself is surrounded by three constrictor muscles arranged one inside the other like a stack of bottomless beakers.

 26.10 Summary

Tonsils and adenoids

- Adenoids are large in young children but become relatively smaller with age
- They may cause nasal obstruction and be involved in the pathogenesis of otitis media with effusion and childhood sleep apnoea
- Tonsils may require removal because of recurrent tonsillitis or peritonsillar abscess in adults and children
- Children with sleep apnoea and obstructive tonsils may also benefit from tonsillectomy
- Unilateral tonsillar enlargement may be due to squamous carcinoma or lymphoma.

Diseases of the oropharynx

Pharyngitis

Viral infection of the pharynx is common and often follows the common cold. Symptomatic relief can be obtained from analgesics with or without decongestants. Sore throat with exudate over the tonsils is a common manifestation of infectious mononucleosis (glandular fever). This disease is due to EBV, which also causes cervical adenopathy and hepatosplenomegaly. Liver function should be tested, and patients with abnormal tests advised to refrain from alcohol for a period of time. Irritation of the pharynx may be due to tobacco smoke and acid reflux. Guidelines exist for the management of sore throat and indications for tonsillectomy (EBM 26.3 and 26.4).

Tonsillitis

This is due to bacterial infection of the tonsils, usually with *Strep. pyogenes*. Patients present with episodic sore throat associated with dysphagia, lymph node enlargement, fever and malaise. Tonsillitis must be differentiated from viral sore throats, which are not usually associated with pyrexia and often form part of a more generalised upper respiratory tract infection. Infectious mononucleosis can easily be confused with tonsillitis. Tonsillitis may be complicated by the development of a peritonsillar abscess (quinsy). This may require incision and drainage. Recurrent tonsillitis whose frequency and severity fulfil consensus-based guidance can be treated successfully by tonsillectomy.

EBM **26.3 Antibiotics for acute sore throat**

- *Antibiotics should not be used to secure symptomatic relief of a sore throat*
- *In severe cases, where the practitioner is concerned about the clinical condition of the patient, antibiotics should not be withheld*
- *Penicillin V 500 mg 6-hourly for 10 days is the preferred dosage*
- *Practitioners should be aware that infectious mononucleosis may present with severe sore throat*
- *Ampicillin-based antibiotics should be avoided in infectious mononucleosis*
- *Sore throat should not be treated with antibiotics specifically to prevent development of rheumatic fever or acute glomerulonephritis.*

SIGN Guideline 117; 2010 Management of sore throat and indications for tonsillectomy.
For further information: www.sign.ac.uk

EBM **26.4 Indications for tonsillectomy**

- *Sore throats due to acute tonsillitis*
- *The episodes of sore throat are disabling and prevent normal functioning*
- *Seven or more well-documented, clinically significant, adequately treated sore throats in the preceding year, or*
- *Five or more such episodes in each of the preceding two years, or*
- *Three or more such episodes in each of the preceding three years.*

SIGN Guideline 117; 2010 Management of sore throat and indications for tonsillectomy.
For further information: www.sign.ac.uk

Snoring and sleep apnoea

Snoring arises because of obstruction within the pharynx during sleep or vibration of the soft palate. In some cases, it is associated

26

with obstructive sleep apnoea. Apnoeic individuals tend to sleep poorly, wake unrefreshed and become drowsy during the day. If significant apnoea is confirmed by overnight monitoring, the use of nocturnal continuous positive airway pressure (CPAP) may be indicated. Simple snoring can be improved by weight loss and reduction of nocturnal alcohol intake. Adenotonsillectomy will cure over 80% of childhood cases of sleep apnoea.

Tumours

B-cell lymphomas occur mostly in adults (with a peak in those aged 50–60 years). There is a smooth enlargement of the affected tonsil. Squamous carcinoma usually presents with ulceration of the tonsil. The traditional association with cigarette smoking is less strong, as more now seem related to prior HPV exposure. Due to the prevalence of HPV infection, the oropharynx in many Western countries is now the most common primary site of squamous carcinoma and in some countries has the fastest rate of increase in incidence of any cancer. HPV-related oropharyngeal tumours have a greater sensitivity to chemoradiotherapy than HPV-negative tumours, and have a better outcome regardless of treatment type. Early disease should receive single-modality treatment. Advanced disease requires combined treatment.

MRI is preferred for the primary site and CT for the neck and chest. PET-CT is recommended to assess response to chemoradiotherapy. HPV testing is recommended when available. When excision of the primary site is recommended, this is often a conservation transoral approach: either transoral laser or transoral robotic intervention. In such cases the neck may be treated surgically, with chemoradiotherapy or expectantly with PET-CT follow-up. PET-CT at 10–12 weeks after chemoradiotherapy results in a similar survival to planned neck dissection, but with considerably fewer patients requiring surgery, hence less morbidity and greater cost efficiency.

Hypopharynx

Anatomy

Below the oropharynx, the aerodigestive tract divides into an air passage (larynx/trachea) and an alimentary passage (oesophagus). The entrance to the air passage is protected by a purse-string mechanism formed when the mobile cartilage of the epiglottis is drawn down over the laryngeal inlet as the aryepiglottic folds shorten. Closure of the false cords forms a second sphincteric layer to protect against aspiration. Glottic closure, conversely, serves chiefly to stop air escaping from the chest, as when sustaining a long note in phonation, straining or lifting (fixing the chest volume). The entry of material into the oesophagus is controlled by the cricopharyngeus ring of muscle. Lateral to the larynx, the pharynx continues inferiorly on both sides into a pair of blind-ended pits known as the *pyriform fossae* (Fig. 26.28).

Physiology of swallowing

Swallowing is achieved by the coordinated contraction and relaxation of muscles. It is initiated by the tongue, which pushes the bolus to the back of the mouth. A solid bolus will then gather at the tongue base, until the tongue propels it off through the pharynx when the swallow reflex fires. The pharyngeal constrictor muscles follow the tail of the bolus, in particularly 'mopping up' any liquid pharyngeal residue. As the laryngeal inlet closes, the

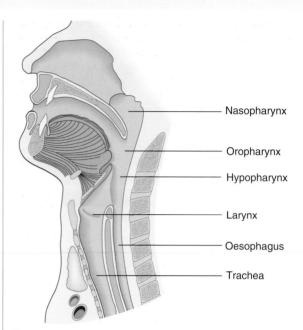

Fig. 26.28 Anatomy of the pharynx and larynx.

larynx itself moves upwards and forwards, widening the mouth of the oesophagus as the cricopharyngeal sphincter relaxes, and coming up over the now descending bolus. The entire sequence takes half a second, at the end of which respiration, which must pause during the swallow sequence, can resume. A much slower, smooth muscle peristaltic wave then carries the bolus down the tubular oesophagus to the stomach.

Assessment

Clinical features

Obstruction of the oesophagus and disorders that interfere with the muscle activity involved in swallowing cause dysphagia. Physical obstruction causes dysphagia that is worse for solids, whereas neurological disorders cause more difficulty with liquids. Hypopharyngeal pain may be felt locally or retrosternally, or may be referred to the ear (see Table 26.1). The level of obstructive dysphagia is always below the level at which the symptom is experienced. Hence, dysphagia localised by the patient in the pharynx requires an assessment down to the gastro-oesophageal junction.

Examination

The pharynx can be assessed in the clinic using a flexible rhinolaryngoscope. An ultra-thin, transnasal, digital video-oesophagoscope can be used to visualise the oesophagus and gastro-oesophageal junction under topical anaesthesia. More detailed images are obtained by the gastroenterology team using a wider bore flexible scope passed transorally, if required, as far as the duodenum.

Imaging

A barium swallow has a relatively limited part to play in swallow dysfunction. It will show structural abnormalities within the pharynx and oesophagus, and also gives some information about the dynamics of swallowing, but is not a first-line investigation for dysphagia. Video recording of small-volume contrast swallows (videofluoroscopy) can be used to provide additional information about the biomechanics of the oropharyngeal phase, and about bolus transit. It is the examination of choice where there is a suspicion of aspiration or misdirected swallow. CT can be used to identify spread of oesophageal lesions into surrounding tissues and to demonstrate lesions causing external compression of the oesophagus.

Diseases of the hypopharynx

Pharyngeal pouch

This is formed by mucosal herniation through the weakest part of the pharyngeal musculature, the posterior midline between the two portions of the inferior constrictor of the pharynx. The cause may be muscular incoordination; it tends to occur in older men. The hallmark symptom is dysphagia for solids, as the pouch tends to fill and compress the tubular oesophagus; but there may also be regurgitation of food, sometimes hours or even days after it was swallowed. In most cases, it is possible to divide the wall between the pouch and the oesophagus anterior to it. A specially designed disposable staple gun is passed transorally via an adjustable endoscope (diverticuloscope). The jaws of the gun simultaneously cut and insert two rows of lateral staples. Once the bar is divided, there is usually only a low shelf between the pouch and the oesophagus, and food no longer builds up under pressure. An alternative is laser division of the cricopharyngeal bar, especially if the pouch is too small to admit the staple gun. Endoscopic techniques may not be possible where transoral access is limited or the pouch is a very large pouch, and excision via an external neck incision may be indicated.

Tumours

Squamous carcinoma may arise from the pharyngeal walls, the epiglottis, the pyriform fossa or the upper oesophagus (postcricoid region). Postcricoid carcinoma is sometimes preceded by the development of a thin membrane in the upper oesophagus, a postcricoid web. This is associated with iron-deficiency anaemia, glossitis and stomatitis (Paterson–Brown–Kelly syndrome). The web itself causes some dysphagia, and treatment of the anaemia can prevent progression to tumour. Other pharyngeal tumours are associated with smoking. Hypopharyngeal tumours are treated by radiotherapy or surgery.

Larynx

Anatomy

The larynx has a cartilaginous framework. Superiorly, it is supported and protected anteriorly by the thyroid cartilage. Inferiorly lies the cricoid cartilage, which connects to the trachea (Fig. 26.29). Within the laryngeal lumen, two soft tissue folds pass from anterior to posterior. The upper folds are the ventricular bands or 'false cords'. The lower pair are the (true) vocal cords, which are responsible for phonation. These consist of a vocal ligament covered with mucosa. The vibrating free edge of the mucosa is important in achieving glottic closure and voice quality.

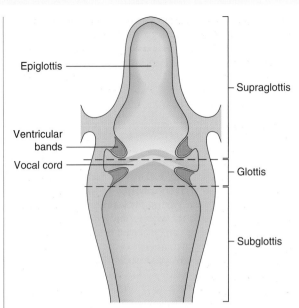

Fig. 26.29 Regions of the larynx

Physiology of voice

Voice production requires an air supply from the lungs, the presence of normally functioning vocal cords to create vibrations, and the tongue and mouth to articulate the vibrating air source into speech.

Assessment

Clinical features

Hoarseness of the voice is the cardinal symptom of laryngeal dysfunction. Patients may also complain of pain locally or referred to the ear (see Table 26.1). The voice is weak and breathy in unilateral vocal cord palsy, but rough and husky in severe laryngitis and laryngeal cancer. Patients with psychogenic dysphonia often have a squeaky voice quality.

Examination

The larynx is nowadays usually inspected in the clinic using a flexible fibreoptic rhinolaryngoscope or videoendoscope (which provides higher definition). Under general anaesthesia, a better view can be obtained using angled rigid endoscopes and operating microscope.

Imaging

CT can be used to assess the spread of laryngeal lesions to surrounding tissues, to assess congenital lesions and the diameter of any suspected upper airway narrowing.

Diseases of the larynx

Congenital disorders

Most congenital abnormalities of the larynx are rare. The most common is laryngomalacia, where the laryngeal inlet—epiglottis and soft tissue of the (aryepiglottic) folds that join it to the arytenoid cartilages—are high, soft and tend to collapse inwards. This

26

causes inspiratory stridor and dyspnoea, which becomes worse during upper respiratory infections. Most children grow out of the problem by the age of 2 years and do not require active intervention. In severe cases, a CO_2 laser is used to divide or debulk the aryepiglottic folds.

Laryngitis

The most common cause of hoarseness is acute inflammation of the vocal cords after an upper respiratory tract infection. Antibiotics are of no value but steam inhalations, voice rest and frequent drinking of small volumes of fluid may be helpful. The common predisposing factors for chronic laryngitis are smoking, acid reflux and excessive voice use. Women smokers with chronic laryngitis may have a fluid build-up deep to the vocal cord epithelium (Reinke's oedema). This can be treated by surgical drainage of the submucosal space at microlaryngoscopy. Other morphological variants of chronic laryngitis include thickened red cords or keratotic plaques (leukoplakia). In heavy voice abusers, vocal nodules at the junction of the anterior third and the posterior two-thirds of the vocal cords may develop. These may respond to speech therapy. If removal becomes necessary, patients must accept the risk of vocal cord scar and the need for intensive postoperative voice therapy to prevent recurrence.

Patients with hoarseness in the absence of a structural or movement disorder at laryngoscopy usually have functional dysphonia, which responds well in most cases to a programme of voice care and voice therapy.

Vocal cord palsy

The palsy is usually unilateral, more often on the left side, due to the intrathoracic course of the recurrent laryngeal nerve. Left vocal cord palsy may be caused by invasion of the recurrent laryngeal nerve by a bronchial carcinoma or mediastinal involvement by other tumours. The right recurrent nerve does not pass down into the chest. Damage to the recurrent laryngeal nerves in the neck may occur as a result of surgery, trauma or neoplastic invasion. Unilateral palsy causes a weak breathy voice. The voice may be improved by the injection lateral to the vocal ligament of hyaluronic acid or calcium hydroxyl apatite under local anaesthetic in the outpatient clinic, or by injection of fat or plastic fillers under general anaesthetic. Bilateral cord palsy most often presents as stridor (airway obstruction). In high (vagal trunk) lesions, dysphagia may be pronounced due to the associated pharyngeal weakness.

Tumours

Carcinoma of the larynx is the most common head and neck cancer, and is almost always squamous. Over 90% of cases occur in smokers, many of whom also drink alcohol to excess. Tumours of the glottis (true vocal cords) tend to present earlier, due to the resulting hoarseness. As the glottis has very few lymphatics, regional nodes are involved late.

Larger lesions may grow in the supraglottic space until they cause airway obstruction, haemoptysis or clinically apparent nodal disease. At least 90% of T1 lesions of the vocal cord are cured, provided the patient gives up smoking. Early laryngeal tumours may also be treated by excision, using a laser. The outlook is less favourable in more advanced tumours. The treatment choices include more radical primary surgery or chemoradiotherapy with salvage

EBM 26.5

Carcinoma of the larynx: treatment

- *Outcomes for early lesions (T1–T2a N0 M0) are not significantly different following external beam radiotherapy, endolaryngeal laser resection or open partial laryngeal surgery*
- *There is only one RCT comparing open surgery and radiotherapy but its interpretation is limited because of concerns about treatment regimens and deficiencies in reporting*
- *A trend towards improved local control of T1b tumours treated with radiotherapy was based on a limited number of published outcomes*
- *Patient self report voice scores are comparable following transoral laser microsurgery and radiation therapy for T1 glottic carcinoma*
- *Most patients with T2b–T3 glottic and T3 supraglottic cancers are suitable for non-surgical larynx preservation therapies. Where expertise and multi-disciplinary rehabilitation services allow, transoral laser microsurgery or open partial surgical procedures ± post-operative radiotherapy may also be used.*

Warner L et al. Radiotherapy versus open surgery versus endolaryngeal surgery (with or without laser) for early laryngeal squamous cell cancer. Cochrane Database Syst Rev. 2014;(12):CD002027.
See also O'Hara J et al. Transoral laser surgery versus radiotherapy for tumour stage 1a or 1b glottic squamous cell carcinoma: systematic review of local control outcomes. J Laryngol Otol. 2013;127:732–8.
D'cruz A et al. Consensus recommendations for management of head and neck cancer in Asian countries. Oral Oncol. 2013;49:872–7.

surgery for treatment failures (EBM 26.5). Operative treatment of the more extensive lesions usually involves total removal of the larynx. Here, the trachea is brought out onto the surface of the neck as an end tracheostomy. Patients can regain speech by generating a vibrating column of air in the pharynx. There are two ways of doing this: air swallowing, or valved speech through a surgically created tracheo-oesophageal puncture. Here, the patient has the advantage of lung-powered phonation. This valve diverts air from the trachea into the pharynx. Once the valve is closed, the air is expelled through the mouth where the articulators (teeth and tongue) use the airflow to generate the sounds of speech. Chemoradiotherapy has the potential to avoid neck breathing in two-thirds of patients, but has a much higher rate of enteral feeding dependency and also a lower survival.

26.11 Summary

Advanced carcinoma of the larynx treatment

- Larynx preservation with chemoradiotherapy (CRT) should be considered for T4 tumours, unless there is tumour invasion through cartilage into the soft tissues of the neck, in which case total laryngectomy yields better outcomes
- Concurrent CRT should be regarded as standard of care for the nonsurgical management of stage III/IV laryngeal cancer because it yields higher laryngeal preservation rates compared with induction chemotherapy followed by RT and RT alone
- Treatment options for patients who are unsuitable for concurrent CRT include altered fractionation RT or RT with concurrent cetuximab
- Postoperative RT is recommended for pT4 laryngeal cancers of any nodal stage, pT1/T2/T3 tumours with N2–N3 nodal stage, and for all patients with close or positive resection margins and/or extracapsular spread
- Cisplatin chemotherapy with postoperative RT improves locoregional control and disease-free survival compared with postoperative RT alone for locally advanced tumours, albeit at the expense of increased mucosal and haematological toxicity and possibly increased deaths.

Neck

Anatomy

The investing layer of deep cervical fascia (Fig. 26.30) covers the deeper structures all around like a collar. Platysma separates the skin from the fascia and runs obliquely upwards and is medially innervated by the cervical branch of the facial nerve. Most neck swellings lie deep to the platysma. Skin flaps are raised in the sub-platysmal plane to maintain the vascular supply to the overlying skin. The sternocleidomastoid muscle (SCM) passes obliquely in the neck from the mastoid process above to the sternoclavicular junction below, supplied by the spinal accessory nerve (XI cranial nerve), and separating the anterior and posterior triangles (see Fig. 26.30).

The marginal mandibular branch of the facial nerve lies deep to the platysma muscle and superficial to the investing layer of the deep fascia that forms the capsule of the submandibular gland. Injury to the nerve leads to an asymmetrical appearance to the mouth, particularly when smiling. The facial artery travels through the submandibular gland before passing over the mandibular ramus into the face. The anterior oral cavity drains into the submandibular group of nodes, which are intimately related to the submandibular gland; the gland needs to be removed during lymph node clearance of this triangle.

Deep to the sternocleidomastoid is the carotid sheath – common carotid artery, internal jugular vein (IJV), vagus nerve. The posterior triangle is formed by the SCM anteriorly, trapezius posteriorly and clavicle inferiorly. The occipital triangle contains the spinal accessory nerve that exits the skull via the jugular foramen, passing lateral and posterior to the IJV in the majority of cases. It penetrates and supplies the SCM at the junction of the upper third and lower two thirds. The nerve exits the posterior aspect of the SCM at the junction of the upper two thirds and the lower third to supply the trapezius muscle. The supraclavicular triangle contains the brachial plexus and the subclavian artery. The plexus is crossed by the supraclavicular nerves, the posterior belly of the omohyoid, the external jugular vein and the transverse cervical artery. On the left side of the neck the thoracic duct ends by opening into the junction of the left subclavian and IJVs. The thyroid gland lies anterior and lateral to the trachea, the isthmus overlying the second to fourth tracheal rings (Fig. 26.31).

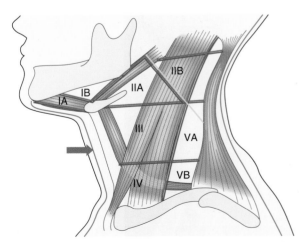

Fig. 26.30 Oncological levels of neck nodes. *Arrow* shows the investing layer of the deep cervical fascia.

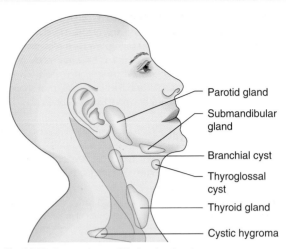

Fig. 26.31 Key structures of the head and neck.

Assessment

Clinical features

Most neck masses are painless, but infection and malignant disease may cause pain. Rapid enlargement makes malignant disease more likely. Salivary gland swellings caused by duct obstruction enlarge when the patient eats; there may also be a bad taste.

Examination

Inspection is usually carried out from the front and palpation from behind to establish the site, size, shape and consistency of the swelling. Fixation to the skin or underlying structures should be established.

Imaging

Plain x-rays can be used to demonstrate salivary calculi. Cystic swellings can be differentiated from solid ones by ultrasound. CT can be used to assess most neck masses and will sometimes reveal lymph node swellings that have not been detected clinically. Both CT and MRI are of value in assessing salivary gland swellings. The introduction of contrast into the duct of a salivary gland (sialogram) is occasionally used to confirm the presence of a calculus or to demonstrate inflammatory changes.

Diseases of the neck

For skin and subcutaneous swellings, see Chapter 18.

Assessment

Careful examination of the upper aerodigestive tract is mandatory. Direct examination of the oral mucosa is followed by transnasal endoscopic examination of the nose, nasopharynx, hypopharynx and larynx. Transnasal oesophagoscopy where available can visualise the tubular oesophagus. Palpation of the tonsils and tongue may reveal an occult tumour.

The most common sources of neck swelling are the lymph nodes (see Table 26.1). Systemic lymph node enlargement and hepatosplenomegaly should be excluded. If clinical findings are unhelpful, the next step depends on the level of suspicion that there is a squamous cancer. Fine-needle aspiration cytology (FNAC) and rigid endoscopy under general anaesthetic with

26

ipsilateral diagnostic tonsillectomy should be considered. PET-CT of the neck is useful at this stage and may precede tonsillectomy. As a last resort, it may be necessary to excise the swelling for histological examination. However, small mobile lymph node swellings can be observed, especially if ultrasound reveals a well-preserved length-to-transverse ratio, i.e., a normal, oval-shaped node. Tumour-infiltrated nodes are more typically spherical.

Thyroglossal cyst

The thyroid gland begins its embryological development in the base of the tongue at the foramen caecum (apex of the junction of anterior two-thirds with posterior one-third of the tongue). It descends into the neck as a bi-lobed diverticulum that remains attached to the tongue by the thyroglossal duct. Normally, the duct disappears completely except as a little remnant often on the left of the midline, the pyramidal lobe. Patency of any portion of the thyroglossal duct leads to the development of a thyroglossal cyst (Fig. 26.32). This is a midline swelling usually situated just above the upper border of the thyroid cartilage. The cyst may contain mucoid-to-purulent fluid, rich in cholesterol, and may be lined by stratified squamous, ciliated respiratory or pseudostratified columnar epithelium. Normal thyroid tissue may be found in the cyst wall. Since the duct or its remnant is attached to the

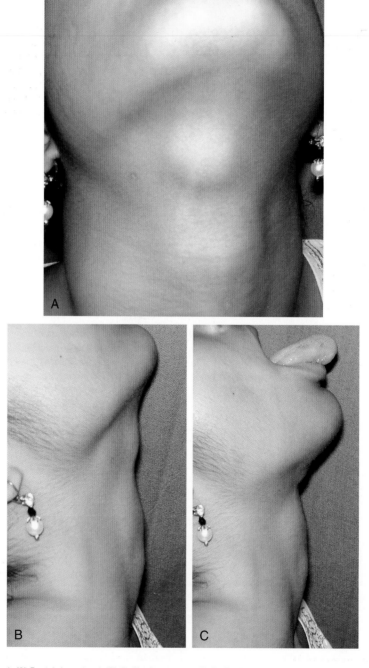

Fig. 26.32 Thyroglossal cyst. (A) Frontal view: at rest. **(B)** Profile view: at rest. **(C)** Profile view: movement with protrusion of the tongue.

foramen caecum, it moves on protrusion of the tongue (a thyroid swelling does not move up on protrusion of the tongue). Also, as a thyroglossal cyst is intimately related to the hyoid bone, it also moves on swallowing. If an infected thyroglossal cyst bursts or is incised for drainage a thyroglossal fistula results. Hence, a thyroglossal fistula is always acquired. With growth of the patient it becomes crescentic with a hood superiorly (convexity facing upwards). This 'hooding' is exaggerated when the patient is asked to swallow.

Occasionally, the thyroid gland fails to migrate as far as the lower neck (misnamed *ectopic thyroid*). Thyroglossal cysts may be differentiated from aberrant thyroid tissue by an ultrasound scan, although the requirement for this appears to be more medicolegal than clinical.

Treatment is by surgical excision (Sistrunk's operation). The central segment of the hyoid bone and the persistent thyroglossal duct in continuity up to the base of the tongue should also be excised with the cyst to reduce the recurrence rate, which can be up to 10%.

Branchial cyst and fistula

Branchial cyst is a cystic swelling arising in connection with a persistent cervical sinus of His, formed due to the fusion of an overgrowing second branchial cleft with the fifth. Although congenital, branchial cysts commonly present as a painless lump in the upper neck in the second decade of life and have no sex predilection (Fig. 26.33). The cyst usually lies 5–10 cm below the angle of mandible. The ectodermal appendages lining the cyst secrete sweat sebum rich in cholesterol, rendering it cystic in consistency with smooth margins and minimal mobility. It seldom transilluminates. Lymphoid tissue is found in the walls. They may become infected and usually require excision (Table 26.5). Resected specimens should always be sent for histology to exclude a focus of squamous carcinoma in the cyst wall.

Branchial fistulae may occur between the skin surface on the anterior border of the lower third of the SCM, and the tonsil or lower pharynx internally. Attachment of the stylopharyngeus muscle moves the tract up on swallowing. Infection often occurs and excision usually requires step ladder incisions to follow the track up the neck.

Table 26.5 Branchial cyst

- Ectodermal appendages secrete sweat sebum rich in cholesterol
- Age: 10–40 years
- M = F
- Painless lump in the upper neck anterior to upper third of sternomastoid
- Smooth cyst with distinct margins with minimal mobility.

Other cystic swellings

Cystic hygroma is a rare, benign lymphangioma of the neck (Fig. 26.34), which usually presents in early life. It can go from the neck into the axilla through the cervicoaxillary canal and therefore the axilla should also be examined. Complete excision is difficult, leading to frequent recurrence. Dermoid cysts may also occur in the upper neck, usually in the midline or submandibular area, in younger children. They contain skin appendages unlike sebaceous cysts. External laryngocoeles occur as a result of herniation of laryngeal mucosa laterally into the neck. They distend with air during the Valsalva manoeuvre and may become infected. Excision is usually required.

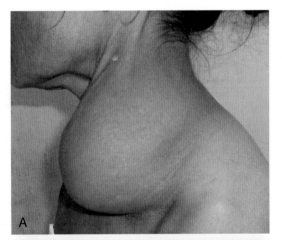

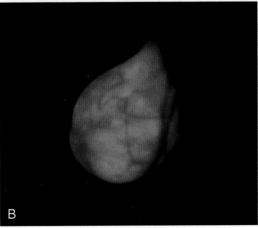

Fig. 26.34 (A) Cystic hygroma. **(B)** Exhibiting brilliant translucence.

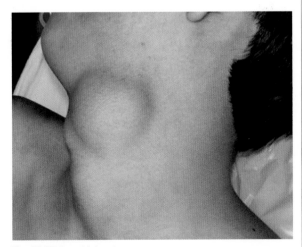

Fig. 26.33 Branchial cyst.

26

Lymph node swellings

Lymph nodes may become enlarged in response to infection or cancer in their area of drainage (Fig. 26.35; see Table 26.1). Primary neoplasms of lymph nodes (lymphomas), tuberculous lymphadenitis and secondary deposits (usually from squamous carcinoma of the head and neck) are commonly seen lymph node swellings in the neck. Secondaries from thyroid carcinoma must be kept in mind. Lymph node enlargement in the lower half of the neck warrants exclusion of a primary in the breast, chest and abdomen (including testis/ovary). Systemic lymph node enlargement (including hepatosplenomegaly) should be looked for.

26.12 Summary

Lymphadenopathy

- Nodes become palpable when their diameter exceeds 1 cm, but impalpable nodes may contain tumour
- Painless neck nodes in patients >45 years are often due to metastases from carcinoma. In most cases, the primary is within the head and neck. A thorough search for a primary lesion must precede biopsy
- Fine-needle aspiration cytology can be diagnostic for secondary carcinoma in lymph nodes from head and neck tumours or for tuberculosis; histology is needed for lymphoma
- In lymphoma:
  - The nodes are often bilaterally enlarged, rubbery, firm and discrete
  - Extranodal disease suggests non-Hodgkin's lymphoma
  - Bone marrow examination and CT are used in staging.

Neck node metastases in head and neck cancer

The status of the regional lymphatics is the key prognostic indicator in patients with head and neck cancer. The Memorial Sloan–Kettering Cancer Center classification of nodal levels divides the neck into five groups or levels (see Fig. 26.30). Prognosis is influenced by the number of positive nodes, the level in the neck, the presence of extracapsular spread, perineural and vascular invasion, previous treatment and resectability (Tables 26.6 and 26.7). Many malignant nodes measure less than 1 cm. Extracapsular spread occurs in nodes as small as 2 mm. These may be missed on conventional cross-sectional imaging. The instance

Table 26.6 TNM staging of cervical nodes

Nx Regional lymph nodes cannot be assessed
N0 No regional lymph node metastases
N1 Metastasis in a single ipsilateral lymph node ≤3 cm in greatest dimension
N2 Metastasis in a single ipsilateral lymph node, >3 cm but ≤6 cm, or in multiple ipsilateral lymph nodes none >6 cm, or in bilateral or contralateral lymph nodes, none >6 cm
N2a Metastasis in a single ipsilateral lymph node, >3 cm but ≤6 cm
N2b Metastasis in multiple ipsilateral lymph nodes, none >6 cm
N2c Metastasis in bilateral or contralateral lymph nodes, none >6 cm
N3 Metastasis in a lymph node >6 cm.

Note: Midline nodes are considered to be ipsilateral nodes.

Table 26.7 Recommended levels of dissection for N0 disease by site

Oral cavity I–III including IIb
Oropharynx I–III including IIb; NB significant chance of contralateral disease
Supraglottis IIa–III
Glottis IIa–III
Subglottis II–IV; VI
Hypopharynx II–IV.

of nodal involvement ranges from less than 1% for early glottic cancers to 80% with pharyngeal cancers. Neck dissection aims to target all relevant involved lymph nodes, but with minimum trauma to functional structures (Table 26.8). There are different recommendations for the management of the neck with no evidence of tumour involvement (N0) and those with detectable disease (N+ neck) (Tables 26.9 and 26.10).

Lymphoma

In Hodgkin's disease, the unique abnormal lymphocyte is the Reed–Sternberg cell (a B lymphocyte). Epstein–Barr virus plays a role in causation. The four main categories of Hodgkin's are nodular sclerosis, mixed cellularity, lymphocyte depleted and lymphocyte predominant. The initial treatment for patients with Hodgkin's

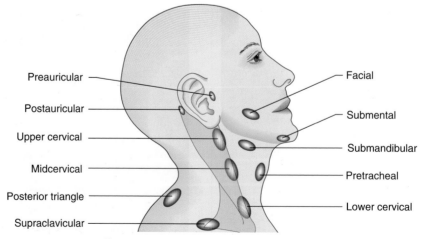

Fig. 26.35 Lymph node groups in the head and neck.

Table 26.8 Classification of neck dissection techniques

RND	Removal of levels I–V, accessory nerve, IJV and sternomastoid muscle
Modified RND	Removal of levels I–V dissected; preservation of one or more of the accessory nerve, IJV or sternomastoid muscle (types I–III, respectively)
Selective neck dissection	Preservation of one or more levels of lymph nodes
Extended RND	Removal of one or more additional lymphatic and/or nonlymphatic structures relative to an RND, e.g., retropharyngeal lymph nodes

IJV, internal jugular vein; RND, radical neck dissection.

Table 26.9 Recommendations for N$_0$ neck

- The levels dissected depend on the primary site. See Table 26.8
- Patients with a clinically N$_0$ neck, with more than 15–20% risk of occult nodal metastases should be offered prophylactic treatment of the neck
- The treatment choice of the N$_0$ neck should be guided by the treatment to the primary site
- If observation is planned for the N$_0$ neck, this should be supplemented by regular ultrasonography to ensure early detection
- All patients with T$_1$ and T$_2$ oral cavity cancer and N$_0$ neck should receive prophylactic neck treatment
- Selective neck dissection is as effective as MRND for controlling regional disease in N$_0$ necks for all primary sites
- Elective neck dissection and elective neck irradiation have equal efficacy in controlling occult neck disease.

MRND, modified radical neck dissection.

Table 26.10 Recommendations for N+ neck

- Management is guided by the treatment to the primary site
- SND is adequate for pN1 neck disease without adverse histological features
- Adjuvant radiation following surgery for patients with adverse histological features improves regional control rates
- Postoperative chemoradiation improves regional control of extracapsular spread and/or microscopically involved surgical margins
- Following chemoradiotherapy, complete responders at 10–12 weeks on PET-CT do not require neck dissection.
- Salvage surgery considered if incomplete or equivocal PET-CT nodal response.

PET-CT, Positron emission tomography combined with computed tomography; SND, selective neck dissection.

lymphoma is based on the stage and histological characteristics of the disease, and the presence or absence of prognostic factors associated with poor outcome. Various combinations of chemo- and radiotherapy are used. Autologous stem cell transplantation may be required for treatment failures. Immunotherapy and allogeneic stem cell transplantation may also be required.

There are about 30 subtypes of non-Hodgkin's lymphoma (NHL), the majority originating in B cells; e.g., diffuse large B cell is aggressive, comprising around 30% of NHL, with average age of onset in the seventh decade. Those demonstrating rearrangement in MYC, an oncogene promoting cellular proliferation, may be resistant to conventional therapy. Double-hit lymphomas, with rearrangements in MYC as well as BCL2 and/or BCL6

oncogenes, also have a poor prognosis. Other NHL variants are follicular (indolent), mantle cell (aggressive or indolent), MALT (indolent), T-cell and NK-cell types.

Tuberculous cervical lymphadenitis

Both bovine and human tuberculosis bacilli may cause cervical lymphadenopathy secondary to tonsil invasion. A painless swelling in the neck may be initially firm but then 'soften' (Fig. 26.36). Despite effective antituberculosis chemotherapy, case-fatality rates of up to 25% are described in both industrialised and resource-poor settings.

Evening rise of temperature, night sweats, anorexia and weight loss may be present. Interferon-γ (IFN-γ) release assays measure immune reactivity to *Mycobacterium tuberculosis*. White blood cells from most people who have been infected release IFN-γ when mixed with *M. tuberculosis* antigens.

Clinically, the disease follows a pattern of progression through various stages:

1. *Acute lymphadenitis*: enlarged tender lymph nodes with fever
2. *Periadenitis*: Nodes matted due to pericapsular inflammation. The pain, tenderness and fever abate
3. *Caseation necrosis and cold abscess:* The necrosis yields a cystic nontender node, the cold abscess. A cold abscess in the neck may also result from spinal TB
4. *Collar-stud abscess*: The cold abscess is deep to the investing layer of deep cervical fascia and emerges where the neurovascular bundles pierce the fascia. The dumb-bell-shaped components superficial and deep to the deep fascia are known as a collar-stud abscess
5. *Discharging sinus*: The skin overlying the collar stud becomes dusky and indurated, eventually giving way as a sinus discharging straw-coloured thin fluid.

Diagnostic work-up involves FNAC of the residual nodal swelling after complete aspiration of the pus. The FNAC smear infrequently demonstrates acid-fast bacilli (AFB). Occasionally, lymph node

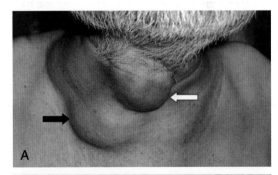

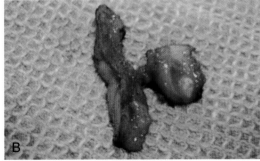

Fig. 26.36 Tuberculous cervical lymphadenitis. (A) Cold abscess, *black arrow*, collar stud abscess, *white arrow*. **(B)** Sinus excised with the underlying caseating lymph node.

26

biopsy is necessary with histopathological examination and AFB culture and sensitivity. Polymerase chain reaction (PCR) may help differentiate other mycobacterial infections. Refractory nodes after antituberculosis treatment may require limited neck dissection.

Tracheostomy

Tracheostomy may be required to relieve acute upper airway obstruction. It is carried out by creating a window in the anterior tracheal wall at the level of the second and third tracheal rings, and introducing a suitable tube. When short-term airway support and the causative pathology allow, the situation is better managed by passing an endotracheal tube. Cricothyroidotomy (Fig. 26.37) provides a rapid short-term solution to airway obstruction and can be carried out with makeshift equipment. Foreign bodies in the upper airway can be displaced by turning a small child upside down and performing a few interscapular back slaps. In a larger individual, if back slaps fail, perform abdominal thrusts by standing behind the patient. Wrap your arms around the chest and clasp

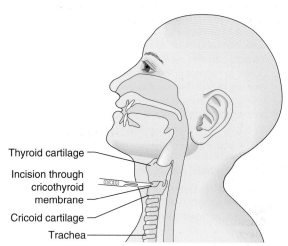

Thyroid cartilage

Incision through cricothyroid membrane

Cricoid cartilage

Trachea

Fig. 26.37 Cricothyrotomy

your hands before exerting sharp pressure in the epigastrium, on the bottom of the diaphragm. This compresses the lungs and exerts pressure on any object lodged (Heimlich's manoeuvre). Tracheostomy may also be of value to reduce the dead space in patients with respiratory disease and to facilitate longer term artificial ventilation.

Salivary gland anatomy

The major salivary glands are the paired parotid, submandibular and sublingual glands. The minor glands are small glands located beneath the mucosa of the upper aerodigestive tract, most concentrated in the palate, nasal cavity and oral cavity. The parotid gland overlies the angle of the mandible and is closely related to the cartilage of the ear canal posteriorly, the zygoma superiorly, the parapharyngeal space medially, and the sternocleidomastoid and posterior digastric muscles inferiorly (Fig. 26.38). The facial nerve trunk exits the stylomastoid foramen and divides into temporozygomatic and cervicofacial divisions. The nerve then runs through the substance of the parotid gland, splitting into its five main branches. The nerve lies superficial to the retromandibular vein, formed by the union of the superficial temporal and maxillary veins. It divides into the external jugular and posterior facial vein in the lower portion of the gland. The 20% of the parotid substance deep to the facial nerve is termed the 'deep lobe', the remaining tissue the 'superficial lobe'. The parasympathetic supply is from the glossopharyngeal nerve (cranial nerve IX). The postsynaptic postganglionic fibres are distributed through the auriculotemporal nerve.

The submandibular gland abuts the body of the mandible superolaterally, the lingual and hypoglossal nerves medially, the mylohyoid muscle anteriorly, and the tail of the parotid gland posteriorly The marginal mandibular branch of the facial nerve runs along the lateral surface of the gland, just deep to the platysma (Fig. 26.39).

Salivary gland disease

The submandibular salivary gland is the source of 80% of salivary gland calculi, most of which are radio-opaque. (Fig. 26.40).

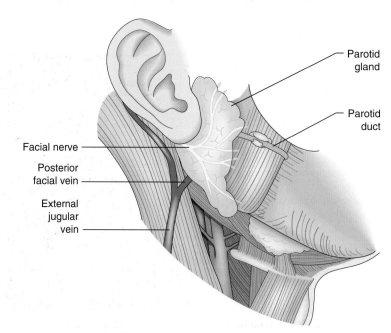

Parotid gland

Parotid duct

Facial nerve

Posterior facial vein

External jugular vein

Fig. 26.38 Anatomy of the parotid gland.

- Sublingual gland
- Submandibular duct

- Lingual nerve
- Mylohyoid muscle
- Submandibular gland

Fig. 26.39 Anatomy of the submandibular salivary gland.

Salivary stagnation, increased alkalinity or calcium content of the saliva, infection or inflammation of the salivary duct or gland, and physical trauma to the salivary duct or gland may predispose to calculus formation. The submandibular gland saliva is susceptible because its saliva is far more alkaline, has a greater concentration of calcium and phosphate, and also carries more mucus.

Submandibular gland swelling results from obstruction of the duct by a stone or inflammation. Some stones may pass spontaneously. Those in the main duct may be removed by opening the duct in the floor of the mouth. Those within the substance of the gland usually require gland excision. Inflammatory changes can occur in the absence of stone and are confirmed by ultrasound or sialography. Chronic sialadenitis may also be an indication for removal of the submandibular gland.

By contrast, most swellings of the parotid gland are (benign) tumours. Since total removal of the parotid gland would be required to treat inflammation, this should be avoided if possible due to the risk of damage to the facial nerve.

26.13 Summary

Salivary gland swellings

- Swellings in the submandibular gland are more often due to calculi, but those in the parotid gland are commonly benign neoplasms
- The most common salivary gland tumours are pleomorphic adenomas
- Parotid swellings generally require removal with a cuff of normal salivary tissue (partial superficial parotidectomy)
- The facial nerve runs through the parotid gland as a series of branches and is at risk during parotid surgery.

Salivary gland tumours

Most salivary glands tumours are slow growing benign lesions; malignant tumours are uncommon.

26.14 Summary

Salivary gland neoplasms

Benign
- Pleomorphic adenoma
- Monomorphic adenoma
- Adenolymphoma (also known as papillary cystadenoma lymphomatosum, Warthin's tumour)

Intermediate
- Oncocytoma
- Mucoepidermoid tumour

Malignant
- Squamous carcinoma
- Adenoid cystic carcinoma
- Adenocarcinoma
- Lymphoma.

26

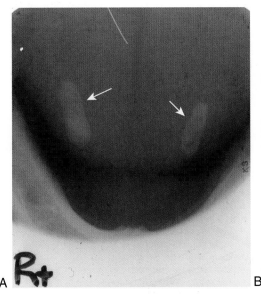

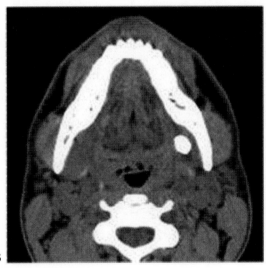

Fig. 26.40 Submandibular salivary calculus. **(A)** X-ray. **(B)** Computed tomography.

The parotid gland is the most common site of origin of salivary neoplasms, almost 80% of which are benign.

Pleomorphic adenoma

Treatment consists of complete excision of the tumour with a cuff of normal tissue, and may require superficial parotidectomy or total parotidectomy based on the location of the tumour in the superficial or deep lobe of the parotid gland. Deep lobe involvement will push the lingual tonsil medially. CT is useful to differentiate deep lobe tumours from other parapharyngeal masses (Fig. 26.41). It is important to note that the tumour should not be enucleated as it may result in a multicentric recurrence.

26.15 Summary

Pleomorphic adenoma

- Most common salivary gland tumour
- Most in parotid gland
- Benign, slow growing
- Potential for malignant transformation
- Lobulated: pseudocapsule with pseudopods (Fig. 26.42)
- Epithelial and mesenchymal elements with fibromyxoid, fibroid stroma
- More common in adult males
- Facial nerve is never involved.

Warthin's tumour

This 'adenolymphoma' is the second most common tumour of the salivary glands.

26.16 Summary

Salivary adenolymphoma/Warthin's

- Almost exclusively parotid
- Mean age = 60 years
- 60% male
- 30% bilateral
- Most in the lower pole of the parotid gland
- Soft or cystic
- Option of watchful waiting may be discussed with patient.

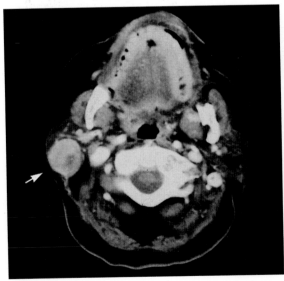
Fig. 26.41 Computed tomography scan showing parotid tumour.

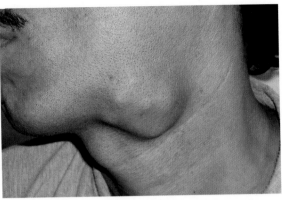
Fig. 26.42 Pleomorphic adenoma of the submandibular gland.

Mucoepidermoid carcinoma

This is the most common salivary gland malignancy. Mucoepidermoid carcinoma (MEC) ranges from a near benign variant to an intermediate or very aggressive high-grade tumour. It has a mix of mucin-producing columnar cells and squamous cells. The grade of the tumour is increased if the lesion is solid and has a high proportion of squamous cells. While superficial parotidectomy with a cuff of normal tissue may be adequate for low-grade, superficial lobe lesions, intermediate and high-grade lesions require total parotidectomy (Table 26.11). Patients with unresectable and metastatic mucoepidermoid carcinoma have poor long-term clinical outcomes; no targeted therapies are available.

Adenoid cystic carcinoma

This tumour can affect any of the salivary glands and is the most common malignant tumour of the submandibular salivary gland. It is locally aggressive and tends to invade the nerves. It has a high propensity to recur, even after several years. Pathological grades are Grade 1 (tubular), Grade 2 (cribriform) and Grade 3 (solid).

Complications of parotidectomy

These are listed in Table 26.12. Among the most common is Frey's syndrome, gustatory sweating due to the aberrant regeneration of sectioned postganglionic parasympathetic cholinergic fibres misdirected to innervate the vessels and sweat glands of the skin overlying the parotid.

Table 26.11 Features suggestive of malignant transformation of a benign salivary gland tumour

- Sudden and rapid increase in size
- Pain
- Prominence of the veins over the swelling
- Change to harder consistency
- Deep tissue fixation
- Overlying skin infiltrated
- Involvement of the facial nerve
- Area of anaesthesia over the skin
- Restriction of jaw movements
- Enlargement of cervical lymph nodes
- Evidence of distant metastases.

Table 26.12 Complications of operations on the parotid gland

- Facial nerve palsy due to neuropraxia/neurotmesis
- Loss of sensation on and around the lower half of the pinna: division of the great auricular nerve
- Soft tissue defect proportional to size of resection
- Gustatory sweating (Frey's syndrome)
- Salivary fistula.

26.17 Summary

Frey's syndrome

- Perspiration and flushing of the cheek during meals
- Typically about 6 weeks postoperatively
- Increases in frequency with the volume of gland resected
- Incidence of gustatory sweating after parotidectomy varies from 2% to 96%
- Minor's starch iodine test: visualise blue-black reaction in the sweating area
- Reduce incidence by raising thick skin flaps; or interposing a submuscular aponeurotic system or sternocleidomastoid flap.

Once the syndrome has developed, it will regress spontaneously in the majority of patients, while in a minority further treatment is required (Table 26.13). Where botulinum toxin A is used to inhibit the release of acetyl choline, the target treatment area is defined by the starch iodine test.

Table 26.13 Treatment of Frey's syndrome

- Antiperspirant preparations
- Local application of anticholinergic drugs such as scopolamine cream or glycopyrrolate cream
- Tympanic neurectomy to section the efferent neural arc
- Interposition of a subcutaneous barrier, e.g., sternocleidomastoid flap, fascia lata or temporal fascia
- Injection of botulinum toxin in the involved skin.

Carotid body tumour

Six genes have been associated with the development of paraganglioma, including *RET*, *VHL* and *NF1*. Paragangliomas may also be hereditary, included as part of genetic syndromes such as von Hippel–Lindau, neurofibromatosis type I, MEN 2A and MEN 2B. Sporadic cases may be caused by germline mutations. The three most common paragangliomas in the head and neck region are carotid body tumour, glomus jugulare and glomus intravagale. The carotid body is located in the adventitia of the posteromedial aspect of the carotid bifurcation. Its chemoreceptors regulate ventilation in response to changes in arterial blood gases and pH.

26.18 Summary

Features of carotid body tumours

- Incidence is higher at high altitudes
- Bilateral in 10%
- Painless, slow-growing lump close to the superior horn of the thyroid cartilage
- Variable history of fainting
- Lesion is mobile only transversely, firm to palpation
- Transmitted pulsation, thrill and audible bruit
- CT: splaying of internal and external carotid arteries (lyre sign) (Fig. 26.43)
- MRI T2-weighted images: 'salt' (high signal foci of haemorrhage/slow flow) and 'pepper' (the low-signal flow voids)

Angiography is useful to define (and possibly embolise) the feeder vessels. Biopsy is hazardous because of the risk of bleeding and formation of a pseudoaneurysm. About 5–10% of these tumours are malignant. A diagnosis of malignancy is based on lymph node or distant metastases as pathology. Histopathological criteria are unreliable to make a diagnosis of malignant carotid body tumour.

Treatment is surgical excision. Operative bleeding and duration of surgery are reduced by preoperative embolisation. Occasionally, vascular repair of the carotid artery is required. Preoperative balloon occlusion studies can be used to assess the cerebral blood flow. The tumour may be excised by dissecting in the sub-adventitial plane. The superior laryngeal nerve, vagus nerve and hypoglossal nerve are at risk during the procedure. In bilateral lesions, operate on the smaller first and counsel the patient that there may be fluctuation in blood pressure following the second side excision due to complete loss of carotid sinus function. It is estimated that malignant paragangliomas have less than a 50% 10-year survival rate; surgery is the treatment of choice as chemotherapy and radiation do not appear to be of significant benefit.

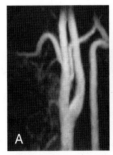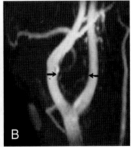

Fig. 26.43 Carotid body tumour. (A). Normal carotid angiogram. **(B)** Splaying of the carotid fork by tumour (*arrows*).

26

John C. McKinley
Issaq Ahmed

Orthopaedic surgery

Chapter Contents

Introduction 528

History 528

Examination 529

Description of deformity 530

Investigations 531

Osteoarthritis: degenerative disease of the joints 532

Inflammatory disorders 533

Bone and joint infection 533

Orthopaedic procedures 535

Paediatric orthopaedic surgery 537

Metabolic bone diseases 538

Musculoskeletal tumours 538

The upper limb 540

The lower limb 541

Trauma and fractures 542

Introduction

Orthopaedic surgery involves the assessment and management of a wide spectrum of common conditions that affect bones, joints and soft tissues. The focus of this chapter is the assessment and management of degenerative and inflammatory joint diseases; bone and joint infection; congenital and developmental (growing skeleton) conditions; soft tissue and bone tumours; and trauma. Assessment almost always begins with history and examination, and is followed frequently by imaging.

History

A diagnosis can often be made with history alone. The cardinal symptoms (Summary 27.1) of the musculoskeletal system are pain, swelling, redness, heat, loss of function and weakness. It is important to determine the onset of these symptoms and their nature: acute versus chronic, monoarticular versus polyarticular,

27.1 Summary

Cardinal symptoms of musculoskeletal system

1. Pain (limb or joint)
   - SOCRATES: Site, Onset, Character, Radiation, Alleviating factors, Timing, Exacerbating factors, Severity
2. Swelling, redness and heat
   - SOCRATES
3. Loss of function: effect on activities of daily living
4. Weakness

27.2 Summary

Red flag symptoms

- History of malignancy
- Weight loss
- Night sweats
- Reduction in appetite
- Night pain
- Pain that is progressive or persistent
- Pain in children

small versus large joints and precipitation factors (e.g., medications, trauma). Red flag symptoms (Summary 27.2) are important to exclude if any sinister diagnosis is contemplated. Other particular points in the history include those listed in Summaries 27.1 and 27.2.

Age

This often distinguishes degenerative conditions (elderly) from those related to an underlying congenital, birth-related or developmental problem (young), and different types of bone tumours. Back pain could be due to disc prolapse or ankylosing spondylitis in young adults, or due to metastasis or degenerative spondylosis in the elderly.

Birth and developmental history

There may be a direct link between events around the time of birth and conditions such as upper limb weakness (traction injury to the brachial plexus), cerebral palsy (hypoxia) and dysplastic disease of the hip (more common in a breech delivery or first child). Abnormalities in the development of the growing skeleton may result in a range of conditions, some of which are associated with visible deformity. Sometimes, such apparent deformity is just a stage of normal development. For example, some children go through a phase of being bow-legged and anxious parents need to be reassured that this is a normal physiological variation and not a disease.

Dominant hand

This is particularly relevant to upper limb conditions and has a bearing on the management of disorders of the upper extremities.

Occupation

Degenerative processes may be a consequence of, or at least exacerbated by, occupation or repetitive strain injuries, which can occur in certain occupations. The need to return a patient to employment or a certain skill will also greatly affect the way and urgency with which a condition is treated.

Trauma

Many conditions follow a clearly defined episode of trauma, the nature and mechanism of which can help establish the diagnosis. For example, sudden injury to the knee, with acute swelling followed by instability, is highly suggestive of anterior cruciate ligament (ACL) rupture. It is important to ascertain that the history of trauma is significant, since some patients associate trauma with the onset of symptoms of diseases such as tuberculosis and bone tumours.

Details of previous treatment

The condition may have been treated by means of physiotherapy, traction, acupuncture, osteopathy, steroid injection and drugs over many years in primary care prior to referral to an orthopaedic surgeon. Previous surgical interventions performed on the same joint or limb may affect both the current options for surgery and the chance of success.

Past medical history

If operative intervention is planned, general fitness for anaesthesia and surgery must be carefully assessed and the patient medically optimised. The consequences of other comorbidities must be considered.

Drug history

With regard to analgesia, changing the dose or preparation may result in significant relief of symptoms. Drugs such as warfarin or antiplatelet medication may need to be stopped prior to surgery. Some immunosuppressive drugs increase the risk of infection; smoking and nonsteroidal anti-inflammatories can slow bone healing.

Examination

Examination should include all the other systems (e.g., cardiovascular, neurological, skin), as well as the specific limb and joint. Café au lait spots of neurofibromatosis may be associated with congenital pseudoarthrosis of the tibia or scoliosis. It is important to assess the joint above and below and check limb alignment, as hip pathology can present with knee pain and hind foot pathology may be exacerbated by a varus or valgus knee. Musculoskeletal examination should always involve look, feel, and measuring both passive and active movement after assessing for any joint deformity. It is particularly important to note whether any joint deformity is passively correctable or fixed.

Look

In lower limb conditions, observe the patient's use of a stick, their ability to get out of a chair unaided and their gait. Observe any joint or limb asymmetry, muscle wasting, scars, sinus, skin colour changes, malalignment or shortening. The patient may voluntarily assume the position of a joint at a particular angle, which may not necessarily be a fixed deformity. A joint deformity is present only if the opposite movement is not possible. Therefore, it is better to refer to the position of the joint on observation as an attitude rather than a deformity. An attitude of flexion, adduction and internal rotation of the hip with apparent shortening would be present in a posterior dislocation of the hip joint (Fig. 27.1).

Feel

Palpate around the joint or limb. Establish areas of tenderness and try to relate these to anatomical structures (e.g., tendons, joint lines, etc.). Establish the presence of any swelling and whether this is fluctuant or solid (Table 27.1). A thickened irregular bone associated with a puckered adherent scar or discharging sinus would be diagnostic of underlying osteomyelitis (Fig. 27.2).

27

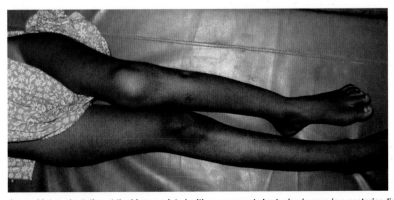

Fig. 27.1 Flexion, adduction and internal rotation at the hip associated with an apparent shortening is seen in a posterior dislocation of the hip joint.

Table 27.1 Features describing a lump or swelling: three groups starting with SCTF

S	Size	Shape	Surface
C	Colour	Consistency	Contour
T	Temperature	Tenderness	Transilluminable
F	Fluctuance	Fixity	Fields

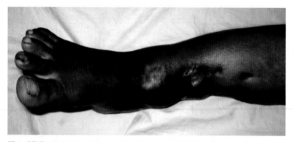

Fig. 27.2 A thickened irregular bone associated with a puckered adherent scar or discharging sinus would be diagnostic of underlying osteomyelitis.

A detailed neurological assessment is important in spinal disorders. Test the neurovascular status of the limb (motor power, deep tendon reflexes, sensation to light touch and pinprick, and peripheral pulses) and compare this to the other side.

Move (active and passive)

Ask the patient to actively move the affected part through a full range of movement, check for any deformity in the joint and observe for limitations of movement, pain, or apparent weakness.

Some deformities may not be revealed. A flexion deformity of the hip may be missed due to a compensatory lumbar lordosis (Fig. 27.3). Thomas's test is performed to reveal flexion deformity of the hip. On flexing the uninvolved opposite hip to obliterate the lumbar lordosis, the pelvis becomes tilted, thereby revealing the flexion deformity. Similarly, abduction and adduction deformities of the hip may be missed due to tilting of the pelvis and scoliosis. After recording the deformities, move the joint passively through its full range of movement, stopping in response to pain, stiffness or crepitus. Test power of relevant muscles and apply stress tests to the ligaments, looking for instability.

There are specific provocative tests for most joints that are performed depending on the initial findings. Examples include testing for shoulder impingement (Hawkin's test), asking the patient to stand on one leg to test the power of the abductor muscles of the hip (Trendelenburg test) and stressing the ACL of the knee to look for a rupture (anterior drawer test).

Description of deformity

With patients in the anatomical position (i.e., lying on their back with their palms pointing up to the ceiling), limb deformities are described relative to the midline. When the distal part of the limb or deformity is away from the midline it is termed *valgus* and when it is towards the midline it is referred to as *varus*. For example, when the ankles are away from the midline there is a genu valgum or a knock-knee deformity (Fig. 27.4). In a genu varum or bow-leg deformity, the knees are away but the ankles are towards the midline. It is possible to have genu varum on one side and genu valgum on the other limb, known as a wind swept or tackle deformity. Hyperextension of the knee joint is known as *recurvatum* (Fig. 27.5).

The three types of spinal deformity are:

- *Kyphosis*: forward flexion ('the kyphotic kisses his knees') or hunch back
- *Lordosis*: the opposite, extension or bent-over-backwards deformity; this represents the normal alignment of the lumbar and cervical spine
- *Scoliosis*: a sideward deformity that is normally associated with a degree of rotation.

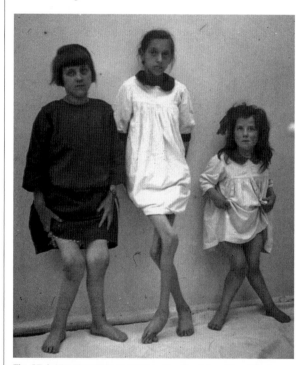

Fig. 27.4 Historical slide of children, showing deformities of the knees. All the children show valgus knee, i.e., knock-kneed, deformities.

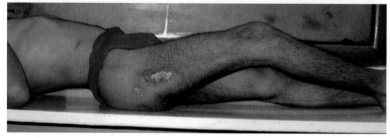

Fig. 27.3 Tuberculosis of hip joint with flexion deformity of the hip joint associated with increased lumbar lordosis. Note the healed scar of a sinus.

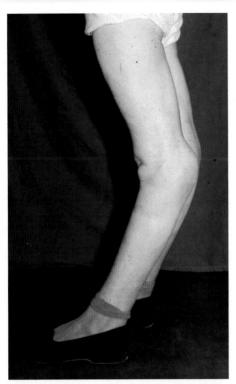

Fig. 27.5 A recurvatum deformity of the knees with hyperextension.

Investigations

Plain x-rays

Two views in orthogonal planes including the joint above and below are generally used to evaluate almost all bone pathology and are performed weight-bearing whenever possible. Oblique views are used for fractures of the scaphoid or acetabulum, and are also performed to look for spondylolysis of the spine due to any break in the pars interarticularis, which may result in slippage of the vertebrae (spondylolisthesis). Alignment (the degree of varus or valgus deformity), as well as true bone length, can be quantified. X-rays are also used routinely to confirm the correct alignment of bones, joints or prostheses after surgery.

Ultrasound

This is used frequently to evaluate soft tissue pathology (e.g., tendon rupture, bleed into soft tissues, joint fluid, other muscular or tendinous pathology) and to guide biopsy or injection. As a dynamic technique, it can be used to visualise the movements of tendons and muscles under direct vision.

Nerve conduction tests and electromyography

These are used to evaluate nerve entrapment syndromes such as carpal tunnel or cubital tunnel syndrome, nerve injuries, neuropathies and abnormalities of muscular contraction.

Computed tomography

Computed tomography (CT) provides excellent images of bone anatomy (Fig. 27.6) and can be used to provide three-dimensional images to help in the reconstruction of complex fractures. The thin axial slices are particularly useful as a guide for obtaining biopsy specimens.

Magnetic resonance imaging

Magnetic resonance imaging (MRI) provides excellent images of soft tissue, joint (Fig. 27.7) and bone pathology without exposure to radiation. It is widely used in virtually all branches of orthopaedics, being especially useful for diagnosis of meniscal and ligamentous injuries of the knee joint, musculoskeletal infections, in determining the extent of tumours and for preoperative planning.

Bone scans

These can be used to assess a number of bone conditions, including infection and tumours (Fig. 27.8). A DEXA scan is used to quantify osteoporosis in the elderly and postmenopausal women.

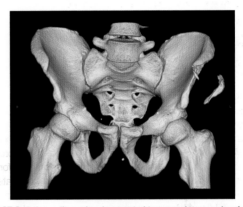

Fig. 27.6 A three-dimensional computed tomography scan showing an iliac wing fracture.

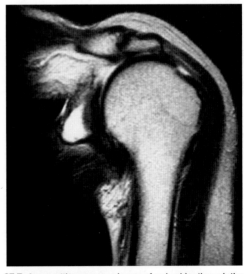

Fig. 27.7 A magnetic resonance image of a shoulder through the level of the acromioclavicular joint and the glenohumeral joint.

27

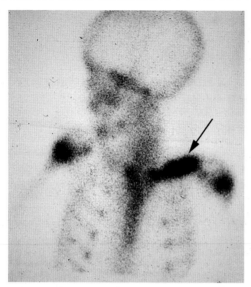

Fig. 27.8 An example of a bone scan showing increased uptake of radioactive tracer in the clavicle (arrowed): in this case, indicative of infection. There are also increased areas of uptake in the shoulders and sternum.

Osteoarthritis: degenerative disease of the joints

Osteoarthritis (OA) of a joint may occur as a primary idiopathic condition or secondary to problems such as malalignment, intra-articular fractures or over-stressing (obesity, overuse). In some patients, there is a strong genetic component. OA may occur in any joint (shoulder, elbow, wrist and hands) but predominantly affects those that are weight-bearing (hip and knee). Idiopathic OA is generally of slow onset and affects the elderly. Secondary OA can affect the young and may develop quite rapidly when a joint injury leads to loss of articular cartilage. On plain x-ray (Fig. 27.9), OA is associated with:

- Joint space loss due to thinning of articular cartilage
- Sclerosis of the joint surface, with the development of increased density of the bone just under the joint space
- Osteophytes
- Cystic change.

Medical management of OA

The treatment of OA may be conservative or operative (Table 27.2). The former focuses on the use of drugs and physical methods of pain and stress relief to the joint.

Drug therapy

Simple analgesics, such as paracetamol with or without the inclusion of nonsteroidal antiinflammatory drugs (NSAIDs, are the mainstay of treatment. More powerful analgesics, such as codeine or morphine, may be introduced if simple analgesics prove inadequate.

Off-loading

This involves the use of aids, such as a walking stick and weight loss, aimed at reducing the forces passing through the joint. In the obese, weight loss is helpful as the load across a joint is 3–6-times body weight. Various insoles and braces are commonly used to off-load joints and are fitted by an orthotist.

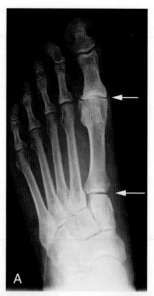

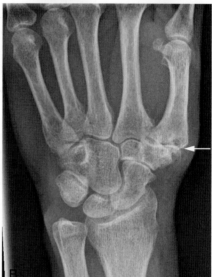

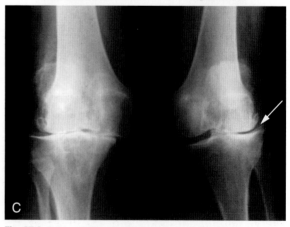

Fig. 27.9 Osteoarthritis can affect any joint. (A) The first toe metatarsophalangeal and tarsometatarsal joints (arrowed) are clearly arthritic as a result of osteoarthritic change. (B) Similarly, the carpometacarpal joint (arrowed) at the base of the thumb can be affected. (C) Bilateral knee osteoarthritis. The left knee (on the right-hand side in the illustration) shows predominantly lateral wear (arrowed) and has a valgus deformity. The right knee has osteoarthritis of both medial and lateral compartments.

Table 27.2 Management options for osteoarthritis	
Nonoperative	**Operative**
Analgesia	Osteotomy
Physiotherapy	Joint debridement
Orthotics	Excisional osteotomy
Injections	Joint replacement (arthoplasty)
Lifestyle modifications	Joint fusion (arthrodesis)

Injections

Introducing a mix of a corticosteroid and local anaesthetic into the joint may reduce inflammation and ease pain. Injections of compounds of hyaluronic acid are increasingly used and are designed to supplement the natural joint levels of hyaluronic acid essential to normal functioning of articular cartilage. They work best in early OA but may have only a temporary effect in late-stage disease.

Other conservative treatments

Physiotherapy and hydrotherapy both have a part to play in the control of symptoms, especially in early disease. Building up lost muscle bulk (frequently lost due to reduced activity) provides the joint with an increased degree of muscular control and may lead to considerable symptom improvement. Other treatment modalities, such as acupuncture, are recognised to have a role in the management of pain associated with OA.

Surgical management of OA

The main operative interventions include osteotomy, joint replacement (arthroplasty) and fusion of the joint (arthrodesis). These procedures are described in the section on orthopaedic procedures.

Inflammatory disorders

Rheumatoid arthritis

Rheumatoid arthritis (RA) is the most common chronic inflammatory disease. It affects all ethnic groups and the peak incidence is in women between the ages of 30 and 50 years.

The pathogenesis of RA is not fully understood, but it is currently thought that genetically-susceptible individuals develop the disease in response to an unidentified, possibly infectious, trigger, which induces an immune activation and cross-reactivity with endogenous antigens, leading to chronic inflammation in the joints and other tissues. There is a strong genetic association with *HLA-DR4* and *DR1*. Smoking is associated with more severe disease.

Characteristic clinical features of RA are: symmetrical joint pain, stiffness, and swelling affecting the small joints of the hand and feet, wrists, elbows and knees. There is usually early morning stiffness with synovial swelling and hypertrophy. Distinctive changes seen on radiographs include soft tissue swelling, periarticular osteoporosis, symmetrical joint space narrowing, juxta-articular erosions/osteopenia and joint subluxation/dislocation leading to deformity.

Cervical spine involvement occurs at the atlantoaxial joint resulting in possible instability and awareness of this is important for the anaesthetists during endotracheal intubation. Extra-articular and systemic features include fever, fatigue, weight loss and anaemia. Diagnosis is usually based on clinical findings along with blood tests

(normocytic anaemia, raised erythrocyte sedimentation rate [ESR], rheumatoid factor positive in 75% of patients) and radiographs. Early diagnosis and start of disease-modifying antirheumatic drugs (DMARDs; methotrexate or sulfasalazine) may prevent destruction of joints and deformities. In resistant cases biological therapy (anti-TNF [tumour necrosis factor] or anti-B-cell therapy) may be used.

Surgery is indicated for progressive disease resistant to medical management and ranges from tendon repair or reconstruction, synovectomy, joint replacement or arthrodesis.

Ankylosing spondylitis

Ankylosing spondylitis is a chronic inflammatory disorder characterised by inflammation of the sacroiliac joints and spine, ultimately leading to spinal fusion. The onset is usually during young adulthood (age 20–30 years) and the disease is more common in men (3:1). Clinical features include early morning lower back pain and stiffness, which improves with exercise. Diminished range of spinal movement in all directions leading to characteristic stooped posture with loss of lumbar lordosis, hyperextension of the neck, and flexion of the hips and knees. There is variable involvement of peripheral joints and nonarticular structures.

Diagnosis is usually made clinically, but 90% of patients are positive for the HLA-B27 antigen. Characteristic findings on x-ray of the spine include ligament calcification (syndesmophytes) with bony ankylosis resulting in a 'bamboo spine' appearance. MRI can be used for diagnosis in the early stages.

These patients should be referred and managed jointly with a rheumatologist. Treatment usually consists of pain relief with anti-inflammatories and physiotherapy, with a specific focus on back exercises. In cases of resistant disease DMARDs or anti-TNF therapy are considered. Surgery can involve joint replacement and in the case of significant spinal deformity a spinal osteotomy may be considered.

Bone and joint infection

Osteomyelitis

Infection of the bone and its marrow is known as osteomyelitis (osteo = bone, and myelitis = inflammation of marrow). Osteomyelitis is common in tropical areas and is caused by haematogenous transmission of microorganisms.

Acute osteomyelitis

Primarily a disease of childhood, these infections present with acute pain, swelling, loss of function (reluctance to use the limb, presenting as pseudoparalysis), and often follow a bout of respiratory or skin infection. The infection begins at the metaphyseal ends of long bones, commonly of the lower limb. In children, 90% of cases are due to *Staphylococcus aureus*. By contrast, adults may present with rare and unexpected organisms as a result of other comorbidity, HIV, immunosuppressant therapy, indwelling prosthetic material (e.g., renal dialysis catheters) or intravenous drug abuse.

The diagnosis can be made on clinical suspicion but MRI has a high sensitivity and specificity. The importance of obtaining blood cultures, aspirations or bone samples prior to starting antibiotics cannot be overemphasised. X-rays may be normal in the first 1 or 2 weeks but later show periosteal reaction.

The treatment for acute osteomyelitis involves urgent admission and commencement of intravenous antibiotics for 2 weeks followed by oral therapy for a total duration of 6 weeks.

27

Chronic osteomyelitis

Persistent bone infection despite treatment can lead to chronic osteomyelitis. This may be due to poor antibiotic delivery to necrotic bone or antibiotic-resistant microorganisms, particularly in patients with prosthetic implants. Eventually the pieces of dead bone surrounded by infected granulation tissue separate from the host bone to form sequestrum. There is an attempt by the host to form new bone or involucrum as a result of the periosteal reaction. The sequestrum acts as a reservoir of infection and may lie dormant for many years before reactivating. Underlying pus may come out through the involucrum creating channels or cloacae eventually discharging out of the skin, forming a sinus.

Clinically a palpable thickened, irregular bone with discharging sinus whose tract is fixed to the underlying bone is diagnostic of chronic osteomyelitis. The treatment of chronic osteomyelitis is a combination of long-term antibiotic treatment, pain relief and lifestyle changes (e.g., smoking cessation) along with surgery. Surgery usually involves drainage and 'sequestrectomy' of the devitalised dead pieces of bone followed by reconstruction.

Septic arthritis

Acute haematogenous pyogenic infection of the joint usually occurs in infants. The hip is the most commonly involved joint. High-grade fever and swelling around the joint with loss of limb function distal to the joint are the common clinical features. However, children may only present with an unexplained limp. Inflammatory markers (C-reactive protein and ESR) along with white cell count are usually elevated. An ultrasound scan, particularly of the hip in children, is helpful to look for an effusion before proceeding to aspiration. In most cases, aspiration of pus from the joint confirms the diagnosis, necessitating a formal arthrotomy to drain the pus. If less obvious, the fluid should be sent for urgent Gram stain before commencing antibiotics. Intravenous antibiotic cover for the initial 2 weeks followed by oral antibiotics for a total duration of 6 weeks is the usual treatment.

Musculoskeletal tuberculosis

Tuberculosis (TB) is prevalent in certain developing countries and is of concern in developed countries due to immunosuppression from HIV infections. Patients often present with low-grade fever, evening rise of temperature, and loss of appetite and weight along with signs and symptoms of the part affected.

The most common site of musculoskeletal TB is the spine ('caries spine') followed by involvement of large joints, although any joint can be involved. The treatment of TB as recommended by the WHO includes 6–9 months of chemotherapy with a combination of drugs given as an initial intensive phase of 2 months and a subsequent continuation phase. The first-line drugs include isoniazid, rifampicin, ethambutol and pyrazinamide, of which the first two drugs are not withdrawn during the continuation phase.

Spinal tuberculosis

Patients with spinal TB ('Pott's spine') present with pain and muscle spasm, and have different presentations in different regions of the spine. Patients with cervical spine involvement can present with torticollis or may support their chin on their hands (Rust's sign). Thoracic spine caries may have a military attitude while lumbar spine involvement may have a lordotic (Alderman's) gait.

Spinal TB most commonly affects the anterior part of the vertebral bodies adjacent to a common intervertebral disc, the area having a common blood supply (Fig. 27.10). Collapse of the anterior part of the vertebral body due to the destructive pathology may lead to a kyphotic deformity. Neurological deficits ('Pott's paraplegia') usually result from involvement of the mid-thoracic spine where the spinal canal is narrow. The 'cold abscess' formed in spinal TB tracks away from the deep-seated underlying pathology along planes of least resistance such as the neurovascular bundle or fascia covering muscles. It is therefore not as red, warm and tender as a pyogenic abscess.

The treatment of spinal TB includes antitubercular therapy and bed rest in the initial period followed by braces, typically the 'Taylor's brace' or anterior spinal hyperextension (ASH) brace for the thoracic spine. The sterno-occipito-mandibular immobilisation (SOMI) brace or four-post collar is used for the cervical spine and a Halo vest for craniovertebral TB. The healing in spinal TB occurs by fibrous or bony ankylosis. Usually cold abscesses are not drained because they heal well with antitubercular drugs. A large cold abscess (Fig. 27.11), however, may be aspirated or

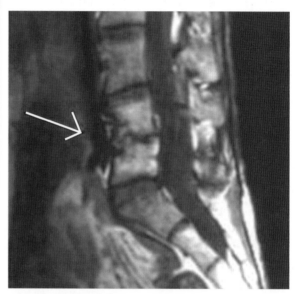

Fig. 27.10 Typically the paradiscal site on either sides of the disc is involved in spinal tuberculosis.

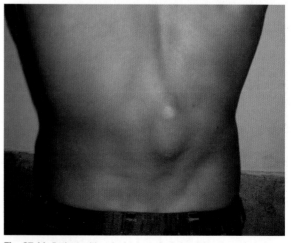

Fig. 27.11 Patient with spinal tuberculosis involving the anteriorly placed vertebral body presenting with a 'cold abscess' on the back.

drained using an antigravity method to prevent formation of a non-healing sinus tract. Pott's paraplegia may require surgical debridement and spinal stabilisation.

Tuberculous hip

The hip is the most common large joint to be involved in TB. It has the following stages:

- *Stage of synovitis*. The joint is swollen and distended to its maximum capacity, resulting in the typical attitude of flexion, abduction and external rotation of the joint with an apparent lengthening of the limb
- *Stage of early arthritis*. Cavitation and destruction of the femoral head and acetabulum results in pain, spasm and night cries. The attitude of flexion, adduction and internal rotation is adopted by the patient with an apparent shortening of the limb. There is less than a centimetre of true shortening due to the destruction of the joint
- *Stage of late arthritis*. Further destruction of the acetabulum results in a significant true shortening of the limb as the femoral head is pulled proximally into the damaged 'migrating' acetabulum (Fig. 27.12).

The treatment of hip TB includes antitubercular therapy along with traction of the hip to relieve the pain and correct the deformities. Healing occurs by fibrosis, resulting in fibrous ankylosis that permits only a minimum range of painful movements. Surgical treatment includes excisional arthroplasty or removal of the femoral head, which eventually results in a short limb but a painless mobile hip allowing patients to sit cross-legged or squat as per their local customs and social needs. Total hip replacement after adequate antitubercular therapy is becoming popular but has the risk of reactivation of the infection.

Tuberculous knee

TB of the knee joint usually commences in the synovial lining of the joint or in the adjoining bones. There may be swelling in the knee joint due to synovitis and a thickened synovium, resulting in a 'doughy' feel proximal to the medial femoral condyle under the thin vastus medialis, which is the first muscle to be 'wasted' in the

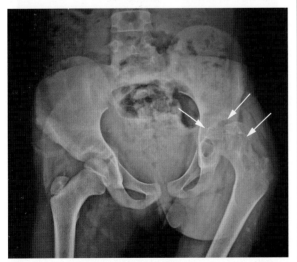

Fig. 27.12 Tubercular arthritis of the hip showing lytic areas within the head of the femur and acetabulum. The damaged osteopenic acetabulum has migrated superiorly and the femur is lying adducted with a subluxed head (*arrowed*).

disease process. There may be a flexion deformity of the knee initially, which later progresses to a typical triple deformity of flexion, external rotation and posterior subluxation. Treatment follows the same principles as for involvement of the hip. The painful arthritic joint may need to be arthrodesed into a stable painless knee.

Poliomyelitis

The incidence of poliomyelitis has decreased with the widespread campaign for vaccination against the polio virus. However, it is not uncommon to see post-polio patients who present with limb length discrepancies, joint contractures and secondary OA.

Orthopaedic procedures

The majority of orthopaedic operations fall into the following categories: the same principles apply to whatever bone or joint is involved.

Arthroscopy

Arthroscopy or keyhole surgery has become an important part of the orthopaedic armamentarium since it was developed in the 1970s. This is a form of minimally invasive surgery where a camera or arthroscope is placed through a small portal and the procedure is performed through a second portal using shavers, burr and other instruments. This initially became popular in the knee for resection of meniscal tears, but is now commonly used in most joints. The techniques have been refined and now tendon repairs and ligament reconstruction are common using specialised bone anchors and sutures.

Arthrodesis

In arthrodesis (or fusion), the diseased residual articular cartilage is removed down to bleeding cancellous bone before the joint is rigidly fixed, resulting in complete loss of movement (Fig. 27.13).

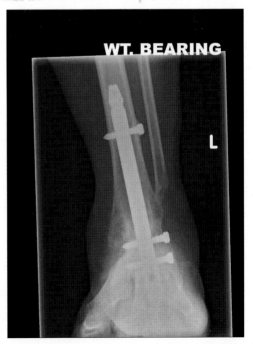

Fig. 27.13 An arthrodesis of the ankle and subtalar joint. The joint has been excised and the bone surfaces have been brought together. An intramedullary nail has been used to hold the position.

27

Small joint fusions of toes and fingers are the most common examples. Fusion of a large joint, such as the hip or knee, will have a significant effect on mobility and will add additional stress on the joints above and below. However, knee arthrodesis may be the only possible salvage procedure in failed infected knee arthroplasty.

Osteotomy

An osteotomy describes an operation in which a bone is broken in order to lengthen, shorten or re-align it. This is useful in the younger more active patient, in whom joint replacement may not meet the patient's expectations. The aim is to change the axis of the joint, so that a portion of the joint surface that has thus far been protected from wear and tear now forms the weight-bearing area. For example, with respect to the knee, although there may be severe OA of the medial compartment in conjunction with a varus (bow-legged) deformity, the lateral compartment may have well-preserved articular cartilage. Over-correcting the varus deformity by means of osteotomy (removing wedges of bone from the tibia), so that body weight is now largely transmitted through the lateral compartment, may lead to significant improvement in symptoms, thus delaying the need for joint replacement.

Arthroplasty

Arthroplasty means 're-forming' of a joint, and is the term used for a joint replacement. Hip, knee, ankle and shoulder replacements are the most common procedures, although almost any joint can now be partially or completely replaced in a number of different ways with varying degrees of success. Indications for different joint replacement vary but the main ones include pain affecting the patient's functional abilities and quality of life (including sleep), worsening joint contractures, and deformities (particularly in inflammatory arthritis) and failure of conservative management.

Successful joint replacement surgery is associated with low revision rates for prosthetic failure of less than 5% at 10–15 years. However rare complications such as dislocation (in hip replacements), infection, stiffness and fractures around the implants due to osteoporosis remain a concern.

Hemiarthroplasty

In this operation, only one-half of the joint is replaced, leaving half of the joint intact. It is normally the natural socket, for example, the acetabulum, that is left untouched. The most common example is following fracture of the femoral neck in the elderly where only the head of the femur is replaced and the acetabulum is untouched. Such patients usually have low demand on the joint, and the hemiarthroplasty (Fig. 27.14) gives adequate function without risking many of the complexities of a total hip replacement in the elderly.

Total joint replacement

This entails resurfacing of both sides of a joint. The choice of materials for the weight-bearing surfaces varies, depending on the joint and prosthesis in question. A metallic femoral head against a high-density polyethylene acetabular liner is most commonly used, although other prostheses involving metal and ceramic surfaces

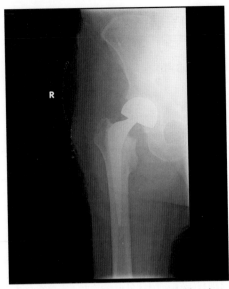

Fig. 27.14 An example of a hemiarthroplasty of the hip, where only the femoral part of the hip joint has been replaced. This type of procedure is commonly used after a displaced intracapsular fracture of the neck of femur in the elderly.

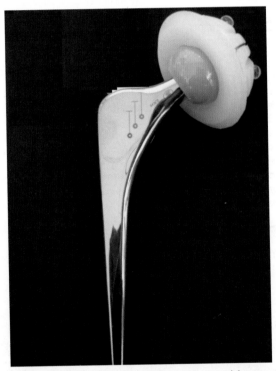

Fig. 27.15 A total hip arthroplasty design showing a modular ceramic femoral head articulating against an ultra-high-molecular-weight polyethylene acetabular cup.

have been developed for use in younger patients (Fig. 27.15). Fixation of the implants may be with cement, or by encouraging bone to grow into or onto the surface of the implant. In small joints, such as those of the fingers and hand in patients with rheumatoid arthritis, silastic prosthesis may be used as a buffer or spacer between the two joint surfaces.

Interposition arthroplasty

The joint is excised and the residual space is filled with autogenous or allograft material. For example, the trapezium in the hand can be excised and the space filled with a rolled-up tendon, such as palmaris longus.

Excision arthroplasty

The joint surfaces are excised, giving a 'joint' formed of scar tissue resulting from fibrosis. For example, in Keller's procedure, the first metatarsophalangeal joint is excised to treat hallux rigidus and in the Girdlestone's operation, the femoral head is excised. The hip heals in a shortened position and patients require a significant shoe raise to equalise the length of their legs, but the joint is relatively pain free and mobile. This would be regarded as a salvage procedure after, for example, removal of an infected hip prosthesis or in TB of the hip.

Paediatric orthopaedic surgery

The growing child presents particular challenges, and certain disease processes may only occur at certain stages of childhood. Surgery must be planned carefully so as not to interfere with the growth plates.

Developmental dysplasia of the hip (DDH)

This is more common in first-born children, females and breech deliveries. It is due to inadequate development of the hip joint (Fig. 27.16), and presents with varying severity. When diagnosed in the newborn, milder forms, in which the femoral head has a tendency to sublux from the acetabulum, are best treated using a 'harness device' that allows freedom of movement while holding the femoral head in the joint. More severe forms, where there is actually fixed dislocation, may require operative reduction and occasionally osteotomies. All newborn babies should be screened for this condition at birth and at 6 weeks for hip instability. Two tests that are commonly performed are the Ortolani and Barlow test.

Perthes' disease

This is a self-limiting disease due to avascular necrosis of a portion of the developing femoral head. The cause is unknown but the disease tends to occur between 4 and 10 years of age and is more common in males. An early stage of inflammation and synovitis is followed by a regenerative stage, in which the necrotic area is replaced by viable bone (reossification). Clinically, the onset is slow and the child complains of pain and limping. Treatment aims to relieve pain and prevent deformity while the femoral head is healing. Prognosis depends on the age of onset, degree of involvement of the femoral head and adequacy of treatment; in general, the older the child, the worse the outcome.

Cerebral palsy (CP)

This is a disorder of movement and posture due to a defect in the developing brain. CP is usually caused by adverse birth events, such as hypoxia and infection, and comes in a variety of forms (spastic, athetoid, ataxic, mixed) and extents: monoplegia (one limb; rare), hemiplegia (one side of the body affected), diplegia (both lower limbs affected), tetraplegia and quadriplegia. Different gait patterns such as scissoring crouch, in-toeing or pigeon gait may be seen in cerebral palsy. Contractures can be treated with regular stretching, botulinum toxin, tendon release or muscle transfer. Bony abnormalities may require osteotomy.

Slipped upper femoral epiphysis (SUFE)

The femoral head epiphysis weakens and the head slips, resulting in the upward and anterior displacement of the femoral neck. SUFE is of unknown aetiology. It usually develops between 10 and 16 years of age, and is most common in boys at the time of their growth spurt; it is found more frequently in the short, overweight, hypogonadal or hypothyroid child, suggesting a hormonal influence. It is a bilateral condition in 25% of cases. It frequently presents with referred pain to the knee and is thus commonly misdiagnosed as a knee problem. The condition may present as a chronic slip that occurs over a few months, or acutely after a seemingly minor episode of trauma. Treatment involves pinning of the slip in situ using a screw. The contralateral side is at risk and in some cases prophylactically fixed. There is a risk of avascular necrosis in severe slips.

Congenital club foot (congenital talipes equinovarus or CTEV)

This is an idiopathic fixed deformity of the foot, which is frequently bilateral. There may be a genetic component and it is twice as common in males. The foot is shaped like a golf club with an outer convex and inner concave border, and has an adducted forefoot with an inverted heel in equinus or plantar flexion.

The idiopathic club foot should be differentiated from a similar-shaped foot seen in spina bifida (examination of the back is essential to rule it out), cerebral palsy and arthrogryposis multiplex congenita (doll-like creaseless skin due to underlying fibrotic muscles). Ponseti's technique of manipulation and serial casting, and if required a tenotomy of the tight tendoachilles, has drastically reduced the requirement of a major surgical correction. Orthotic devices are required to maintain correction.

Neglected club foot is sometimes seen in developing countries and patients may present in late adulthood due to painful arthritic changes (Fig. 27.17). Correction of such deformities may require staged surgical procedure and triple arthrodesis of subtalar, talonavicular and calcaneocuboid joints.

27

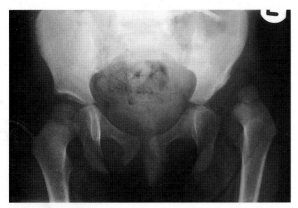

Fig. 27.16 Dysplastic disease of the hip, showing a dislocated left hip.

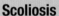

Fig. 27.17 A neglected club-shaped congenital talipes equinovarus foot in an adult, with callosities due to abnormal weight bearing on the convex outer border of the foot (*arrow*).

Scoliosis

This can be divided into structural and nonstructural. 'Nonstructural' scoliosis is secondary to some other problem (e.g., inequality of leg length, lumbar disc prolapse) and disappears when the underlying cause is removed. Nonstructural scoliosis disappears on making the patient sit down or bend forwards (Adam's test). Structural scoliosis is a fixed deformity of the spine caused by a variety of conditions, although 90% of childhood cases are idiopathic. Unlike the nonstructural form, there is an accompanying rotational deformity. The usual presentation of idiopathic scoliosis is between 10 and 13 years of age, and the condition is more common in females. It is usually asymptomatic, with the curve being noticed by the child's parents. Painful scoliosis should be investigated for a potential underlying cause (e.g., tumour). The treatment of scoliosis is complex but involves spinal bracing and surgical intervention.

Angular deformities

Physiological genu varum (bow legs) is often seen in very early childhood. It often corrects and tends to genu valgum (knock knees) between 18 months and 3 years; this then corrects by 4–7 years. It is important not to forget alternative diagnoses, such as rickets and Blount's disease (idiopathic abnormality of the upper medial tibial epiphysis), which is more common in the developing world.

Metabolic bone diseases

Rickets and osteomalacia

Rickets in children and osteomalacia in adults, due to the nutritional deficiency of vitamin D, is frequently seen in developing countries, although the incidence is increasing in the Western world due to poor nutrition and lack of sun light exposure. Failure of adequate calcium supplementation in patients taking antiepileptic medications may result in osteomalacia.

A low serum calcium and phosphorus and elevated serum alkaline phosphatase (ALP) along with radiological evidence of 'cupping, fraying and splaying' of the metaphysis is diagnostic of rickets (Fig. 27.18).

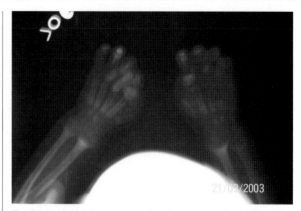

Fig. 27.18 Trumpet-shaped 'cupping, fraying and splaying' of metaphysis of distal end of forearm bones in rickets cause widening of the wrists.

Supplementation of vitamin D and calcium improves the biochemical abnormalities along with the radiological changes of a white line of mineralisation of healed rickets, unless there is vitamin D-resistant or renal rickets.

Osteoporosis

Osteoporosis represents a reduction in bone density due to a higher rate of bone resorption compared to bone formation. The physiological peak bone mass attained in early adulthood decreases in the elderly, more so after menopause in women. Thyroid disorders, Cushing's syndrome and steroid intake increase the degree of osteoporosis.

A DEXA scan quantifies the degree of osteoporosis. Calcium supplementation along with bisphosphonates, nasal calcitonin spray or parathyroid hormone (teriparatide) are used to treat severe osteoporosis.

Musculoskeletal tumours

Musculoskeletal tumours may arise from cartilage, skeletal muscle, synovium or bone, and may be benign or malignant. They are rare, and usually present with deep-seated pain that often continues into the night, or a soft tissue swelling. There may be a history of incidental trauma, to which the symptoms are frequently attributed. High-grade tumours may have a short history (of several months), whereas the more benign lesions have a prolonged course. Clues to malignancy include rapid growth, fracture through the pathological bone, destruction of the bone cortex and invasion into the soft tissues.

Bone tumours may be classified according to cell type (Box 27.1). Radiologically, tumours can also be classified depending on their site within the bone:
- Epiphyseal lesions:
  - Giant cell tumour
  - Chondroblastoma
- Metaphyseal lesions:
  - Osteochondroma
  - Osteosarcoma
- Diaphyseal lesions:
  - Ewing's sarcoma
  - Adamantinoma.

Once a bone tumour is suspected, the patient should be referred immediately to the regional specialist treatment centre

Box 27.1 Classification of bone-forming tumours

Bone-forming tumours
- Benign: osteoid osteoma, osteoblastoma
- Malignant: osteosarcoma

Cartilage-forming tumours
- Benign: osteochondroma, enchondroma, chondroblastoma, chondromyxoid fibroma
- Malignant: chondrosarcoma

Giant cell tumours
- Benign giant cell tumour
- Malignant giant cell tumour

Marrow tumours
- Malignant: Ewing's sarcoma, plasma cell tumour, multiple myeloma, lymphoma

Tumour-like lesions
- Bone cysts: simple bone cyst, aneurysmal bone cyst
- Eosinophilic granuloma
- Fibrous cortical defect

for biopsy, staging and definitive treatment. Over the last decade, advances in adjuvant treatment (chemotherapy prior to and following surgery) have resulted in considerable improvements in long-term prognosis.

The most common tumours affecting the bone are skeletal metastasis arising from primary breast, prostate, lung, gastrointestinal or kidney tumours. The most common primary bone tumour is multiple myeloma, seen in the elderly. Some of the common bone tumours are described here.

Osteoid osteoma

This tumour occurs in young adults and presents with characteristic night pain relieved by salicylates. The lesion consists of a nidus surrounded by dense sclerotic bone, which needs to be excised.

Chondroblastoma

It is also known as *Codman's tumour* and occurs in young adults. The cartilaginous benign tumour advances across the physeal growth plate towards the epiphysis and needs to be removed by curettage and bone grafting.

Osteochondroma

This benign cartilaginous tumour known as *exostosis* may be solitary or multiple. The multiple varieties are believed to be a developmental lesion of the bone known as *diaphyseal achlasis*. The solitary exostosis may be sessile or pendunculated, with a narrow bony base and a cap made of hyaline cartilage. The pendunculated variety grows away from the joint, giving a 'coat hanger' appearance. These painless lesions can develop pain due to overlying adventitious bursitis, stretching of an overlying nerve, fracture through the lesion or with malignant transformation into a chondrosarcoma, which is very rare in solitary lesions (1%) but more common in multiple lesions (5–10%). Rapid growth in size or pain may be a sign of malignant transformation, which may

be missed in the lesions of the axial skeleton, resulting in large-sized tumours within the pelvis or around the scapula. Radiologically, the tumours seem smaller than the clinically palpable lesion since the cartilaginous cap is radiolucent. Calcification in the cartilaginous cap is suggestive of malignant transformation. Treatment consists of excision of the tumour extraperiosteally to prevent recurrence.

Giant cell tumour

Giant cell tumour or osteoclastoma is a benign tumour with potential for local aggression and recurrence. Histopathology shows the characteristic feature of multinucleated giant cells scattered on a background of stromal cells. The classic radiological appearance is of a 'soap bubble' within the epiphyseal large lytic lesion. Treatment consists of various possibilities ranging from curettage, extended curettage, curettage supplemented with cryotherapy using liquid nitrogen or chemical using phenol, curettage and bone cement, curettage and bone grafting, and excision of tumour with reconstruction by arthrodesis or arthroplasty.

Simple bone cyst

This lesion, also known as *unicameral bone* or *solitary cyst*, is a true cyst with a lining membrane inside the bone cavity filled with amber-coloured fluid. The cyst appears in childhood, is asymptomatic, and detected after a pathological fracture or as an incidental finding during routine x-ray. In children, it may grow from the metaphysis near the growth plate towards the diaphysis as it becomes latent. On x-ray, it appears as a centrally located lytic lesion larger longitudinally than transversely within the metaphysis. After a fracture a typical 'fallen leaf fragment' sign is seen but the lesion usually heals spontaneously. Treatment of large or symptomatic cysts includes aspiration and steroid injection. Rarely, curettage and bone grafting is required.

Osteosarcoma

This is a highly malignant bone tumour arising within the metaphysis, usually seen in children just prior to skeletal maturity around the time of closure of the growth plate. The patient typically presents with night pain. The x-ray appearance of the raised periosteal reaction of 'Codman's triangle' is not pathognomonic of this condition. However, a sunburst or sunray appearance is characteristic and results from new bone formation along the tumourous blood vessels. Histopathology shows spindle cells with a pink-staining osteoid matrix. Neoadjuvant chemotherapy is given to decrease the size of the tumour before excision or amputation is undertaken. Limb salvage and tumour prosthesis can be contemplated if the lesion has not become 'extra compartmental' and not infiltrated into the neurovascular bundle.

Ewing's sarcoma

This malignant tumour arises from the endothelial cells of the marrow and is common in children between the age of 10 and 20 years. The child may present with fever and x-ray shows a lamellated periosteal reaction like an 'onion peel' within the diaphysis of the long bones, similar to chronic osteomyelitis. Histopathology reveals sheets of small dark polyhedral cells with no particular arrangement typical of a malignant round cell tumour. Treatment includes preoperative chemotherapy followed by wide excision if accessible or radiotherapy if inaccessible.

27

The upper limb

The shoulder

Anterior dislocation

Anterior shoulder dislocation is the most common form of dislocation, and can be associated with or without fracture (Fig. 27.19). The cause of an anterior dislocation is often traumatic. Treatment involves immediate reduction with analgesia and sedation using Kocher's, Milche's or Hippocratic methods. Patients require to be immobilised in a sling and a check radiograph is mandatory to confirm reduction and exclude a fracture. Instability following shoulder dislocation is common in young males and in this group of patients an arthroscopic examination and stabilisation may be required if there is a high risk of recurrence.

Impingement syndrome

This is a very common cause of shoulder pain. The syndrome describes pain in the subacromial space when the humerus is elevated or internally rotated. During forward flexion, the supraspinatus tendon and bursa become entrapped between the anteroinferior corner of the acromion, leading to so-called *impingement pain*. Steroid injections and physiotherapy may be effective. If there is a bony spur at the undersurface of the acromion that is contributing to the impingement, this can be removed arthroscopically (subacromial decompression).

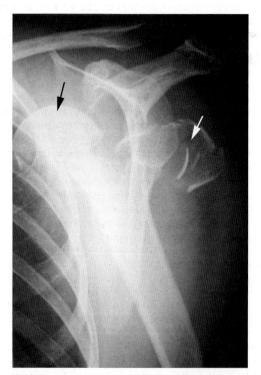

Fig. 27.19 Fracture dislocation of the humeral head. The head of the humerus is fractured from the shaft and is lying dislocated from the glenoid cavity (*black arrow*) and the greater tuberosity is a separate fragment (*white arrow*).

Rotator cuff disease

Rotator cuff disease is a degenerative process affecting the tendons that make up the rotator cuff (supraspinatus, infraspinatus, subscapularis and teres minor). The avascular region near the insertion of the supraspinatus tendon can be particularly affected. Complete or partial tears may be present in up to 50% of the population over 60 years of age, but most are asymptomatic. Acute rotator cuff tears may occur as a result of trauma or chronic impingement. Patients most commonly present with pain around the shoulder and weakness, particularly on shoulder abduction. Treatment options include conservative management with physiotherapy and corticosteroid injections or surgery (arthroscopic repair with a subacromial decompression).

Osteoarthritis

Arthritic changes can affect the glenohumeral or acromioclavicular joints, and may give rise to prolonged pain associated with shoulder movements. Acromioclavicular joint OA is treated with either injection or excision of the joint. OA of the glenohumeral joint may be secondary to avascular necrosis of the humeral head or as a result of previous fracture of the proximal humerus. If conservative methods fail, glenohumeral joint OA can be treated with either a total shoulder replacement or resurfacing procedure.

The elbow

Tennis and golfers' elbow

The most common pathologies to affect the elbow are inflammation of the lateral (tennis) or medial (golfers') epicondyle at the point of insertion of the muscle mass (epicondylitis). The mainstays of treatment are bracing and strapping, injections and physiotherapy. If these fail, operative release of the tendinous insertion may be indicated.

Rheumatoid elbow

Options include a synovectomy, with debridement of the joint and excision of the radial head; interposition and covering the joint surfaces of the elbow with fascia; and total elbow replacement.

The hand and wrist

Wrist disease

The cause of pain around the wrist can be a challenging diagnosis to make. Common causes include those secondary to trauma such as a distal radius fracture (Colles' fracture) or a scaphoid fracture (see 'Trauma' section); degenerative causes such as RA or OA, and those secondary to inflammation affecting the tendon sheaths such as de Quervain's disease, which affects the abductor pollicis longus and extensor pollicis brevis tendons.

Carpal tunnel disease

The median nerve is compressed, either by the tunnel itself or by its contents; for example, by a synovial swelling or increased fluid. Symptoms include pain, 'pins and needles' or sensory loss in the distribution of the median nerve (a variable area of supply normally including the palmar aspect of the thumb, index and middle fingers, with a variable amount of the ring finger involved). Treatment options include night splinting and injection or surgical decompression of the tunnel by releasing the flexor retinaculum overlying the median nerve. This can be done as an open procedure or with an endoscope.

Trigger finger

Thickening of the flexor tendon causes it to jam under the pulley system that would normally allow the tendon to slide backwards and forwards. Injection around the tendon or release of the pulley results in a cure of the condition.

Dupuytren's disease

Thickening of the palmar fascia draws the fingers (predominantly the fourth followed by the fifth) into a flexed and deformed position, resulting in disability and loss of function. It is more common in diabetics and epileptics, and can often be associated with previous trauma to the area affected. The condition mainly affects men over the age of 40 years. Surgery is considered if there is significant disability affecting the fingers. This involves dissecting and removing the thickened fascial bands, either dividing the thickened tissue (fasciotomy), dissecting and removing the thickened fascial bands alone (fasciectomy) or with the overlying skin (dermofasciectomy), taking great care to preserve the associated nerves and blood vessels. In severe cases, amputation of the affected finger may be the best line of treatment.

The lower limb

The hip joint

The main problems are the late complications of young persons' diseases of the hip and OA. Treatment ranges from conservative methods through osteotomy to joint-replacement surgery. Where a remnant of articular surface remains intact, osteotomies may be extremely useful to realign usable portions of cartilage against each other.

Avascular necrosis of the femoral head

This typically presents with severe pain, often at night, and initial x-rays may appear normal in the early stages. MRI is usually diagnostic. If the head has not collapsed, it is usually decompressed via a channel drilled up the femoral neck (core decompression). If the head has collapsed, then total joint arthroplasty may be the treatment of choice.

Hip arthroscopy

Recent developments in hip arthroscopy have led to a greater understanding of the nature of adolescent and adult hip pathologies and their management, particularly in athletes and other young individuals with hip injuries. It remains to be seen whether early diagnosis and treatment of acetabular labral tears or lesions of the cartilage using this technique will curb the progression of OA.

The knee joint

History

The history often points to the likely diagnosis. Inability to carry on playing sport immediately after an injury hints to a ligament rupture. Rapid swelling within a few minutes or hours suggests a major injury within the knee. A large haemarthrosis occurring within the first few hours after an injury indicates a major ligament tear, a peripheral tear of the meniscus or an osteochondral fracture. All of these conditions require further evaluation. Ligament injuries may present in clinic with a history of preceding injury and subsequent instability. Often, this is a feeling of an inability to trust the knee on trying to move from side to side, although the knee may feel stable when the person is running in a straight line. Regular episodes of giving way are thought to accelerate the development of OA. Patterns of injury do tend to coexist and may be related to certain mechanisms of injury.

Meniscal injuries

These are relatively common and occur more frequently in men. Damage to these fibrocartilaginous structures can be acute (normal menisci, sports-related injury, younger patients) or chronic (abnormal menisci, repetitive injuries, elderly patients). The medial meniscus is more commonly affected than the lateral due to its decreased mobility in relation to the capsule. However, a lateral meniscal injury will more likely lead to degenerative changes due to the convex shape of the lateral tibial plateau.

The position of the tear is of clinical relevance in terms of the ability to heal due to varying blood supply, which enters at its periphery. The more peripheral the tear, the greater the chance of repair.

The diagnosis is usually made on the basis of clinical history of pain, swelling, clicking or locking, and occasionally giving way. Joint line tenderness, a locked knee (inability to extend the knee), effusion or a meniscal cyst may be seen. A positive McMurrays or Apley's test is suggestive of a tear in up to 70% of cases. The diagnosis is confirmed by MRI or arthroscopy.

Treatment involves rest, ice, compression, elevation (RICE), analgesia and physiotherapy. Arthoscopic surgery in those cases that are resistant to conservative management or in cases where the knee is locked involves either repair or partial menisectomy.

Ligamentous injuries

Ligament injuries of the knee are very common. They are often associated with a twisting injury or a direct blow to the medial or lateral aspect of the knee. They can occur in isolation as a sprain or rupture, or in combination with other ligamentous or meniscal tears. The pain is often diffuse and extends to beyond the joint. Rapidly developing effusions are often associated with ligament injuries due to their vascularity.

Medial collateral ligament injuries are by far the most common ligament injured within the knee. They can occur in isolation or be associated with an ACL or meniscal injury. The mechanism is often a lateral blow (valgus stress). Diagnosis is usually obvious, with a history of trauma, tenderness and bruising medially, and valgus stress testing positive. MRI can confirm the diagnosis. Management involves RICE, physiotherapy, and in some cases an immobilisation brace can be used. Surgery is indicated in chronic injuries or acute high-grade injuries.

ACL injury is the second most common ligament injury in the knee. Its injury rate is higher in women than in men (4.5:1), and this is thought to be due to neuromuscular forces and control, landing biomechanics and anatomical and genetic factors. The injury is often the result of a noncontact pivoting mechanism. It is not uncommon that the patient feels a 'pop' in the knee and present with an immediate haemarthosis. The Lachmann test is the most sensitive examination for acute ACL injuries. MRI helps to confirm the diagnosis and exclude other associated ligamentous

27

or meniscal injuries. Treatment decisions are individualised on the basis of age, activity level, instability and associated injuries. Initial management consists of physiotherapy to regain a range of movement and reduce swelling. Surgical treatment involves arthroscopic-assisted reconstruction of the ligament using either hamstring tendons (semitendonosis and gracilis) or patella tendon.

The foot and ankle

Sprains of the ankle are very common. Most recover, but damage to the supporting lateral ligaments may lead to recurrent instability and 'giving way' of the ankle. This may be associated with damage to the cartilage in the ankle. Arthritis may occur in any of the joints of the foot; ankle arthritis is increasingly treated with an ankle replacement, but other joints are generally fused or treated nonoperatively.

Foot deformities frequently occur. The most common are pes planus (flat feet with loss of the medial arch) and pes cavus (excessive arching of the foot), leading to chronic foot pain and difficulty in walking. The most common forefoot deformity is hallux valgus (more commonly known as a *bunion*), in which the great toe is deviated in a valgus direction at the metatarsophalangeal joint. Treatment is generally with a metatarsal osteotomy to realign the toe. Hallux rigidus is OA of the first metatarsophalangeal joint and can be treated with insoles, a fusion or a joint replacement. Frequently, the lesser toes may be deformed and are straightened using tendon transfers or fusions. Nerve entrapments are sometimes seen; Morton's neuroma (compression of the digital plantar nerve) and tarsal tunnel syndrome (tibial nerve compression) are the most common.

Trauma and fractures

General approach

The initial assessment and resuscitation of the (multiply) injured patient follows the Advanced Trauma Life Support (ATLS) guidelines (Box 27.2). Management of the injured patient requires a team approach, and often entails joint care by a number of different specialties, from the time of initial resuscitation in the Accident and Emergency department right through to the definitive treatment of each injury. Certain patterns of orthopaedic injuries can be anticipated. For example, patients who fall from a height and land on their feet may be expected to have sustained a fracture to the calcaneus, tibial plateau, hip and pelvis. At impact, patients tend to fall forward, often leading to spinal fractures and head injuries.

 Box 27.2 Advanced trauma life-support guidelines

Primary survey

A. Airway with C-spine control
B. Breathing and ventilation
C. Circulation and haemorrhage control
D. Disability (neurological evaluation)
E. Exposure and environment

Secondary survey

Once the resuscitation efforts are well established and the vital signs are normalising, the secondary survey can begin. This involves a complete history and physical examination, including the reassessment of all vital signs.

Examination

Careful examination of each injured limb includes:

- *Skin.* Ascertain whether any skin breaks communicate with an underlying fracture
- *Circulation.* The most common cause of absent pulses is kinking or compression of the artery by the fracture. Often, reduction of the fracture (realigning the fracture into the anatomical position) or application of traction results in the return of perfusion. Supracondylar fractures of the humerus and femur are likely to result in vascular compromise due to pressure on the brachial or popliteal artery by a displaced fragment of bone
- *Nerves.* Certain injuries may have a high associated risk of neurological injury, manifest by loss of power and/or sensation. For example, the axillary nerve is at risk from shoulder fracture dislocation and its integrity should be documented prior to reduction (see Fig. 27.19)
- *Joint above and below.* Often fractures can involve the joint immediately above or below. A complete examination of these joints is required as it may influence definitive treatment of the injury.

Joint dislocation

Reduction of the joint must be performed as soon as possible, either in the Accident and Emergency department under sedation and/or regional anaesthetic blocks (e.g., distal radius fracture), or in the operating theatre under general anaesthesia. In some cases when closed reduction fails, open surgical reduction is performed.

Fracture management

Classification

Fractures are usually classified by:

- Whether they are in communication with the skin surface (open or compound) or not (closed)
- Their appearance on x-ray: for example, comminuted (in multiple pieces; Fig. 27.20), spiral (where the fracture curves in a large spiral around the long axis of the bone) or transverse (straight across the bone; Fig. 27.21). This appearance usually correlates with the mechanism of injury; a twisting injury tends to cause a spiral fracture, for example
- Anatomical site: for example, intra-articular (involving the joint surface; Fig. 27.22), metaphyseal, epiphyseal or diaphyseal.

Children

Fractures often behave differently in children. Because their bones are more pliable, children may suffer from greenstick fractures, in which the cortex of the bone does not break but bends instead. There may be buckling of a single cortex of the bone (torus fracture). Injuries around the physis or growth plate (Salter–Harris classification; Fig. 27.23) may lead to growth arrest or deformities due to damage of the growth plate. Generally, fractures heal much more quickly in children.

Principles of fracture healing

There are many differing ways of treating fractures. However, they all have the same fundamental objectives: namely, the close approximation of uncontaminated, well-vascularised bone ends in a stable configuration that will maximise bone and soft tissue

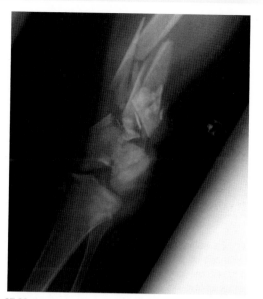

Fig. 27.20 A comminuted fracture of the distal femur also involving the knee joint. The femur can be seen to have broken into multiple (comminuted) fragments.

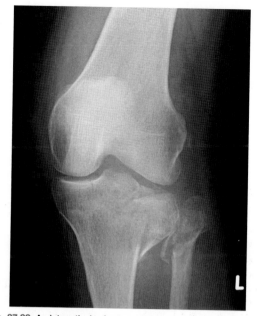

Fig. 27.22 An intraarticular fracture of the lateral tibial plateau of the knee.

Nonunion

Nonunion of a fracture is a complete arrest of the process of union in which continuation of immobilisation fails to achieve union. If the causes of delayed union are not recognised and treated, the fracture may result in nonunion. Loss of bone following an open fracture, muscle interposition between the fracture ends or retraction of fractured ends due to the pull of muscles, such as patellar or olecranon fractures, may result in nonunion. Infection after open fracture may result in infected nonunion.

Treatment of nonunion should ensure good contact of the fracture ends with proper stabilisation and bone grafting. Ilizarov's method of distraction osteogenesis involving controlled distraction of the nonunion site converts the fibroblasts of the scar tissue at the nonunion site into bone. The circular frame of the Ilizarov fixator allows axial micromotion at the fracture site which helps fracture union, contrary to the previous practice of rigid fixation.

Malunion

Fracture ends may unite in a malposition, resulting in unacceptable angulation, rotation or shortening (Fig. 27.24). It is important to recognise unsatisfactory reduction of the fracture at the time of surgery or possible loss of reduction during the period of immobilisation. In children, angular deformities remodel well; however, rotational malunion does not remodel. Unacceptable malunion requires corrective osteotomy.

Open fractures

Open fractures frequently result from high-velocity road traffic accidents and farmyard injuries, and may be grossly contaminated. These injuries should be managed with input from a plastic surgeon. Definitive treatment involves:

- Removal of all the damaged and dead tissue
- Thorough cleaning of the wound, with at least 3–6 L of fluid depending on the degree of contamination ('the solution to pollution is dilution')

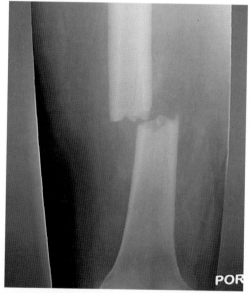

Fig. 27.21 A transverse fracture of the femoral shaft with over 50% displacement.

healing without deformity or loss of function. In general, the fracture-healing process takes approximately 8–10 weeks in adults but can take longer depending on the severity of the injury and whether it is an open fracture.

Delayed union

Some fractures may not unite within the expected time frame and clinically there is tenderness at the fracture site. Delayed union may be due to incorrect splintage, intact adjacent bone in the leg or forearm, or infection following open fractures, and is more common in certain sites, such as the distal femur and tibia. However continuation of immobilisation results in union, albeit 'delayed'.

27

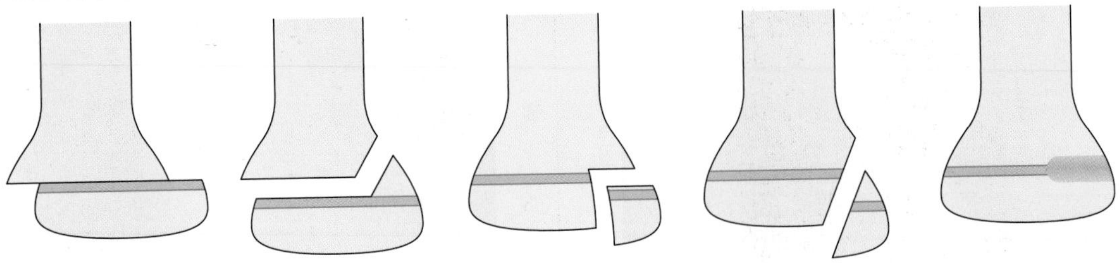

I	II	III	IV	V
Epiphyseal slip only	Fracture through epiphyseal plate with a fragment of metaphysis attached	Fracture through the epiphysis extending into epiphyseal plate	Fracture of epiphysis and metaphysis, crossing the epiphyseal plate	Damage to the epiphyseal plate

Fig. 27.23 The Salter–Harris classification of fractures.

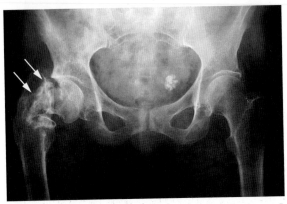

Fig. 27.24 This fracture has healed in a malunited position (arrowed) and would be called a malunion.

- Intravenous antibiotics
- Stabilisation of the fracture to realign the bones to their anatomical position. Depending on the degree of contamination and soft tissue coverage, this may be by definitive or temporary fixation. Temporary external fixators are often secured by means of pins to the bones on either side of the fracture site to allow access to the wound while imparting stability
- Soft tissue coverage, which can be immediate or delayed and can involve direct closure, skin grafts or more sophisticated procedures such as skin, muscle or musculocutaneous flaps.

Intraarticular fractures

It is essential that the joint surface be reconstructed as accurately as possible to minimise the progression of secondary OA. In certain fractures of the humeral and femoral heads, joint replacement may be the best option.

Conservative treatment

Closed fractures with good healing potential are usually treated with external stabilisation using a simple bandage, plaster of Paris (POP) or a synthetic lightweight cast. In some cases where there is significant swelling the initial cast should not encircle the whole circumference of the limb. Use of a 'back slab' of plaster allows the limb to swell and avoids the potential risk of compartment syndrome. Once the acute swelling has settled, the cast can be completed to become a circumferential (full) cast. Displaced fractures often require manipulation under some form of anaesthetic prior to immobilisation in POP.

Compartment syndrome

The diagnosis of compartment syndrome must be considered in any patient with an injury to the limb who complains of increasing pain in the limb, which is refractory to analgesia, out of proportion or worse on passive stretch. Paralysis, paraesthesia, and absent pulses are very late signs. If compartment syndrome is suspected or cannot be excluded, the POP must be split down to skin immediately, even if the fracture position is lost. A pressure transducer can be inserted into the muscle compartments to monitor the pressures, particularly in obtunded patients. Compartment syndrome is diagnosed if the absolute compartmental pressure is greater than 30 mmHg or if the diastolic blood pressure minus the compartmental pressure is less than 30 mmHg (Delta P). Missed compartment syndrome has devastating consequences for the patient, cannot be rectified and is a common cause of medicolegal litigation. If splitting the POP fails to relieve the symptoms of a compartment syndrome very quickly, then urgent surgical decompression of the compartment is required.

Volkman's ischaemic contracture

Arterial injuries or compartment syndrome may result in ischaemic contracture of muscles. Ischaemic injury to the nerves can produce sensory and motor paralysis, which may be partial or complete. The contracted muscles in the forearm lead to claw hand and in the leg cause clawing of the toes. Volkman's sign is based on constant length phenomenon of the contracted muscles wherein the clawed fingers can be stretched out by passive flexion of the wrist. Nonoperative treatment includes either a turnbuckle splint or progressive corrective splints to gradually stretch out the contracted muscles. Surgical release of contracted soft tissues and muscle sliding is used to correct the residual deformities.

Operative treatment

This involves the use of devices that are broadly divided into those that remain external to the skin and those that are internal (screws, plates and nails; Fig. 27.25). The details of their use are beyond

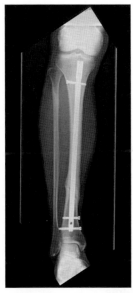

Fig. 27.25 The use of an intramedullary nail to fix a tibial fracture.

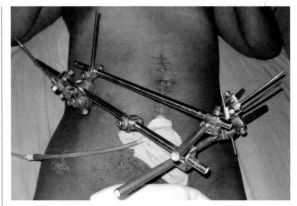

Fig. 27.27 'Damage control' by application of an external fixator in pelvis fractures can be life saving. Note the associated laparotomy wound and suprapubic catheter in this polytrauma patient.

Pelvic fractures

Fractures of the pelvis are common in patients who have suffered high-energy trauma as result of a road traffic injury. More than 2 L of blood may be lost in pelvic fractures without any external evidence of bleeding, necessitating immediate intravenous administration of crystalloids until blood is available. Pelvic compression–distraction should not be attempted more than once by a senior clinician to clinically assess the fracture. A pelvic harness or external fixator (Fig. 27.27) may be life saving for the patient, since the stability provided prevents displacement of the fractured bones and can tamponade any further bleeding. Each time the patient is shifted, movements at the unstable fracture site results in dislodgement of the formed clots, leading to a vicious cycle of consumption coagulopathy.

Fractures of the femoral neck

These are generally seen in the elderly with osteoporotic bone, as a result of low-energy falls and can often result from an underlying medical condition. They are extremely common and utilise very considerable health-service resources. Such fractures are divided into:

- *Extracapsular*, occurring outside the margins of the joint capsule, particularly the metaphyseal trochanteric area of the femur
- *Intracapsular*, involving the femoral neck within the capsule.
- This differentiation is important because blood reaches the femoral head via the capsule and runs along the femoral neck. Extracapsular fractures are normally reduced and stabilised using a pin and plate system, commonly known as a *dynamic hip screw* (DHS), which allows sliding and impaction of the fracture site as the patient walks (see Fig. 27.24).

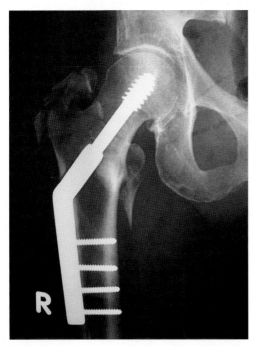

Fig. 27.26 A dynamic hip screw, a device used to secure hip fractures where the hip fracture is extracapsular as shown. The device is dynamic, as the screw can collapse down as the fracture heals.

the scope of this book but depend on fracture type, site and morphology. Some devices are 'dynamic', in that they allow controlled collapse of the fracture, leading to compression of the bone ends and early weight bearing (Fig. 27.26).

Some specific fractures

Detailed treatment of individual fractures is beyond the scope of this book. However, some common fractures and their management principles are discussed here.

Undisplaced intracapsular fractures are pinned in the hope that the blood supply to the femoral head has been preserved and avascular necrosis of the femoral head will not develop. Treatment of displaced intracapsular fractures is a challenge and it still remains 'an unsolved fracture'. Attempt is made to retain the femoral head in a young patient since hip replacement may wear out, requiring revision surgery. Accurate reduction of a displaced intracapsular fracture may require opening the capsule for visualisation of the fracture, further jeopardising the blood supply. In the older patient the preferred treatment is to perform either a

27

hemiarthroplasty or a total hip replacement. These allow immediate weight bearing and a more predictable recovery.

Colles' fractures

This is a type of distal radius fracture, commonly seen in the osteoporotic elderly and is usually sustained as a result of falling onto an outstretched hand. Patients present with pain and swelling, with a dinner fork deformity due to the dorsal displacement of the distal fragment. Treatment involves manipulation under regional anaesthesia (Bier's block) and application of a cast. Surgery is usually performed in intraarticular fractures or fractures that have redisplaced, and involves fixation with either k-wires, a plate or external fixation. Colles' fracture can cause compression of the median nerve or a delayed rupture of the extensor pollicis longus tendon. Smith's fracture is similar but has volar displacement of the distal fragment. Other more specific fracture patterns of distal radius fractures may be seen in young adults.

Forearm fractures

The principle behind all forearm fractures (Fig. 27.28) is that it is difficult to fracture one bone and have displacement and shortening without there being another injury to the other bone in the forearm or to the proximal or distal joint. The fracture(s) may occur at any point along the length of the radius and ulna. Although in the

child it may be permissible to treat these conservatively, in the adult midshaft fractures are almost invariably fixed into anatomical alignment using open reduction and plate fixation. Correct anatomical alignment is essential to allow correct pronation and supination of the forearm.

Scaphoid fractures

These may present with subtle symptoms and signs: typically, pain and tenderness in the anatomical snuffbox following a fall on the outstretched hand. Initial x-rays may fail to demonstrate the fracture and, if clinical suspicion is high, it is wise to immobilise the wrist and repeat the x-ray with anteroposterior, lateral and oblique views at 2 weeks. If suspicion is still high but the x-rays appear normal, further imaging (MRI) should be performed. The scaphoid gains its blood supply for the proximal portion through blood vessels that pass from the distal to proximal pole. Thus, a displaced fracture in the proximal portion of the scaphoid may disrupt the blood supply and lead to nonunion or avascular necrosis, leading to secondary arthritic change.

Ankle fractures

These can involve any portion of the distal tibia or fibula. Technically, the fractures involving the actual articular surface of the distal tibia are known as tibial plafond fractures, whereas fractures involving either the medial or lateral malleoli (and certain

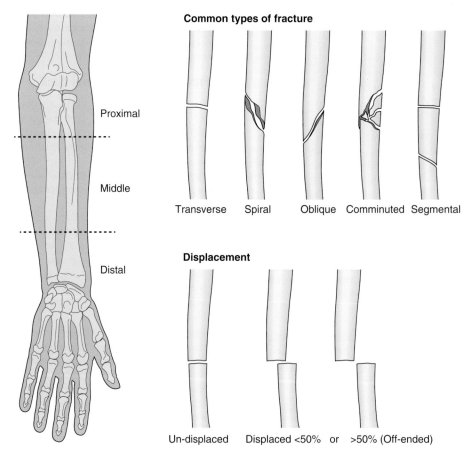

Fig. 27.28 The location and description of many common fracture types.

combinations of fibula injury) are ankle fractures. The types and classification of ankle fracture are complex. The degree of displacement and/or the threat to joint stability will determine whether the fracture can be treated conservatively or requires internal fixation. Stable injuries have a good prognosis almost irrespective of treatment and are managed in plaster cast for around 6 weeks. Internal fixation of unstable fractures is carried out for those injuries that have a high likelihood of displacing in cast or resulting in delayed or nonunion.

Tibial plateau fractures

These are intraarticular fractures of the knee joint involving the tibial plateau in varying forms. Treatment depends on age, the patient's functional level and the degree of displacement. A large proportion of these fractures will require internal fixation to achieve the best clinical result. Complications include knee stiffness and development of OA due to malunion if accurate reduction is not achieved.

Appendix

Laboratory reference ranges

Table A1 Urea and electrolytes in venous blood

Analysis	Reference range SI units	Reference range Non-SI units
Sodium	135–145 mmol/L	135–145 meq/L
Potassium (plasma)	3.3–4.7 mmol/L	3.3–4.7 meq/L
Potassium (serum)	3.6–5.1 mmol/L	3.6–5.1 meq/L
Chloride	95–107 mmol/L	95–107 meq/L
Urea	2.5–6.6 mmol/L	15–40 mg/dL
Creatinine	60–120 μmol/L	0.68–1.36 mg/dL

Table A2 Arterial blood analysis

Analysis	Reference range SI units	Reference range Non-SI units
Bicarbonate	21–29 mmol/L	21–29 meq/L
Hydrogen ion	37–45 nmol/L	pH 7.35–7.43
Pa_{CO_2}	4.5–6.0 kPa	34–45 mmHg
Pa_{O_2}	12–15 kPa	90–113 mmHg
Oxygen saturation	>97%	

Table A3 Other common analytes in venous blood in adults

Analyte	Reference range SI units	Reference range Non-SI units
Alanine aminotransferase (ALT)	10–50 U/L	–
Albumin	35–50 g/L	3.5–5.0 g/dL
Alkaline phosphatase	40–125 U/L	–
Amylase	<100 U/L	–
Aspartate aminotransferase (AST)	10–45 U/L	–
Bilirubin (total)	3–16 μmol/L	0.18–0.94 mg/dL
Calcium (total)	2.1–2.6 mmol/L	4.2–5.2 meq/L or 8.50–10.50 mg/dL
C-reactive protein	<5 mg/L Highly sensitive CRP assays also exist which measure lower values and may be useful in estimating cardiovascular risk	
Gamma-glutamyl transferase (GGT)	Male 10–55 U/L Female 5–35 U/L	–
Glucose (fasting)	3.6–5.8 mmol/L	65–104 mg/dL
Glycated haemoglobin (HbA$_{1c}$)	4.0–6.0% 20–42 mmol/mol Hb	–
Lactate	0.6–2.4 mmol/L	5.40–21.6 mg/dL
Lactate dehydrogenase (total)	208–460 U/L	–
Osmolality	280–296 mmol/kg	–
Osmolarity	280–296 mosm/L	–
Phosphate (fasting)	0.8–1.4 mmol/L	2.48–4.34 mg/dL
Protein (total)	60–80 g/L	6–8 g/dL

Table A4 Haematological values

Analysis	Reference range	
	SI units	Non-SI units
Coagulation screen		
Prothrombin time	10.5–13.5 s	–
Activated partial thromboplastin time	26–36 s	–
D-dimers		
To detect disseminated intravascular coagulation	<200 µg/L	<200 ng/mL
To detect venous thromboembolism	<500 µg/L	<500 ng/mL
Fibrinogen	1.5–4.0 g/L	0.15–0.4 g/dL
Haemoglobin		
Male	130–180 g/L	13–18 g/dL
Female	115–165 g/L	11.5–16.5 g/dL
Leucocytes (adults)	$4.0–11.0 \times 10^9$/L	$4.0–11.0 \times 10^3$/mm^3
Differential white cell count		
Neutrophil granulocytes	$2.0–7.5 \times 10^9$/L	$2.0–7.5 \times 10^3$/mm^3
Lymphocytes	$1.5–4.0 \times 10^9$/L	$1.5–4.0 \times 10^3$/mm^3
Monocytes	$0.2–0.8 \times 10^9$/L	$0.2–0.8 \times 10^3$/mm^3
Eosinophil granulocytes	$0.04–0.4 \times 10^9$/L	$0.04–0.4 \times 10^3$/mm^3
Basophil granulocytes	$0.01–0.1 \times 10^9$/L	$0.01–0.1 \times 10^3$/mm^3
Mean cell volume (MCV)	78–98 fL	–
Packed cell volume (PCV) or haematocrit		
Male	0.40–0.54	–
Female	0.37–0.47	–
Platelets	$150–350 \times 10^9$/L	$150–350 \times 10^3$/mm^3
Reticulocytes (adults)	$25–85 \times 10^9$/L	$25–85 \times 10^3$/mm^3

Index

Note: Page numbers followed by *f* indicate figures, *t* indicate tables, and *b* indicate boxes.

A

AAA. *See* Abdominal aortic aneurysm (AAA)
Abbreviated injury scale (AIS), 100
ABC approach, 24
ABCDE, 104–105
Abdomen
  acute *see* Acute abdomen
  auscultation in, 166–167
  burst, 135–136, 135*f*
  divisions of, 164, 164*f*
  examination of, 253–254
  guarding, 160
  inspection of, 165–167
  pain *see* Abdominal pain
  palpation of, 165–166
  percussion in, 166
Abdominal aortic aneurysm (AAA), 393–394
  asymptomatic, 393–394
  clinical features of, 393
  endovascular aneurysm repair in, 394–396, 395–396*f*, 396*b*
  epidemiology of, 393
  open, repair, 394, 395*f*
  ruptured, 394
  screening for, 393, 393*b*, 394*f*
  symptomatic, 394
Abdominal hernia, 148–158
  complications of, 157–158
  external, 156
  inguinal *see* Inguinal hernia
  internal, 157, 157*f*
  management of complicated, 158
  ventral, 155, 155*f*
Abdominal injury, identification and management of, 109, 109*t*
Abdominal pain, 161*b*, 182
  characteristics of, 164*t*
  movement of, 165, 165*f*
  nature of, 164
  onset of, 164
  pathophysiology of, 159–161
  progression of, 165
  radiation of, 164
  severity of, 164
  site of, 164
  somatic, 159–161
  specific clinical signs in, 167
  visceral, 161 *see also* Acute abdomen
Abdominal paracentesis, 120, 120*f*
Abdominal procedures, 118–120. *See also specific procedures*
Abdominal quadrants, 164, 164*f*
Abdominal tuberculosis, 266, 267*f*
Abdominal wall, 147–158

Abdominal x-ray
  for bowel obstruction, 264, 265*f*
  for gallstones, 225
Abducens nerve(CN VI), 462, 465
Aberrations of normal development and involution (ANDI), breast disease and, 331, 331*t*
ABO antigens, 32, 32*t*
ABO incompatibility, 32
Abortion, 63
Abrasions, 301–302, 426
Abscesses, 57–58
  appendix, 177*b*
  brain, 473, 473*f*
  breast, 334, 334*f*
  cerebellar pyogenic, 474*f*
  cold, 534, 534*f*
  in Crohn's disease, 256
  in crypt, 259, 259*f*
  intraabdominal, 173, 174*f*
  liver
    amoebic, 212, 212*f*
    pyogenic, 211–212
  pancreatic, 240
  pelvic, 174*f*
  perianal *see* Perianal abscess
  pericolic, 268–269
  spleen, 250
  in ulcerative colitis, 256
Absorbable sutures, 113
AC regimen, 344, 346*b*
Accessory nerve (CN XI), 462
Accessory nipples, 326
Acetylcholine, 181
Achalasia, 188, 188*f*
Achlasia, diaphyseal, 539
Acid
  gastric, 181
    hypersecretion, 193–194
  ingestion of, 190
Acid-base balance, 17, 17*f*
Acidosis, 15
  lactic, 18
  metabolic, 17–18, 18*b*
  respiratory, 18, 19*b*
Acinar cell carcinoma, of pancreas, 244
Acoustic neuroma, right, 477*f*
Acquired cardiac disease, 411–419
Acquired coagulopathy, 79
Acquired haemolytic anaemias, 249
Acral lentiginous melanoma, 321, 322*f*
Acromegaly, 363–364
ACTH. *See* Adrenocorticotrophic hormone (ACTH)
Actinic keratosis, 319, 319*f*
Active movement, orthopaedic examination, 530

Acupuncture, for osteoarthritis, 533
Acute abdomen, 159–178
  aetiology of, 159
  appendicitis *see* Appendicitis
  causes of, 160*t*
  clinical assessment of, 163–172
  definition of, 159
  examination of, 165, 166*t*
  gynaecological causes of, 177–178, 178*b*
  history, 164, 164*t*
  investigations for, 167
  management of, 172
  nonspecific abdominal pain in, 177
  pathogenesis of, 161–163
  peritoneal investigations for, 170–171
Acute alcohol withdrawal syndrome, 134
Acute cholangitis, 211*b*
Acute coagulopathy of trauma (ACoT), 26
Acute embolus, in acute limb ischaemia, 391, 391*f*
Acute inflammatory response, 3, 4*t*
Acute limb ischaemia, 389–396
  aetiology of, 389, 390*t*
  classification of, 390, 390*t*
  clinical features of, 390, 390*f*
  intraarterial drug administration for, 392
  management of, 390–391
  symptoms and signs of, 390*t*
Acute lymphadenitis, 523
Acute mesenteric ischaemia, 389
Acute normovolaemic haemodilution, 39
Acute osteomyelitis, 533
'Acute-phase protein response', 7, 8*t*
Acute rejection, 488
Acute renal failure
  perioperative implications, 78
  postoperative, 133
Acute respiratory distress syndrome (ARDS), 132, 132*f*
  massive transfusion complications, 38*t*
Acute suppurative otitis media, 505, 505*b*
Acute suppurative peritonitis, 172
Acute toxic confusion state, 134
Acute transfusion reaction, management of, 37*f*
Acute tubular necrosis (ATN), 23
  burns and, 313
  recovery from, 134
Acute volume replacement, 38
Adenocarcinoma
  of appendix, 255
  bladder, 444

Adenocarcinoma (*Continued*)
  colorectal *see* Colorectal adenocarcinoma
  gastric, 198
  of pancreas, 243–244, 246*b*
    aetiology of, 243
    clinical features of, 244, 244*t*
    curative management for, 245
    multidisciplinary management (MDM) planning for, 245–246, 245*f*
    palliative treatment of, 245–246
    pathology of, 243–244
  of small bowel, 261
Adenohypophysis, 363
  tumours of, 363–364, 363*f*, 364*b*
Adenoid cystic carcinoma, 526
Adenoids, 510, 515*b*
Adenolymphoma, 526, 526*b*
Adenoma-carcinoma progression, 87*f*
Adenomas
  adrenal, 368
  colorectal, 272–274
  liver cell, 217–218
  pituitary, 363, 364*f*
  primary hyperparathyroidism and, 360
  renal, 434
  toxic, 357
Adenomatous polyps, gastric, 198
Adenomyomatosis, 225
ADH. *See* Antidiuretic hormone (ADH)
Adhesion molecules, 3
Adjuvant chemotherapy
  for breast cancer, 344–345, 345*t*, 346*b*
  for colorectal cancer, 281, 281*b*
Adjuvant treatment/therapy
  for breast cancer, 344, 345*b*, 345*t*
  for colorectal cancer, 280–281
Adrenal cortex, 365–366
  adrenal feminisation and, 369
  adrenogenital syndrome and, 369
  Cushing's syndrome *see* Cushing's syndrome
  function, 365–366, 365–366*f*
  hyperaldosteronism *see* Hyperaldosteronism
  tumours of, 370–371
Adrenal feminisation, 369
Adrenal gland, 364–372, 365*f*
  cortex *see* Adrenal cortex
  development of, 364–365
  medulla *see* Adrenal medulla
  pathologies, 372*b*
  surgical anatomy of, 364–365, 365*f*
Adrenal hormones, 4*t*

Adrenal incidentaloma, 371, 371b
Adrenal medulla, 369
  adrenalectomy and, 372
  incidentaloma, 371, 371b
  non-endocrine tumours, 370–371
  phaeochromocytoma and, 369–370, 370b, 370f
Adrenal virilism, 369
Adrenalectomy, 372
  indications for, 372
  patient information and, 372
  replacement therapy in, 372
  technique of, 372
Adrenaline
  in cardiogenic shock, 28
  for practical procedures, 113
α-adrenergic receptors, 441
Adrenocorticotrophic hormone (ACTH), 363
  Cushing's syndrome and, 366–369
  metabolic response to injury, 6f
Adrenogenital syndrome, 369
Advanced Trauma Life Support (ATLS), 102
  guidelines, 542, 542b
Aeroallergens, 508
Afferent arm of immune response, 487
Afferent nerve impulses, 4
Aflatoxin, 218
Age
  breast cancer and, 336, 336f
  breast disease evaluation and, 327
  effect on burn prognosis, 312
  effect on wound healing, 304
Air conduction, 503
Airway
  changing tracheostomy tube in, 116
  endotracheal intubation of, 115–116, 115f
  laryngeal mask, 115, 115f
  maintaining, 114, 114f
  obstruction, postoperative care for, 129
  postoperative care for, 128
  in resuscitation, 104
  in shock, 24
  surgical, 116, 117f see also Ventilation
Airway, breathing, circulation (ABC) approach, 24
Alanine transaminase (ALT), 236
Alberti regimen, 77, 77t
Alcohol
  colorectal cancer and, 276
  oral cancer and, 511
  portal hypertension and, 213
  preoperative assessment, 66
Alcohol-associated pancreatitis, 235
Alderman's gait, 534
Aldosterone, 366f, 366b
  fluid and electrolyte balance, 9–10
  hypersecretion of, 369
  metabolic response to injury, 5
Alfacalcidol, 362
Alkaline, ingestion of, 190
Alkaline phosphatase, 208
Alkalosis
  metabolic, 18, 18b
  respiratory, 18, 19b
Allergic reaction, transfusion reactions, 35t
Allergies, preoperative assessment and, 67
Allocation concealment, in randomised controlled trial, 138
Allograft rejection, patterns of, 488–489, 488t
Altmeier procedure, 295
Alveolus, carcinoma of, 514f, 514b
Amaurosis fugax, 387
Ambu bag, 114–115

Ambulatory manometry, 184–185, 186f
Amelanotic melanoma, 321
American Joint Committee on Cancer (AJCC) staging, for colorectal cancer, 281t
Amine precursor uptake and decarboxylation (APUD) cells, 372
Amino acids, 7
Amoebiasis, colonic, 266
Amoebic liver abscess, 212, 212f
Amoeboma, 266
Ampulla of Vater, 244
Ampullary tumours, 244
Amputation
  in arterial reconstruction, 385, 386f
  empirical therapy, 55t
Amyand's hernia, 148
Amylase
  acute abdomen and, 167
  in pancreatitis, 235–236
  perforated peptic ulcer and, 196
Anabolic flow phase, 3
Anabolism, 8–9
Anaemia
  after peptic ulcer surgery, 197
  perioperative implications, 79
  tolerance of, 33
Anaesthesia, 79
  complications of, 130–136
  epidural, 80
  local, 79–80, 112–113
  local infiltration, 80
  pain assessment, 82
  peripheral nerve block, 80
  postoperative analgesia, 82–83
  previous, 68
  in respiratory disease, 76
  spinal, 80
  topical, 81–82
Anal canal, 283, 284f
  epithelium, 283–284, 284f
  lymphatic drainage, 285
Anal cancer, 293–294, 293f, 294b
  assessment of, 293
  clinical features of, 293, 293f
  management of, 294
  staging of, 293–294, 294t
Anal continence, 285b
Anal cushions, 284–285
Anal fissure. See Fissure-in-ano
Anal glands, 284, 285f
Anal incontinence, 296–297, 297b
  aetiology of, 296, 296t
  assessment of, 296
  clinical features of, 296
  management
    conservative, 296–297
    surgical, 297
Anal intraepithelial neoplasia (AIN), 293, 293f
Anal polyp, fibroepithelial, 292
Anal skin tags, 292
Anal sphincters, 283, 284f
  chemical relaxation of, 289
  implantable artificial, 297
  repair, 297
Analgesia
  for acute abdomen, 166
  epidural, 82
  multimodal, 82
  postoperative, 83b
    in respiratory disease, 76
    strategy, 82–83
Anaphylactic shock, 20, 28
Anaphylaxis, management of, 28t
Anaplastic carcinoma, 358–359
Anastomotic leak, 272
Anatomic bypass, 383, 383f
Anderson-Hynes pyeloplasty, 440f
Androgenic steroids, 366b

Androgens, 8–9
Aneurysmal SAH, management of, 467–468
Aneurysms, 392–393
  abdominal aortic see Abdominal aortic aneurysm (AAA)
  aetiology of, 392–393
  aortic see Aortic aneurysm
  atherosclerotic, 392
  clipping in, 467, 467f, 467b
  coiling in, 467, 467b, 467f
  false, 393, 393f, 418
  femoral, 396
  iliac, 396
  left ventricular, 414–415
  morphology of, 393
  mycotic, 392–393
  saccular intracranial, 466
  site of, 392
  of splenic artery, 250
  true, 393, 393f
  tubulosaccular, 417–418, 418f
  in vascular access, 408
Angell's sign, 457
Angina
  perioperative implications, 73
  surgery for, 411–415
Angiodysplasia, 271
Angiography
  in acute abdomen, 170
  coronary, 412, 413f see also Computed tomographic (CT) angiography; Magnetic resonance angiography (MRA)
Angiosarcoma, 325
  hepatic, 219, 219f
Angiotensin, 4t
Angiotensin-converting enzyme (ACE), 5
Angiotensin-converting enzyme (ACE) inhibitors, 75
Angular deformities, 538
Angular dermoids, 483
Anion gap, 17–18
Ankle, orthopaedic surgery for, 542
Ankle/brachial pressure index, in critical limb ischaemia, 379
Ankle fractures, 546–547
Ankylosing spondylitis, 533
Annular pancreas, 234
Anorectal disorders, 285–292
Anorectal sepsis, 290b
Anorectum, 283–298
Anorexia, causes of, 43, 43t
Antecubital fossa, 120
Anterior circulation, in brain, 462
Anterior cruciate ligament (ACL), injury, 541–542
Anterior drawer test, 530
Anterior spinal hyperextension, 534–535
Anthracyclines, breast cancer and, 344, 348
Anti-HER2 therapy, 345, 345b, 348
Antibacterial agents, topical, 314
Antibiotic prophylaxis, 52, 52t, 52b, 72–73, 72t, 72b
  antibiotic choice, 52
  carriage of resistant organisms and, 52
  for cholecystectomy, 228, 228b
  dose, 52
  for immunosuppressed patients, 52
  timing of, 52
  wounds, 304–305
Antibiotics, 48–59
  for breast infections, 334t
  effect on commensals, 48
  endocarditis, 415
  for lymphoedema, 406
  policy, principles of, 54t
  in septic shock, 26, 27b
  for sore throat, 515b
  for surgical infections, 53–54, 54t

Antibody-mediated rejection, 488
Antibody screening, pretransfusion, 32
Antibody therapies, 490
Anticoagulants
  perioperative implications, 78–79
  preoperative assessment, 67
Antidepressants, preoperative assessment and, 67
Antidiuretic hormone (ADH), metabolic response to injury, 5
Antigen presentation, 488, 488f
Antioxidants, 3
Antiplatelet therapy, preoperative assessment and, 67
Antiproliferative agents, 489–490
Antireflux surgery, 186–187, 186b
Antithyroid drugs, 355
Antrectomy, for duodenal cancer, 195
Anuria, 430
Anus
  anatomy of, 283–285
  innervation, 283
  itching, 297
  musculature, 283, 284f
  pain, causes of, 285b
  stretching of, 289
Anxiolytic medication, preoperative, 73
Aorta, coarctation of, 420, 421f
Aortic aneurysm, 417–418
  abdominal see Abdominal aortic aneurysm (AAA)
  aortic dissection, 418, 418f
  aortoannulo ectasia, 418
  assessment, 419, 419f
  false, 418f
  surgery, 419
  tubulosaccular, 417–418, 418f
Aortic dissection, 418, 418f
Aortic valve
  regurgitation, 416
  stenosis, 416, 416f
  surgical outcomes, 416
Aortoannulo ectasia, 418
Aortobifemoral bypass, 383t
APACHE II score, for pancreatitis, 236, 237f
Aphthous ulcers, 511
Apnoea, sleep, 515–516
Apocrine sweat glands, 301, 316
Appendicectomy, 176, 176b
Appendicitis, 255
  acute, 174–177, 176–177b
    aetiology of, 174
    anatomy of, 174, 174f
    clinical features of, 175–177
      variations in, 175
    complications of, 176
    differential diagnosis of, 175t
    epidemiology of, 174
    examination of, 175
    history of, 175
    investigations of, 176, 176f
    management of, 176
    pathogenesis of, 175
    prognosis of, 177
  gangrenous, 176
Appendix, 174, 174f
  abscess, 177b
  anatomy of, 253
  disorders of, 255
  function of, 253
  mass, 176–177, 177b
  perforation of, 175
  tumours of, 255, 255b
APUD cells, 372
Apudomas, 372
Arachnoid, 462
Arm claudication, in atherosclerosis, 386
Aromatase inhibitors, breast cancer and, 345

Arrhythmias
significance of, in perioperative period, 69t
surgery complications of, 133
Arterial anastomosis, 494, 495f
Arterial blood gas analysis, 17, 17t, 421t
preoperative, 70, 70t
in shock, 24
Arterial blood sampling, 124
Arterial catheter, 75t
Arterial disease
clinical features of, 375, 377b
haemodynamic mechanism of, 375
mechanism of injury, 375–376, 378f
pathophysiology of, 375–376, 377f
of upper limb, 386–389
see also Atherosclerosis
Arterial oxygen content, 65
Arterial reconstruction
complications of, 384–385
indications for, 382
principles of, 382–384
Arteriolar vasoconstriction, 21
Arteriovenous malformations, 468, 468–469f
Arthritis
of foot and ankle, 542
in tuberculous hip, 535f
Arthrodesis, 535–536, 535f
Arthroplasty, 536
excision, 537
interposition, 537
Arthroscopy
hip, 541
in orthopaedic surgery, 535–536
Aryepiglottic folds, 517–518
Asbestos exposure, 424–425
Ascaris lumbricoides, 266
Ascaris worms, 235
Ascites, in portal hypertension, 216–217, 217f
Aseptic peritonitis, 172
Aseptic techniques, 50, 112, 113t
Asiatic cholangiohepatitis, 231
Aspiration, pleural, 118, 118f
Aspirin, as protective agent, for colorectal cancer, 276, 276b
Asthma, 66, 83
Astrocytomas, 479
Asymptomatic AAA, 393–394
Asymptomatic carotid disease, 388
AT regimen, 346b
Atelectasis, 131
Atheroembolism, 375
in atherosclerosis, 386
Atheroma, 269
Atherosclerosis
clinical features of, 375, 377b
mechanism of injury, 375–376, 378f
pathophysiology of, 375–376, 377f
Atlanto-axial subluxation, 79
Atonic myogenic bladder, 453
Atrial fibrillation, surgery complications of, 133
Atrial natriuretic peptide (ANP), 10
Atrial septal defect, 420
Attic, 502
Atticoantral disease, 505–506
Atypical lobular hyperplasia (ALH), 337–338
Audiometry, 503, 503–504f
Auerbach's plexus, 181, 252, 271
Auscultation, abdominal, 166–167
Autoimmune thyroiditis, 354
Autonomic neuropathy, in critical limb ischaemia, 380
Autonomy, 60, 61b
Autosomal polyposis syndromes, 276
Avascular necrosis, of femoral head, 541
Axillary lymph nodes, 326, 327–328f, 328, 339, 339f

Axillary surgery, for operable breast cancer, 343–344
Axillary vein thrombosis, 405
Axonal injury, diffuse, 473
Azathioprine, 489
Azygous veins, 179

B
B-cell activation, 488
B-lymphocytes, 50
Back-table preparation
liver transplantation and, 497
pancreas transplantation and, 498–499, 498f
renal transplantation and, 494
Bacteraemia, 20b
Bacterial contamination, 35t
Bacterial factors, infections and, 48, 49f
Bacterial infections
intracranial, 473–474, 474f
in pancreatitis, 235
Bacterial overgrowth, 254
Bacteriology, in acute abdomen, 168
Bacteroides species, 54t
Balanced solutions, intravenous fluids, 13
Balanitis, 455
Balanitis xerotica obliterans (BXO), 456
Balloon angioplasty (BAP), in critical limb ischaemia, 381f, 382, 382b
Balloon dilatation, oesophageal sphincter, 188
Balloon tamponade, variceal bleeding, 215, 215f
Banff 07 diagnostic criteria, 488, 488t
Bariatric surgery, 203–205, 205b
complications of, 205
obesity and related comorbidities, 204–205
Barium enema, 126
Barium meal, 184f
Barium sulphate, 126
Barium swallow, 126, 516–517
Barrett's oesophagus, 186–187, 186b
Barron's rubber band, for haemorrhoids, 286–287, 287f
Basal cell carcinoma, 320, 320f
Basal germinal cells, 317t
Basal metabolic rate (BMR), 7
Bassini's herniorrhaphy, modified, 152
Bat ears, 504
Bell's palsy, 507, 507b
Beneficence, 60, 61b
Benign disease, breast cancer and, 336
Benign naevi (moles), 318–319, 318f
Benign paroxysmal positional vertigo, 506
Benign prostatic hyperplasia (BPH), 445–449
clinical features, 446
investigations, 446–447
management, 447–448
open prostatectomy, 449
pathology, 445–446
Better Blood Transfusion programmes, 39
Bezoars, 203, 203f
Bicarbonate, 9
Bier's block, 546
Bile acids, 220
Bile duct, 219–232
carcinoma of, 231–232, 232f
congenital abnormalities, 221–222
injury to, as cholecystectomy complication, 228
physiology, 220–221
stricture, 229–230, 230f
Bile leakage, as cholecystectomy complication, 229
Bile salts, 220–221, 221b
Biliary atresia, 221

Biliary colic, 163, 223
Biliary cyst, 211, 211f
Biliary hamartoma, 217
Biliary pain, atypical, 230
Biliary system, anatomy of, 219–220, 220f
Biliary tract, 206–232
tumours of, 231–232
Billroth I gastrectomy, 195
Biochemical investigations, 433–434
for jaundice, 208
Biochemistry, preoperative assessment and, 69
'Biological' dressings, 314
Biological valve prostheses, 415f
Biopsy
core see Core biopsy
intracranial tumours and, 479
liver, 210
open see Open biopsy
sentinel lymph node see Sentinel lymph node biopsy
Birth history, orthopaedic surgery, 528–529
Bladder
anatomy, 441
atonic myogenic, 453
chronic outflow obstruction, 452
diverticula, 445–446
emptying, 453 see also Micturition
hypersensitive, 452
neck obstruction, 441b
storage, 442
thimble, 439
trauma, 442–443
tumours see Bladder tumoursLower urinary tract
Bladder tumours, 444–445
clinical features, 444, 444f
invasive, 445
investigations, 444, 445f
management, 444–445
pathology, 444
prognosis, 445
staging, 443f, 444
superficial, 444–445
Blast injury, 99
Bleeding
as cholecystectomy complication, 228
in diverticular disease, 269
nose, 508–509, 509b, 509t, 509f
peptic ulcer, 196–197
variceal, 215–216, 215t, 215f, 215–216b see also Haemorrhage
Blinding, in randomised controlled trial, 138
Blisters, 312
α-blockers, 448
β-blockers, in perioperative management, of cardiovascular disease, 75
Blood
administration of, 33–34, 34b
components, 29–31, 30f
flow-conserving measures, 5–7
preoperative donation, 35
salvage, intraoperative, 39
urinary, 429, 430t
volume in hypovolaemic shock, 25
Blood borne viruses, preoperative assessment and, 70–71
Blood buffers, 17
Blood culture, venepuncture for, 121, 121b
Blood donation, 29
Blood gas analysis
for acute abdomen, 167
see also Arterial blood gas analysis
Blood glucose, 168
Blood grouping, 32

Blood pressure
in shock, 25 see also Hypertension; Hypotension
Blood supply
in brain, 462, 463f
influence on wound healing, 304
Blood tests
acute abdomen, 167
gastrointestinal bleeding, 197
oesophagus, stomach and duodenum, 182
urological surgery, 430
Blood transfusion, 68
acute volume replacement, 38
administration of blood, 33–34, 34b
adverse effects of, 34–35, 34f, 36t
autologous, 35–36
Better Blood Transfusion programmes, 39
burns and, 313
cardiopulmonary bypass, 38
errors, 35b
future trends, 39
indications, 33, 33b
massive, 38, 38t
methods to reduce need for, 38–39
pretransfusion testing, 32–33
reducing the need for, 39
intraoperative measures, 39
postoperative measures, 39
preoperative measures, 39
requirements in special settings, 36–38
surgical ward postoperative care for, 130
Blood vessels, metabolic response to injury, 3, 4f
Blue naevi, 319
Blummer's shelf, 182
Blunt trauma, 99
BMPR1A gene, 275
Boas's sign, 167, 223
Body mass index (BMI), 40–42, 41b, 203
Boerhaave's syndrome, 183f, 189
Bolam case, 63
Bone and joint infection, orthopaedic surgery for, 533–535
Bone conduction, 503
Bone cyst, simple, 539
Bone disease, and breast cancer, 348–349
Bone scans, 449–450
orthopaedic surgery, 531, 532f
Botulinum toxin, 188
Bow legs, 538
Bowel preparation, for surgery, 278
Bowel sounds, 166–167
Bowen's disease, 319
Brachialgia, 483–484
Brachytherapy, 450
oesophageal cancer, 193
Bradycardia, surgery complications of, 133
Brain
abscess, 473, 473f
anterior circulation in, 462
blood supply in, 462, 463f
death, 491, 493t
injury, 470 see also Head injury
metastases, 349, 477, 478f
oedema, 473–474
posterior circulation of, 462
surgical anatomy and physiology of, 461–462
Brain herniation syndromes, 463
false localising signs and, 464–465
Brain tissue metabolism, 465
Brainstem
death, 493t
glioma, 480f
Branchial cyst, 521, 521t, 521f
Branchial fistula, 521

Bravo capsule, 184–185, 185f
BRCA1/BRCA2 genes, 337
Breast, 326–350
  anatomy of, 326, 327f
  asymmetry, 326
  benign conditions of, 331, 331t
  cancer *see* Breast cancer
  cancer types and, 338
  congenital abnormalities of, 326
  disease *see* Breast disease
  hormonal control of breast
    development and function, 326
  lumpiness and, 331–333
  male, 349–350
  miscellaneous tumours of, 349
  nodularity and, 332, 332f
  pain *see* Mastalgia
  physiology of, 326
  reconstruction, 347, 347f
Breast cancer, 335–349
  clinical examination of, 327–328,
    327–328f
  complications of treatment, 346
  curability of, 340
  epidemiology of, 335, 336t
  follow-up and, 347
  growth factor receptors and, 338
  hormone receptors and, 338
  imaging in, 328–329, 329b
  invasive, 338
  male, 350
  mammographic features of, 339, 339f
  management, 337
    of locally advanced, 342f, 347–348,
      347t, 347f, 348b
    of metastatic or advanced, 348,
      348b
    of operable breast cancer, 343
      breast conservation and, 343,
        343–344b
      local therapy and, 343–344
      in situ breast cancer, 343
      systemic therapy and, 344, 345b
  mortality rates in, 339b
  noninvasive, 336t, 337–338,
    337–338f
  in pregnancy, 346
  presentation of, 341–343, 341–343f
  prognosis of, 340–341, 341f
  psychological aspects of, 346
  risk factors for, 336–337
  screening for, 338–339, 339b
  spread of, 326
  staging of, 339–340, 340t
  types of, 337–338
Breast-conserving surgery, for operable
    breast cancer, 343
Breast disease
  aberrations of normal development
    and involution (ANDI), related to,
    331, 331t
  atypical hyperplasia and, 332–333,
    336
  benign neoplasms and, 333–334,
    334b
  clinical examination of, 327–328,
    327–328f
  of cyclical change, 331–332
  duct papilloma and, 333, 333f
  fine-needle aspiration cytology
    (FNAC), core biopsy and,
    329–330
  history of, 327
  imaging and, 328–329
  infection, 334–335, 334t, 335b
  investigations, accuracy of, 330, 330t
  lipoma and, 333
  patient with, assessment of, 326–330,
    327f
  phyllodes tumour and, 333–334, 333f
  regional nodes, assessment of, 328,
    328f

Breast disease (*Continued*)
  skin-associated infection and, 335,
    335f
Breathing
  postoperative care for, 128
  in resuscitation, 104
  in shock, 24
Breslow staging, malignant melanoma,
  322
British Committee for Standards in
    Haematology, 33–34
Bronchial obstruction, 129
Bronchiectasis, 427
Bronchogenic carcinoma, 421–422,
  422f, 422b
Bronchospasm, 129
Bubonocoele, 150
Buccal mucosa, carcinoma, 514f, 514b
Buerger's disease, in arterial
    reconstruction, 384–385, 385b
Buffalo hump, 367
Buffers, blood, 17
Bullectomy, 426
Bunion, 542
Bupivacaine, 80t
Burns, 308–315, 312b
  classification of, 309–312, 310f
  consequences of, 311b
  depth of, 310–312, 311f
  first aid for, 312, 312t
  general effects of, 308
  hypovolaemic shock and, 313, 313t
  local effects of, 308, 310t
  management of, 312–315
  mechanisms of, 308
  prognosis, 312
  size of, 309, 310–311f
  wounds, 301–302
Burst abdomen, 135–136, 135f
Bypass grafting, in arterial
    reconstruction, 383, 383f, 383t
Bypass surgery
  in critical limb ischaemia, 382, 382b
  gastric, 204f, 205

C

Caecum, 253
  perforation of, 264
Calcified tissue, 126
Calcineurin inhibitors (CNIs), 490
Calcitonin, 351–352
Calcium, 16
  acute abdomen and, 168
  serum, 168
Calcium oxalate stones, 436
Calcium phosphate stones, 436
Calculi
  radiolucent, 437
  salivary gland, 519, 524–525
  urinary tract, 436–438
Calot's triangle, 220
Calprotectin, fecal, 254
Calvaria, 461
Cancer, 86–97
  adjuvant treatment of, 95–96
  advanced, palliation of, 96
  biology of, 86–89, 86b
  carcinogenesis of, 87–88, 87f, 88b
  cell cycle and, 86, 86b
  cell replication and, 86, 87f
  counselling of, 96
  diagnostic investigations of, 92–93,
    92t, 92–93f
  dying from, 96–97
  estimate of cure of, 89, 89f
  follow-up for, 96, 96b
  GP for, consultation with, 92
  immunosuppression and, 490–491
  inherited, screening for, 90–91
  invasion of, 88–89, 88f, 89t
  investigations for, 92–93
  local effects of, 91

Cancer (*Continued*)
  management of, 90–97, 91f, 91t
  metastasis of, 88–89, 88–89f, 89t
  natural history of, 89
  prognosis of, 96
  referral for, 92
  screening of, 90–91, 90–91b, 90f, 91t
  staging investigations of, 93, 93f, 93b
  symptoms of, 91–92, 92b
  systemic effects of, 91–92
  treatment of, 93–96, 95–96b
Cancer cachexia, 91–92
Candida infection
  Candida albicans, 57
  sepsis, empirical therapy for, 55t
Cannulae, parenteral nutrition, 45
Cannulation
  central venous, 123b, 123f
  of internal jugular vein, 122–123, 123f
  of subclavian vein, 123, 123f
Capacity, 61
Capecitabine, 280–281
Caput medusae, 213–214
Carbimazole, 355
Carbohydrate metabolism, 7, 9b
Carbolic acid, 48
Carbon dioxide, 21
Carcinogenesis, 87–88, 87f, 88b
Carcinoid syndrome, 373–374
Carcinoid tumours, 202, 255, 373–374,
    373t, 424
  large bowel, 282
  small bowel, 261, 262f
Carcinoma in situ, ductal, 337–338,
    337–338f, 343b
Carcinomas
  adrenal, 368
  anaplastic, 358–359
  basal cell, 320, 320f
  bile ducts, 231–232, 232f
  bladder, 231
  bronchogenic *see* Bronchogenic
    carcinoma
  buccal mucosa, 514f, 514b
  floor of the mouth, 514,
    514b, 515f
  follicular, 358, 358f
  gastric, 198–199
  hard palate, 515, 515b
  hepatocellular, 218, 218b
  larynx, 518, 518b
  lip, 511, 513b, 513f
  medullary, 359–360
  mucoepidermoid, 526, 526f
  papillary, 358
  penile, 456, 456f
  renal, 435–436, 435f
  renal pelvis, 436
  squamous cell *see* Squamous cell
    carcinoma
Cardiac catheterisation, 410t
Cardiac complications, 132
Cardiac disease
  acquired, 411–419
  congenital, 411–419
Cardiac failure, surgery complications of,
  133
Cardiac investigations, preoperative
    assessment, 69, 69t
Cardiac output (CO), 20
  in cardiogenic shock, 28
Cardiac tamponade, 105
  with penetrating trauma, 419
Cardiac transplantation, 428
Cardiac valvular disease, 415
  assessment of, 415
  surgical management of,
    415, 415f
Cardinal symptoms, of musculoskeletal
    system, 528, 528b
Cardiogenic shock, 20–21, 28, 102
Cardioplegia, 409–410

Cardiopulmonary bypass (CPB), 409,
    410–411f
  blood transfusion, 38
Cardiopulmonary exercise testing, 70
Cardiothoracic surgery, 409–428
  complications, 411
  mortality, 409
  pathophysiological assessment, 409,
    410t
  postoperative care, 410–411
  recovery time, 411, 412f
  risk, assessment of, 409
  stroke, 409
  surgical technique, 409–410 *see also*
    specific techniques
Cardiovascular disease
  perioperative implications of,
    73–75
  perioperative management of, 75, 75t,
    75b
Cardiovascular system
  effect of shock on, 23, 24b
  obesity and, 67t
  preoperative assessment and, 65–66,
    69b
Care pathways, 140b
  complications and, 140b
  guidelines and, 140
Caroli's disease, 222
Carotid arteries
  disease *see* Carotid artery disease
  internal, 462
Carotid artery disease, 387–388, 387f
Carotid artery stenting (CAS), 388, 388f
Carotid body tumour, 527, 527f, 527b
Carotid endarterectomy (CEA), 388,
    388b, 389f
Carotid sheath, 519
Carpal tunnel disease, 540–541
Carpal tunnel syndrome, 486
Case-control study, 139
Case reports, 139–140
Case series, 139–140
Caseation necrosis, 523
Cast, in urine, 168
Castration, 450
Catabolic flow phase, 3
Catabolism, 7–8, 9b
Catastrophic haemorrhage, 103
Catecholamines, 369
  carbohydrate metabolism, 7
  fat metabolism, 7
Catheters
  arterial, 75t
  cardiac, 410t
  central venous, 75t
  nasobiliary, 229
  parenteral nutrition, 46, 46t
  pulmonary artery, 75t
  surgical ward postoperative care for,
    130
  urinary, 56, 56f, 432f
Cauda equina syndrome, 484
Caval filters, for venous
    thromboembolism, 404
Cavernomas, 469, 470f
Cavernous haemangiomas,
    211, 217
CD4 T cells, 488
CD8 T cells, 488
Cell cycle, cancer and, 86, 86b
Cell-mediated immunity, 248
Cell replication, cancer and, 86, 87f
Cell salvage, 36
Cellular function, in shock, 22, 23f
Cellulitis, 305, 315, 510f
Central cord syndrome, 473
Central infection, 334–335
Central nervous system
  procedures, 125–126 *see also*
    specific procedures
  vascular disorders of, 469b

Central pontine myelinolysis, 15
Central venous access, trauma and, 104
Central venous cannulation, 123b, 123f
Central venous catheter, 75t
    insertion of, 122–123, 122b
    peripherally-inserted, 123–124
Cerebellar impaction, 464
Cerebellar pyogenic abscess, 474f
Cerebellopontine angle, MRI of, 504f
Cerebral blood flow, 462
Cerebral complications, 134
Cerebral oedema, 15
Cerebral palsy (CP), 537
Cerebral perfusion pressure (CPP), 463
Cerebrospinal fluid
    drainage, 482, 482f
    surgical anatomy and physiology of,
        462
Cerebrovascular accidents (CVAs), 134
Cerebrovascular disease, 465–469,
    469b
Cerumen, 504
Cervical cancer, 453
Cervical cytology, 90, 90f
Cervical intraepithelial neoplasia (CIN),
    293
Cervical lymphadenopathy, 512–513,
    513t
Cervical spine
    spinal degenerative disease,
        483–486, 484–485f, 486b
    trauma, 473
Cervical sympathectomy, 428
Cetuximab, 281
Chagas' disease, 188
Cheilitis, 513b
Chemotherapy
    adjuvant see Adjuvant chemotherapy
    breast cancer, 346b, 348
    for cancer, 95
    complications of, 346
    gastric cancer, 201, 201b
        palliative, 201, 202b
    hepatocellular carcinoma, 218
    oesophageal cancer, 192
Chenodeoxycholic acid, 220
Chest infection, treatment of, 55t
Chest pain, 188
Chest wall deformities, 428
Chest wound, sucking, 425
Chest x-ray, 410t, 421t
    in acute abdomen, 168, 168f
    oesophageal perforation, 189
    oesophagus, stomach, and
        duodenum, 183, 183f
    preoperative, 70
Chiari II malformation, 481
Child-Turcotte-Pugh (CTP) grading
    system, 214, 214t
Childbirth, incontinence after,
    452–453
Childhood rectal prolapse, 295
Children
    acute abdomen in
        causes of, 160t
        examination of, 165
    appendicitis in, 175
    fractures in, 542
    informed consent and, 62
    otitis media in, 505b
    renal tumours in, 435t
Chin-lift manoeuvre, 114, 114f
Chlamydial infection, 178
Chloride, 9
Cholangiocarcinoma, 218
    bile duct, 231, 232f
    pancreatic, 244
Cholangiohepatitis, Asiatic, 231
Cholangitis
    acute, 211b, 230–231
    primary sclerosing, 231
    treatment of, 55t

Cholecystectomy, 227b
    cholecystitis, 224
    complications of, 226b, 228
        intraoperative, 228
    for gallstones, 225, 225b
    laparoscopic, 225–227, 226–227f
    open, 226, 226f
    timing of, 224b
Cholecystitis
    acute, 223, 224b
    chronic, 223–224
    complications of, 223
    management, 224
    treatment of, 55t
Cholecystokinin (CCK), 181, 221, 233
Choledochal cysts, 208, 221–222,
    221–222f
Choledocholithiasis, 223–224
Choledochotomy, 227–228
Cholestatic jaundice, 208
Cholesteatoma, 505–506
Cholesterol stones, 222
Cholesterosis, 224–225
Cholic acid, 220
Chondroblastoma, 539
Chronic allograft damage, 488–489
Chronic atrophic gastritis, 199
Chronic disc degeneration, 484
Chronic lower limb arterial disease,
    376–385
Chronic obstructive pulmonary disease
    (COPD), 66, 130
Chronic osteomyelitis, 534
Chronic renal failure
    dialysis-dependent patients, 77–78
    nondialysis-dependent patients, 78
    perioperative implications of, 77–78,
        77t
Chronic venous insufficiency (CVI),
    400–401
    assessment of, 401
    compression therapy for, 401, 402f
    elastic compression hosiery for, 401
    examination of, 401
    history of, 401
    investigations in, 401
    management of, 401
    medical therapy for, 401
    pathophysiology, 400, 400t, 400f
    surgical and endovenous therapy for,
        401, 402b
Chronic venous ulceration (CVU), 400,
    400t, 400f
Chvostek's sign, 360t
Chyme, 181
Cingulate gyral herniation, 463, 464f
Circle of Willis, 462, 463f
Circulation
    injured limb, 542
    postoperative care for, 128
    in resuscitation, 104
    in shock, 24–25, 25f
Circulatory overload, transfusion-
    associated, 35t
Circumcision, 455
Cirrhosis
    perioperative implications, 78
    portal hypertension, 213
C-kit gene, 261
Clean-contaminated operations, 52t, 72t
Clean-contaminated procedures, 304
Clean operations, 52t, 72t
Clean procedures, 304
Cleveland Clinic Incontinence Score, 296
Clingfilm, 312
Clinical audit, 141, 141b, 141f
Clinical effectiveness, 141
Clinical governance, 140–141, 140f
Clipping, aneurysmal SAH and, 467,
    467f, 467b
Clitoris, 454–455
Clonorchis sinensis, 231

Clopidogrel, preoperative assessment
    and, 67
Closed-loop obstruction, 163, 163f
Clostridium difficile
    infection, 54t, 56–57
    reducing, 59
    treatment of, 57
Clostridium perfringens, 58
Clostridium spp., 54t
Clostridium tetani, 58–59
Clotting factor deficiency, 26
CO transfer, 421t
Coagulase-negative staphylococci, 54t
Coagulation
    abnormal, perioperative implications
        of, 78–79, 78t
    inherited disorders of, 79
    response to injury, 8
    screen, 68, 69t
Coagulopathy
    acquired, 79
    massive transfusion complications,
        38t
    perioperative implications of, 78
Coarctation of, aorta, 420, 421f
Cocaine, 81–82
Cochlea, 502–503
Cochrane Collaboration, 137
Cochrane review, 137, 140b
Codman's tumour, 539
Coeliac axis, 201f
Coeliac disease, 254
'Coffee bean' sign, 270, 271f
Cognitive impairment, informed consent
    and, 62
Cohort study, 139
Coiling, aneurysmal SAH and, 467,
    467b, 467f
Cold abscess, 523, 534, 534f
Cold storage, organ preservation and,
    491
Colic, in acute abdomen, 163
Colitis
    ischaemic, 269, 270f
        gangrenous, 269
    microscopic, 271
    pseudomembranous, 56–57, 271
Collagenous colitis, 271
Collar-stud abscess, 523
Colles' fractures, 546
Colloid particles, 3
Colloids, 13, 313b
Colonic amoebiasis, 266
Colonic diverticular disease, 266–269,
    267–268f, 268b
    bleeding in, 269
    complications of, 267–268, 268t
    diverticulitis in, 268
    fistula in, 269
    perforation in, 268–269
    stricture formation and obstruction in,
        269
Colonoscopy
    for colorectal adenocarcinoma, 277,
        277f
    for ulcerative colitis, 259–260, 260f
Colorectal adenocarcinoma, 275–277,
    276b, 276f, 282b
    aetiology of, 275–277
    clinical features of, 277
    investigations for, 277, 277–278f
    management of, 278–282
        adjuvant therapy for, 280–281
        palliative therapy for, 281
        pathology and staging in, 279–280,
            280–281t, 280f
        prognosis in, 282
        surgery for, 278–279, 279b, 279f
    population screening for, 277
    preoperative staging for, 277, 278f
Colorectal adenoma, 272–274, 273f,
    275b

Colorectal adenoma-carcinoma
    progression, 88f
Colorectal resection, for colorectal
    cancer, 279
Colour flow Doppler (duplex) ultrasound
    (CDU), in carotid artery disease,
    387, 387f
Colovesical fistula, 269
Commensals, 48, 49f
Commissural fibres, 461–462
Common bile duct, exploration of,
    227–228, 227b
Common hepatic duct, 219–220
Compartment syndrome, 392, 392f, 544
Complement, 50
Complement-dependent cytotoxicity
    cross match (CDC-XM), 489
Compliance, 503
Complicated DVT, 404
Compression therapy, for chronic
    venous insufficiency, 401, 402f
Computed tomographic (CT)
    angiography, neurosurgery, 465
Computed tomography (CT), 126, 421t,
    431–432, 437f
    acute abdomen, 170, 172f
    appendicitis, 176, 176f
    chronic pancreatitis, 242f
    gastric cancer staging, 200
    gastrointestinal tract, 254
    jaundice, 210
    larynx, 517
    neurosurgery, 465
    oesophageal perforation, 189, 190f
    oesophagus, stomach and
        duodenum, 184
    orthopaedic surgery, 531, 531f
    parotid tumour, 526, 526f
    temporal bone, 504
    trauma, 106
Conductive deafness, 503, 503f
Confidentiality, 62
Confusion, postoperative, 134
Congenital cardiac disease, 411–419
Congenital club foot, 537, 538f
Congenital disorders, of larynx, 517–518
Congenital hydrocoele, 459
Congenital hypertrophy of the retinal
    pigment epithelium (CHRPE),
    274
Congenital nonhaemolytic
    hyperbilirubinaemia, 207–208
Congenital talipes equinovarus, 537,
    538f
Coning, 464
Connective tissue, tumours of,
    324–325
Conn's syndrome, 369
Constipation
    and faecal incontinence, 296–297
    idiopathic slow-transit, 272
    and rectal prolapse, 295
Contaminated operations, 52t, 72t
Contaminated procedures, 304
Continuing professional development
    (CPD), 141–143
Continuous positive airway pressure
    (CPAP), 28
Continuous suture, for practical
    procedures, 114
Contrast radiology, in acute abdomen,
    169–170, 169b, 170–171f
Contrast studies, 126
Contrast swallow/meal
    oesophageal perforation, 189
    oesophagus, stomach and
        duodenum, 183, 184f
Core biopsy, breast disease and, 329,
    330f
Coronary angiography, 412, 413f
Coronary artery disease (CAD), 411–415
    assessment, 412, 412–413f

Coronary artery disease (CAD)
(Continued)
coronary bypass, 413–414, 413f,
414b
indications for surgery, 412
results, 414, 414b
surgery for complications of,
414–415, 414b
Coronary bypass, 413–414, 413f, 414b
Coronary circulation, 412, 412f
Corpus luteum, ruptured, 177
Corrosive oesophagitis, 190–191, 190f
Cortical control, impaired, 453
Cortical grey matter, 461–462
Corticosteroids
for Crohn's disease, 258
immunosuppression, 489, 490t
Corticosterone, 365–366
Corticotrophin-releasing factor (CRF),
363
Cortisol, 366b
Cushing's syndrome and, 366–369
fat metabolism, 7
Courvoisier's law, 224, 244, 244t
Courvoisier's sign, 244
Cowden's disease, 275
Cranial cavity, 462
Cranial dermal sinuses, 483
Cranial dural AVFs, 468, 469f
Cranial melioidosis, 473–474
Cranial nerves
surgical anatomy and physiology of,
462
tumours, 476
Craniopharyngiomas, 477, 478f
Craniosynostosis, 483, 483f
Craniotomy, subdural haematoma and,
472
C-reactive protein, 167
Creatinine, 430
Cremation, 63
Crepitus, 182
Creutzfeldt-Jakob disease, 52
Cricothyroidotomy, 524, 524f
needle, 116
surgical, 116, 117f
Critical appraisal, 141, 141b, 142f
Critical limb ischaemia, 379–381, 380f
ankle/brachial pressure index in, 379
autonomic neuropathy in, 380
balloon angioplasty in, 382, 382b
bypass surgery in, 382, 382b
diabetic foot in, 379
diabetic vascular disease in, 379
examination findings in, 379
management of, 381
endovascular, 381–382, 381f
medical, 381
motor neuropathy in, 380
pulse status in, 379
rest pain in, 379
sensory neuropathy in, 379
Crohn's disease, 255–259
clinical features of, 256–257, 256t,
257f
fulminant, 256, 257f
indications for surgery in, 259b
investigations of, 257, 257–258f
management of, 258–259
medical, 258
surgical, 258–259, 258b
pathology of, 255–256, 256f
Cronkhite-Canada syndrome, 275
Cross-matching
preoperative, 69
pretransfusion, 32
transplantation surgery, 489
Crush injuries, 301–302
Crushing mechanisms, blunt trauma
and, 99
Cryoprecipitate, 31
Cryptoglandular infection, 290

Cryptorchidism, 456–457
Crystalloids, 12–13, 13f, 313b
Cullen's sign, 167
Curling's ulcers, 194, 314
Cushing's disease, 364
Cushing's syndrome, 366–369
cancer and, 92
causes of, 366t
clinical features of, 367, 367f
investigations of, 366t, 368, 368f
management of, 368–369
types of, 367f
Cushing's ulcers, 194
Cyanosis, 128–129, 419–420
Cyclical mastalgia, 331t
Cyclosporin (CYA), 490
Cystadenoma, 255
Cystectomy, bladder tumours, 439,
445b
Cystic artery, 220
Cystic duct, 220
Cystic hygroma, 521, 521f
Cystitis
postoperative, 133
tuberculous, 439
Cysts, 316
branchial, 521, 521t, 521f
breast, 329f, 331–332f, 332
dermoid, 316, 316f, 521
epidermoid, 316
of the epididymis, 459
pilar, 316
retention, 511
sebaceous, 316, 316f
simple bone, 539
simple renal, 434
thyroglossal, 520–521, 520f
Cytokines
acute inflammatory response, 3, 4t
infection and, 50
'Cytopathic shock', 22

D
Damage Control Resuscitation, 105
Damage control surgery, 105, 107–108,
108–109b
Day surgery, 83–85
admission for, 85, 85f
clinical effectiveness of, 84b
cost-effectiveness of, 84b
discharge criteria, 85, 85t
facilities, 83–84
patient pathway, 84, 84f, 85t
preassessment in, 84b
principles of, 85b
De Quervain's disease, 354
Deafness, 506, 506t
conductive, 503f
sensorineural, 503, 504f
Death certificate, 63–64
Debridement, in burns, 314
Declaration of Helsinki, 64
Decontamination, hand, 50, 51f
Deep cervical fascia, 519
Deep partial-thickness burns, 310
Deep venous thrombosis (DVT)
aetiology of, 402–403
complicated, 404
diagnosis of, 403, 403f
epidemiology of, 402
management of, 404
pathology of, 402
prevention of, 134, 403–404
surgery complications of, 134
treatment for, 134
uncomplicated, 404
Deformity, description of, 530,
530–531b
Degenerative disease of the joints,
532–533
Degloving injuries, 301–302
Dehiscence, wound, 135–136, 135f

Dehydroepiandrosterone sulphate
(DHA-S), 366b
Delayed cerebral deficit, aneurysmal
SAH and, 467
Delayed graft function, 488b, 495
Delayed-type hypersensitivity (DTH), 488
Delayed union, of fractures, 543
Delirium tremens, surgery complications
of, 134
Delorme's procedure, 295
Dermal sarcoma, 325
Dermal sinuses, cranial, 483
Dermatofibroma, 318
Dermatofibrosarcoma protruberans
(DFSP), 325, 325f
Dermis, 301
Dermoid cysts, 178, 316, 316f, 521
Dermoids, angular, 483
Desmoid tumour, 147
Detrusor hypertrophy, 452
Detrusor muscle
hypertrophy, 445–446
myectomy, 453–454
Detrusor-sphincter dyssynergia, 453
Developing countries, breast cancer in,
336
Developmental dysplasia of the hip
(DDH), 537, 537f
Developmental history, orthopaedic
surgery, 528–529
Deviated nasal septum, 508, 508f
Devitalised skin flaps, 305, 306f
Dexamethasone, for brain oedema,
473–474
Dexamethasone test, Cushing's
syndrome and, 368, 368f
Dextrose, 12–13, 12t
Dextrose-saline solutions, 13
Diabetes insipidus, 364
Diabetes mellitus
comorbidity of, 76
effect on wound healing, 304
perioperative implications of, 76–77
perioperative management of, 76, 77t
Diabetic foot
in critical limb ischaemia, 379
infections, 58
Diabetic vascular disease, in critical limb
ischaemia, 379
Diagnosis of brain death (DBD), 491
Dialysis, transplantation surgery versus,
487b
Dialysis-dependent patients,
perioperative implications of,
77–78
Diaphragm, shoulder and, shared
sensory innervation of, 161f
Diaphragmatic herniation, 157, 157f
Diaphyseal achlasis, 539
Diarrhoea
after peptic ulcer surgery, 195
in enteral nutrition, 44
fluid loss from, 12
Diarrhoeal illness, 254
Diet
breast cancer and, 336
colorectal cancer and, 276
faecal incontinence and, 296–297
gastric cancer and, 198
Dietary fibre, 276
Diethylcarbamazine, 407
Dieulafoy's lesion, 203
Diffuse axonal injury, 473
Diffuse oesophageal spasm, 188–189
Dimercaptosuccinic acid (DMSA), 432
Dipstick testing, 168
Direct arteriovenous communications
(fistulae), 468
Direct inguinal hernia, 151
clinical features of, 151
management of, 152–153, 153–154f
Dirty operations, 52t, 72t

Discectomy, 486
Discharging sinus, 523
Disinfection, thermal, 51
Dislocation
joint, 542
shoulder, 540, 540f
Disseminated intravascular coagulation
(DIC), 3
Distal small bowel obstruction, 264
Diuretics, 134
Diverticula
bladder, 445–446, 446f
duodenal, 203
Diverticulitis, 203, 268
Diverticuloscope, 517
Diverticulosis, jejunal, 263, 263f
Dominant hand, in orthopaedic surgery,
529
Donor organ, recipient's immune
response to, 487–488
Dopamine, 364
Doppler, oesophageal, 75t
Dormia basket, 229
Dorsal root, of spinal cord, 462
Drains, surgical ward postoperative care
for, 130
Drapes, 112
Dressings, in burns, 314
Drugs
abnormal micturition and, 453
history, orthopaedic surgery and, 529
Drug therapy
for osteoarthritis, 532
in perioperative management, of
cardiovascular disease, 75
preoperative assessment and, 66–67
Duct ectasia, 332, 333f
Duct papillomas, 333, 333f
Ductal carcinoma in situ (DCIS),
337–338, 337–338f, 343b
Ductus arteriosus, patent, 420
Dukes' staging, of colorectal cancer,
280, 280t
Dumping, 195
Duodenal ileus, 203
persistent, 240
Duodenal switch, 204
Duodenal ulcers, 193, 193f
clinical features, 194
management
medical, 194–195, 195b
surgical, 195
perforation, 195, 196f
Duodenum, 179–205
diagnosis, 193–194
diverticula, 203
examination, 182
history, 181–182
investigations, 182–186
management, 193–194
obstruction, 203
surgical anatomy, 179, 180f
symptoms, 181–182
tuberculosis, 203
DVT. See Deep venous thrombosis
(DVT)
Dynamic hip screw, 545
Dynamic ultrasound, for sportsman's
hernia, 153
Dysoxia, 22
Dyspepsia, 182, 182b
Dysphagia, 181, 182t, 516
Dysphasia, 478
Dysphonia, functional, 518
Dysplasia, gastric, 199
Dysplasia-associated lesion or mass
(DALM), 261
Dysuria, 429

E
Ear, 502–507
anatomy, 502–503, 502f

Ear (*Continued*)
  assessment, 503–504
  clinical features, 503
  diseases
    external auditory meatus, 504–505
    facial nerve, 507
    inner ear, 506–507
    middle ear, 505–506
    pinna, 504
  examination, 503–504
  external, 502, 502*f*
  inner, 502–503
  middle, 502, 502*f*
  physiology, 503
Early deaths, trauma and, 98
Early gastric cancer, 199
Early goal-directed therapy (EGDT),
    septic shock, 27, 27*b*
Ebb phase, 3
E-cadherin gene, 199
Eccrine sweat glands, 301
Echinococcus granulosus, 213
Echinococcus multilocularis, 213
Echocardiography
  cardiothoracic surgery, 410*t*
  preoperative, 69–70
  transthoracic, 415
Ectasia, aortoannulo, 418
Ectopic pregnancy, ruptured, 177–178
Ectopic thyroid, misnamed, 521
Ectopic ureter, 453
Eczema, of nipples, 341–343, 343*f*
Efferent arm, of immune response, 488
Effort thrombosis, 405
Eisenmenger's syndrome, 419–420
Ejaculation, 455
Elastic compression hosiery, for chronic
    venous insufficiency, 401
Elbow, orthopaedic surgery in, 540
Elderly patients, appendicitis in, 175
Electrical burns, 312
Electrocardiography (ECG)
  cardiothoracic surgery, 410*t*, 421*t*
  exercise, 412
  preoperative, 69–70
Electrolyte
  abnormalities, 14–18
  balance, 9–11, 10*f*
    normal, 9–11, 10*f*
  daily requirement, 11*t*
  loss
    assessing in the surgical patient, 11
    daily, 11*t*
Electromyography, for orthopaedic
    surgery, 531
Elephantiasis, of lower limb, 406–407,
    407*f*
Embolectomy, for acute embolus, 391,
    391*f*
Embolus
  in acute limb ischaemia, 391*f*
  versus thrombosis in situ, 390*t*
Emergency room thoracotomy (ERT),
    110–111, 110*f*
Emergency surgery, preoperative
    assessment for, 71
Emotional state, 453
Emphysema, 426–427
Emphysematous pyelonephritis, 438
Empyema, 427, 427*f*
Encephalopathy, metabolic, 15
Encysted hydrocoele of the cord, 459*f*
'End-of-life' issues, 63
End-stage renal failure (ESRF), 487,
    487*b*
Endarterectomy, in arterial
    reconstruction, 382, 382*f*
Endocarditis, 415–416
Endocrine function, in pancreas,
    233–234, 242
Endocrine response to surgery, 4, 4*t*
Endocrine surgery, 351–374

Endogenous acid, 17–18
Endoluminal ultrasound
  gastric cancer staging, 200
  oesophagus, stomach and
    duodenum, 184, 185*f*
Endolymph, 502–503
Endolymphatic hydrops, 506–507
Endoscopic investigations, in acute
    abdomen, 170
Endoscopic prostatectomy, 448–449
Endoscopic retrograde
    cholangiopancreatography
    (ERCP), 235, 238*b*
  for jaundice, 210
Endoscopic treatment
  for acute pancreatitis, 238
  for chronic pancreatitis, 242
  for gastrointestinal bleeding, 197
  for infected pancreatic necrosis, 242
Endoscopic ultrasound, 423
Endoscopic variceal ligation (EVL),
    215
Endoscopy
  oesophagus, stomach and
    duodenum, 183
  variceal bleeding, 215
Endothelium, metabolic response to
    injury, 3, 4*f*
Endotoxin, 48
Endovascular aneurysm repair (EVAR),
    394–396, 395–396*f*, 396*b*
Endovascular surgery, 375–408
Endovenous LASER ablation (EVLA), in
    varicose veins, 398
Endovenous therapy, for chronic venous
    insufficiency, 401, 402*b*
Energy
  expenditure, 7*f*, 8*t*
  metabolism, increased in metabolic
    response to injury, 7, 7*f*
  requirements, 42, 42*t*
  reserves, 40
Enhanced recovery after surgery (ERAS),
    8–9
Entamoeba histolytica, 212
Enteral feeding, for pancreatitis, 238
Enteral nutrition, 42–43, 44*b*
  complications of, 44
  methods of administration, 43–44
  oral route, 43
  routes of, 43*f*
  vs. parenteral nutrition, 43*b*
Enteritis, radiation, 263
Enterococci, 54*t*
Enterocystoma, 147
Enterogastric reflex, 181
Enterohepatic circulation,
    220–221, 221*f*
Enteroteratoma, 147
Epidermis, 301, 306
Epidermoid cyst, 316, 316*f*
Epididymis, 458
Epididymo-orchitis, 457
Epidural anaesthesia, 80, 81*f*, 81*t*
Epidural analgesia, 82
Epigastric hernia, 155–156
Epilepsy
  functional neurosurgery and, 483
  perioperative implications, 79*t*
Epispadias, 455
Epistaxis, 508–509, 509*b*, 509*t*, 509*f*
Epithelial hyperplasia, 332–333
Epley's particle repositioning
    manoeuvre, 506
Epstein-Barr virus, 522–523
Erb's sign, 360*t*
Erythema, in burns, 312
Erythrocyte sedimentation rate (ESR),
    430
Erythroplasia of Queyrat, 319
Eschar, 308
Escharotomy, 314

Escherichia coli
  antibiotics for, 54*t*
  peritonitis and, 173
Estimated blood volume (EBV), 25
ET regimen, 346*b*
Ethics, 60–85
  committees, 64
  principles in, 60–61, 61*t*
  sources of further information on, 63*t*
  specific topics in, 63–64
Ethmoid labyrinth, 509
Eustachian tube, 502
Euthanasia, 63
Euvolaemic hypernatraemia, 15*b*
Evaporative dressings, 314
Evidence
  gold standard of, 137*b*
  levels of, 137–140, 138*t*
Evidence-based medicine, 137, 137*b*
Evidence-based practice, 137–144,
    143*b*
Ewing's sarcoma, 539
Excision arthroplasty, 537
Excision of lumps and swellings, 126
Exercise
  colorectal cancer and, 276
  preoperative assessment and, 66
Exercise electrocardiography(ECG), 412
Exocrine function, in pancreas, 233
Exophthalmos, 355, 356*f*
Exostosis, 539
Explicit consent, 62
Extended Focused Assessment with
    Sonography for Trauma (FAST),
    106
Extended spectrum β-lactamase
    (ESBLs), 52
External auditory meatus, diseases of,
    504–505
External beam radiotherapy (EBRT), 450
External ear, 502, 502*f*
External genitalia, 454–460, 454*f*
External hernias, 156
External laryngocoeles, 521
Extraanatomic bypass, in arterial
    reconstruction, 383–384, 384*f*
Extracapsular fractures, 545
Extracellular fluid (ECF), 9
  increased volume, 15*b*
  low volume, 15*b*
Extracorporeal shockwave lithotripsy
    (ESWL), 437
Extradural haematoma, 472, 472*f*

F

Facial artery, 519
Facial nerve (CN VII), 462, 502–503, 519
  disorders of, 507
Facial palsy, 507
Factor VIII concentrates, 31
Factor IX concentrates, 31
Faecal immunological test, 277
Fairness, 61
Fallot's tetralogy, 420–421
False aneurysms, 393, 393*f*, 418
False localising signs, 464–465
Familial adenomatous polyposis (FAP),
    274, 274*f*
FAST (Focused Abdominal Scans for
    Trauma), 170
Fasting, perioperative, 73, 73*b*
Fat metabolism, 7
Febrile non-haemolytic transfusion
    reactions, 35*t*
FEC regimen, 346*b*
Feel, orthopaedic examination,
    529–530, 530*t*, 530*f*
Female, urethral catheterisation in,
    124–125
Feminisation, adrenal, 369
Femoral aneurysms, 396
Femoral canal, 153

Femoral head, avascular necrosis of,
    541
Femoral hernia, 153–155
  clinical features of, 154
  surgical anatomy of, 153, 155*f*
  surgical repair of, 154–155, 155*b*
Femoral neck fractures, 545–546
Femoral ring, 155*f*
Femoral vein, trauma and, 104
Femorodistal bypass, 383*t*
Femoropopliteal bypass, 383*t*
FEV₁ (forced expiratory volume in 1
    second), 421*t*
Fever, postoperative, 136, 136*b*
Fibrin sealant, 39
Fibrinogen, deficiency, 26
Fibroadenoma, breast, 331, 331*f*
Fibroepithelial anal polyp, 292
Fibro-epithelial polyps, 318
Fibrosarcoma, 147, 325
Fibrosis, retroperitoneal, 430, 441*b*,
    445*f*
Fibrotic lung disease, 66
Filariasis, 406–407, 407*f*
Fine-needle aspiration cytology (FNAC)
  breast disease and, 329–330
  nipples and, 329–330
First aid, for burns, 312, 312*t*
Fissure-in-ano, 288–289, 288*f*, 289*b*
  clinical features of, 288
  management of, 289
Fistula-in-ano, 290–292, 292*b*
  assessment of, 290–291, 291*f*
  categories of, 291*f*
  clinical features of, 290–291
  management of, 291–292, 292*f*
Fistula(e), 147
  in acute pancreatitis, 240–241
  branchial, 521
  in Crohn's disease, 256
  in diverticular disease, 269
  intestinal, 272
  mammary duct, 335, 335*f*
Fistulation, and gallstones, 223
Fitness, operative, 64–65
Flail chest, 104
Flamazine, 314
Flame burns, 312
Flavine adenine dinucleotide (FADH), 22
Fleming, Alexander, 48
Flexible oesophagogastroduo-
    denoscopy, 183
Flexible sigmoidoscopy, in acute
    abdomen, 170
Floor of the mouth, carcinoma, 514,
    514*b*, 515*f*
Flora, normal, 49*f*
Florey, Howard, 48
Flow cytometry cross-match (FC-XM),
    489
Flow phase, 3
Fludrocortisone acetate, 372
Fluid
  balance, 9–18
    abnormalities, 14–18
    normal, 9–11, 10*f*
    surgical ward postoperative care
    for, 130
  loss
    assessing in the surgical patient,
    11–12, 11*t*
    causes of, 5*t*
    insensible, 9
    sources of, 11*t*
  resuscitation, in hypovolaemic shock,
    25
Fluid-conserving measures, 5
Fluid management, 428
Fluid resuscitation
  in burns, 313
  in pancreatitis, 237
18-Fluoro-deoxyglucose (FDG), 184

5-Fluorouracil (5-FU), 280–281
Focal neurological deficit, 478
Focal nodular hyperplasia (FNH), 217, 217f
Focused Assessment with Sonography for Trauma (FAST), 106
Follicle-stimulating hormone (FSH), 363
Follicular carcinoma, 358, 358f
Foot, orthopaedic surgery for, 542
Foramen magnum, 461
Foramina, 461
Foraminal (tonsillar) herniation, 464, 464f
Forced expiratory volume in one second (FEV$_1$), 421t
Forced expire volume, 70t
Forced vital capacity (FVC), 70t, 421t
Forearm fractures, 546, 546f
Foreign bodies
  obstruction by, 129
  oesophageal, 181
Foreskin, 455
Fournier's gangrene, 58, 315
Fractures
  ankle, 546–547
  in children, 542
  classification of, 542, 543f
  Colles', 546
  compartment syndrome, 544
  conservative treatment, 544
  delayed union, 543
  examination of, 542
  femoral neck, 545–546
  forearm, 546, 546f
  healing principles, 542–543
  intraarticular, 544
  malunion, 543, 544f
  management, 542
  nonunion, 543
  open, 543–544
  operative treatment, 544–545, 545f
  orthopaedic surgery and, 542–547
  pelvic, 545, 545f
  scaphoid, 546
  skull, 472
  tibial plateau, 547
  Volkman's ischaemic contracture, 544
Frank-Starling curve, 25f
Frantz tumour of the pancreas, 244, 244f
Free fatty acids (FFAs), 7
Free tissue transfer, 307, 308f
Fresh frozen plasma (FFP), 26, 31
Frey's syndrome, 526–527, 527t, 527b
Frontal sinus, 509
Full blood count (FBC), 167
  preoperative, 68
Full-thickness burns, 310–311
Full-thickness rectal prolapse, 295
Full-thickness skin grafts, 306
Fulminant Crohn's colitis, 256, 257f
Functional dysphonia, 518
Functional neurosurgery, 483
Fundoplication, 186, 187f, 188
Fungal infections, 57
Funiculitis, 458
FVC (forced vital capacity), 70t, 421t

G
Gallbladder, 219–232
  agenesis of, 221
  carcinoma of, 231
  congenital abnormalities, 221–222
  physiology of, 220–221
  strawberry, 224–225
Gallstone ileus, 225
Gallstone pancreatitis, 235, 236f
Gallstones, 222–231, 223b
  common clinical syndromes associated with, 223–224
  nonsurgical treatment of, 230
  pathogenesis of, 222–223
  pathological effects of, 223

Gallstones (Continued)
  retained, 229, 229f
  surgical treatment of, 225b
  ultrasonography, 208
Gamma glutamyl transferase (GGT), 167
Ganglioneuromas, 370
Gangrene, 58f
  Fournier's see Fournier's gangrene
  gas see Gas gangrene
Gangrenous appendicitis, 176
Gangrenous ischaemic colitis, 269
Gardner's syndrome, 147
Gas gangrene, 55t, 58
Gas transfer factor, 70t
Gastrectomy
  gastric cancer, 200, 201f
  peptic ulceration, 195f
  sleeve, 204f, 205
Gastric banding, 204, 204f
Gastric bypass, 204f, 205
Gastric cancer, 198f, 202b
  advanced, 199–200
    factors affecting, 199–200, 200b
  carcinoma, 198–199, 198f
  clinical features of, 200
  diagnosis, 200
  early, 199
  palliation, 201–202, 202b, 202f
  prognosis, 202, 202t
  staging, 200, 200t
  treatment, 200–201, 201f, 201–202b
Gastric dysplasia, 199
Gastric emptying, 181
  studies, 185–186
Gastric erosions, burns, 314
Gastric inhibitory peptide, 181
Gastric outlet obstruction, 197
Gastric polyps, 198
Gastric secretions, 181
Gastric ulcers, 193
  clinical features of, 194
  management
    medical, 194–195
    surgical, 195, 195f
  perforation, 195
Gastrin, 181
Gastrinomas, 194, 247
Gastritis, 203
  chronic atrophic, 199
Gastroenteritis, 175
Gastroenterostomy, 198
Gastrografin, 126
Gastrointestinal bleeding
  in acute pancreatitis, 240, 241f
  causes of, 196t
  peptic ulceration, 196–197
Gastrointestinal ischaemia, 240–241
Gastrointestinal stromal tumours (GISTs), 198, 261, 282
Gastrointestinal symptoms, clinical assessment of, 252b
Gastrointestinal tract
  effect of shock on, 23–24, 24b
  fluid losses from, 12, 12t
Gastrooesophageal reflux disease (GORD), 186–187, 186–187b
Gastroplasty, vertical banded, 205
Gastrostomy, 43–44, 43f
  for pseudocysts, 240f
Gelofusine, 12t
General Medical Council, doctor registered with, duties of, 61t
General precautions, 112
Genes, high risk, breast cancer and, 337
Genetic factors, peptic ulceration, 194
Genetic susceptibility, colorectal cancer and, 276–277
Genetic testing, breast cancer and, 337
Genetics, breast cancer and, 337
Genitourinary tuberculosis, 438–439
Gentamicin, 53

Genu valgum, 538
Genu varum, 538
Geographical variation, breast cancer and, 336
Giant cell tumour, 539
Giant hairy naevi, 318
Gilbert's syndrome, 207–208
Gingivitis, 511
Girdlestone's operation, 537
Glandular fever, 515
Glasgow Coma Score (GCS), 100, 100t
  neurosurgery and, 470, 471f
Glasgow Prognostic score, for pancreatitis, 236, 237f
Gleason score, 449
Gliomas, 476, 476f
Glomerular filtration rate (GFR), 430
Glossopharyngeal nerve (CN IX), 462
Glottic closure, 516
Gloves, for practical procedures, 112
Glucagon, 233–234
  in carbohydrate metabolism, 7
  in fat metabolism, 7
Gluconeogenesis, 7
Glucose
  parenteral nutrition, 46
  storage in liver, 206–207
'Glue ear', 505
Glycerol, 7
  fat metabolism, 7
Glycogenolysis, 7
Glycolysis, 22, 22f
Glycoproteins, 363
Glycosuria, 430
Goitre, 353, 354b
  clinical features of, 353, 353f
  non-toxic nodular, 353–354, 354f
  retrosternal, 353, 354f
  thyrotoxic, 354
  toxic multinodular, 357
'Golden hour', 98
Golfers' elbow, 540
Gonadotrophin-releasing hormone (GnRH), 363
Goodsall's law, 290–291, 291f
Gout, 436
Gowns, for practical procedures, 112
Graafian follicle, 177
Graciloplasty, anal incontinence, 297
Graft, blockage of, in arterial reconstruction, 384
Graft-versus-host disease (GVHD), 35t
Graves' disease, 355, 356f
Grey Turner's sign, 167
Group O blood, 32
Growth factors, 338
Growth hormone (GH), 363
  excess, 363
  in fat metabolism, 7
  involvement in anabolism, 8–9
Gunshot wounds, 301–302, 305
Gut functional disorder, nonmechanical, 264–266, 265t
Gynaecomastia, 349–350, 350f

H
Haemaccel, 12t
Haemangioendothelioma, hepatic, 219
Haemangiomas
  cavernous, 211, 217
  infantile, 323–324
  involuting, 324
  noninvoluting, 324
  renal, 434
  sclerosing, 318
Haematemesis, 196–197
Haematocoele, 458
Haematological investigations, for jaundice, 208
Haematology, preoperative, 68–69
Haematoma
  extradural, 472, 472f

Haematoma (Continued)
  intracerebral, 472
  perianal, 292
  of rectus sheath, 147
  retroperitoneal, 109, 109t
  subdural, 472, 472b, 472f
  in wound infection, 135
Haematuria, 429, 430t, 444f
Haemodialysis, vascular access for, 407–408
Haemodilution
  isovolaemic, 35
  normovolaemic, 39
Haemodynamic therapy, perioperative, 75
Haemoglobin, low, red cell transfusion in, 33b
Haemolytic anaemias, acquired, 249
Haemolytic jaundice, 208
Haemolytic transfusion reaction
  acute, 35t
  delayed, 36t
Haemophilia A, 79
Haemophilia B, 79
Haemophilus influenzae, 54t
Haemopoiesis, 248
Haemorrhage
  blood component use in, 36–38
  as cholecystectomy complication, 228
  hypovolaemic shock, 25
  in ischaemic steal syndrome, 408
  massive, 25, 104
  peptic ulcer, 196–197, 196f, 197f
  post-thyroidectomy and, 359
  postoperative care for, 129
  typhoid fever and, 266
Haemorrhagic diatheses, 304
Haemorrhagic shock, 38, 102
Haemorrhoidal artery ligation operation (HALO), 287
Haemorrhoidal cushions, 284–285
Haemorrhoidectomy, 287
Haemorrhoidopexy, 287
Haemorrhoids, 285–287, 287b
  classification of, 286, 286f
  clinical features of, 285–286
  examination of, 286
  history of, 286
  management of, 286
  nonoperative approaches in, 286–287, 287f
  thrombosis, 286
Haemostatic resuscitation, 105
Haemothorax, massive, 104
Hair cells, 503
Hair follicles, 301
Hallux rigidus, 542
Hallux valgus, 542
Halo naevus, 319
Hamartomas, 275
  biliary, 217
Hand
  atheroembolism, 386
  dominant, in orthopaedic surgery, 529
  orthopaedic surgery in, 540–541
Hand decontamination, 50, 51f
Hand hygiene, 304
Hard palate, carcinoma, 515, 515b
Hartmann's pouch, 220
Hartmann's procedure
  for colorectal cancer, 279
  for diverticular disease, 268–269
Hashimoto's disease, 354
Hawkin's test, 530
Head, neck node metastases in, 522
Head injury, 470
  assessment of, 470
  management of, 470
Healthcare-associated infections, 59, 59b, 59f
Hearing loss, 503

Heart
chambers, 410f
transplantation, 428
trauma, 419
valve disease, 415
Heart failure, 74, 74t
Heart transplantation, 499–501, 501b
complications in, 500
indications to, 499–500
and lung transplantation, combined, 500–501
operative procedure of, 500
outcome of, 501
patient assessment in, 499–500
postoperative management of, 500
Heartburn, 181–182, 187
Height, breast cancer and, 337
Heimlich's manoeuvre, 524
Helicobacter pylori, 193–194
eradication of, 194–195, 195b
and gastric cancer, 198, 198b
tests for, 183
Heller's myotomy, 188
Hemi-azygous veins, 179
Hemiarthroplasty, 536, 536f
Hemicolectomy, 279
Hemilivers, 206, 207f
Hemiparesis, 478
Hemithyroidectomy, 359
Hepatic acinus, 206
Hepatic artery, 206
Hepatic ducts, 219–220
Hepatic mucinous cystic neoplasm, 219
Hepatitis, perioperative implications of, 78
Hepatobiliary system, effect of shock on, 24
Hepatobiliary triangle, 220
Hepatocellular carcinoma, 218, 218b
Hepatocellular jaundice, 208
Hepatocytes, 206
Hepatoma, 218, 218b
HER receptors, 338
testing for, 338
Hereditary diffuse gastric cancer, 199, 200b
Hereditary pancreatitis, 241
Hereditary spherocytosis, 208, 249
Hernia, 147–158, 148b, 149f
abdominal *see* Abdominal hernia
hiatus *see* Hiatus hernia
irreducibility in, 157
obstruction in, 157
strangulation in, 157–158
Herniography, 153
Hernioplasty, 152
Herniorrhaphy, modified Bassini's, 152
Herniotomy, 152
Herpes zoster infection, 507
Hesselbach's triangle, 151
Hiatus hernia, 157, 187–188, 187f
clinical features of, 187–188
management of, 188
rolling, 187, 187f
sliding, 187, 187f
Hiccups
hiatus hernia, 188
postoperative, 130
Hickman catheter, 45
Hidradenitis suppurativa, 316, 316f
High-output congestive cardiac failure, in ischaemic steal syndrome, 408
High-protein oedema, 405f
Hinchey classification, of diverticular disease, 267–268, 268t
Hip arthroscopy, 541
Hip joint
orthopaedic surgery in, 541
tuberculous, 535, 535f
Hippocampal sclerosis, 483
Hirschsprung's disease, 271–272
Histamine, 181

Histiocytoma, 318
HLA (human leucocyte antigen), 487
Hoarseness, 517–518
Hodgkin's disease, 522–523
Hogarth-Pringle manoeuvre, 228
Hormonal treatment, of metastatic breast cancer, 348, 348t
Hormone replacement therapy (HRT), 67
breast cancer risk, 336–337, 336t
Hormones
involvement in anabolism, 8–9
metabolic response to injury, 8
role in breast cancer, 338
Hormone therapy, 450
adjuvant, breast cancer and, 345, 345t, 346b
complications of, 346
Horseshoe kidneys, 434
Host defence systems, 48–50, 49f
Hounsfield Unit, 126
Howell-Jolly bodies, 248
Human albumin solution (HAS), 12t, 31
Human epidermal growth factor receptors (HER), 338
Human immunodeficiency virus (HIV)
anal cancer risk, 293
perianal abscess and, 289
Human leucocyte antigen (HLA), 487
Human papillomavirus (HPV)
anal cancer risk, 293
oral cavity cancer and, 511
oropharyngeal tumours and, 516
Human Tetanus Immunoglobulin (HTIG), 59
Human Tissue Act, 63
Humoral immunity, 248
Hutchinson's melanotic freckle, 321, 321f
Hydatid disease, 213, 213f
Hydrocephalus, 481–482
aetiology of, 481–482, 481f
clinical features of, 481–482, 482f
management of, 482, 482f
prognosis for, 482
Hydrocoele, 458–459, 459f, 459t
Hydrocolloid dressings, 314
Hydrocortisone, replacement therapy for, 364
Hydrogel dressings, 314
Hydronephrosis, idiopathic, 446, 446f
Hydrotherapy, for osteoarthritis, 533
1->-hydroxyvitamin D₃, 362
Hyperacute rejection, 488
Hyperaldosteronism, 369
primary (Conn's syndrome), 369
secondary, 369
Hyperamylasaemia, 168t
Hyperbilirubinaemia, congenital nonhaemolytic, 207–208
Hypercalcaemia, 235, 360, 361t
acute abdomen and, 168
cancer and, 92
in metastatic breast cancer, 349
Hypergastrinaemia, 194
Hyperglycaemia, 7, 76
Hyperkalaemia, 15–16, 17t
massive transfusion complications, 38t
Hyperlipidaemia, 235
Hypernatraemia, 14–15, 15b
euvolaemic, 15b
hypervolaemic, 15b
hypovolaemic, 15, 15b
Hyperparathyroidism, 361t
peptic ulceration and, 194
primary, 360–362
secondary, 362
tertiary, 362
Hyperplastic polyposis syndrome, 275
Hyperprolactinaemia, 364
Hyperpyrexia, malignant, 68
Hypersplenism, 249

Hypertension
paroxysmal, 370
perioperative implications of, 75
Hyperthyroidism, 355, 356t
primary thyrotoxicosis and, 355, 356f
toxic multinodular goitre, toxic adenoma and, 357
Hypertonic saline solution, 13
Hypertrophy
detrusor, 452
juvenile, 331
Hyperventilation, 11
Hypervolaemic hypernatraemia, 15b
Hypoadrenalism, 66–67
Hypoalbuminaemia, 66
Hypocalcaemia, 38t, 360, 361t
Hypochloraemia, 18
Hypoglossal nerve (CN XII), 462
Hypoglycaemia, 76
cancer and, 92
Hypokalaemia, 16, 16b
hyperaldosteronism, 369
massive transfusion complication, 38t
parenteral nutrition, 46–47
Hypomagnesaemia, 16–17
Hyponatraemia, 15, 15b
Hypoparathyroidism, 360, 360t, 362
Hypopharynx, 516–517
Hypophosphataemia, 46–47
Hypophysectomy, surgical, 364, 364f
Hypophysial stalk, 363
Hypospadias, 455, 455f
Hypotension, treatment of, 14
Hypothermia, 38t
Hypothermic machine perfusion, organ preservation and, 491
Hypothyroidism, 360
Hypovolaemia
metabolic response to injury, 5–7, 5t
postoperative, treatment of, 14
Hypovolaemic shock, 19, 19t, 102
as acute lung injury cause, 25, 26t
burns and, 313, 313t
causes of, 19t
Hypoxaemia, 23
postoperative, 130–131, 131b

I
Idiopathic club foot, 537
Idiopathic hydronephrosis, 446, 446f
Idiopathic slow-transit constipation, 272
Idiopathic thrombocytopenic purpura (ITP), 249
Ileal conduit, 446f
Ileofemoral bypass, 383t
Ileostomy, 272
Ileotransverse anastomosis, 279
Ileus, 166–167
chronic duodenal, 203
gallstone, 225
paralytic, 162, 264
Iliac aneurysms, 396
Imaging, 126–127
Immediate deaths, trauma and, 98
Immune response, 491b
afferent arm of, 487–488
to donor organ, recipient's, 487–488, 488b
efferent arm of, 488
Immunisation
postsplenectomy, 251
tetanus, 58–59
Immunity, spleen and, 248
Immunoglobulin preparations, 30f, 31–32, 31t
Immunology, in transplantation surgery, 487–491
Immunosuppressed patients, prophylaxis for, 52
Immunosuppression
in Crohn's disease, 258
general risks of, 490–491

Immunosuppression (*Continued*)
new therapies for, 490
transplantation surgery and, 489, 489f
Impingement syndrome, 540
Implantation dermoid cysts, 316
Implied consent, 62
Impotence, 456
Incidentaloma, adrenal, 371, 371b
Incised wounds, 301–302
Incisional hernia, 156, 156–157f
Incompatibility, blood group, 495–496
Incontinence
management, 453
neurogenic disorders, 453–454
structural disorders, 452–453
urinary, 430
'Increased anion gap acidosis', 17–18
Indirect inguinal hernia, 150–151
clinical features of, 150–151, 151f
management of, 152, 152f
Infarction, in acute abdomen, 162–163, 162t
clinical features of, 162–163
Infections, 48–59
bacterial factors, 48
biology of, 48–50, 49f
breast disease, 334–335, 334t, 335b
as cholecystectomy complication, 228
diabetes and, 76
effect on wound healing, 304
empirical therapy for, 55t
following trauma, 58
hepatic, 211
host defence systems, 48–50
immunosuppression and, 490
importance of, 48
intracranial, 473–475, 473f
management of surgical, 53–54, 57b
antibiotic therapy of, 53–54
diagnosis of, 53
parenteral nutrition complications, 46
prevention of, 50–52, 52b
protection of, 237
pulmonary, 131–132
skin, 315–316, 335, 335f
surgical management of, 57–59
susceptibility to, classification of operations, 52t
transfusion-transmitted, 34, 36t
in vascular access, 408
Infective warts, 317f
Inferior mesenteric arteries, 253, 254f, 269
Inferior thyroid artery, 351
Inferior thyroid veins, 179
Inflammation
in acute abdomen, 161–162, 161t
rejection process and, 487
Inflammatory bowel disease, 255–261
colorectal cancer and, 276
Inflammatory disorders, orthopaedic surgery for, 533
Inflammatory phase, wound healing, 302
Inflammatory response
acute, 3, 4t
inhibition of, in pancreatitis, 237
Informed consent, 61–62, 62b
in children, 62
explicit, 62
general considerations in, 61–62
implied, 62
in mental illness, 62
in transient/irreversible cognitive impairment, 62
Inguinal canal, 149
Inguinal hernia, 148–153, 155b
direct, 151
femoral hernia, 151f, 153–155
indirect, 150–151
management of, 151–153, 152–153f, 152–153b

Inguinal hernia (Continued)
sliding, 148
sportsman's hernia, 153
surgical anatomy of, 149–150, 150f
Inguinal ligament, 153
Inherited disorders of coagulation, 79
Injections, for osteoarthritis, 533
Injury severity, 99–100
Injury severity score (ISS), 100
Inner ear, 502–503, 506–507
Inotropes, 25
Insensible fluid loss, 11
Insulin, 233–234
administration of, methods of, 77, 77t
involvement in anabolism, 8–9
Insulin-like growth factors, 8–9
Insulinomas, 247, 247t
Intensity modulated radiotherapy, 450
Intensive care, 410–411
Intention, secondary, wound healing by, 303f
Intention-to-treat analysis (ITT), 139
Intercostal drainage tube, removal of, 117–118
Intercostal tube drainage, 116–117, 118f
Intercurrent disease, effect on wound healing, 304
Interleukin-1 (IL-1), 3, 4t
Interleukin-6 (IL-6), 3, 4t
Interleukin-8 (IL-8), 3, 4t
Interleukin-10 (IL-10), 3, 4t
Intermittent claudication, 376–379
arterial reconstruction in, 382
clinical features of, 378–379, 379f
differential diagnosis of, 378t
endovascular management of, 381–382
epidemiology of, 376–378
pathology of, 380f
symptoms of, 380f
Internal carotid arteries, 462
Internal hernia, 157, 157f
Internal inguinal ring, 149, 149f
Internal jugular vein
cannulation, 122–123, 123f
trauma and, 104
Internal thoracic artery (ITA), coronary bypass, 413, 413f
International Prostate Symptom Score (IPSS), 446–447, 447t
Interposition arthroplasty, 537
Intersphincteric abscess, 290
Interstitial lung disease, 427
Interventional radiology (IR), of trauma, 106
Intestinal failure, 42, 44
Intestinal fistula, 12
Intestinal ischaemia, 272
Intestinal metaplasia, 199
Intestinal obstruction, fluid loss, 12
Intestinal stoma, 272, 272f
Intestinal tuberculosis, 266, 267f
Intraabdominal abscess, 173
Intraabdominal viscus, perforation, 163
Intraarterial digital subtraction angiography (IA-DSA)
in carotid artery disease, 387
in cerebrovascular disease, 466f
Intraarterial drug, administration of, acute limb ischaemia, 392
Intracapsular fractures, 545
Intracellular fluid, 10f
Intracerebral haematoma, 472
Intracerebral haemorrhage (ICH), primary, 468, 468b
common cause of, 465
Intracranial infections, 473–475, 473f
Intracranial mass lesions, 463, 463f
Intracranial pressure (ICP), 462–465, 463f, 465b
head injury and, 470
intracranial tumours and, 475–480

Intracranial pressure (ICP) (Continued)
raised, 478
Intracranial tumours, 475–480, 479b
clinical features of, 478
diagnosis of, 476f, 478–479
management of, 479, 479b
paediatric neurooncology in, 479–480, 480f
Intraductal papillary mucinous neoplasm (IPMN), 243
Intraoperative blood salvage, 39
Intraosseous access, trauma and, 104
Intravenous fluid administration, 12, 12t
composition of fluid, 12t
treatment of hypovolaemia/hypotension, 14, 14b
types of, 12–13
Intravenous pyelography, 170
Intravenous thrombolysis, 388
Intravenous urography (IVU), 431, 431f
Intravesical chemotherapy, 445b
Intrinsic factor, 181
Invasion, of cancer, 88–89, 88f, 89t
Investigations
acute abdomen, 167
appendicitis, acute, 176, 176f
benign prostatic hyperplasia, 446–447
bladder tumours, 444, 445f
cancer, 92–93
cardiac, 69, 69t
chronic venous insufficiency, 401
colorectal adenocarcinoma, 277, 277–278f
Crohn's disease, 257, 257–258f
large intestine, 254
lymphoedema, 406
neurosurgery, 465
oesophageal perforation, 189
oesophagus, stomach and duodenum, 182–186
orthopaedic surgery, 531
for pancreatic cancer, 245–246, 245f
preoperative, 68, 68b
prostate carcinoma, 449–450
subarachnoid haemorrhage (SAH), 466
ulcerative colitis, 259–260, 260f
urological surgery, 430–434
Involuting (RICH) haemangiomas, 324
Irinotecan, 281
Iron overload, 36t
Irreducible hernia, 157
Irreversible cognitive impairment, informed consent and, 62
Irritable bowel syndrome, 270
Ischaemia
chronic mesenteric, 263–264
large intestinal, 269–272
Ischaemia reperfusion injury (IRI), 487
Ischaemic colitis, 269, 270f
Ischaemic heart disease, 411
see also Coronary artery disease (CAD)
Ischaemic heart disease, perioperative implications of, 73
Ischaemic steal syndrome (ISS), in vascular access, 408
Ischaemic stricture, of colon, 269–270, 270f
Ischiorectal abscess, 290
Islets of Langerhans, 233–234
Isotope scans, 421t
Isotopic liver scanning, for jaundice, 210
Isovolaemic haemodilution, 35–36
Ivor Lewis two-phase oesophagectomy, 191, 192f

J
Jaboulay's procedure, 458–459
Japanese Research Society of Gastric Cancer (JRSGC), 200

Jaundice, 207–211, 208f, 211b
cholestatic, 208
diagnosis, 208–211, 209–210f
haemolytic, 208
hepatocellular, 208
history, 208
obstructive, 207–208
perioperative implications, 78
progressive, 240
types of, 209f
Jaw-thrust manoeuvre, 114, 114f
Jejunal diverticulosis, 263, 263f
Jejunal obstruction, proximal, 264
Jejunostomy, 43–44, 44f
for pseudocysts, 240f
Jejunum, 252
Joint
dislocation, 542
injured limb, 542
Justice, 61, 61b
Juvenile fibroadenoma, 331, 331f
Juvenile hypertrophy, 331, 331t
Juvenile polyposis syndrome (JPS), 275

K
Kaolin, 424
Kaplan-Meier equations, 89, 89f
Kaposi's sarcoma, 325
Kasabach-Merritt syndrome, 324
Kasai operation, 221
Keller's procedure, 537
Keratin horn, 319, 319f
Keratinocytes, 301, 314
Keratoacanthoma, 318, 318f
Kernohan's notch, 465
Ketamine, 83
Ketoacidosis, 76
17-Ketosteroids, 8–9
Kidney-ureter-bladder (KUB), 431
Kidneys
adenocarcinoma, 444, 445b
anatomy of, 434–436, 434f
benign tumours, 434
decompression, 437–438
developmental anomalies, 434
horseshoe, 434
hypoperfusion, 133
palpation, 430f, 459
putty, 438
Klebsiella spp., 54t
Knee joint, orthopaedic surgery in, 541–542
history, 541
ligamentous injuries, 541–542
meniscal injuries, 541
Knock knees, 538
Kyphosis, 530

L
Labia, 454–455
β-Lactam antibiotics, 56
Lactating infection, breast and, 334, 334f
Lactic acid, 22
Lactic acidosis, 18b
Laerdal bag, 114–115
Lag phase, wound healing, 303f
Lamina, 461
Laminectomy, 486
Laparoscopic surgery
colorectal surgery, 94–95, 95b
for hernia, 152, 154f
in kidney transplantation, 492–493
Laparoscopy
in acute abdomen, 170–171, 173f
in appendicitis, 176
gastric cancer staging, 200, 200f
in jaundice, 210
Laparotomy, for trauma, 109
Large intestine
anatomy of, 253, 254f
clinical history taking for, 253

Large intestine (Continued)
examination of, 253–254
function of, 253
investigations of, 254
ischaemia in, 269–272
malignant tumours of, 275–282
microcirculation of, 254–255
neoplastic disorders of, 266–272
obstruction of, 264–266
polyps and polyposis syndromes of, 272–275, 273t
principles of operative intestinal surgery for, 254–255
Laryngeal nerve damage, thyroidectomy, 359–360
Laryngitis, 518
Laryngoceoeles, external, 521
Larynx, 517–518
anatomy, 516–517f, 517
assessment, 517
carcinoma of, 518, 518b
diseases, 517–518
oedema, airway obstruction, 129
spasm, airway obstruction, 129
Laser prostatectomy, 448, 448b
Late deaths, trauma and, 98
Le Veen shunt, 217f
Left thoracolaparotomy, 191
Left ventricular aneurysm, 414–415
Lentigo maligna, 321, 321f
Leukoplakia, 511, 511f, 518
Levator ani, 283, 284f
Lichtenstein open tension-free repair, 152, 153f
Lidocaine, 80t
for practical procedures, 113
Ligamentous injuries, orthopaedic surgery in, 541–542
Limb fitting, in amputation, 385
Lip cancer, 511, 513b, 513f
Lipase, 235–236
Lipoma, 324, 333
Lipopolysaccharide (LPS), 48
Liposarcoma, 325
Lister, Joseph, 48
Lithium, 67
Little's area, 507
Littre's hernia, 148
Liver, 206–232
abscess
amoebic, 212, 212f
pyogenic, 211–212
anatomy of, 206–207, 207b, 207f
segmental, 206
biopsy, jaundice, 210
blood supply, 206–207, 207f
congenital abnormalities of, 211, 211f
cysts, 211, 211f
function of, 206–207
infections and infestations, 211
metastases, 349
percussion of, 166
resection of, 219
trauma to, 211–213
tumours, 217–219
metastatic, 219
Liver cell adenoma, 217–218
Liver function tests
for acute abdomen, 167
preoperative, 69
Liver transplantation, 219, 496–498, 498b
complications in, 497
indications for, 496, 496t
living donation for, 494, 497
operative procedure for, 497, 497f
outcome of, 497–498
patient assessment in, 496, 496t
postoperative management of, 497
Living donation for liver transplantation (LDLT), 494

LKB1 gene, 261–262
Lobectomy, 359
Lobular carcinoma in situ (LCIS), 337–338, 338*f*
Lobular intraepithelial neoplasia (LIN), 337–338, 338*f*
Local anaesthesia, 112–113
  agents for, 79–80, 80*t*
Local treatments, in metastatic breast cancer, 348–349
Locally advanced breast cancer (LABC), 342*f*, 347–348, 347*t*, 347*f*, 348*b*
Lockwood approach, 155
Long-term steroid therapy, 66–67
Look, orthopaedic surgery, 529, 529*f*
Lordosis, 530
Lord's procedure, 289, 458–459
Lotheissen's approach, 155
Low-protein oedema, 405*f*
Lower limbs
  arterial disease, chronic, 376–385
  arteries and veins of, anatomy of, 376*f*
  orthopaedic surgery in, 541–542
Lower urinary tract, 441–452
  anatomy, 441*f*
  physiology, 441–442
  trauma, 442–444, 442*f*
  vesicoureteral reflux, 450–451
Ludwig's angina, 511
Lumbar hernia, 156
Lumbar puncture, 125–126
Lumpiness, breast and, 331*f*, 332
Lumps
  breast, 332
  excision of, 126
Lung(s)
  closing volume, 131
  infection, 131–132
  resection, 422*b*
  transplantation *see* Lung transplantation
  volume, 131
Lung transplantation, 499–501, 501*b*
  complications in, 500
  and heart transplantation, combined, 500–501
  indications to, 499–500
  operative procedure of, 500
  outcome of, 501
  patient assessment in, 499–500
  postoperative management of, 500
Luteinizing hormone (LH), 363
Lymph nodes
  anal cancer, 293–294
  assessment in breast disease, 326–330
  axillary, 326, 327–328*f*, 328, 339, 339*f*
  cervical, 512–513, 513*t*, 522*f*
  dissection, gastric cancer of, 200*b*
  enlargement, 519–520
  swellings, 522
Lymphadenitis
  acute, 523
  tuberculous, 266
    cervical, 523–524, 523*f*
Lymphadenopathy, 182, 522*b*
  cervical, 512–513, 513*t*
Lymphocoeles, 495
Lymphocytic colitis, 271
Lymphoedema, 405–406
  clinical features of, 406
  investigation of, 406
  management of, 406
  pathophysiology of, 405–406, 405*f*
  primary, 406
  secondary, 406
  types of, 405*f*
Lymphomas, 250, 282
  breast, 349

Lymphomas (*Continued*)
  gastric, 202
  neck, 522–523
  small bowel, 261
  thyroid gland, 359
Lysozyme, 50
Lytle's repair, 152

M

Maastricht criteria, organ preservation and, 491, 493*t*
Macrocirculation, 21, 21*t*
Macrophages, 50
MAG-3 (radio-labelled mercaptoacetyltriglycine), 432, 433*f*
Magnesium, 16–17
Magnesium ammonium phosphate stones, 436
Magnetic resonance angiography (MRA), 465
  in carotid artery disease, 387, 387*f*
Magnetic resonance cholangiopancreatography (MRCP), for jaundice, 209–210, 210*f*
Magnetic resonance imaging (MRI), 127, 421*t*
  breast disease, 329, 329*b*
  cerebellopontine angle, 504*f*
  ear, 504
  intracranial tumours, 478–479
  jaundice, 210, 210*f*
  neurosurgery and, 465
  of oropharyngeal tumours, 516
  in orthopaedic surgery, 531, 531*f*
  trauma, 106
Major histocompatibility complex (MHC), 487
Male
  breast, 349–350
  breast cancer, 350
  urethral catheterisation in, 124, 125*f*
Malignancy, immunosuppression and, 490–491
Malignant hyperpyrexia, 68
Malignant melanoma (MM), 320–322, 322–323*b*, 323*t*
  acral lentiginous, 321, 322*f*
  amelanotic, 321
  Hutchinson's melanotic freckle, 321, 321*f*
  management of, 322–323, 322*f*, 323*b*
  nodular, 321
  other types of, 321
  prognosis in, 324*t*
  sentinel lymph node biopsy, 320
  spread of, 321–322
  staging for, 323, 323–324*t*
  subungual, 321
  superficial spreading, 321, 321*f*
Malignant paraganglioma, 371*f*
Malleus, 502, 502*f*
Mallory-Weiss tear, 189
Malnutrition, 40, 41*f*
  preoperative assessment, 66
Malpighian bodies, 248
MALT lymphomas, 202
Malunion, of fractures, 543, 544*f*
Mammary duct fistula, 335, 335*f*
Mammography, 328
  breast cancer, features of, 339, 339*f*
  breast screening by, 338–339, 339*f*
Manometry, oesophagus, stomach and duodenum, 184–185, 185–186*f*
Marjolin's ulcer, 320, 321*f*
Marrow infiltration, in metastatic breast cancer, 349
Massive blood transfusion, 30, 38, 38*t*
Mastalgia
  cyclical, 331*t*
  noncyclical, 332, 332*f*

Mastectomy, 344*b*
  modified radical, 344
Mastitis
  periductal, 334
  tubercular, 335
Mastoidectomy, 505–506
Matrix metalloproteinase (MMP) inhibitors, 96
Maturation phase, wound healing, 302–303
Maxillary sinuses, 509
Maximal surgical blood ordering schedule (MSBOS), 33, 33*b*
McBurney's point, 174, 174*f*
McEvedy approach, 155
McKeown three-phase oesophagectomy, 193
Mean arterial blood pressure (MAP), 19
Mean arterial pressure (MAP), 463
Meatal stenosis, 456
Mechanical thrombectomy, 388
Mechanical valve prostheses, 415*f*
Meckel's diverticulum, 147–148, 262–263
Medial collateral ligament injuries, 541
Mediastinoscopy, 423
Mediastinotomy, 423
Mediastinum, 425
  infection, 425
  mass lesions, 425, 425*f*
  video-assisted thoracic surgery, 425
Medical negligence, 63
Medullary cancers, 338
Medullary carcinoma, 359–360
Medulloblastoma, 480*f*
Megacolon, acquired, 272
Meissner's plexus, 181, 252, 271
Melaena, 196–197, 253
Melanocyte-stimulating hormone (MSH), 368–369
Melanocytes, 316, 317*t*, 318, 319*b*
Melanotic freckle, Hutchinson's, 321, 321*f*
Meleney's gangrene, 315, 315*f*
Melioidosis, cranial, 473–474
Memorial Sloan-Kettering Cancer Center classification, 522
Ménétrier's disease, 203
Ménière's disease, 506–507
Meninges, 462
Meningiomas, 476, 476*f*
Meningitis, 474–475
Meniscal injuries, orthopaedic surgery for, 541
Menstrual cycle, 332
Menstrual factor, of breast cancer, 336
Mental illness, informed consent and, 62
Meralgia paraesthetica, 486
Mercedes-Benz incision, 497, 497*f*
Mesenteric angina, 263
Mesenteric angiography, 170
Mesenteric artery disease, 389
Mesenteric ischaemia, chronic, 263–264
Mesh repair, for hernia, 152, 152*b*, 153*f*
Mesothelioma, 424–425
Meta-analysis, 138, 140*b*
Metabolic acidosis, 17–18, 18*b*
Metabolic alkalosis, 18, 18*b*
Metabolic bone diseases, orthopaedic surgery for, 538
Metabolic complications
  parenteral nutrition, 46–47
  primary thyrotoxicosis, 355
Metabolic encephalopathy, 15
Metabolic response to injury, 3–9
  consequences of, 5–9, 5*b*, 6*f*
  factors associated with, 9*t*
  factors mediating, 3–4, 5*b*

Metabolic response to injury (*Continued*)
  factors modifying, 9, 9*t*
  features of, 3
  maintenance fluid requirements, 13–14, 14*t*
  urinary changes in, 7*b*
Metabolism, calcium, 360
Metaplasia, intestinal, 199
Metastases, 88–89, 88–89*f*, 89*t*, 349*b*
  brain, 349, 477, 478*f*
  breast cancer, 348, 348*b*, 348*t*
  liver, 349
  pancreatic, 244
  surgery for, 96, 96*b*
Metastatic disease, 424, 424*f*
Metastatic signature, 88
Methicillin-resistant *Staphylococcus aureus* (MRSA), 54*t*, 59*f*
  preoperative screening, 50, 50*b*, 71
  reducing, 59
Methicillin-sensitive *Staphylococcus aureus*, 54*t*
Microcirculation
  of large intestine, 254–255
  in shock, 21, 21*f*
Microdiscectomy, 486
Microlithiasis, 235
Microscopic colitis, 271
Micturating cystourethrogram (MCU), 432, 433*f*
Micturition, 454*b*
  cycle, 442
  disorders of, 429
  neurological control of, 441–442
Middle ear, 502, 502*f*, 505–506
Minimally invasive oesophagectomy, 192
Minnesota tube, 119
Mirizzi's syndrome, 229
Miscellaneous benign perianal lumps, 292
Mitral valve disease, 416–417
  regurgitation, 417
  stenosis, 416–417, 417*f*
  surgical outcomes, 417
Mittelschmerz, 177
Model for end stage liver disease (MELD) score, 496, 496*t*
Modified Bassini's herniorrhaphy, 152
Moles, benign naevi, 318–319, 318*f*
Molluscum sebaceum, 318, 318*f*
Monoamine oxidation inhibitors (MAOIs), 67
Monoclonal antibodies, 258
Mons pubis, 454–455
Moon face, 367*f*
Mortality, cardiothoracic surgery, 409
Morton's neuroma, 542
Motor neuropathy, in critical limb ischaemia, 380
Mouth
  diseases, 511–515
  ulcers, 511
Movement, orthopaedic examination, 530
Movement disorders, functional neurosurgery and, 483
Mucinous cancers, 338
Mucinous cystic neoplasm, 243, 243*f*
Mucocoele, 223, 255
Mucoepidermoid carcinoma, 526, 526*t*
Mucosa-associated lymphoid tissue (MALT) lymphomas, 202
Mucosal disease, 505
Mucosal rectal prolapse, 295
Mucous retention cysts, 511
Mucus, 181
Multidisciplinary management (MDM) planning, for pancreatic cancer, 245–246, 245*f*
Multimodal analgesia, 82

Multiple endocrine neoplasia (MEN), 372
type I, 247–248, 373
type II, 373
Multiple endocrine neoplasia syndromes, 373, 373t
Multiple injury, 98–111
Multiple organ dysfunction syndrome, 236–237
Multiple sclerosis, perioperative implications of, 79t
Multislice computed tomography (MSCT), 126
Murphy's sign, 167, 223
Muscles, tumours of, 324–325
Musculoskeletal disease, perioperative implications of, 79
Musculoskeletal system, symptoms of, 528, 528b
Musculoskeletal tuberculosis, 534
Musculoskeletal tumours, orthopaedic surgery for, 538–539, 539b
Mutations, cancer and, 86, 87t
MUYTH-associated polyposis (MAP), 275
Myasthenia gravis, perioperative implications of, 79t
Mycophenolate mofetil (MMF), 490
Mycophenolic acid (MPA), 490
Myelomeningocoele, 481
Myenteric plexus, 181
Myocardial infarction (MI)
cardiogenic shock, 28
perioperative implications, 73, 73t
surgery complications of, 133
ventricular septal defect after, 414
Myocardial ischaemia, 133
Myocardial preservation, 409–410
Myotomy
achalasia, 188
pouches, 189
Myringoplasty, 505
Myringotomy, 505, 506f

N

Naevi, 318–319, 318f
blue, 319
giant hairy, 318
halo, 319
types of, 319
Nasal septum, 507, 507f
Nasobiliary, catheter, 229
Nasogastric tubes
feeding via, 43
fine-bore, 119
insertion of, 118–119, 119f
surgical ward postoperative care for, 130
Nasojejunal tubes, feeding via, 43
Nasopharynx, 510
Natal cleft, 297–298
National Comprehensive Cancer Network (NCCN), 140
National Institute for Health and Care Excellence (NICE) guidelines, 140
for dyspepsia, 182b
Natural braided sutures, 113
Nausea, postoperative.
See Postoperative nausea and vomiting (PONV)
Near-total thyroidectomy, 359
Neck, 519–527
anatomy, 519, 519f
assessment, 519
cancer, 522
diseases, 519–524
dissection, 522–523t
node metastases, 522
swellings, 519–521
Necrotising fasciitis, 58, 58f, 315, 315f
Needle cricothyroidotomy, 116
Needle pericardiocentesis, 124, 124f

Needles, for practical procedures, 112
Neglected club foot, 537, 538f
Negligence, 63
Neoadjuvant therapy, 94, 95f
breast cancer and, 345–346
Neonates, choledochal cysts, 222
Neoplasms
in small intestine, 261
see also Tumours see also specific neoplasms
Neostigmine, 128–129, 133
Nephroblastomas, 434–435, 435t
Nerve conduction tests, 531
Nerves
damage from thyroidectomy, 352t, 359–360
injured limb, 542
tumours of, 324
Nervous system, in shock, 23
Neural transplantation, 483
Neurilemmoma, 324, 324f
Neuroblastomas, 370–371, 435t
Neurocysticercosis, 474, 475f
Neurofibroma, 324, 324f
Neurofibromatosis, 324, 324f
type 2, 485f
Neurogenic shock, 20–21, 102
Neurohypophysis, 364, 365f
Neurooncology, paediatric, 479–480, 480f
Neuropathic pain, 83, 83b
Neuropathy, diabetes and, 76
Neuropsychiatric disturbances, 134
Neurosurgery, 461–486
functional, 483
investigations in, 465
physiology, 461–462
surgical anatomy, 461–462
Neurotrauma, 470–473, 473b
assessment of, 470
contusions and, 472
diffuse axonal injury and, 473
extradural haematoma and, 472, 472f
intracerebral haematoma and, 472
management of, 470–471, 472b
neurological examination for, 470
skull fracture and, 472
subdural haematoma and, 472, 472b, 472f
traumatic spinal injury and, 473
Neutrophils, 50
Nicotinamide adenine dinucleotide (NADH), 22
Nimodipine, 467b
Nipples
accessory, 326
discharge, 330, 330t, 333f, 341–343, 341–342f
eczema of, 341–343, 343f
fine-needle aspiration cytology and, 329–330
Paget's disease of, 341–343, 342f
Nissen fundoplication, 186–187, 187f
Nitrates, 198
Nitrogen
intake, 8
loss, 8, 8t
requirements, 42
Nocturia, 429
Nodular hyperplasia, thyroid gland and, 353
Nodular melanoma, 321
Nodularity, breast and, 331f, 332
Nonabsorbable sutures, 113
Nondialysis-dependent patients, perioperative implications of, 78
Non-Hodgkin's lymphomas, 261, 523
Non-invasive ventilation (NIV), 76
Noninvoluting haemangiomas, 324
Nonlactating infection, breast and, 334–335

Nonmalfeasance, 60–61, 61b
Nonmechanical gut functional disorder, 264–266, 265t
Nonspecific abdominal pain, 177
Non-steroidal anti-inflammatory drugs (NSAIDs)
for colorectal adenocarcinoma, 276, 276b
peptic ulceration and, 194
postoperative analgesia, 83
Non-toxic nodular goitre, 353–354, 354f
Nonunion, of fractures, 543
Noradrenaline, 369
Normothermic perfusion, organ preservation and, 491
Normovolaemic haemodilution, acute, 39
Nose, 507–509
anatomy, 507, 507f
assessment, 507–508
clinical features, 507
diseases, 508–509
examination, 507
imaging, 507–508, 508f
obstruction, 507
physiology, 507
polyps, 508, 508f
Notara's procedure, 289
NSAIDs. See Non-steroidal anti-inflammatory drugs (NSAIDs)
Nuclear imaging, urological surgery, 432
Nucleus pulposus, 483–484
Nuss procedure, 428
Nutcracker oesophagus, 189
Nutrition
causes of inadequate intake, 42
requirements, 42
surgical ward postoperative care for, 130
Nutritional disorders, 40. See also specific disorders
Nutritional management, in burns, 313
Nutritional status, 42b
assessment, 40–41, 41f
effect on wound healing, 304
preoperative assessment and, 66
Nutritional support, 40–47, 41f
in acute pancreatitis, 238, 238b
methods of providing, 42–47
monitoring of, 47 see also Enteral nutrition; Parenteral nutrition

O

Obesity
morbid, 203
preoperative assessment, 66, 67t
surgery for, 203–204 see also Bariatric surgery
Observation, orthopaedic examination, 529, 529f
Obstruction
in acute abdomen, 163–164
biliary, 224
duodenal, 203–205
pelviureteric junction, 439, 440f
peptic ulceration, 197
in small and large bowel, 264–266, 265f
causes of, 264t
distal small, 264
in diverticular disease, 269
proximal jejunal in, 264
urinary tract, 439–441, 439t
Obstructive jaundice, 207–208
Obstructive shock, 102
Obturator hernia, 156
Occipital triangle, 519
Occlusive dressings, burns, 314
Occupation, orthopaedic surgery, 529
Oculomotor nerve (CN III), 462
Odynophagia, 181

Oedema
brain, 473–474
cerebral, 15
formation, 3, 11
types of, 405f see also Lymphoedema
Oesophageal carcinoma, 181, 191–193, 193b
clinical features of, 191
investigations for, 191
management of, 191
palliation, 192–193, 193f
postoperative care, 192, 192b
radiotherapy and chemotherapy, 192
surgical resection, 191–192
Oesophageal Doppler, 75t
Oesophageal tamponade, 119–120
Oesophagectomy, 191–192, 192f
Oesophagitis
corrosive, 190–191, 190f
hiatus hernia, 188
odynophagia, 181
Oesophagogastroduodenoscopy, flexible, 183
Oesophagus, 179–205
diagnosis, 186–191
diffuse spasm, 188–189
examination, 182
history, 181–182
investigations, 182–186
management, 186–191
nutcracker, 189
perforation, 189–190, 190f
pouch, 189
sphincters, 179
stricture, 181
surgical anatomy, 179–180, 180f
surgical physiology of, 181
symptoms, 181–182
tumours, 191–193
see also Oesophageal carcinoma
variceal bleeding, 215–216, 215t, 215f, 215–216b
Oestrogen, 338
Oestrogen receptors (ERs), 338
Off-loading, for osteoarthritis, 532
Olfactory nerve, 462
Oliguria, 5, 430
Oophorectomy, 345
Open AAA repair, 394, 395f
Open biopsy, breast disease and, 330
Open fractures, 543–544
Open pneumothorax, 104
Operative fitness, 64–65
Ophthalmopathy, thyroid-associated, 355, 356f
Opioid regimens, 83
strong, 83
weak, 83
Optic nerve (CN II), 462
Oral analgesia, 83b
Oral cavity, 510–515
Oral cavity cancer
alveolus, 514f, 514b
assessment, 511–513, 511–512f
buccal mucosa, 514f, 514b
floor of the mouth, 514, 514b, 515f
hard palate, 515, 515b
lip, 511, 513b, 513f
retromolar trigone, 514
tongue, 513–514, 513f, 514b
Oral contraceptives, 67
Oral intake, burns and, 313
Oral supplements, 43
Orange peel appearance, of skin, 342f, 347
Orbital cellulitis, 510f
Orchiectomy, 450
Organ donation, 491–494, 492f, 494b
after circulatory death, 491, 491b, 493t
deceased, 491, 493t
donor contraindications to, 493t

Organ donation (Continued)
extended criteria donors and, 491
living, 491–494
organ preservation and, 491
Organ failure, burns and, 313–314
Organ preservation, 491
Oropharynx, 515–516
Orthopaedic surgery, 528–547
age and, 528
for bone and joint infection, 533–535
description of deformity, 530, 530–531f
examination for, 529–530, 529–530f, 530t
history, 528–529, 528b
for inflammatory disorders, 533
investigations, 531
in knee joint, 541–542
in lower limb, 541–542
for metabolic bone diseases, 538
for musculoskeletal tumours, 538–539, 539b
occupation, 529
paediatric, 537–538
procedures, 535–537
in upper limb, 540–541
Ossiculoplasty, 505
Osteitis fibrosa cystica, 361
Osteoarthritis, 532–533, 532f
conservative treatments for, 533
medical management of, 532–533, 533t
shoulder, 540
surgical management of, 533
Osteochondroma, 539
Osteoclastoma, 539
Osteoid osteoma, 539
Osteomalacia, 538
Osteomyelitis, 533
Osteoporosis, 538
Osteosarcoma, 539
Osteotomy, 536
Otalgia, 503, 503t
Otitis externa, 504–505
Otitis media, 506b
acute suppurative, 505, 505b
chronic suppurative, 505–506
with effusion, 505
Otosclerosis, 506
Ovarian cyst, 178
Over-hydration, parenteral nutrition, 46
Overflow incontinence, 430
Oxygen, delivery, 23f, 65
Oxygen transport parameters, 21t
Oxytocin, 364

P
Pacemakers, perioperative implications of, 75
Packed red blood cells (PRBC), 25–26
Paediatric neurooncology in, 479–480, 480f
Paediatric orthopaedic surgery, 537–538
Paget's disease of the nipple, 341–343, 342f
Pain
anal, 285b
atypical biliary, 230
control, postoperative, 428
neuropathic, 83
pancreatic, 234
postoperative, assessment, 82
on swallowing, 181
urinary tract symptoms, 429
Palliation
gastric cancer, 201–202, 202b, 202f
oesophageal cancer, 192–193, 193f
Palliative treatment, of pancreatic cancer, 245–246
Palpation
abdominal, 165–166

Palpation (Continued)
orthopaedic examination, 529, 530t, 530f
Palpitations, 188
Pancolitis, 261
Pancreas, 233–251
abscess in, 240
adenocarcinoma of, 243–244, 243f
cancer see Pancreatic cancer
congenital disorders of, 234
endocrine function in, 233–234, 242
exocrine function in, 233
infected acute necrotic collection in, 238–239
neoplasms of, 243–246
pain in, 234
pseudocysts in, 240, 240f, 242
surgical anatomy of, 233, 234f
surgical physiology of, 233–234
Pancreas graft, 499, 499f
Pancreas transplantation, 498–499, 499b
indications to, 498
operative procedure of, 498–499
outcome of, 499
patient assessment in, 498, 498f
Pancreatic cancer, 245–246, 245f
Pancreatic ductal adenocarcinoma, 243, 243f
Pancreatic function, suppression of, 237
Pancreatic hormones, 4t
Pancreatic neuroendocrine tumours (pNET), 246–248, 247t
clinical features of, 247t
functioning, 246
gastrinoma, 247, 247t
glucagonoma, 247t
insulinoma, 247, 247t
miscellaneous, 247
multiple endocrine neoplasia type 1, 247–248
nonfunctioning, 246, 247f
nonsyndromic, 247t
somatostatinoma, 247t
VIPoma, 247, 247t
Pancreaticoduodenectomy, 245, 246f
Pancreaticojejunostomy, pancreatic, 242, 242f
Pancreatitis, 234–243
acute, 235–241, 241b
aetiology of, 235–241
assessment of severity of, 236–237, 237t
causes of, 235t
clinical features of, 235
complications of, 238–241, 239t
diagnosis of, 235–236
differentiation between gallstone- and alcohol associated pancreatitis in, 236
ERCP in, 238b
management of, 237–238
nutritional support for, 238b
prognosis of, 241
prophylactic antibiotics for, 238b
scoring systems in, 237t
sphincterotomy in, 238b
chronic, 241–242
aetiology of, 241
clinical features of, 241
hereditary pancreatitis in, 241
investigations and diagnosis of, 241–242, 242f
management of, 242
pathophysiology of, 241
surgical treatment of, 242, 242f
topical, 243
Papillary carcinoma, 358
Papillomas, 317–318 see also Warts
Papillotomy, endoscopic, 229, 230f
Paracentesis, abdominal, 120, 120f
Paracetamol, 83

Paraganglionoma, malignant, 371f
Paralytic ileus, 12, 162, 264
Paranasal sinuses, 507, 509–510
anatomy, 509, 509f
diseases, 509–510
Paraphimosis, 455
Parastomal hernia, 156
Parathormone (PTH), 360–361
Parathyroid glands, 351, 360–363
calcium metabolism and, 360
surgical anatomy and, 360
Parathyroidectomy, 362–363
Paraumbilical hernia, 156, 156f
Parenteral analgesia, 83, 83b
Parenteral nutrition, 42–44, 46b
administration of, 45, 45f
composition of, 45
indications for, 44–45
for pancreatitis, 238
peripheral venous nutrition, 47
standard regimen, 45t
vs. enteral nutrition, 43b
Parietal cells, 181
Parietal peritoneum, 159–160
Parkland formula, 313b
Parotid gland, 524, 524f
Parotidectomy, complications of, 526–527, 527t
Paroxysmal hypertension, 370
Partial-thickness burns
deep, 310
superficial, 310
Passive movement, orthopaedic examination, 530
Past medical history
gastrointestinal bleeding, 197
orthopaedic surgery and, 529
Pasteur, Louis, 49
Patent ductus arteriosus, 420
Paterson-Brown-Kelly syndrome, 517
Patient-controlled analgesia, 83
Patient pathway, 84, 84f, 84b, 85t
Peak expiratory flow rate (PEFR), 70t
Pectineal ligament of Astley Cooper, 153
Pectus carinatum, 428
Pectus excavatum, 428
Pedicles, 461
Pelvic floor muscles, 452–453
Pelvic fractures, 545, 545f
Pelvic inflammatory disease, 55t
Pelvis, abscess in, 174f
Pelviureteric junction obstruction, 439
Penetrating trauma, 99
Penicillin, 48
Pepsin, 181
Pepsinogen, 181
Peptic ulceration/ulcer, 193–194, 196b
aetiology of, 193–194
clinical features of, 194
complications operative intervention, 195–197
acute haemorrhage, 196–197
obstruction, 197
perforation, 195–196, 196f
contrast radiology in, 169
diagnosis of, 194
management of, 194–195
medical, 194–195
surgical, 195
pathology, 193
perforated, 169
special forms, 194
stress, 194
Zollinger-Ellison syndrome, 194
Per protocol (PP) analysis, 139
Percussion, abdominal, 166
Percutaneous coronary intervention (PCI), 412
Percutaneous drainage/debridement, of infected pancreatic necrosis, 239

Percutaneous nephrolithotomy (PCNL), 437
Percutaneous transhepatic cholangiography (PTC), 210
Perforation, 163, 163f
clinical features of, 163
in diverticular disease, 268–269
oesophagus, 189–190
peptic ulcers, 195–196, 196f
Periadenitis, 523
Perianal abscess, 289–290, 289f
clinical features of, 290
management of, 290
Periareolar infection, 334–335, 334t, 335f
Pericardial constriction, 419, 420f
Pericardial effusion, 419
Pericardiocentesis, needle, 124, 124f
Pericolic abscess, 268–269
Peridiverticulitis, 267–268
Periductal mastitis, 334
Perilymph, 502–503
Perineal rectosigmoidectomy, 295
Perioperative management, principles of, 71b
Peripheral nerve block, 80, 82t
Peripheral nerve lesions, 486
Peripheral nonlactating abscesses, 334t, 335
Peripheral venous access, trauma and, 104
Peripheral venous cannulation, 121–122
Peripheral venous nutrition, 47
Peristalsis, intestinal, 162
Peristalsis, oesophageal, 181
Peritoneal dialysis catheter, 120, 120f
Peritoneal lavage, 170
Peritoneum
parietal, 159–160
visceral, 161
Peritonitis, 162
in acute abdomen, 172–173
acute suppurative, 172
aseptic, 172
classification of, 162t
clinical features of, 162
intraabdominal abscess, 173, 174f
postoperative, 173
primary, 173
spontaneous bacterial, 173
tuberculosis in, 266
Permissive hypotension, 105, 105b
Persistent vitello-intestinal duct, 147, 148f
Personal protective equipment (PPE), 51
Personality disintegration, intracranial tumours and, 478
Perthes' disease, 537
Peutz-Jeghers syndrome, 261–263
clinical features of, 262, 262f
management and surveillance of, 262
pathology of, 262
Peyer's patches, 252–253
Peyronie's disease, 456
pH studies, oesophagus, stomach and duodenum, 184–185, 185–186f
Phaeochromocytoma, 369–370, 370b, 370f
Phantom pain, in amputation, 385
Pharmacomechanical thrombectomy, for venous thromboembolism, 404
Pharyngeal pouch, 181, 189, 517
Pharyngitis, 515
Pharynx, 516f
Phenol, 48
Phimosis, 455
Phosphate, 17
Phreno-oesophageal ligament, 179
Phrygian cap, 221
Phyllodes tumours, 333–334, 333f
Physical activity, breast cancer and, 337

Physiotherapy
  for osteoarthritis, 533
  pre- and postoperative, in respiratory disease, 76
Phytobezoars, 203
Pia, 462
Piggyback procedure, 497, 497f
Pigment stones, 222–223
Pilar cyst, 316
Piles. See Haemorrhoids
Pilonidal disease, 297–298, 298b, 298f
Pinna, 502, 502f, 504
Pituitary gland, 363–364
  anterior, 363
    tumours of, 363–364, 363f, 364b
  disease, 368–369
  posterior, 364, 365f
  surgical anatomy of, 363, 363f
Pituitary hormones, 4t
Pituitary stalk, 363
Pituitary tumours, 477, 477f
Plantar warts, 317, 317f
Plasma, 9–10
Plasma products, 31–32
Plastic surgery, 301–325
Plateau phase, wound healing, 303f
Platelet-derived growth factor receptor alpha gene (PDGFRA), 261
Platelets
  donation, 30
  dysfunction, 26
'Platinum 10 minutes', 98
Pleomorphic adenoma, 526, 526f, 526b
Pleural aspiration, 118, 118f
Pleural effusion
  in metastatic breast cancer, 349
  postoperative, 132, 132f
Pleurectomy, 426
Pleurodesis, 426
Pleuropneumonectomy, 424–425
Pleuropulmonary infection, 427–428
Plummer-Vinson syndrome, 182
'Pneumaturia', 269
Pneumonectomy, 423
Pneumothorax, 425–426, 426f
  postoperative, 132
Poliomyelitis, 535
Polycystic disease
  kidney, 434
  liver, 211
Polygeline gelatin, 12t
Polymerase chain reaction (PCR), 50b
Polymerase proof-reading associated polyposis (PPAP), 275
Polypectomy
  for colorectal adenoma, 273–274, 274f
  for early polyp cancers, 278
Polypeptides, 363
Polyposis syndrome, 272–275, 273t
Polyps
  gastric, 198
  in large intestine, 272–275, 273t
  nose, 508, 508f
Polythene bags, 314
Popliteal aneurysms, 396
Porphobilinogen, urinary, 168
Porphyria, 168
Porta hepatis, 206
Portal hypertension, 213–217, 217b
  ascites, 216–217, 217f
  causes of, 214t
  clinical features of, 214, 214t
  effects of, 213–214
  posthepatic, 214
  segmental, 249
  variceal bleeding, 215–216, 215t, 215f, 215–216b
Portal vein, 206
  thrombosis, 213
Portal venous system, 213, 214f
Portosystemic shunting, 213–214, 214f

Portosystemic shunting (Continued)
  emergency, and variceal bleeding, 215–216
Positron emission tomography (PET), 127, 421t, 423, 423t
  gastric cancer staging, 200
  gastrointestinal tract, 254
  jaundice, 210
  oesophagus, stomach and duodenum, 184
Post-transplant lymphoproliferative disorders (PTLDs), 490–491
Postcholecystectomy syndrome, 230
Postcricoid carcinoma, 517
Posterior circulation, of brain, 462
Posterior triangle, 519
Posterolateral protrusion, 483–484
Posthitis, 456
Postischaemic syndrome, in acute limb ischaemia, 392
Postmicturition dribble incontinence, 452
Postmortem examination, 64
Postoperative analgesia, 82–83, 82f
Postoperative care, 128–136
  complications of, 130–136, 136b
    airway obstruction, 129
    cardiac, 132
    cerebral, 134
    general, 130
    haemorrhage, 129
    pulmonary, 130
    timeline, 129f
    urinary, 133–134
    venous thrombosis and pulmonary embolism, 134–135
    wound, 135–136
  complications of, peritonitis, 173
  immediate, 128–129, 129b
  optimal, 128b
  surgical ward, 129–130
Postoperative nausea and vomiting (PONV), 68, 83, 130
Postsurgical infection, neurosurgery and, 474
Potassium
  abnormalities, 15–16
    loss, 11
  homeostasis, 69
  hyperaldosteronism and, 369
  supplements, postoperative, 130
'Pott's paraplegia', 534
'Pott's spine', 534
Pouches, 189
Povidone-iodine, 314
PPomas, 247
Preferred Reporting Items for Systematic Reviews and Meta-analyses (PRISMA) statement, 138, 140b
Pregnancy
  after treatment, for breast cancer, 346
  appendicitis in, 175
  breast cancer in, 336, 346
  ectopic see Ectopic pregnancy
  haemorrhoids in, 285
  preoperative assessment and, 67, 67t
  test, acute abdomen and, 168
Prehn's sign, 457
Preoperative assessment, 64–83, 68b
  alcohol, 66
  allergies, 67
  cardiovascular system, 65–66
  drug therapy, 66–67
  for emergency surgery, 71
  exercise, 66
  investigation, 68, 68b
  MRSA screening for, 71
  nutritional status, 66
  obesity, 66
  operative fitness, 64–65
  oxygen delivery, 65
  pregnancy, 67

Preoperative assessment (Continued)
  previous operations and anaesthetics, 68
  respiratory system, 66
  risk, 64–65, 65f
  smoking, 66, 66t
  systematic, 65–69
Prepuce, 455
Presbycusis, 506
Pressure garments, burns, 315
Previous treatment, orthopaedic surgery and, 529
Priapism, 456
Prilocaine, 80t
Primary access, for haemodialysis, 407
Primary hyperparathyroidism, 360–362, 361t, 362b, 362f
Primary lymphoedema, 406
Primary sclerosing cholangitis, 231
Primitive neuroectodermal tumours (PNET), 479, 480f
Principalism, 60–61, 61b
Prion diseases
  prevention of, 52 see also Creutzfeldt-Jakob disease
Probiotic therapy, for pancreatitis, 238
Processus vaginalis, 149, 459
Procidentia, 294
Proctocolectomy
  for familial adenomatous polyposis (FAP), 274
  for ulcerative colitis, 261
Proctoscopy, 286
Professional development, 137–144
  continuing, 141–143
Profundaplasty, 382f
Progesterone, role in breast cancer, 338
Progesterone receptors (PgRs), 338
Prolactin-inhibiting factor (PIF), 363
Prolactin (PRL), 363
Prolapse, rectal. See Rectal prolapse
Proliferative phase, wound healing, 302
Prophylactic antibiotics, for pancreatitis, 238b
Prostate carcinoma, 449–450
  clinical features, 449
  epidemiology, 449
  investigations, 449–450
  management, 450, 450b
  pathology, 436t, 449
  prognosis, 450, 450b
Prostate-specific antigen (PSA), 449t
Prostatectomy
  incontinence after, 452
  laser, 448
  open, 449
Prosthetic devices
  and anal sphincters, 297
  heart valves, 415, 415f
  infections of, 57
Prosthetic grafts, infections of, in arterial reconstruction, 384
Protease inhibitors, 3
Protein
  metabolism, 7–8, 8t, 9b
  normal dietary intake, 8
  requirements, 42, 42t
Proteinuria, 430
Proteus spp., 54t
Prothrombin complex concentrates, 31
Prothrombin time, 24
Proton pump inhibitors, 181–182
Pruritus ani, 297
Pseudoaneurysm, in vascular access, 408
Pseudocholinesterase deficiency, 68
Pseudocysts, pancreatic, 240, 240f
Pseudomembranous colitis, 56–57, 271
Pseudomonas aeruginosa, 54t
Pseudomonas infections, 55t
Pseudomyxoma peritonei, 255

Pseudoobstruction, intestinal, 265–266, 265t
Psoas stretch sign, 175
Psychiatric drugs, preoperative assessment and, 67
Psychological aspects, of breast cancer, 346
Puborectalis sling, 283, 284f
Pulmonary artery catheter, 75t
Pulmonary collapse, 131
Pulmonary complications, 130
Pulmonary embolism, surgery complications, 134–135, 135f
Pulmonary function tests, 70, 70t, 421t
Pulmonary infection, 131–132
Pulmonary metastases, 424, 424f
Pulmonary transplantation, 428
Pulmonary tuberculosis, 427–428
Pulse oximetry, 24
Pulse status, in critical limb ischaemia, 379
Punch biopsy, breast disease and, 329
Purpura, posttransfusion, 36t
Putty kidney, 438
Pyelonephritis, 55
  acute, 438–441
Pyeloplasty, 439–441, 440f
Pylorus, 179
Pyogenic liver abscess, 211–212
Pyrexia, 11
Pyriform fossae, 516
Pyruvate dehydrogenase, 22

Q
Quality improvement, 141, 141b
Quinsy, 515

R
Radial artery, coronary bypass, 413–414
Radiation
  breast cancer and, 336
  see also Radiotherapy
Radiation enteritis, 263
Radio-labelled mercaptoacetyltriglycine (MAG-3), 432, 433f
Radioactive iodine, 355
Radiofrequency ablation (RFA), in varicose veins, 398
Radiography, 126
  of trauma, 106
Radioisotope imaging, 127
Radiology, in pancreatitis, 236, 236f
Radiolucent calculi, 437
Radiotherapy
  adjuvant, 95
  anal cancer, 294
  breast cancer, 343b, 344
  colorectal cancer, 280–281, 281b
  complications of, 346
  oesophageal cancer, 192
  organ-confined disease, 450
  paediatric neurooncology, 480
  palliative, gastric cancer, 201
  pituitary gland, 364
Ramsay-Hunt syndrome, 507
Randomisation, in randomised controlled trial, 138
Randomised controlled trial, 138–139, 140b
Ranson's score, 236, 237t
Ranulas, 511
Rathke's pouch, 363
Raynaud's phenomenon, in arterial reconstruction, 385, 385t
Rebleeding, aneurysmal SAH and, 467
Rebound tenderness, 165
Receptive relaxation, 181
Recipient operation
  complications in, 499, 499t

Recipient operation (*Continued*)
liver transplantation and, 497, 497f
pancreas transplantation and, 499
postoperative management of, 499
renal transplantation and, 494–495
Reconstructive ladder, 301, 302f
Reconstructive plastic surgery, 301
Recovery, cardiothoracic surgery, 411
Rectal examination, 167, 174f
Rectal prolapse, 294–296, 295f, 296b
assessment of, 295
clinical features of, 295
management of, 295
solitary rectal ulcer syndrome, 295–296
Rectopexy, 295
Rectum, 253
Rectus muscle, disorders of, 147
Rectus sheath, haematoma of, 147
Recurrent laryngeal nerve, 351
damage from thyroidectomy, 360
Red blood cells
in additive solution, 29–30
response to injury, 8
serology, 32, 32t
synthesis, 8
Red cell transfusion trigger, 68b
Red flag symptoms, of musculoskeletal system, 528, 528b
5α reductase inhibitors, 448
Reed-Sternberg cell, 522–523
Refeeding syndrome, 17
Regurgitation, 182, 187
Rehabilitation, in amputation, 385
Reinke's oedema, 518
Renal adenomas, 434
Renal artery disease, 388–389, 389b
Renal artery stenosis, 495
Renal carcinoma, 436b
Renal cell carcinoma, 435–436, 435f, 436t
Renal colic, 163
Renal cysts, simple, 434
Renal disease, 76
Renal failure
acute *see* Acute renal failure
burns and, 313
chronic *see* Chronic renal failure
postoperative, 133–134
in shock, 23
Renal obstruction, 170
Renal tract, effect of shock on, 23, 24b
Renal transplantation, 487b, 494–496, 496b
complications in, 495
indications for, 494
living donor, 491–494, 493t
operative procedure of, 494–495, 495f
outcome of, 495
patient assessment in, 494, 494t
postoperative management of, 495
recent developments in, 495–496
Renin, 4t, 5
Renin-angiotensin-aldosterone system, 6f
Renin-angiotensin system, 5, 6f
Reperfusion injury, 392
Reperfusion injury, ischaemia, 487
Replacement therapy
in adrenalectomy, 372
in pituitary gland, 364
Research governance, 64
Resection
bronchogenic carcinoma, 423, 424t
of liver, 219
Respiratory acidosis, 18, 19b
Respiratory alkalosis, 18, 19b
Respiratory disease, perioperative implications of, 75–76
Respiratory failure, 132

Respiratory system
associated injury of burns in, 312
complications in, due to burns, 313
effect of shock on, 23, 24b
obesity and, 67t
preoperative assessment and, 66
Respiratory tract infections, 56
Rest pain, in critical limb ischaemia, 379
Resuscitation, 102–105, 105b
active, and variceal bleeding, 215
acute haemorrhage, 196–197
ATMIST handover and, 102, 103t
definition of, 102
fluid, 105
haemostatic, 105
primary survey of, 102–103, 103t
secondary survey of, 103
tertiary survey of, 103
RET oncogene, 271
Retention cysts, 511
Retractile testis, 456
Retrograde ejaculation, 448–449
Retrograde pyelography (RGP), 432, 432f
Retromolar trigone, 514
Retroperitoneal fibrosis, 430, 441b, 445f
Retroperitoneal haematoma, 109, 109t
Retrosternal goitre, 353, 354f
Revised trauma score (RTS), 100, 100t
Rhabdomyosarcoma, 325
Rhesus antigens (RH), 32
Rheumatoid arthritis, 533
perioperative implications, 79t
Rheumatoid elbow, 540
Rhinitis, chronic, 508
Rhinolaryngoscope, 516
Rib notching, 421f
Richter's hernia, 148
Rickets, 538, 538f
Riedel's thyroiditis, 354–355
Ringer's lactate, 12t, 13
Rinne's test, 503
Risk
assessment of, cardiothoracic surgery, 409
preoperative assessment, 64–65, 65f
Rodent ulcer, 320, 320f
Rokitansky-Aschoff sinuses, 225
Rotational thromboelastometry (ROTEM), 26
Rotator cuff disease, 540
Round worm infestation, 266
Rovsing's sign, 167, 175
Rubber band ligation, for haemorrhoids, 286–287, 287f
Rule of nines, burns, 309, 310f
Ruptured AAA, 394, 395f
Rust's sign, 534
Rutherford Morris incision, 494

S

Saccular intracranial aneurysms, 466
Sacral nerve stimulation, 297
Safety, for vascular procedures, 121
Saline
dextrose solutions, 13
hypertonic, 13
Saliva
as barrier, 50
daily production of, 181
Salivary gland
anatomy, 524–527
disease, 524–525
swellings, 525b
tumours, 525–526, 525b
Salivary stagnation, 524–525
Salpingitis, acute, 178
Salter-Harris classification, 542, 544f
Saphenous thrill, 154
Saphenous vein, venous cut-down of, 122, 122f

Sarcomas, 324–325
in breast, 349
Satiety, early, 43
Scalds, 312
Scaphoid fractures, 546
Scars
abnormal, 303–304
thyroidectomy, 360
Schwannomas, 476–477, 477f
Sciatica, 483–484
Scintigraphic renography, 432
Sclerosing haemangioma, 318
Sclerotherapy, variceal bleeding, 215
Scoliosis, 530, 538
perioperative implications, 79t
Screening, for breast cancer, 338–339, 339b
Scrotum, 456
Sebaceous cysts, 316, 316f, 335
Sebaceous glands, 301
Seborrhoeic keratosis, 317–318, 317f
Secondary access, for haemodialysis, 407
Secondary lymphoedema, 406
Secretions, management of, 428
Segmental portal hypertension, 249
Seizures
epilepsy and, 483
intracranial tumours and, 478
Semen analysis, 433
Semi-occlusive dressings, burns, 314
Seminomas, 457
Sengstaken-Blakemore tube, 119
Sengstaken tube, 119
Senile warts, 317–318, 317f
Sensation, burns, 312
Sensorineural deafness, 503, 504f
Sensory neuropathy, in critical limb ischaemia, 379
Sentinel lymph node biopsy, 94b
for breast disease, 330
for malignant melanoma, 320
Sentinel pile, 288
Sepsis, 20b
anorectal, 290b
burns and, 314
care pathway for, 54t
catheter-related, 46t
diagnosis of, 53
early goal-directed therapy, 27
interrelationship between SIRS, infection and, 20f
screening, 53t
treatment of, 55t
umbilical, 147
Septic arthritis, 534
Septic shock, 19–20, 20f, 26–28, 27b, 102
cellular function, 22, 23f
empirical therapy for, 55t
microcirculation, 21
Septicaemia
burns and, 314
empirical therapy for, 55t
Serious Hazards of Transfusion (SHOT) scheme, 33, 34f, 34b
Serous cystic neoplasm, pancreatic, 244
Sham surgery, 139, 139b
Sharp, for practical procedures, 112
Shearing mechanisms, blunt trauma and, 99
Shock, 18–28, 19b, 102, 102b
burns and, 313–314, 313t
classification of, 19–20, 20b
clinical assessment of, 24t
definition of, 18–19, 102
effect of, on individual organ systems, 23
management of, 24–28, 102
pathophysiology of, 20–21
postoperative, 133 *see also specific types*

Short bowel syndrome, 42
Shoulder, 540
anterior dislocation, 540, 540f
impingement syndrome, 540
osteoarthritis, 540
rotator cuff disease, 540
shared sensory innervation of, 161f
Shouldice (Toronto) repair, for hernia, 152
Sialogram, 519
Sickle-cell anaemia, perioperative implications of, 79t
Sickle tests, for acute abdomen, 168
Siderocytes, 243
Sigmoid cancer, 94f
Sigmoid colon, 253
volvulus in, 270–271, 271f
Silver sulfadiazine cream, 314
Simple bone cyst, 539
Simple renal cysts, 434
Sinus bradycardia, surgery complications, 133
Sinus tachycardia, surgery complications, 133
Sinusitis, 509, 510f
Sirolimus, 490
Sister Joseph Nodule, 182
Sistrunk's operation, 521
Skeletal muscle
response to injury, 7
wasting, 40
Skin
benign lesions of, 317–319
blood supply, 304
cancer *see* Malignant melanoma (MM); Skin cancer
functions of, 301
grafts, 306
infections, 315–316, 335, 335f
injured limb, 542
lesions, 315–325
malignant lesions of, 319–320
as mechanical barrier, 50
premalignant lesions, 319
preparation of, for surgery, 51
structure of, 301, 302f
suturing, 113–114, 114t
swellings, 315b
tumours of, 316, 317t
Skin appendages, 301
Skin cancer, 319–320
immunosuppression and, 490–491
malignant melanoma *see* Malignant melanoma (MM)
Skin flaps, 306–307, 307–309f
devitalised, 305, 306f
Skull
fibrous dysplasia and, 475, 476f
fracture, 472
malformations of, 482–483
surgical anatomy and physiology of, 461
tumours, 475, 479b
Skull base, 461
Sleep apnoea, 515–516
Sleeve gastrectomy, 204f, 205
Slipped upper femoral epiphysis (SUFE), 537
Slow-transit constipation, idiopathic, 272
SMAD4 gene, 275
Small bowel ischaemia, 263
clinical features of, 263
investigations and diagnosis of, 263
management of, 263
Small intestine, 252–282
anastomoses, 254–255
anatomy of, 252–253, 253f
disorders of, 261–264
function of, 252–253
mucosa of, 253
neoplasms in, 261
obstruction of, 264–266

Small intestine (Continued)
  causes of, 264t
  principles of operative intestinal
    surgery for, 254–255
Smoking
  colorectal cancer and, 276
  Crohn's disease and, 255
  oral cavity tumours and, 511
  peptic ulceration and, 194
  preoperative assessment, 66, 66t
Snoring, 515–516
Sodium, 10
  abnormalities, 14–15
  retention, response to injury, 5
Sodium chloride, 13
Soft tissue lesions, 315–325
Solar keratosis, 319, 319f
Solid pseudopapillary tumour, of
    pancreas, 244, 244f
Solitary cyst, 539
Solitary rectal ulcer syndrome, 295–296
Solitary thyroid nodules, 355, 355b, 356f
Somatic pain, 159–161
Somatostatin, 181
Somatostatinoma, 247
Sorafenib, 218
Sore throat, 515b
Spermatic cord, 149–150
Sphenoid sinus, 509
Spherocytosis, hereditary, 208, 249
Sphincter of Oddi, 230, 230f
Sphincterotomy
  anal fissure, 289
  pancreatitis, 238, 238b
Spigelian hernia, 156
Spina bifida aperta, 481
Spinal anaesthesia, 80, 81f
Spinal cord
  compression, 349
  surgical anatomy and physiology of,
    462
Spinal degenerative disease, 483–486,
    484–485f, 486b
Spinal dural AVFs, 468, 469f
Spinal dysraphism, 480–481, 481f
  closed, 481
  open, 481
Spinal tuberculosis, 534–535, 534f
Spine
  decompression, 486
  fusion, 486
  surgical anatomy and physiology of,
    461
Spirometer, incentive, 56, 57f
Spleen, 248–251
  circulatory filtration for, 248
  cysts of, 250
  haemopoiesis, 248
  immunological function of, 248
  infarction of, 250
  physiology of, 248
  surgical anatomy of, 248
Splenectomy
  effects of, 251
  indications for, 248–251, 249t
  traumatic, 250–251, 250t
Split-thickness skin grafts, 306
Spondylitis, perioperative implications of,
    79t
Spondylosis, 484
Spontaneous bacterial peritonitis, 173
Spontaneous pneumothorax, 426
Sportsman's hernia, 153
Sprains, of ankle, 542
Squamous cancer, of large bowel, 282
Squamous cell carcinoma, 320, 320f
  bladder, 456
  ear canal, 505
  oesophageal, 191
  pinna, 504, 505f
Squamous cell papillomas, 317, 317f
Squamous disease, 505–506

Staging, cancer
  anal cancer, 293–294, 294t
  bladder, 444
  breast cancer, 339–340
  bronchogenic carcinoma, 423, 423t
  colorectal cancer, 277, 278f
  laparoscopy, oesophagus, stomach
    and duodenum, 184
  malignant melanoma, 323, 323–324t
  oesophageal carcinoma, 191
Stapedectomy, 506
Stapes, 502, 506
Staphylococci, coagulase-negative, 54t
Staphylococcus aureus
  methicillin-resistant see Methicillin-
    resistant Staphylococcus aureus
    (MRSA)
  methicillin-sensitive, 54t
  skin infections due to, 315
  in vascular access, 408
Starvation, 7–8, 40
  acute, 8
  chronic, 8
Station manometry, 184–185
Steatohepatitis, and portal hypertension,
    213
Stenosis, in vascular access, 408
Stenting
  for critical limb ischaemia, 381f, 382
  for gastric cancer, 201
  for oesophageal cancer, 193, 193f
Sternal protuberance, 428
Sternal retraction, 428
Sterno-occipito-mandibular
    immobilisation (SOMI) brace,
    534–535
Sternocleidomastoid muscle, 519
Steroid therapy, long-term, 66–67
Stoma, intestinal, 272, 272f
Stomach, 179–205
  examination, 182
  history, 181–182
  investigations, 182–186
  neoplasia, 198–202, 198–199f
  secretions, 181
  surgical anatomy, 179, 180f
  surgical physiology of, 181
  symptoms, 181–182
Stomatitis, 511
Strawberry gallbladder, 224–225
Streptococci, 314
Streptococcus pneumoniae, 54t
Streptococcus pyogenes, 54t
Stress incontinence, 430
Stress response, 11
Stricture
  in diverticular disease, 269
  ischaemic, of colon, 269–270
Stroke, 387, 409, 465
Stromal tumours, gastrointestinal, 282
Strong opioids, 83
Struvite stones, 436
Subacute thyroiditis, 354
Subarachnoid haemorrhage (SAH),
    465–466, 466f, 466t
  grading of, 466
  investigations of, 466
  management of, 467–468
  rebleeding and, 467
  saccular intracranial aneurysms and,
    466
Subclavian steal, in atherosclerosis, 386,
    386f
Subclavian vein
  cannulation, 123, 123f
  thrombosis, 405
  trauma and, 104
Subdural haematoma, 472, 472b, 472f
Subfalcine herniation, 463, 464f
Submandibular gland, 524, 525f
  swelling, 525, 525f
Submucosal plexus, 181

Substrate cycling, 7
Subtotal thyroidectomy, 359
Subungual melanoma, 321
Succinylated gelatin, 12t
Superficial partial-thickness burns, 310
Superficial spreading melanoma
    (SSMM), 321, 321f
Superficial thrombophlebitis, 398–400
Superior mediastinal syndrome, 46
Superior mesenteric arteries,
    253, 254f
Superior thyroid artery, 351
Superior vena cava
  access to, 45
  thrombosis, 404–405
Supraclavicular triangle, 519
Supralevator abscess, 290
Suprapubic catheterisation, 125, 125f
Surgery
  complications of, 130–136, 136b
    airway obstruction, 129
    cardiac, 132
    cerebral, 134
    general, 130
    haemorrhage, 129
    pulmonary, 130
    timeline, 129f
    urinary, 133–134
    venous thrombosis and pulmonary
      embolism, 134–135
    wound, 135–136
  day see Day surgery
  endocrine response to, 4, 4t
  vascular and endovascular, 375–408
Surgical instruments, sterilisation, 51
Surgical site infection, 55
  classification of, 55b
  diagnosis of, 55
  prevention of, 55
  treatment of, 55
Surgical thrombectomy, for venous
    thromboembolism, 404
Surgical ward care, 129–130
  blood transfusion, 130
  fluid balance, 130
  general, 129–130
  nutrition, 130
  tubes, drains and catheters, 130
Sutures, of skull, 461
  premature closure of, 482
Suturing, 113–114
  absorbable sutures for, 113
  materials for, 113
  nonabsorbable sutures for, 113
  skin, 113–114, 114t
Swallowing
  pain on, 181
  physiology of, 516
Sweat glands, 301
Sweating, 11
Swellings
  excision of, 126
  neck, 519–521
  parotid gland, 526
  salivary gland, 525b
  skin, 315b
  submandibular gland, 525, 525f
Swimming, 505
Swollen limb, differential diagnosis of,
    406b
Sympathectomy, cervical, 428
Sympathetic nervous system, 355
  metabolic response to injury, 4
Symptomatic AAA, 394
Synergistic bacterial gangrene, 58
Synthetic braided materials, 113
Synthetic monofilament materials, 113
Systematic review, 138, 140b
Systemic inflammatory response
    syndrome (SIRS), 20b, 50
  interrelationship between sepsis,
    septic shock and, 19, 20f

Systemic inflammatory response
    syndrome (SIRS) (Continued)
  in pancreatitis, 236–237
Systemic vascular resistance (SVR), 20

T
Tachycardia, surgery complications, 133
Tachypnoea, 23
Tacrolimus, 490, 490b
Talipes equinovarus, congenital, 537,
    538f
Tamoxifen, 345
Tapeworms, 213
Tarsal tunnel syndrome, 542
Taxanes, 344, 348
'Taylor's brace', 534–535
^{99m}Tc-labelled methylene
    diphosphonate (MDP), 432
T-cell activation, 488
T-cell receptor
  binding, 488
  costimulation, 488
T cells, 50
Tears, as barrier, 50
Technetium-labelled diethylenetriamine
    pentaacetic acid (Tc-DTPA), 432,
    433f
Temozolomide, 281
Temporal bone imaging, 504
Temporal lobe epilepsy, 483
Tenesmus, 253
Tennis elbow, 540
Tension-free vaginal tapes (TVT),
    453–454
Tension pneumothorax, 104,
    425, 426f
Teratomas, 458, 458b, 479
Terminal ileum, 254
Tertiary access, for haemodialysis, 407
Testosterone, 450, 450b
Tetanospasmin, 58–59
Tetanus, 58–59
Tetralogy of Fallot, 420–421
Thalamic cavernoma, 470f
Thallium isotope scan, 410t
Therapeutic drug monitoring, 53
"Therapeutic privilege,", 62
Thermal disinfection, 51
Thermogenesis, 7
Thimble bladder, 439
Third-space losses, 5, 11
Thomas's test, 530
Thoracic aortic aneurysms, 418f
Thoracic outlet syndrome, in acute limb
    ischaemia, 392
Thoracic procedures, 116–118
Thoracic surgery, 421–428
  assessment of, 421, 421t
  bronchogenic carcinoma, 421–422,
    422b, 422f, 422f see also
    specific procedures
Thoracolaparotomy, left, 191
Thoracotomy, for trauma, 110
Throat, sore, 515b
Thromboangiitis obliterans, in arterial
    reconstruction, 384–385, 385b
Thrombocythaemia, 68
Thrombocytopenia, 26, 68
  massive transfusion complications,
    38t
  platelets in, 30
Thromboelastography (TEG), 26
Thromboembolism, 376
  risk of, 8
  venous see Venous
    thromboembolism
Thrombogenesis, 402
Thrombolysis, for venous
    thromboembolism, 404
Thrombophlebitis, parenteral nutrition
    complications, 46
Thromboprophylaxis, 72, 72t

Thrombosis
  in arterial disease, 375
  parenteral nutrition complications, 46
  portal vein, 213
  in situ
    in acute limb ischaemia, 391–392
    embolus *versus*, 390*t*
  in vascular access, 408
Thymoma, 425, 425*f*
Thyroglossal cysts, 520–521, 520*f*
Thyroglossal duct, 351
Thyroid gland, 351–360, 352*f*
  anatomy of, 351, 352*f*
  cancers, 357–358, 357*t*, 357*b*
  development of, 351
  disease, assessment of, 352–353, 353*f*
  enlargement of *see* Goitre
  function of, 351–352, 353*f*
  solitary nodules, 355, 355*b*, 356*f*
  strap muscles and, 351
Thyroid nodules, solitary, 355, 355*b*, 356*f*
Thyroid receptor antibodies (TRAbs), 355
Thyroid-stimulating hormone (TSH), 351–352
Thyroidectomy, 359
  goitre and, 353
  primary thyrotoxicosis and, 355
Thyroiditis, 354–355
  autoimmune, 354
  Riedel's, 354–355
  subacute, 354
Thyrotoxic goitre, 354
Thyrotoxicosis, primary, 355
Thyrotropin-releasing hormone (TRH), 351–352, 363
Thyroxine (T$_4$), 351
Tibial plateau fractures, 547
Tinel's sign, 486
Tinnitus, 503
Tissue factor, 3
Tissue typing, transplantation surgery and, 489
TNM staging
  anal cancer, 294*t*
  bladder tumours, 444
  breast cancer, 339–340, 340*t*
  cervical nodes, 522*t*
  colorectal cancer, 280, 280*t*
  gallbladder carcinoma, 231
  gastric cancer, 200*t*
  lung cancer, 424*t*
  melanoma, 323*t*
  renal cell carcinoma, 436*t*
Tobacco, oral cancer and, 511
Tongue
  carcinoma, 513–514, 513*f*, 514*b*
  obstruction by, 129
Tonsillar herniation, foraminal, 464, 464*f*
Tonsillectomy, indications for, 515*b*
Tonsillitis, 515
Tonsils, 515*b*
Topical anaesthesia, 81–82
Topical antibacterial agents, 314
Toronto repair, for hernia, 152
Torus fracture, 542
Total joint replacement, 536, 536*f*
Total parenteral nutrition. *See* Parenteral nutrition
Total thyroidectomy, 359
Toupet repair, 186–187
Toxic adenoma, 357
Toxic multinodular goitre, 357
Tracheal compression, 129
Tracheostomy, 524, 524*f*
  tube, changing, 116
Tranexamic acid, 26, 105, 105*b*
Trans-hiatal oesophagectomy, 191
Transaminase, serum, 24

Transanal endoscopic microsurgery (TEM), for colorectal cancer, 273–274
Transcutaneous ultrasonography, 126–127
Transfer to hospital, of patients with burns, 312
Transfusion-related acute lung injury (TRALI), 35*t*, 37*f*
Transient/irreversible cognitive impairment, informed consent and, 62
Transient ischaemic attack (TIA), 387
  neurosurgery and, 465
Transitional cell carcinoma, 444, 445*f*
  bladder, 444
Transoesophageal echocardiography, 419*f*
Transplantation surgery, 487–501
  dialysis *versus*, 487*b*
  heart *see* Heart transplantation
  immunology in, 487–491
  liver *see* Liver transplantation
  lung *see* Lung transplantation
  organ donation and, 491–494
  pancreas *see* Pancreas transplantation
  pancreatic islet, 499
  renal *see* Renal transplantation
Transrectal ultrasonography (TRUS), 430–431
Transtentorial (uncal) herniation, 463–464, 464*f*
Transurethral resection of bladder tumour (TURBT), 444
Transurethral resection of the prostate (TURP), 448
Transverse colon, 253
Trastuzumab, 345, 345*b*
Trauma, 98–111, 99*b*
  in acute limb ischaemia, 392
  airway management in, 103–104
  blunt, 99
  cardiac, 419
  centres, 101
  critical decision-making in, 106–107, 107*b*
  deaths, temporal distribution of, 98–99
  division of, by physiology, 107, 107*f*
  in extremis, 107, 108*f*
  general approach to, 542
  imaging of, 105–106, 106*b*
  importance of, 98
  infections following, 58
  junctional zone, 111, 111*f*
  to liver, 211–213
  management of, 111*b*
  mechanism of injury of, 99, 99*b*
  miscellaneous, 99
  nasal, 508
  orthopaedic surgery and, 529, 542–547
  pancreatitis from, 234
  penetrating, 99
  pinna, 504
  scoring systems of, 100, 100*b*
  surgery for, 107–111, 111*b*
  surgical access to, 110
  surgical strategy to, 110
  system, 101, 101*b*
  team, 101, 101*t*
  vascular access in, 104
Trauma related injury severity score (TRISS), 100
Traumatic spinal injury, 473
Trench mouth, 511
Trendelenburg test, 530
Triangular intrahepatic portosystemic stent shunting (TIPSS), for variceal bleeding, 216, 216*f*
TRICC trial, 33

Trichobezoars, 203, 203*f*
Tricholemmal cyst, 316
Tricuspid valve disease, 417
Tricyclic antidepressants, preoperative assessment and, 67
Trigeminal nerve (CN V), 462
Trigger finger, 541
Triglycerides, 7
Triiodothyronine (T$_3$), 351
Triple assessment, breast disease and, 330
Trochlear nerve (CN IV), 462
Troisier's sign, 182
Tropical pancreatitis, 243
Trousseau's sign, 244, 244*t*, 360*t*
True aneurysms, 393, 393*f*
Trypanosoma cruzi, 188
Trypsin, 233
T-tube drainage, of the common bile duct, 228*f*, 229
Tubercular epididymo-orchitis, 458
Tubercular mastitis, 335
Tuberculomas, 474, 475*f*
Tuberculosis
  abdominal, 266, 267*f*
  duodenal, 203
  genitourinary, 438–439
  intestinal, 266, 267*f*
  musculoskeletal, 534
  peritonitis, 266
  spinal, 534–535, 534*f*
Tuberculous cervical lymphadenitis, 523–524, 523*f*
Tuberculous cystitis, 439
Tuberculous hip, 535, 535*f*
Tuberculous knee, 535
Tuberculous lymphadenitis, 266
Tuberculous meningitis, 474, 474*f*
Tubotympanic disease, 505
Tubular cancers, 338
Tubulosaccular aneurysm, 417–418, 418*f*
Tumour necrosis factor alpha (TNF-c), 3, 4*t*
Tumours
  of adrenal cortex, 366
  of anterior pituitary, 363–364, 363*f*, 364*b*
  appendiceal, 255, 255*b*
  benign, 87–88, 94
  of biliary tract, 231–232
  bladder *see* Bladder tumours
  carotid body, 527, 527*f*, 527*b*
  of connective tissues, 324–325
  external auditory meatus, 505
  gastric, 198–202, 198*f*
  hypopharynx, 517
  intracranial, 475–480, 479*b*
  of large intestines, 275–282
  laryngeal, 518
  liver, 217–219
    metastatic, 219
  malignant, 87–88, 94–95, 94–95*b*
    of thyroid, 357–358, 357*t*, 357*b*
  of muscles, 324–325
  musculoskeletal, 538–539, 539*b*
  nasopharyngeal, 510, 510*b*
  of nerves, 324
  non-endocrine adrenal medullary, 370–371
  oesophagus, 191–193
  operable breast, 343, 343*b*
  oral cavity, 511–513
  oropharynx, 516
  of pancreas, 244
  paranasal sinuses, 509–510, 510*f*
  pinna, 504, 505*f*
  pituitary, 477, 477*f*
  renal, 434*t*
  salivary gland, 525–526, 525*b*
  skin, 316, 317*t*
  umbilical, 147

Tumours (*Continued*)
  urothelial, 445*b*
  vascular, 323–324
  Wilms', 434, 435*t*
Turbinate bones, 507
Turcot's syndrome, 275
TURP syndrome, 448
Tylosis palmarum, 191
Tympanic bone, 502, 502*f*
Tympanic membrane, 502
Tympanometry, 503
Typhoid fever, 266

U
Ulcerative colitis, 259–261
  cancer surveillance in, 261
  clinical features of, 256*t*, 259
  investigations of, 259–260, 260*f*
  management of, 260–261
    medical, 260
    surgical, 260–261, 261*b*
  pathology of, 259
Ulnar nerve compression, at elbow, 486
Ultrasonography, 126–127
  abdominal, 421*t*
  abdominal aortic aneurysm, 393, 394*f*
  acute abdomen, 170
  breast disease, 329, 329*f*
  endoluminal *see* Endoluminal ultrasound
  gallstones, 225, 225*f*
  jaundice, 208
  orthopaedic surgery, 531
  trauma, 106
Ultrasound. *See* Ultrasonography
Ultrasound-guided foam sclerotherapy (UGFS), for varicose veins, 398, 399*f*
Umbilical hernia, 156
Umbilicus, 147
  developmental abnormalities of, 147
  sepsis, 147
  tumours, 147
Uncal herniation, transtentorial, 463–464, 464*f*
Uncinate process, 507
Uncomplicated DVT, 404
Under-hydration, parenteral nutrition, 46
Undescended testes, 456–457
Unicameral cysts, 539
Unstable angina, perioperative implications of, 73
'Unsteadiness', 503
Upper limb
  arterial disease of, 386–389
    aetiology of, 386, 386*f*
    carotid artery disease, 387–388
    cerebrovascular disease, 387
    management of, 387
    overview of, 386
    renal artery disease, 388–389
    vertebrobasilar disease, 388
  orthopaedic surgery in, 540–541
Upper urinary tract, 434–438
  anatomy of, 434–436, 434*f*
  benign tumours, 434
  calculi, 436–438
  developmental anomalies, 434
  emphysematous pyelonephritis, 438
  genitourinary tuberculosis, 438–439
  horseshoe kidneys, 434
  nephroblastomas, 434–435, 435*t*
  obstruction, 439–441
  pelviureteric junction obstruction, 439–441
  physiology of, 434
  polycystic kidney disease, 434
  radiolucent calculi, 437
  renal cell carcinoma, 435–436, 435*f*, 436*t*

Upper urinary tract (*Continued*)
  renal cysts, simple, 434
  urothelial cell cancer, 436
    see also Kidneys; Ureters
Urachus, 147
Urea and electrolytes (U&Es), 167
  preoperative assessment and, 69
Ureteric colic, 163
Ureterosigmoidostomy, bladder
    tumours, 445
Ureters, anatomy of, 434–436, 434f
Urethra
  anatomy, 454–455, 454f
  obstruction, 451–452, 451f
  trauma, 443–444 *see also* Lower
    urinary tract
Urethral catheterisation, 124–125
Urethral rupture, 443f
Urge incontinence, 430
Uric acid stones, 436
Urinalysis, for acute abdomen, 168
Urinary cellular markers, 430
Urinary complications, 133–134
Urinary frequency, 439
Urinary leak, renal transplantation and,
    495
Urinary porphobilinogen, 168
Urinary procedures, 124–125 *see also*
    specific procedures
Urinary retention, 448, 448b
  postoperative, 133, 133f
Urinary tract
  calculi, 436–438
  obstruction, 439–441
  stones, 434
  symptoms, 429–430 *see also* Lower
    urinary tract; Upper urinary tract
Urinary tract infections, 55–56
  postoperative, 133
  treatment of, 55t
Urine
  blood in, 429, 430t
  investigations, 430–434
Urine output, in renal failure, 134
Urodynamic studies, 433, 433f
Urological surgery, 429–460
  assessment, 429–434
  examination, 430, 430f
  investigations, 430–434
  nuclear imaging, 432
Urothelial tumours, 445b

V

Vagotomy, 195
Vagus nerve (CN X), 462
Valvular heart disease, perioperative
    implications, 74, 74f
Vancomycin, 53
Variceal bleeding, 215–216, 215t, 215f,
    215–216b
Varicocoele, 459–460, 459–460f

Varicose veins, 397–398
  aetiology of, 397
  clinical features of, 397
  complications of, 397
  cosmetic issues, 397
  epidemiology of, 397
  examination and investigation of,
    397–398
  management of, 398
    conservative, 398
    endovenous treatment in,
      398, 399f
    surgery in, 398, 398f
  symptoms of, 397
  treatment of, indications for, 397
Vascular access, for haemodialysis,
    407–408
  assessing, 407–408
  complications of, 408
  methods of, 407, 407t
  planning and preoperative
    assessment in, 407
  primary, 407
  secondary, 407
  tertiary, 407
Vascular diseases/disorders
  of central nervous system, 469b
  diabetes and, 76
Vascular procedures, 120–124 *see also*
    specific procedures
Vascular surgery, 375–408
Vasoactive drugs, 26t
Vasoactive intestinal peptide, 181
Vasogenic shock, 102
Vasopressors, 25
Venepuncture, 120–121, 121f
Venous cut-down, 122, 122f
Venous disease
  pathophysiology of, 396–401
  physiology of, 397, 397f
Venous gangrene, 403–404
Venous stenting, for venous
    thromboembolism, 404
Venous thromboembolism, 402–404
  aetiology of, 402–403
  diagnosis of, 403, 403f
  epidemiology of, 402
  management of, 404
  pathophysiology of, 402
  prevention of, 403–404
  prophylaxis, 71–72, 71b
  risk of, 72t
  venous gangrene in, 403–404
    see also Deep venous
    thrombosis (DVT); Pulmonary
    embolism
Ventilation
  burns, 312
  by mask, 114–115
  postoperative, in respiratory disease,
    76

Ventral hernia, 155, 155f
Ventral root, of spinal cord, 462
Ventricular aneurysm, left, 414–415
Ventricular septal defect (VSD), post-
    myocardial infarction, 414
Ventriculoperitoneal shunt (VP), 474f,
    482f
Verruca plantaris, 317, 317f
Verruca vulgaris, 317f
Vertebral column, 483–486
Vertical banded gastroplasty, 205
Vertigo, 503, 506–507
Vesicoureteral reflux, 450–451
Vesicovaginal fistula, 452–453
Vestibular neuronitis, 506
Vestibulo-cochlear nerve (CN VIII), 462
Video-assisted thoracic surgery, 425
Videothoracoscopy, 423
VIPoma, 247, 247t
Viral infection, 235
Viral warts, 317, 317f
Virchow's node, 182
Virchow's triad, 134, 402
Virilism, adrenal, 369
Virtual crossmatch, 489
Visceral pain, 161
Visceral peritoneum, 161
Viscus
  obstruction, 163–164
  perforation, 162–163, 172
Vitamin C, 304
Vitamin K, 79
Vitello-intestinal duct, persistent, 147,
    148f
Vocal cords, 517
  palsy, 518
Voice, physiology of, 517
Volkman's ischaemic contracture, 544
Volume replacement, acute, 38
Volvulus, 163f, 270–271, 271f
  caecal, 270–271
Vomiting, 182
  in enteral feeding, 44
  postoperative *see* Postoperative
    nausea and vomiting (PONV)
Von Hippel-Lindau syndrome, 244, 246
von Recklinghausen's disease, 324,
    324f
von Willebrand's disease, 79

W

Walking test, 421t
Walled-off pancreatic necrosis,
    239–240, 239f
Warfarin
  perioperative implications, 78–79
  preoperative assessment, 67
Warthin's tumour, 526, 526b
Warts, 317
  anal, 292
  infective, 317f

Warts (*Continued*)
  papillomas, 317–318
  plantar, 317, 317f
  senile, 317–318, 317f
Water
  abnormalities, 14–15
  depletion, 14
  excess, 14
  retention, response to injury, 5
Watson repair, 186–187
Wax, ear, 504
Weak opioids, 83
Weber's test, 503
Weight, breast cancer and, 337
Weight loss, 40–42, 41f
  in chronic pancreatitis, 241
Whipple's procedure, 245, 246f
White cell count, 68
Wilms' tumour, 434, 435t
World Federation of Neurosurgical
    Societies (WFNS) grading, 466,
    466t
"Worm colic,", 266
Wound healing
  classification of, 304b
  factors influencing, 304, 305b
  phases of, 303f, 303t
  principles of, 302–303
Wound infection, 304–305
  classification of, 304–305
  clinical features of, 305
  management of, 305, 305b
  prevention of, 305
  surgery complications, 135, 135f
  treatment of, 55t
Wounds, 301–307
  chest *see* Chest wound
  dehiscence, 135–136, 135f
  devitalised skin flaps, 305, 306f
  involvement of other structures,
    305
  primary closure, 305b
  with skin loss, 306–307
  surgery complications of,
    135–136
  types of, 301–302
Wrist disease, orthopaedic surgery in,
    540

X

X-rays
  acute abdomen, 168–169, 168–169f,
    169t
  neurosurgery, 465
  orthopaedic surgery, 531
  urological examination, 431
Xenografts, 314

Z

Zinc, 304
Zollinger-Ellison syndrome, 194, 247